White and Pharoah's

ORAL RADIOLOGY

Principles and Interpretation

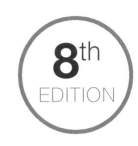

8th EDITION

White and Pharoah's

ORAL RADIOLOGY
Principles and Interpretation

SANJAY M. MALLYA, BDS, MDS, PhD
Diplomate, American Board of Oral and Maxillofacial Radiology;
Associate Professor and Chair
Section of Oral and Maxillofacial Radiology
School of Dentistry
University of California, Los Angeles
Los Angeles, California

ERNEST W.N. LAM, DMD, MSc, PhD, FRCD(C)
Diplomate, American Board of Oral and Maxillofacial Radiology;
Professor and the Dr. Lloyd & Mrs. Kay Chapman Chair in Clinical Science,
Associate Dean, Graduate Education
Oral and Maxillofacial Radiology
Faculty of Dentistry
The University of Toronto
Toronto, Ontario, Canada

ELSEVIER

ELSEVIER

3251 Riverport Lane
St. Louis, Missouri 63043

Previous editions copyrighted 2014, 2009, 2004, 2000, 1994, 1987, 1982 by Elsevier Inc.

Library of Congress Control Number: 2018950312

Content Strategist: Alexandra Mortimer
Content Development Specialist: Caroline Dorey-Stein
Publishing Services Manager: Julie Eddy
Senior Project Manager: Rachel E. McMullen
Design Direction: Patrick Ferguson

Printed in the United States of America

Last digit is the print number: 9   8   7   6   5   4   3

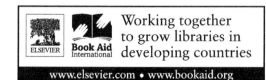

To our teachers and mentors, and our students, both past and present.

CONTRIBUTORS

Mariam T. Baghdady, BDS, MSc, PhD, FRCD(C)
Diplomate, American Board of Oral and
    Maxillofacial Radiology;
Assistant Professor, Oral and Maxillofacial
    Radiology
Department of Diagnostic Sciences
Faculty of Dentistry
Kuwait University
Safat, Kuwait;
Assistant Professor (affiliate)
Oral and Maxillofacial Radiology
Faculty of Dentistry
University of Toronto
Toronto, Ontario, Canada

Laurie C. Carter, DDS, PhD
Professor and Director of Oral and
    Maxillofacial Radiology,
Director, Advanced Dental Education
Department of Oral Diagnostic Sciences
School of Dentistry
Virginia Commonwealth University
Richmond, Virginia

Edwin Chang, DDS, MSc, FRCD(C)
Diplomate, American Board of Oral and
    Maxillofacial Radiology;
Oral and Maxillofacial Radiology
Faculty of Dentistry
University of Toronto
Toronto, Ontario, Canada

Fatima M. Jadu, BDS, MSc, PhD, FRCD(C)
Diplomate, American Board of Oral and
    Maxillofacial Radiology;
Associate Professor
Department of Oral Radiology
King Abdulaziz University
Faculty of Dentistry
Jeddah, Saudi Arabia

Mel L. Kantor, DDS, MPH, PhD
Diplomate, American Board of Oral and
    Maxillofacial Radiology;
Oliver M. Ramsey Endowed Chair in Health
    Sciences
Institute for Health Sciences
University of Wisconsin-Eau Claire
Eau Claire, Wisconsin

Ernest W.N. Lam, DMD, MSc, PhD, FRCD(C)
Diplomate, American Board of Oral and
    Maxillofacial Radiology;
Professor and the Dr. Lloyd & Mrs. Kay
    Chapman Chair in Clinical Science,
Associate Dean, Clinical Education
Oral and Maxillofacial Radiology
Faculty of Dentistry
The University of Toronto
Toronto, Ontario, Canada

Sanjay M. Mallya, BDS, MDS, PhD
Diplomate, American Board of Oral and
    Maxillofacial Radiology;
Associate Professor and Chair
Section of Oral and Maxillofacial Radiology
School of Dentistry
University of California, Los Angeles
Los Angeles, California

André Mol, DDS, MS, PhD
Diplomate, American Board of Oral and
    Maxillofacial Radiology;
Associate Professor
Department of Diagnostic Sciences
University of North Carolina at Chapel Hill
School of Dentistry
Chapel Hill, North Carolina

Carol Anne Murdoch-Kinch, DDS, PhD
Diplomate, American Board of Oral and
    Maxillofacial Radiology;
The Dr. Walter H. Swartz Professor of
    Integrated Special Care Dentistry
Associate Dean for Academic Affairs
School of Dentistry
University of Michigan
Ann Arbor, Michigan

Susanne E. Perschbacher, DDS, MSc, FRCD(C)
Diplomate, American Board of Oral and
    Maxillofacial Radiology;
Assistant Professor
Oral and Maxillofacial Radiology
Faculty of Dentistry
University of Toronto
Toronto, Ontario, Canada

Anitha Potluri, BDS, DMD, MDsc
Diplomate, American Board of Oral and
    Maxillofacial Radiology;
Associate Professor and Chair
Department of Diagnostic Sciences,
Director of Oral and Maxillofacial Radiology
School of Dental Medicine
University of Pittsburgh
Pittsburgh, Pennsylvania

Aruna Ramesh, BDS, DMD, MS
Diplomate, American Board of Oral and
    Maxillofacial Radiology;
Chair and Associate Professor
Department of Diagnostic Sciences
Tufts University School of Dental Medicine
Boston, Massachusetts

William C. Scarfe, BDS, FRACDS, MS
Diplomate, American Board of Oral and
    Maxillofacial Radiology;
Professor and Director
Division of Radiology and Imaging Science,
Department of Surgical/Hospital Dentistry
University of Louisville School of Dentistry
Louisville, Kentucky

Aditya Tadinada, DDS, MS, MDS
Diplomate, American Board of Oral and
    Maxillofacial Radiology;
Assistant Professor
Oral and Maxillofacial Radiology
School of Dental Medicine
University of Connecticut
Farmington, Connecticut

Sotirios Tetradis, DDS, PhD
Diplomate, American Board of Oral and
    Maxillofacial Radiology;
Senior Associate Dean and Professor
UCLA School of Dentistry
Los Angeles, California

Daniel P. Turgeon, DMD, MSc, FRCD(C)
Diplomate, American Board of Oral and
    Maxillofacial Radiology;
Assistant Professor
Département de Stomatologie
Faculté de Médecine Dentaire
Université de Montréal
Montréal, Quebec, Canada

Robert E. Wood, DDS, PhD, FRCD(C)
Diplomate, American Board of Forensic
    Odontology;
Head, Department of Dental Oncology
Princess Margaret Hospital;
Associate Professor
Oral and Maxillofacial Radiology
Faculty of Dentistry
University of Toronto
Toronto, Ontario, Canada

We take on our roles as the new editors of this textbook with enthusiasm and energy. The previous seven editions, under the leadership of Professors Paul W. Goaz, Stuart C. White, and Michael J. Pharoah, presented the science of diagnostic oral and maxillofacial radiology to dental students worldwide for over three decades. We hope that our contributions continue this textbook's tradition of excellence and provide our readers with exceptional educational content that is current and scientifically based. The book encompasses the full scope of oral and maxillofacial radiology for the dental student and serves as a comprehensive resource for graduate students and dental practitioners.

Radiologic imaging is an integral component of diagnosis and treatment planning in general and specialty dental practices. Dentists have access to a variety of imaging modalities, either in their offices, or at imaging centers and hospitals. To optimally apply diagnostic imaging in patient care, dentists must understand the basic principles of radiographic image formation and interpretation. To this end, the book provides foundational knowledge, and related guidelines and regulations for the safe and effective use of x-rays, as well as in-depth knowledge on conventional and advanced imaging techniques used to evaluate oral and maxillofacial disease. This new edition also provides us the opportunity to discuss the latest developments in our field. With advances in digital dentistry, information from multiple digital sources is being combined to guide treatment planning or to fabricate appliances and restorations. Oral and maxillofacial radiology often forms the backbone of such integrated data. A new chapter—*Beyond Three-Dimensional Imaging*—introduces advanced applications of 3D imaging, including additive manufacturing. Since the last edition, several professional organizations have published imaging guidelines, technical reports and position statements that impact the practice of oral and maxillofacial radiology. This edition has been updated to incorporate new recommendations for quality assurance and updated guidelines for use of cone beam computed tomography in dentistry.

Dentists must be familiar with the key radiographic features of diseases of the maxillofacial region. This book provides comprehensive coverage of radiographic manifestations and the differential interpretation of diseases affecting the teeth, jaws, paranasal sinuses, salivary glands, and temporomandibular joints. The chapters emphasize the biological foundations of disease as they relate to their radiologic interpretation. To enhance integration of basic and clinical sciences, we include a new chapter that consolidates diseases affecting the structure of bone. Where applicable, radiographic appearances of disease are illustrated using not only conventional, 2-dimensional imaging but also advanced imaging, providing knowledge that is applicable in general and specialty dental practices.

The book also offers supplemental resources to instructors via the companion Evolve website (http://evolve.elsevier.com), including test banks and the image collection.

Our goal is to make the study of oral and maxillofacial radiology stimulating and exciting.

Sanjay M. Mallya, BDS, MDS, PhD
Ernest W.N. Lam, DMD, MSc, PhD, FRCD(C)

ACKNOWLEDGMENTS

We thank our colleagues who have contributed as chapter authors. We appreciate their willingness to share their expertise and knowledge with our readers. This edition welcomes five new authors: Drs. Edwin Chang, Aruna Ramesh, Anitha Potluri, Aditya Tadinada, and Daniel Turgeon.

We thank Mr. John Harvey for creating the new illustrations of the disease processes that may be found in the latter chapters of the book.

We thank Drs. Freny Karjodkar, Matheus Oliveira, and Nandita Shenoy for providing region-specific information that adds to the book's global reach. We appreciate the effort of individuals who assisted in proofreading the chapters during the production phase: Drs. Katya Archambault, William Boggess, Karan Dharia, Akrivoula Soundia, Holly Vreeburg, Matthew Whiteley, and Kaycee Walton.

We are particularly thankful to our colleagues and students, and our readers worldwide, who have contacted us to suggest improvements or when they have uncovered an error. Among these individuals are: Drs. Mansur Ahmad, Ulkem Aydin, Hannah Duong, Rumpa Ganguly, Mohammed Husain, Sung Kim, Tore Larheim, Peter Mah, Mohadeseh Markazimoghadam, Susan White, Matheus Oliviera, and Kaycee Walton.

We thank the staff team from Elsevier whose tireless efforts helped keep the book's author and editorial team on track to meet production milestones: Caroline Dorey-Stein, Kathy Falk, Jennifer Flynn-Briggs, Lucia Gunzel, Alexandra Mortimer, Ramkumar Bashyam, and Rachel McMullen.

Finally, we thank Drs. Stuart White and Michael Pharoah for generously sharing their vast experience as the former editors of this book. Their feedback and advice have been invaluable.

Sanjay M. Mallya, BDS, MDS, PhD
Ernest W.N. Lam, DMD, MSc, PhD, FRCD(C)

CONTENTS

Physics

Sanjay M. Mallya

One atom says to a friend, "I think I lost an electron." The friend replies, "Are you sure?" "Yes," says the first atom, "I'm positive."

Radiologic examination is an integral component of the dentist's diagnostic armamentarium. Dentists often make radiographic images of patients to obtain additional information beyond that available from a clinical examination or their patient's history. Information from these images is combined with the clinical examination and history to make a diagnosis and formulate an appropriate treatment plan. This chapter provides basic knowledge on the nature of radiation, the operation of an x-ray machine, and the interactions of x-radiation with matter, with an emphasis on diagnostic x-radiation. This foundational knowledge is important for the safe and effective use of x-rays in dentistry.

COMPOSITION OF MATTER

Matter is anything that has mass and occupies space. The atom is the basic unit of all matter and consists of a nucleus containing protons and neutrons, and electrons that are bound to the nucleus by electrostatic forces. The classic view of the atom, the Bohr model, considers the structure of atoms like a solar system, with negatively charged electrons that travel in discrete orbits around a central, positively charged nucleus (Fig. 1.1A). The contemporary view, the quantum mechanical model, assigns electrons into complex three-dimensional orbitals with energy sublevels (see Fig. 1.1B).

Atomic Structure
Nucleus
In all atoms except hydrogen, the nucleus consists of positively charged protons and neutral neutrons. A hydrogen nucleus contains a single proton. The number of protons in the nucleus, its atomic number (Z), is unique to each element. Each of 118 known elements has a unique atomic number. The total number of protons and neutrons in the nucleus of an atom is its atomic mass (A). The ratio of neutrons to protons determines the stability of the nucleus and is the basis of radioactive decay.

Electron Orbitals
Electrons are negatively charged particles that exist in the extranuclear space and are bound to the nucleus by electrostatic attraction. The *Bohr model* considers that electrons exist in discrete orbits or "shells" denoted as K, L, M, N, O, and P, with the K-shell being closest to the nucleus

(see Fig. 1.1A). The shells are also described by a quantum number 1, 2, 3 …, with 1 being the quantum number for the K-shell. Each shell can hold a maximum of $2n^2$ electrons, where n is the quantum number of the shell.

The *quantum mechanical model* describes the electrons within three-dimensional orbitals, or electron clouds (see Fig. 1.1B). The electron orbitals are described based on their distance from the nucleus (*principal quantum number*; $n = 1, 2, 3 …$) and their shape (designated s, p, d, f, g, h, and i). Only two electrons may occupy an orbital. The electron orbitals in order of filling are 1s, 2s, 2p, 3s, 3p, 3d, 4s, 4p, 4d, 4f … and so forth. The Bohr model and the quantum mechanical model both provide an adequate basis to conceptually understand diagnostic x-ray production and interactions.

The energy needed to overcome the electrostatic force that binds an electron to the nucleus is termed the electron binding energy. The electron binding energy is related to the atomic number and the orbital type. Elements with a large atomic number (high Z) have more protons in their nucleus and thus bind electrons in any given orbital more tightly than smaller Z elements. Within a given atom, electrons in the inner orbitals are more tightly bound than the more distant outer orbitals. Electron binding energy is the conceptual basis to understand ionization, which occurs when matter is exposed to x-rays.

Ionization
When the number of electrons in an atom is equal to the number of protons in its nucleus, the atom is electrically neutral. If a neutral atom loses an electron, it becomes a positive ion, and the free electron becomes a negative ion. This process of forming an ion pair is termed ionization. To ionize an atom, sufficient external energy must be provided to overcome the electrostatic forces, and free the electron from the nucleus. High-energy particles, x-rays, and ultraviolet radiation have sufficient energy to displace electrons from their orbitals and ionize atoms. Such radiations are referred to as ionizing radiations. In contrast, visible light, infrared and microwave radiations, and radio waves do not have sufficient energy to remove bound electrons from their orbitals and are nonionizing radiations.

NATURE OF RADIATION

Radiation is the transmission of energy through space and matter. It may occur in two forms: (1) electromagnetic and (2) particulate (Table 1.1). Practical applications of these radiations in healthcare are listed.

- Diagnostic imaging with projection radiography and computed tomography use x-rays, a category of electromagnetic radiation that is ionizing in nature.
- Magnetic resonance imaging (MRI, Chapter 13) uses electromagnetic radiations of significantly lower energies than x-rays and at energies that are nonionizing.
- Some radiopharmaceuticals used in diagnostic nuclear medicine emit particulate radiation. For example, ^{18}F-fluorodeoxyglucose (^{18}F-FDG) emits positrons, a key step in imaging with positron emission tomography (PET; Chapter 13).
- High-energy electromagnetic radiations (gamma rays, γ) and high-energy particulate radiations (electron beams and protons) are used in cancer therapy.

TABLE 1.1   Particulate Radiation

Particle	Symbol	Elementary Charge[a]	Rest Mass (amu)
Alpha	α	+2	4.00154
Beta$^+$ (positron)	β^+	+1	0.000549
Beta$^-$ (electron)	β^-	−1	0.000549
Electron	e^-	−1	0.000549
Neutron	n^0	0	1.008665
Proton	p	+1	1.007276

[a]Elementary charge of 1 equals that the charge of a proton or the opposite of an electron.
amu, Atomic mass units, where 1 amu = $\frac{1}{12}$ the mass of a neutral carbon-12 atom.

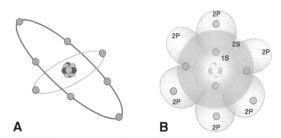

Fig. 1.1 (A) Schematic view of the Bohr model of the oxygen atom showing a nucleus with electrons that travel around the nucleus in circular orbits. (B) Schematic view of the quantum mechanical model of the oxygen atom. The central nucleus is surrounded by an electron cloud that represents probability plots of the location of the electron in a complex arrangement.

Electromagnetic Radiation

Electromagnetic radiation is the movement of energy through space as a combination of electric and magnetic fields. It is generated when the velocity of an electrically charged particle is altered. γ-Rays, x-rays, ultraviolet rays, visible light, infrared radiation (heat), microwaves, and radio waves all are examples of electromagnetic radiation (Fig. 1.2). γ-Rays originate in the nuclei of radioactive atoms. They typically have greater energy than x-rays. In contrast, x-rays are produced outside the nucleus and result from the interaction of electrons with large atomic nuclei, as in x-ray machines. The higher-energy types of radiation in the electromagnetic spectrum—ultraviolet rays, x-rays, and γ-rays—are capable of ionizing matter. Some properties of electromagnetic radiation are best explained by quantum theory, whereas others are most successfully described by wave theory.

Quantum theory considers electromagnetic radiation as small discrete bundles of energy called **photons**. Each photon travels at the speed of light and contains a specific amount of energy, expressed with the unit **electron volt** (eV).

The wave theory of electromagnetic radiation maintains that radiation is propagated in the form of waves, similar to the waves resulting from a disturbance in water. Such waves consist of electric and magnetic fields oriented in planes at right angles to one another that oscillate perpendicular to the direction of motion (Fig. 1.3). All electromagnetic waves travel at the velocity of light ($c = 3.0 \times 10^8$ m/s) in a vacuum. Waves are described in terms of their wavelength (λ, meters) and frequency (ν, cycles per second, hertz).

Both theories are used to describe properties of electromagnetic radiation. Quantum theory has been successful in correlating experimental data on the interaction of radiation with atoms, the photoelectric effect, and the production of x-rays. Wave theory is more useful for considering radiation in bulk when millions of quanta are being examined, as in experiments dealing with refraction, reflection, diffraction, interference, and polarization. Considering the value of both theories to understand the properties of electromagnetic radiation energy, wavelength, and frequency are all used to describe these radiations. In practical use, high-energy photons such as x-rays and γ-rays are typically characterized by their energy (eVs), medium-energy photons (e.g., visible light and ultraviolet waves) are typically characterized by their wavelength (nanometers), and low-energy photons (e.g., AM and FM radio waves) are typically characterized by their frequency (KHz and MHz).

Box 1.1 shows the relationships between photon energy, wavelength, and frequency.

Particulate Radiation

Small atoms have approximately equal numbers of protons and neutrons, whereas larger atoms tend to have more neutrons than protons. Larger

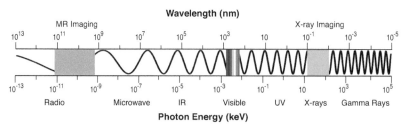

Fig. 1.2 Electromagnetic spectrum showing the relationship between photon wavelength and energy and the physical properties of various portions of the spectrum. Photons with shorter wavelengths have higher energy. Photons used in dental radiography *(blue)* have energies of 10 to 120 keV. Magnetic resonance *(MR)* imaging uses radio waves *(orange)*. *IR,* Infrared radiation; *UV,* ultraviolet radiation.

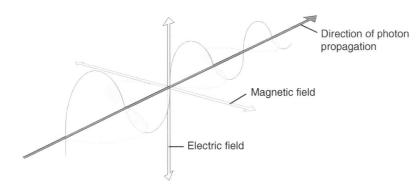

Direction of photon
propagation

Magnetic field

Electric field

Fig. 1.3 Electric and magnetic fields associated with electromagnetic radiation.

BOX 1.1 **Relationship Between Energy (E) and Wavelength (λ) of Electromagnetic Radiation**

$$E = h \times \frac{c}{\lambda}$$

simplified as

$$E = \frac{1.24}{\lambda}$$

$$E \propto \frac{1}{\lambda}$$

E is energy (kiloelectron volts, keV)
h is the Planck constant (6.626×10^{-34} joule-seconds or 4.13×10^{-15} eV-s)
c is the velocity of light $= 3 \times 10^8$ m/s
λ is wavelength (nanometers, nm)

Key point: **Inverse relationship between energy and wavelength of an electromagnetic radiation**

atoms are unstable because of the unequal distribution of protons and neutrons, and they may break up, releasing α (alpha) or β (beta) particles or γ (gamma) rays. This process is called **radioactivity**. When a radioactive atom releases an α or a β particle, the atom is transmuted into another element. Another type of radioactivity is γ decay, producing γ-rays. They result as part of a decay chain where a nucleus converts from an excited state to a lower level ground state; this often happens after a nucleus emits an α or β particle or after nuclear fission or fusion.

Examples of radioactive decay that are important in healthcare are listed.

- An unstable atom with an excess of protons may decay by converting a proton into a neutron, a β^+ particle (positron), and a neutrino. Positrons quickly annihilate with electrons to form two γ-rays. This reaction is the basis for PET imaging (see Chapter 13).
- An unstable atom with an excess of neutrons may decay by converting a neutron into a proton, a β^- particle, and a neutrino. β^- particles are identical to electrons. High-speed β^- particles are able to penetrate up to 1.5 cm in tissue. β^- particles from radioactive iodine-131 are used for treatment of some thyroid cancers.
- α particles are helium nuclei consisting of two protons and two neutrons. They result from the radioactive decay of many large atomic number elements. Because of their double positive charge and heavy mass, α particles densely ionize matter through which they pass and penetrate only a few micrometers of body tissues. This limited range has prompted use of alpha emitters such as radium-223 in targeted radiation therapy for bone metastasis.

The capacity of particulate radiation to ionize atoms depends on its mass, velocity, and charge. The rate of loss of energy from a particle as it moves along its track through matter (tissue) is its linear energy transfer (LET). The greater the physical size of the particle, the higher its charge, and the lower its velocity, the greater its LET. For example, α particles, with their high mass compared with an electron, high charge,

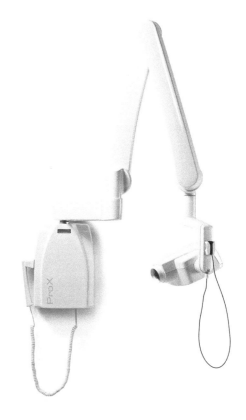

Fig. 1.4 Example of an intraoral wall-mounted x-ray unit, the Planmeca ProX. (Courtesy Planmeca USA, Inc. Roselle, Illinois.)

and low velocity, are densely ionizing, lose their kinetic energy rapidly, and have a high LET. β^- particles are much less densely ionizing because of their lighter mass and lower charge; they have a lower LET. High LET radiations concentrate their ionization along a short path, whereas low LET radiations produce ion pairs much more sparsely over a longer path length.

X-RAY MACHINE

X-ray machines produce x-rays that pass through a patient's tissues and strike a digital receptor or film to make a radiographic image. The primary components of an x-ray machine are the x-ray tube and its power supply, positioned within the tube head. For intraoral x-ray units, the tube head is typically supported by an arm that is usually mounted on a wall (Fig. 1.4). A control panel allows the operator to adjust the duration of the exposure, and often the energy and exposure rate, of the x-ray beam. An electrical insulating material, usually oil, surrounds the tube and transformers. Often, the tube is recessed within the tube head to increase the source-to-object distance and minimize distortion (Fig. 1.5; also see Chapter 6).

X-Ray Tube

An x-ray tube is composed of a cathode and an anode situated within an evacuated glass envelope or tube (Fig. 1.6). To produce x-rays, electrons stream from the filament in the cathode to the target in the anode, where the energy from some of the electrons is converted into x-rays.

Cathode

The cathode (Figs. 1.7B and 1.8) in an x-ray tube consists of a filament and a focusing cup. The filament is the source of electrons within the x-ray tube. It is a coil of tungsten wire approximately 2 mm in diameter and 1 cm or less in length. Filaments typically contain approximately 1% thorium, which greatly increases the release of electrons from the heated wire. The filament is heated to incandescence with a low-voltage source and emits electrons at a rate proportional to the temperature of the filament.

The filament lies in a focusing cup (see Fig. 1.7B; see also Fig. 1.8), a negatively charged concave molybdenum bowl. The parabolic shape of the focusing cup electrostatically focuses the electrons emitted by the filament into a narrow beam directed at a small rectangular area

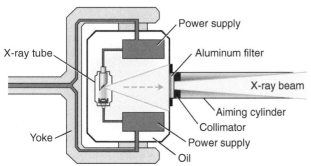

Fig. 1.5 Tube head showing a recessed x-ray tube, components of the power supply, and oil that conducts heat away from the x-ray tube. Path of useful x-ray beam *(blue)* from the anode, through the glass wall of the x-ray tube, oil, and finally an aluminum filter. The beam size is restricted by the metal tube housing and collimator. Low-energy photons are preferentially removed by the aluminum filter.

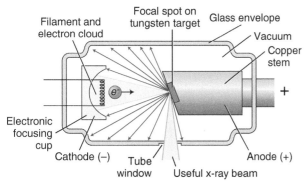

Fig. 1.6 X-ray tube with the major components labeled. The path of the electron beam is shown in *yellow*. X-rays produced at the target travel in all directions. The useful x-ray beam is shown in *blue*.

on the anode called the focal spot (see Figs. 1.7C and 1.8). The electrons move to the focal spot because they are both repelled by the negatively charged cathode and attracted to the positively charged anode. The x-ray tube is evacuated to prevent collision of the fast-moving electrons with gas molecules, which would significantly reduce their speed. The vacuum also prevents oxidation, or "burnout," of the filament.

Anode

The anode in an x-ray tube consists of a tungsten target embedded in a copper stem (see Figs. 1.6 and 1.7C). The purpose of the target in an x-ray tube is to convert the kinetic energy of the colliding electrons into x-ray photons. The conversion of the kinetic energy of the electrons into x-ray photons is an inefficient process, with more than 99% of the electron kinetic energy converted to heat.

The target is made of tungsten, an element that has several characteristics of an ideal target material, including the following:
- **High atomic number** (74), allows for efficient x-ray production.
- **High melting point** (3422°C), to withstand heat produced during x-ray production.
- **High thermal conductivity** (173 W m^{-1} K^{-1}), to dissipate the heat produced away from the target.
- **Low vapor pressure** at the working temperatures of an x-ray tube, to help maintain vacuum in the tube at high operating temperatures.

The tungsten target is typically embedded in a large block of copper which functions as a thermal conductor to remove heat from the tungsten, reducing the risk of the target melting.

The focal spot is the area on the target to which the focusing cup directs the electrons and from which x-rays are produced. The size of the focal spot is an important technical parameter of image quality—a smaller focal spot yields a sharper image (see Chapter 6). A limitation to reducing focal spot size is the heat generated. To overcome this limitation, x-ray tubes use one of the two anode configurations.

Stationary anode: In this configuration, the target is placed at an angle to the electron beam (see Fig. 1.8). Typically, the target is inclined approximately 20 degrees to the central ray of the x-ray beam. When viewed through the aiming ring, the area from which the photons of the useful x-ray beam originate appears smaller, making the effective focal spot smaller than the actual focal spot size. This allows production of x-rays from a larger area, allowing better heat distribution while maintaining the image quality benefits of a small focal spot. In the example shown in Fig. 1.8, the effective focal spot is approximately 1 mm × 1 mm, as opposed to the actual focal spot, which is approximately 1 mm × 3 mm. This smaller effective focal spot results in a small apparent source of x-rays and an increase in the sharpness of the image (see Figs. 6.1 and 6.2), with a larger actual focal spot size to improve heat dissipation.

Rotating anode: In this design, the tungsten target is in the form of a beveled disk that rotates during the period of x-ray production (Fig. 1.9). As a result, the electrons strike successive areas of the target disk, distributing the heat over this extended area of the disk. However, at any given time, x-rays are produced from a small spot on the target. X-ray tubes with rotating anode can be used with longer exposures and with higher tube currents of 100 to 500 milliamperes (mA), which is 10 to 50 times that possible with stationary targets. The target and rotor (armature) of the motor lie within the x-ray tube, and the stator coils (which drive the rotor at approximately 3000 revolutions per minute) lie outside the tube. Such rotating anodes are not used in intraoral dental x-ray machines but are occasionally used in cephalometric units; are usually used in cone beam machines; and are always used in multidetector computed tomography x-ray machines, which require high radiation output for longer, sustained exposures.

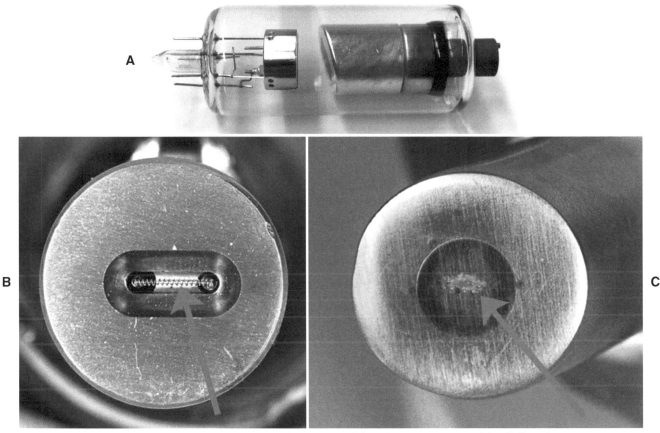

Fig. 1.7 (A) Dental stationary x-ray tube with cathode on left and copper anode on right. (B) Focusing cup containing a filament *(arrow)* in the cathode. (C) Copper anode with tungsten inset. Note the elongated actual focal spot area *(arrow)* on the tungsten target of the anode. ([B] and [C], Courtesy John DeArmond, Tellico Plains, Tennessee.)

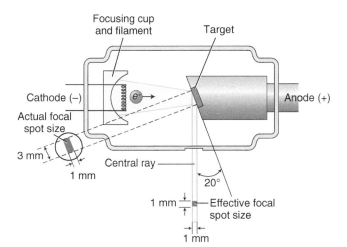

Fig. 1.8 The angle of the target to the central ray of the x-ray beam has a strong influence on the apparent size of the focal spot. The projected effective focal spot (seen below the target) is much smaller than the actual focal spot size (projected to the left). This provides a beam that has a small effective focal spot size to produce images with high resolution, while allowing for heat generated at the anode to be dissipated over the larger area.

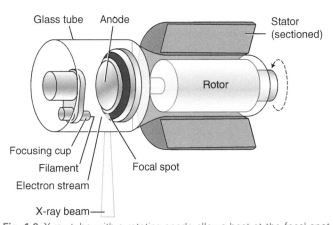

Fig. 1.9 X-ray tube with a rotating anode allows heat at the focal spot to spread out over a large surface area *(dark band)*. Current applied to the stator induces rapid rotation of the rotor and the anode. The path of the electron beam is shown in *yellow*, and the useful x-ray beam is shown in *blue*.

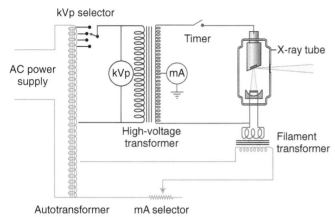

Fig. 1.10 Schematic of dental x-ray machine circuitry and x-ray tube with the major components labeled. The operator selects the desired kVp from the autotransformer. The voltage is greatly increased by the high-voltage step-up transformer and applied to the x-ray tube. The kVp dial measures the voltage on the low-voltage side of the transformer but is scaled to display the corresponding voltage in the tube circuit. The timer closes the tube circuit for the desired exposure time interval. The mA dial measures the current flowing through the tube circuit. The filament circuit heats the cathode filament and is regulated by the mA selector. *AC,* Alternate current.

Power Supply

The x-ray tube and two transformers lie within an electrically grounded metal housing called the head of the x-ray machine. The primary functions of the power supply transformers of an x-ray machine are to:
* Provide a low-voltage current to heat the x-ray tube filament (Fig. 1.10, filament transformer).
* Generate a high potential difference to accelerate electrons from the cathode to the focal spot on the anode (see Fig. 1.10, high-voltage transformer).

X-Ray Tube Controls
Tube Current (Milliamperes, mA)
During x-ray production, electrons produced at the filament are attracted to the anode. This flow of electrons from the cathode to the anode generates a current across the x-ray tube and is called the tube current. The magnitude of this current is regulated by the milliampere control (see Fig. 1.10, mA selector), which adjusts the resistance and the current flow through the filament, thereby regulating the number of electrons produced. For many intraoral dental x-ray units, the mA setting is fixed, typically at 7 to 10 mA. Some units offer the flexibility of a selection of mA settings, ranging from 2 to 10 mA.

Tube Voltage (Kilovoltage, kV)
A high voltage is required between the anode and cathode to give electrons sufficient energy to generate x-rays. The kilovolt peak (kVp) selector adjusts the high-voltage transformer to boost the peak voltage of the incoming line current (110 or 220 V). Typically, intraoral, panoramic, and cephalometric machines operate between 50 and 90 kVp (50,000 to 90,000 V), whereas computed tomographic machines operate at 90 to 120 kVp, and higher.

Alternating Current X-ray Generators: For an incoming line with alternating current (AC), the polarity of the line current alternates (60 cycles per second in North America; Fig. 1.11A), and the polarity of the x-ray tube alternates at the same frequency (see Fig. 1.11B). When

the polarity of the voltage applied across the tube causes the target anode to be positive and the filament to be negative, the electrons around the filament accelerate toward the positive target, and x-rays are produced (see Fig. 1.11C). When the voltage across the cathode and anode is highest, the efficiency of x-ray production is highest, and thus the intensity of x-ray pulses peaks at the center of each cycle (see Fig. 1.11C).

During the following half (or negative half) of each cycle, the filament becomes positive, and the target becomes negative (see Fig. 1.11B). At these times, the electrons do not flow across the gap between the two elements of the tube, and no x-rays are generated. When an x-ray tube is powered with 60-cycle AC, 60 pulses of x-rays are generated each second, each having a duration of $\frac{1}{120}$ second. Thus, when using a power supply with AC, x-ray production is limited to half the AC cycle. Such x-ray units are referred to as self-rectified or half-wave rectified. Many conventional dental x-ray machines are self-rectified.

Constant Potential (Direct Current) X-ray Generators: Some dental x-ray manufacturers produce machines that replace the conventional 60-cycle AC, half-wave rectified power supply with a high-frequency power supply that provides an almost direct current (see Fig. 1.11D). This results in an essentially constant potential between the anode and cathode (see Fig. 1.11E), and x-rays are produced through the entire cycle. This almost constant voltage yields x-rays with a narrow spectrum of energies, and the mean energy of the x-ray beam produced by these x-ray machines is higher than the mean energy from a conventional half-wave rectified machine operated at the same voltage.

Practical implications with the use of constant potential intraoral x-ray units are as follows:
* Because x-ray production occurs during the entire voltage cycle, constant potential units require shorter exposure times to produce the same number of x-ray photons, minimizing patient motion.
* The intensity of x-ray photons produced is more consistent and reliable, especially with short exposure times. This is of practical importance when using digital receptors that require less radiation.
* When operated at the same kVp, the x-ray beam produced by constant potential units has a higher mean energy, which decreases radiographic image contrast. To offset this effect, constant potential x-ray units are typically operated at a slightly lower kVp, typically 60 to 65 kVp.
* The narrower spectrum of energies, with fewer lower-energy photons, lowers the patient radiation dose by 35% to 40%, compared with conventional AC x-ray generators.

Timer

A timer is built into the high-voltage circuit to control the duration of the x-ray exposure (see Fig. 1.10). The electronic timer controls the length of time that high voltage is applied to the tube and thus the time during which x-rays are produced. However, before the high voltage is applied across the tube, the filament must be brought to operating temperature to ensure an adequate rate of electron emission. Subjecting the filament to continuous heating at normal operating current shortens its life. To minimize filament damage, the timing circuit first sends a current through the filament for approximately half a second to bring it to the proper operating temperature and then applies power to the high-voltage circuit. In some circuit designs, a continuous low-level current passing through the filament maintains it at a safe low temperature, further shortening the delay to preheat the filament. For these reasons, an x-ray machine may be left on continuously during working hours.

Some x-ray machine timers display the exposure time in fractions of a second. In some intraoral units, the exposure times are preset for different anatomic areas of the jaws. In some units, the exposure time

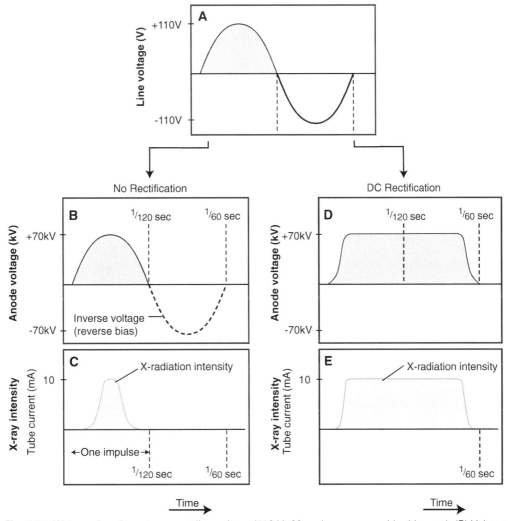

Fig. 1.11 (A) Incoming alternate current line voltage (110 V, 60 cycles per second in this case). (B) Voltage at the anode varies from zero up to the kVp setting (70 kVp in this case). (C) The intensity of radiation produced at the anode *(blue)* is strongly dependent on the anode voltage and is highest when the tube voltage is at its peak. (D) Incoming constant potential (110 V in this case) that is maintained through the operation cycle. (E) Voltage at the anode varies from zero up to the kVp setting (70 kVp in this case). Note that the increase and decrease of the potential difference at the start and end of the cycle is rapid. The intensity of radiation produced at the anode *(blue)* is higher with considerably less heterogeneity of photon energy. (Modified from Johns HE, Cunningham JR. *The Physics of Radiology.* 3rd ed. Springfield, IL: Charles C Thomas; 1974.)

is expressed as number of pulses in an exposure (e.g., 3, 6, 9, 15). The number of pulses divided by 60 (the frequency of the power source) gives the exposure time in seconds. A setting of 30 pulses means that there will be 30 pulses of radiation, equivalent to a 0.5-second exposure (Box 1.2).

Tube Rating and Duty Cycle

X-ray tubes produce heat at the target while in operation. The heat buildup at the anode is measured in heat units (HU), where HU = kVp × mA × seconds. The heat storage capacity for anodes of dental diagnostic tubes is approximately 20 kHU. Heat is removed from the target by conduction to the copper anode and then to the surrounding oil and tube housing and by convection to the atmosphere.

Each x-ray machine comes with a tube rating chart that describes the longest exposure time the tube can be energized for a range of voltages (kVp) and tube current (mA) values without risk of damage

---

BOX 1.2   Practical Applications of Exposure Controls

In many intraoral x-ray units, the mA setting, kVp setting, or both is fixed. If the mA setting is variable, the operator should select the highest mA value available and operate the machine at this setting; this allows the shortest exposure time and minimizes the chance of patient movement.

If tube voltage can be adjusted on an intraoral radiographic unit, the operator may choose to operate at a fixed voltage, typically 65–70 kVp. This protocol simplifies selecting the proper patient exposure settings by using just exposure time as the means to adjust for anatomic location within the mouth and patient size.

The kVp setting is often used to compensate for patient tissue thickness, particularly for panoramic and cephalometric radiography. A rule of thumb is to vary the setting by 2 kVp/cm of tissue thickness.

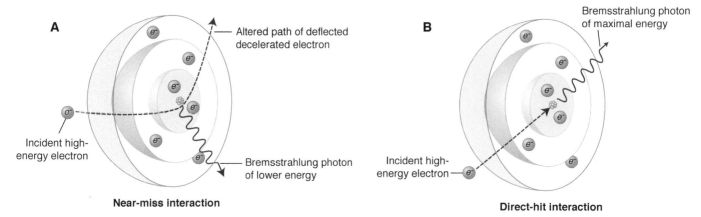

Fig. 1.12 Bremsstrahlung radiation is produced most often by the passage of an electron near a nucleus, which results in electrons being deflected and decelerated (A) or, less frequently, by the direct hit of an electron on a nucleus in the target (B). For the sake of clarity, this diagram and other similar figures in this chapter show only the 1s, 2s, or 3s orbitals.

to the target from overheating. These tube ratings generally do not restrict tube use for intraoral radiography. Duty cycle relates to the frequency with which successive exposures can be made without overheating the anode. The interval between successive exposures must be long enough for heat dissipation. This characteristic is a function of the size of the anode, the exposure kVp and mA, and the method used to cool the tube. A duty cycle of 1:60 indicates that one could make a 1-second exposure every 60 seconds.

PRODUCTION OF X RAYS

Most high-speed electrons traveling from the filament to the target interact with target electrons and release their energy as heat. Occasionally, the electron's kinetic energy is converted into x-ray photons by the formation of bremsstrahlung radiation and characteristic radiation.

Bremsstrahlung Radiation

Bremsstrahlung photons are the primary source of radiation from an x-ray tube. *Bremsstrahlung* means "braking radiation" in German, and these photons are produced by the sudden stopping or slowing of high-speed electrons by tungsten nuclei in the target as follows:

Most high-speed electrons pass by tungsten nuclei with near or wide misses (Fig. 1.12A). In these interactions, the electron is attracted toward the positively charged nuclei, its path is altered toward the nucleus, and it loses some of its velocity. This deceleration causes the electron to lose kinetic energy that is given off in the form of x-ray photons. The closer the high-speed electron approaches the nuclei, the greater the electrostatic attraction between the nucleus and the electron, and the resulting bremsstrahlung photons have higher energy. The efficiency of this process is proportional to the square of the atomic number of the target; high Z metals are more effective in deflecting the path of the incident electrons, and this is the basis for selection of tungsten (Z = 74) as a target material.

Occasionally, electrons from the filament directly hit the nucleus of a target atom. When this happens, all the kinetic energy of the electron is transformed into a single x-ray photon (see Fig. 1.12B). The energy of the resultant photon (in keV) is numerically equal to the energy of the electron (i.e., the voltage applied across the x-ray tube at that instant).

Bremsstrahlung interactions generate x-ray photons with a continuous spectrum of energy. The energy of an x-ray beam is usually described by identifying the peak operating voltage (in kVp). For example, a

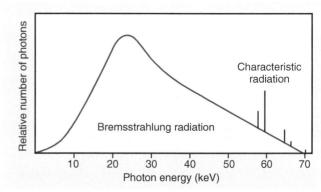

Fig. 1.13 Spectrum of photons emitted from an x-ray machine operating at 70 kVp. The vast preponderance of radiation is bremsstrahlung *(blue)*, with a minor addition of characteristic radiation.

dental x-ray machine operating at a peak voltage of 70 kVp applies a voltage of up to 70 kVp across the tube. This tube therefore produces a continuous spectrum of x-ray photons with energies ranging to a maximum of 70 keV (Fig. 1.13). The reasons for this continuous spectrum are as follows:

- The continuously varying voltage difference between the target and filament causes the electrons striking the target to have varying levels of kinetic energy.
- The bombarding electrons pass at varying distances around tungsten nuclei and are thus deflected to varying extents. As a result, they give up varying amounts of energy in the form of bremsstrahlung photons.
- Most electrons participate in multiple bremsstrahlung interactions in the target before losing all their kinetic energy. Consequently, an electron carries differing amounts of energy after successive interactions with tungsten nuclei.

Characteristic Radiation

Characteristic radiation contributes only a small fraction of the photons in an x-ray beam. It is made when an incident electron ejects an inner electron from the tungsten atom. When this happens, an electron from an outer orbital is quickly attracted to the void in the deficient inner orbital (Fig. 1.14). When the outer orbital electron replaces the displaced

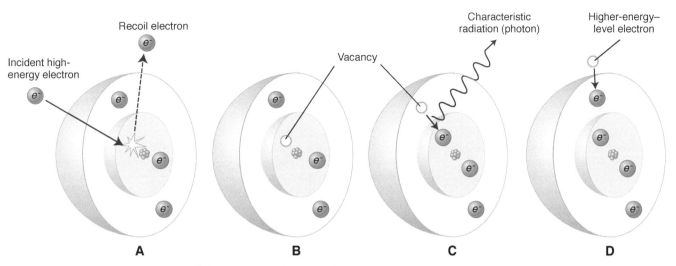

Fig. 1.14 Production of characteristic radiation. An incident electron (A) ejects an electron from an inner orbital creating an electron vacancy (B). (C) An electron from an outer orbital fills this vacancy, and a photon is emitted with energy equal to the difference in energy levels between the two orbitals. (D) Electrons from various orbitals may be involved, giving rise to other characteristic photons. The energies of the photons released are characteristic of the energy transitions for the target atom.

electron, a photon is emitted with energy equivalent to the difference in the binding energies of the two orbitals. The energies of characteristic photons are discrete because they represent the difference of the energy levels of specific electron orbitals and are characteristic of the target atoms. The production of characteristic radiation has no practical implications for dentomaxillofacial radiography.

FACTORS CONTROLLING THE X-RAY BEAM

An x-ray beam may be modified by altering the beam exposure duration (timer), exposure rate (mA), energy (kVp and filtration), shape (collimation), or intensity (target-patient distance).

Exposure Time (s)

Changing the exposure time—typically measured in fractions of a second—modifies the duration of the exposure and thus the number of photons generated (Fig. 1.15). When the exposure time is doubled, the number of photons generated at all energies in the x-ray emission spectrum is doubled. The range of photon energies is unchanged. Practically, it is desirable to keep the exposure time as short as possible to minimize blurring from patient motion.

Milliamperage Setting (mA, Tube Current)

Like the effects of exposure time, the quantity of radiation produced by an x-ray tube (i.e., the number of photons that reach the patient) is directly proportional to the milliamperage setting (mA setting; Fig. 1.16). As the mA setting is increased, more power is applied to the filament, which heats up and releases more electrons that collide with the target to produce radiation. Thus, as with exposure time, doubling the mA setting will double the number of photons produced. The product of mA setting and exposure time (**mA × s**, or **mAs**) is often used as a single parameter to denote the total number of photons produced. For instance, a machine operating at 10 mA for 1 second (**10 × 1 = 10 mAs**) produces the same number of photons when operated at 20 mA for 0.5 second (**20 × 0.5 = 10 mAs**). The term beam quantity refers to the number of photons in an x-ray beam. Linearity and reproducibility of the mA and s settings are often included in the quality assurance programs for x-ray units, including those used in dental and maxillofacial imaging.

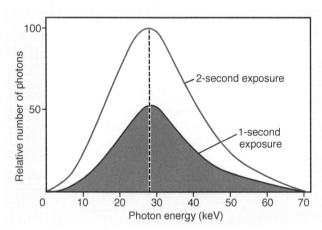

Fig. 1.15 Spectrum of photon energies generated in an x-ray machine showing that as exposure time increases (kVp and mA settings held constant), so does the total number of photons. The mean energies (*dotted line*, approximately 29 keV in this example) and maximal energies (70 keV in this example) of the beams are unchanged.

Tube Voltage Peak (kVp)

Increasing the kVp increases the potential difference between the cathode and the anode, increasing the kinetic energy of the electrons as they move toward the target. The greater the energy of an electron, the greater the probability it will be converted into x-ray photons at the target. Increasing the kVp of an x-ray machine increases:
- The number of photons generated.
- The mean energy of the photons.
- The maximal energy of the photons (Fig. 1.17).
  The term beam quality refers to the mean energy of an x-ray beam.

Filtration

Although an x-ray beam consists of a continuous spectrum of x-ray photon energies, only photons with sufficient energy to penetrate through anatomic structures and reach the image receptor (digital or film) are useful for diagnostic radiology. Low-energy photons that cannot reach the receptor contribute to patient risk but do not offer any benefit. Consequently, it is desirable to remove these low-energy photons from the beam. This removal can be accomplished in part by placing a metallic disk (filter) in the beam path. A filter preferentially removes low-energy photons from the beam but allows high-energy photons that contribute to making an image to pass through (Fig. 1.18).

Inherent filtration consists of the materials that x-ray photons encounter as they travel from the focal spot on the target to form the usable beam outside the tube enclosure. These materials include the glass wall of the x-ray tube, the insulating oil that surrounds many dental tubes, and the barrier material that prevents the oil from escaping through the x-ray port. The inherent filtration of most x-ray machines ranges from the equivalent of 0.5 to 2 mm of aluminum.

Added filtration may be supplied in the form of aluminum disks placed over the port in the head of the x-ray machine. Total filtration is the sum of the inherent and added filtration. Federal regulations in the United States require the total filtration in the path of a dental x-ray beam to be equal to the equivalent of 1.5 mm of aluminum for a machine operating at up to 70 kVp and 2.5 mm of aluminum for machines operating at higher voltages (see Chapter 3).

Collimation

A collimator is a metallic barrier with an aperture in the middle used to shape and restrict the size of the x-ray beam and the volume of tissue irradiated (Fig. 1.19). Round and rectangular collimators are most frequently used in intraoral radiography. Dental x-ray beams are usually collimated to a circle 2.75 inches (7 cm) in diameter at the patient's face. A round collimator (see Fig. 1.19A) is a thick plate of metal with a circular opening centered over the port in the x-ray head through which the x-ray beam emerges. Typically, round collimators are built into open-ended aiming cylinders. Rectangular collimators (see Fig. 1.19B) further limit the size of the beam to just larger than the intraoral receptor, further reducing patient exposure. Some types of receptor-holding instruments also provide rectangular collimation of the x-ray beam (see Chapters 3 and 7).

Collimators also improve image quality. When an x-ray beam is directed at a patient, the hard and soft tissues absorb approximately

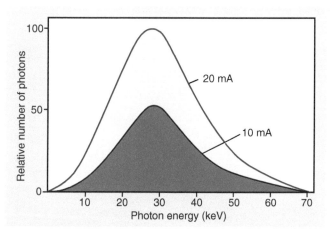

Fig. 1.16 Spectrum of photon energies generated in an x-ray machine showing that as the mA setting increases (kVp and exposure time held constant), so does the total number of photons. The mean energies and maximal energies of the beams are unchanged. Note similarity to the effect of exposure time; see Fig. 1.15.

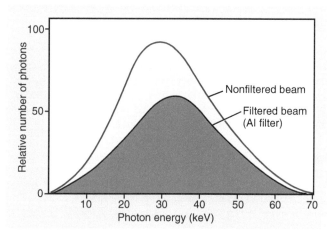

Fig. 1.18 Spectrum of filtered x-ray beam generated in an x-ray machine showing that an aluminum filter preferentially removes low-energy photons, reducing the beam intensity, while increasing the mean energy of the residual beam. Compare with Figs. 1.15–1.17.

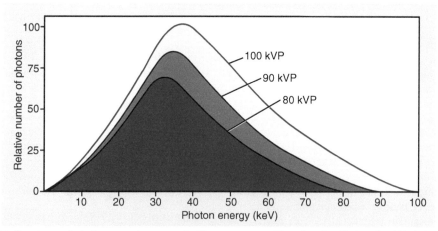

Fig. 1.17 Spectrum of photon energies generated in an x-ray machine showing that as the kVp is increased (mA and s held constant), there is a corresponding increase in the mean energy of the beam, the total number of photons emitted, and the maximal energy of the photons. Compare with Figs. 1.15 and 1.16.

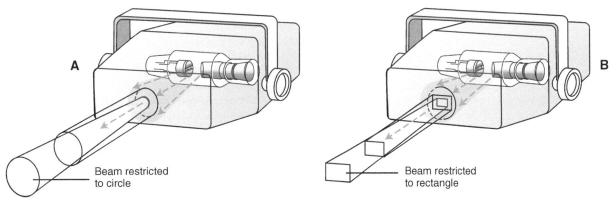

Fig. 1.19 Collimation of an x-ray beam *(blue)* is achieved by restricting its useful size. (A) Circular collimator. (B) Rectangular collimator restricts area of exposure to just larger than the detector size and thereby reduces unnecessary patient exposure.

90% of the photons and approximately 10% pass through the patient to reach the image receptor (film, or digital receptor). Many of the absorbed photons generate scattered radiation within the exposed tissues by a process called Compton scattering (see later in chapter). These scattered photons travel in all directions, and some reach the receptor and degrade image quality. Collimating the x-ray beam thus reduces the exposed volume and thereby the number of scattered photons reaching the image receptor, resulting in reduced patient exposure and improved images.

Inverse Square Law

The intensity of an x-ray beam (the number of photons per cross-sectional area per unit of exposure time) varies with distance from the focal spot. For a given beam, the intensity is inversely proportional to the square of the distance from the source (Fig. 1.20). The reason for this decrease in intensity is that an x-ray beam spreads out as it moves from its source. The relationship is as follows:

$$\frac{I_1}{I_2} = \frac{(D_2)^2}{(D_1)^2}$$

where I is intensity and D is distance. If a dose of 4 Gy is measured at 1 m, a dose of 1 Gy would be found at 2 m and a dose of 0.25 Gy would be found at 4 m.

Practical Applications

- Changing the distance between the x-ray tube and the patient, such as by switching from a machine with a short aiming tube to one with a long aiming tube, has a marked effect on beam intensity. Such a change requires a corresponding modification of the kVp or mA to maintain the same intensity at the image receptor.
- Increasing operator distance from the x-ray source is an effective method to minimize operator dose (see Chapter 3).

INTERACTIONS OF X RAYS WITH MATTER

In dental and maxillofacial imaging, the x-ray beam enters the face of a patient, interacts with hard and soft tissues, and strikes a digital sensor or film. The incident beam contains photons of many energies but is spatially homogeneous. That is, the intensity of the beam is essentially uniform from the center of the beam outward. As the beam goes through the patient, it is reduced in intensity (attenuated). This attenuation results from absorption of individual photons in the beam by atoms in the tissues or by photons being scattered out of the beam. In absorption interactions, photons interact with tissue atoms and cease to exist.

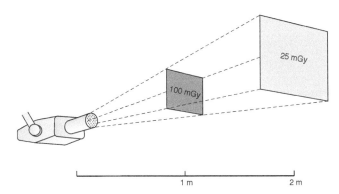

Fig. 1.20 Intensity of an x-ray beam is inversely proportional to the square of the distance between the source and the point of measure. When the distance from the focal spot is doubled, the intensity of the beam decreases to one quarter.

In scattering interactions, photons also interact with tissue atoms but then move off in another direction. The frequency of these interactions depends on the type of tissue exposed (e.g., bone vs. soft tissue). Bone is more likely to absorb x-ray photons, whereas soft tissues are more likely to let them pass through. Although the incident beam striking the patient is spatially homogeneous, the remnant beam—the attenuated beam that exits the patient—is spatially heterogeneous because of differential absorption by the anatomic structures through which it has passed. This differential exposure of the film or digital sensor forms a radiographic image.

There are three means of beam attenuation in a diagnostic x-ray beam (Table 1.2):

- Photoelectric absorption
- Compton scattering
- Coherent scattering

In addition, approximately 9% of the primary photons pass through the patient's tissues without interaction and strike the sensor to form an image (Fig. 1.21 and Table 1.3).

PHOTOELECTRIC ABSORPTION

Photoelectric absorption is critical in diagnostic imaging because it is the basis of image radiographic formation. This process occurs when an incident photon interacts with an electron in an inner orbital of an atom in the patient. The incident photon loses all its energy to the electron and ceases to exist. The energy absorbed by the electron is expended to overcome the binding energy, and the remainder energy remains as the kinetic energy of the electron as it escapes the confines of its orbital (Fig. 1.22). The kinetic energy imparted to the electron (termed recoil electron or photoelectron) is equal to the energy of the incident photon minus the binding energy of the electron. In the case of atoms with low atomic numbers (e.g., atoms in most biologic molecules), the binding energy is small and the photoelectron acquires most of the energy of the incident photon. Photoelectrons ejected during photoelectric absorption travel only short distances in the absorber before they give up their energy through secondary ionizations.

Most photoelectric interactions occur in the 1s orbital because the density of the electron cloud is greatest in this region, and there is a higher probability of interaction. Approximately 27% of interactions in a dental x-ray beam exposure involve photoelectric absorption.

The photoelectric interaction causes ionization of the atom because of the loss of an electron. This electron deficiency (usually in the 1s orbital) is instantly filled, usually by a 2s or 2p electron, with the release of characteristic radiation (see Fig. 1.14). Whatever the orbital of the replacement electron, the characteristic photons generated are of such low energy that they are absorbed within the patient and do not fog the receptor.

The probability of photoelectric interaction is directly proportional to the third power of the atomic number (Z) of the absorber, and inversely proportional to the third power of the energy of the incident photon (E).

$$\text{Probablity of photoelectric interaction} \propto \frac{Z^3}{E^3}$$

The practical implications of photoelectric interaction are listed in Box 1.3.

Compton Scatter

Compton scatter occurs when a photon interacts with an outer orbital electron (Fig. 1.23). Approximately 57% of interactions in a dental x-ray beam exposure involve Compton scatter. In this interaction, the incident photon collides with an outer orbital electron, which receives kinetic energy and recoils from the point of impact. The path of the incident photon is deflected by this interaction and is scattered in a new direction. The energy of this scattered photon equals the energy of the incident photon minus the sum of the kinetic energy gained by the recoil electron and its binding energy. In the diagnostic energy range, most of the energy is retained by the scattered photon which can then cause additional ionizations, often at tissue sites outside the circumference of the incident beam. When these scattered photons reach the image receptor, they cause degradation of the image.

As with photoelectric absorption, Compton scatter results in the loss of an electron and ionization of the absorbing atom. Additional ionizations are caused by the scattered photons and the recoil electrons as they course through the patient's tissues. The probability of a Compton interaction is inversely proportional to the photon energy and is independent of atomic number. The probability of Compton scatter is dependent on the electron density of the absorber, which is relatively constant in tissue.

The practical implications of Compton scatter are listed in Box 1.4.

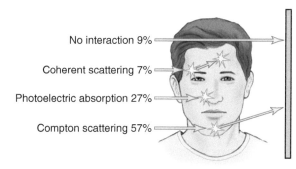

No interaction 9%

Coherent scattering 7%

Photoelectric absorption 27%

Compton scattering 57%

Fig. 1.21 Photons in an x-ray beam interact with the object primarily by Compton scattering (57% of primary interactions), in which case the scattered photon may strike the film and degrade the radiographic image by causing fog. The next most frequent interaction is photoelectric absorption (27%), in which the photons cease to exist. A radiographic image is produced by photons passing through low atomic number structures (soft tissue) and preferentially undergoing photoelectric absorption by high atomic number structures (bone, teeth, and metallic restorations). Relatively few photons undergo coherent scattering (7%) within the object or pass through the object without interaction (9%) and expose the image receptor.

TABLE 1.2 Interactions of Photons From a Diagnostic X-Ray Beam

Interaction	Ionization	Scatter	Practical Implications
Photoelectric absorption	Yes	No	Basis of radiographic image formation
Compton scatter	Yes	Yes	Scatter radiation can degrade image, expose personnel and patient
Coherent scatter	No	No	Minimal contribution to scatter

TABLE 1.3 Fate of 1 Million Incident Photons in Bite-wing Projection

Interaction	Fate of Incident Photon	Primary Photons	Scattered Photons[a]	Total[b]
Coherent scattering	Scatters from atom	74,453	78,117	152,570
Photoelectric absorption	Ejects inner electron and ceases to exist; releases characteristic photon	268,104	261,041	529,145
Compton scattering	Ejects outer electron, both scatter	565,939	549,360	1,115,300
No interaction	Passes through patient	91,504	379,350	470,855
Total		1,000,000	1,267,868	2,267,869

[a]The fate of scattered photons resulting from primary Compton, photoelectric, and coherent interactions.
[b]The sum of the total number of photoelectric interactions and photons that exit the patient equals the total number of incident photons.
From SJ Gibbs, personal communication, 1986.

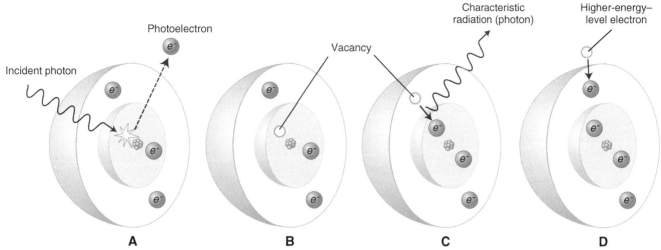

Fig. 1.22 Photoelectric absorption. (A) Photoelectric absorption occurs when an incident photon gives up all of its energy to an inner electron, which is ejected from the atom (a photoelectron). The incident electron ceases to exist at this point. (B) The ionized atom now has an electron vacancy in the inner orbital. (C) An electron from a higher energy level fills the vacancy and emits characteristic radiation. (D) All orbitals are subsequently filled, completing the energy exchange.

BOX 1.3 Practical Implications of Photoelectric Effect

Differential absorption in various tissues and objects (restorations for example) provides radiographic contrast. Because the effective atomic number of compact bone ($Z = 13.8$) is greater than that of soft tissue ($Z = 7.4$), the probability of photoelectric interaction of x-ray photons in bone is approximately 6.5 times greater than in an equal thickness of soft tissue ($13.8^3/7.4^3 = 6.5$). This marked difference in the absorption of x-ray photons by the soft and hard tissues makes the production of a radiographic image possible. This differential photoelectric absorption of x-ray photons in enamel, dentin, pulp, bone, and soft tissue is what we observe as different degrees of radiopacity on the radiographic image.

Causes ionization and potential for biological damage.

BOX 1.4 Practical Implications of Compton Scatter

Scattered photons travel in all directions and may exit the patient and strike the image receptor. These photons carry no useful information and degrade the image by reducing contrast.

Scattered photons that exit the patient can expose the operator.

Scattered photons travel varying distances within the patient's tissues and cause ionizations. This internal scatter increases patient radiation dose and often exposes organs and tissues outside of and distant from the path of the primary beam.

Coherent Scatter

Coherent scatter (also known as Rayleigh, classical, or elastic scatter) may occur when a low-energy incident photon (<10 keV) interacts with a whole atom. The incident photon causes it to become momentarily excited (Fig. 1.24). The incident photon then ceases to exist. The excited atom quickly returns to the ground state and generates another x-ray photon with the same energy as the incident photon. Usually the secondary photon is emitted in a different direction than the path of the incident photon. The net effect is that the direction of the incident x-ray photon is altered (scattered). Coherent scattering accounts for

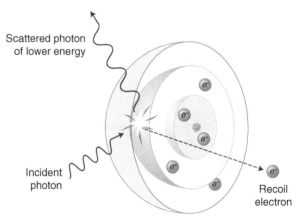

Fig. 1.23 Compton scattering occurs when an incident photon interacts with an outer electron, producing a scattered photon of lower energy than the incident photon and a recoil electron ejected from the target atom. The new scattered photon travels in a different direction from the incident photon.

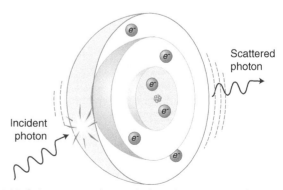

Fig. 1.24 Coherent scattering results from the interaction of a low-energy incident photon with a whole atom, causing it to be momentarily excited. After this interaction, the atom quickly returns to the ground state and emits a scattered photon of the same energy but at a different angle from the path of the incident photon.

only approximately 7% of the total number of interactions in a dental exposure (see Table 1.3). Because no energy is transferred to the biologic atom and no ionizations are caused, the biologic effects of coherent scatter are insignificant. Because coherent scatter occurs primarily in the lower energy range, the scattered photon has insufficient energy to reach the image receptor, and thus coherent scatter has minimal impact on image degradation.

Beam Attenuation

As an x-ray beam travels through matter, its intensity is reduced primarily through photoelectric absorption and Compton scattering. The extent of beam attenuation depends primarily on the energy of the beam and the thickness and density of the attenuating material. High-energy x-ray photons have a greater probability of penetrating matter, whereas lower-energy photons have a greater probability of being attenuated. The higher the kVp setting, the greater the penetrability of the resulting beam through matter. A useful way to characterize the penetrating quality of an x-ray beam is by its half-value layer (HVL). The HVL is the thickness of an absorber, such as aluminum, that reduces the number of x-ray photons by 50%. As the mean energy of an x-ray beam increases, so does the amount of material required to reduce the beam intensity by half (its HVL). The HVLs of several materials have been established for a wide range of photon energies. This allows medical physicists to calculate the thickness of material required and design appropriate shielding in diagnostic radiology facilities.

The reduction of beam intensity also depends on physical characteristics of the absorber. Higher-density materials attenuate more because of more photoelectric absorption and more Compton scattering with increasing density. In addition, increasing the thickness of an absorber increases the number of interactions. A monochromatic beam of photons, a beam in which all the photons have the same energy, provides a useful example. When only the primary (not scattered) photons are considered, a constant fraction of the beam is attenuated as the beam moves through each unit thickness of an absorber. For example, if 1.5 cm of water reduces a beam intensity by 50%, the next 1.5 cm reduces the beam intensity by another 50% (to 25% of the original intensity), and so on. This is an exponential pattern of absorption (Fig. 1.25). The HVL described earlier is a measure of beam energy describing the amount of an absorber that reduces the beam intensity by half; in the preceding example, the HVL is 1.5 cm of water.

In contrast to the previous example using a monoenergetic x-ray beam, there is a wide range of photon energies in an x-ray beam. Low-energy photons are much more likely than high-energy photons to be attenuated. Thus the superficial layers of an absorber remove the low-energy photons but transmit many of the higher-energy photons. As an x-ray beam passes through this material, the intensity of the beam decreases from preferential removal of low-energy photons. Because the transmitted photons are predominantly higher energy, the mean energy of the residual beam increases. The term beam hardening is used to describe this increase in the mean energy of the beam by preferential removal of lower-energy photons.

As the energy of an x-ray beam increases, so does the transmission of the beam through an absorber. However, when the energy of the incident photon is increased to match the binding energy of the 1s orbital electrons of the absorber, the probability of photoelectric absorption increases sharply and the number of absorbed photons is greatly increased. This is called K-edge absorption. The probability that a photon will interact with an orbital electron is greatest when the energy of the photon equals the binding energy of the electron; it decreases as the photon energy increases. Photons with energy less than the binding energy of 1s orbital electrons interact by photoelectric absorption only with electrons in the 2s or 2p orbitals and in orbitals even farther from

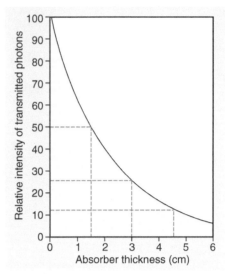

Fig. **1.25** Intensity of an energetically homogeneous x-ray beam declines exponentially as it travels through an absorber. In this instance, the half-value layer of the beam is 1.5 cm of absorber (i.e., every 1.5 cm of the absorber reduces the intensity of the beam by half). The curve for a heterogeneous x-ray beam (e.g., a dental x-ray beam) does not drop quite as precipitously because of the preferential removal of low-energy photons by the absorber and the increased mean energy of the resulting beam.

the nucleus. Rare earth elements are sometimes used as filters because their 1s orbital binding energies, or K edges (e.g., 50.24 keV for gadolinium), greatly increase the absorption of high-energy photons. This is desirable because these high-energy photons degrade image contrast and are not as likely as mid-energy photons that primarily contribute to a radiographic image.

DOSIMETRY

Table 1.4 presents some frequently used units of radiation and radiation detriment. Contemporary literature uses radiation measurement units from the SI system (*Système International d'Unités*), and these will be used in this book. Traditional units and their conversion have been included for reference.

Exposure

Exposure is a measure of the capacity of x-rays or γ-rays to ionize air. It is measured as the amount of charge per mass of air—coulombs/kg. It is a measure of the intensity of the radiation field as opposed to the amount of radiation absorbed, although there is a direct relationship. The roentgen has been largely replaced by the SI equivalent unit of air kerma.
Traditional unit: roentgen (R)
$1 \text{ R} = 2.58 \times 10^{-4} \text{ C/kg}$
One R will produce 2.08×10^8 ion pairs in 1 cm³ of air.

Air Kerma

When radiation interacts with matter via photoelectric absorption and Compton scattering, it transfers energy to electrons of the absorber. The kerma, an acronym for *k*inetic *e*nergy *r*eleased in *ma*tter, measures the kinetic energy transferred from photons to electrons and is expressed in units of dose (gray [Gy]), where 1 Gy equals 1 J/kg. Kerma is the sum of the initial kinetic energies of all the charged particles liberated by uncharged ionizing radiation (e.g., x-rays) in a sample of matter divided by the mass of the sample. Kerma values made in air are called

TABLE 1.4 Summary of Radiation Quantities and Units

Quantity	Description	SI Unit	Traditional Unit	Conversion
Exposure	Amount of ionization of air by x- or γ-rays	coulomb/kg (C/kg)	roentgen (R)	1 C/kg = 3876 R
Kerma	Kinetic energy transferred to charged particles	gray (Gy)	—	—
Absorbed dose	Total energy absorbed by a mass	gray (Gy)	rad	1 Gy = 100 rad
Equivalent dose	Absorbed dose weighted by biologic effectiveness of radiation type used	sievert (Sv)	rem	1 Sv = 100 rem
Effective dose	Sum of equivalent doses weighted by radiosensitivity of exposed tissue or organ	sievert (Sv)	—	—
Radioactivity	Rate of radioactive decay	becquerel (Bq)	curie (Ci)	1 Bq = 2.7×10^{-11} Ci

air kerma. The kerma is rapidly replacing exposure measured in coulombs/kg or R. An exposure of 1 R results in an air kerma of approximately 8.77 mGy.

Absorbed Dose

Absorbed dose is a measure of the total energy absorbed by any type of ionizing radiation per unit of mass of any type of matter. It varies with the type and energy of radiation and the type of matter absorbing the energy.

SI unit: gray, where 1 Gy = 1 J/kg
Traditional unit: rad (radiation absorbed dose)
1 rad = 100 ergs/g of absorber
1 Gy = 100 rad.

Equivalent (Radiation-Weighted) Dose

The equivalent dose (H_T) is used to compare the biologic effects of different types of radiation on a tissue or organ. Particulate radiations have a high LET and are more damaging to tissue than is radiation with low LET, such as x-rays. Thus deposition of 1 Gy of α particles causes much more biologic damage than 1 Gy of x-ray photons. The equivalent dose considers not only the absorbed dose but also this relative biologic effectiveness of the incident radiation using a radiation-weighting factor (W_R). The W_R of photons, the reference, is 1. The W_R of 5-keV neutrons and high-energy protons is 5, and the W_R of α particles is 20. The equivalent dose (H_T) is computed as the product of the radiation-weighting factor (W_R) and the absorbed dose averaged over a tissue or organ (D_T).

$$H_T = W_R \times D_T$$

SI Unit: Sievert (Sv)
For x-rays, 1 Sv = 1 Gy
Traditional unit: rem (roentgen equivalent mammal)
1 Sv = 100 rems

Effective Dose

The effective dose (E) is used to estimate the risk in humans. It is hard to compare the risk from a dental exposure with, for example, the risk from a radiographic chest examination because different tissues with different radiosensitivities are exposed. To allow such comparisons, the effective dose is a calculation that considers the relative biologic effectiveness of different types of radiation *and* the radiosensitivity of different tissues exposed in terms of the risk for stochastic effects of radiation (cancer induction and heritable effects). Tissue weighting factors (W_T) have been developed to factor individual tissue radiosensitivity (Table 1.5). E is the sum of the products of the equivalent dose to each organ or tissue (H_T) and the tissue weighting factor (W_T)

$$E = \sum W_T \times H_T$$

TABLE 1.5 Tissue Weighting Factors[a]

Tissue	Tissue Weighting Factor (W_T)
Bone marrow, colon, lung, stomach, breast, remainder tissues[b]	0.12
Gonads	0.08
Bladder, esophagus, liver, thyroid	0.04
Bone surface, brain, salivary glands, skin	0.01

[a]ICRP Publication 103: The 2007 Recommendations of the International Commission on Radiological Protection.
Adrenals, extrathoracic region, gallbladder, heart, kidneys, lymphatic nodes, muscle, oral mucosa, pancreas, prostate, small intestine, spleen, thymus, uterus/cervix.

SI Unit: Sievert (Sv)
Traditional unit: rem (roentgen equivalent mammal)
1 Sv = 100 rems

Radioactivity

The measurement of radioactivity (A) describes the decay rate of a sample of radioactive material. Although not directly applicable to dentomaxillofacial radiography, diagnostic nuclear medicine examinations indicate the amount of radiopharmaceutical delivered to the patient using the following units.
SI Unit: becquerel (Bq)
1 Bq = 1 disintegration per second (dps)
Traditional unit: curie (Ci)
1 Ci = 3.7×10^{10} dps
1 Bq = 2.7×10^{-11} Ci
1 mCi = 37 megaBq

BIBLIOGRAPHY

Bushberg JT. *The Essential Physics of Medical Imaging.* 3rd ed. Philadelphia: Lippincott Williams & Wilkins; 2012.
Bushong SC. *Radiologic Science for Technologists: Physics, Biology, and Protection.* 11th ed. St Louis: Mosby; 2017.
Greene B. *The Elegant Universe.* 1st ed. New York: Vintage; 1999.
Sacks O. *Uncle Tungsten: Memories of a Chemical Boyhood.* New York: Vintage; 2002.
The 2007 recommendations of the International Commission on Radiological Protection. IRCP Publication 103. *Ann ICRP.* 2007;37:1–332.

2

Biologic Effects of Ionizing Radiation

Sanjay M. Mallya

Photons from a diagnostic or therapeutic x-ray beam interact with the patient's tissues, causing ionization of biologic molecules. These initial interactions occur almost instantaneously, within 10^{-13} seconds after exposure. Subsequent modification of biologic molecules follows within seconds to hours, and the damage from these modifications may manifest in hours, days, years, and even generations, depending on the extent and type of damage. This chapter provides basic knowledge to understand the biologic effects of diagnostic and therapeutic radiation, with special emphasis on maxillofacial tissue effects.

CHEMICAL AND BIOCHEMICAL CONSEQUENCES OF RADIATION ABSORPTION

Biologic effects of ionizing radiation occur through direct and indirect actions (Fig. 2.1). In *direct actions*, the photon directly interacts with and ionizes a biologic macromolecule. The free electrons produced by the ionization interaction *(secondary electrons)* may also interact directly with biologic macromolecules. In contrast, in *indirect actions*, photons and secondary electrons interact with water and the products of water ionizations cause biologic damage. Direct and indirect actions both yield unstable *free radicals*—atoms or molecules with an unpaired electron in the valence orbital. Free radicals are extremely reactive and have very short lives. Free radicals play a dominant role in producing molecular changes in biologic molecules.

Direct Actions

In direct actions, biologic molecules (denoted RH, where *R* is the molecule and *H* is a hydrogen atom) absorb energy from ionizing radiation and within 10^{-10} seconds form unstable free radicals. These free radicals quickly re-form into stable configurations by dissociation (breaking apart) or cross-linking (joining of two molecules).

$$x - radiation + RH \rightarrow R^\bullet + H^+ + e^-$$

$$R^\bullet \rightarrow X + Y^\bullet (Dissociation)$$

$$R^\bullet + S^\bullet \rightarrow RS (Cross - linking)$$

Because the altered biologic molecules differ structurally and functionally from the original molecules, the consequence is a biologic change in the irradiated organism. *Direct actions dominate with high linear energy transfer (LET) radiations and are less predominant with low-LET radiations such as x- and γ-rays.*

Indirect Actions

In indirect actions, the initial interaction of a photon occurs with a water molecule—which constitutes approximately 70% of mammalian cells. *Indirect actions are the predominant mode of x-radiation–induced biologic damage.* Ionizing radiation initiates a complex series of chemical changes in water, collectively referred to as radiolysis of water. The initial series of interactions of x-ray photon with water produce hydrogen ($\mathbf{H^\bullet}$) and hydroxyl ($\mathbf{OH^\bullet}$) free radicals that interact with biologic macromolecules. *The hydroxyl radical is highly reactive and is estimated to cause two-thirds of the biologic damage to mammalian cells from x-rays.* The resulting organic free radicals are unstable and transform into stable, altered molecules, as described in the previous section on direct effects. These altered molecules have different chemical and biologic properties from the original molecules.

$$x - radiation + H_2O \rightarrow H^\bullet + OH^\bullet$$

$$R - H + OH^\bullet \rightarrow R^\bullet + H_2O$$

$$R - H + H^\bullet \rightarrow R^\bullet + H_2$$

The presence of dissolved oxygen, as is the case in normal tissues, significantly modifies the species of free radicals formed during water radiolysis. In the presence of oxygen, hydroperoxyl and hydrogen peroxide are formed—these are strong oxidizing agents that contribute significantly to indirect actions.

$$H^\bullet + O_2 \rightarrow HO_2^\bullet$$

$$HO_2^\bullet + HO_2^\bullet \rightarrow H_2O_2 + O_2$$

Deoxyribonucleic Acid and Chromosomal Damage and Damage Response

Damage to a cell's deoxyribonucleic acid (DNA) is the primary cause of radiation-induced cell death, heritable mutations, and carcinogenesis. Ionizing radiations, via production of free radicals, produce many different types of alterations in DNA, including:
- Base damage
- Single-strand breaks
- Double-strand breaks
- DNA-DNA and DNA-protein cross-links

Mammalian cells have evolved intricate mechanisms to respond to DNA damage. These include sensor molecules that recognize specific DNA damage types and signal transduction pathways that activate or upregulate DNA repair mechanisms. The *base excision repair* and *nucleotide excision repair* mechanisms efficiently repair most base damages, single-strand breaks, and DNA cross-links. A DNA double-strand break is the most important damage type and is believed to be the detrimental event for cell killing, tumor-induction, and heritable effects of ionizing radiation. DNA double-strand breaks are repaired by either *nonhomologous end-joining* or *homologous recombination*. Nonhomologous end-joining is an error-prone mechanism and accounts

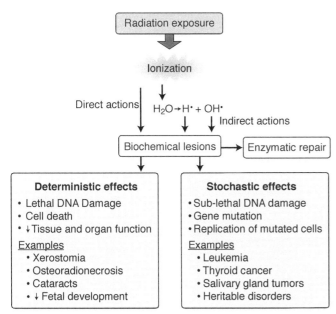

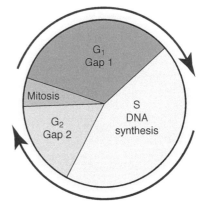

Fig. 2.3 Cell cycle. A proliferating cell moves in the cycle from mitosis phase when chromosomes are condensed and visible to gap 1 (G₁) to the period of deoxyribonucleic acid *(DNA)* synthesis (S) to gap 2 (G₂) to the next mitosis. Cells are most radiosensitive in the G₂ and mitosis phase, less sensitive in the G₁ phase, and least sensitive during the latter part of the S phase.

Fig. 2.1 Overview of events after exposure of humans to ionizing radiation. The initial ionization, direct and indirect actions, and initial molecular changes in organic molecules occur in less than a second. The enzymatic repair or development of further biochemical lesions occurs in minutes to hours. The deterministic and stochastic effects occur over a time scale of months to decades to generations. *DNA*, Deoxyribonucleic acid.

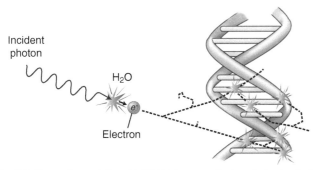

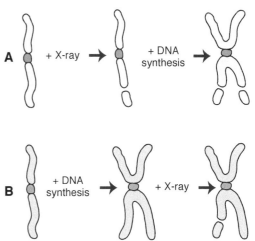

Fig. 2.4 Chromosome aberrations. (A) Irradiation before deoxyribonucleic acid *(DNA)* synthesis results in a double-arm (chromosome) aberration because the damage is replicated in the next S phase and becomes visible in the next mitosis phase. (B) Irradiation of a cell after DNA synthesis results in a single-arm (chromatid) aberration.

Fig. 2.2 Deoxyribonucleic acid *(DNA)* damage cluster. A single photon may cause multiple ionizations in DNA, resulting in a cluster of DNA damage. In this instance, an incident photon causes ionization of a water molecule, and the recoil electron causes a cluster of damage to multiple sites in a DNA molecule. Such cluster damage is difficult to repair and is believed to be responsible for most radiation cell killing, carcinogenesis, and heritable effects.

for many of the ionizing radiation-induced mutations. Ionizing radiation may also cause clustered DNA damage—two or more closely spaced damages (base damages, strand breaks) occurring within two turns of the DNA helix (Fig. 2.2). The energy deposition pattern from a single x-ray photon may cause these damage clusters, which are thought to be critical lesions for cell killing and mutagenesis.

The DNA in the nucleus of eukaryotes is distributed into chromosomes. Each chromosome is a long DNA molecule associated with proteins that fold and pack the DNA into a compact structure. Human somatic cells have 46 chromosomes. During the S phase of the cell cycle (Fig. 2.3), the chromosomes are duplicated and the two daughter sister chromatids are held together at a region called the centromere. During mitosis, the sister chromatids separate at the centromere and are segregated into the daughter cells. This process is tightly regulated to ensure

that each daughter cell receives the appropriate chromosomal complement. A DNA double-strand break causes a breach in the integrity of the chromosome. If the breaks rejoin with fidelity to re-create the original intact chromosome, the damage will go unrecognized. However, failure to rejoin or incorrect rejoining of broken chromosomal ends will result in aberrations.

When a DNA strand break occurs prior to chromosomal duplication (G1 and early S phase of the cell cycle; Fig. 2.3), the break is replicated and both sister chromatids will carry the damage. Resultant aberrations are termed chromosome aberrations (Fig. 2.4A). If the cell is irradiated after chromosomal duplication, the break will occur in only one of the sister chromatids and generate a chromatid aberration (see Fig. 2.4B). The frequency of aberrations is generally proportional to the radiation dose received. Some aberrations are lethal to the cell—*ring chromosome, dicentric chromosome,* and *anaphase bridge* (Fig. 2.5A–C)—and cause cell death during mitosis. Other types of aberrations are nonlethal and include *translocations* and *small deletions* (see Fig. 2.5D and E). These

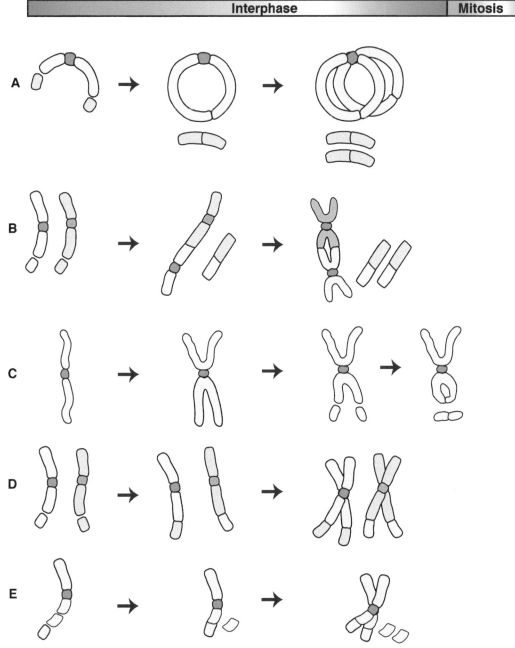

Fig. 2.5 Chromosome and chromatid aberrations. (A) Ring formation plus acentric fragment. (B) Dicentric formation. (C) Anaphase bridge formation. (D) Translocation and (E) deletion. The occurrence of the breakage and fusion events relative to the cell cycle phase is denoted by the bar on the top.

nonlethal aberrations may cause tumor induction and heritable effects of radiation.

STOCHASTIC AND DETERMINISTIC EFFECTS

There are two fundamental categories of radiation-induced biologic effects—stochastic and deterministic. The differences between these effects are summarized in Table 2.1. The characterizing difference between these two categories is the dose threshold for its occurrence. Stochastic effects do not exhibit a dose threshold, whereas deterministic effects manifest only when the radiation dose exceeds a certain threshold.

Diagnostic radiation doses place the patient at risk for stochastic effects but **not** deterministic effects.

Stochastic Effects

One outcome of radiation-induced DNA damage is that the cell survives but with mutation of its DNA. Stochastic effects are the consequence of such sublethal changes in the DNA of an individual cell. The manifestation of a stochastic effect is dependent on the individual cell type damaged. For example, heritable effects will manifest only if the mutation occurred in a germ cell. Causation of a stochastic effect is also dependent on the specific DNA mutation induced. For example, for carcinogenesis

TABLE 2.1 Comparison of Stochastic and Deterministic Effects of Radiation

	Stochastic Effects	Deterministic Effects
Caused by	Sublethal DNA damage	Cell killing
Threshold dose	No	Yes
	There is no minimum threshold dose. Effect can be caused by any dose of radiation	Effect occurs only when the threshold dose is exceeded
Severity of clinical effects and dose	Severity of clinical effects is independent of dose; all-or-none response—an individual either manifests effect or does not	Severity of clinical effects is proportional to dose; the higher the dose, the more severe the effect
Relationship between dose and effect	Frequency of effect proportional to dose; the higher the dose, the higher the risk of manifesting the effect	Probability of effect independent of dose; most individuals manifest effect when threshold dose is exceeded
Caused by doses used in diagnostic radiology	Yes	No
Examples	Radiation-induced cancer Heritable effects Radiation-induced skin cancer	Osteoradionecrosis Radiation-induced cataract formation Radiation-induced skin burns

DNA, Deoxyribonucleic acid.

to occur, the mutation must confer that specific cell with a selective growth advantage.

Stochastic effects are considered to occur without a dose threshold. This belief is shaped by our current understanding of the molecular mechanisms of DNA damage repair.

- A single x-ray photon has the potential to cause a DNA mutation. Thus even the smallest radiation dose could cause a heritable effect or cancer.
- As radiation dose increases, the number of radiation-induced DNA damage sites in increased and the risk of subsequent disease-causing mutation is higher. Thus, *the probability of a stochastic effect increases with dose.*

Radiation-Induced Cancer

Carcinogenesis is a multistep process in which a cell accumulates DNA mutations that provide it with a selective growth advantage. These mutations may occur sporadically or may be caused by exogenous insults such as chemicals and ionizing radiation. There is strong evidence that ionizing radiation causes cancer and is the most important adverse effect of diagnostic radiation. Our current understanding of the molecular mechanistic basis for radiation-induced cancer builds on experimental studies of cultured cells and animals, and human populations that were exposed to ionizing radiation, either accidentally or for medical purposes. In particular, the human population studies have provided insights into tissue sensitivities and risk estimates for carcinogenesis. Such populations include radium dial painters, children irradiated to treat scalp infections, women who underwent repeated fluoroscopies to monitor tuberculosis,

BOX 2.1 General Features of Radiation-Induced Cancer

- Radiation-induced cancers are clinically and histologically indistinguishable from sporadically occurring or chemical-induced cancers.
- Certain tissues, for example the female breast and the thyroid gland, are more sensitive to the carcinogenic effects of ionizing radiation.
- There is a long latent period, ranging from years to decades, between radiation exposure and the occurrence of cancer.
- The risk of radiation-induced tumor induction is approximately threefold higher in children than in adults.

and survivors of the atomic bomb explosions and the radiation accident in Chernobyl. The general conclusions that emerge from these studies are listed in Box 2.1.

Radiation-induced cancer in tissues at risk from diagnostic maxillofacial radiography are discussed next.

Leukemia. The incidence of leukemia (other than chronic lymphocytic leukemia) increases after exposure of the bone marrow to radiation. The risks are highest in children, peaking at approximately 7 years and ceasing after approximately 30 years.

Thyroid cancer. The incidence of thyroid carcinomas, predominantly papillary thyroid carcinomas, increases in humans after radiation exposure. There is strong dependence on age at exposure—susceptibility to radiation-induced thyroid cancer is higher in children than adults. There is little evidence for a dose response for individuals exposed during adulthood. Females are 2 to 3 times more susceptible than males to radiogenic and spontaneous thyroid cancers.

Salivary gland tumors. The incidence of salivary gland tumors, both benign and malignant, is increased in patients treated with irradiation for diseases of the head and neck and in Japanese atomic bomb survivors. Most of the tumors were benign, with Warthin tumor being the most frequent. Among the malignant tumors, the frequency of mucoepidermoid tumor was highest.

An association between tumors of the salivary glands and dental radiography has been shown, although this association is likely a consequence of more dental radiographs made to investigate the symptoms of an existing tumor, rather than the dental radiation doses inducing tumors.

Breast cancer. The female breast is highly sensitive to radiation-induced cancer. Studies from several cohorts demonstrate a linear relationship between risk and dose. The risk is significantly higher when exposed before age 20.

Brain and nervous system cancers. Patients exposed to diagnostic x-ray examinations in utero and to therapeutic doses in childhood or as adults (average midbrain dose of approximately 1 Gy) show excess numbers of malignant and benign brain tumors. Case-control studies have shown an association between intracranial meningiomas and previous medical or dental radiography. However, this association is likely due to more dental radiographs that were made in response to facial pain referred from the tumor rather than the radiation causing more meningiomas.

Heritable Effects

Heritable effects are changes seen in the offspring of irradiated individuals. They are the consequence of DNA damage in germ cells. At low levels of exposure, such as encountered in dentistry, they are far less important than carcinogenesis. Our knowledge of heritable effects of radiation on humans comes largely from the atomic bomb survivors. To date, no such radiation-related genetic damage has been demonstrated.

TABLE 2.2   Casarett's Categorization of Cell Types by Radiosensitivity

| Radiosensitivity | Category | CHARACTERISTICS | | Examples |
		Cell Division	Differentiation Status	
High	I. Vegetative intermitotic	Rapid	Undifferentiated	Basal cells of oral mucosa, bone marrow stem cells
↑	II. Differentiating intermitotic	Regular	Some differentiation	Myelocytes, spermatocytes
Intermediate	III. Multipotent connective tissue			Fibroblasts, endothelial cells
↓	IV. Reverting postmitotic	Not regular, but can be stimulated to divide	Fully differentiated	Hepatocytes
Low	V. Fixed postmitotic	No	Highly differentiated	Neurons, muscle cells

Modified from Rubin P, Casarett GW. *Clinical Radiation Pathology*. Philadelphia: W.B. Saunders; 1968.

No increase has occurred in adverse pregnancy outcome, leukemia or other cancers, or impairment of growth and development in the children of atomic bomb survivors. Similarly, studies of the children of patients who received radiotherapy show no detectable increase in the frequency of genetic diseases. These findings do not exclude the possibility that such damage occurs at a very low frequency.

Deterministic Effects

Deterministic effects of radiation are caused by cell killing and are the consequences of cell death on the function of a tissue or organ. Deterministic effects manifest only when the radiation exposure to an organ or tissue exceeds a threshold level. The magnitude of this threshold dose is dependent on the tissue type. At doses below the threshold, the effect does not occur. Most individuals who receive doses higher than the threshold will develop the effect. The severity of this effect is proportional to the dose: the higher the dose, the more severe the effect. Diagnostic radiologic examinations are designed to keep the dose below the threshold dose, and thus deterministic effects are not encountered in diagnostic maxillofacial radiography. However, dentists will frequently encounter patients undergoing radiation therapy for head and neck malignancies. These therapeutic protocols deliver doses that exceed the threshold for various tissues, and these effects are described in the next section.

Cell Killing

Mitotic death. The predominant mode of radiation-induced cell killing is *mitotic death (or mitotic catastrophe)*, resulting from lethal chromosomal and chromatid aberrations (see Fig. 2.5). A cell's sensitivity to this mode of death is determined by its mitotic rate and degree of differentiation. This relationship is referred to as the law of Bergonié and Tribondeau, in honor of the radiobiologists that first described this principle.

$$\text{Cell radiosensitivity to killing} \propto \frac{\text{Mitotic rate}}{\text{Degree of differentiation}}$$

This rule predicts that rapidly dividing cells will be more radiosensitive and postmitotic specialized cells will be most radioresistant; it holds true for most cell types. Building on the work of Bergonié and Tribondeau, Casarett described discrete cell type categories based on their radiosensitivity (Table 2.2). This classification system helps to understand sensitivity of individual tissues and organs to manifest deterministic effects.

Apoptosis. Lymphocytes are the most radiosensitive mammalian cell and are an exception to the law of Bergonié and Tribondeau. Likewise, serous acini of the salivary glands are highly radiosensitive, although they do not divide rapidly. In these cell types, *apoptosis* is the predominant

BOX 2.2   Relative Radiosensitivity of Various Organs

High	Intermediate	Low
Lymphoid organs	Fine vasculature	Neurons
Bone marrow	Growing cartilage	Muscle
Testes	Growing bone	
Intestines	Salivary glands	
Mucosal lining	Lungs	
	Kidney	
	Liver	

mode of radiation-induced death. In this mechanism, radiation damage induces a programmed cascade of events that rapidly causes cell death within hours after radiation exposure. Unlike mitotic death, apoptotic death does not require the cell to undergo mitosis, and the cell dies in interphase. There is strong evidence that the initial signals for apoptosis are triggered by radiation-induced DNA damage. The tumor suppressor gene *p53* is a major regulator of apoptosis.

Recent evidence from cultured cells has demonstrated a *bystander effect*, in which cells that are in the proximity of irradiated cells, but not directly exposed, exhibit radiation-induced damage. The contribution of this effect to cell death in vivo is yet undetermined.

Radiosensitivity of a tissue or organ is dependent on the radiation dose and the sensitivity of its constituent cell types (Box 2.2). Manifestation of a deterministic effect reflects the consequences of cell death on function of the irradiated tissue or organ. Short-term effects may become apparent in hours to days and are consequent to a reduction in the number of mature cells in the tissues. The long-term deterministic effects (develop in months and years after exposure) are primarily caused by death of replicating cells, replacement with fibrous tissue, and damage to the fine vasculature.

Deterministic Radiation Effects on Embryos and Fetuses

Embryos and fetuses are considerably more radiosensitive than are adults because most embryonic cells are relatively undifferentiated and rapidly mitotic. The effects of radiation on embryos and fetuses have been extensively studied in animals, predominantly rodents. Data on effects on human embryos and fetuses are derived from studies of survivors of the atomic bomb, exposed in utero, and from children of women exposed to diagnostic or therapeutic radiation during pregnancy. The general conclusions from these studies are summarized as follows.

- The effects are dependent on the dose and gestational age during irradiation.

- Irradiation during preimplantation (0 to 9 days in humans) causes embryonic death. The threshold for this effect is estimated to be 100 mGy—approximately 14,000 times more than the fetal dose from dental radiographic examinations. In comparison, the dose to an embryo and fetus from natural background radiation is approximately 0.5 to 1 mSv during the 9 months of gestation.
- In humans, fetal irradiation is associated with microcephaly (irradiation at 8 to 15 weeks gestation) and mental retardation (irradiated at 8 to 25 weeks' gestation). The threshold dose for these effects is 0.3 Gy—approximately 42,000 times higher than fetal doses from dentomaxillofacial radiographic examinations.

Cataracts

Ionizing radiation damage to the lens of the eye induces cataracts—clouding or opacification of the lens. Recently, the International Commission on Radiological Protection (ICRP) proposed a lower dose threshold for cataract induction—0.5 Gy for low LET radiations such as x-rays, replacing previous estimates of 2 Gy. The National Council on Radiation Protection and Measurements (NCRP) estimates of the threshold dose are slightly higher, at 1 to 2 Gy, for vision-impairing cataracts. The absorbed dose in the lens of the eye during dentomaxillofacial radiographic examinations ranges from 0.02 to 0.4 mGy—at least 1250 times lower than the conservative estimate from ICRP.

RADIOTHERAPY INVOLVING THE ORAL CAVITY

Dentists are likely to manage patients who are undergoing radiation therapy or have received such treatment for management of head and neck malignancies. Often, the radiotherapy approach is combined with surgery and chemotherapy.

The radiation treatment is administered as many daily small doses (fractions). Such fractionation of the total x-ray dose provides greater tumor destruction than is possible with a large single dose. Fractionation also allows increased cellular repair of surrounding normal tissues that are unavoidably exposed. Fractionation also increases the mean oxygen tension in an irradiated tumor, rendering the tumor cells more radiosensitive. This results from killing rapidly dividing tumor cells and shrinking the tumor mass after the first few fractions, reducing the distance that oxygen must diffuse from the fine vasculature through the tumor to reach the remaining viable tumor cells. Typically, 2 Gy is delivered daily for a weekly exposure of 10 Gy. The radiotherapy course continues for 6 to 7 weeks until a total of 60 to 70 Gy is administered. Fig. 2.6 summarizes the temporal sequence of occurrence of oral complications from this therapy. In recent years, a new three-dimensional technique called intensity-modulated radiotherapy (IMRT) has been used to control the dose distribution with high accuracy, minimizing exposure to adjacent normal tissues.

Oral Mucosa

The oral mucosa contains a basal layer composed of rapidly dividing, radiosensitive progenitor cells. By the end of the second week of therapy, the cell death induces an inflammatory response and the mucous membranes begin to show areas of redness and inflammation (mucositis). During therapy, the irradiated mucous membrane separates from the underlying connective tissue and forms a white-to-yellow pseudomembrane (the desquamated epithelial layer) (Fig. 2.7). At the end of therapy, the mucositis is usually most severe, discomfort is at a maximum, and food intake is difficult. Good oral hygiene minimizes infection. Topical anesthetics may be required at mealtimes. Secondary yeast infection by *Candida albicans* is a common complication and may require treatment.

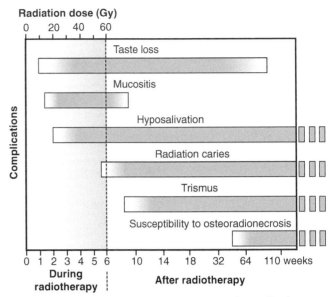

Fig. 2.6 Oral complications. Typical time course of complications seen during and after a course of radiation therapy to the head and neck. *Shaded area* in first 6 weeks represents accumulated dose. *Shading within bars* indicates severity of complication. Note recovery of taste and healing of mucositis. Changes persisting after 2 years pose lifelong risks. (Adapted from Kielbassa AM, Hinkelbein W, Hellwig E, Meyer-Lückel H. Radiation-related damage to dentition. *Lancet Oncol.* 2006;7:326–335.)

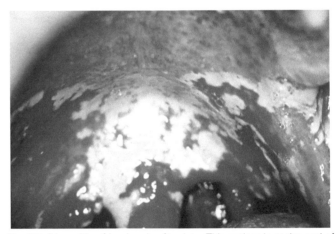

Fig. 2.7 Mucositis of hard and soft palate. This patient is at the end of a course of radiotherapy and demonstrates an inflammatory response in the oral mucosa and areas of white pseudomembrane, areas where the oral epithelium separated from the underlying connective tissue.

Following completion of radiotherapy, the mucosa heals rapidly. Healing is usually complete by approximately 2 months. However, fibrosis of the underling connective tissue causes the mucosa to become atrophic, thin, and relatively avascular. These atrophic changes complicate denture wearing because they may cause oral ulcerations of the compromised tissue. Ulcers may also result from radiation necrosis or tumor recurrence. A biopsy may be required to make the differentiation.

Taste Buds

Taste buds are sensitive to radiation. Doses in the therapeutic range cause a loss of taste acuity during the second or third week of radiotherapy, and taste acuity usually decreases by a factor of 1000 to 10,000 during the treatment period. Bitter and acid flavors are more severely affected when the posterior two-thirds of the tongue is irradiated, and salt and sweet flavors are affected more when the anterior third of the tongue is irradiated. Alterations in the saliva may partly account for this reduction. Taste loss is reversible, and recovery takes 2 to 4 months.

Salivary Glands

Salivary glands are highly sensitive to radiation, despite their relatively differentiated constituent cells. This is likely due to radiation-induced apoptosis of salivary acinar cells. Radiation therapy protocols attempt to limit the cumulative dose to the parotid to approximately 25 Gy, so that salivary function can be restored post therapy. This dose limit is 39 Gy for submandibular glands, which are more radioresistant than the parotid. Within the first week of radiation therapy, patients experience an approximately 50% decrease in salivary flow, attributed to apoptosis of the acinar cells. The salivary flow gradually decreases to less than 10% within 1 year. Late changes in the gland include fibrosis and decreased vascularity, impacting regaining salivary gland function. The residual gland function, is dose dependent. At doses less than 45 Gy, only 5% of patients experience permanent loss of function, determined at 5 years post therapy. At doses of 60 Gy and greater, this fraction increases to 50%. Use of IMRT has helped to spare the contralateral salivary glands and thus minimize the loss of salivary function.

The loss of saliva production results in xerostomia, a debilitating consequence with significant impact on quality of life. Xerostomic patients have trouble with chewing and swallowing. The biochemical properties of the saliva produced are different—the saliva has a lower pH, an average of 5.5 in irradiated patients compared with 6.5 in unexposed individuals. This pH is low enough to initiate decalcification of normal enamel. The buffering capacity of saliva is also decreased. Various saliva substitutes are available to help restore function.

Radiation Caries

Radiation caries is a rampant form of dental decay that may occur in patients with radiation-induced xerostomia. Caries results from changes in the salivary glands and saliva, including reduced flow, decreased pH, reduced buffering capacity, increased viscosity, and an altered flora. Patients receiving radiation therapy to oral structures have increases in *Streptococcus mutans, Lactobacillus,* and *Candida.* The residual saliva in individuals with xerostomia also has a low concentration of Ca^{2+} ion; this results in greater solubility of tooth structure and reduced remineralization. Because of the reduced or absent cleansing action of normal saliva, debris accumulates quickly.

Clinically, three patterns of radiation caries exist. The most common is widespread superficial lesions attacking buccal, occlusal, incisal, and palatal surfaces (Fig. 2.8). Another type involves primarily the cementum and dentin in the cervical region. These lesions may progress around the teeth circumferentially and result in loss of the crown. The third type appears as a dark pigmentation of the entire crown. The incisal edges may be markedly worn. Combinations of all these lesions develop in some patients. The location, rapid course, and widespread attack distinguish radiation caries. There is also evidence that radiation caries is more likely to lead to periapical inflammatory lesions if the periapical bone received a high dose of radiation.

The best method to reduce radiation caries is daily application of a viscous topical 1% neutral sodium fluoride gel in custom-made applicator trays. The best results are achieved from a combination of restorative dental procedures, excellent oral hygiene, a diet restricted in cariogenic foods, and topical applications of sodium fluoride. Patient cooperation in maintaining oral hygiene is extremely important because radiation caries is a lifelong threat. Teeth with gross caries or periodontal involvement are often extracted before irradiation.

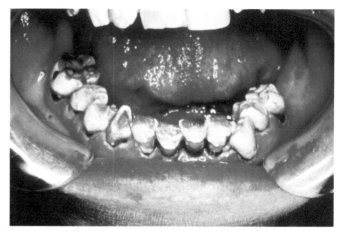

Fig. 2.8 Radiation caries. Note the extensive loss of structure on the occlusal surface of the mandibular teeth resulting from radiation-induced xerostomia.

Teeth

The effect on teeth depends on the stage of tooth development. If exposure occurs at early development, irradiation may destroy the tooth bud. In partially developed teeth irradiation may inhibit cellular differentiation, causing malformations and arresting general growth. Such exposure may retard or abort root formation, but the eruptive mechanism of teeth is relatively radiation resistant. Irradiated teeth with altered root formation typically erupt, even if rootless. In general, the severity of the damage is dose dependent. Children receiving radiation therapy to the jaws may show defects in the permanent dentition, such as retarded root development, dwarfed teeth, or failure to form one or more teeth (Fig. 2.9).

Bone

The primary damage to mature bone results from radiation-induced damage to the vasculature of the periosteum and cortical bone. Osteoradionecrosis (ORN) is a late complication of radiation therapy and occurs when an area of irradiated bone becomes devitalized. ORN is formally defined as "an area of exposed irradiated bone tissue that fails to heal over a period of three months, without residual or recurrent tumor; and when other causes of osteonecrosis have been excluded" (Fig. 2.10). A widely-accepted model is that radiation-induced microvascular changes create a state of hypoxia, hypovascularity, and hypocellularity, thereby disturbing normal bone homeostasis, and leading to a chronic, nonhealing wound. Radiation-induced fibrosis also contributes to ORN development. Radiation-induced cell damage triggers a cascade of chronic inflammation and deregulated fibroblastic activity around the blood vessel walls, exacerbating a chronic fibrotic response in both the bone and the overlying mucosa.

ORN typically manifests 6 to 12 months following radiation treatment but can develop anytime, from months to years following radiation therapy. The incidence of ORN is approximately 5% to 7% for conventional radiotherapy, IMRT, and brachytherapy. ORN is more frequent in the mandible than in the maxilla, likely due to the relatively lower vascularity in the mandible. ORN risk is dose dependent and increases 11-fold when the dose to the bone exceeds 66 Gy. When the dose is less than 60 Gy, ORN is unlikely, and it rarely occurs if the dose is less than 50 Gy. Important risk factors of clinical significance include carious teeth, periodontal disease, and trauma from dental extractions or ill-fitting dentures. Widening of

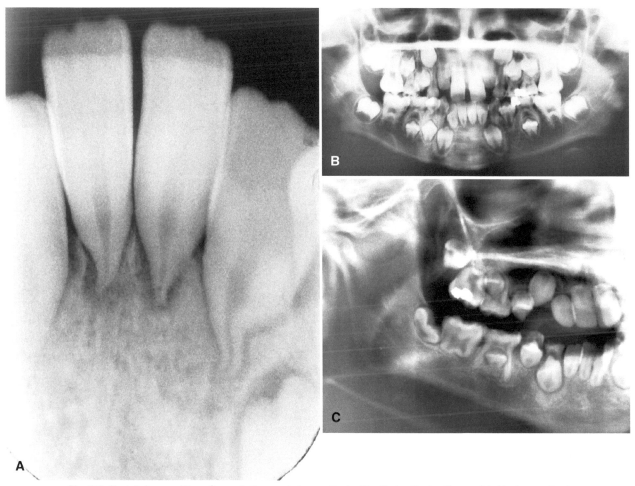

Fig. 2.9 Dental abnormalities after radiotherapy in two patients. The first patient, a 9-year-old girl who received 35 Gy at age 4 years because of Hodgkin disease, had severe stunting of the incisor roots with premature closure of the apices at 8 years (A) and retarded development of the mandibular second premolar crowns with stunting of the mandibular incisor, canine, and premolar roots at 9 years (B). The second patient (C), a 10-year-old boy who received 41 Gy to the jaws at age 4 years, had severely stunted root development of all permanent teeth with a normal primary molar. ([A] and [B], Courtesy Mr. P. N. Hirschmann, Leeds, UK. [C], Courtesy Dr. James Eischen, San Diego, California.)

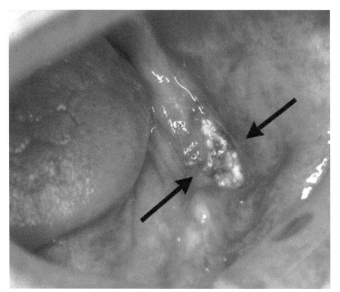

Fig. 2.10 Osteoradionecrosis presenting as an area of exposed bone in the irradiation field. Note the loss of oral mucosa (arrows).

the periodontal ligament space along the mandibular tooth roots is a common finding in the irradiated mandible but requires no management if the adjacent bone is not lytic. As the disease progresses, bone destruction becomes radiographically evident as patchy radiolucent areas with radiodense islands of necrotic bone, or sequestrum. The bone destruction may be severe enough to cause pathologic fracture (Fig. 2.11A and B).

Preradiotherapy dental care is important to minimize ORN risk. Carious teeth must be restored before radiation therapy. Preventive measures of good oral hygiene and daily topical fluoride application must be emphasized. Teeth with extensive caries or with poor periodontal support may be extracted, allowing 2 to 3 weeks for the extraction wounds to heal before beginning radiation therapy.

Posttherapy management is equally important. Periodic oral examinations and radiographs will allow early detection of caries and periapical inflammation. The radiation dose from such diagnostic exposures is negligible compared with the amount received during therapy and should not deter making radiographs when indicated. Extractions in an area of irradiated bone must performed with minimal surgical trauma. Dentures may need to be adjusted to minimize the risk of denture sores.

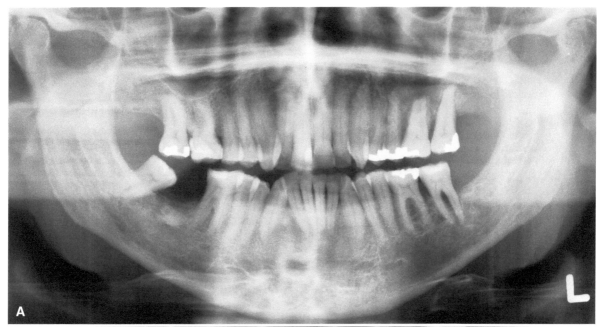

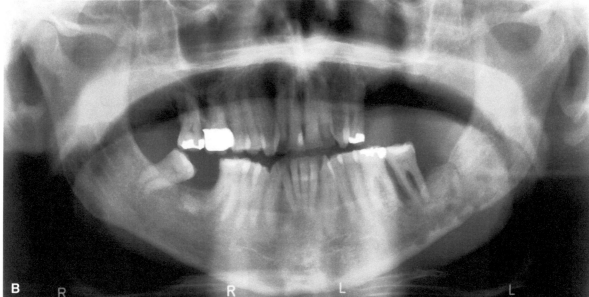

Fig. 2.11 (A) Panoramic radiograph taken to evaluate the teeth and jaws in a postradiation therapy patient shows presence of mild periodontal bone loss. (B) Panoramic radiograph of same patient taken 3 years later shows extensive bone destruction in the left posterior mandible body-angle region, extending to the inferior mandibular cortex.

Musculature

Radiation may cause inflammation and fibrosis, resulting in contracture and trismus in the muscles of mastication. The masseter or pterygoid muscles usually are involved. Restriction in mouth opening usually starts approximately 2 months after radiotherapy is completed and progresses thereafter. Exercises for mouth opening are helpful to minimize trismus.

BIBLIOGRAPHY

Hall EJ, Giaccia AJ. *Radiobiology for the Radiologist*. 7th ed. Philadelphia: Lippincott Williams & Wilkins; 2011.

Joiner M, van der Kogel A. *Basic Clinical Radiobiology*. 4th ed. London: Hodder Arnold; 2002.

National Research Council. *Health Risks from Exposure to Low Levels of Ionizing Radiation: BEIR VII Phase*. Washington, DC: The National Academies Press; 2006.

Radiation-Induced Cancer

Hall EJ. Is there a place for quantitative risk assessment? *J Radiol Prot.* 2009;29(0):A171–A184.

Hanahan D, Weinberg Robert A. Hallmarks of cancer: the next generation. *Cell.* 2011;144(5):646–674.

Mossman KL. The LNT debate in radiation protection: Science vs. Policy. *Dose Response.* 2012;10(2):190–202.

Ozasa K, Shimizu Y, Suyama A, et al. Studies of the mortality of atomic bomb survivors, Report 14, 1950-2003: an overview of cancer and noncancer diseases. *Radiat Res.* 2012;177:229–243.

Preston DL, Shimizu Y, Pierce DA, et al. Studies of mortality of atomic bomb survivors. Report 13: solid cancer and noncancer disease mortality: 1950-1997. *Radiat Res.* 2003;160:381–407.

Ron E, Saftlas AF. Head and neck radiation carcinogenesis: epidemiologic evidence. *Otolaryngol Head Neck Surg.* 1996;115(5):403–408.

Tetradis S, White SC, Service SK. Dental X-rays and risk of meningioma; the Jury is still out. *J Evid Based Dent Pract.* 2012;12(3):174–177.

Heritable Effects

United Nations Scientific Committee on the Effects of Atomic Radiation. Hereditary effects of radiation; 2001. http://www.unscear.org/unscear/en/publications/2001.html. Accessed January 10, 2018.

Cell Killing

Eriksson D, Stigbrand T. Radiation-induced cell death mechanisms. *Tumour Biol.* 2010;31(4):363–372.

Hall EJ. The bystander effect. *Health Phys.* 2003;85(1):31–35.

Deterministic Radiation Effects on Embryo and Fetus

Kelaranta A, Ekholm M, Toroi P, et al. Radiation exposure to foetus and breasts from dental X-ray examinations: effect of lead shields. *Dentomaxillofac Radiol.* 2016;45(1):20150095.

Wagner LK, Lester RG, Saldana LR. Exposure of the pregnant patient to diagnostic radiations. *A Guide to Medical Manangement.* Madison, Wis: Medical Physics Publishing; 1997.

Cataracts

Dauer LT, Ainsbury EA, Dynlacht J, et al. Guidance on radiation dose limits for the lens of the eye: overview of the recommendations in NCRP Commentary No. 26. *Int J Radiat Biol.* 2017;93(10):1–9.

Neriishi K, Nakashima E, Akahoshi M, et al. Radiation dose and cataract surgery incidence in atomic bomb survivors, 1986–2005. *Radiology.* 2012;265:167–174.

Radiotherapy Involving the Oral Cavity

Chan KC, Perschbacher SE, Lam EW, et al. Mandibular changes on panoramic imaging after head and neck radiotherapy. *Oral Surg Oral Med Oral Pathol Oral Radiol.* 2016;121(6):666–672.

Chung EM, Sung EC. Dental management of chemoradiation patients. *J Calif Dent Assoc.* 2006;34:735–742.

Dahllof G. Craniofacial growth in children treated for malignant diseases. *Acta Odontol Scand.* 1998;56:378.

Delanian S, Lefaix JL. The radiation-induced fibroatrophic process: therapeutic perspective via the antioxidant pathway. *Radiother Oncol.* 2004;73(2):119–131.

Jacobson AS, Buchbinder D, Hu K, et al. Paradigm shifts in the management of osteoradionecrosis of the mandible. *Oral Oncol.* 2010;46:795–801.

Kielbassa AM, Hinkelbein W, Hellwig E, et al. Radiation-related damage to dentition. *Lancet Oncol.* 2006;7:326–335.

Mallya SM, Tetradis S. Imaging of radiation- and medication-related osteonecrosis. *Radiol Clin North Am.* 2018;56:77–89.

Marx RE. Osteoradionecrosis: a new concept of its pathophysiology. *J Oral Maxillofac Surg.* 1983;41(5):283–288.

Schwartz HC, Kagan AR. Osteoradionecrosis of the mandible: scientific basis for clinical staging. *Am J Clin Oncol.* 2002;25(2):168–171.

3

Safety and Protection

Sanjay M. Mallya

Dentists must be prepared to intelligently discuss with patients the benefits and possible hazards involved with the use of x-rays and to describe the steps taken to reduce these hazards. This chapter considers sources of exposure, estimates of risks from dental radiography, and means to minimize exposure from radiographic examinations.

SOURCES OF RADIATION EXPOSURE

The general population is exposed to radiation primarily from natural background and medical sources (Table 3.1). These exposure sources provide a useful contextual framework to understand the magnitude of diagnostic radiation exposure.

Background Radiation

All life on earth has evolved in a continuous exposure to natural background radiation (Fig. 3.1; see Table 3.1). Background radiation from space and various terrestrial sources yields an average annual effective dose of approximately 3.1 mSv in the United States. There is considerable variation in background radiation exposure depending on geographic location—the global average is 2.4 mSv/year, and the typical global range is 1 to 13 mSv.

Radon and Its Progeny

Radon-222 is a radioactive element produced as an intermediate step in the decay of uranium-238, one of the most significant naturally occurring radioactive elements in the earth's crust. Radon, a gas, is released from the ground and enters homes and buildings. Radon-222 and its decay product polonium-218 emit α particles. Radon and its decay products may become attached to dust particles that can be inhaled and deposited on the bronchial epithelium in the respiratory tract. Radon is estimated to be responsible for approximately 73% of the background exposure of the world's population. Exposure to this quantity of radiation may cause 10,000 to 20,000 lung cancer deaths per year in the United States, mostly in smokers.

Space Radiation

Radiation from space comes from the sun or cosmic rays. It is composed primarily of protons, helium nuclei, and nuclei of heavier elements, as well as other particles generated by the interactions of primary space radiation with the earth's atmosphere. Exposure from space radiation is primarily a function of altitude, almost doubling with each 2000-m increase in elevation because less atmosphere is present to attenuate the radiation. At sea level, the exposure from space radiation is approximately 0.33 mSv/year; at an elevation of 1600 m (approximately 1 mile, the elevation of Denver, Colorado), it is approximately 0.50 mSv/

year. Space radiation contributes approximately 11% of background exposure.

Internal Radionuclides

Another source of background radiation is radionuclides that are ingested. The greatest internal exposure comes from foods containing uranium and thorium and their decay products, primarily potassium-40 but also rubidium-87, carbon-14, tritium, and others. The total exposure from ingestion contributes approximately 9% of background exposure.

Terrestrial Radiation

The final source of background radiation comes from exposure from radioactive nuclides in the soil, primarily potassium-40 and the radioactive decay products of uranium-238 and thorium-232. Most of the γ-radiation from these sources comes from the top 20 cm of soil. Indoor exposure from radionuclides is close to the exposure occurring outdoors because the shielding provided by structural materials balances the exposure from radioactive nuclides contained within these shielding materials. Terrestrial exposure contributes approximately 7% of background exposure.

Medical Exposure

Humans have contributed many additional sources of radiation (Fig. 3.2). The largest of these sources is medical imaging, with much smaller contributions from consumer products and other minor sources.

Approximately 3.6 billion x-ray and nuclear medicine examinations are performed annually worldwide; approximately 14% of these are dental radiographic examinations. More recent estimates suggest that medical exposure in developed countries has grown rapidly in recent decades, particularly computed tomography (CT) of the chest and abdomen and increased use of cardiac nuclear medicine studies. It is estimated that in the United States, the average exposure from medical diagnostic radiation is approximately 3.1 mSv, equivalent to natural background exposure. CT examinations (see Chapter 13) contribute more than half of medical radiation exposure. The distribution of medical exposures is highly skewed, with older and sicker individuals receiving most medical exposures. Dental x-ray examinations, although made relatively frequently, comprise only 0.26% of the total exposure from medical imaging.

Consumer Products

Consumer products contain some of the most interesting and unsuspected sources. This group includes, in order of importance, radiation exposure from cigarette smoking, building materials, air travel, mining and agriculture, and combustion of fossil fuels. With increasing air

TABLE 3.1 Average Annual Effective Dose of Ionizing Radiation

Source	DOSE (mSv) US[a]	DOSE (mSv) Global[b]
Natural background		
Radon	2.3	1.3
Space	0.3	0.4
Internal radionuclides	0.3	0.3
Terrestrial	0.2	0.5
Subtotal background	*3.1*	*2.4*
Medical		
Computed tomography	1.5	0.57
Interventional fluoroscopy	0.4	
Conventional radiography and fluoroscopy	0.3	
Dental	0.007	0.002
Nuclear medicine	0.8	0.03
Subtotal medical	*3.0*	*0.6*
Consumer products and other	0.1	0.01
Grand total	*6.2*	*3.0*

[a]Data from National Council on Radiation Protection and Measurements. *Ionizing Radiation Exposure of the Population of the United States.* Bethesda, MD: National Council on Radiation Protection and Measurements; 2009. NCRP Report 160.
[b]Calculated from doses reported by United Nations Scientific Committee on the Effects of Atomic Radiation, UNSCEAR 2008 Report to the General Assembly, http://www.unscear.org/unscear/en/publications/2008_1.html.

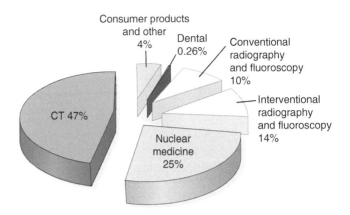

Medical, consumer products and other 3.1 mSv/year

Fig. 3.2 Sources of Radiation in the United States From Medical Examinations and Consumer Products. The average person in the United States receives approximately as much radiation from medical and consumer products sources (3.1 mSv/year) as from natural background exposure. Most medical x-ray exposures come from computed tomography *(CT)*, nuclear medicine (primarily cardiac imaging), fluoroscopy, and conventional radiography. Exposures from dental examinations and from occupational, fallout, and nuclear power sources are small. Although individuals with exposures from natural background are fairly evenly distributed in the population, most medically exposed individuals are relatively old and sick.

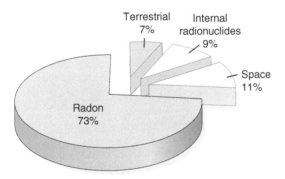

Background 3.1 mSv/year

Fig. 3.1 Natural Background Radiation Contributes 3.1 mSv on Average Per Year. Most exposure comes from radon, but there are significant contributions from space, ingested radionuclides, and terrestrial sources, including external radionuclides in the soil and building materials. (Data from National Council on Radiation Protection and Measurements. *Ionizing Radiation Exposure of the Population of the United States.* Bethesda, MD: National Council on Radiation Protection and Measurements; 2009. NCRP Report 160,)

Other Sources

Other sources of exposure affect caregivers or others in contact with patients receiving nuclear medicine treatments; people who work in nuclear power generation; individuals involved in areas of industrial, medical, educational, or research activities; workers in medical and dental x-ray facilities; workers in airport baggage inspection systems; and commercial flight personnel. All these sources of radiation combined contribute only approximately 0.1% of the total average annual exposure.

DENTOMAXILLOFACIAL RADIOLOGY: RISK AND DOSES

The basic principle of diagnostic imaging is that the benefit to the patient far outweighs the radiation-associated risks. To satisfy this principle, doses from dentomaxillofacial radiographic examination must be:

- Optimized to produce a diagnostically acceptable image, and
- Less than the threshold needed to cause any deterministic effects, and
- Minimized to keep the risk of stochastic effects within an acceptable range

Estimating Cancer Risk From Diagnostic Dentomaxillofacial Radiology

The principal risk of dentomaxillofacial radiography is the unlikely chance of radiation-induced cancer. Cancer is a common disease, affecting approximately 40% of people at some time during their lives and accounting for approximately 20% of all deaths. There is convincing evidence from studies of humans and research animals that links radiation exposure to cancer formation (both solid tumors and leukemias). Human epidemiologic studies of individuals exposed to ionizing radiations either by accident or by intention include survivors of the atomic bombings in Hiroshima and Nagasaki, patients exposed during diagnostic

travel, cosmic radiation becomes a more significant contributor to exposure. Typically, an airline flight of 5 hours at a cruising altitude of 12 km results in an exposure of 25 μSv. Other minor sources of exposure from consumer products include dental porcelain, television receivers, and smoke alarms. In total, consumer products contribute only approximately 1.6% of the total average annual exposure.

and therapeutic procedures, and occupation- or environment-related exposures. In general, these studies demonstrate reasonable evidence that cancer risk increases linearly with protracted radiation exposures greater than 100 mSv. However, there is great uncertainty regarding the extrapolation of these risks with exposures less than 100 mSv, the dose range of most diagnostic radiographic procedures. Scientific investigation of the uncertainties of low-dose radiation effects are challenging. Epidemiologic studies designed to address the ambiguities of cancer risk from low-dose radiation would require large sample sizes and are impractical to conduct. These uncertainties have resulted in controversy with regard to the application of this knowledge to develop radiation protection guidelines and policy.

The current paradigm of radiation protection is based on the linear no-threshold (LNT) hypothesis, which predicts that there is a linear relationship between dose and the risk of inducing a new cancer, even at very low doses (Fig. 3.3). This hypothesis considers that there is no threshold or "safe dose" below which there is no added cancer risk. Several lines of evidence indicate that the LNT model is scientifically plausible. Complex damage to DNA, the basis of cancer formation, may occur with even one x-ray photon (see Fig. 2.2). Although sophisticated DNA repair mechanisms exist, some types of complex damage to DNA may be beyond the cell's capability to repair with fidelity. Thus even the smallest dose carries a risk, although minimal, of cancer induction. Epidemiologic data do not exclude a risk at very low doses.

The LNT model is not a demonstrated scientific fact, and its assumptions for low-dose effects have been contested. For example, there is evidence of cellular adaptive responses—stress responses induced by low-dose radiation that augment a cell's response to subsequent higher doses. These studies have prompted suggestions that low-dose radiation may have a protective effect (referred to as *hormesis*), that the risks are lower than those predicted by the LNT model, and that there is a threshold dose that must be exceeded to induce cancer. On the other hand, studies of cultured cells have suggested the presence of *bystander effects*, in which biologic effects occur in cells that are not directly irradiated. Such off-target effects could potentially yield a supralinear response, and the risk may potentially be higher than predicted by the LNT model.

Despite its uncertainties in the low-dose range, policymakers need guidance to set dose limits for individuals exposed in the low-dose range, including from diagnostic imaging procedures and from occupational exposure. Most radiation protection organizations believe that it is prudent to assume that risk is proportional to dose and that there is no safe threshold. Opponents of the LNT model argue that applying an overly conservative approach results in an inappropriate fear, which may compromise the full diagnostic benefits of imaging and increase costs for implementation of radiation protection programs. However, in the absence of data that conclusively support alternate models, the LNT model is considered to be the most appropriate approach to radiation risk assessment from a policy perspective. *The radiation safety practices described in this text have considered recommendations that are based on the LNT hypothesis.*

Patient Doses From Diagnostic Dentomaxillofacial Radiology

Radiation doses to the patient from radiographic imaging are usually reported as effective dose, a measure of the stochastic risks. Table 3.2 and Fig. 3.4 show typical effective doses from common dentomaxillofacial and medical radiographic examinations, and the equivalent exposure in terms of days of natural background radiation. These effective doses consider the absorbed doses to various organs from a specific radiographic procedure, and the relative sensitivity of the exposed organ to stochastic effects of radiation. Typically, the doses are measured using an anthropomorphic phantom or may be modeled by computational simulation. However, effective dose does not consider age, gender, and individual susceptibility factors and thus is not intended to represent an individual's radiation dose from that procedure. Nevertheless, effective dose is a convenient measure to compare the relative risks from different radiographic examinations and to convey the relative magnitude of the risk to patients. To assist healthcare providers and patients categorize the magnitude of radiation-associated risks, the American College of Radiology developed a categorization of relative radiation levels (Table 3.3). These levels categorize exposure based on a range of effective doses and also consider that cancer risks associated with pediatric radiation exposures are higher than for adults.

Communicating Radiation Risks to Patients

Although most patients readily accept dental radiographs as part of their diagnosis, some have anxiety about radiation exposure for themselves or members of their families—usually their children. It is important to speak clearly and confidently with your patients to address these concerns. With all the discussion of radiation risks in the general media

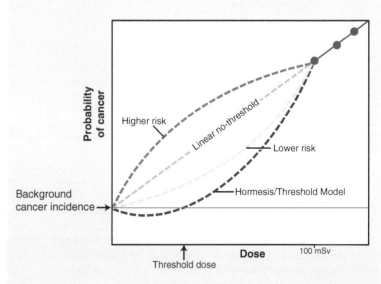

Fig. 3.3 Modeling Low-Dose Cancer Risk. Doses of radiation higher than approximately 100 mSv *(green dots)* result in a dose-dependent increase in the cancer rate. The linear no-threshold model (LNT) posits that at doses less than 100 mSv, there is a linear relationship between dose and risk *(orange dashed line)* and that there is no threshold dose below which there is no additional risk. Alternate models propose that risk may be higher or lower than those predicted by the LNT model, and that low doses may have a protective effect with a threshold dose. The LNT model is currently accepted as the approach to develop radiation protection guidelines.

TABLE 3.2 Typical Effective Dose From Radiographic Examinations

Examination	Median Effective Dose	Equivalent Background Exposure[a]
Intraoral[b]		
Rectangular collimation		
Posterior bite-wings: PSP or F-speed film	5 µSv	0.6 day
Full-mouth: PSP or F-speed film	40 µSv	5 days
Full-mouth: CCD sensor (estimated)	20 µSv	2.5 days
Round collimation		
Full-mouth: D-speed film	400 µSv	48 days
Full-mouth: PSP or F-speed film	200 µSv	24 days
Full-mouth: CCD sensor (estimated)	100 µSv	12 days
Extraoral		
Panoramic[b]	20 µSv	2.5 days
Cephalometric[b]	5 µSv	0.6 day
Chest[c]	100 µSv	12 days
Cone beam CT[b]		
Small field of view (<6 cm)	50 µSv	6 days
Medium field of view (dentoalveolar, full arch)	100 µSv	12 days
Large field of view (craniofacial)	120 µSv	15 days
Multidetector CT		
Maxillofacial[b]	650 µSv	2 months
Head[c]	2 mSv	8 months
Chest[c]	7 mSv	2 years
Abdomen and pelvis, with and without contrast[c]	20 mSv	7 years

[a]Approximate equivalent background exposure is calculated based on an estimated background radiation dose of 3.1 mSv/year. Exposures more than the equivalent of 3 days are rounded off to the nearest day, month, or year.
[b]Median dose from dentomaxillofacial radiography with typical exposure protocols is calculated from data collated from multiple published studies. Doses in the range of 10–1000 µSv are rounded off to the nearest multiple of 10.
[c]American College of Radiology, https://www.acr.org/~/media/ACR/Images/Quality-Safety/eNews/2015-September/Dose_chart.png?la=en
CCD, Charge-coupled device; *CT*, computed tomography; *PSP*, photostimulable phosphor.

and the availability of information via the internet, it is completely reasonable that an individual may be concerned.

- Allow the patient to fully express his or her thoughts. Do not interrupt the patient's comments or belittle the patient's concerns. Acknowledge their concerns and indicate that you understand their apprehension.
- Tell the patient why you need radiographs as part of the patient's personal diagnosis—such as the detection of interproximal caries, the extent of bone loss from periodontal disease suggested by probing, periapical infections suggested by pain, or any anticipated findings specific to the patient's condition that are important and can be attained only by radiologic investigation. Assure new patients that you will contact their previous dentist to obtain previous radiographs that may assist you in their diagnosis.
- Reassure the patient that you make efforts to minimize their radiation dose. Describe the many measures you take to reduce patient exposure, such as using fast film or digital sensors, rectangular collimation, and thyroid collars. With these assurances, including that you will make only the exposures you specifically need for the patient's benefit, most patients will appreciate your attention to their concerns and accept radiographs.
- Convey the relative magnitude of the dose that the patient is likely to receive. Table 3.2 provides information on typical effective doses from dentomaxillofacial radiography. However, these doses are not easily comprehended by patients. Rather, convey the relative magnitude of the dose in terms of equivalent days, months, or years of natural background radiation (see Fig. 3.3). To help the patient place the risk in perspective, compare the magnitude of these risks with other sources of radiation exposure such as an airline flight or other common imaging procedures. Note that dentomaxillofacial radiography delivers negligible to minimal doses, relative to other medical imaging procedures.
- Often patients who are pregnant may require radiographic examination. Dental practices should implement a policy to identify pregnancy in patients who are of childbearing age. This can be accomplished by reviewing the patient's menstrual history and by direct inquiry of whether the patient thinks that she may be pregnant. Routine radiographic evaluation of asymptomatic pregnant patients may be deferred until after pregnancy. When radiographs are needed for management of a pregnant patient, emphasize that the diagnostic and treatment planning benefits are crucial to maintain oral health, and that dental disease and its sequelae could have an adverse impact of the health of the unborn child. If the patient is concerned about the potential adverse effects of diagnostic radiation on the fetus, emphasize that the fetal doses from dentomaxillofacial radiography are approximately 42,000-fold lower than the threshold dose for deterministic effects on the embryo and fetus (see Chapter 2).

IMPLEMENTING RADIATION PROTECTION

Guiding Principles

There are three guiding principles in radiation protection:
1. Justification
2. Optimization
3. Dose limitation

The principle of justification means the dentist should identify situations where the benefit to a patient from the diagnostic exposure

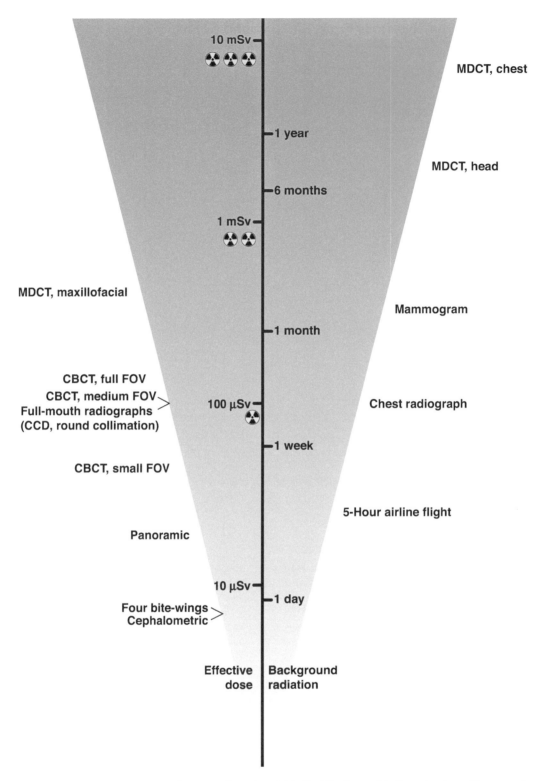

Fig. 3.4 Radiation Doses From Common Dental and Medical Radiographic Examinations. The central axis (log scale) shows the effective dose and the equivalent period of background radiation exposure. The radiation symbols adjacent to the dose identify the relative radiation level categories (see Table 3.3). *CBCT,* Cone beam computed tomography; *FOV,* field of view; *MDCT,* multi detector computed tomography.

likely exceeds the risk of harm. In practice, this principle influences which patients are selected for radiographic examinations and what examinations are chosen. These matters are considered in Chapter 17.

The principle of optimization holds that dentists should use every reasonable means to reduce unnecessary exposure to their patients, their staff, and themselves. This philosophy of radiation protection is often referred to as the principle of ALARA (*As Low As Reasonably Achievable*). ALARA holds that exposures to ionizing radiation should be kept as low as reasonably achievable, with economic and social factors being taken into account. The means to accomplish this end are

TABLE 3.3 Relative Radiation Level Designations, American College of Radiology

Relative Radiation Level	Adult Effective Dose Range	Pediatric Effective Dose Range
☢	<100 µSv	<30 µSv
☢☢	100 µSv to 1 mSv	30 µSv to 300 µSv
☢☢☢	1–10 mSv	300 µSv–3 mSv
☢☢☢☢	10–30 mSv	3–10 mSv
☢☢☢☢☢	30–100 mSv	10–30 mSv

From ACR Appropriateness Criteria, Radiation Dose Assessment, https://www.acr.org/Quality-Safety/Appropriateness-Criteria

BOX 3.1 Means for Reducing X-Ray Exposure

Use Good Clinical Judgment and Apply Evidence-Based Imaging Guidelines
- Make radiographs when they are likely to contribute to diagnosis and treatment planning
- Use selection criteria to assist in determining type and frequency of radiographic examinations

Use Best Practices in Radiographic Imaging
- Optimize your exposure settings to the patient's size and anatomic area to be imaged
- Intraoral radiography
  - Use E/F-speed film or digital sensors
  - Use holders to support film or digital sensors
  - Use rectangular collimation
  - Make exposures with 60–70 kVp
  - Use thyroid collars
- Panoramic radiography
  - Use rare-earth screens for film imaging or use digital systems
- Cephalometric radiography
  - Use rare-earth screens for film imaging or use digital systems
  - Use a thyroid collar, if it will not obstruct anatomic landmarks for cephalometry
- Cone beam computed tomography (CBCT)
  - Restrict the field of view to cover the region of interest
- Film-based imaging
  - Use time-temperature processing rather than "sight" processing, or use an automatic processor

Use Best Practices in Personnel Protection
- Stand behind a protective barrier or at least 6 feet (2 m) away from patient and away from the x-ray machine when making exposure
- For handheld devices, ensure the protective backscatter shield is in place

considered by dentists every day in their practices and are discussed later in this chapter (Box 3.1).

The principle of dose limitation provides dose limits for occupational and public exposures to ensure that no individuals are exposed to unacceptably high doses. This principle applies to dentists and their staff who are exposed occupationally but not to patients because there are no dose limits for individuals exposed for diagnostic purposes. Many of the steps described in the following sections that optimize exposures of the patient also reduce exposure to dentists and their staff.

The dentist in each facility is responsible for the design and conduct of the radiation protection program. In this section, methods of exposure and dose reduction are described that can be used in dental radiography. Each subsection begins with a recommendation of the American Dental Association (ADA) Council on Scientific Affairs. This recommendation is followed by a discussion of ways in which the recommendation can be satisfied. All methods that reduce exposure to patients also reduce exposure to the dental staff and usually improve the quality of the radiographs made.

Patient Protection
Patient Selection Criteria

Radiographic screening for the purpose of detecting disease before clinical examination should not be performed. A thorough clinical examination, consideration of the patient history, review of any prior radiographs, caries risk assessment and consideration of both the dental and the general health needs of the patient should precede radiographic examination (ADA 2012).

The most effective approach to reduce unnecessary exposure is to reduce unnecessary radiographic examinations. Radiographs should be made only when they are likely to provide additional information that is likely to contribute to the diagnosis and treatment plan. The ADA has published radiographic selection criteria—clinical or historical findings that identify patients for whom a high probability exists that a radiographic examination would provide information affecting their treatment or prognosis. These criteria satisfy the principle of justification and are considered in Chapter 17.

When a decision is made to obtain a radiograph, the dentist should obtain the lowest dose image that would provide the necessary diagnostic information. Table 3.2 shows that there is a wide range of patient exposures from various dental examinations.

Conducting the Examination

When the dentist has determined that a radiographic examination is justified (using patient selection criteria), the specific radiographic protocol or the principle of optimization greatly influences patient exposure to radiation. Considerations for designing an optimal radiographic study include choice of equipment, choice of exposure settings, operation of equipment, and processing and interpreting the radiographic image.

Film and Digital Imaging

Good radiologic practice includes use of the fastest image receptor compatible with the diagnostic task (F-speed film or digital) (ADA 2012).

Intraoral dental x-ray film is available in two speed groups: D and E/F (see Chapter 5). Clinically, film of speed group E/F is approximately twice as fast (sensitive) as film of group D and thus requires only half the exposure (see Fig. 5.30). Fast films are effective for exposure reduction. Multiple studies have found that E/F-speed film provides the same useful density range, latitude, contrast, and image quality as D-speed films without sacrifice of diagnostic information. Current digital sensors (see Chapter 4) offer equal or greater dose savings than does E/F-speed film, and comparable diagnostic utility.

Intensifying Screens and Film

Rare-earth intensifying screens are recommended ... combined with high-speed film of 400 or greater (ADA 2006).

Contemporary intensifying screens used in extraoral radiography use the rare-earth elements gadolinium and lanthanum (see Chapter 5). Compared with the older calcium tungstate screens, rare-earth screens are more efficient in converting x-ray photons to light and decrease patient exposure by 55% in panoramic and cephalometric radiography.

Film-based panoramic and cephalometric imaging is being replaced with imaging using storage phosphors or charge-coupled device (CCD) sensors. However, unlike with intraoral radiography, dose reduction with these digital technologies is minimal.

Source-to-Skin Distance

Use of long source-to-skin distances of 40 cm, rather than short distances of 20 cm, decreases exposure by 10 to 25 percent. Distances between 20 cm and 40 cm are appropriate, but the longer distances are optimal (ADA 2006).

Two standard focal source-to-skin distances have evolved over the years for use in intraoral radiography—20 cm (8 inches) and 40 cm (16 inches). With a longer source-to-skin distance, the x-ray beam is less divergent, reducing the exposed tissue volume (Fig. 3.5). The use of a longer source-to-object distance also decreases image magnification (see Fig. 7.3).

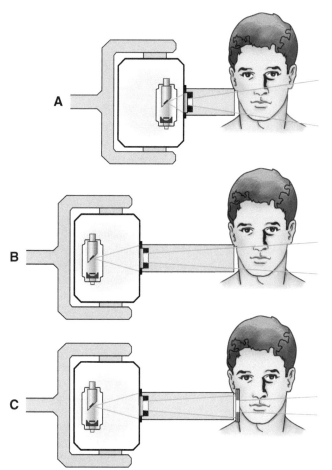

Fig. 3.5 Effect of Source-to-Skin Distance and Collimation on the Volume of Tissue Irradiated. A larger volume of irradiated tissue results with use of a short source-to-skin distance (A) compared with use of a longer source-to-skin distance (B), which produces a less divergent beam. Using a rectangular collimator between the round position-indicating device and the patient (C) results in a smaller, less divergent beam and a smaller volume of tissue irradiated than in A or B.

Rectangular Collimation

Since a rectangular collimator decreases the radiation dose by up to five-fold as compared with a circular one, radiographic equipment should provide rectangular collimation for exposure of periapical and bitewing radiographs (ADA 2012).

In the United States, the Code of Federal Regulations (21CFR1020) and most state regulations require that the x-ray beam used in intraoral radiography be collimated so that the field of radiation at the patient's skin surface is no more than 7 cm (2.75 inches) in diameter. The area of this circular field size is almost 3 times larger than the area of No. 2 intraoral film (3.2 cm × 4.1 cm) or digital sensor. Consequently, further limiting the size of the x-ray beam to the size of the image receptor significantly reduces unnecessary patient exposure. If the tissue volume exposed is decreased, the amount of scattered radiation is decreased, image fogging is decreased, and the resultant image has improved diagnostic quality. Rectangular collimation reduces the area of the patient's skin surface exposed by 60% over that of a round collimated (7-cm diameter) beam (Fig. 3.6A).

There are several means to limit the size of the x-ray beam. A simple approach is to use a rectangular collimator assembled onto the receptor holder (see Fig. 3.6B). This device can be used without modifying the round aiming cylinder of the x-ray tube. A second approach is to use a rectangular collimator that attaches to the aiming cylinder of the radiographic tube housing (see Fig. 3.6C) and also incorporates a position-indicating device (PID). Use of a PID that centers the rectangular collimated beam over the receptor will minimize partial exposure errors (cone-cut). The third approach is to replace the manufacturer's cylindrical collimator with a rectangular collimator that attaches to the tube housing. These rectangular collimators are also provided with PIDs that attach to the end of the rectangular collimator and facilitate accurate positioning of the beam over the receptor (see Fig. 3.6C).

Filtration

The x-ray beam emitted from the radiographic tube consists of a spectrum of x-ray photons. Low-energy photons, which have little penetrating power, are absorbed mainly by the patient and do not contribute to the information on the image. The purpose of filtration is to preferentially remove these low-energy x-ray photons from the x-ray beam (see Chapter 1, Fig. 1.18). Filtration results in decreased patient exposure with no loss of radiographic information.

When an x-ray beam is filtered with 3 mm of aluminum, the surface exposure is reduced to approximately 20% of the exposure with no filtration. Federal regulations in the United States require the total filtration in the path of a dental x-ray beam to be equal to the equivalent of 1.5 mm of aluminum for a machine operating at 50 to 70 kVp and 2.5 mm of aluminum for machines operating at higher voltages.

Protective Aprons and Thyroid Collars

The thyroid gland is more susceptible to radiation exposure during dental radiographic exams given its anatomic position, particularly in children. Protective thyroid collars and collimation substantially reduce radiation exposure to the thyroid during dental radiographic procedures. Because every precaution should be taken to minimize radiation exposure, protective thyroid collars should be used whenever possible (ADA 2012).

The American Thyroid Association recommends the reduction of thyroidal radiation exposure as much as possible without compromising the clinical goals of dental radiographic examinations.

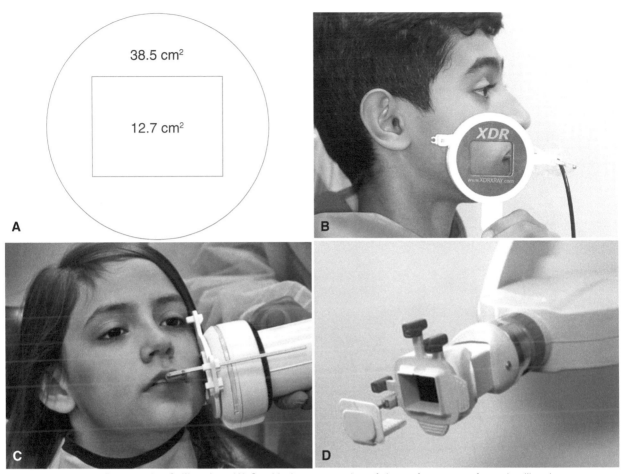

Fig. 3.6 Rectangular Collimation. (A) Graphical representation of the surface areas of round collimation (7-cm diameter) and rectangular collimation (size 2 receptor). The rectangular collimated area is approximately 66% less than the round collimation field. (B) The XDR collimator, a metallic shield placed in the path of the beam limits the size of the exposure field to an area just larger than the film or sensor. (C) The Tru-Image x-ray positioning system includes rectangular collimation that is attached to the end of the standard aiming cylinder. It includes a magnetic alignment ring to facilitate accurate positioning of the beam over the receptor. (D) A rectangular lead-lined collimator that attaches to the x-ray tube housing, replacing the standard aiming ring. The collimator is used with a receptor holder to facilitate beam alignment to the receptor. (C, Courtesy Interactive Diagnostic Imaging: http://www.idixray.com. D, Courtesy Margraf Dental Manufacturing, Inc., www.margrafdental.com.)

The function of protective aprons and thyroid collars (Fig. 3.7) is to reduce radiation exposure of the gonads and thyroid gland. There is reason to be concerned about radiation exposure to the thyroid gland. Multiple studies, including studies performed after the explosion of the Chernobyl reactor, have shown that the thyroid gland in children is highly sensitive to radiation-induced cancer. It is important to protect the thyroid glands of children during radiographic examinations. The best ways to accomplish this aim are to use thyroid collars, in addition to fast receptors and rectangular collimation. Thyroid collars should be used for intraoral radiography because it does not mask essential anatomic details captured on the image. In cephalometric radiography, the thyroid collar typically does not compromise identification of anatomic landmarks for most cephalometric analyses. However, the thyroid collar does not allow for adequate evaluation of the cervical vertebrae, for example to assess skeletal maturity.

The National Council on Radiation Protection and Measurements (NCRP) and ADA concluded that protective aprons to cover the gonads are unnecessary because it is far more important to place emphasis on reducing exposure of the primary beam to facial structures than to reduce the already negligible gonadal exposure. *The ADA guidelines state that if all other means to reduce radiation exposure are applied, including use of patient selection criteria, fast receptors (E/F-speed film or digital sensors), and rectangular collimators, then protection of the gonads in unnecessary.* Indeed, recent research has shown that the risk of heritable effects from dental exposure is insignificant (see Chapter 2). However, many states in the United States currently require the use of protective aprons. In recent years, lead-free aprons have been developed for radiation protection. These aprons include materials with high atomic numbers and low densities, such as antimony, tin, tungsten, or bismuth, to provide beam attenuation. These aprons typically attenuate approximately 98% as much as conventional aprons but weigh only approximately 60% as much. Furthermore, they are recyclable and can be safely disposed as nonhazardous waste.

Film and Sensor Holders

Film holders that align the film precisely with the collimated beam are recommended for periapical and bitewing radiographs (ADA 2006).

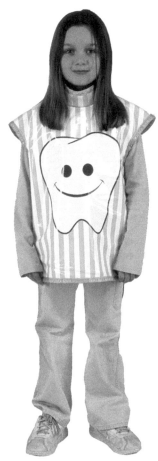

Fig. 3.7 Protective Apron With a Thyroid Collar. Children are more sensitive to radiation than are adults, and so the use of leaded aprons with thyroid collars is especially important for this population. (Courtesy Dentsply Rinn, www.rinncorp.com.)

Film or digital receptor holders should be used when intraoral radiographs are made because they improve the alignment of the film, or digital sensor, with teeth and the x-ray machine. Their use results in a significant reduction in unacceptable images and thus avoidable retakes. The use of film and sensor holders allows the operator to control the position and alignment of the film or sensor with respect to the teeth and jaws. This is especially important when used with the paralleling technique (see Chapter 6). In these cases, it is often desirable to position the receptor away from the teeth so as to get the best image and reduce patient discomfort. This requires the use of a film or sensor holder. Most such devices have an external guide that shows the operator where to align the aiming cylinder. As a result, the x-ray beam is properly directed toward the receptors; this greatly reduces the chance of the beam partially missing the image receptor (a "cone-cut") and reduces image distortion (see Chapter 6). As discussed earlier, many film holder assemblies include a collimator to restrict the beam to the size of the image receptor.

Kilovoltage

The optimal operating potential of dental x-ray units is between 60 and 70 kVp (ADA 2012).

Kilovoltage (kVp) influences fimage contrast and patient dose. At lower kVp, the image contrast is increased, which could potentially enhance diagnosis. At higher kVp, the patient radiation dose is decreased. Most intraoral x-ray units operate at 60 to 70 kVp, which provides adequate diagnostic quality with reduced radiation dose. Constant-potential (fully rectified), high-frequency, and direct current (DC) dental x-ray units can produce radiographs with lower kilovoltage and at reduced levels of radiation. The surface exposure required to produce a comparable radiographic density using a constant-potential unit is approximately 25% less than that of a conventional self-rectified unit operating at the same kilovoltage. Currently, several manufacturers produce DC units.

Milliampere-Seconds

The operator should set the amperage and time settings for exposure of dental radiographs of optimal quality (ADA 2006).

Of the three settings on an x-ray machine (tube voltage, milliamperage, and exposure time), exposure time is the most crucial factor in influencing diagnostic quality. In terms of exposure, optimal image quality means that the radiograph is of diagnostic density, neither overexposed (too dark) nor underexposed (too light). Both overexposed and underexposed radiographs result in repeat exposures, leading to needless additional patient exposure. Image density is controlled by the quantity of x-rays produced, which is best controlled by the combination of milliamperage and exposure time, termed milliampere-seconds (mAs) (see Chapter 1). Typically, a radiograph of correct density demonstrates very faint soft tissue outlines, and a gray scale that adequately distinguishes enamel, dentin, cortical bone, and trabecular bone. If the x-ray machine has a variable milliampere control, it should be set at the highest mA setting. Proper exposure times should be determined empirically when using optimal film processing conditions (see Chapter 5) or manufacturer's recommendations for digital sensors. A chart showing optimal exposure times for each region of the arch in children and adults should be mounted by each x-ray machine. Because film-processing conditions are standardized and the mA and kVp settings are fixed, the only decision the dentist or the assistant needs to make is to select the proper exposure time for the age of the patient (less for young patients) and the region of the mouth being imaged (less in the anterior region).

Film Processing

All film should be processed following the film and processer manufacturer recommendations. Poor processing technique, including sight-developing, most often results in underdeveloped films, forcing the x-ray operator to increase the dose to compensate, resulting in patient and personnel being exposed to unnecessary radiation (ADA 2012).

A major cause of unnecessary patient exposure is the practice of overexposing films and compensating by underdevelopment. This procedure results in both unnecessary exposure of the patient and films that are of inferior diagnostic quality because of incomplete development. Time-temperature processing is the best way to ensure optimal film quality (see Chapter 5). To help ensure optimal image quality, the dental assistant should follow the film manufacturer's recommendation for processing solutions.

The use of automatic film processing machines has become widespread, with more than 90% of dentists using such processors. They should be used in a darkroom. Although some units have daylight loaders, allowing film to be placed in the machine in room light, such loaders are difficult to keep clean and free of contamination. However, film processors can increase patient exposure if not correctly maintained. Approximately 30% of retakes of film-based radiographs are because of incorrect film density related to processor variability. Using a

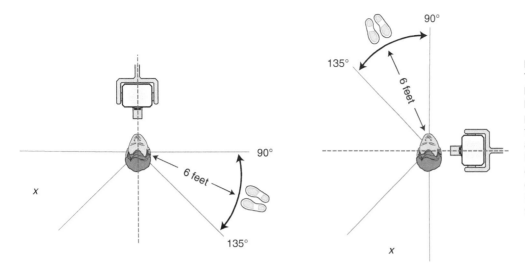

Fig. 3.8 Position-and-Distance Rule. The operator may be exposed from leakage radiation from the x-ray tube head, scattered radiation from the patient, and primary photons passing through the patient. If no barrier is available, the operator should stand at least 6 feet from the patient, at an angle of 90 to 135 degrees to the central ray of the x-ray beam, when the exposure is made because this region receives the least overall exposure.

comprehensive maintenance program can reduce this retake rate significantly, resulting in a substantial savings in both patient exposure and operating costs.

Interpreting the Images

The dentist should view radiographs under appropriate conditions for analysis and diagnosis (ADA 2006).

Radiographs are best viewed in a semi-darkened room with light transmitted through the films; all extraneous light should be eliminated. In addition, radiographs should be studied with the aid of a magnifying glass to detect even the smallest change in image density. Similarly, digital images are best interpreted on a computer screen in a darkened environment. Software features such as density and contrast enhancement, and magnification are useful for viewing all features of the radiographic image.

Personnel Protection

Dentists and their staff who operate radiographic equipment are occupationally exposed to radiation. This includes potential exposure from the primary beam and scattered radiation. Personnel must follow appropriate procedures to reduce the chance of occupational exposure.

Barriers

Operators of radiographic equipment should use barrier protection when possible, and barriers should contain a leaded glass window to enable the operator to view the patient during exposure. When shielding is not possible, the operator should stand at least two meters from the tube head and out of the path of the primary beam (ADA 2006).

Dentists should consult with a qualified expert to design and construct dental offices and clinics to meet the radiation shielding requirements specified by their state and national regulations. Primary barriers such as walls or mobile lead barriers provide the most effective method to protect the operator from primary and scattered radiation. The exposure switch should be located behind this barrier. The barrier should have a leaded window and allow the operator to maintain visual and verbal contact with the patient during the exposure.

If the office design does not permit the operator to leave the room or use an appropriate barrier, then strict adherence to the position-and-distance rule is required. The operator should stand at least 6 feet

(2 m) from the patient, at an angle of 90 to 135 degrees to the central ray of the x-ray beam (Fig. 3.8). When applied, this rule not only takes advantage of the inverse square law to reduce x-ray exposure to the operator but also takes advantage of the fact that in this position the patient's head absorbs most scatter radiation. All practitioners should check their state's regulations for use of ionizing radiation regarding operator position during x-ray exposures. The operator should never hold films or sensors in place. Film or sensor-holding instruments should be used (see earlier section on rectangular collimation). If correct film placement and retention are still not possible, a parent or other individual responsible for the patient should be asked to hold the sensor in place and be afforded adequate protection with a protective apron. Under no circumstances should this person be one of the office staff. The operator or the patient should not hold the radiographic tube housing during the exposure, except for specifically designed handheld intraoral radiographic units. Suspension arms should be adequately maintained to prevent housing movement and drift.

In addition to shielding the operator, radiation regulations also specify requirements for shielding of the walls to minimize radiation dose to nonoccupationally exposed individuals (e.g., the office receptionist in the adjacent office). The NCRP recommendation states that walls must be of sufficient density or thickness so that the exposure to these nonoccupationally exposed individuals is less than 0.02 mGy/week (1 mGy/year). In most instances, it is not necessary to line the walls with lead to meet this requirement. Walls constructed of gypsum wallboard (drywall or sheet rock), brick, or concrete are adequate for the average dental office.

Handheld Radiographic Devices

The use of handheld portable x-ray units for intraoral radiography requires special consideration. These battery-operated devices are designed to be held by the operator during use. To minimize exposure to the operator, a backscatter shield is incorporated into the device at the end of the collimator ring and provides a zone where scattered radiation is negligible. For optimal operator protection, the device must be held in a horizontal position, oriented perpendicular to the operator, and with backscatter shield placed close to the patient. Angling of the device changes the zone of protection and can expose the operator to scatter radiation. In this situation, it may be necessary for the patient to angle his or her head instead. In the United States, handheld devices have been approved for use by the Food and Drug Administration. Some states have additional regulatory requirements related to dose

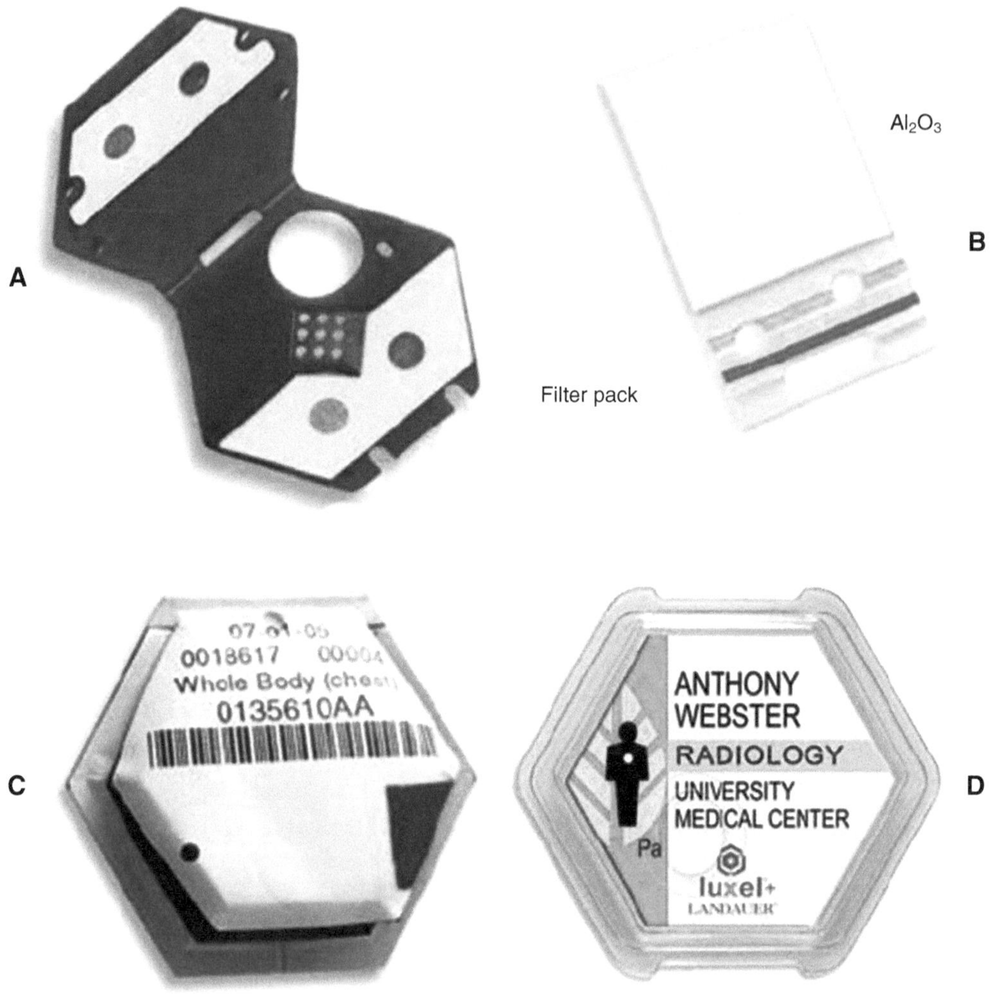

Fig. 3.9 A personal optically stimulated luminescence dosimeter. (A) Filter pack containing an open window and plastic, aluminum, and copper filters. (B) Strip of Al_2-O_3, which is sensitive to radiation. (C and D). The filter pack and Al_2-O_3, are packaged into blister pack and worn by an operator. The amount and ratio of light output during the stimulation process from the regions of the Al_2-O_3 under the filters allows determination of the energy and dose of radiation to which the badge was exposed. (Courtesy Landauer, Inc., Glenwood, IL.)

monitoring or personnel protective equipment that must be worn by the operators of these devices.

Personnel Monitoring Devices

The ADA recommends that workers who may receive an annual dose greater than 1 mSv should wear personal dosimeters to monitor their exposure levels.

Pregnant dental personnel operating x-ray equipment should use personal dosimeters, regardless of anticipated exposure levels (ADA 2012).

Personnel-monitoring devices are used to ensure that staff consistently follow office radiation safety rules such as those described previously. These devices provide a means to measure the operator's occupational radiation dose. The requirement to use personnel dosimeters is specified by state and national regulations. In the United States, the code of federal regulations requires that personnel likely to receive more than 10% of the annual dose limit be monitored. There are additional considerations in managing exposure of pregnant, occupationally exposed personnel. The US Code of Federal Regulations requires that pregnant personnel be monitored if the dose to the embryo and fetus is likely to exceed 1 mSv during the entire period of pregnancy. Personnel monitoring is an effective approach to identify undesirable change in work habits and help to respond to office staff members who may be apprehensive about the risks from occupational radiation exposure.

Several companies in the United States offer dosimetry-monitoring services. The monitoring devices are worn clipped to clothing on the front of the chest. A widely used technology for personnel monitoring is the optically stimulated luminescent dosimeter (OSLD). The device consists of a strip of crystalline aluminum oxide (Al_2O_3:C) that luminesces in proportion to the amount of radiation exposure (Fig. 3.9). The device is sent to a service, typically at monthly intervals, where the accumulated dose is measured and reported back to the dental clinic (Fig. 3.10). Another technology for personnel monitoring is based on direct ion storage. The device incorporates the dosimeter with a USB interface allowing the end user to directly perform the dose reading via the internet. Both these technologies are sensitive to a dose as low as 10 μSv of x-rays.

Dose Limits

Recognizing the harmful effects of radiation, and the potential risks involved with its use, several national, regional, and international organizations establish guidelines for limits on the amount of radiation received by occupationally exposed individuals and by the public (Table 3.4). These limits pertain to planned exposure situations, not to background radiation, and do not include radiation received for diagnostic or therapeutic purposes. Since their initial establishment in the 1930s, these dose limits have been revised downward several times, adapting to new knowledge on the harmful effects of radiation and the increased ability to use radiation more efficiently.

LANDAUER®

SAMPLE ORGANIZATION
RADIATION SAFETY OFFICER
2 SCIENCE ROAD
GLENWOOD, IL 60425

Landauer, Inc. 2 Science Road   Glenwood, Illinois 60425-1586
Telephone: (708) 755-7000   Facsimile: (708) 755-7016
www.landauerinc.com

RADIATION DOSIMETRY REPORT

luxel®

ACCOUNT NO.	SERIES CODE	ANALYTICAL WORK ORDER	REPORT DATE	DOSIMETER RECEIVED	REPORT TIME IN WORK DAYS	PAGE NO.
103702	RAD	992150087	06/13/03	06/09/03	4	1

PARTICIPANT NUMBER	NAME (ID NUMBER / BIRTH DATE / SEX)	DOSIMETER	USE	RADIATION QUALITY	DOSE EQUIVALENT (MREM) FOR PERIODS SHOWN BELOW — DEEP DDE	EYE LDE	SHALLOW SDE	YEAR TO DATE DOSE EQUIVALENT (MREM) — DEEP DDE	EYE LDE	SHALLOW SDE	LIFETIME DOSE EQUIVALENT (MREM) — DEEP DDE	EYE LDE	SHALLOW SDE	RECORDS FOR YEAR	INCEPTION DATE (MM/YY)
FOR MONITORING PERIOD:					05/01/03 - 05/31/03			2003							
0000H	CONTROL	J	CNTRL		M	M	M							5	07/97
	CONTROL	P	CNTRL		M	M	M								07/97
	CONTROL	U	CNTRL				M								07/97
00189	ADAMS, HEATHER 336235619 08/31/1968 F	P	WHBODY		M	M	M	9	10	12	29	31	42	5	07/01
00191	ADDISON, JOHN 471563287 10/04/1968 M	J	WHBODY	PN	90	90	90	100	100	100	200	200	200	5	07/01
		P		P	60	60	60	70	70	70	170	170	170		
				NF	30	30	30	30	30	30	30	30	30		
00202	HARRIS, KATHY 587582144 06/09/1960 F	P	WHBODY		M	M	M	M	M	M	M	M	M	5	02/02
		U	RFINGR				M			30			30		02/02
00005	MEYER, STEVE 982778955 07/15/1964 M	P	COLLAR	PL	119	119	113							5	08/97
		P	WAIST	P	10	11	11								08/97
			ASSIGN		19	119	113	33	185	174	1387	2308	2320		
			NOTE		ASSIGNED DOSE BASED ON EDE 1 CALCULATION										
		U	RFINGR				140			690			2180		08/97
00203	STEVENS, LEE 335478977 08/25/1951 M	P	WHBODY		ABSENT			M	M	M	M	M	M	4	07/02
		U	RFINGR		ABSENT					M			M		07/02
00204	WALKER, JANE 416995421 03/21/1947 F	P	WHBODY		3	3	3	12	11	11	22	21	21	5	11/02
00188	WEBSTER, ROBERT 355381469 05/15/1972 M	P	WHBODY NOTE		40 CALCULATED	40	40	200	200	200	240	240	240	5	07/01

M: MINIMAL REPORTING SERVICE OF 1 MREM
ELECTRONIC MEDIA TO FOLLOW THIS REPORT

QUALITY CONTROL RELEASE: LMR   1 - PR   6774 - PT131 - N1   -21587

NVLAP LAB CODE 100518-0**

Fig. 3.10 Sample radiation dosimetry report showing exposure received by various individuals during the month reported as well as type of dosimeter, its location, and the dose distribution. The report also shows totals for the year to date and lifetime exposure. (Courtesy Landauer, Inc., Glenwood, IL.)

The International Commission on Radiological Protection (ICRP) is an independent, international organization that develops and disseminates recommendations and guidance on protection against ionizing radiation. Its recommendations are adopted or modified to establish radiation regulatory requirements in several countries worldwide. In the United States the NCRP, chartered by the US Congress, formulates guidance and recommendations on radiation protection and radiation measurements. The NCRP-recommended dose limits are incorporated into federal regulations (Title 10 of the Code of Federal Regulations, Part 20, Standards for protection against radiation). The current occupational exposure limits have been established to ensure that no individuals will have deterministic effects and that the probability for stochastic effects is as low as reasonably and economically feasible.

Occupational dose limits: Dentists and their staff who make diagnostic radiographs are considered as occupationally exposed individuals and thus should be familiar with regulatory dose limits in their region or country. The ICRP-established dose limit for occupationally exposed individuals is 20 mSv of whole-body radiation exposure per year. Although this level of exposure is considered to present only a minimal risk, every effort should be made to keep the radiation dose to all individuals as low as practical. The dental profession does well in limiting occupational exposure. The average dose for individuals occupationally exposed in the operation of dental x-ray equipment is 0.2 mSv—1% of the allowable dose limit. The section on protection of personnel describes approaches to minimize radiation dose to occupationally exposed staff.

Public dose limits: Support staff members (e.g., receptionists and auxiliary staff who do not perform radiography) and patients are subject to dose limits for members of the general public. The recommended limits for exposure to the public do not include natural background radiation and radiation received for individual medical and dental care. There are no limits on the exposure a patient can receive from diagnostic examinations, interventional procedures, or radiation therapy; this is because these exposures are made intentionally for the direct benefit of the recipient. Individual circumstances make the setting of limits inappropriate.

Increasing concern for minimizing patient exposure has led multiple institutions, including the NCRP, to issue diagnostic reference levels (DRLs) for medical and dental diagnostic imaging. DRL exposure values represent the acceptable upper limits for patient exposure (75th percentile of general practice), whereas achievable doses represent the median dose (50th percentile) in general practice. The NCRP recommends a DRL of 1.6 mGy entrance skin dose for intraoral periapical and bite-wing radiography. The NCRP further recommends an achievable dose of 1.2 mGy for intraoral radiography.

Quality Assurance

Quality assurance protocols for the x-ray machine, imaging receptor, film processing, dark room, and patient shielding should be developed and implemented for each dental health care setting (ADA 2012).

Quality assurance is defined as a program for periodic assessment of the performance of all parts of the radiologic procedure. It is intended to ensure that a dental office consistently produces high-quality images with minimum exposure to patients and personnel (see Chapter 15).

TABLE 3.4 Recommended Dose Limits for Human Exposure to Ionizing Radiation

	NCRP[a]	ICRP[b]
Occupational Exposure		
Annual effective dose	50 mSv/year	20 mSv, averaged over defined 5-year periods
Cumulative effective dose	10 mSv × age	100 mSv in 5 years *and* should not exceed 50 mSv[c] in any single year
Annual equivalent dose		
Lens of eye	Absorbed dose of 50 mGy	20 mSv, averaged over defined 5-year periods, *and* exposure in any single year should not exceed 50 mSv
Skin	500 mSv	500 mSv
Hands and feet		
Pregnant workers	0.5 mSv/month to embryo-fetus	1 mSv to the embryo/fetus after declaration of pregnancy
Public Exposure[d]		
Annual effective dose	1 mSv (continuous or frequent exposure) 5 mSv (infrequent exposure)	1 mSv
Annual equivalent dose in:		
Lens of eye	15 mSv	15 mSv
Skin	50 mSv	50 mSv

[a]Recommendations from the National Council on Radiation Protection and Measurement. Report No. 116, Limitation of exposure to ionizing radiation, 1993. NCRP Commentary No. 26, Guidance on radiation dose limits for the lens of the eye, 2016.
[b]Recommendations of the International Commission on Radiological Protection. IRCP Publication 103. *Ann ICRP*. 2007;37:1–332. ICRP Statement on Tissue Reactions and Early and Late Effects of Radiation in Normal Tissues and Organs—Threshold Doses for Tissue Reactions in a Radiation Protection Context. ICRP Publication 118. *Ann ICRP*. 2012;41:1–322.
[c]The Atomic Energy Regulatory Board, Government of India, has set a lower dose limit of 30 mSv in any single year.
[d]Dose limits for public exposure do not include exposure from diagnostic or therapeutic radiation.
ICRP, The International Commission on Radiological Protection; *NCRP*, The National Council on Radiation Protection and Measurements.

Studies have indicated that dentists may be needlessly exposing their patients to compensate for improper exposure techniques, film processing practices, and darkroom procedures. One study reported that only 33% of panoramic radiographs that accompanied biopsy specimens were of acceptable diagnostic quality. However, when demands were placed on dentists to improve their techniques, the number of unsatisfactory radiographs was significantly reduced. Two studies by a dental insurance carrier demonstrated that after claims were rejected for unsatisfactory radiographs and the dentist was made aware of the errors and ways in which they could be corrected, the number of satisfactory radiographs submitted doubled. This study suggests that when the dentist is presented with guidelines for quality assurance, along with proper motivation,

patient exposure can be dramatically reduced. Commercial mail-in devices are available to dentists and radiation protection agencies to measure dental image quality and dose of their radiographs.

Some states require dental offices to establish written guidelines for quality assurance and to maintain written records of quality assurance tests. Regardless of requirements, each dental office should establish maintenance and monitoring procedures, as outlined in Chapter 16.

Continuing Education

Practitioners should remain informed about safety updates and the availability of new equipment, supplies and techniques that could farther improve the diagnostic quality of radiographs and decrease radiation exposure (ADA 2006).

Individuals who administer ionizing radiation must be familiar with the magnitude of exposure encountered in medicine, dentistry, and everyday life; the possible risks associated with such exposure; and the methods used to affect exposure and dose reduction. Although this chapter presents some of this information, acquiring knowledge and developing and maintaining skills is a lifelong process.

BIBLIOGRAPHY

Acharya S, Pai KM, Acharya S. Repeat film analysis and its implications for quality assurance in dental radiology: an institutional case study. *Contemp Clin Dent*. 2015;6:392–395.

American Dental Association Council on Scientific Affairs. The use of dental radiographs: update and recommendations. *J Am Dent Assoc*. 2006;137:1304–1312.

American Dental Association Council on Scientific Affairs. Dental radiographic examinations: recommendations for patient selection and limiting radiation exposure; Revised 2012. http://www.ada.org/sections/professionalResources/pdfs/Dental_Radiographic_Examinations_2012.pdf.

Code of Federal Regulations, Title 10, Chapter I, Part 20. Standards for protection against radiation; https://www.ecfr.gov/cgi-bin.

Committee to Assess Health Risks from Exposure to Low Levels of Ionizing Radiations. *Health Risks From Exposure to Low Levels of Ionizing Radiation: BEIR VII*. Washington, DC: National Academy Press; 2006.

Dental radiographs: benefits and safety. *J Am Dent Assoc*. 2011;142:1101.

Environmental Protection Agency. Calculate your radiation dose; http://www.epa.gov/radiation/understand/calculate.html.

Hall EJ. Is there a place for quantitative risk assessment? *J Radiol Prot*. 2009;29(0):A171–A184.

Hall EJ, Giaccia AJ. *Radiobiology for the Radiologist*. 6th ed. Baltimore: Lippincott Williams & Wilkins; 2006.

Horner K, Rushton VE, Walker A, et al. European guidelines on radiation protection in dental radiology: the safe use of radiographs in dental practice. *Radiat Protect*. 2004;136:1–115.

Mossman KL. The LNT debate in radiation protection: science vs. policy. *Dose Response*. 2012;10(2):190–202.

National Council on Radiation Protection and Measurements. *Control of Radon in Houses, NCRP Report 103*. Bethesda, MD: National Council on Radiation Protection and Measurements; 1989.

National Council on Radiation Protection and Measurements. *Quality Assurance for Diagnostic Imaging, NCRP Report 99*. Bethesda, MD: National Council on Radiation Protection and Measurements; 1990.

National Council on Radiation Protection and Measurements. *Limitation of Exposure to Ionizing Radiation, NCRP Report 116*. Bethesda, MD: National Council on Radiation Protection and Measurements; 1993.

National Council on Radiation Protection and Measurements. *Dental X-Ray Protection, NCRP Report 145*. Bethesda, MD: National Council on Radiation Protection and Measurements; 2003.

National Council on Radiation Protection and Measurements. *Ionizing Radiation Exposure of the Population of the United States, NCRP Report 160*. Bethesda, MD: National Council on Radiation Protection and Measurements; 2009.

National Council on Radiation Protection and Measurements. *Reference Levels and Achievable Doses in Medical and Dental Imaging: Recommendations for the United States, NCRP Report 172*. Bethesda, MD: National Council on Radiation Protection and Measurements; 2012.

Nationwide Evaluation of X-Ray Trends (NEXT): tabulation and graphical summary of the 1999 dental radiography survey, CRCPD Publication E-03-6; Bethesda, MD, 2003, Center for Devices and Radiological Health, U.S. Food and Drug Administration.

Preston RJ. Radiation biology: concepts for radiation protection. *Health Phys*. 2005;88:545–556.

Sansare K, Khanna V, Karjodkar F. Utility of thyroid collars in cephalometric radiography. *Dentomaxillofac Radiol*. 2011;40(8):471–475.

SEDENTEXCT. Guidelines on CBCT for dental and maxillofacial radiology; http://www.sedentexct.eu/.

Sources and effects of ionizing radiation, UNSCEAR 2008 report: volumes I and II; New York, 2008. UNSCEAR (United Nations Publications vol I released in 2010 and vol II released in 2011). https://unp.un.org/details.aspx?pid=20417 and https://unp.un.org/Details.aspx?pid=21556.

The 2007 recommendations of the International Commission on Radiological Protection. IRCP Publication 103. *Ann ICRP*. 2007;37:1–332.

4

Digital Imaging

André Mol

The advent of digital imaging has revolutionized radiology. This revolution is the result of both technologic innovation in image acquisition processes and the development of networked computing systems for image retrieval and transmission. Dentistry has seen a steady increase in the use of these technologies, improvement of software interfaces, and introduction of new products. Numerous forces have driven the shift from film to digital systems. The detrimental effects of inadequate film processing on diagnostic quality and the difficulty of maintaining high-quality chemical processing are well documented. Digital imaging does not require chemical processing, thus eliminating hazardous wastes in the form of processing chemicals and lead foil from film. Images can be electronically transferred to other health care providers without any alteration of the original image quality. In addition, digital intraoral receptors require less radiation than film, thus reducing patient exposure. Finally, digital imaging allows enhancements, measurements, and corrections not available with film.

Digital systems do have a few disadvantages compared with film. The initial expense of setting up a digital imaging system is relatively high. Certain components, such as the electronic x-ray receptor used in some intraoral systems, are susceptible to rough handling and are costly to replace. Because digital systems use evolving technologies, there is a risk—perhaps even a likelihood—of systems becoming obsolete or manufacturers going out of business. The latter is true for most electronic devices, including computers.

Computers play a vital role in most dental practices, and that role is expanding as various functions—including appointment scheduling, procedure billing, and patient charting—are integrated into seamless practice management software solutions. This has made the adoption of digital imaging in dentistry easier, and for many dental practices digital imaging is the preferred technology. This chapter describes the characteristics of digital images, image receptors, display options, and storage devices and discusses digital image processing.

ANALOG VERSUS DIGITAL

The term *digital* in digital imaging refers to the numeric format of the image content and its discreteness. Conventional film imaging can be considered an analog medium in which differences in the size and distribution of black metallic silver result in a continuous density spectrum. Digital images are numeric and discrete in two ways, in terms

of (1) the spatial distribution of the picture elements (pixels) and (2) the different shades of gray of each of the pixels. A digital image consists of a large collection of individual pixels organized in a matrix of rows and columns (Fig. 4.1). Each pixel has a row and column coordinate that uniquely identify its location in the matrix. The formation of a digital image requires several steps, beginning with analog processes. At each pixel of an electronic detector, the absorption of x-rays generates a small voltage. More x-rays generate a higher voltage and vice versa. At each pixel, the voltage can fluctuate between a minimum and maximum value and is therefore an analog signal (Fig. 4.2A).

Production of a digital image requires a process called analog-to-digital conversion (ADC). ADC consists of two steps: (1) sampling and (2) quantization. Sampling means that a small range of voltage values are grouped together as a single value (see Fig. 4.2B). Narrow sampling better mimics the original signal but leads to larger memory requirements for the resulting digital image (see Fig. 4.2C). Once sampled, the signal is quantized, which means that every sampled signal is assigned a value. These values are stored in the computer and represent the image. For the clinician to see the image, the computer organizes the pixels in their proper locations and displays a shade of gray that corresponds to the number that was assigned during the quantization step.

To understand the strengths and weaknesses of digital radiography, one must establish which elements of the radiographic imaging chain stay the same and which change. The imaging chain can be conceptualized as a series of interconnecting links beginning with the generation of x-rays. Exposure factors, patient factors, and the projection geometry determine how the x-ray beam is attenuated. A portion of the unattenuated x-ray beam is captured by the image receptor to form a latent image. This latent image is processed and converted into a real image, which is viewed and interpreted by the clinician. The use of digital detectors changes the way in which we acquire, store, retrieve, and display images. However, besides an adjustment of the exposure time, digital detectors do not fundamentally change the way in which x-rays are selectively attenuated by the tissues of the patient. The physics of the interaction of x-rays with matter and the effects of the projection geometry on the appearance of the radiographic image are unaltered and remain critically important for understanding image content and optimizing image quality. Elements in this part of the imaging chain that limit diagnostic performance affect both film-based radiography and digital radiography.

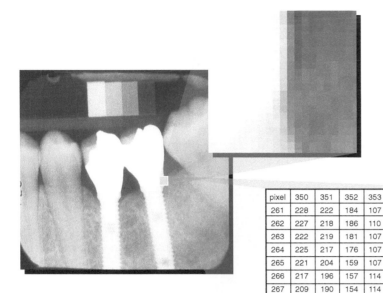

pixel	350	351	352	353	354	355	356	357
261	228	222	184	107	76	92	90	98
262	227	218	186	110	90	104	103	98
263	222	219	181	107	97	107	102	104
264	225	217	176	107	98	100	100	107
265	221	204	159	107	105	101	107	102
266	217	196	157	114	105	104	106	100
267	209	190	154	114	107	103	97	100
268	202	195	166	118	102	102	92	94
269	197	196	168	122	98	102	90	94
270	195	190	166	130	104	105	92	97
271	199	190	172	144	111	107	100	106
272	201	193	177	160	120	103	112	106
273	203	195	181	166	129	102	111	106
274	201	200	186	172	133	110	112	102

Fig. 4.1 A digital image is made up of a large number of discrete picture elements (pixels). The pixels are so small that the image appears smooth at normal magnification. The location of each pixel is uniquely identified by row and column coordinates within the image matrix. The value assigned to a pixel represents the intensity (gray level) of the image at that location.

DIGITAL IMAGE RECEPTORS

Digital image receptors encompass numerous different technologies and come in many different sizes and shapes. Different and sometimes confusing names are in use to identify these receptors in medicine and dentistry. The most useful distinction is that between two main technologies:

- *Solid-state technology.* Although solid-state detectors can be subdivided further, these detectors have in common certain physical properties and the ability to generate a digital image in the computer without any other external device. In medicine, the use of solid-state detectors is referred to as digital radiography (DR). In dentistry, intraoral solid-state detectors are often called *sensors.*
- *Photostimulable phosphor (PSP) technology.* This technology consists of a phosphor-coated plate in which a latent image is formed after x-ray exposure. The latent image is converted to a digital image by a scanning device through stimulation by laser light. This technology is sometimes referred to as *storage phosphor* on the basis of the notion that the image information is temporarily stored within the phosphor. Other times the term *image plates* is used to differentiate them from film and solid-state detectors. The use of PSP plates in medical radiology is referred to as *computed radiography* (CR).

SOLID-STATE DETECTORS

Solid-state detectors collect the charge generated by x-rays in a solid semiconducting material (Fig. 4.3). The key clinical feature of these detectors is the rapid availability of the image after exposure. The matrix and its associated readout and amplifying electronics of intraoral detectors are enclosed within a plastic housing to protect them from the oral environment. These elements of the detector consume part of the real estate of the sensor so that the active area is smaller than its total surface area. Sensor bulk, although reduced by continued miniaturization of the electronic components, is a potential drawback of intraoral solid-state detectors. In addition, most detectors incorporate an electronic cable to transfer data to the computer. The presence of a cable can make positioning of the sensor more challenging and requires some adaptation. It also results in increased vulnerability of the device to fail due to wear of the cable connections from normal use. Manufacturers have addressed these issues in various ways. Some manufacturers have changed the location of the cable attachment to the corner of the sensor. Others offer sensors with magnetic connectors, induction connectors, or reinforced cables to reduce accidental damage to the device. Wireless radiofrequency transmission also has been introduced to eliminate the cable altogether. Wireless transmission frees the detector from a direct tether to the computer, but it necessitates some additional electronic components, thus increasing the overall bulk of the sensor.

Many manufacturers produce detectors with varying active sensor areas roughly corresponding to the different sizes of intraoral film. Detectors without flaws are relatively expensive to produce, and the expense of the detector increases with increasing matrix size (total number of pixels). Pixel size ranges from less than 20 μm to 70 μm. Three types of solid-state sensors are in common use.

Charge-Coupled Device

The charge-coupled device (CCD), introduced to dentistry in 1987, was the first digital image receptor to be adapted for intraoral imaging. The CCD uses a thin wafer of silicon as the basis for image recording. The silicon crystals are formed in a pixel matrix (Fig. 4.4). When exposed to radiation, the covalent bonds between silicon atoms are broken, producing electron-hole pairs (Fig. 4.5). The number of electron-hole pairs that are formed in an area is proportional to the amount of x-ray exposure that area receives. The electrons are attracted toward the most positive potential in the device, where they create "charge packets." Each packet corresponds to one pixel. The pattern of charge packets formed from the individual pixels in the matrix represents the latent image

(Fig. 4.6). The image is read by transferring each row of pixel charges from one pixel to the next in "bucket brigade" fashion. As a charge reaches the end of its row, it is transferred to a readout amplifier and transmitted as a voltage to the analog-to-digital converter located within or connected to the computer. Voltages from each pixel are sampled and assigned a numeric value representing a gray level (ADC). Because CCD detectors are more sensitive to light than to x-rays, most manufacturers use a layer of scintillating material coated directly on the CCD surface or coupled to the surface by a fiberoptic plate. This scintillating material increases the x-ray absorption efficiency of the detector. Gadolinium oxybromide compounds similar to those used in rare earth radiographic screens and cesium iodide are examples of scintillators that have been used for this purpose.

CCDs have also been made in linear arrays a few pixels wide and many pixels long for panoramic and cephalometric imaging. In the case of panoramic units, the CCD is fixed in position opposite to the x-ray source with the long axis of the array oriented parallel to the fan-shaped x-ray beam. Some manufacturers provide CCD sensors that may be retrofitted to older panoramic units. In contrast to film imaging, the mechanics for cephalometric imaging are different. Construction of a single CCD of a size that could simultaneously capture the area of a full skull would be prohibitively expensive. Combining a linear CCD array and a slit-shaped x-ray beam with a scanning motion permits scanning of the skull over several seconds. One disadvantage of this approach is the increased possibility of patient movement artifacts during the several seconds required to complete a scan.

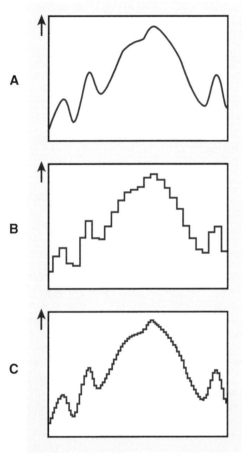

Fig. 4.2 (A) Illustration of an analog voltage signal generated by a detector. (B) Sampling of the analog signal discards part of the signal. (C) Sampling at a higher frequency preserves more of the original signal.

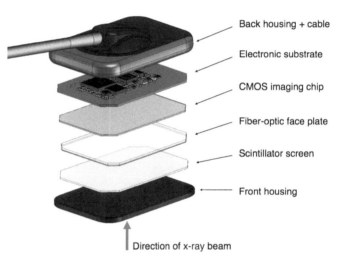

Fig. 4.3 Exploded View of Complementary Metal Oxide Semiconductor (CMOS) Sensor. The front and back housings form a watertight and light-tight barrier to protect the sensor components. The scintillator screen fluoresces when exposed to x-rays and forms a visible light radiographic image. The fiberoptic faceplate couples the scintillator screen to the CMOS chip to reduce image noise. The CMOS imaging chip captures the light from the scintillator and creates a charge in each pixel proportional to the exposure. The sensor electronics read the charge in each pixel and transmit it to a computer. (Courtesy XDR Radiology, Los Angeles, CA, https://www.xdrradiology.com.)

Fig. 4.4 (A) Basic structure of a charge-coupled device. The electrodes are insulated from an n-p silicon sandwich. The surface of the silicon typically incorporates a scintillating material to improve x-ray capture efficiency and fiberoptics to improve resolution. One pixel uses three electrodes. (B) Excess electrons from the n-type layer diffuse into the p-type layer, whereas excess holes in the p-type layer diffuse into the n-type layer. The resulting charge imbalance creates an electric field in the silicon with a maximum just inside the n-type layer.

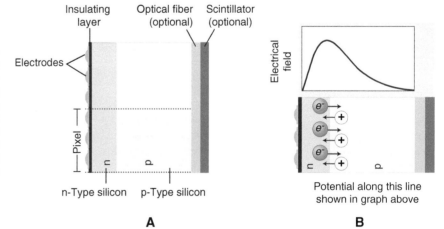

Complementary Metal Oxide Semiconductors

Complementary metal oxide semiconductor (CMOS) technology is the basis for typical consumer-grade digital cameras. These detectors are also silicon-based semiconductors but are fundamentally different from CCDs in the way that pixel charges are read. Each pixel is isolated from its neighboring pixels and is directly connected to a transistor. Similar to the CCD, electron-hole pairs are generated within the pixel in proportion to the amount of x-ray energy that is absorbed. This charge is transferred to the transistor as a small voltage. The voltage in each transistor can be addressed separately, read by a frame grabber, and stored and displayed as a digital gray value. CMOS technology is widely used in the construction of computer central processing unit chips and digital camera detectors, and the technology is less expensive than that used in the manufacture of CCDs. Most manufacturers currently use this technology for intraoral imaging applications (Fig. 4.7).

Flat-Panel Detectors

Flat-panel detectors are used for medical imaging but have also been used in several extraoral imaging devices. The detectors can provide relatively large matrix areas with pixel sizes less than 100 μm; this allows direct digital imaging of larger areas of the body, including the head. Two approaches have been taken in selecting x-ray–sensitive materials for flat-panel detectors. Indirect detectors are sensitive to visible light, and an intensifying screen (gadolinium oxysulfide or cesium iodide) is used to convert x-ray energy to light. The performance of these devices is determined by the thickness of the intensifying screen. Thicker screens are more efficient but allow greater diffusion of light photons, leading to less sharp images. Direct detectors use a photoconductor material (selenium) with properties similar to silicon and a higher atomic number, which permits more efficient absorption of x-rays. Under the influence

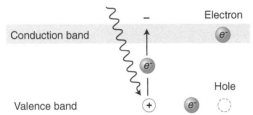

Fig. 4.5 X-ray or light photons impart energy to electrons in the valence band, releasing them into the conduction band. This generates an "electron hole" charge pair.

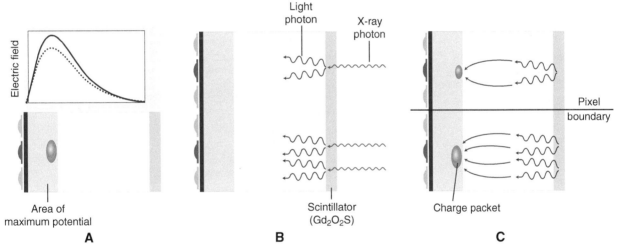

Fig. 4.6 (A) Before exposure, the central electrode of each pixel is turned on, creating an area of maximal potential or a potential well. (B) X-ray photons are absorbed in the scintillating material and converted to light photons. Light photons are absorbed in the silicon through photoelectric absorption. (C) Electrons released from the valence band collect selectively near the n-p layer interface in the area of maximum potential to form a charge packet. During charge-coupled device readout, the electrical potential of the pixel electrodes is sequentially modulated to shift the charge packet from pixel to pixel.

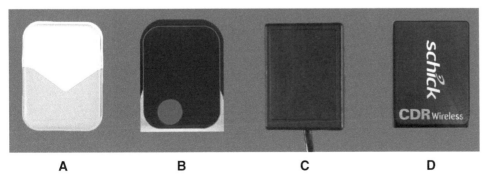

Fig. 4.7 (A) Kodak (courtesy Carestream Health, Inc., exclusive manufacturer of Kodak dental systems) No. 2 film. (B) Soredex (Milwaukee, WI) OpTime No. 2 PSP plate (outlined in red) placed on a barrier envelope to demonstrate packaged size. (C) Gendex (Hatfield, PA) No. 2 charge-coupled device sensor. (D) Schick (Sirona Dental Inc., Charlotte, NC) No. 2 complementary metal oxide semiconductor wireless sensor.

of an applied electrical field, the electrons that are freed during x-ray exposure of the selenium are conducted in a direct line to an underlying thin film transistor (TFT) detector element. Direct detectors using selenium ($Z = 34$) provide higher resolution but are less efficient compared to indirect detectors using intensifying screens with gadolinium ($Z = 64$) or cesium ($Z = 55$). The electrical energy generated in flat-panel detectors is proportional to the x-ray exposure and is stored at each pixel in a capacitor. The energy is released and read out by applying appropriate row and column voltages to a particular pixel's transistor. Flat-panel detectors are relatively expensive and currently limited to specialized imaging tasks, such as cone beam computed tomography (CBCT).

PHOTOSTIMULABLE PHOSPHOR

PSP plates absorb and store energy from x-rays and release this energy as light (phosphorescence) when stimulated by another light of an appropriate wavelength. To the extent that the stimulating light and phosphorescent light wavelengths differ, the two may be distinguished, and the phosphorescence can be quantified as a measure of the amount of x-ray energy that the material has absorbed.

The PSP material used for radiographic imaging is "europium-doped" barium fluorohalide. Barium in combination with iodine, chlorine, or bromine forms a crystal lattice. The addition of europium (Eu+2) creates imperfections in this lattice. When exposed to a sufficiently energetic source of radiation, valence electrons in europium can absorb energy and move into the conduction band. These electrons migrate to nearby halogen vacancies (F-centers) in the fluorohalide lattice and may become trapped there in a metastable state. While in this state, the number of trapped electrons is proportional to x-ray exposure and represents a latent image. When stimulated by red light of around 600 nm, the barium fluorohalide releases trapped electrons to the conduction band. When an electron returns to the Eu+3 ion, energy is released as light in the green spectrum between 300 and 500 nm (Fig. 4.8). Fiberoptics conduct the light from the PSP plate to a photomultiplier tube. The photomultiplier tube converts this light into electrical energy. A red filter at the photomultiplier tube selectively removes the stimulating laser light, and the remaining green light is detected and converted to

a varying voltage. The variations in voltage output from the photomultiplier tube correspond to variations in stimulated light intensity from the latent image. The voltage signal is quantified by an analog-to-digital converter and stored and displayed as a digital image. In practice, the barium fluorohalide material is combined with a polymer and spread in a thin layer on a base material to create a PSP plate. For intraoral radiography, a polyester base similar to radiographic film is used.

When they are manufactured in standard intraoral sizes, these plates provide handling characteristics similar to intraoral film. PSP plates are also made in sizes commonly used for panoramic and cephalometric imaging. Some PSP processors accommodate a full range of intraoral and extraoral plate sizes. Other processors are limited to intraoral or extraoral formats.

Before exposure, PSP plates must be erased to eliminate residual images from prior exposures. This erasure is accomplished by flooding the plate with a bright light. Current PSP systems integrate automatic plate erasing within the scanner. Plates can also be erased by placing them on a dental viewbox with the phosphor side of the plates facing the light for 1 or 2 minutes. More intense light sources can be used for shorter periods of time. Inadequate plate erasure results in double images and usually renders the image undiagnostic. Erased plates are placed in light-tight containers before exposure. In the case of intraoral plates, sealable polyvinyl envelopes that are impervious to oral fluids and light are used for packaging. For large-format plates, conventional cassettes without intensifying screens are used. After exposure, plates should be processed as soon as possible because trapped electrons spontaneously release over time. The rate of loss of electrons is greatest shortly after exposure. The rate varies depending on the composition of the storage phosphor and the environmental temperature. Some phosphors lose 23% of their trapped electrons after 30 minutes and 30% after 1 hour. Because loss of trapped electrons is uniform across the plate surface, early loss of charge does not typically result in clinically meaningful image deterioration. However, underexposed images may have noticeable image degradation in the form of increased image noise. Adequately exposed images may be stored for 12 to 24 hours and retain acceptable image quality. A more important source of latent image fading is exposure to ambient light during plate preparation for processing. A semidark environment is recommended for plate handling. The more intense the

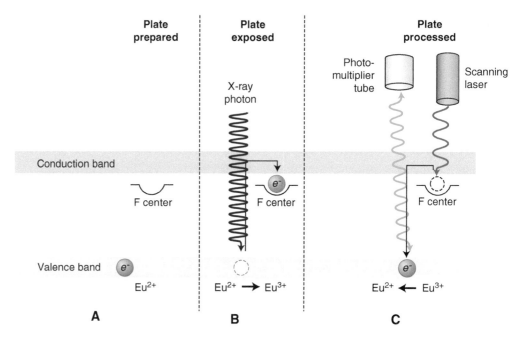

Fig. 4.8 Photostimulable Phosphor (PSP) Image Formation. (A) Initially, the PSP plate is flooded with white light to return all electrons to the valence band. (B) Exposure to x-rays imparts energy to europium valence electrons, moving them into the conduction band. Some electrons become trapped at "F centers." (C) A red scanning laser imparts energy to electrons at the F centers, promoting them to the conduction band, from which many return to the valence band. With the electron's return to the valence band, energy is released in the form of light photons in the green spectrum. This light is detected by a photomultiplier tube or diode with a red filter to screen out the scanning laser light.

background light and the longer the exposure of the plate to this light, the greater the loss of trapped electrons and the more degraded the resultant image. Red safelights found in most darkrooms are not safe for exposed PSP plates, which are most sensitive to the red light spectrum.

Photostimulable Phosphor Scanners

A number of approaches have been adopted for "reading" the latent images on PSP plates. Soredex (Milwaukee, WI) in its Digora and OpTime systems and Air Techniques (Melville, NY) in its ScanX system use a rapidly rotating multifaceted mirror that reflects a beam of red laser light. As the mirror revolves, the laser light sweeps across the plate. The plate is advanced, and the adjacent line of phosphor is scanned. The direction of the laser scanning the plate is termed the *fast scan direction*. The direction of plate advancement is termed the *slow scan direction*.

These scanners, as well as the Carestream (Atlanta, GA) CS 7600 scanner and the Planmeca (Helsinki, Finland) ProScanner, also include automatic plate clearance after scanning. Automatic plate clearance improves work flow and reduces potential plate damage from manual erasing. The mechanism used for plate intake in the Soredex OpTime scanner requires a metal disk on the back of the plate. This disk also serves as a marker to indicate when a plate was exposed backward. Carestream and Planmeca use radio-frequency identification (RFID) technology to link patient information to the plates. This prevents plates from being scanned into the wrong patient file. The RFID chip also serves to alert the operator when a plate is accidentally exposed backward.

Current PSP scanners all use individual plate loading. An alternative approach to plate reading involves a rapidly rotating drum that can hold multiple plates. Although some of these systems are likely still being used, they are no longer produced by the leading manufactures.

DIGITAL DETECTOR CHARACTERISTICS

Contrast Resolution

Contrast resolution is the ability to distinguish different densities in the radiographic image; this is a function of the interaction of the following factors:
- Attenuation characteristics of the tissues imaged
- Capacity of the imaging system to distinguish differences in numbers of x-ray photons and translate them into gray values
- Ability of the computer display to portray differences between gray levels
- Ability of the observer to recognize those differences

Current digital detectors capture data at 8, 10, 12, or 16 bits. The bit depth is a power of 2 (Fig. 4.9). This means that the detector can theoretically capture 256 (2^8) to 65,536 (2^{16}) different attenuation levels. In practice, the actual number of meaningful attenuation levels that can be captured is limited by inaccuracies in image acquisition—that is, noise. Regardless of the number of attenuation differences that a detector can capture, conventional computer monitors are capable of displaying a gray scale of only 8 bits. Because operating systems such as Windows reserve many gray levels for the display of system information, the actual number of gray levels that can be displayed on a monitor is 242. A more important limiting factor is the human visual system, which is capable of distinguishing only about 60 gray levels at any time under ideal viewing conditions. Considering the typical viewing environment in the dental operatory, the actual number of gray levels that can be distinguished decreases to less than 30. Human visual limitations are also present for film viewing; however, the luminance (brightness) of a typical radiograph viewbox is much greater than that of a typical computer display. Therefore the ambient lighting of the room in which

Fig. 4.9 Contrast Resolution. Examples of gray-scale ramps representing distinct gray levels from black to white. Bit depth controls the number of possible gray levels in the image. The actual number of distinct gray levels that are displayed depends on the output device and image processing. The perceived number of gray levels is influenced by viewing conditions and the visual acuity of the observer. (A) 6 bits/pixel = 64 gray levels. (B) 5 bits/pixel = 32 gray levels. (C) 4 bits/pixel = 16 gray levels. (D) 3 bits/pixel = 8 gray levels.

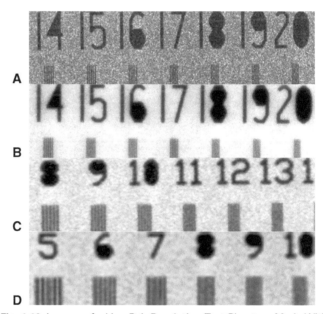

Fig. 4.10 Images of a Line-Pair Resolution Test Phantom Made With Various Receptors. (A) Kodak (Atlanta, GA) InSight film. (B) Trophy RVGui (Kodak) high-resolution charge-coupled device. (C) Gendex (Hatfield, PA) DenOptix photostimulable phosphor (PSP) scanned at 600 dots per inch (DPI). (D) Gendex DenOptix PSP scanned at 300 DPI.

the image is viewed theoretically has a lower impact on film than on digital displays.

Spatial Resolution

Spatial resolution is the capacity for distinguishing fine detail in an image. Resolution is often measured and reported in units of line pairs per millimeter. Test objects consisting of sets of very fine radiopaque lines separated from each other by spaces equal to the width of a line are constructed with a variety of line widths (Fig. 4.10). A line and its associated space are called a line pair (lp). At least two columns of pixels are required to resolve a line pair, one for the bright line and one for the dark space. Typical observers are able to distinguish about 6 lp/mm without benefit of magnification. Intraoral film is capable of providing more than 20 lp/mm of resolution. Unless a film image is magnified, the observer will be unable to appreciate the extent of the detail in the image.

BOX 4.1 Conversion Between Pixel Size and Theoretical Limit of Resolution

	THEORETICAL LIMIT OF RESOLUTION	
Pixel Size (µm)	Line Pairs per Millimeter (lp/mm)	Dots or Points per Inch (DPI or PPI)
20	25	1270
50	10	508
A	$1000/(A \times 2)$	25,400/A
$1000/(B \times 2)$	B	$B \times 2 \times 25.4$
25,400/C	$C/(2 \times 25.4)$	C

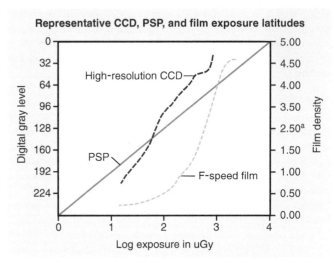

Representative CCD, PSP, and film exposure latitudes

[a]An optical density of 2.5 is generally considered the upper limit of useful clinical density in the absence of special illumination or "hot lighting" of films.

Fig. 4.11 Representative Exposure Latitudes of Charge-Coupled Device *(CCD)*, Photostimulable Phosphor *(PSP)*, and Intraoral Film Sensors. The clinically useful optical density of film has an upper limit of 2.5. Use of a more intense viewbox or "hot lighting" can extend the upper end of the usable density range and expand useful film latitude. PSP plates are unique in responding linearly to exposure.

With solid-state digital imaging systems, the theoretic resolution limit is determined by the pixel size: the smaller the size of the pixel, the higher the maximally attainable resolution. A sensor with 20-µm pixels can obtain a maximum theoretical resolution of 25 lp/mm: One line pair requires two pixels, in this case 2×20 µm, which equals 40 µm. Thus the maximal resolution would be 1 lp/40 µm, which is equal to 25 lp/mm (Box 4.1). Alternatively, resolution can be expressed in dots per inch (DPI) or points per inch (PPI). At best, there is one dot or point per pixel. Thus if the pixel size is 20 µm, there is one dot or point per 20 µm. This is equal to 1270 DPI or PPI because there are 25,400 µm in 1 inch (25,400/20 = 1270). However, in practice, actual detector resolution is lower than these theoretical limits for a variety of reasons, including: (1) electronic noise; (2) diffusion of photons in the scintillator coating; and (3) potentially imperfect optical coupling between the scintillator, the fiberoptic screen (when present), and the photodetector. Currently the highest-resolution intraoral solid-state detector for dentistry has a measured resolution of approximately 20 lp/mm; however, this does not mean that this level of resolution is obtained clinically. Clinical spatial resolution depends not only on detector characteristics but also on the size of the focal spot, the source-to-object distance, and the object-to-image distance (see Chapter 6).

Resolution in PSP systems is influenced by the thickness of the phosphor material. Thicker phosphor layers cause more diffusion and yield a lower resolution. A thicker layer enhances x-ray absorption efficiency, resulting in a faster image receptor. Resolution is also inversely proportional to the diameter of the laser beam. Effective beam diameter is increased by vibration in the rotating mirror and drum scanner designs. Slow scan motion influences resolution by the increment of plate advancement. This increment may be adjusted to increase or reduce resolution in some systems. Current PSP systems are capable of providing more than 10 lp/mm of resolution.

Software displays of all digital images permit magnification of images. A periapical image filling the display of a computer monitor may be magnified by a factor of 10 times or more. At this level of magnification, the image takes on a building-block pattern or pixelated appearance, and the limits of resolution of the imaging system are evident.

Detector Latitude

The ability of an image receptor to capture a range of x-ray exposures is termed *latitude*. A desirable quality in intraoral image receptors is the ability to record a broad range of tissue attenuation differences—from gingiva to enamel. At the same time, subtle differences in attenuation within these tissues should be visually apparent. The useful range of densities in film radiography is two orders of magnitude, from 0.5 to 2.5. The dynamic range of film actually extends for more than four orders of magnitude, but densities of 3 and 4, which transmit only 1/1000 to 1/10,000 of the incident light, require intensified illumination or hot lighting to be distinguished from a density of 2.5. Such devices

are not commonly used in general practice. The latitude of CCD and CMOS detectors is similar to the latitude of film and can be extended with digital enhancement of contrast and brightness. PSP receptors enjoy larger latitudes and have a linear response to five orders of magnitude of x-ray exposure (Fig. 4.11).

Detector Sensitivity

The sensitivity, or speed, of a detector is its ability to respond to small amounts of radiation. Intraoral film speed is classified according to speed group based on criteria developed by the International Organization for Standardization. Extraoral screen-film combinations use a classification system developed by Eastman Kodak. Currently there are no classification standards for dental digital x-ray receptors. As a result, the reported sensitivity of systems by equipment manufacturers is difficult to compare and the performance that can be achieved in routine practice may be exaggerated. The useful sensitivity of digital receptors is affected by numerous factors, including detector efficiency, pixel size, and system noise. Current PSP systems for intraoral imaging allow dose reductions of about 50% compared with F-speed film with similar diagnostic performance. Subjectively, most observers prefer intraoral PSP images with a higher level of x-ray exposure. Paradoxically, patient doses may increase if the level of x-ray exposure is determined by image criteria that are based on the subjective perception of "attractiveness." Additionally, patient exposure may increase with CCD systems because of the ease of making repeat exposures. In general, solid-state detectors require less exposure than PSP systems or film. CCD and PSP systems for extraoral imaging require exposures similar to exposures needed for 200-speed screen-film systems.

DIGITAL IMAGE VIEWING

Electronic Displays

Flat-panel and laptop displays use TFT technology, similar to what is used in flat-panel detectors. The process involves sending signals to the transistor associated with each pixel, which causes the associated liquid crystal display (LCD) to transmit light of an intensity proportional to the transistor voltage. Subpixels composed of red, green, and blue phosphors are subjected to varied voltages and in combination create a pixel output of a particular hue and intensity. The output of laptop displays is limited in intensity and does not have the dynamic range or contrast found in conventional desktop LCD displays. The viewing angle of laptop displays is also limited, and the observer must be positioned squarely in front of the display for optimum viewing quality. Current laptop displays are of sufficient quality to be used for typical dental diagnostic tasks. Desktop versions of TFT LCD displays have overcome problems of brightness and viewing angle but consume more power and thus are not suited for laptop configurations. Most modern flat-panel displays have sufficient brightness and contrast and have viewing angles of 160 degrees. Most flat-panel displays incorporate a digital video interface, which allows direct display of digital information without digital-to-analog conversion. These displays virtually eliminate signal loss and distortion from digital-to-analog conversion.

Display Considerations

The display of digital images on electronic devices is a straightforward engineering issue. Positioning an image in the context of other diagnostic and demographic information and in useful relationships with other images is a more complex challenge that may vary according to diagnostic task, practice pattern, and practitioner preference. These challenges are answered with varying degrees of success by image display software. The quality, capabilities, and ease of use of display software vary from vendor to vendor. Even with the same software, the display of images can vary dramatically depending on how the software handles resizing of windows or the size and resolutions of different displays. For instance, on some displays it may be impossible to view a full-mouth series of images on a single screen at normal magnification (100%). Software may permit reduction in image size or scrolling around the window to compensate for smaller display areas. These approaches are not as fast or flexible as shifting a film mount around on a viewbox. The visibility of electronic displays is degraded by many of the same elements that degrade viewing of film images. Bright background illumination from windows or other sources of ambient light reduces visual contrast sensitivity. Light reflecting off a monitor surface may reduce the visibility of image contrast further. Images are best viewed in an environment in which lighting is subdued and indirect.

In using electronic displays for viewing digital images or other patient related information, the design and layout of the practice must be such that access to protected health information (PHI) by other patients or unauthorized individuals is prevented. In the United States, this is necessary to comply with the Health Insurance Portability and Accountability Act (HIPAA). This can be challenging in practices that use an open bay layout.

HARD COPIES

The need to print digital images for sharing with other clinicians or with third parties is decreasing rapidly as digital technology has become mainstream. However, when digital image sharing is not feasible, digital image printing is an economical solution for making digital radiographs transferable. Any time a digital image is modified, including the process of printing it in hard copy, there must be sufficient assurance that the image retains relevant diagnostic information. The requirements for quality vary with the diagnostic task at hand. For instance, assessment of the impaction status of a third molar puts a lower demand on the image quality than caries detection. There is limited scientific evidence to support the diagnostic efficacy of printed images. The large number of variables that influence the quality of the printed image (e.g., printing technology, printer quality, printer settings, and type of media) makes the printing process a much more complicated process than it initially appears to be. When images must be printed, it is imperative to use a printing system that is designed for its intended use and to follow the manufacturer's recommendations. It is always preferable to transfer images digitally when possible. The main types of printing technologies available for image printing include laser, inkjet, and dye sublimation with the use of either film or paper.

Film Printers

Radiologists have traditionally relied on film images for common interpretive tasks. High-quality film printers that use laser or dye sublimation technologies are expensive, and low-cost alternatives have less diagnostic quality. Current film transparencies produced with inkjet technology appear to be suboptimal for tasks such as caries diagnosis.

Paper Printers

Although printing on film allows radiographs to be evaluated in a traditional manner with the transmitted light of a viewbox, paper-printed digital radiographs require reflective light from a normally lit room. Because most dental operatories are not well equipped to control the ambient light level for viewing film images on a viewbox, paper-printed digital radiographs offer a substantial advantage. By printing digital radiographs on paper, the dentist is able to use technologies developed for the digital photography domain.

Photographic printers vary widely in price and quality. Although more costly models usually provide higher resolution, printer resolution is only one of many factors determining the final quality of the printed image. Inkjet printers are the most dominant in the market and offer the most economical alternative. Dye sublimation printers provide excellent image quality but are generally more expensive.

For any printing technology, the printing resolution is usually defined as the number of DPI the printer can print. A printer with a higher DPI number is capable of laying the ink down more tightly than a printer with a lower DPI number. As a result, printers with a higher DPI number can print smaller objects and thus are said to have higher resolution. The resolution of the digital radiograph can never be increased by a printer that prints at a higher resolution than that of the image itself. Printing digital radiographs at a lower resolution may reduce the final resolution of the image unless the printed size of the image is increased. Spatial resolution is preserved as long as the image prints pixel for pixel.

The same cannot be said of contrast resolution, which is always reduced by the printing process. The reason for this reduction in contrast resolution is that the printer is not printing with shades of gray but instead is printing varying numbers of black dots. Typically, an 8×8 pixel page array is assigned to each image pixel (Fig. 4.12). The number of elements in the array that are filled with a black ink dot determines the relative gray level of the array. The 8×8 array provides for 0 to 64 ink dots or 65 gray values. With an 8×8 dot array, it may not be possible to print all pixels of an image on a single page. For instance, a PSP panoramic image with a physical size of 15 cm × 30 cm might be scanned at 150 DPI. For each pixel of this image to print within the same dimensions, a printer resolution of 1200 DPI (8×150) is required. If the maximal resolution of the printer is 1200 DPI, images with higher resolutions must be printed at a larger size to obtain full spatial resolution. Likewise, a bite-wing image scanned at 300 DPI must be printed at twice its physical size of 30 mm × 40 mm to preserve the original resolution. Resizing of an image to fit on a printed page leads to interpolation of pixels and can result in a significant loss of resolution.

A final drawback of paper prints is the limited contrast ratio owing to the physics of the reflective process used for viewing images. The darkest inks absorb at most 96% of the incident visible light. If the paper were able to reflect 100% of the incident light, the maximum reflective contrast ratio achievable would be only 25:1.

IMAGE PROCESSING

Any operation that acts to improve, restore, analyze, or in some way change a digital image is a form of image processing. The use of digital imaging in dental radiography involves various image processing operations. Some of these operations are integrated in the image acquisition and image management software and are hidden from the user. Others are controlled by the user with the intention to improve the quality of the image or to analyze its contents. The fact that some of the image processing steps are hidden from the user may have consequences that have no analog in film. One such consequence is the difficulty in assessing underexposure or overexposure in digital radiographs. For film, this condition is readily apparent, but a suboptimally exposed digital image rarely appears too light or too dark because image processing usually includes automatic gray-scale leveling. Other metrics, such as the data histogram or noise measurements, should be employed.

Image Restoration

When the raw image data enter the computer, they are usually not yet ready for storage or display. A number of preprocessing steps must be performed to correct the image for known defects and to adjust the image intensities so that they are suitable for viewing. For example, some of the pixels in a CCD sensor are always defective. The image is

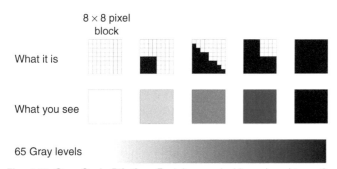

Fig. 4.12 Gray Scale Printing. Each image pixel is assigned to an 8 × 8 pixel array on the printed page. From 0 to 64 *black ink dots* can be used to fill each array, resulting in 65 potential gray levels. This means that an 8-bit (256 gray levels) image is reduced to 6 bits with a concomitant loss of contrast resolution during the printing process.

restored by substituting the gray values of the defective pixels with some weighted average of the gray values from the surrounding pixels. Depending on the quality of the sensor and the choices made by the manufacturer, various other operations may be applied to the image before it becomes visible on the display. These operations are executed very rapidly and are unnoticed by the user. Most preprocessing operations are set by the manufacturer and cannot be changed.

Image Enhancement

The term *image enhancement* implies that the adjusted image is an improved version of the original one. Most image enhancement operations are applied to make the image visually more appealing (subjective enhancement). This can be accomplished by increasing contrast, optimizing brightness, improving sharpness, and reducing noise. Subjective image enhancement does not improve the accuracy of image interpretation. Image enhancement operations are often task-specific: what benefits one diagnostic task may reduce the image quality for another task. For example, increasing contrast between enamel and dentin for caries detection may make it more difficult to identify the contour of the alveolar crest. Image enhancement operations are also dependent on viewer preference.

Brightness and Contrast

Digital radiographs do not always use the full range of available gray values effectively. They can be relatively dark or light, and they can show too much contrast in certain areas or not enough. Although the brightness and contrast can be judged visually, the image histogram is a convenient tool to determine which of the available gray values the image is using (Fig. 4.13). The minimum and maximum values and the shape of the histogram indicate the potential benefit of brightness- and contrast-enhancement operations.

Digital imaging software commonly includes a histogram tool and tools for the adjustment of brightness and contrast. Some tools also allow adjustment of the gamma value. Changing the gamma value of an image selectively enhances image contrast in either the brighter or the darker areas of the image. Adjustment of brightness, contrast, and gamma value changes the original intensity values of the image (input) to new values (output). The operator can choose to make these changes permanent or to restore the image to its original settings. Fig. 4.14 is a graphic representation of the relationship between input values (horizontal axis) and output values (vertical axis) with the corresponding images and their histograms. Digital imaging software usually also includes tools for histogram equalization and gray-scale inversion.

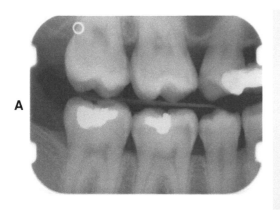
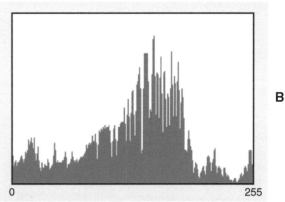

Fig. 4.13 Digital image (A) with image histogram (B). Horizontal axis represents image gray levels (8 bits = 256 levels); vertical axis represents number of pixels. Each *bar* indicates the number of pixels in the image with that particular gray level.

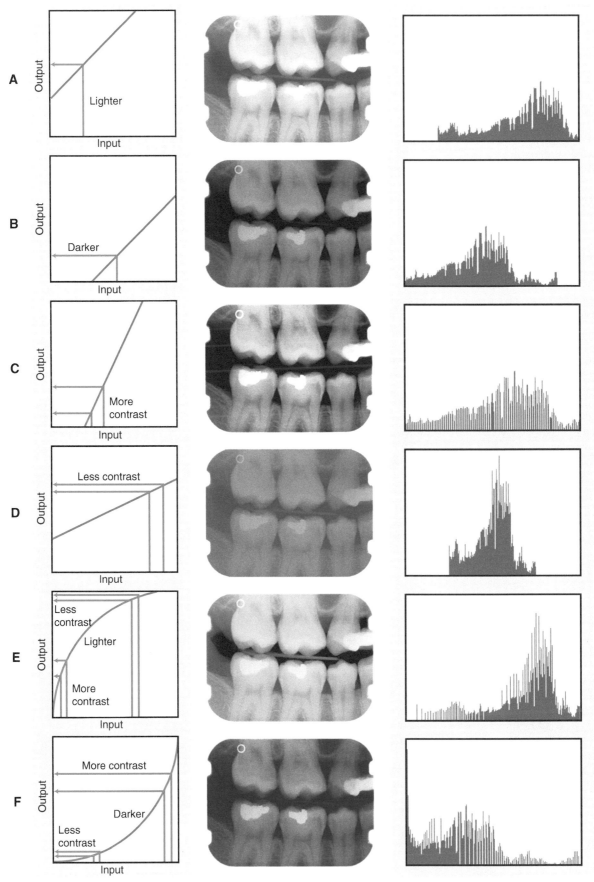

Fig. 4.14 Effect of brightness, contrast, and gamma adjustment as illustrated by image transformation graphs *(left column)*, digital images *(middle column)*, and image histograms *(right column)*. The image adjustments are relative to those of Fig. 4.13. (A) Increase in brightness. (B) Decrease in brightness. (C) Increase in contrast. (D) Decrease in contrast. (E) Increase in gamma. (F) Decrease in gamma.

Histogram equalization is an enhancement operation that increases contrast between the image intensities abundantly present within the image while reducing contrast between image intensities that are used only sparsely. The actual effect of histogram equalization depends on the image content and may sometimes lead to unexpected degradation of image quality. Gray-scale inversion changes a radiographic positive image into a radiographic negative image. Although this may affect the subjective perception of the image content, the altered appearance is foreign to interpretive practice and is little used.

The effect of contrast enhancement on the diagnostic value of digital radiographs is controversial. Some studies show substantial benefits of contrast enhancement operations, whereas others have found only limited value or no improvement at all. The effect of contrast enhancement cannot be predicted easily. The key to successful image enhancement is to enhance relevant radiographic signs selectively without simultaneously enhancing distracting features.

Sharpening and Smoothing

The purpose of sharpening and smoothing filters is to improve image quality by removing blur or noise. Noise represents random intensity variation and is often categorized as high-frequency noise (small-scale intensity variations) or low-frequency noise (gradual or large-scale intensity variations). Speckling is a special type of high-frequency noise that is characterized by isolated small regions surrounded by lighter or darker regions. Filters that smooth an image are sometimes called noise or despeckling filters because they are designed to remove high-frequency noise. Filters that sharpen an image either remove low-frequency noise or enhance boundaries between regions with different intensities (edge enhancement). For the purposeful application of filters, it is important to know what type of noise the filters reduce and how that affects radiographic features of interest. Without this knowledge, important radiographic features may degrade or disappear as noise is removed. Similarly, edge enhancement of radiographic features of interest may enhance noise or enhance local contrast to the extent that it simulates disease. Sharpening and smoothing filters may make the dental radiographic images subjectively more appealing; however, there is no scientific evidence suggesting an increase in diagnostic value. The indiscriminate use of filters made available in most imaging software packages should be avoided if there is no scientific support for their clinical usefulness.

Color

Most digital systems on the market provide opportunities for color conversion of gray-scale images, also called pseudocolor. Humans can distinguish many more colors than shades of gray. Transforming the gray values of a digital image into various colors theoretically could enhance the detection of objects within the image; however, this works only if all the gray values representing an object are unique for that object. Because this is rarely the case, boundaries between objects may change, and new boundaries may be created. In most cases, these changes distract the observer from seeing the real content of the image and result in degraded image interpretation. Therefore color conversion of radiographs is neither diagnostically nor educationally useful. Some useful applications of color do exist. When objects can be uniquely identified on the basis of a set of image features, color can be used to label or highlight these objects. The development of such criteria is a complex task, and only a few successful studies have been reported in the literature.

Digital Subtraction Radiography

When two images of the same object are registered and the image intensities of corresponding pixels are subtracted, a uniform difference image is produced. If there is a change in the radiographic attenuation between the baseline and follow-up examinations, this change shows up as a brighter area when the change represents gain and as a darker area when the change represents loss, such as loss of enamel and dentin owing to caries or loss of alveolar bone height with periodontitis. The strength of digital subtraction radiography (DSR) is that it cancels out the complex anatomic background against which this change occurs and reveals subtle changes. However, for DSR to be diagnostically useful, the baseline projection geometry and image intensities must be closely reproduced—a requirement that is difficult to achieve clinically.

IMAGE ANALYSIS

Image analysis operations are designed to extract diagnostically relevant information from the image. This information can range from simple linear measurements to fully automated diagnosis. The use of image analysis tools brings with it the responsibility to understand their limitations. The accuracy and precision of a measurement are limited by the extent to which the image is a truthful and reproducible representation of the patient and by the operator's ability to make an exact measurement.

Measurement

Digital imaging software provides numerous tools for image analysis. Digital rulers, densitometers, and various other tools are readily available. These tools are usually digital equivalents of existing tools used in endodontics, orthodontics, periodontology, implantology, and other areas of dentistry (Fig. 4.15). Digital imaging has also added new tools that were not available with film-based radiography. The size and image intensity of any area within a digital radiograph can be measured. Tools are also being developed for measuring the complexity of the trabecular bone pattern. Such measurements can be useful as screening tools for osteoporosis assessment and for detecting other diseases.

Diagnosis

One of the most challenging areas of research is the development of tools and procedures that automate the detection, classification, and quantification of radiographic signs of disease. The rationale for the

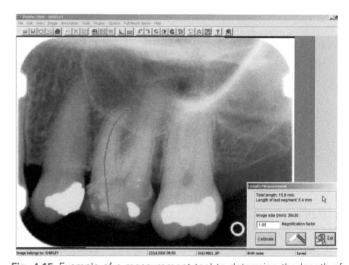

Fig. 4.15 Example of a measurement tool to determine the length of the crown and mesiobuccal root of the first molar. The measurement has been calibrated for a magnification factor of 1.05. The digital measurement tool is more versatile than the analog ruler; however, for both types of measurement tools, the apparent length remains dependent on the projection geometry.

use of such methods is early and accurate disease detection through use of reproducible and objective criteria. The development of automated image analysis operations is very complex and requires a thorough understanding of anatomy, pathology, and radiographic image formation. The three basic steps of image analysis are segmentation, feature extraction, and object classification. Of these, segmentation is the most critical step. The goal of segmentation is to simplify the image and reduce it to its basic components. This involves subdividing the image, thus separating objects from the background. Objects of interest are defined by the diagnostic task (e.g., a tooth, a carious lesion, a bone level, or an implant). When image segmentation results in the detection of an object, a variety of features can be measured that assist in determining what the object represents. Such features may include measures of size and shape, relative location, average density, homogeneity, and texture. A unique set of values for a certain combination of features can lead to classification of the object. Automated cephalometric landmark identification is an example of this technology. Other dental examples include caries detection, classification of periodontal disease, and detection and quantification of periapical bone lesions. The success of many of these applications is highly dependent on specific imaging parameters; very few provide reliable results when used clinically. This situation underscores the complexity of the radiographic image interpretation process.

IMAGE STORAGE

The use of digital imaging in dentistry requires an image archiving and management system very different from that used for film radiography. Storage of diagnostic images on magnetic or optical media raises new issues that must be considered, such as capacity, reliability, data integrity, and security. The file size of dental digital radiographs varies considerably, ranging from approximately 200 kilobytes for intraoral images to 6 megabytes for extraoral images. Storage and retrieval of these images in an average-sized dental practice is not a trivial issue. The development of new storage media and the continuing decrease in the price of a unit of storage has alleviated the capacity issue in dental radiography.

The simplicity with which digital images can be modified through image processing poses a potential risk with respect to ensuring the integrity of the diagnostic information. Once in a digital format, critical image data can be deleted or modified. It is important that the software prevents the user from permanently deleting or modifying original image data, whether intentionally or unintentionally. Not all software programs provide such a safeguard. As the use of digital imaging in dentistry continues to expand, the implementation of standards for preserving original image data becomes urgent. It is also imperative that images and other important patient-related information are duplicated to prevent permanent loss of data in case of a hardware or software malfunction. The use of computers for storing critical patient information mandates the design and use of a backup protocol. Box 4.2 shows some issues that must be considered when a backup protocol is designed. Backup media suitable for external storage of digital radiographs include external hard drives, digital tapes, CDs, and DVDs. The use of cloud-based software is rapidly gaining popularity because it offers a seamless solution for primary and secondary storage with the ability to access the data from any location. These solutions need to be HIPAA-compliant and require reliable, secure, and sufficiently fast network connections.

Image Compression

The purpose of image compression is to reduce the size of digital image files for archiving or transmission. In particular, storing extraoral images in a busy clinic may pose a challenge to storage capacity and speed of

BOX 4.2 Digital Image Backup Considerations

- Type of backup media
- Time and method of backup
- Backup interval
- Storage location of backup media
- Recovery time
- Recovery reliability
- Security
- Future compatibility of backup technology

image access. The purpose of file compression is to reduce the file size significantly while preserving critical image information.

Compression methods are generally classified as lossless or lossy. Lossless methods do not discard any image data, and an exact copy of the image is reproduced after decompression. Most compression techniques take advantage of redundancies in the image, which can be expressed in simpler terms. The maximum compression rate for lossless compression is usually less than 3:1. Lossy compression methods achieve higher levels of compression by discarding image data; empiric evidence suggests that this does not affect the diagnostic quality of an image. Compression rates of 12:1 and 14:1 were shown to have no appreciable effect on caries diagnosis. For determining endodontic file length, a rate of 25:1 was diagnostically equivalent to the uncompressed image. A compression rate of 28:1 was acceptable for the subjective evaluation of image quality and the detection of artificial lesions in panoramic radiographs.

Version 3.1 of the Digital Imaging and Communications in Medicine (DICOM) standard adopted Joint Photographic Experts Group (JPEG) as the compression method, which provides a range of compression levels. Other types of image compression methods, such as wavelet compression, are being investigated for their use in medical imaging. Although low and medium levels of lossy compression appear to have little effect on the diagnostic value of dental images, lossy compression should be used with caution and only after its effect for specific diagnostic tasks has been evaluated. With the continuing increase in the capacity of storage media and the widespread use of high-speed data communication lines, lossy compression of dental radiographs is rapidly becoming obsolete. At the same time, new digital image receptors are generating images with more and more pixels and more bits per pixel, thus increasing storage needs. Image compression negates to some extent the gain from such high-end detectors. Diagnostic criteria should dictate the need for high-resolution detectors and use of image compression. Current evidence suggests that detector quality and moderate image compression have a limited impact on diagnostic outcomes.

SYSTEMS COMPATIBILITY

The development of digital imaging systems for dental radiography has largely been driven by industry. Manufacturers have adopted and developed technologies according to individual needs and philosophies. As a result, image formats among systems from different vendors are not standardized, and image archival, retrieval, and display systems are often incompatible. Despite the proprietary nature of imaging software, it is possible to transfer images from one vendor's system to the other. Most systems provide image export and import tools using a variety of generic image formats, such as JPEG and tagged image file format

(TIFF). However, the process of transferring images through export-import procedures is cumbersome. It requires many steps, and the operator needs to ensure that the right images are imported into the proper patient folder. Also, it cannot be assumed that the display and calibration of imported and native images will be the same.

Exporting and importing is not the method of choice when digital imaging is going to be used on a large scale. It has long been recognized that the adoption of a standard for transferring images and associated information between digital imaging devices in medicine and dentistry is necessary. The American College of Radiology and the National Electrical Manufacturers Association formed a joint committee to develop a standard for digital imaging systems. Numerous professional organizations have contributed to this complex development process, which has resulted in the current DICOM standard. Various dental organizations, including the American Dental Association, are playing an active role in defining aspects of the DICOM standard related to dentistry. The DICOM standard is not a static set of rules dictating to manufacturers how to build imaging devices. Rather, it is an evolving document addressing the interoperability of medical and dental imaging and information systems. Manufacturers of digital imaging systems for dental radiography are responding to the call to adopt the DICOM standard. Currently most systems conform to the DICOM standard, although some may not conform to every aspect of the standard. The successful adoption of digital imaging in dentistry requires interoperability of all devices. It is likely that manufacturers do not want to be left behind and that the market will weed out the systems that are noncompliant. Dentists using different vendors with DICOM-compliant imaging devices are able to exchange images seamlessly. The exchange of any data that are considered PHI must be done in a secure HIPAA-compliant manner.

CLINICAL CONSIDERATIONS

Some fundamental differences from film in the clinical handling of digital receptors should be noted (Tables 4.1 and 4.2). Because digital receptors are intended to be reusable, they must be handled with greater care than their film counterparts. In certain situations film may be intentionally damaged through bending to accommodate patient anatomy. This situation never occurs with digital receptors, as bending sensors would damage them. Instead, allowances must be made for sensor rigidity, such as placement of the sensor toward the midline to allow for greater clearance or to modify beam angulation to account for the smaller imaging area of digital sensors. Examples of common image artifacts found on images made with solid-state or PSP systems are presented in Box 4.3. PSP plates are susceptible to bending and scratching during handling—defects that induce permanent artifacts in the receptor. These artifacts obscure information of potential diagnostic importance and may necessitate disposal of the receptor and repeat imaging of the patient. Because of the inability of digital detectors to be bent to accommodate patient anatomy, new imaging strategies must be used for some patients. It may not be possible to capture the distal surface of the canine on premolar views consistently. An additional projection may be required to visualize this surface adequately.

A significant potential problem with PSP systems is the inability to distinguish images from plates that have been exposed backward. In contrast to film packets, which incorporate a lead foil with a characteristic embossed pattern that results in an underexposed image of the anatomy with the pattern artifact when exposed backward, PSP images have little x-ray attenuation from the polyester base. It is much too easy for inattentive radiographers to mount these digital images on the contralateral position from their true side. One can imagine the liability that could occur from diagnosing and treating disease on the opposite side of the actual lesion. The Soredex OpTime system has addressed this issue by

incorporating a round metal disk on the back of intraoral plates (see Fig. 4.7). This marker becomes visible on the image if the imaging plate is exposed backward. The appearance of the marker on the image does not fully obscure the anatomic information, and these images can be "mirrored" with imaging software tools without the need for repeated exposure. Carestream and Planmeca use RFID technology in their PSP plates, which also serves to identify plates that have been exposed backward.

Infection control is also an issue with digital receptors. Digital receptors cannot be sterilized by conventional means. They may be disinfected by wiping with mild agents such as isopropyl alcohol but should not be immersed in disinfecting solutions. The adage that "you can autoclave a digital receptor … once" stems from the fact that heat ruins electronic components in CCD and CMOS sensors and distorts the polyester base of PSP plates. Although each of the preceding concerns is of potential importance, the advantage of eliminating chemical processing in digital systems should not be overlooked. The time required to monitor and maintain a film processor properly is significant. Too often insufficient attention is paid to this critical aspect of film radiography. Digital systems may not save the time gained by eliminating film processing, but they do eliminate the loss in diagnostic quality that occurs when insufficient time and effort are spent on film processing quality assurance.

CONCLUSION

Although film remains an acceptable means to acquire and display dental radiographic image, the adoption of digital imaging is now widespread and will be the sole technology of the future. Comparison of imaging systems based on technical properties like resolution, contrast, and latitude is somewhat confounded by a lack of standardization in the assessment of these characteristics. From a diagnostic standpoint, most studies suggest that digital performance is not clinically different from film for typical diagnostic tasks, such as caries diagnosis. The "look and feel" of digital displays is distinctly different from film viewing, and some practitioners may find this difference disconcerting. A basic understanding of computers and a mastery of common computing skills are essential for viewing digital images. Beyond this, learning the peculiarities and vagaries of a particular acquisition and display software takes time and may not be intuitive. Multiple mouse clicks through multiple menus may be required to view a full-mouth series of images. This activity may modestly increase the time required to complete the interpretative process.

In selecting an imaging system, other issues should be considered. Digital images avoid environmental pollutants encountered with film processing, but what about the environmental impact associated with the disposal of broken or obsolete electronic equipment? The initial financial outlay for digital imaging hardware makes these systems more expensive than film. Manufacturers point out that the costs of film or digital systems should be amortized over the life of the equipment and consumables; however, the life expectancy of newer digital systems is speculative. Mishandling of digital system components can catastrophically shorten any projected life expectancy. Additionally, what price should we place on the ability to transmit images instantly and to integrate them into a fully electronic record? There are no universal answers to these questions. They must be asked and answered according to the needs and objectives of individual dental practices. As practice patterns and technology change with time, the answers will also change. Although the details of the image in our crystal ball have yet to resolve, the trends of increasing adoption of digital imaging and continuing technologic innovation make the future of digital imaging in dentistry certain.

TABLE 4.1   Clinical Comparison of Intraoral Imaging Alternatives

Imaging Step	Film	CCD/CMOS	PSP
Receptor preparation	None	1. Place protective plastic sleeve over receptor envelope 2. Receptor must be connected to computer and patient-identifying information entered for acquisition/archiving software	1. "Erase" plates. 2. Package plates in protective plastic
Receptor placement	1. Numerous generic film-holding devices are available 2. Film may be bent to accommodate anatomy	1. Specialized receptor holder specific for manufacturer's receptor may limit options 2. Receptor inflexibility and bulk limit placement options 3. Receptor cable must be carefully routed out of patient's mouth 4. Patient discomfort more likely than with film or PSP	1. Many receptor holders used for film may be adapted for PSP plates 2. Bending of receptor may irreversibly damage it
Exposure	1. Simple exposure	1. Computer must be activated before exposure	1. Simple exposure
Processing	1. Dark, light-safe environment in form of darkroom or daylight loader required 2. Processor chemistry must be prepared or replenished 3. Chemical temperature must be warmed, or processing time must be adjusted to accommodate temperature 4. Films must be removed from wrapper; lead foil must be separated for recycling	1. Image acquisition and display almost immediate	1. Dimly lit environment to prevent loss of image information 2. Processor must be programmed with patient information so that the images are stored properly Alternatively, plates can be preprogrammed with patient information using RFID 3. Processor must be programmed with detector information so that the images are preprocessed 4. Protective wrapper must be removed from plates
Display preparation	1. Films may be placed in a variety of film mounts 2. Mounts must be labeled with patient-identifying information	1. Software may be configured to place image in appropriate position in digital mount when exposures are made in a predetermined sequence; otherwise images must be individually placed in the mount	1. Images must be individually placed in mount 2. Images may have to be digitally rotated to achieve proper orientation
Display	1. A room with subdued lighting and a masked viewbox are optimal 2. Any light source (including the operatory window or ceiling light) permits quick evaluation of the image	The same considerations apply to all digital receptor types: 1. A room with subdued lighting is optimal for interpretation activities 2. Computer and display with appropriate software are necessary; viewing is restricted to the location of the computer 3. Laptop computers increase flexibility of computer placement but may reduce display quality 4. Size of display restricts the numbers of images that may be viewed simultaneously; more time is required to open/close or expand/contract images when interpreting a series of images	
Image duplication	1. Quality of duplication is always inferior to original and is sometimes nondiagnostic	1. Electronic copies may be stored on various media without loss of image quality 2. Output on film or paper is inferior and is often nondiagnostic unless appropriate combinations of expensive printers and papers or film are used	

CCD, Charge-coupled device; CMOS, complementary metal oxide semiconductor; PSP, photostimulable phosphor; RFID, radio-frequency identification.

TABLE 4.2 Comparison of Physical Properties of Film, Charge-Coupled Devices, Complementary Metallic Oxide Semiconductors, and Photostimulable Phosphor Receptors

Feature	Technical Comment	Clinical Comment
Spatial resolution	Intraoral systems: Film > CCD = CMOS > PSP Panoramic systems: Film = CCD = PSP Cephalometric systems: Film > CCD = PSP	Limits of resolution for digital systems are readily appreciated when magnifying these images. With magnification, a "blocky" or "pixelated" appearance is evident. Resolution of panoramic systems is limited by mechanical motion to about 5 lp/mm
Exposure latitude	PSP $\gg$ CCD $\geq$ CMOS > film	Because of the wide latitude of PSP and the automatic brightness and contrast "optimization" by image acquisition software, use of more x-ray exposure than is necessary is possible
Receptor dimensions	For equivalent imaged area, film = PSP < CCD = CMOS	"Active area" of CCD and CMOS receptors is smaller than surface area because of other electronic components within the plastic housing
Time for image acquisition	CCD = CMOS $\ll$ PSP = film	Rapid image acquisition may be important for endodontic procedures or during implant placement
Image quality	Subjective quality is best with film when carefully exposed and well processed	Digital and film imaging are not significantly different when used for common diagnostic tasks
Image adjustment/processing	Improves appearance of digital images	Takes time; may not improve diagnostic performance
Cost	Initial costs of digital systems are greater than those of film. Subsequent costs vary greatly depending on receptor wear and tear or abuse	Manufacturers' estimates of life expectancy of reusable receptors may be overly optimistic
Reliability	Mechanical problems affect digital PSP and film systems. Software reliability varies greatly among manufacturers. Changes in unrelated computer components and software can cause digital systems to malfunction	Digital systems fail when problems occur with receptors during image acquisition or with computers during image processing, archiving, and display
Image storage and retrieval	Data backup is critical for digital systems	Films can be misfiled and lost or be damaged by poor storage conditions. Digital data can be lost as a result of failures in power supplies or storage media and operator error
Transmitting images to others	Rapidly done with digital images	Facilitates communication between colleagues or with insurance companies

CCD, Charge-coupled device; CMOS, complementary metal oxide semiconductor; lp, line pairs; PSP, photostimulable phosphor.

BOX 4.3 Common Problems in Digital Image Receptor Exposure, Processing, and Handling

Enrique Platin

Noisy Images

Although the brightness of these images has been adjusted to display similar average gray values, notice the noisy appearance of the underexposed periapical radiograph (Fig. 4.16A, 0.032 s) compared with the properly exposed radiograph (see Fig. 4.16B, 0.32 s).

Two PSP bite-wing radiographs (Fig. 4.17). Image A was processed properly and image B was exposed to excessive ambient light prior to scanning, causing it to fade. Exposed PSP plates must be protected from ambient light prior to scanning to prevent trapped electrons being released from their meta-stable state.

Nonuniform Image Density

Partial exposure of PSP plates to excessive ambient light before scanning results in nonuniform image density (Fig. 4.18A). This happens when plates are overlapped while exposed to ambient light (see Fig. 4.18B).

Distorted Images

Bending of PSP plates during intraoral placement: moderate bending (Fig. 4.19A), retake of image A (see Fig. 4.19B), severe bending (see Fig. 4.19C), and retake of image C (see Fig. 4.19D).

Double Images

PSP double image on incisor periapical radiograph resulting from incomplete erasure of previous image of posterior periapical region (Fig. 4.20A) and retake of image (see Fig. 4.20B).

Another example of a double image resulting from incomplete erasure of a PSP receptor: posterior periapical radiograph with double image (Fig. 4.21A), and retake of image A (see Fig. 4.21B).

Damaged Image Receptors

Scratched phosphor surface mimicking root canal filling (Fig. 4.22A) and retake of image (see Fig. 4.22B).

Image artifacts resulting from excessive bending of the PSP plate (Fig. 4.23A). Excessive bending has resulted in permanent damage to the phosphor plate (see Fig. 4.23B).

PSP circular artifact as a result of plate damage (Fig. 4.24A). The plate shows localized swelling of the protective coating as a result of ethylene oxide gas used to disinfect the plates (see Fig. 4.24B). Most likely a pinhole was present in the protective coating allowing the gas to infiltrate and separate the protective coating from the phosphor layer.

PSP image artifact resulting from exposure of the plate to liquid disinfectant (Fig. 4.25A). The disinfectant caused damage to the protective coating and the phosphor layer (see Fig. 4.25B). Plates should be protected from harsh disinfectants.

BOX 4.3   Common Problems in Digital Image Receptor Exposure, Processing, and Handling—cont'd

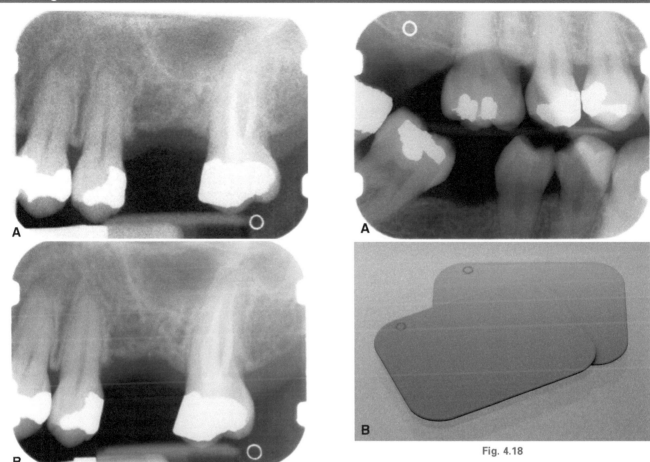

Fig. 4.16

Fig. 4.18

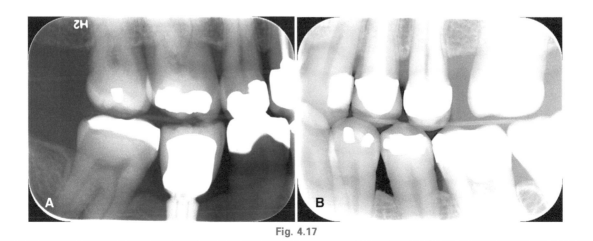

Fig. 4.17

Continued

BOX 4.3   Common Problems in Digital Image Receptor Exposure, Processing, and Handling—cont'd

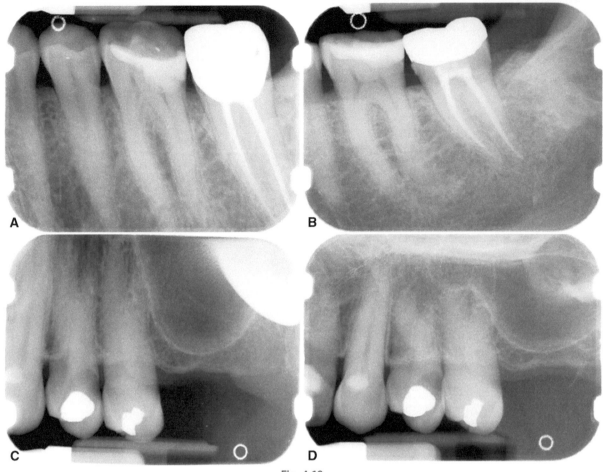

Fig. 4.19

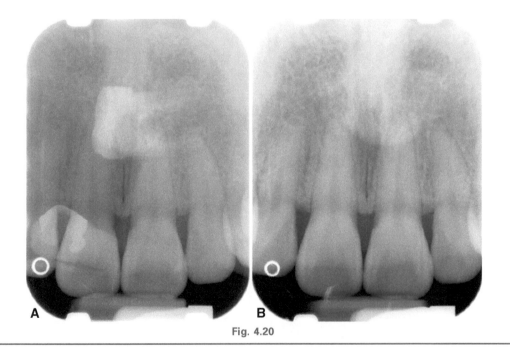

Fig. 4.20

BOX 4.3   Common Problems in Digital Image Receptor Exposure, Processing, and Handling—cont'd

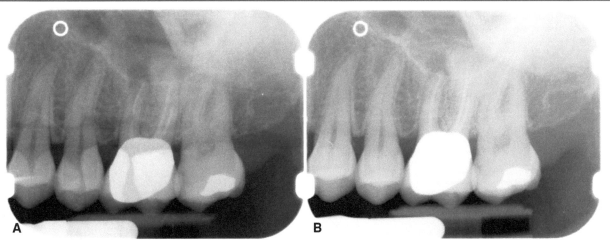

Fig. 4.21

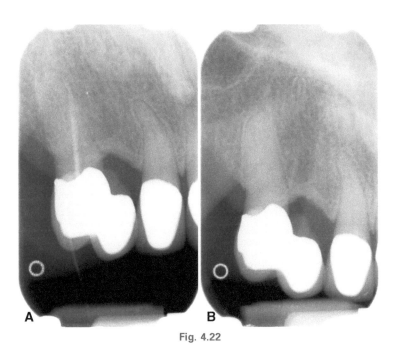

Fig. 4.22

Malfunctioning CCD sensor resulting from incorrect exposure or misinterpretation of the incoming data by the processing software (Fig. 4.26A and B). The sensor was not damaged.

Improper Use of Image Processing

Straight radiopaque line artifact on PSP image as a result of dust on the lens of the scanner's photomultiplier (Fig. 4.27). After removal of the scanner cover, the lens can be cleaned according to manufacturer's recommendations.

Improper use of image processing tools, such as filters, may result in false-positive findings. An edge enhancement filter was applied to the panoramic image, which produced radiolucencies at restoration edges simulating recurrent caries (Fig. 4.28A). These radiolucencies are not present in a follow-up intraoral image (see Fig. 4.28B).

Effect of Image Scanning Resolution

Settings for the resolution of PSP scanning may have a significant impact on image quality. Scanning at 150 DPI (Fig. 4.29A) produces an image that lacks detail and appears pixelated when magnified. Scanning at 300 DPI provides increased detail through higher resolution (see Fig. 4.29B). Box 4.1 shows how to convert from DPI (scanner) to lp/mm (image resolution).

Continued

BOX 4.3   Common Problems in Digital Image Receptor Exposure, Processing, and Handling—cont'd

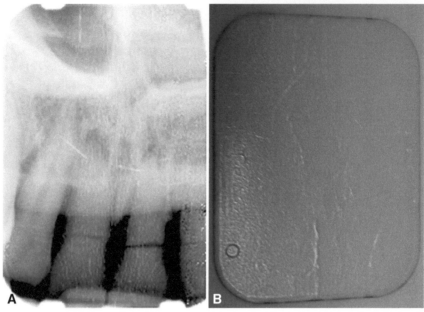

Fig. 4.23

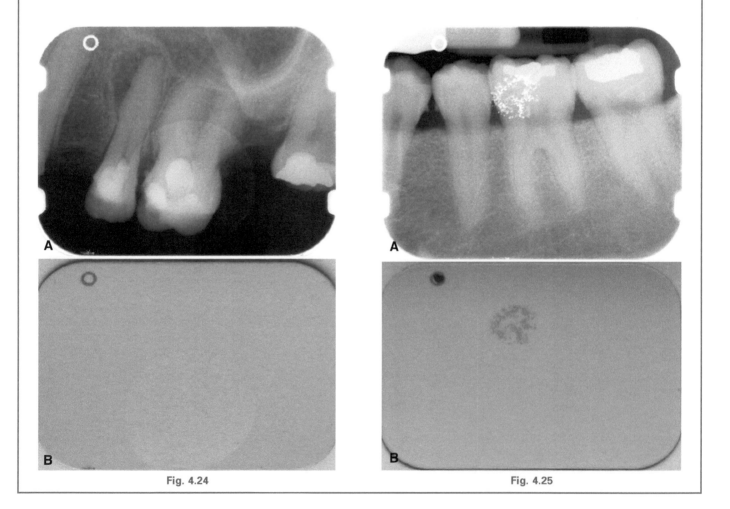

Fig. 4.24   Fig. 4.25

BOX 4.3 Common Problems in Digital Image Receptor Exposure, Processing, and Handling—cont'd

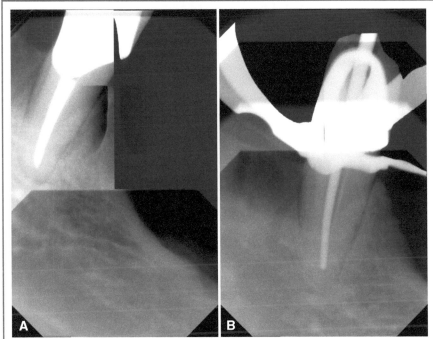

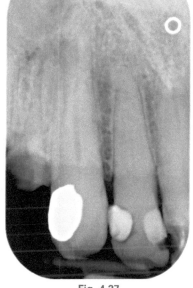

Fig. 4.26

Fig. 4.27

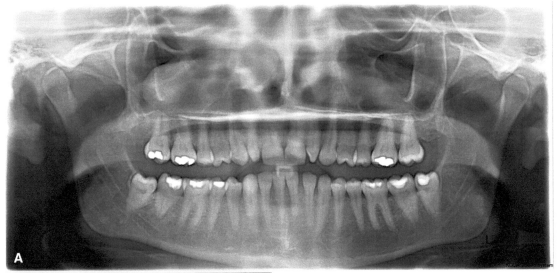

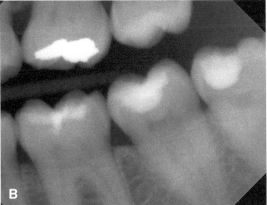

Fig. 4.28

Continued

BOX 4.3   Common Problems in Digital Image Receptor Exposure, Processing, and Handling—cont'd

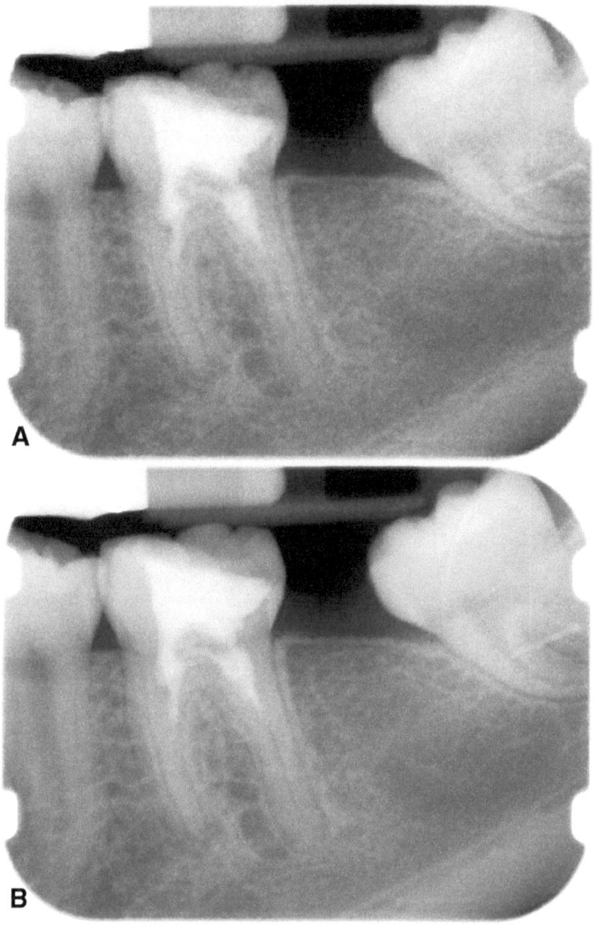

Fig. 4.29

CCD, Charge-coupled device; *PSP*, photostimulable phosphor.

BIBLIOGRAPHY

Digital Detectors and Displays

Abreu M Jr, Mol A, Ludlow JB. Performance of RVGui sensor and Kodak Ektaspeed Plus film for proximal caries detection. *Oral Surg Oral Med Oral Pathol Oral Radiol Endod.* 2001;91:381–385.

Butt A, Mahoney M, Savage NW. The impact of computer display performance on the quality of digital radiographs: a review. *Aust Dent J.* 2012;57(suppl 1):16–23.

Couture RA, Hildebolt C. Quantitative dental radiography with a new photostimulable phosphor system. *Oral Surg Oral Med Oral Pathol Oral Radiol Endod.* 2000;89:498–508.

Hildebolt CF, Couture RA, Whiting BR. Dental photostimulable phosphor radiography. *Dent Clin North Am.* 2000;44:273–297.

Mol A, Yoon DC. Guide to digital radiographic imaging. *J Calif Dent Assoc.* 2015;43:503–511.

Sanderink GC, Miles DA. Intraoral detectors: CCD, CMOS, TFT, and other devices. *Dent Clin North Am.* 2000;44:249–255.

Vandenberghe B, Jacobs R, Bosmans H. Modern dental imaging: a review of the current technology and clinical applications in dental practice. *Eur Radiol.* 2010;20:2637–2655.

Van der Stelt PF. Principles of digital imaging. *Dent Clin North Am.* 2000;44:237–248.

Image Processing

Analoui M. Radiographic image enhancement, I: spatial domain techniques. *Dentomaxillofac Radiol.* 2001;30:1–9.

Analoui M. Radiographic digital image enhancement, II: transform domain techniques. *Dentomaxillofac Radiol.* 2001;30:65–77.

Gonzalez R, Wood R. *Digital Image Processing.* 3rd ed. Upper Saddle River, NJ: Prentice Hall; 2007.

Mol A. Image processing tools for dental applications. *Dent Clin North Am.* 2000;44:299–318.

Russ JC. *The Image Process Handbook.* 5th ed. Boca Raton, FL.: CRC Press; 2006.

Clinical Considerations

Wenzel A. A review of dentists' use of digital radiography and caries diagnosis with digital systems. *Dentomaxillofac Radiol.* 2006;35:307–314.

Wenzel A, Møystad A. Work flow with digital intraoral radiography: a systematic review. *Acta Odontol Scand.* 2010;68:106–114.

5

Film Imaging

Sanjay M. Mallya

A beam of x-ray photons that passes through the dental arches is reduced in intensity (attenuated) by absorption and scattering of photons out of the primary beam. The pattern of the photons that exits the patient, the remnant beam, conveys information about the patient's anatomy. For this information to be useful diagnostically, the remnant beam must be recorded on an image receptor. The image receptor most often used in dental radiography is x-ray film. This chapter describes x-ray film and film processing and the use of intensifying screens. Digital radiographic receptors are described in Chapter 4.

X-RAY FILM

Composition

X-ray film has two principal components: (1) emulsion and (2) base. The emulsion is sensitive to x-rays and visible light and records the radiographic image. The base is a plastic support onto which the emulsion is coated (Fig. 5.1).

Emulsion

The two principal components of emulsion are silver halide grains, which are sensitive to x-radiation and visible light, and a vehicle gelatinous matrix in which the crystals are suspended. The silver halide grains are composed primarily of crystals of silver bromide. The silver halide grains in INSIGHT film and Ultra-speed film (Carestream Dental, a division of Carestream Health, Inc., Atlanta, Georgia) are flat, tabular crystals with a mean diameter of approximately 1.8 μm (Fig. 5.2). The tabular grains are oriented parallel with the film surface to offer a large cross-sectional area to the x-ray beam. INSIGHT film has approximately twice the number of silver grains so that it requires only half the exposure of Ultra-speed film.

The silver halide grains are suspended in a surrounding vehicle that is applied to both sides of the supporting base. During film processing (described later in this chapter) the vehicle absorbs processing solutions, allowing the chemicals to reach and react with the silver halide grains. An additional layer of vehicle is added to the film emulsion as an overcoat (see Fig. 5.2). This barrier helps to protect the film from damage by scratching, contamination, or pressure from rollers when an automatic processor is used.

Film emulsions are sensitive to both x-ray photons and visible light. Film intended to be exposed by x-rays is called direct exposure film. All intraoral dental film is direct exposure film. Screen film is used with intensifying screens (described later in this chapter) that emit visible light. Screen film and intensifying screens are used for extraoral projections, such as panoramic and cephalometric radiographs.

Base

The function of the film base is to support the emulsion. The base for dental x-ray film is made of polyester polyethylene terephthalate, which provides the proper degree of flexibility to allow easy handling of the film. The film base must also withstand exposure to processing solutions without becoming distorted. The base is uniformly translucent and casts no pattern on the resultant radiograph.

Intraoral X-Ray Film

Intraoral dental x-ray film is made as a double-emulsion film (i.e., both sides of the base are coated with an emulsion). With a double layer of emulsion, less radiation is required to produce an image. Direct exposure film is used for intraoral examinations because it provides higher resolution images than screen-film combinations. Some diagnostic tasks, such as detection of incipient caries or early periapical disease, require this higher resolution.

One corner of each dental film has a small, raised dot that is used for film orientation (Fig. 5.3). The manufacturer orients the film in the packet so that the convex side of the dot is toward the front of the packet and faces the x-ray tube. The side of the film with the depression is thus oriented toward the patient's tongue. After the film has been exposed and processed, the dot is used to orient the patient's right- and left-side images properly. When mounting radiographs, each film is oriented with the convex side of the dot toward the viewer, and on the basis of the features of the teeth and anatomic landmarks in the adjacent bone, the films are arranged in their normal sequential relationship in the mount.

Intraoral x-ray film packets contain either one or two sheets of film (Fig. 5.4). When double film packs are used, the second film serves as a duplicate record that can be sent to insurance companies or to a colleague. The film is encased in a protective black paper wrapper and then in an outer moisture-resistant paper or plastic wrapping. The outer wrapping clearly indicates the location of the raised dot and identifies which side of the film should be directed toward the x-ray tube.

A thin lead foil backing with an embossed pattern is between the wrappers in the film packet. The foil is positioned in the film packet behind the film (see Fig. 5.4), away from the tube. This lead foil serves several purposes.

- It shields the film from backscatter (secondary) radiation, which fogs the film and reduces image contrast (image quality).
- It reduces patient exposure by absorbing some of the residual x-ray beam.
- Most importantly, if the film packet is placed backward in the patient's mouth so that the tube side of the film is facing away from the x-ray machine, the lead foil will be positioned between the subject and the film. In this circumstance, most of the radiation is absorbed by the lead foil, and the resulting radiograph is light and shows the embossed pattern in the lead foil (Fig. 5.5). This combination of a light film with the characteristic pattern indicates that the film packet was exposed backward in the patient's mouth and that the patient's right side–left side designation indicated by the film dot is reversed.

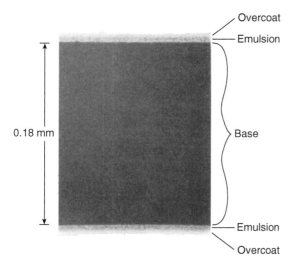

Fig. 5.1 Scanning electron micrograph of INSIGHT dental x-ray film (original magnification 300×). Note the overcoat, emulsion, and base on this double-emulsion film. (Courtesy Carestream Dental, a division of Carestream Health, Inc., Atlanta, Georgia.)

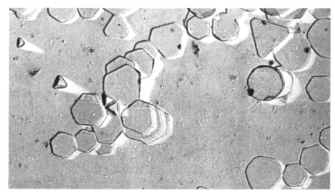

Fig. 5.2 Scanning electron micrograph of emulsion of INSIGHT film showing flat tabular silver bromide crystals, which capture incident photons. (Courtesy Carestream Dental, a division of Carestream Health, Inc., Atlanta, Georgia.)

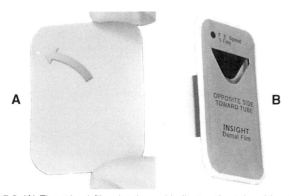

Fig. 5.3 (A) The raised film dot *(arrow)* indicates the tube side of the film and identifies the patient's right and left sides. (B) The location of this dot is clearly marked with a *black circle* on the outside of every film packet. (Courtesy of Carestream Dental, a division of Carestream Health, Inc., Atlanta, Georgia.)

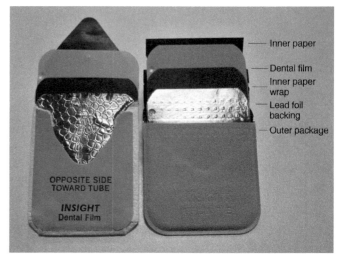

Fig. 5.4 Moisture-proof and lightproof packets, paper on the left and vinyl on right, contain an opening tab on the side opposite the tube. Inside is an interleaf paper wrapper that is folded around the film as well as a sheet of lead foil. Film is packaged with one or two sheets of film. The foil is positioned between the back side of the packet and the paper wrapper. In this position, it absorbs radiation that has passed through the film and prevents scatter radiation from blurring the image. If the film packet is inadvertently placed backward in the patient's mouth, the mottled image of the foil shows on the resultant image. (Courtesy of Carestream Dental, a division of Carestream Health, Inc., Atlanta, Georgia.)

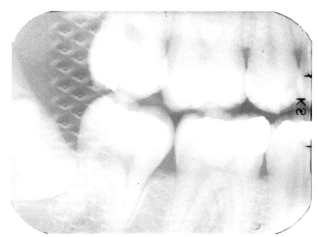

Fig. 5.5 Placing a film backward in the patient's mouth when the exposure was made results in a radiograph that is too light and shows the characteristic markings caused by exposure through the lead foil in the film packaging. In such an image, the left and right sides of the patient are reversed when using the dot as the orientation guide.

Periapical View

Periapical views record the crowns, roots, and surrounding bone. Film packs come in three sizes (Fig. 5.6):

- Size 0 for small children (22 mm × 35 mm)
- Size 1, which is relatively narrow and used for views of the anterior teeth (24 mm × 40 mm)
- Size 2, the standard film size used for adults (30.5 mm × 40.5 mm)

Bite-Wing View

Bite-wing (interproximal) views record the coronal portions of the maxillary and mandibular teeth in one image. They are used to detect

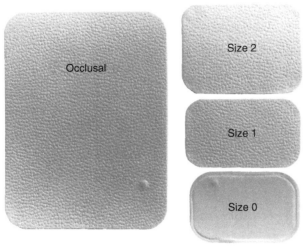

Fig. 5.6 Dental X-Ray Film Is Commonly Supplied in Various Sizes. *Left,* Occlusal film. *Top right,* Size 2 for adult posterior film. *Middle right,* Size 1 for adult anterior film. *Bottom right,* Size 0 for child-size film (in vinyl wrapping).

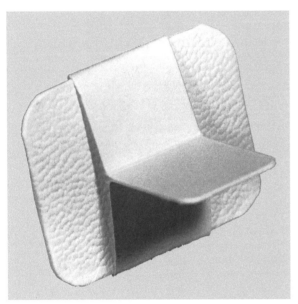

Fig. 5.7 Paper loop placed around a size 2 adult film to support the film when the patient bites on the tab for a bite-wing projection. This projection reveals the tooth crowns and alveolar crests.

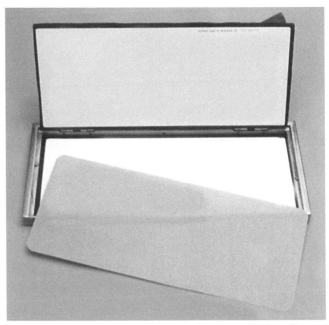

Fig. 5.8 Cassette for 8-Inch × 10-Inch Film Along With a Sheet of Screen Film. When the cassette is closed, the film is supported in close contact between the two white intensifying screens seen on the inside of the cassette. These intensifying screens absorb most of the incident x-ray beam and then fluoresce and expose the film.

interproximal caries and evaluate the height of alveolar bone. Size 2 film is normally used in adults; the smaller size 1 is preferred in children. In small children, size 0 may be used. A relatively long size 3 is also available.

Bite-wing films often have a paper tab projecting from the middle of the film on which the patient bites to support the film (Fig. 5.7). This tab is rarely visualized on the image and does not interfere with the diagnostic quality of the image. Film-holding instruments for bite-wing projections also are available.

Occlusal View

Occlusal film, size 4, is more than 3 times larger than size 2 film (see Fig. 5.7). It is used to show larger areas of the maxilla or mandible than may be seen on a periapical film. These films also are used to obtain right-angle views to the usual periapical view. The name derives from

the fact that the film is held in position by having the patient bite lightly on it to support it between the occlusal surfaces of the teeth (see Chapter 7).

Screen Film

The extraoral projections used most frequently in dentistry are panoramic and cephalometric views. For these projections, screen film is used with intensifying screens (described later in this chapter) to reduce patient exposure (Fig. 5.8). Screen film is different from dental intraoral film. It is designed to be sensitive to visible light because it is placed between two intensifying screens when an exposure is made. The intensifying screens absorb x-rays and emit visible light, which exposes the film. Silver halide crystals are inherently sensitive to ultraviolet (UV) and blue light (300 to 500 nm) and thus are sensitive to screens that emit UV and blue light. When film is used with screens that emit green light, the silver halide crystals are coated with sensitizing dyes to increase absorption. It is important to use the appropriate screen-film combination recommended by the screen and film manufacturer so that the emission characteristics of the screen match the absorption characteristics of the film.

Contemporary screen films use tabular-shaped (flat) grains of silver halide (Fig. 5.9) to capture the image. The tabular grains are oriented with their relatively large, flat surfaces facing the radiation source, providing a larger cross section (target) and resulting in increased speed without loss of sharpness. To increase the sharpness of images, some manufacturers add an absorbing dye in the film emulsion. This dye reduces light from one screen crossing through the film to reach the emulsion on the opposite side. EVG film (Enhanced Visualization, Green sensitive) from Carestream Dental is an example of this type of film.

INTENSIFYING SCREENS

Early in the history of radiography, scientists discovered that various inorganic salts or phosphors fluoresce (emit visible light) when exposed

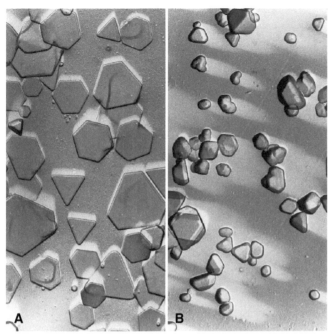

Fig. 5.9 Tablet grains of silver halide in an emulsion of T-MAT film (A) are larger and flatter than the smaller, thicker crystals in an emulsion of older conventional film (B). The flat surfaces of the tablet grains are oriented parallel with the film surface, facing the radiation source. (Courtesy of Carestream Dental, a division of Carestream Health, Inc.)

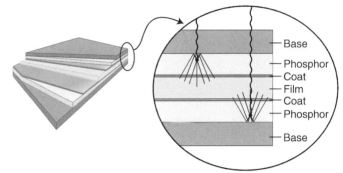

Fig. 5.10 Image on the *left* shows a schematic of two intensifying screens enclosing a film *(yellow)*. An intensifying screen is composed of a supporting base *(purple)*, a layer containing the phosphors *(light blue)*, and a protective coat *(orange)*. The detailed view on the *right* shows x-ray photons entering at the top, traveling through the base, and striking phosphors in the base. The phosphors emit visible light, exposing the film. Some visible light photons may reflect off the reflecting layer of the base.

TABLE 5.1 **Rare Earth Elements Used in Intensifying Screens**	
Emission	**Phosphor**
Green	Gadolinium oxysulfide, terbium activated
Blue and ultraviolet	Yttrium tantalite, niobium activated

to an x-ray beam. The intensity of this fluorescence is proportional to the x-ray energy absorbed. These phosphors are incorporated into intensifying screens for use with screen film. The sum of the effects of the x-rays and the visible light emitted by the screen phosphors exposes the film in an intensifying cassette (see Fig. 5.8).

Function

The presence of intensifying screens creates an image receptor system that is 10 to 60 times more sensitive to x-rays than is the film alone. Consequently, use of intensifying screens substantially reduces the dose of x-radiation to the patient. Intensifying screens are used with films for virtually all extraoral radiography, including panoramic, cephalo-metric, and skull projections. However, the use of an intensifying screen decreases image resolution.

Intensifying screens are not used intraorally with periapical or occlusal films because their use would reduce the resolution of the resulting image below that necessary for detailed evaluation of dental disease.

Composition

Intensifying screens are made of a base-supporting material, a phosphor layer, and a protective polymeric coat (Fig. 5.10). In all dental applications, intensifying screens are used in pairs, one on each side of the film, and they are positioned inside a cassette (see Fig. 5.8). The purpose of a cassette is to hold each intensifying screen in close contact with the x-ray film to maximize the sharpness of the image.

Base

The base material of most intensifying screens is some form of polyester plastic that is approximately 0.25 mm thick. The base provides mechanical support for the other layers. In some intensifying screens, the base also is reflective; thus it reflects light emitted from the phosphor layer back toward the x-ray film (see Fig. 5.10). This reflective base increases the

light exposing the film but also results in some image "unsharpness" because of the divergence of light rays reflected back to the film.

Phosphor Layer

The phosphor layer is composed of phosphorescent crystals suspended in a polymeric binder. When the crystals absorb x-ray photons, they fluoresce (see Fig. 5.10). The phosphor crystals often contain rare earth elements, most commonly lanthanum and gadolinium. Their fluorescence can be increased by the addition of small amounts of elements, such as thulium, niobium, or terbium. Common phosphor combinations used in intensifying screens are shown in Table 5.1. Rare earth screens convert each absorbed x-ray photon into approximately 4000 lower-energy, visible light (green or blue) photons. These visible photons expose the film.

Different phosphors fluoresce in different portions of the spectrum. For example, light emission from Lanex rare-earth intensifying screens ranges from 375 to 600 nm and peaks sharply at 545 nm (green). Fig. 5.11 shows the spectral emission of a rare-earth screen and the spectral sensitivity of an appropriate film. Other intensifying screens have a major peak at 350 nm (UV) and at 450 nm (blue). It is important to match green-emitting screens with green-sensitive films and blue-emitting screens with blue-sensitive films.

Intensifying screens are described in terms of their speed—their ability to convert x-ray photons to visible light photons. Fast screens have large phosphor crystals and efficiently convert x-ray photons to visible light but produce images with lower resolution. As the size of the crystals or the thickness of the screen decreases, the speed of the screen also declines, but image sharpness increases. Fast screens also have a thicker phosphor layer and a reflective layer, but these properties also decrease sharpness. In deciding on the combination to use, the practitioner must consider the resolution requirements of the task for which the image will be used. Screen-film combinations are rated for

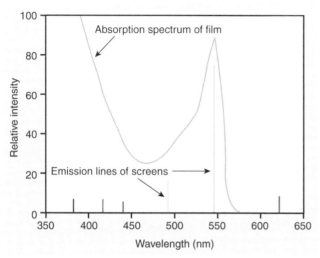

Fig. 5.11 Relative sensitivity of T-MAT film *(orange line)* and emission lines (shown in their visual colors) of Carestream Dental LANEX and EV screens (gadolinium oxysulfide, terbium activated). Intensifying screens emit light as a series of relatively narrow line emissions. The maximal emission of the screen at 545 nm *(green)* corresponds well to a high-sensitivity region of the film. (Data from Carestream Dental, a division of Carestream Health, Inc.)

speed, a measure of the amount of radiation required for a proper exposure. For dental extraoral diagnostic tasks, it is recommended to use screen-film combinations that have a speed of 400 or faster.

Protective Coat

A protective polymer coat (≤15 μm thick) is placed over the phosphor layer to protect the phosphor and to provide a surface that can be cleaned. The intensifying screens should be routinely cleaned because any debris, spots, or scratches may cause light spots on the resultant radiograph.

FORMATION OF THE LATENT IMAGE

When a beam of photons exits the patient and exposes an x-ray film (either direct exposure film or screen film exposed by light photons), it chemically changes the photosensitive silver halide crystals in the film emulsion. These chemically altered silver bromide crystals constitute the latent (invisible) image on the film. Before exposure, film emulsion consists of photosensitive crystals containing primarily silver bromide (Fig. 5.12A). These silver halide crystals also contain a few free silver ions (interstitial silver ions) and trace amounts of sulfur compounds bound to the surface of the crystals. Along with physical irregularities in the crystal produced by iodide ions, sulfur compounds create sensitivity sites, sites in the crystals that are sensitive to radiation. Each crystal

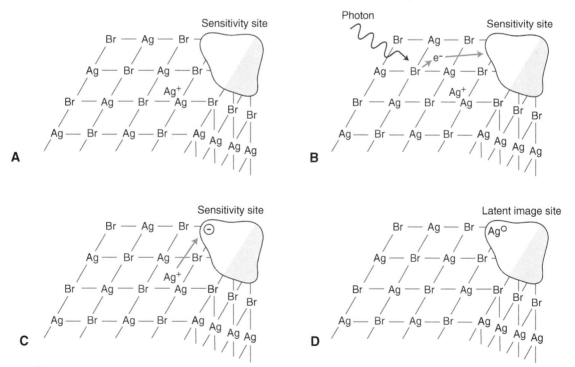

Fig. 5.12 (A) A silver bromide crystal in the emulsion of an x-ray film contains mostly silver and bromide ions in a crystal lattice. There are also free interstitial silver ions and areas of trace chemicals that form sensitivity sites. (B) Exposure of the crystal to photons in an x-ray beam results in the release of electrons, usually by interaction of the photon with a bromide ion. The recoil electrons have sufficient kinetic energy to move about in the crystal. When electrons reach a sensitivity site, they impart a negative charge to this region. (C) Free interstitial silver ions (with a positive charge) are attracted to the negatively charged sensitivity site. (D) When the silver ions reach the sensitivity site, they acquire an electron and become neutral silver atoms. These silver atoms now constitute a latent image site. The collection of latent image sites over the entire film constitutes the latent image. Developer causes the neutral silver atoms at the latent image sites to initiate the conversion of all the silver ions in the crystal into one large grain of metallic silver. The bromine dissolves in the developer.

has many sensitivity sites. When the silver halide crystals are irradiated, x-ray photons release electrons from the bromide ions (see Fig. 5.12B). The free electrons move through the crystal until they reach a sensitivity site, where they become trapped and impart a negative charge to the site. The negatively charged sensitivity site attracts positively charged free interstitial silver ions (see Fig. 5.12C). When a silver ion reaches the negatively charged sensitivity site, it is reduced and forms a neutral atom of metallic silver (see Fig. 5.12D). The sites containing these neutral silver atoms are now called latent image sites. This process occurs numerous times within a crystal. The overall distribution of crystals with latent image sites in a film after exposure constitutes the latent image. Processing the exposed film in developer and fixer converts the latent image into the visible radiographic image.

PROCESSING SOLUTIONS

Film processing involves the following procedures:
1. Immerse exposed film in developer.
2. Rinse developer off film in water bath.
3. Immerse film in fixer.
4. Wash film in water bath to remove fixer.
5. Dry film and mount for viewing.

Following exposure, each grain of silver halide in film emulsion (Fig. 5.13A) contains neutral silver atoms at their latent image sites (see Fig. 5.13B). These latent image sites render the crystals sensitive to development and image formation. Developer converts silver bromide crystals with neutral silver atoms deposited at the latent image sites into black, solid silver metallic grains (see Fig. 5.13C). These solid silver grains block light from a viewbox. Fixer removes unexposed, undeveloped silver bromide crystals (crystals without latent image sites), leaving the film clear in unexposed areas (see Fig. 5.13D). Thus the radiographic image is composed of light (radiopaque) areas, where few photons reached the film, and dark (radiolucent) areas of the film that were struck by many photons.

Developing Solution

The developer reduces all silver ions in the exposed crystals of silver halide (crystals with a latent image) to metallic silver grains (see Fig.

5.13). To produce a diagnostic image, this reduction process must be restricted to crystals containing latent image sites; to accomplish this, the reducing agents used as developers are catalyzed by the neutral silver atoms at the latent image sites (see Fig. 5.13B). Individual crystals are developed completely or not at all during the recommended developing times (see Fig. 5.13C). Variations in density on the processed radiographs are the result of different ratios of developed (exposed) and undeveloped (unexposed) crystals. Areas with many exposed crystals are darker because of their higher concentration of black metallic silver grains after development.

When an exposed film is developed, the developer initially has no visible effect (Fig. 5.14). After this initial phase, the density increases, rapidly at first and then more slowly. Eventually, all the exposed crystals develop (are converted to black metallic silver), and the developing agent starts to reduce the unexposed crystals. The development of unexposed crystals results in chemical fog on the film. The interval between maximal density and fogging explains why a properly exposed film does not become overdeveloped, although it may be in contact with the developer longer than the recommended interval.

The chemical components of the developing solution and their functions are described in Table 5.2.

Developer Replenisher

The developing solution of both manual and automatic developers should be replenished with fresh solution each morning to prolong the life of the used developer. The recommended amount to be added daily is 8 ounces of fresh developer (replenisher) per gallon of developing solution. This assumes the development of an average of 30 periapical or 5 panoramic films per day. Some of the used solution may need to be removed to make room for the replenisher.

Rinsing

After development, the film emulsion swells and becomes saturated with developer. At this point, the films are rinsed in water for 30 seconds with continuous, gentle agitation before they are placed in the fixer. Rinsing dilutes the developer, slowing the development process. It also removes the alkali activator, preventing neutralization of the acid fixer. This rinsing process is typical for manual processing but is not used with most automatic processors.

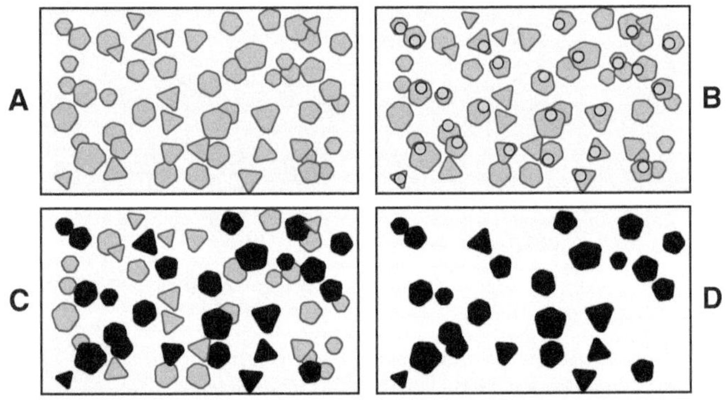

Fig. 5.13 Emulsion Changes During Film Processing. (A) Before exposure, many silver bromide crystals *(gray)* are present in the emulsion. (B) After exposure, the exposed crystals containing neutral silver atoms at latent image sites *(orange dots* within some crystals) constitute the latent image. (C) The developer converts the exposed crystals containing neutral silver atoms at the latent image sites into solid grains of metallic silver *(black)*. (D) The fixer dissolves the unexposed, undeveloped silver bromide crystals, leaving only the solid silver grains that form the radiographic image.

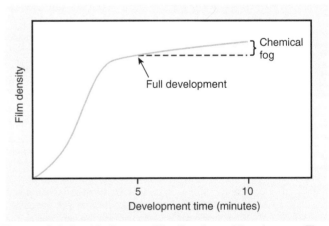

Fig. 5.14 Relationship Between Film Density and Development Time. The density of film increases quickly initially in the developer. After full development, the density continues to increase slowly because of chemical fog.

TABLE 5.2 Components and Function of Radiographic Developer Solution

Component	Ingredient	Function
Developer	Phenidone	Serves as the first electron donor that converts silver ions to metallic silver at the latent image site. This electron transfer generates the oxidized form of phenidone
	Hydroquinone	Hydroquinone provides an electron to reduce the oxidized phenidone back to its original active state so that it can continue to reduce silver halide grains to metallic silver
Activator	Sodium hydroxide or potassium hydroxide	Maintains an alkaline pH (approximately 10) for activity of developer. Causes the gelatin to swell so that the developing agents can diffuse more rapidly into the emulsion to reach silver bromide crystals
Preservative	Sodium sulfite	Antioxidant that extends life of developing solution. Combines with oxidized developer to produce a compound that subsequently stains images brown if not washed out
Restrainer	Bromine-containing compounds	Restrains development of unexposed silver halide crystals. Acts as antifog agents and increases contrast

TABLE 5.3 Components and Function of Radiographic Fixer Solution

Component	Ingredient	Function
Clearing agent	Ammonium thiosulfate	Dissolves the unexposed silver halide grains Excessive fixation (hours) results in a gradual loss of film density because the grains of silver slowly dissolve in the fixing solution
Acidifier	Acetic acid	Maintain an acidic pH (approximately 4–4.5) Promotes good diffusion of thiosulfate into the emulsion and of silver thiosulfate complex out of the emulsion Inactivates any residual developing agents
Preservative	Ammonium sulfite	Prevents oxidation of ammonium thiosulfate, which is unstable in the acidic environment
Hardener	Aluminum sulfate	Complexes with the gelatin during fixing to prevent damage to the gelatin overcoat during subsequent handling

Fixing Solution

Fixing solution removes undeveloped silver halide crystals from the emulsion (see Fig. 5.13D). If these crystals are not removed, the image on the resultant radiograph is dark and nondiagnostic (Fig. 5.15). Fixer also hardens and shrinks the film emulsion.

The chemical components of the developing solution and their functions are described in Table 5.3. As with developer, fixer should be replenished daily at the rate of 8 ounces per gallon.

Washing

After fixing, the processed film is washed in water to remove all thiosulfate ions and silver thiosulfate complexes. Washing efficiency declines rapidly when the water temperature decreases to less than 60°F. Any silver compound or thiosulfate that remains because of improper washing discolors and causes stains, which are most apparent in the radiopaque (light) areas.

DARKROOM AND EQUIPMENT

A conventional darkroom with manual wet processing tanks should be convenient to the x-ray machines and dental operatories and should be at least 4 feet × 5 feet (1.2 m × 1.5 m).

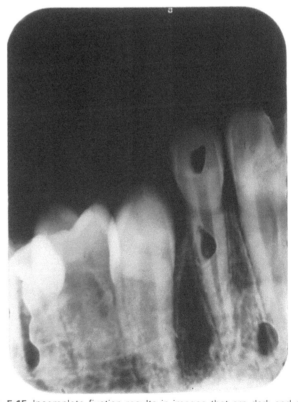

Fig. 5.15 Incomplete fixation results in images that are dark and discolored, making them nondiagnostic. This film was also poorly positioned in the patient's mouth, cutting off most apices of the teeth. Staining may also be caused by using depleted developer or fixer or using contaminated solutions.

DARKROOM

One of the most important requirements is that the darkroom be lightproof. If it is not, stray light can cause film fogging and loss of image contrast. To make the darkroom lightproof, a light-tight door or doorless maze (if space permits) is used. The door should have a lock to prevent accidental opening, which might allow an unexpected flood of light that can ruin opened films. The darkroom must also be well ventilated to provide a comfortable working environment and to exhaust moisture from drying films. In addition, a comfortable room temperature helps to maintain optimal conditions for developing, fixing, and washing solutions.

Safelights

The processing room should have both white illumination and safelights. A safelight is low-intensity illumination of relatively long wavelength (red) that does not rapidly affect open film but permits one to see well enough to work in the area (Fig. 5.16). To minimize the fogging effect

of prolonged exposure, the safelight should have a frosted 15-W bulb or a clear 7.5-W bulb and should be mounted at least 4 feet above the surface where opened films are handled.

X-ray films are very sensitive to the blue-green region of the spectrum and are less sensitive to red wavelengths. The red GBX-2 filter is recommended as a safelight in darkrooms where either intraoral or extraoral films are handled because this filter transmits light only at the red end of the spectrum (Fig. 5.17). Film handling under a safelight should be limited to approximately 5 minutes because film emulsion shows some sensitivity to light from a safelight with prolonged exposure. The older ML-2 filters (yellow light) are not appropriate for fast intraoral dental film or extraoral panoramic or cephalometric film.

Manual Processing Tanks

Dental offices that use automatic film processors should maintain the capability to manually process film. The tank must have hot and cold running water and a means of maintaining the temperature between 60°F and 75°F. A practical size for a dental office is a master tank

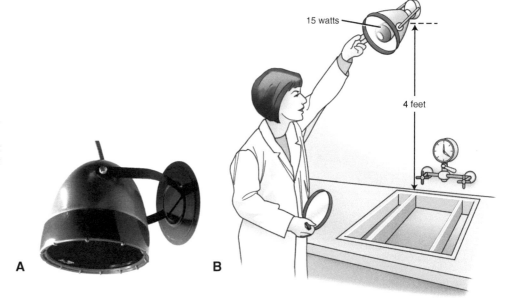

Fig. 5.16 (A) A safelight may be mounted on the wall or ceiling in the darkroom and should be at least 4 feet from the work surface. (B) The safelight uses a GBX-2 filter and 15-W bulb.

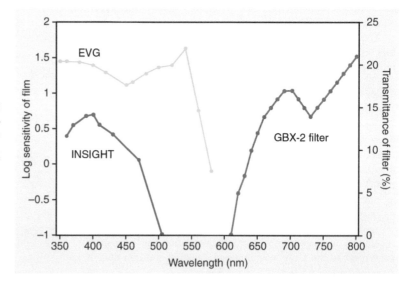

Fig. 5.17 Spectral sensitivities of EVG film *(green line)* and INSIGHT film *(blue line)* shown with the transmission characteristics of a GBX-2 filter *(red line)*. The films are more sensitive in the blue-green portion of the spectrum (shorter than 600 nm), whereas the GBX-2 filter transmits primarily at the red end of the spectrum (longer than 600 nm).

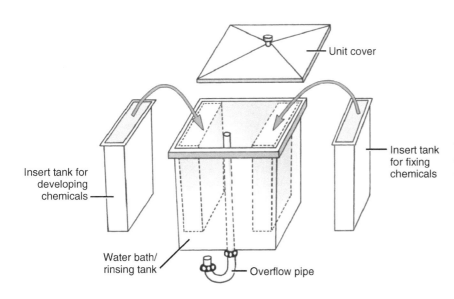

Fig. 5.18 Processing Tank. The developing and fixing tanks are inserted into a bath of running water with an overflow drain. The water bath may be maintained at a stable and optimal temperature for film processing.

approximately 20 cm × 25 cm (8 inches × 10 inches) that can serve as a water jacket for two removable inserts that fit inside (Fig. 5.18). The insert tanks usually hold 3.8 L (1 gallon) of developer or fixer and are placed within the outer, larger master tank. The outer tank holds the water for maintaining the temperature of the developer and fixer in the insert tanks and for washing films. The developer customarily is placed in the insert tank on the left side of the master tank, and the fixer is placed in the insert tank on the right. All three tanks should be made of stainless steel, which does not react with the processing solutions and is easy to clean. The master tank should have a cover to reduce oxidation of the processing solutions, protect the developing film from accidental exposure to light, and minimize evaporation of the processing solutions.

Thermometer

The temperature of the developing, fixing, and washing solutions should be closely controlled. A thermometer can be left in the water circulating through the master tank to monitor the temperature and ensure that the water temperature regulator is working properly. The most desirable thermometers clip onto the side of the tank. Thermometers may contain alcohol or metal, but they should not contain mercury because they could break and contaminate the processor or solutions.

Timer

The x-ray film must be exposed to the processing chemicals for specific intervals. An interval timer is indispensable for controlling development and fixation times.

Drying Racks

Two or three drying racks can be mounted on a convenient wall for film hangers. Drip trays are placed underneath the racks to catch water that may run off the wet films. An electric fan can be used to circulate the air and speed the drying of films, but it should not be pointed directly at the films.

MANUAL PROCESSING PROCEDURES

Manual processing of film requires the following nine steps:
1. *Replenish solutions.* The first step in manual tank processing is to replenish the developer and fixer. Check the solution levels to ensure

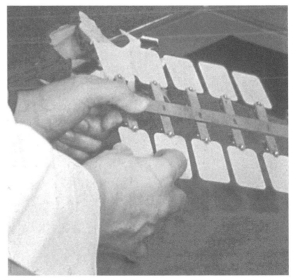

Fig. 5.19 Films Are Mounted Securely on Film Clips. Film is always held by its edges to avoid fingerprints on the image. (Courtesy C. L. Crabtree, DDS, Bureau of Radiological Health, Rockville, MD.)

that the developer and fixer cover the films on the top clips of the film hangers.
2. *Stir solutions.* Stir the developer and fixing solution to mix the chemicals and equalize the temperature throughout the tanks. To prevent cross-contamination, use a separate paddle for each solution. It is best to label one paddle for the developer and the other for the fixer.
3. *Mount films on hangers.* Using only safelight illumination in the darkroom, remove the exposed film from its lightproof packet or cassette. Hold the films by their edges only to avoid damage to the film surface. Clip the bare film onto a film hanger, one film to a clip (Fig. 5.19). Label the film racks with the patient's name and the exposure date.

4. *Set timer.* Check the temperature of the developer, and set the interval timer to the time indicated by the manufacturer for the solution temperature, typically:

Temperature (°F)	Development Time (Minutes)
68	5
70	4½
72	4
76	3
80	2½

Processing films at either higher or lower temperatures and for longer or shorter times than recommended by the manufacturer reduces the contrast of the processed film.

5. *Develop.* Start the timer mechanism, and immerse the hanger and films immediately in the developer. Agitate the hanger mildly for 5 to 10 seconds to remove air bubbles from the film. Do not agitate the film during development.

6. *Rinse.* After development, remove the film hanger from the developer, draining excess into the water bath, and place in the running water bath for 30 seconds. Agitate the films continuously in the rinse water to remove excess developer, thus slowing development and minimizing contamination of the fixer.

7. *Fix.* Place the hanger and film in the fixer solution for 2 to 4 minutes and agitate for 5 of every 30 seconds. Agitation eliminates bubbles and brings fresh fixer into contact with the emulsion. When the films are removed, drain the excess fixer into the wash bath.

8. *Wash.* After fixation of the films is complete, place the hanger in running water for at least 10 minutes to remove residual processing solutions. After the films have been washed, remove surface moisture by gently shaking excess water from the films and hanger.

9. *Dry.* Dry the films in circulating, moderately warm air. After drying, the films are ready to mount.

RAPID-PROCESSING CHEMICALS

Rapid-processing solutions typically develop films in 15 seconds and fix them in 15 seconds at room temperature. They have the same general formulation as conventional processing solutions but often contain a higher concentration of hydroquinone. They also have a more alkaline pH than conventional solutions, which causes the emulsion to swell more, thus providing greater access to developer. These solutions are especially advantageous in endodontics and in emergency situations, when short processing time is essential. Although the resultant images may be satisfactory, they often do not achieve the same degree of contrast as films processed conventionally, and they may discolor over time if not fully washed. After viewing, rapidly processed films are placed in conventional fixing solution for 4 minutes and washed for 10 minutes; this improves the contrast and helps to keep them stable in storage. Conventional solutions are preferred for most routine use.

CHANGING SOLUTIONS

All processing solutions deteriorate as a result of continued use and exposure to air. Although regular replenishment of the developer and fixer prolongs their useful life, the accumulation of reaction products eventually causes these solutions to cease functioning properly. Exhaustion of the developer results from oxidation of the developing agents, depletion of the hydroquinone, and buildup of bromide. With regular replenishment, solutions may last 3 or 4 weeks before they must be changed.

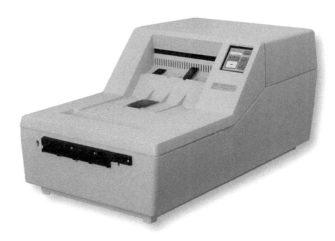

Fig. 5.20 Dent-X 810 AR Film Automatic Film Processor. The operator opens the film packet in a darkroom and inserts the film into the opening on the left end of the machine. The exposed film is carried on a roller apparatus through processing solutions, and the processed and dried film is returned through the upper right opening in 4.5 minutes. (Courtesy ImageWorks, Elmsford, NY.)

A simple procedure can help to determine when solutions should be changed. A double film packet is exposed on one projection for the first patient radiographed after new solutions have been prepared. One film is placed in the patient's chart, and the other is mounted on a corner of a viewbox in the darkroom. As successive films are processed, they are compared with this reference film. Loss of image contrast and density become evident as the solutions deteriorate, indicating when it is time to change them. The fixer is changed when the developer is changed.

AUTOMATIC FILM PROCESSING

Equipment that automates all processing steps is available (Fig. 5.20). Although automatic processing has numerous advantages, the most important is the time saved. Depending on the equipment and the temperature of operation, an automatic processor requires only 4 to 6 minutes to develop, fix, wash, and dry a film. Many dental automatic processors have a light-shielded (daylight loading) compartment in which the operator can unwrap films and feed them into the machine without working in a darkroom. However, special care must be taken to maintain infection control when using these daylight-loading compartments (see Chapter 16).

When extraoral films are processed, the light-shielded compartment is removed to provide room for feeding the larger film into the processor. Another attractive feature of the automatic system is that the density and contrast of the radiographs tend to be consistent. However, because of the higher temperature of the developer and the artifacts caused by rollers, the quality of films processed automatically often is not as high as the quality of films carefully developed manually. With automatically processed films, if more grain is evident in the final image, the correct choice of processing solutions may be able to help minimize the issue.

Whether automatic processing equipment is appropriate for a specific practice depends on the dentist and the nature and volume of the practice. The equipment is expensive and must be cleaned frequently, as described by the processor manufacturer. In addition, automated equipment may break down, and conventional darkroom equipment may still be needed as a backup system.

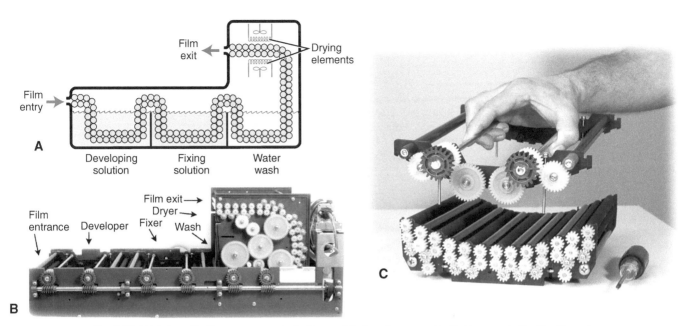

Fig. 5.21 (A) Automatic film processors typically consist of a roller assembly that transports the film through developing, fixing, washing, and drying stations. (B) Assembly of film transport mechanism. (C) One roller assembly. (B and C, Courtesy ImageWorks, Elmsford, NY.)

Mechanism

Automatic processors have an in-line arrangement consisting of a transport mechanism that picks up exposed, unwrapped film and passes it through the developing, fixing, washing, and drying sections (Fig. 5.21). The transport system most often used is a series of rollers driven by a motor that operates through gears, belts, or chains. The rollers often consist of independent assemblies of multiple rollers in a rack, with one rack for each step in the operation. Although these assemblies are designed and positioned so that the film crosses over from one roller to the next, the operator may remove them independently for cleaning and repairing.

The primary function of the rollers is to move the film through the developing solutions, but they also serve at least three other purposes. First, their motion helps to keep the solutions agitated, which contributes to the uniformity of processing. Second, in the developer, fixer, and water tanks, the rollers press on the film emulsion, forcing some solution out of the emulsion. The emulsions rapidly fill again with solution, thus promoting solution exchange. Finally, the top rollers at the crossover point between the developer and fixer tanks remove developing solution, minimizing carryover of developer into the fixer tank. This feature helps to maintain the uniformity of processing chemicals.

The chemical compositions of the developer and fixer are modified to operate at higher temperatures than the temperatures used for manual processing and to meet the more rapid development, fixing, washing, and drying requirements of automatic processing. The quality of the fixer is very important. High-quality fixers contain an additional hardener that helps the emulsion withstand the rigors of the transport system and improves transport. Poor-quality fixers containing no hardener produce more film artifacts, and film may slip and jam during transport.

Operation

Successful operation of an automatic processor requires standardized procedures and regular maintenance. The processor and surrounding area should always be kept clean so that no chemicals contaminate hands or films. The solution level and temperature should be checked each morning before films are processed. Hands should be dry when handling film, and films should be touched on their edges only. The better processors have automatic replenishment systems. A daily, weekly, and quarterly maintenance routine (see Chapter 16) should be followed, including cleaning the rollers and other working parts. It is vital to run a large roller transport cleanup film daily through the processor to clean the top and bottom rollers.

ESTABLISHING CORRECT EXPOSURE TIMES

When radiographs are first made with a new x-ray machine, it is important to examine the exposure guidelines that come with the machine. Typically, such guidelines provide a table listing the various anatomic regions (incisors, premolars, or molars), patient size (adult or child), and the length of the aiming cylinder. For each of these combinations, there is a suggested exposure time. It is also important to start out using fresh processing chemicals and optimal processing conditions as previously described. After the first images are made on patients, it may be necessary to adjust exposure time. If optimal film processing techniques are being followed and the images are consistently dark, exposure times should be decreased until optimal images are obtained. If images are consistently light, exposure times should be increased. When the optimal times have been determined, these values should be posted by the control panel.

MANAGEMENT OF RADIOGRAPHIC WASTES

To prevent environmental damage, many communities and states have passed laws governing the disposal of wastes. In the United States, such laws often derive from the federal Resource Conservation and Recovery Act of 1976. Although dental radiographic waste constitutes only a small potential hazard, it should be discarded properly. The primary ingredient of concern in processing solutions is the dissolved silver found in used fixer. Another material of concern is the lead foil found in film packets.

IMAGE CHARACTERISTICS

Processing an exposed x-ray film causes it to become dark in the exposed area. The degree and pattern of film darkening depend on numerous factors, including the energy and intensity of the x-ray beam, composition of the subject imaged, film emulsion used, and characteristics of film processing. This section describes the major imaging characteristics of x-ray film.

Radiographic Density

When a film is exposed by an x-ray beam (or by light, in the case of screen-film combinations) and then processed, the silver halide crystals in the emulsion that were struck by the photons are converted to grains of metallic silver. These silver grains block the transmission of light from a viewbox and give the film its dark appearance. The degree of darkening or opacity of an exposed film is referred to as optical density, defined as follows:

$$\text{Optical density} = \log_{10}\frac{I_0}{I_t}$$

where I_0 is the intensity of incident light (e.g., from a viewbox) and I_t is the intensity of the light transmitted through the film. With an optical density of 0, 100% of the light is transmitted; with a density of 1, 10% of the light is transmitted; with a density of 2, 1% of the light is transmitted; and so on.

A plot of the relationship between film optical density and exposure is called a characteristic curve, or Hurter-Driffield curve (see Fig. 5.21). It usually is shown as the relationship between the optical density of the film and the logarithm of the corresponding exposure. As exposure of the film increases, its optical density increases. A film is of greatest diagnostic value when the structures of interest are imaged on the relatively straight portion of the graph, between 0.6 and 3.0 optical density units. The characteristic curves of films reveal much information about film contrast, speed, and latitude.

An unexposed film, when processed, shows some density. This appearance is caused by the inherent density of the base and added tint and the development of a few unexposed silver halide crystals. This minimal density is called base plus fog and typically is 0.2 to 0.3. Radiographic density is influenced by exposure and the thickness and density of the imaged structure.

Exposure

The overall film density depends on the number of photons absorbed by the film emulsion. Increasing the milliamperage (mA), peak kilovoltage (kVp), or exposure time increases the number of photons reaching the film and thus increases the density of the radiograph. Reducing the distance between the focal spot and film also increases film density.

Subject Thickness

The thicker the subject, the more the beam is attenuated, and the lighter the resultant image (Fig. 5.22). If exposure factors intended for adults are used on children or edentulous patients, the resultant films are dark because a smaller amount of absorbing tissue is in the path of the x-ray beam. The dentist should vary exposure time according to the patient's size to produce radiographs of optimal density.

Subject Density

Variations in the density of the subject exert a profound influence on the image. The greater the density of a structure within the subject, the

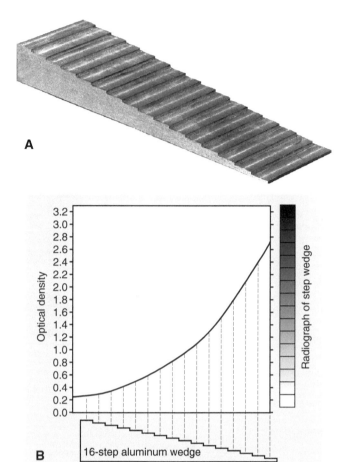

Fig. 5.22 (A) Aluminum step wedge. (B) Graph of the optical density of a radiograph made by exposing the step wedge. As the thickness of the aluminum decreases, more photons are passed through the wedge and are available to expose the film, and the image becomes progressively darker.

greater the attenuation of the x-ray beam directed through that subject or area. In the oral cavity, the relative densities of various natural structures, in order of decreasing density, are enamel, dentin and cementum, bone, muscle, fat, and air. Metallic objects (e.g., restorations) are far denser than enamel and hence better photon absorbers. Because an x-ray beam is differentially attenuated by these absorbers, the resultant beam carries information that is recorded on the radiographic film as light and dark areas. Dense objects (which are strong absorbers) cause the radiographic image to be light and are said to be radiopaque. Objects with low densities are weak absorbers. They allow most photons to pass through, and they cast a dark area on the film that corresponds to the radiolucent object.

Radiographic Contrast

Radiographic contrast is a general term that describes the range of densities on a radiograph. It is defined as the difference in densities between light and dark regions on a radiograph. An image that shows both light areas and dark areas has high contrast; this also is referred to as a short grayscale of contrast because few shades of gray are present between the black-and-white images on the film. Alternatively, a radiographic image composed only of light gray and dark gray zones has low contrast, also referred to as having a long grayscale of contrast (Fig. 5.23). The radiographic contrast of an image is the result of the

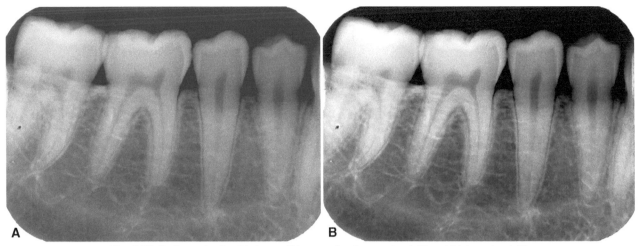

Fig. 5.23 Radiograph of a dried mandible revealing low contrast (A) and high contrast (B).

interplay of subject contrast, film contrast, scattered radiation, and beam energy.

Subject Contrast

Subject contrast is the range of characteristics of the subject that influences radiographic contrast. It is influenced largely by the subject's thickness, density, and atomic number. The subject contrast of a patient's head and neck exposed in a lateral cephalometric view is high. The dense regions of the bone and teeth absorb most of the incident radiation, whereas the soft tissue facial profile transmits most of the radiation.

Subject contrast also is influenced by beam energy and intensity. The energy of the x-ray beam, selected by the kVp, influences image contrast. Fig. 5.24 shows an aluminum step wedge exposed to x-ray beams of differing energies. Because increasing the kVp increases the overall density of the image, the exposure time has been adjusted so that the density of the middle step in each case is approximately the same. As the kVp of the x-ray beam increases, subject contrast decreases. Similarly, when relatively low kVp energies are used, subject contrast increases. A kVp in the range of 60 to 80 is optimal for dental imaging. At higher kVp, the exposure time is reduced, but the loss of contrast may be objectionable because subtle changes may be obscured. Changing the time or mA of the exposure (and holding the kVp constant) also influences subject contrast. If the film is excessively light or dark, contrast of anatomic structures is diminished.

Film Contrast

Film contrast describes the inherent capacity of radiographic films to display differences in subject contrast (i.e., variations in the intensity of the remnant beam). A high-contrast film reveals areas of small difference in subject contrast more clearly than a low-contrast film does. Film contrast usually is measured as the average slope of the diagnostically useful portion of the characteristic curve (Fig. 5.25): the greater the slope of the curve in this region, the greater the film contrast. In Fig. 5.25, film *A* has a higher contrast than film *B*. When the slope of the curve in the useful range is greater than 1, the film exaggerates subject contrast. This desirable feature, which is found in most diagnostic film, allows visualization of structures that differ only slightly in density. For example, the remnant beam in the region of a tooth pulp chamber is more intense (greater exposure) than the beam from the surrounding

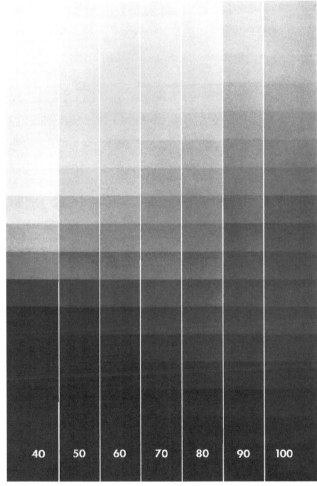

Fig. 5.24 Seven radiographs of a step wedge made at 40 to 100 peak kilovoltage (kVp) shown side by side. As the kVp increased, the milliamperage was reduced to maintain an approximately uniform middle-step density. Note the long grayscale (low contrast) image with high kVp and the short scale (high contrast) image when using low kVp. (Courtesy of Carestream Dental, a division of Carestream Health, Inc.)

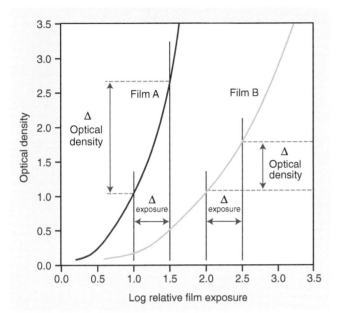

Fig. 5.25 Characteristic curves of two films demonstrating the greater inherent contrast of film *A* compared with film *B*. The slope of film *A* is greater than the slope of film *B*; film *A* shows a greater change in optical density than film *B* for a constant change in exposure. The fact that film *A* is faster than film *B* in this figure is unrelated to film contrast.

enamel crown. A high-contrast film shows a greater contrast (difference in optical density) between these structures than a low-contrast film. As can be seen in Fig. 5.26, film contrast also depends on the density range being examined. With dental direct exposure film, the slope of the curve continually increases with increasing exposure. As a result, properly exposed films have more contrast than underexposed (light) films. Films used with intensifying screens typically have a slope in the range of 2 to 3.

Film processing is another factor that influences film contrast. Film contrast is maximized by optimal film processing conditions. Incomplete or excessive development diminishes contrast of anatomic structures. In addition, storage at too high a temperature, exposure to excessively bright safelights, and light leaks in the darkroom degrade film contrast.

Fog on an x-ray film results in increased film density arising from causes other than exposure to the remnant beam and reduces film contrast. Common causes of film fog are improper safelighting, storage of film at too high a temperature, expired film, exhausted processing chemicals, and development of film at an excessive temperature or for a prolonged period. Film fog can be reduced by proper film processing and storage.

Scattered Radiation

Scattered radiation results from photons that have interacted with the subject by Compton or coherent interactions. These interactions cause the emission of photons that travel in directions other than that of the primary beam. This scattered radiation causes fogging of a radiograph—an overall darkening of the image—and results in loss of radiographic contrast. In most dental applications, the best means of reducing scattered radiation are to use a relatively low kVp and to collimate the beam to the size of the receptor to prevent scatter from an area outside the region of the image.

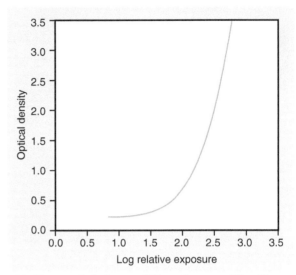

Fig. 5.26 **Characteristic Curve of Direct Exposure Film.** The contrast (slope of the curve) is greater in the high-density region than in the low-density region.

TABLE 5.4   Intraoral Film Speed Classification Per ISO 3665 and ISO 5799

Film Speed Group	Speed Range (Reciprocal Roentgens[a])
C	No longer listed because it is no longer offered
D	14–27.9
E	28–55.9
F	56–111.9

[a]Reciprocal roentgens are the reciprocal of the exposure in roentgens required to obtain a film with an optical density of 1.0 above base plus fog after processing. ISO 3665, Third edition, 2011-09-01. Data from National Council on Radiation Protection and Measurements, Report No. 145, Appendix E, 2004. *ISO,* International Organization for Standardization.

Radiographic Speed

Radiographic speed refers to the amount of radiation required to produce an image of a standard density. Film speed frequently is expressed as the reciprocal of the exposure (in roentgens) required to produce an optical density of 1 above base plus fog. A fast film requires a relatively low exposure to produce a density of 1, whereas a slower film requires a longer exposure for the processed film to have the same density. Film speed is controlled largely by the size of the silver halide grains and their silver content.

The speed of dental intraoral x-ray film is indicated by a letter designating a particular group (Table 5.4). Currently used intraoral x-ray films have a speed rating of D or E/F (i.e., it is right on the border between the E- and F-speed categories). Only films with a D or faster speed rating are appropriate for intraoral radiography. E/F-speed film is preferred because it requires approximately half the exposure time and thus half the radiation dose of D-speed film. In the United States the most widely used films are ULTRA-speed (D-speed) and INSIGHT (E/F speed). INSIGHT F-speed film is faster than Ultra-speed D-speed film because it has double the amount of tabular crystal grains. The characteristic curves in Fig. 5.27 show that INSIGHT film (curve on the left) is faster than Ultra-speed film (curve on the right) because

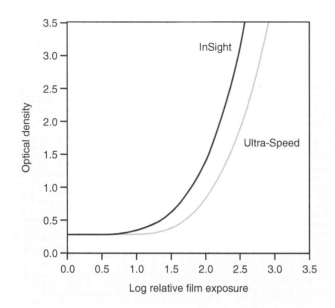

Fig. 5.27 Characteristic Curves for INSIGHT and Ultra-Speed Film. INSIGHT film is faster and has essentially the same contrast (slope) as Ultra-speed film. INSIGHT film requires only half as much patient exposure and is the preferred film. (Courtesy of Carestream Dental, a division of Carestream Health, Inc.)

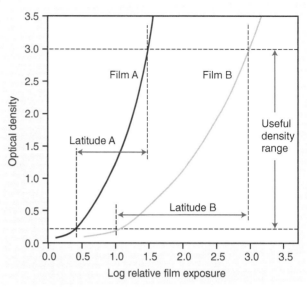

Fig. 5.28 Characteristic curves for two films demonstrating greater inherent latitude of film *B* compared with film *A*. The slope of film *B* is less steep than the slope of film *A*; film *B* records a greater range of exposures within the useful density range than film *A*.

less exposure is required to produce the same level of density, although the two films have similar contrast.

Film Latitude

Film latitude is a measure of the range of exposures that can be recorded as distinguishable densities on a film. A film optimized to display wide latitude records a wide range of subject contrasts. A film with a characteristic curve that has a long straight-line portion and a shallow slope has wide latitude (Fig. 5.28). As a consequence, wide variations in the amount of radiation exiting the subject can be recorded. Films with wide latitude have lower contrast than films with a narrow latitude. Wide-latitude films are useful when both the osseous structures of the skull and the soft tissues of the facial region must be recorded.

Radiographic Noise

Radiographic noise is the appearance of uneven density of a uniformly exposed radiographic film. It is seen on a small area of film as localized variations in density. The primary causes of noise are radiographic mottle and radiographic artifact. Radiographic mottle is uneven density resulting from the physical structure of the film or intensifying screens. Radiographic artifacts are defects caused by errors in film handling, such as fingerprints or bends in the film, or errors in film processing, such as splashing developer or fixer on a film or marks or scratches from rough handling.

On intraoral dental film, mottle may be seen as film graininess, which is caused by the visibility of silver grains in the film emulsion, especially when magnification is used to examine an image. Film graininess is most evident when high-temperature processing is used.

Radiographic mottle is also evident when the film is used with fast intensifying screens. Two important causes of the phenomenon are quantum mottle and screen structure mottle. Quantum mottle is caused by a fluctuation in the number of photons per unit of the beam cross-sectional area absorbed by the intensifying screen. Screen structure mottle is graininess caused by screen phosphors. Quantum mottle and screen structure mottle are each most evident when fast film-screen combinations are used.

Radiographic Sharpness and Resolution

Sharpness is the ability of a radiograph to precisely define an edge (e.g., the dentin-enamel junction, or a thin trabecular plate). Resolution, or resolving power, is the ability of a radiograph to record separate structures that are close together. It usually is measured by radiographing an object made up of a series of thin lead strips with alternating radiolucent spaces of the same thickness. The groups of lines and spaces are arranged in the test target in order of increasing numbers of lines and spaces per millimeter (Fig. 5.29). The resolving power is measured as the highest number of line pairs (a line pair being the image of an absorber and the adjacent lucent space) per millimeter that can be distinguished on the resultant radiograph when examined with low-power magnification. Typically, direct exposure films used for intraoral radiography can delineate 20 lp/mm (line pairs per millimeter) or more. Screen-film combinations for panoramic and cephalometric radiography resolve approximately 5 lp/mm.

Radiographic blur is the loss of sharpness. It can be caused by image receptor (film and screen) blurring, motion blurring, or geometric blurring.

Image Receptor Blurring

With intraoral dental x-ray film, the size and number of the silver grains in the film emulsion determines image sharpness: the finer the grain size, the finer the sharpness. In general, slow-speed films have fine grains, and faster films have larger grains.

Use of intensifying screens in extraoral radiography has an adverse effect on image sharpness. Some degree of sharpness is lost because visible light and UV radiation emitted by the screen spread out beyond the point of origin and expose a film area larger than the phosphor crystal (see Fig. 5.10). The spreading light causes a blurring of fine detail on the radiograph. Intensifying screens with large crystals are

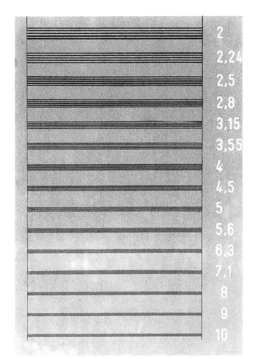

Fig. 5.29 Radiograph of a resolving power target consisting of groups of radiopaque lines and radiolucent spaces. Numbers at each group indicate the number of line pairs per millimeter represented by the group.

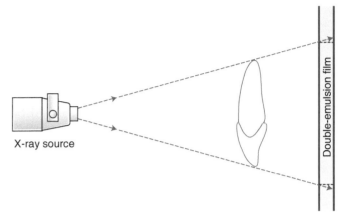

Fig. 5.30 Parallax unsharpness results when double-emulsion film is used because of the slightly greater magnification of the object on the side of the film away from the x-ray source. Parallax unsharpness is a minor problem in clinical practice.

relatively fast, but image sharpness is diminished. Fast intensifying screens have a relatively thick phosphor layer, which contributes to dispersion of light and loss of image sharpness. Diffusion of light from a screen can be minimized and image sharpness maximized by ensuring as close a contact as possible between the intensifying screen and the film.

The presence of an image on each side of a double-emulsion film also causes a loss of image sharpness through parallax (Fig. 5.30). Parallax results from the apparent change in position or size of a subject when it is viewed from different perspectives. Because dental film has a double coating of emulsion and the x-ray beam is divergent, the images recorded on each emulsion vary slightly in size. When intensifying screens are used, parallax distortion contributes to image unsharpness because light from one screen may cross the film base and reach the emulsion on the opposite side. This problem can be solved by incorporating dyes into the base that absorb the light emitted by the screens.

Motion Blurring

Image sharpness also can be lost through movement of the film or subject during exposure. Movement of the x-ray source in effect enlarges the focal spot and diminishes image sharpness. Patient movement can be minimized by stabilizing the patient's head with the chair headrest during exposure. Use of a higher mA and correspondingly shorter exposure times also helps to resolve this problem.

Geometric Blurring

Several geometric factors influence image sharpness. Loss of image sharpness results in part because photons are not emitted from a point source (focal spot) on the target in the x-ray tube. The larger the focal spot, the greater the loss of image sharpness. In addition, image sharpness is improved by increasing the distance between the focal spot and the

object and reducing the distance between the object and the image receptor. Various means of optimizing projection geometry are discussed in Chapter 6.

Image Quality

Image quality describes the subjective judgment by the clinician of the overall appearance of a radiograph. It combines the features of density, contrast, latitude, sharpness, resolution, and perhaps other parameters. Various mathematic approaches have been used to evaluate these parameters further, but a thorough discussion of them is beyond the scope of this text. The detective quantum efficiency (DQE) is a basic measure of the efficiency of an imaging system. It encompasses image contrast, blur, speed, and noise. Often a system can be optimized for one of these parameters, but this usually is achieved at the expense of others. For instance, a fast system typically has a high level of noise. However, even with these and other sophisticated approaches, more information is needed for complete understanding of all the factors responsible for the subjective impression of image quality.

COMMON CAUSES OF FAULTY RADIOGRAPHS

Although film processing can produce radiographs of excellent quality, inattention to detail may lead to many problems and images that are diagnostically suboptimal. Poor radiographs contribute to a loss of diagnostic information and loss of professional and patient time. Box 5.1 presents a list of common causes of faulty radiographs. The steps necessary for correction are self-evident.

MOUNTING RADIOGRAPHS

Film-based radiographs must be preserved and maintained in a satisfactory condition. Periapical, interproximal, and occlusal films are best handled and stored in a film mount (Fig. 5.39). The operator can handle them with greater ease, and there is less chance of damaging the emulsion. Mounts are made of plastic or cardboard and may have a clear plastic window that covers and protects the film. However, the window may have scratches or imperfections that interfere with radiographic interpretation. The operator can arrange several films from the same individual

BOX 5.1   Common Problems in Film Exposure and Development

Light Radiographs (Fig. 5.31)
Processing Errors
Underdevelopment (temperature too low; time too short; thermometer inaccurate)
Depleted developer solution
Diluted or contaminated developer
Excessive fixation (hours)

Underexposure
Insufficient mA
Insufficient kVp
Insufficient exposure time
Film-source distance too long
Film packet reversed in mouth (see Fig. 5.5)

Dark Radiographs (Fig. 5.32)
Processing Errors
Overdevelopment (temperature too high; time too long)
Developer concentration too high
Inadequate time in fixer
Accidental exposure to light
Improper safelighting
Storage of films without shielding, at too high a temperature, or past expiration date

Overexposure
Excessive mA
Excessive kVp
Excessive exposure time
Film-source distance too short

Insufficient Contrast (Fig. 5.33)
Underdevelopment
Underexposure
Excessive kVp
Excessive film fog

Film Fog (Fig. 5.34)
Improper safelighting (improper filter; excessive bulb wattage; inadequate distance between safelight and work surface; prolonged exposure to safelight)

Light leaks (cracked safelight filter; light leaks from doors, vents, or other sources)
Overdevelopment
Contaminated solutions
Deteriorated film (stored at high temperature; stored at high humidity; exposed to radiation; past expiration date)

Dark Spots or Lines (Fig. 5.35)
Fingerprint contamination
Protective wrapping paper sticking to film surface
Film in contact with tank or another film during fixation
Film contaminated with developer before processing
Excessive bending of film
Static discharge to film before processing
Excessive roller pressure during automatic processing
Dirty rollers in automatic processing

Light Spots (Fig. 5.36)
Film contaminated with fixer before processing
Film in contact with tank or another film during development

Yellow or Brown Stains (see Fig. 5.15)
Depleted developer
Depleted fixer
Insufficient washing
Contaminated solutions

Blurring (Fig. 5.37)
Movement of patient
Movement of film (film not stabilized)

Partial Images (Fig. 5.38)
Top of film not immersed in developing solution
Misalignment of x-ray tube head ("cone-cut")

Emulsion Peel
Abrasion of image during processing
Excessive time in wash water

kVp, Peak kilovoltage; *mA,* milliamperage.

in a film mount in the proper anatomic relationship. This facilitates correlation of the clinical and radiographic examinations. Opaque mounts are best because they prevent stray light from the viewbox from reaching the viewer's eyes.

The preferred method of positioning periapical and occlusal films in the film mount is to arrange them so that the images of the teeth are in the anatomic position and have the same relationship to the viewer as when the viewer faces the patient. The radiographs of the teeth in the right quadrants should be placed in the left side of the mount, and the radiographs of the teeth of the left quadrants should be placed in the right side. This system, advocated by the American Dental Association, allows the examiner's gaze to shift from radiograph to tooth without crossing the midline. The alternative arrangement, with the images of the right quadrants on the right side of the mount and the images of the left quadrant on the left side, is not recommended.

DUPLICATING RADIOGRAPHS

Occasionally, film radiographs must be duplicated; this is best accomplished with duplicating film. The film to be duplicated is placed against the emulsion side of the duplicating film, and the two films are held in position by a glass-topped cassette or photographic printing frame. The films are exposed to light, which passes through the clear areas of the original radiograph and exposes the duplicating film. The duplicating film is processed in conventional x-ray processing solutions. In contrast to conventional x-ray film, duplicating film gives a positive image. Thus areas exposed to light come out clear, as on the original radiograph. Duplication typically results in images with less resolution and more contrast than the original radiograph. The best images are obtained when a circular, UV light source is used. In contrast to the usual negative film, images on duplicating film that are too dark or too light are underexposed or overexposed, respectively.

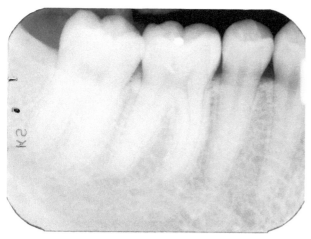

Fig. 5.31 Radiograph That Is Too Light Because of Inadequate Processing or Insufficient Exposure.

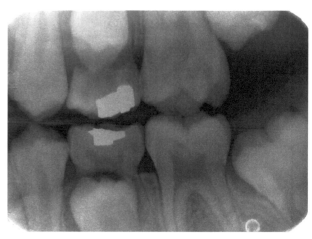

Fig. 5.33 Radiograph With Insufficient Contrast, Showing Gray Enamel and Gray Pulp Chambers.

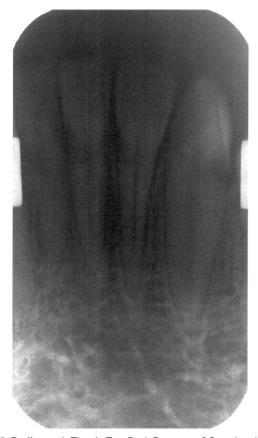

Fig. 5.32 Radiograph That Is Too Dark Because of Overdevelopment or Overexposure.

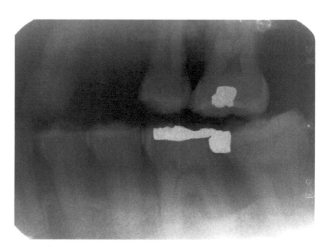

Fig. 5.34 Fogged Radiograph Marked by Darkening and Lack of Image Detail.

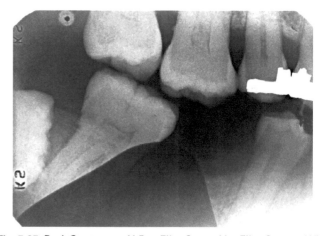

Fig. 5.35 Dark Spot on an X-Ray Film Caused by Film Contact With the Tank Wall During Fixation. This contact prevented the fixer from dissolving the unexposed silver bromide crystals on the emulsion in contact with the tank wall.

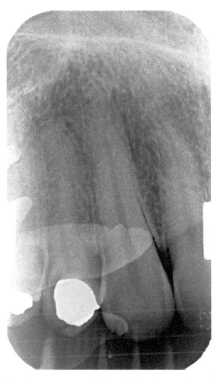

Fig. 5.36 Light Spots on an X-Ray Film Caused by Film Contact With Drops of Fixer Before Processing. The fixer removed the unexposed silver bromide grains on one emulsion but did not affect the opposite side, so there is still an image.

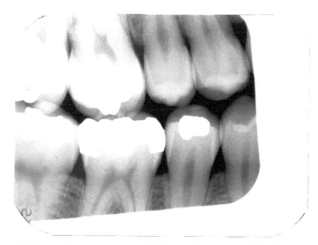

Fig. 5.38 Partial Image Caused by Poor Alignment of the Tube Head With the Film Rectangular Collimator.

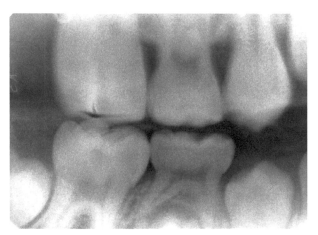

Fig. 5.37 Blurred Radiograph Caused by Movement of the Patient During Exposure.

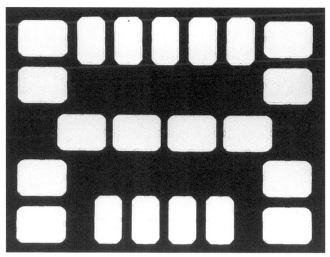

Fig. 5.39 Film mount for holding nine narrow anterior periapical views, eight posterior periapical views, and four bite-wing views. An opaque film mount blocks extraneous light from a viewbox when examining the radiographs.

BIBLIOGRAPHY

American Dental Association Council on Scientific Affairs. Dental radiographic examinations: recommendations for patient selection and limiting radiation exposure; Revised 2012. http://www.ada.org/sections/professionalResources/pdfs/Dental_Radiographic_Examinations_2012.pdf.

Baghele ON, Phadke S, Deshpande AA, et al. A simplified model for biomedical waste management in dental practices - a pilot project at Thane, India. *Eur J Gen Dent.* 2013;2:235–240. Available from: http://www.ejgd.org/text.asp?2013/2/3/235/115992.

Bushberg JT. *The Essential Physics of Medical Imaging.* 3rd ed. Baltimore: Lippincott Williams & Wilkins; 2012.

Bushong SC. *Radiologic Science for Technologists: Physics, Biology, and Protection.* 9th ed. St Louis: Mosby; 2009.

Castro VM, Katz JO, Hardman PK, et al. In vitro comparison of conventional film and direct digital imaging in the detection of approximal caries. *Dentomaxillofac Radiol.* 2007;36:138–142.

de Carvalho FP, da Silveira MM, Frazao MA, et al. Effects of developer exhaustion on DFL Contrast FV-58 and Kodak Insight dental films. *Dentomaxillofac Radiol.* 2011;40:358–361.

Fitterman AS, Brayer FC, Cumbo PE. Processing chemistry for medical imaging, Technical and Scientific Monograph No. 5, N-327; 1995. Rochester, NY, Eastman Kodak.

Ludlow JB, Platin E, Mol A. Characteristics of Kodak InSight, an F-speed intraoral film. *Oral Surg Oral Med Oral Pathol Oral Radiol Endod.* 2001;91:120–129.

Madalli VB, Annigeri RG, Basavaraddi SM. The evaluation of effect of developer age in the detection of approximal caries using three speed dental x-ray films: an in-vitro study. *J Clin Diagn Res.* 2014;8:236–239.

Mees DEK, James TH. *The Theory of the Photographic Process.* New York: Macmillan; 1977.

Nair MK, Nair UP. An in-vitro evaluation of Kodak InSight and Ektaspeed Plus film with a CMOS detector for natural proximal caries: ROC analysis. *Caries Res.* 2001;35:354–359.

Pontual AA, de Melo DP, de Almeida SM, et al. Comparison of digital systems and conventional dental film for the detection of approximal enamel caries. *Dentomaxillofac Radiol.* 2010;39:431–436.

Syriopoulos K, Velders XL, Sanderink GC, et al. Sensitometric evaluation of four dental x-ray films using five processing solutions. *Dentomaxillofac Radiol.* 1999;28:73–79.

Thunthy KH, Ireland EJ. A comparison of the visibility of caries on Kodak F-speed (InSight) and D-speed (Ultra-Speed) films. *LDA J.* 2001;60:31–32.

US Food and Drug Administration. Dental Radiography: Doses and Film Speed. https://www.fda.gov/Radiation-EmittingProducts/RadiationSafety/NationwideEvaluationofX-RayTrendsNEXT/ucm116524.htm.

6

Projection Geometry

Sanjay M. Mallya

A conventional radiograph is made with a stationary x-ray source and displays a two-dimensional image of an anatomic region. Such images are often called plain or projection views (in contrast to ultrasound, computed tomography [CT], magnetic resonance imaging, or nuclear medicine). In plain views, the entire volume of tissue between the x-ray source and the image receptor (digital sensor or film) is projected onto a two-dimensional image. Intraoral radiographs (periapical, bite-wing, and occlusal radiographs; Chapter 7) and cephalometric and skull radiographs (Chapter 8) are examples of projection views commonly made in general and specialty dental practices.

Radiography provides an image of the internal anatomy that is not visible on clinical examination. To interpret a radiograph the clinician must use his or her knowledge of normal anatomy to mentally reconstruct a three-dimensional image of the anatomic structures using information from one or more two-dimensional views. Using high-quality radiographs greatly facilitates this task. The term image quality refers to the reliability of the image to represent the true state of the anatomic region examined. Parameters that define radiographic image quality include image sharpness, spatial resolution, contrast resolution, magnification, and distortion. For optimal diagnosis, the radiographic imaging system should make an image that has minimal magnification and distortion, and with a contrast and spatial resolution that is adequate for the intended diagnostic task.

The five basic principles of projection geometry (Box 6.1) are based on the effects of focal spot size and relative positions of the object and image receptor (digital sensor or film) on image clarity, magnification, and distortion. Clinicians use these principles to maximize radiographic image quality and facilitate accurate radiographic diagnoses.

IMAGE SHARPNESS AND RESOLUTION

Several geometric considerations contribute to image sharpness and spatial resolution. Sharpness measures how well a boundary between two areas of differing radiodensity is revealed. Image spatial resolution measures how well a radiograph reveals small objects that are close together. Although sharpness and spatial resolution are two distinct parameters, they are interdependent, being influenced by the same geometric variables. For clinical diagnosis, it is desirable to optimize conditions that result in images with the optimal sharpness and resolution.

When x-rays are produced at the target in an x-ray tube, they originate from all points within the area of the focal spot. Because these rays originate from different points and travel in straight lines, their projections of an object do not superimpose at the same location on an image

receptor. As a result, the image of the edge of an object is slightly blurred rather than sharp and distinct. Fig. 6.1 shows the path of photons that originate at the margins of the focal spot and provide an image of the edges of an object. The resulting blurred zone at the edge of the image causes a loss in image sharpness, and is referred to as *geometric unsharpness* or *penumbra*. The larger the focal spot area, the wider the zone of geometric unsharpness.

There are three means to maximize image sharpness:

1. *Use as small an effective focal spot as practical.* The effective focal spot sizes in dental x-ray machines ranges from 0.4 to 0.7 mm. Using an x-ray unit with a smaller focal spot size adds to image sharpness. As described in Chapter 1, the size of the effective focal spot is a function of the angle of the target with respect to the long axis of the electron beam. A large angle distributes the electron beam over a larger surface and decreases the heat generated per unit of target area, thus prolonging tube life; however, this results in a larger radiation source and loss of image clarity (Fig. 6.2). A small angle has a greater wearing effect on the target but results in a smaller source and increased image sharpness.

2. *Increase the distance between the source and the object by using a long, open-ended cylinder.* Increasing the source-to-object distance reduces geometric unsharpness by reducing the divergence of the x-ray beam (Fig. 6.3). A longer source-to-object distance yields photons whose paths are almost parallel at the object and minimizes unsharpness. To facilitate making images with a longer source-to-object distance, many manufacturers locate the x-ray tube recessed within the x-ray tube housing. The benefits of using a source-to-object distance support the use of long, open-ended cylinders as aiming devices on dental x-ray machines. For intraoral x-ray units, the distance from the source to the edge of the aiming rim ranges from 8 inches to 16 inches.

3. *Minimize the distance between the object and the image receptor.* As the object-to-image receptor distance is reduced, the divergence of x-ray photons at the object is less, resulting in a decrease in the width of the unsharp zone (Fig. 6.4).

IMAGE SIZE DISTORTION

Image size distortion (magnification) is the increase in size of the image on the radiograph compared with the actual size of the object. The divergent paths of photons in an x-ray beam cause enlargement of the image on a radiograph. Image size distortion results from the relative distances of the source-to-object and object-to-image receptor (see Figs. 6.3 and 6.4). Increasing the source-to-object distance and decreasing the object-to-image receptor distance minimizes image magnification. The use of a long, open-ended cylinder as an aiming device on an x-ray

BOX 6.1   Basic Principles of Projection Geometry for Radiography

1. The focal spot should be as small as possible.
2. The source-receptor distance should be as long as possible.
3. The object-receptor distance should be as small as possible.
4. The receptor should be parallel to the long axis of the object.
5. The central beam should be perpendicular to the object and the receptor.

machine thus reduces the magnification of images on a periapical view. As previously mentioned, this technique also improves image sharpness by increasing the distance between the focal spot and the object. The principle of maintaining a long source-to-object distance is applied during cephalometric radiography, where the distance between the source to midsagittal plane is 60 inches to yield images with minimal magnification.

When imaging the facial bones, a posteroanterior projection is preferable, to position the facial bones closer to the receptor and minimize their magnification.

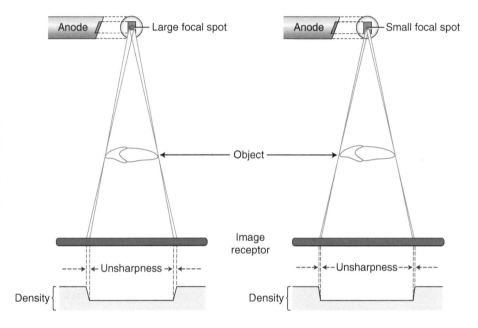

Fig. 6.1 Photons originating at different places on the focal spot *(red)* result in a zone of unsharpness on the radiograph. The density of the image changes from a high background value to a low value in the area of an edge of enamel, dentin, or bone. On the left, a large focal spot size results in a wide zone of unsharpness compared with a small focal spot size on the right, which results in a sharper image (narrow zone of unsharpness).

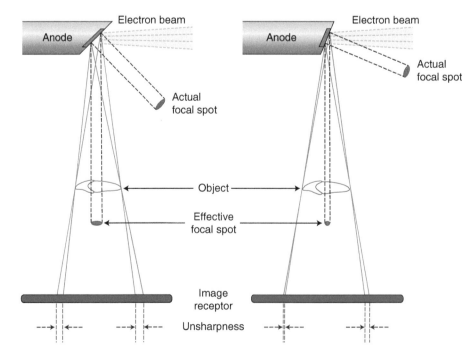

Fig. 6.2 As the angle of the target becomes closer to perpendicular to the long axis of the electron beam (as shown on the *right*) the actual focal spot becomes smaller, which decreases heat dissipation and tube life. The more perpendicular angle also decreases the effective focal spot size, increasing the sharpness of the resulting image.

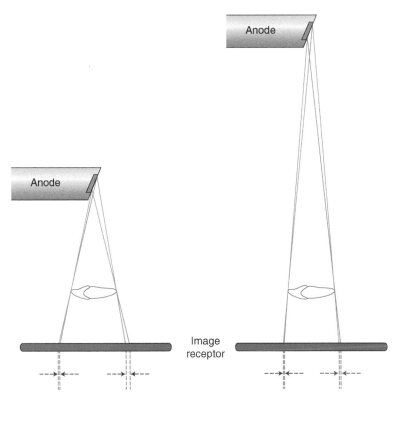

Fig. 6.3 Increasing the distance between the source and the object results in an image with increased sharpness and less magnification of the object as seen on the right.

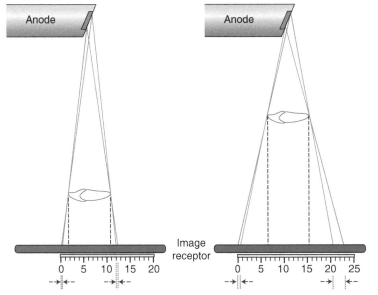

Fig. 6.4 Decreasing the distance between the object and the image receptor increases the sharpness and results in less magnification of the object as seen on the left.

IMAGE SHAPE DISTORTION

Image shape distortion is the result of unequal magnification of different parts of the same object. This situation arises when not all the parts of an object are at the same source-to-object distance. The physical shape of the object may often prevent its optimal orientation, resulting in some shape distortion. Such a phenomenon is seen by the differences in appearance of the image on a radiograph compared with the true shape. To minimize shape distortion, the practitioner should align the x-ray tube, object, and image receptor according to the following guidelines:

1. *Position the image receptor parallel to the long axis of the object.* Image shape distortion is minimized when the long axes of the image

receptor and tooth are parallel. Fig. 6.5 shows that the central ray of the x-ray beam is perpendicular to the image receptor, but the object is not parallel to the image receptor. The resultant image is distorted because of the unequal distances of the various parts of the object from the image receptor. This type of shape distortion is called foreshortening because it causes the radiographic image to be shorter than the object. Fig. 6.6 shows the situation when the x-ray beam is oriented at right angles to the object but not to the image receptor; this results in elongation, with the object appearing longer on the image receptor than its actual length.

2. *Orient the central ray perpendicular to the object and image receptor.* Image shape distortion occurs if the object and image receptor are

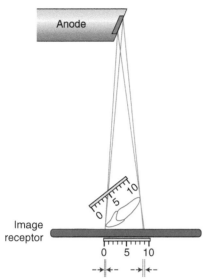

Fig. 6.5 Foreshortening of a radiographic image results when the central ray is perpendicular to the image receptor but the object is not parallel with the image receptor.

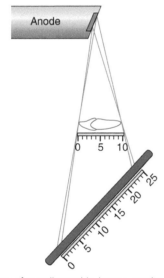

Fig. 6.6 Elongation of a radiographic image results when the central ray is perpendicular to the object but not to the image receptor.

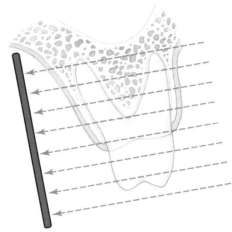

Fig. 6.7 The central ray should be perpendicular to the long axes of both the tooth and the image receptor. If the direction of the x-ray beam is not at right angles to the long axis of the tooth, the appearance of the tooth is distorted, typically by apparent elongation of the length of the palatal roots of upper molars and distortion of the relationship of the height of the alveolar crest relative to the cementoenamel junction.

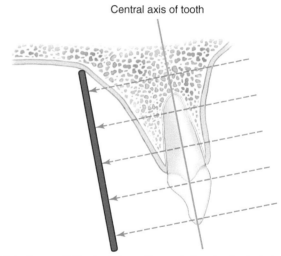

Fig. 6.8 In the paralleling technique, the central ray is directed at a right angle to the central axes of the object and the image receptor. This technique requires a device to support the film in position.

parallel, but the central ray is not directed at right angles to each. This distortion is most evident on maxillary molar views (Fig. 6.7), where the divergence of the buccal and palatal roots precludes placing all roots parallel to the receptor, and the palatal roots appears disproportionately longer than the buccal roots.

The practitioner can prevent shape distortion errors by aligning the object and image receptor parallel with each other and the central ray perpendicular to both.

PARALLELING AND BISECTING-ANGLE TECHNIQUES

The clinical objective of intraoral periapical radiography is to produce images of the dentoalveolar structures with minimal size and shape distortion.

The paralleling technique is the preferred method for making intraoral radiographs. This technique seeks to minimize distortion by placing the image receptor parallel to the long axis of the tooth, and directs the central x-ray beam perpendicular to both the long axis of the tooth and the receptor (Fig. 6.8) and best incorporates the imaging principles described in the first three sections of this chapter (see Box 6.1).

To achieve this parallel orientation, the practitioner often must position the image receptor toward the middle of the oral cavity, away from the teeth. Although this allows the teeth and image receptor to be parallel, it increases the object-to-receptor distance and results in some image magnification and geometric unsharpness. To overcome these limitations, the paralleling technique also uses a relatively long open-ended aiming cylinder ("cone") to increase the source-to-object distance. This "cone" directs only the most central and parallel rays of the beam to the image receptor and teeth and reduces image

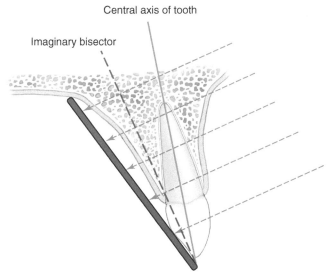

Central axis of tooth

Imaginary bisector

Fig. 6.9 In the bisecting-angle technique, the central ray is directed at a right angle to the imaginary plane that bisects the angle formed by the image receptor and the central axis of the object. This method produces an image that is the same length as the object but results in some image distortion.

magnification, while increasing image sharpness. To facilitate the parallel position of the receptor, image-receptor holders are used to support the image receptor in the patient's mouth (see Chapter 7).

A second method to minimize image distortion and magnification in intraoral radiography is the bisecting-angle technique (Fig. 6.9). In this method, the image receptor is placed as close to the teeth as possible without deforming it. However, when the image receptor is in this position, it is not parallel to the long axes of the teeth. This arrangement inherently causes distortion. Nevertheless, by directing the central ray perpendicular to an imaginary plane that bisects the angle between the teeth and the image receptor, the practitioner can make the length of the tooth's image on the image receptor correspond to the actual length of the tooth. This angle between a tooth and the image receptor is especially apparent when teeth are radiographed in the maxilla or anterior mandible. Although the projected length of a tooth is correct, these images display a distorted image of the position of alveolar crest with respect to the cementoenamel junction of a tooth. In recent years, the bisecting-angle technique is used less frequently for general periapical radiography as use of the paralleling technique has increased.

OBJECT LOCALIZATION

Most often, conventional periapical and bite-wing radiographs are the first radiographic images made of the teeth and supporting bone. An inherent limitation of plain radiography is the two-dimensional nature of the image. Often, the dentist needs to derive three-dimensional information that describes the spatial relationship of the structures imaged. For example, the dentist may need to determine the location of an impacted tooth, or a foreign object within the jaw. Three approaches are frequently used to obtain such three-dimensional information (Box 6.2). The first two approaches combine information from two or more conventional projection radiographs to decipher the three-dimensional spatial location of an object, and are discussed in detail in this chapter. The third approach requires imaging the patient with a three-dimensional imaging modality such as cone beam computed tomography (CBCT) or multidetector computed tomography (MDCT). Dentists must be familiar with the application of the first two approaches—these techniques are valuable

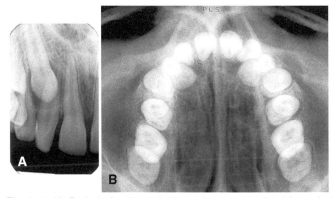

Fig. 6.10 (A) Periapical radiograph shows impacted canine lying apical to roots of lateral incisor and first premolar. (B) Maxillary cross-sectional occlusal view shows that the canine lies palatal to the roots of the lateral incisor and first premolar.

because CT imaging may not be easily accessible or even necessary if the dentist already has multiple periapical views of the region of interest.

Examine two images projected at right angles to each other. In this approach, the clinician identifies the position of the object of interest relative to surrounding anatomic landmarks on both projections, and combines information from both projections to spatially locate the object. For radiography of the teeth and supporting structures, the two projections used are periapical and cross-sectional occlusal radiographs (see Chapter 7).

Fig. 6.10 demonstrates application of this method to spatially define the relationships of an impacted maxillary canine to the adjacent teeth. The periapical radiograph localizes the impacted canine in the mesiodistal and superoinferior dimensions, and the maxillary occlusal radiograph provides information in the mesiodistal and buccolingual dimensions. The combined information allows the clinician to locate the impacted tooth in all three dimensions, which is necessary for planning the surgical approach to expose the canine crown for subsequent orthodontic tooth movement.

This approach is best suited for the mandible, where making cross-sectional occlusal radiographs is easier. On a maxillary cross-sectional occlusal view, the superimposition of features in the anterior part of the skull frequently obscures the area of interest.

The principle of obtaining two projections at right angles can also be applied to cephalometric radiography—the combined analysis of lateral- and posteroanterior projections provides information on skeletal relationships in all three planes.

Use the tube-shift technique employing conventional periapical views. A second approach to identify the spatial position of an object is the tube-shift technique. Other names for this procedure are the buccal-object rule and Clark's rule (Clark described this method in 1910). The rationale for this procedure derives from the manner in which the relative positions of radiographic images of two separate objects change when the projection angle at which the images were made is changed.

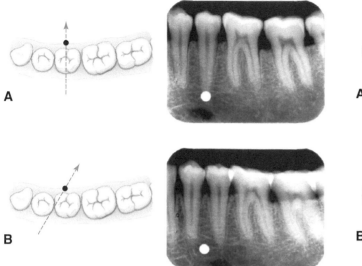

Fig. 6.11 The Position of an Object May Be Determined With Respect to Reference Structures with Use of the Tube Shift Technique. (A) A radiopaque object on the lingual surface of the mandible *(black dot)* may appear apical to the second premolar. (B) When another radiograph is made of this region angulated from the mesial, the object appears to have moved mesially with respect to the second premolar apex ("same lingual" in the acronym SLOB).

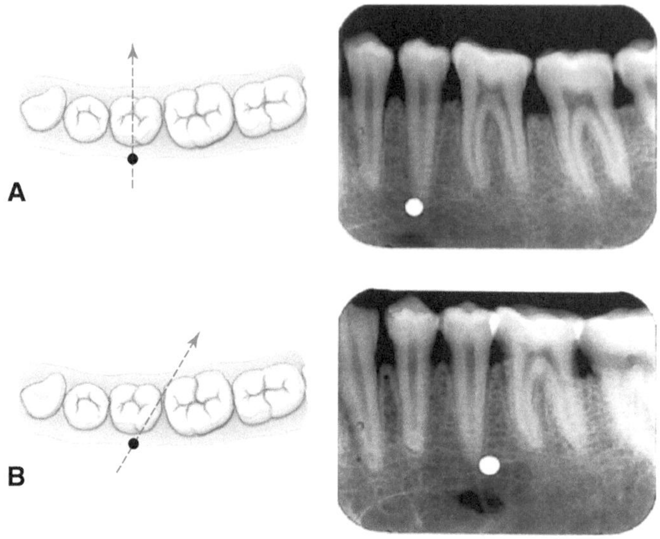

Fig. 6.12 The Position of an Object Can Be Determined With Respect to Reference Structures with Use of the Tube Shift Technique. (A) An object on the buccal surface of the mandible may appear apical to the second premolar. (B) When another radiograph is made of this region angulated from the mesial, the object appears to have moved distally with respect to the second premolar apex ("opposite buccal" in the acronym SLOB).

Fig. 6.11 shows two radiographs of an object, located lingual to the premolar, exposed at different angles. Compare the positions of the object in question on each radiograph with a reference structure—for example the apex of the second premolar. In the first radiograph, the object is superimposed over the apex of the second premolar. The x-ray tube head is then shifted and directed from a more mesial angulation. In the resultant radiograph, the image of the object in question has moved mesially with respect to the apex of the second premolar. **When an object lies lingual to the reference object, its image appears to move in the direction of the tube shift.**

Fig. 6.12 shows two radiographs of an object, now located buccal to the premolar. In the first projection, the object is superimposed over the apex of the second premolar. When the x-ray tube is moved mesially, the image of the object appears to move distal relative to the apex of the second premolar. **When the object lies buccal to the reference object, its image appears to move in the direction of opposite to the tube shift.**

The application of this principle can be easily remembered by the acronym *SLOB*: *s*ame *l*ingual, *o*pposite *b*uccal. Thus, if the object in question appears to move in the *same* direction with respect to the reference structures as does the x-ray tube, it is on the *lingual* aspect of the reference object; if it appears to move in the *opposite* direction as the x-ray tube, it is on the *buccal* aspect. If it does not move with respect to the reference object, it lies at the same depth (in the same vertical plane) as the reference object. The application of this method works equally well when the x-ray tube is moved vertically, instead of horizontally. In this case, the movement of the object's image in the vertical plane (superior or inferior to the reference structure) is evaluated.

A conventional full-mouth radiographic series consists of images of an anatomic region taken at different angles. Dentists can use this principle to decipher the location of anatomic structures. For example, the mental foramen is often superimposed over the apex of the adjacent premolar, and may mimic a periapical radiolucency. However, the projection of the adjacent radiograph, taken at a different angle, will demonstrate movement of the radiolucency away from the apex, and

allows it differentiation from a true periapical radiolucency. Likewise, the same principle can be applied to examine superimposition of the incisive foramen over the apex of a maxillary central incisor.

This technique assists in determining the position of impacted teeth, the presence of foreign objects, and identification of multiple pulp canals. Fig. 6.13 shows two periapical radiographs of the mandibular molar region taken at slightly different horizontal angulations. In the first projection (see Fig. 6.13A), the object of interest (impacted second premolar) is superimposed over the furcation and mesial root of the mandibular permanent first molar. The second projection (see Fig. 6.13B), represents movement of the x-ray tube toward the mesial, and the image of the impacted premolar is now superimposed over the distal root (image has moved distally, opposite to the direction of tube movement). Applying the *SLOB* rule indicates that the impacted premolar is located *buccal* to the roots of the mandibular first molar. Also note the distal movement of the image of the orthodontic bracket anchored on the buccal surface of the molar.

The dentist may have two radiographs of a region of the dentition that were made at different angles, but no record exists of the orientation of the x-ray machine. Comparison of the anatomy displayed on the images helps distinguish changes in horizontal or vertical angulation. The relative positions of osseous landmarks with respect to the teeth help identify changes in horizontal or vertical angulation. Fig. 6.14 shows the inferior border of the zygomatic process of the maxilla over the molars. This structure lies buccal to the teeth and appears to move mesially as the x-ray beam is oriented more from the distal. Similarly, as the angulation of the beam is increased vertically, the zygomatic process is projected occlusally over the teeth.

EGGSHELL EFFECT

Plain radiographs—images that project a three-dimensional volume onto a two-dimensional receptor—may produce an eggshell effect of corticated structures (Fig. 6.15A). Fig. 6.15B shows a schematic view

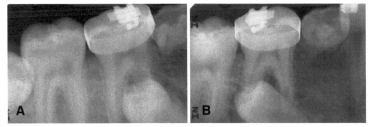

Fig. 6.13 Application of the Tube Shift Technique to Localize an Impacted Premolar. (A) Periapical radiograph of the mandibular molar region showing an impacted second premolar superimposed over the mesial root and furcation. (B) Another radiograph of this region angulated from the mesial; the impacted premolar appears to have moved distally with respect to the mandibular molar roots and indicates a relative buccal position.

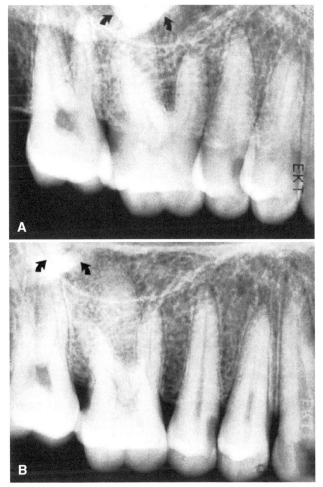

Fig. 6.14 The Position of the Maxillary Zygomatic Process in Relation to the Roots of the Molars Can Help in Identifying the Orientation of Views. (A) The inferior border of the zygomatic process lies over the palatal root of the first molar. (B) The inferior border of the zygomatic process lies posterior to the palatal root of the first molar. This difference in position of the zygomatic process in relation to the palatal root indicates that when the image in A was made, the beam was oriented more from the posterior than when the image in B was made. The same conclusion can be reached independently by examining the roots of the first molar. The palatal root is superimposed over the distobuccal root in the image in A, but it lies between the two buccal roots in the image in B.

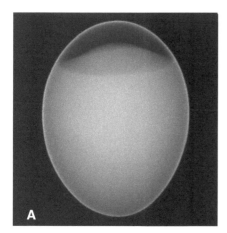 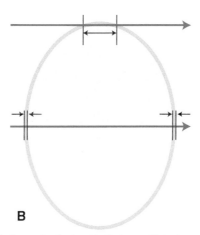 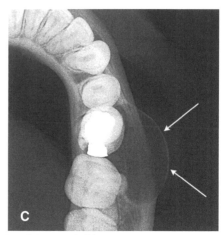

Fig. 6.15 Eggshell Effect. (A) Radiograph of a hard-boiled egg. Note how the rim of the eggshell is opaque even though it is uniform in thickness. (B) Schematic view of the egg being exposed to an x-ray beam. The top photon has a tangential path through the apex of the egg and a longer path through the shell of the egg than the lower photon. As a result, photons traveling through the periphery of a curved surface are more attenuated than the photons traveling at right angles to the surface. (C) An expansile lesion on the buccal surface of the mandible on a cross-sectional occlusal view. The expanded cortex is more opaque than the region inside the border as a result of the eggshell effect.

of an egg being exposed to an x-ray beam. The top photon has a tangential path through the apex of the egg and a much longer path through the shell of the egg than does the lower photon, which strikes the egg at right angles to the surface and travels through two thicknesses of the shell. As a result, photons traveling through the periphery of a curved surface are more attenuated than photons traveling at right angles to the surface. Fig. 6.15C shows an expansile lesion on the buccal surface of the mandible on an occlusal view. The periphery of the expanded cortex is more opaque than the region inside the expanded border. The cortical bone is not thicker on the cortex than over the rest of the lesion, but rather the x-ray beam is more attenuated in this region because of the longer path length of photons through the bony cortex on the periphery. This eggshell effect accounts for why normal structures such as the lamina dura, the border of the maxillary sinuses and nasal fossa, and abnormal structures, including the corticated walls of cysts and benign tumors, are well demonstrated on plain radiographs. Soft tissue masses, such as the nose and tongue, do not show an eggshell effect because they are uniform rather than being composed of a dense layer surrounding a more lucent interior.

BIBLIOGRAPHY

Buccal-Object Rule
Clark CA. A method of ascertaining the relative position of unerupted teeth by means of film radiographs. *Proc R Soc Med Odontol Sect.* 1910;3:87–90.
Gutmann JL, Endo C. Clark's rule vis a vis the buccal object rule: its evolution and application in endodontics. *J Hist Dent.* 2011;59(1):12–15.
Jacobs SG. Radiographic localization of unerupted maxillary anterior teeth using the vertical tube shift technique: the history and application of the

method with some case reports. *Am J Orthod Dentofac Orthop.* 1999;116:415–423.
Jacobs SG. Radiographic localization of unerupted teeth: further findings about the vertical tube shift method and other localization techniques. *Am J Orthod Dentofac Orthop.* 2000;118:439–447.
Katz JO, Langlais RP, Underhill TE, et al. Localization of paraoral soft tissue calcifications: the known object rule. *Oral Surg Oral Med Oral Pathol.* 1989;67:459–463.
Khabbaz MG, Serefoglou MH. The application of the buccal object rule for the determination of calcified root canals. *Int Endod J.* 1996;29:284–287.
Ludlow JB. The buccal object rule. *Dentomaxillofac Radiol.* 1999;28:258.
Richards AG. The buccal object rule. *Dent Radiogr Photogr.* 1980;53:37–56.
Richards AG. The buccal object rule. http://www.unc.edu/~jbl/BuccalObjectRule.html.

Paralleling Technique
Forsberg J. A comparison of the paralleling and bisecting-angle radiographic techniques in endodontics. *Int Endod J.* 1987;20:177–182.
Forsberg J. Radiographic reproduction of endodontic "working length" comparing the paralleling and the bisecting-angle techniques. *Oral Surg Oral Med Oral Pathol.* 1987;64:353–360.
Forsberg J, Halse A. Radiographic simulation of a periapical lesion comparing the paralleling and the bisecting-angle techniques. *Int Endod J.* 1994;27:133–138.
Rushton VE, Horner K. A comparative study of radiographic quality with five periapical techniques in general dental practice. *Dentomaxillofac Radiol.* 1994;23:37–45.
Rushton VE, Horner K. The acceptability of five periapical radiographic techniques to dentists and patients. *Br Dent J.* 1994;177:325–331.
Schulze RK, d'Hoedt B. A method to calculate angular disparities between object and receptor in "paralleling technique". *Dentomaxillofac Radiol.* 2002;31:32–38.

7

Intraoral Projections

Sanjay M. Mallya

Intraoral radiographic imaging examinations are the backbone of diagnostic imaging for the general dentist. Intraoral images can be divided into three categories:

- Periapical projections, which show the entire length of the tooth and the surrounding bone
- Bitewing projections, which show only the crowns of teeth and the adjacent alveolar crests
- Occlusal projections, which show an area of teeth and bone larger than periapical images

A full-mouth radiographic series consists of periapical and bitewing projections (Fig. 7.1; Box 7.1). These projections, when well exposed and properly processed (if film-based), can provide valuable diagnostic information to complement the clinical examination. As with any clinical procedure, the operator must clearly understand the goals of diagnostic imaging and the criteria for evaluating the quality of performance.

Radiographic images should be made only when the historical or clinical findings identify a need for the additional diagnostic information that can be provided by a radiograph. The imaging modality selected and the frequency of such examinations will vary with the individual circumstances of each patient (see Chapter 17).

CRITERIA OF QUALITY

Every radiographic examination should produce images of optimal diagnostic quality, incorporating the following features:

- *Radiographs should record the complete areas of interest on the image.* Periapical radiographs must show the full length of the roots and at least 2 mm of periapical bone. If evidence of an abnormality is present, the area of the entire abnormality plus some surrounding normal bone should be shown by the radiographic examination. When this is not possible to achieve on a periapical radiograph, an appropriate radiographic examination must be designed considering the diagnostic objectives. These additional projections may include occlusal and panoramic radiographs and cone beam computed tomography, as indicated (see Chapters 9, 10, 11, and 17). Bitewing examinations should demonstrate each posterior proximal surface at least once. Overlap of adjacent proximal tooth surfaces should be less than one third of the enamel thickness.
- *Radiographs should have the least possible amount of distortion.* Most distortion is caused by improper angulation of the x-ray beam rather than by the curvature of the structures being examined or inappropriate positioning of the receptor. Close attention to proper positioning of the receptor and x-ray tube, as described in the principles of projection geometry (Chapter 6), results in diagnostically useful images.
- *Images should have optimal density and contrast to facilitate interpretation.* Radiographic exposure settings, including peak kilovoltage

(kVp), the milliamperage (mA), and exposure time (s) are crucial parameters that influence density and contrast for both digital- and film-based radiography. When film-based imaging is used, faulty processing can adversely affect the quality of a properly exposed radiograph (see Chapter 5). Likewise, improper application of digital image enhancements such as contrast and sharpening may produce artifacts that compromise diagnostic interpretation (see Chapter 4).

When evaluating radiographic images, the practitioner must assess whether the initial diagnostic objectives of the examination are adequately met and whether there is a need to retake specific views. For example, a single projection in a full-mouth radiographic series may fail to open a contact or show a periapical region. However, retakes are not necessary if that missing information is available on another view.

PERIAPICAL RADIOGRAPHY

Periapical radiographs are commonly used in dentistry and show the entire length of the tooth and the surrounding bone. The diagnostic objectives of periapical radiographs are summarized in Box 7.2.

Two intraoral projection techniques are commonly used for periapical radiography: (1) the *paralleling technique* and (2) the *bisecting-angle* technique. Both techniques can be applied to digital- and film-based imaging. The paralleling technique is preferred because it provides images with less distortion of the dentition. When anatomic configuration (e.g., palate and floor of the mouth) precludes strict adherence to the paralleling concept, slight modifications may have to be made. If the anatomic constraints are extreme, the principles of the bisecting-angle technique may be used to accomplish the required receptor placement and determine the vertical angulation of the tube.

The term *image receptor* refers to any medium used to capture an image, including film, charge-coupled devices (CCDs), complementary metal oxide semiconductor (CMOS) sensors, or storage phosphor plates. The principles for making projection radiographs are the same for each of these receptor types; thus this chapter uses the general term *receptor* to refer any of the image receptors.

Paralleling Technique

The central principle of the paralleling technique (also called the *right-angle technique* or *long-cone technique*) is that the x-ray receptor is supported parallel to the long axis of the teeth and the central ray of the x-ray beam is directed at right angles to the teeth and receptor (Fig. 7.2). This orientation of the receptor, teeth, and central ray minimizes geometric distortion and presents the teeth and supporting bone in their true anatomic relationships.

Due to anatomic constraints, this parallel orientation places image receptor toward the middle of the oral cavity, away from the teeth. This

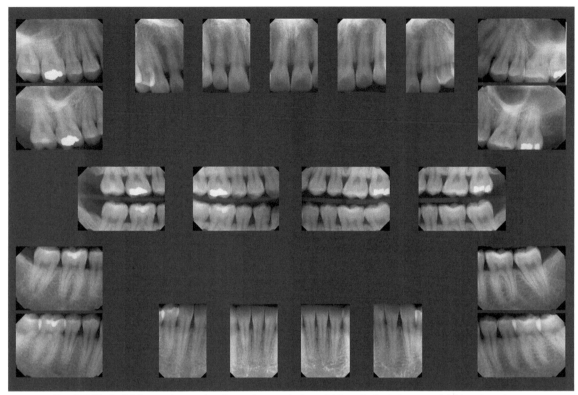

Fig. 7.1 Typical full-mouth set of radiographs consisting of 17 periapical views and 4 bitewing views.

Receptor-Holding Instruments

Receptor holders facilitate the positioning of the receptor in the patient's mouth. These holders stabilize the receptor to a bite block (Fig. 7.4). When the patient bites gently on this bite block, it places the receptor parallel to the tooth's long axis. Many of these receptor holders are specific for various brands of digital sensors, storage phosphor plates, or film. It is also important to use a receptor-holding instrument that has an external guiding ring. This guiding ring is used to align the x-ray collimator; it ensures that the receptor is centered in the beam behind the teeth of interest and that the x-ray beam is perpendicular to the receptor and teeth (see Fig. 7.4). Rectangular collimators should be used to reduce the patient's exposure to radiation (see Chapter 3).

increases the object-to-receptor distance and results in higher image magnification and poor geometric sharpness. To compensate for the resultant distortion and lack of sharpness, the paralleling technique is used with a relatively long source-to-object distance (Fig. 7.3). The paralleling technique can be used effectively with film, CCD, or CMOS sensors or with storage phosphor plates.

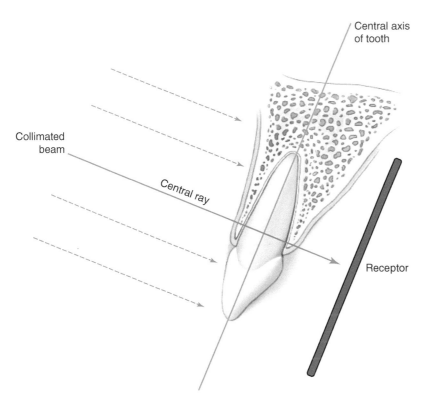

Central axis of tooth

Collimated beam

Central ray

Receptor

Fig. 7.2 Paralleling technique illustrates the parallelism between the long axis of the tooth and the receptor. The central ray is directed perpendicular to each. This technique minimizes image distortion but requires a receptor holder.

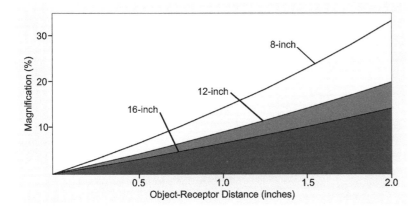

Fig. 7.3 Graph showing change in image magnification with change in the object-receptor distance, using source-object distances of 8 inches, 12 inches, and 16 inches. Magnification caused by an increased object-receptor can be minimized by increasing the source-object distance.

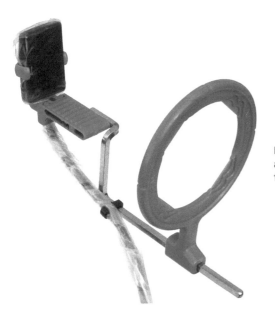

Fig. 7.4 Receptor-holding instruments. XCP instrument for anterior views shown with sensor and cord wrapped in disposable sensor cover for infection control and to protect the sensor from saliva. (Courtesy Dentsply Rinn, Elgin, IL.)

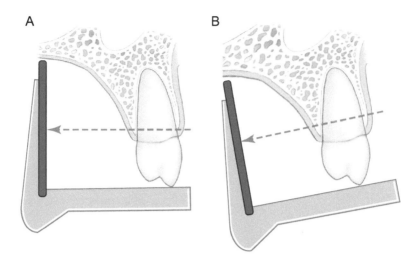

Fig. 7.5 Anatomic constraints in using the paralleling technique. (A) Optimal position of the receptor parallel to the long axis of the tooth. (B) A shallow palate limits placement of the receptor parallel to the tooth. Note that the x-ray beam is perpendicular to the receptor but not the tooth, resulting in distortion.

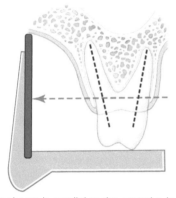

Fig. 7.6 The x-ray beam is parallel to the central axis of the tooth and the receptor. Note that the x-ray beam is at different angles to the buccal and palatal root of the molar, resulting in unequal distortion. Increasing the source-object distance by using a long cone will limit this distortion.

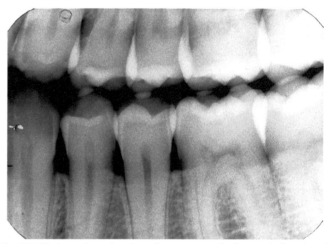

Fig. 7.7 Horizontal overlapping of crowns results from misdirection of the central ray in the horizontal plane.

Receptor Placement

For the best images, the receptor should be positioned parallel to the teeth and deep into the lingual vestibule or palatal vault; this is particularly important when rigid sensors are used because they are bulkier than film. For maxillary projections, the superior border of the receptor generally rests at the height of the palatal vault in the midline. Similarly, for mandibular projections, the receptor should be used to displace the tongue posteriorly or toward the midline to allow the inferior border of the receptor to rest on the floor of the mouth away from the mucosa on the lingual surface of the mandible.

Often anatomic variations do not allow the receptor to be placed deep enough to capture an image of the entire tooth length—for example, a shallow palate (Fig. 7.5), a shallow floor of the mouth, and tori. Another anatomic limitation is that all the roots of a multirooted tooth may not be placed parallel to the receptor, resulting in differential distortion of the roots (Fig. 7.6).

Angulation of the Tube Head

Orient the aiming cylinder of the x-ray machine in the vertical and horizontal planes to align with the aiming ring. The plane of the opening of the cylinder must be parallel to the plane of the aiming ring. The horizontal direction of the beam primarily influences the degree of overlapping of the images of the crowns at the interproximal spaces (Fig. 7.7).

Bisecting Angle Technique

In contemporary dental practice, the bisecting angle technique has been largely replaced by the paralleling technique. Nevertheless the bisecting angle technique may be useful when the operator is unable to apply the paralleling technique because of large rigid sensors or the anatomy of the patient. The bisecting angle technique is based on a simple geometric theorem, Cieszynski's rule of isometry, which states that two triangles are equal when they share one complete side and have two equal angles. Dental radiography applies the theorem as follows. The receptor is positioned as close as possible to the lingual surface of the teeth, resting in the palate or in the floor of the mouth (Fig. 7.8). The plane of the receptor and the long axis of the teeth form an angle with its apex at the incisal edge or occlusal surface. Consider an imaginary line that bisects this angle and direct the central ray of the beam at right angles to this bisector. This creates two triangles with two equal angles and a common side (the imaginary bisector). The hypotenuses of the two triangles represent the actual tooth length and the image length; theoretically they are the same.

To reproduce the length of each root of a multirooted tooth accurately, the central beam must be angled differently for each root. Another limitation of this technique is that the alveolar ridge often projects coronal to its true position and distorts the apparent height of the alveolar bone around the teeth.

Receptor-Holding Instruments

Several methods can be used to support receptors intraorally for bisecting angle projections. The preferred method is to use a receptor-holding bisecting angle instrument with an external device to localize the x-ray beam and guide the appropriate vertical angle. The bisecting angle instrument (BAI, Dentsply Rinn Corporation) uses an angled bite block and secures the receptor at an angle to the tooth. A metal arm attaches to the bite block and anchors an external aiming ring to ensure full coverage of the receptor by the primary x-ray beam. There are several other receptor holders and disposable bite blocks that can be used to support a receptor for this technique. It is undesirable to have the patient support the receptor from the lingual surface with his or her forefinger. Patients often use excessive force and may bend the film or storage phosphor plates, causing distortion of the image. Also, the receptor might slip, resulting in an improper image field. Finally, without an external guide to the position of the receptor, the x-ray beam may miss part of the receptor, resulting in a partial image (cone cut).

Positioning of the Patient

Maxillary projections. The patient should be seated upright in the dental chair with the sagittal plane vertical and the occlusal plane horizontal.

Mandibular projections. The patient should be seated upright in the dental chair with the sagittal plane vertical. The head is tilted back slightly to compensate for the changed occlusal plane when the mouth is opened.

Receptor Placement

Similar to the paralleling technique, the receptor is positioned behind the area of interest, with the apical end against the mucosa on the lingual or palatal surface. The occlusal or incisal edge is oriented against the teeth with an edge of the receptor extending just beyond the teeth. If necessary for the patient's comfort, the anterior corner of a film can be softened by bending it before it is placed against the mucosa. Care must be taken not to bend the film excessively because this may result in considerable image distortion and in pressure defects in the emulsion that are apparent on the processed film. Such bending is less marked with storage phosphor plates, and the rigid structure of the CCD or CMOS sensors cannot be bent to adapt to the arch shape.

Angulation of the Tube Head

Horizontal angulation. When a receptor-holding device with a beam-localizing ring is used, it facilitates alignment with the x-ray beam, so that the central ray is directed through the contacts in the region being examined. If the receptor-holding device does not have a beam-localizing feature, the tube is angled in the horizontal plane to direct the central ray through the contacts. The edge of the x-ray beam collimator cone should be parallel to the buccal surfaces of the teeth being examined.

Vertical angulation. In using the bisecting angle technique, the goal is to aim the central ray of the x-ray beam perpendicular to a plane bisecting the angle between the receptor and the long axis of the tooth. However, if bisecting angle instruments are not used, accurate orientation of the beam is not practically achievable for every single projection to be made. Instead, the clinician uses predetermined angles for specific anatomic regions (Table 7.1). Proper patient positioning is imperative when using

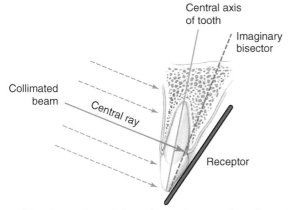

Fig. 7.8 Bisecting angle technique shows the central ray directed at a right angle to the plane that bisects the angle between the long axis of the tooth and the receptor.

TABLE 7.1	Angulation Guidelines for Bisecting-Angle Projections					
	REGION-SPECIFIC SETTINGS					
	NORTH AMERICA		**INDIA[a]**		**BRAZIL[b]**	
Projection	Maxilla	Mandible	Maxilla	Mandible	Maxilla	Mandible
Incisors	+40 degrees	−15 degrees	+45 degrees	−25 degrees	+45 to +55 degrees	−25 to −15 degrees
Canines	+45 degrees	−20 degrees	+45 degrees	−20 degrees	+40 to +50 degrees	−20 to −10 degrees
Premolars	+30 degrees	−10 degrees	+30 degrees	−15 degrees	+30 to +45 degrees	−10 to −5 degrees
Molars	+20 degrees	−5 degrees	+30 degrees	−10 to 0 degrees	+20 to +35 degrees	−5 to 0 degrees

[a]Data courtesy Dr. Freny Karjodkar, from *Essentials of Oral and Maxillofacial Radiology*, 2014, Jaypee Publishers.
[b]Data collated by Prof. Dr. Matheus Lima de Oliveira, UNICAMP—University of Campinas, Piracicaba Dental School.
The occlusal plane is oriented parallel with the floor. By convention, with a positive (+) angulation, the aiming cylinder points downward, and with a negative (−) angulation, it points upward.

these angulations—the patient must be positioned with the occlusal plane parallel to the horizontal plane. The predetermined angles are based on typical human jaw anatomy and are not customized to individual patients. Often the radiographer may need to adjust these angles to account for anatomic variations, such as proclination of the teeth.

Image distortion is likely and limits effective use of the bisecting angle technique. Furthermore, individual divergent roots of multirooted teeth will manifest different extents of distortion.

Diagnostically unacceptable image distortion may require retaking the radiograph with a change in vertical angulation. The pattern of distortion should guide the radiographer to select an appropriate angle. Image foreshortening indicates that the vertical angulation is too high. In contrast, image elongation indicates insufficient vertical angulation.

General Steps for Making Intraoral Radiographs

The following steps describe the overall general procedure to obtain a full-mouth set of radiographs, made using the paralleling technique.

- *Prepare unit for exposure.* Place barriers for universal infection control (see Chapter 16) and have receptors and receptor-holding instruments ready at chairside.
- *Greet and seat the patient.* Position the patient upright in the chair with the back and head well supported, and briefly describe the procedures that are to be performed. Position the dental chair low for maxillary projections and elevated for mandibular projections. Ask the patient to remove eyeglasses and all removable appliances. Jewelry that may be in the path of the x-ray beam, such as nose, lip, and tongue rings should be removed. Drape the patient with a protective apron regardless of whether a single image or a full series is to be made. In the United States, the requirement of protective aprons is regulated by state radiation regulations.
- *Adjust the x-ray unit setting.* Set the x-ray machine for the proper kVp, mA, and exposure time. Generally only the exposure time is adjusted for the various anatomic locations.
- *Wash your hands thoroughly and wear appropriate personal protective equipment.* Wash your hands with soap and water, preferably in front of the patient or at least in an area where the patient can observe or be aware of this step. Put on disposable gloves and a disposable gown or coat.
- *Examine the oral cavity.* Before placing any receptors in the mouth, examine the teeth to estimate their axial inclination, which influences the placement of the receptor. Also note tori or other obstructions that may modify receptor placement. Ensure that all removable appliances and jewelry are removed.
- *Position the x-ray tube head.* Bring the x-ray tube head to the side to be examined so that it is easily accessible for final positioning after the receptor has been placed in the mouth.
- *Position the receptor.* Insert the receptor into the holding device and position the receptor and holding device in the region of the patient's mouth to be examined. Angle the receptor holder such that the film

or sensor is parallel to the occlusal plane. Leading with the apical end of the receptor, rotate it into the oral cavity. This technique avoids the need for the patient to open wide. For maxillary views, place the receptor in the mouth as far from the teeth as possible, near the midline of the palate, where there is the maximal space available. The added space allows the receptor to be oriented parallel to the long axis of the teeth. With the receptor now in the mouth, place it gently on the palate or floor of the mouth. For all bitewing and mandibular periapical images, it is useful to shift the mandible to the side being imaged; this decreases patient discomfort because there is now more room for the sensor on the lingual side of the mandible. After the sensor is positioned, rotate the receptor-holding instrument until the bite block rests on the teeth to be radiographed and place a cotton roll between the bite block and the opposing teeth. The cotton roll helps stabilize the receptor-holding instrument and decreases patient discomfort. Holding the instrument and receptor in place, ask the patient to close the mouth gently. Solid-state receptors (CCD or CMOS sensors) have approximately of 2 to 4 mm of "dead space" between the edge of the plastic casing and the image capture chip, and the captured anatomic region is smaller than the external sensor size. The width of the dead space varies with manufacturer. One manufacturer, XDR Radiology, has a patented technology that provides less dead space toward the mesial imaging end and facilitates imaging of the canine/premolar contact.
- *Position the x-ray tube.* Adjust the vertical and horizontal angulation of the tube head to correspond to the receptor-holding instrument. The end of the aiming ring of the x-ray tube head must be flush or parallel to the guide ring instrument. Alignment is satisfactory when the aiming cylinder covers the port and is within the limits of the face shield. Caution the patient not to move.
- *Make the exposure.* Make the exposure with the preset exposure time. If the receptor is a film or storage phosphor plate, remove the receptor from the patient's mouth after exposure, dry it with a paper towel, remove the infection control sleeve, and place the receptor in an appropriate receptacle outside the exposure area. If the receptor is a CCD or CMOS sensor, you may keep it in the patient's mouth and reposition it for the next view. Ensure patient comfort after each exposure.

Individual Periapical Projections

A typical full-mouth radiographic series consists of 21 images (see Box 7.1 and Fig. 7.1). To facilitate work flow, it is useful to establish a regular sequence of projections in making exposures. It is practical to start with the anterior views because they cause less discomfort for the patient. The following section describes procedural details to make periapical radiographs using the paralleling technique. It describes the field encompassed in the image, the placement of the receptor, the projection of the central ray, and the positioning of the aiming ring.

Text continued on p. 106

PARALLELING TECHNIQUE
Maxillary Central Incisor Projection (Fig. 7.9)

Image Field: The field of view on these radiographs should include both central incisors and their periapical areas (see Fig. 7.9A and B)
Receptor Placement: Place a No. 1 receptor at about the level of the second premolars or first molars to take advantage of the maximal palatal height so that the entire length of the teeth can be projected on it. Have the receptor resting on the palate with its midline centered with the midline of the arch (see Fig. 7.9C). Position the receptor's long axis parallel to the long axis of the maxillary central incisors (see Fig. 7.9D).
Projection of Central Ray: Direct the central ray through the contact point of the central incisors and perpendicular to the plane of the receptors and roots of the teeth (see Fig. 7.9C). Because the axial inclination of the maxillary incisors is about 15 to 20 degrees, the vertical angulation of the tube should be at the same positive angle (see Fig. 7.9E). The tube should have no horizontal angulation (see Fig. 7.9C).
Point of Entry: Direct the point of entry of the central ray high on the lip, in the midline, just below the septum of the nostril (see Fig. 7.9E). If the palatal vault is unusually low or a palatal torus is present, it may be necessary to tilt the receptor holder positively and compromise a completely parallel relationship between the receptor and the teeth to ensure that the periapical region is included on the image.

PARALLELING TECHNIQUE
Maxillary Lateral Projection (Fig. 7.10)

Image Field: This projection should show the lateral incisor and its periapical field centered on the radiograph (see Fig. 7.10A and B). Include the mesial interproximal area with the distal aspect of the central incisor on the radiograph so that no overlap is evident.
Receptor Placement: Place a No. 1 receptor deep in the oral cavity parallel with the long axis and the mesiodistal plane of the maxillary lateral incisor (see Fig. 7.10C and D).
Projection of Central Ray: Direct the central ray through the middle of the lateral incisor (see Fig. 7.10C), with no overlapping of the margins of the crowns at the interproximal space on its mesial aspect. Do not attempt to visualize the distal contact with the canine (see Fig. 7.10B).
Point of Entry: Orient the central ray to enter high on the lip about 1 cm from the midline (see Fig. 7.10E).

PARALLELING TECHNIQUE
Maxillary Canine Projection (Fig. 7.11)

Image Field: This projection should demonstrate the entire canine, with its periapical area, in the midline of the radiograph (see Fig. 7.11A and B). Open the mesial contact area. Ignore the distal contact because it will be visualized on other projections.
Receptor Placement: Place a No. 1 receptor against the palate, well away from the palatal surface of the teeth (see Fig. 7.11C). Orient the receptor packet with its anterior edge at about the middle of the lateral incisor and its long axis parallel with the long axis of the canine (see Fig. 7.11D).
Projection of Central Ray: Position the holding instrument so that it directs the beam through the mesial contact of the canine (see Fig. 7.11C). Do not attempt to open the distal contact.
Point of Entry: Direct the central ray through the canine eminence. The point of entry is at about the intersection of the distal and inferior borders of the ala of the nose (see Fig. 7.11E).

PARALLELING TECHNIQUE
Maxillary Premolar Projection (Fig. 7.12)

Image Field: The radiograph of this region should include the images of the distal half of the canine and the premolars, with room for at least the first molar (see Fig. 7.12A and B).
Receptor Placement: Place a No. 2 receptor in the mouth with the long dimension parallel with the occlusal plane and near the palatal midline (see Fig. 7.12C). The receptor should extend far enough forward to cover the distal half of the canine. It should also include the premolars and the first molar and maybe the mesial portion of the second molar (see Fig. 7.12B). The plane of the receptor should be nearly vertical to correspond with the long axis of the premolar teeth (see Fig. 7.12C). Position the receptor-holding device so that the long axis of the receptor is parallel with the buccal plane of the premolars. This establishes the proper horizontal angulation (see Fig. 7.12C).
Projection of Central Ray: Direct the central ray perpendicular to the receptor (see Fig. 7.12D). The horizontal angulation of the holding instrument should be adjusted to permit the beam to pass through the interproximal area between the first and second premolars (see Fig. 7.12C).
Point of Entry: Place the holding instrument so that the central ray passes through the center of the second premolar root. This point is usually below the pupil of the eye (see Fig. 7.12E).

PARALLELING TECHNIQUE
Maxillary Molar Projection (Fig. 7.13)

Image Field: The radiograph of this region should show the images of the distal half of the second premolar, the three maxillary permanent molars, and some of the tuberosity (see Fig. 7.13A and B). Include the same area on the receptor even if some or all molars are missing. If the third molar is impacted in an area other than the region of the tuberosity, a distal oblique or extraoral projection (e.g., panoramic or oblique lateral jaw view) may be required.
Receptor Placement: When placing the No. 2 receptor for this projection, position the long dimension of the receptor nearly horizontal to minimize brushing the palate and dorsum of the tongue. When the receptor is in the region to be examined, rotate it into position with a firm and definite motion. This maneuver is important in avoiding the gag reflex, and resolute action by the operator enhances the patient's confidence. Place the receptor far enough posterior to cover the first, second, and third molar areas and some of the tuberosity. The anterior border should just cover the distal aspect of the second premolar (see Fig. 7.12B). To cover the molars from crown to apices, place the receptor at the midline of the palate (see Fig. 7.13C). In this position, room should be available to orient the receptor parallel with the molar teeth. The mesial or distal rotation of the receptor-holding device should ensure that the long axis of the receptor is parallel with the mean buccal plane of the molars (to establish the proper horizontal angulation). A shallow palate may require slight tipping of the holding instrument to avoid bending the receptor.
Note: In some cases the size of the mouth (length of the arch) will not allow positioning of the receptor-holding device as far posterior as recommended for the molar projection. However, by placing the receptor-holding device so that half the tube alignment ring or face shield is behind the outer canthus of the eye, the molars and part of the tuberosity usually can be included in the image of the molar projection.
Projection of Central Ray: Direct the central ray perpendicular to the receptor (see Fig. 7.13D). Adjust the horizontal angulation of the receptor-holding device to direct the beam at right angles to the buccal surfaces of the molar teeth (see Fig. 7.13C).
Point of Entry: The point of entry of the central ray should be on the cheek below the outer canthus of the eye and the zygoma at the position of the maxillary second molar (see Fig. 7.13E).

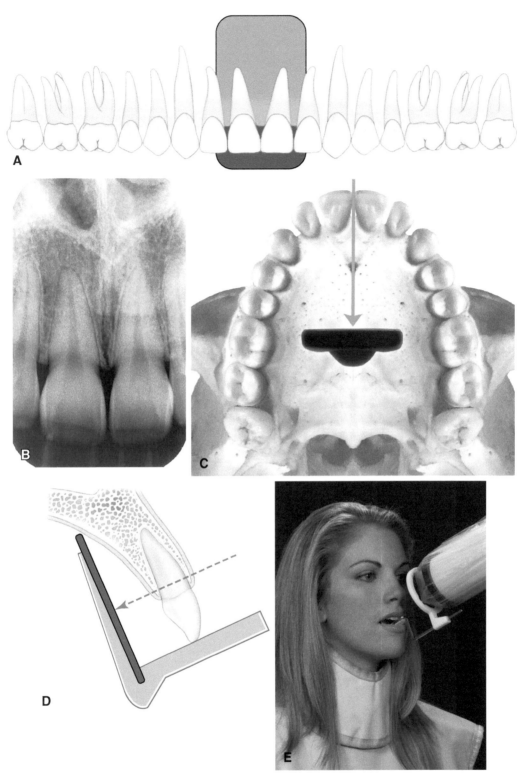

Fig. 7.9 Maxillary central incisor periapical projection. (A) The shaded area outlines the image field. (B) Periapical radiograph of the maxillary central incisor. (C) Position of the receptor in the oral cavity and direction of the x-ray beam *(blue arrow)*. (D) Graphic representation of the image receptor and the x-ray beam relative to the long axis of the central incisor. (E) Position of the patient with the receptor holder in place and the aiming ring aligned for exposure.

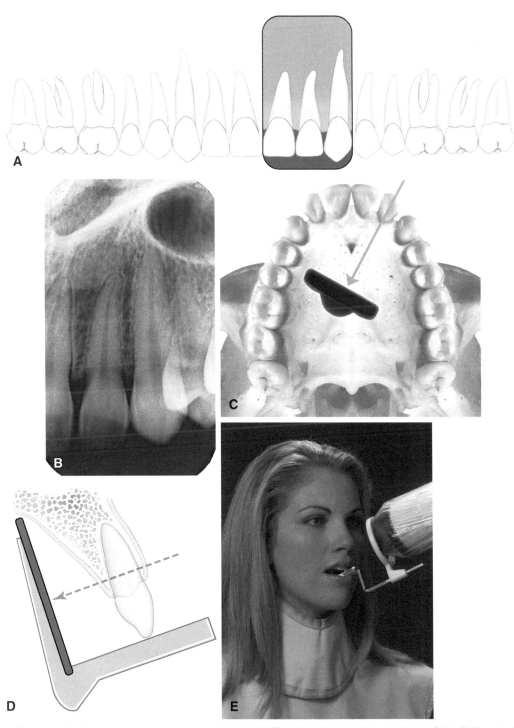

Fig. 7.10 Maxillary lateral incisor periapical projection. (A) The shaded area outlines the image field. (B) Periapical radiograph of the maxillary lateral incisor. (C) Position of the receptor in the oral cavity and direction of the x-ray beam *(blue arrow)*. (D) Graphic representation of the image receptor and the x-ray beam relative to the long axis of the lateral incisor. (E) Position of the patient with the receptor holder in place and the aiming ring aligned for exposure.

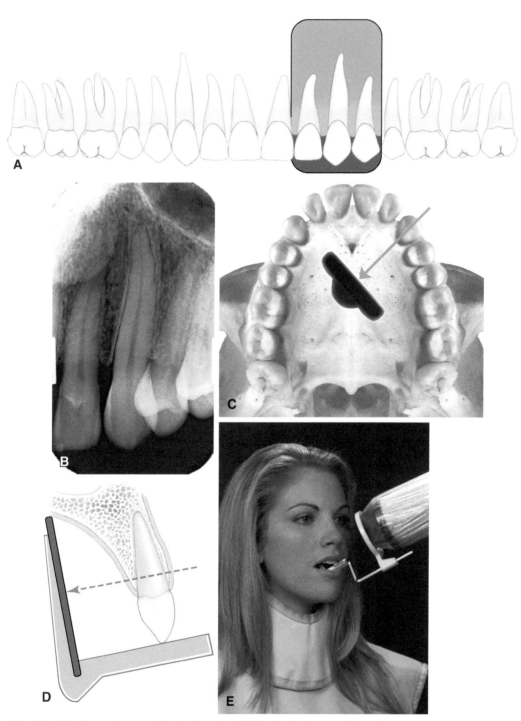

Fig. 7.11 Maxillary canine periapical projection. (A) The shaded area outlines the image field. (B) Periapical radiograph of the maxillary canine. (C) Position of the receptor in the oral cavity and direction of the x-ray beam *(blue arrow)*. (D) Graphic representation of the image receptor and the x-ray beam relative to the long axis of the lateral incisor. (E) Position of the patient with the receptor holder in place and the aiming ring aligned for exposure.

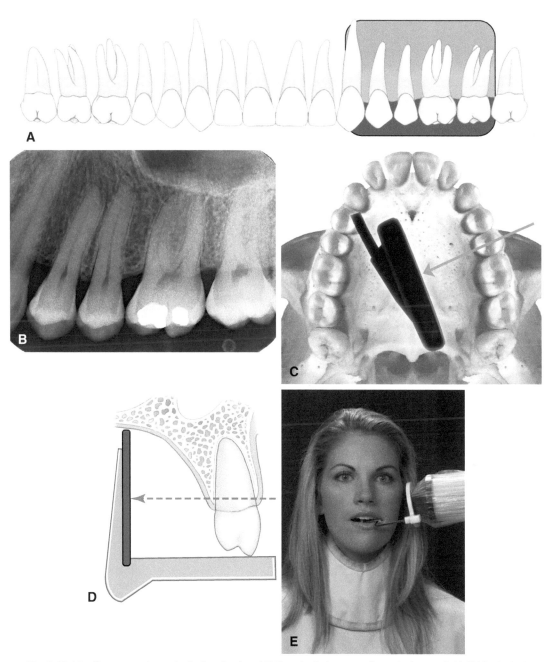

Fig. 7.12 Maxillary premolar periapical projection. (A) The shaded area outlines the image field. (B) Periapical radiograph of the maxillary premolar region. (C) Position of the receptor in the oral cavity and direction of the x-ray beam *(blue arrow)*. (D) Graphic representation of the image receptor and the x-ray beam relative to the long axis of the premolar. (E) Position of the patient with the receptor holder in place and the aiming ring aligned for exposure.

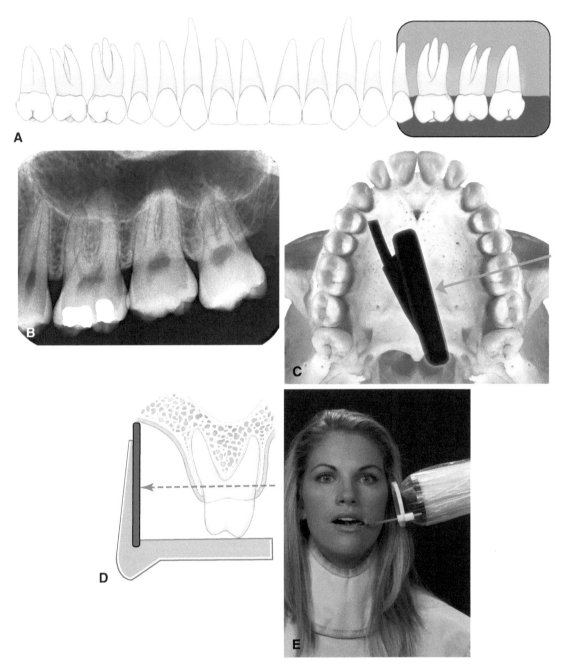

Fig. 7.13 Maxillary molar periapical projection. (A) The shaded area outlines the image field. (B) Periapical radiograph of the maxillary molar region. (C) Position of the receptor in the oral cavity and direction of the x-ray beam *(blue arrow)*. (D) Graphic representation of the image receptor and the x-ray beam relative to the long axis of the molar. (E) Position of the patient with the receptor holder in place and the aiming ring aligned for exposure.

PARALLELING TECHNIQUE
Mandibular Centrolateral Projection (Fig. 7.14)

Image Field: Center the image of the mandibular central and lateral incisors and their periapical areas on the receptor (see Fig. 7.14A and B). Because the space in this area is frequently restricted, use two size 1 receptors for the incisors on each side to provide good coverage with minimal discomfort. In addition, the incisor contact areas are better visualized on two narrower anterior receptors because the angulation of the central ray can be adjusted for the contact area on each side (see Fig. 7.14C).

Receptor Placement: Place the long dimension of the No. 1 receptor vertically behind the central and lateral incisors with the contact area centered and the lower border below the tongue. Position the receptor posteriorly as far as possible, usually between the premolars (see Fig. 7.14C). With the receptor resting gently on the floor of the mouth as the fulcrum, tip the instrument downward until the receptor-holder bite block is resting on the incisors. Instruct the patient to close the mouth slowly. As the patient is closing slowly and the floor of the mouth is relaxing, rotate the instrument with the teeth as the fulcrum to align the receptor to be more parallel with the teeth (see Fig. 7.14D).

Projection of Central Ray: Orient the central ray through the interproximal space between the central and lateral incisors (see Fig. 7.14C).

Point of Entry: The central ray enters below the lower lip and about 1 cm lateral to the midline (see Fig. 7.14E).

PARALLELING TECHNIQUE
Mandibular Canine Projection (Fig. 7.15)

Image Field: This image should show the entire mandibular canine and its periapical area (see Fig. 7.15A and B). Open its mesial contact area. The distal contact is included on other projections.

Receptor Placement: Place a No. 1 receptor packet in the mouth with its long dimension vertical and the canine in the midline of the receptor. Position it as far lingual as the tongue and contralateral alveolar process permit (see Fig. 7.15C), with its long axis parallel and in line with the canine (see Fig. 7.15D). The instrument must be tipped with the bite block on the canine before the patient is asked to close.

Projection of Central Ray: Direct the central ray through the mesial contact of the canine without regard to the distal contact (see Fig. 7.15C).

Point of Entry: The point of entry is nearly perpendicular to the ala of the nose, over the position of the canine, and about 3 cm above the inferior border of the mandible (Fig. 7.15E).

PARALLELING TECHNIQUE
Mandibular Premolar Projection (Fig. 7.16)

Image Field: The radiograph of this area should show the distal half of the canine, the two premolars, and the first molar (see Fig. 7.16A and B).

Receptor Placement: Bring the No. 2 receptor into the mouth with its plane nearly horizontal. Rotate the lead edge to the floor of the mouth between the tongue and the teeth with the anterior border near the midline of the canine. Place the receptor away from the teeth to position it in the deeper portion of the mouth (see Fig. 7.16C). Placing the receptor toward the midline also provides more room for the anterior border of the receptor in the curvature of the jaw as it sweeps anteriorly. Prevent the anterior border from contacting the very sensitive attached gingiva on the lingual surface of the mandible.

Projection of Central Ray: Position the receptor-holding instrument to project the central ray through the second premolar molar area. The vertical angulation should be small, nearly parallel with the occlusal plane, to keep the receptor as nearly parallel with the long axis of the teeth as possible (see Fig. 7.16D). Adjust the horizontal angulation and the placement of the receptor-holding device to direct the beam through the premolar contact points (see Fig. 7.16C).

Point of Entry: The point of entry of the central ray is below the pupil of the eye and about 3 cm above the inferior border of the mandible (see Fig. 7.16E).

PARALLELING TECHNIQUE
Mandibular Molar Projection (Fig. 7.17)

Image Field: The radiograph of this region should include the distal half of the second premolar and the three mandibular permanent molars (see Fig. 7.17A and B). In the case of an impacted third molar or a pathologic condition distal to the third molar, a distal oblique molar projection or even additional extraoral projections (panoramic or lateral ramus) may be required to demonstrate the area adequately. If the molar area is edentulous, place the receptor far enough posterior to include the retromolar area in the examination.

Receptor Placement: Place the No. 2 receptor in the mouth with its plane nearly horizontal. Rotate the inferior edge downward beneath the lateral border of the tongue, displacing it medially. The anterior edge of the receptor should be at about the middle of the second premolar (see Fig. 7.17C). In most cases the tongue forces the receptor near the alveolar process and molars, aligning it parallel with the long axis of the teeth and the line of occlusion.

Projection of Central Ray: Proper placement of the holding instrument directs the central ray through the second molar. Adjust the horizontal angulation to project the beam through the contact areas (see Fig. 7.17C). Because of the slight lingual inclination of the molars, the central ray may have some slight positive angulation (approximately 8 degrees; see Fig. 7.17E).

Point of Entry: Direct the point of entry of the central ray below the outer canthus of the eye about 3 cm above the inferior border of the mandible (see Fig. 7.17E).

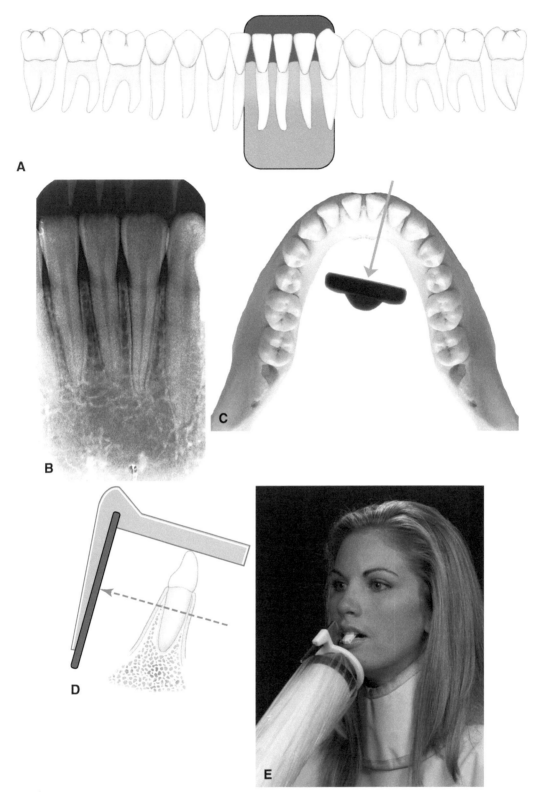

Fig. 7.14 Mandibular centrolateral incisor periapical projection. (A) The shaded area outlines the image field. (B) Periapical radiograph of the mandibular central and lateral incisors. (C) Position of the receptor in the oral cavity and direction of the x-ray beam *(blue arrow)*. (D) Graphic representation of the image receptor and the x-ray beam relative to the long axis of the mandibular incisor. (E) Position of the patient with the receptor holder in place and the aiming ring aligned for exposure.

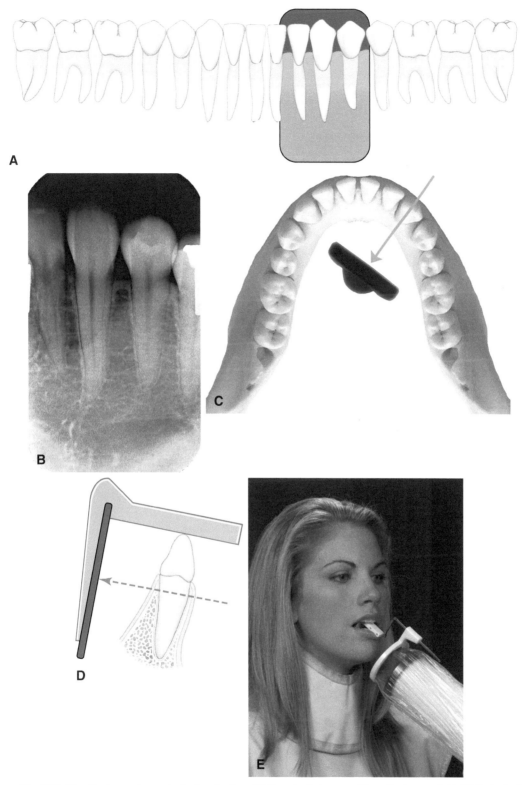

Fig. 7.15 Mandibular canine periapical projection. (A) The shaded area outlines the image field. (B) Periapical radiograph of the mandibular canine. (C) Position of the receptor in the oral cavity and direction of the x-ray beam *(blue arrow)*. (D) Graphic representation of the image receptor and the x-ray beam relative to the long axis of the mandibular canine. (E) Position of the patient with the receptor holder in place and the aiming ring aligned for exposure.

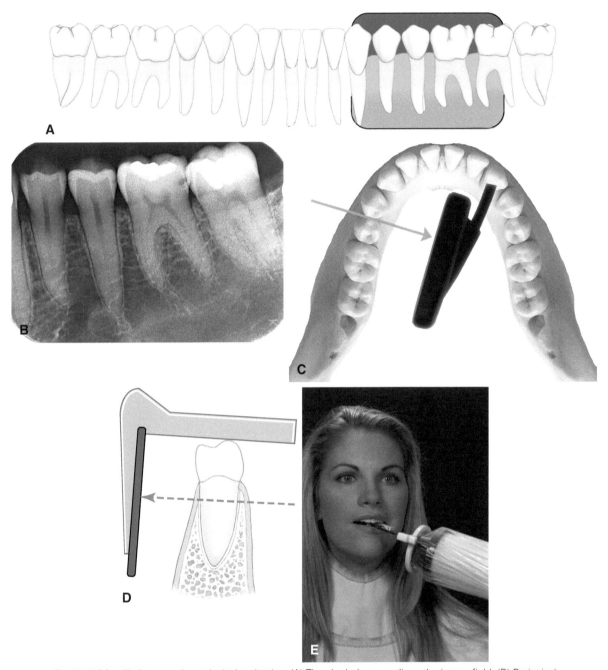

Fig. 7.16 Mandibular premolar periapical projection. (A) The shaded area outlines the image field. (B) Periapical radiograph of the mandibular premolar region. (C) Position of the receptor in the oral cavity and direction of the x-ray beam *(blue arrow)*. (D) Graphic representation of the image receptor and the x-ray beam relative to the long axis of the mandibular premolar. (E) Position of the patient with the receptor holder in place and the aiming ring aligned for exposure.

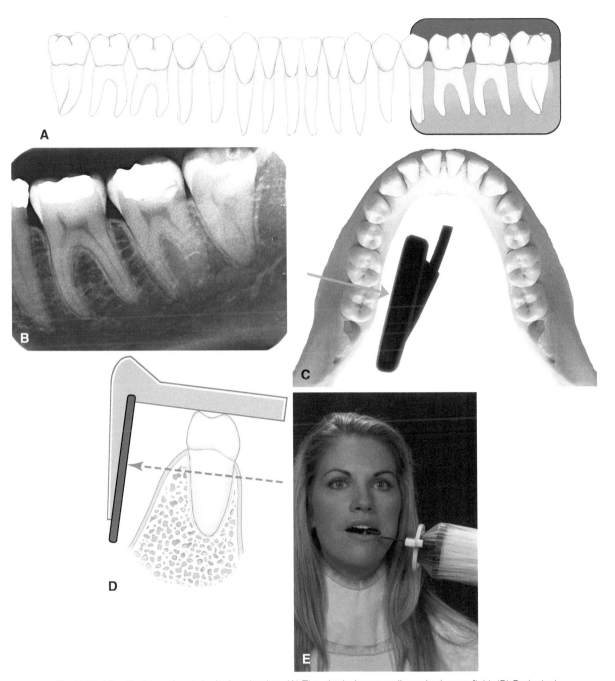

Fig. 7.17 Mandibular molar periapical projection. (A) The shaded area outlines the image field. (B) Periapical radiograph of the mandibular molar region. (C) Position of the receptor in the oral cavity and direction of the x-ray beam *(blue arrow)*. (D) Graphic representation of the image receptor and the x-ray beam relative to the long axis of the mandibular molar. (E) Position of the patient with the receptor holder in place and the aiming ring aligned for exposure.

BITEWING RADIOGRAPHY

Bitewing (also called interproximal) radiographs include the crowns of the maxillary and mandibular teeth and the alveolar crest on the same receptor. The long axis of bitewing receptors usually is oriented horizontally but may be oriented vertically. The beam is directed through the interproximal spaces and parallel with the occlusal plane. The receptor is placed parallel to the buccal and lingual surfaces of the teeth being examined and is perpendicular to the x-ray beam.

The diagnostic objectives of bitewing radiographs are listed in Box 7.3.

Receptor Holding Instruments

Receptor holders are used to position and stabilize the receptor adjacent to the teeth being examined. The bitewing instruments have a bite plate and an external guide ring to aid positioning the tube head (Fig. 7.18). The bite block facilitates positioning of the receptor parallel to the facial surfaces of the teeth being radiographed. Separate bite plates are used for film and storage phosphors, and solid-state digital sensors. The external guide ring helps to align the beam, reduce overlap between proximal surfaces, and reduces the possibility of partially exposing the receptor.

A receptor fitted with a bitewing tab or loop may be used instead of a holding device. These disposable tabs are made of stiff cardboard or plastic, and available for film, storage phosphor plates and digital sensors (Fig. 7.19).

Positioning of the Patient

The patient should be seated upright in the dental chair with the sagittal plane vertical and the occlusal plane horizontal. When receptor holders with external guiding rings are used, the patient's head position is less important. However, when bitewing tabs are used, external guidance to position the x-ray cone is not available; thus standardization of the patient's head position is important.

Receptor Placement

Horizontal bitewing projections. Typically, bitewing radiographs are made with the receptor in a horizontal orientation. Separate views are made for the premolar and molar regions. The receptor is placed in the lingual vestibule adjacent to the teeth to be radiographed, and the receptor bite block or tab is rested onto the mandibular occlusal surface. The receptor is adjusted to be parallel to the buccal surfaces of the teeth being radiographed. The edge of the receptor holders or the tab can be used to assist in this parallel orientation. Once the receptor is positioned, the patient is asked to gently occlude onto the bite block. When using the cardboard bitewing tabs, it is important to direct the patient to close gently to ensure sufficient separation of the maxillary and mandibular teeth.

Two posterior bitewing views, a premolar and a molar, are recommended for each quadrant. However, for children 12 years of age or younger, one bitewing receptor (No. 2) usually suffices. The premolar projection should include the distal half of the canines and the crowns of the premolars. Because the mandibular canines usually are more mesial than the maxillary canines, the mandibular canine is used as the guide for placement of the premolar bitewing receptor. The molar bitewing receptor is placed 1 or 2 mm beyond the most distally erupted molar (maxillary or mandibular). The anterior edge of the receptor is used to guide the position to encompass the appropriate interproximal contacts. When using film or storage phosphor plates, the imaging area of the film or plate is approximately 2 mm from the edge of the packet. When using solid-state sensors, there is approximately of 2- to 4-mm of dead space between the edge of the plastic casing and the image capture chip; this varies with manufacturer. One manufacturer, XDR Radiology, has a patented technology that provides less dead space toward mesial imaging end, and this facilitates imaging of the canine/premolar contact.

Vertical bitewing projections. Vertical bitewing projections are used when the patient has moderate to severe alveolar bone loss. Orienting the length of the receptor vertically increases the likelihood that the residual alveolar crests in the maxilla and the mandible will be recorded on the radiograph (Fig. 7.20). The principles for positioning the receptor and orienting the x-ray beam are otherwise the same as for horizontal bitewing projections. Bite blocks specifically designed for vertical orientation of the sensor are available.

Angulation of the Tube Head

Horizontal angulation. To effectively image the interproximal tooth surface without superimposition, the x-ray beam is directed through the contacts. Some difference may exist in the curvature of the mandibular and maxillary arches. However, when the x-ray beam is accurately directed through the mandibular premolar contacts, overlapping is minimal or absent in the maxillary premolar segment. A few degrees of tolerance are available in the horizontal angulation before overlapping becomes critical. Typically less than one third of the proximal enamel thickness should be overlapped. The contact between the maxillary first and second molars often is angled a few degrees more anteriorly than between the mandibular first and second molars.

When using receptor holders that have an external aiming ring, guide the horizontal position of the x-ray cone to the predetermined direction that passes the x-ray beam through the interproximal spaces. When using bitewing tabs, the horizontal orientation is less straightforward and the operator must ensure accurate horizontal orientation of the tube head to direct the beam through the interproximal spaces and encompass the entire surface of the receptor to prevent cone cuts.

Vertical angulation. The aiming cylinder is positioned about +10 degrees to project the beam parallel with the occlusal plane (occlusal dentinoenamel junction). This orientation minimizes overlapping of the opposing cusps onto the occlusal surface and thus improves the probability of detecting early occlusal lesions at the dentinoenamel junction.

Individual Bitewing Projections

Separate bitewing projections are made of the premolars and molars. The following section describes procedural details to make bitewing radiographs. It describes the field encompassed in the image, the placement of the receptor, the projection of the central ray, and the positioning of the aiming ring.

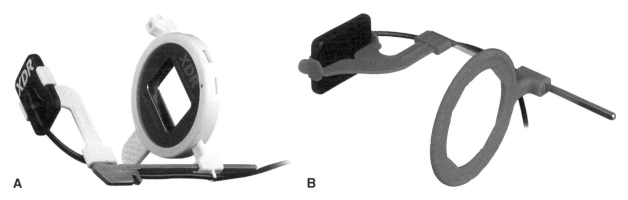

Fig. 7.18 Receptor-holding devices for bitewing radiography. (A) A wired sensor is held in position with a bite block. The aiming ring guides beam alignment and incorporates rectangular collimation to minimize patient radiation dose. (Courtesy XDR Radiology, Los Angeles, CA.) (B) XCP Bitewing Holder, with external localizing ring to guide position of the aiming tube of the x-ray machine to ensure that the entire receptor is in the x-ray beam. (Courtesy Dentsply Rinn, Elgin, IL.) Disposable barriers have been removed to show the detector and wire.

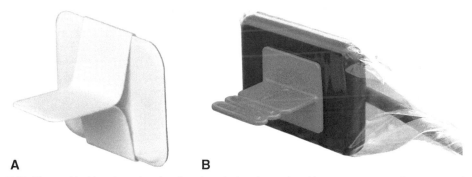

Fig. 7.19 Disposable bitewing tabs showing the tab that the patient bites on to support the receptor during exposure. (A) Cardboard loop for film and storage phosphor plates. (B) Plastic adhesive tab for use with solid-state sensors. Image shows use with the infection-control sleeve over the sensor and wire. (Courtesy Dentsply Rinn, Elgin, IL.)

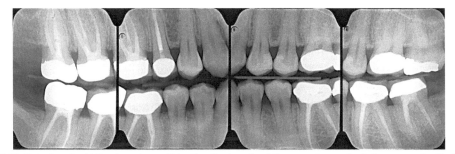

Fig. 7.20 Set of vertical bitewing views. Orienting the length of the receptor vertically increases the likelihood that the residual alveolar crests in the maxilla and the mandible will be recorded on the radiograph even in patients with extensive alveolar bone loss.

PREMOLAR BITEWING PROJECTION (FIG. 7.21)

Image Field: This projection should cover the distal portion of the mandibular canine anteriorly and show equally the crowns of the maxillary and mandibular premolar teeth (see Fig. 7.21A and B).

Receptor Placement: Place the receptor between the tongue and the teeth, far enough from the lingual surface of the teeth to prevent interference by the palate on closing. The receptor should be parallel to the long axes of the teeth (see Fig. 7.21C). The anterior border of the receptor should extend beyond the contact area between the mandibular canine and the first premolar (see Fig. 7.21D). Hold the receptor in place until the patient's mouth is completely closed. Holding the receptor while closing prevents it from being displaced distally.

Projection of Central Ray: Adjust the horizontal angulation of the cone to project the central ray to the center of the receptor through the premolar contact areas (see Fig. 7.21D). To compensate for the slight inclination of the receptor against the palatal mucosa, the vertical angulation should be about +5 degrees. (In the drawing, the mandibular teeth are shown in dashed lines.)

Point of Entry: Identify the point of entry by retracting the cheek and determining that the central ray will enter the line of occlusion at the point of contact between the second premolar and the first molar (see Fig. 7.21E).

MOLAR BITEWING PROJECTION (FIG. 7.22)

Image Field: This projection should show the distal surface of the most posterior erupted molar and equally the crowns of the maxillary and mandibular molars (see Fig. 7.22A and B). Because the maxillary and mandibular molar contact areas may not be open from the same horizontal angulation, they may not be visible on one image. In this case, it may be desirable to open the maxillary molar contacts because the mandibular molar contacts usually are open on the periapical receptors.

Receptor Placement: Place the receptor between the tongue and teeth as far lingual as practical to avoid contacting the sensitive attached gingiva (see Fig. 7.22C). The distal margin of the receptor should extend 1 to 2 mm beyond the most posterior erupted molar (see Fig. 7.22D). When using the XCP, adjust the horizontal angulation by placing the guide bar parallel with the direction of the central ray to open the contact area between the first and second molars.

Projection of Central Ray: Project the central ray to the center of the receptor and through the contact of the first and second maxillary molars (see Fig. 7.22D). Angle the central ray slightly from the anterior because the molar contacts usually are not oriented at right angles to the buccal surfaces of these teeth. A vertical angulation of +10 degrees is recommended.

Point of Entry: The central ray should enter the cheek below the lateral canthus of the eye at the level of the occlusal plane (see Fig. 7.22E).

BOX 7.4 Diagnostic Objectives of Occlusal Radiography

- To locate supernumerary, unerupted, and impacted teeth
- To localize foreign bodies in the jaws and floor of the mouth
- To identify and determine the full extent of disease (e.g., cysts, osteomyelitis, malignancies) in the jaws, palate, and floor of the mouth
- To evaluate and monitor changes in the midpalatal suture during orthodontic palatal expansion. To detect and locate sialoliths in the ducts of sublingual and submandibular glands
- To evaluate the integrity of the anterior, medial, and lateral outlines of the maxillary sinus
- To aid in the examination of patients with trismus, who can open their mouths only a few millimeters; this condition precludes intraoral radiography, which may be impossible or at least extremely painful for the patient
- To obtain information about the location, nature, extent, and displacement of fractures of the mandible and maxilla

OCCLUSAL RADIOGRAPHY

An occlusal radiograph displays a relatively large segment of a dental arch. It may include the palate or floor of the mouth and a reasonable extent of the contiguous lateral structures. Occlusal radiographs also are useful when patients are unable to open wide enough for periapical images or for other reasons cannot accept periapical receptors. Because occlusal radiographs are exposed at a steep angulation, they may be used with conventional periapical images to determine the location of objects in all three dimensions.

The diagnostic objectives of occlusal radiographs are listed in Box 7.4. With the growth of cone beam computed tomography (CBCT) in dentistry, many of these diagnostic objectives are now accomplished with CBCT imaging rather than occlusal radiography. Nevertheless occlusal radiographs continue to be used where access to CBCT imaging may be limited.

To make an occlusal radiograph, a large receptor (7.7 cm × 5.8 cm [3 inches × 2.3 inches]) is inserted between the occlusal surfaces of the teeth. Occlusal receptors are made of film or storage phosphor plates. CCD or CMOS sensors of this size are not manufactured. As its name implies, the receptor lies in the plane of occlusion. The "tube" side of this receptor is positioned toward the jaw to be examined, and the x-ray beam is directed through the jaw to the receptor. Because of its size, the receptor allows examination of relatively large portions of the jaw. Standardized projections are used, which stipulate a desired relationship between the central ray, receptor, and region being examined. However, the clinician should feel free to modify these relationships to meet a specific clinical requirement.

Individual Occlusal Projections

The following section describes procedural details to make specific occlusal radiographic projections. It describes the field encompassed in the image, the placement of the receptor, the projection of the central ray, and the positioning of the aiming ring.

Text continued on p. 115

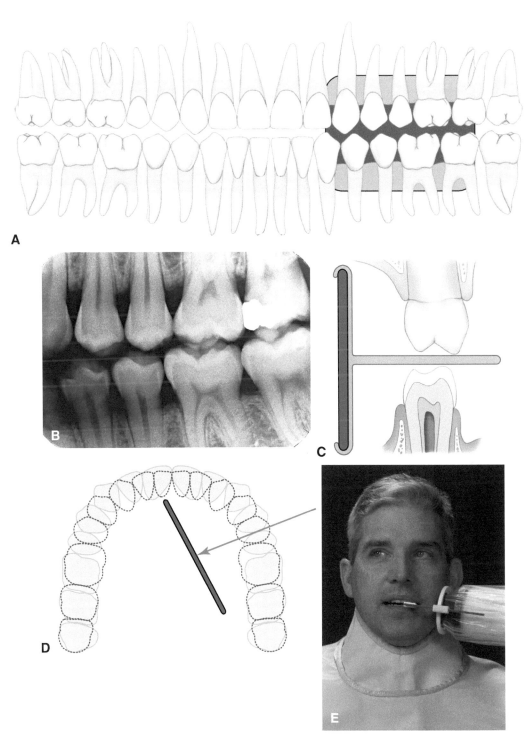

Fig. 7.21 Premolar bitewing projection. (A) The shaded area outlines the image field. (B) Bitewing radiograph of the premolar region. (C and D) Graphic representations of the image receptor and the x-ray beam relative to the crowns of the maxillary and mandibular premolar. (E) Position of the patient with the receptor holder in place and the aiming ring aligned for exposure.

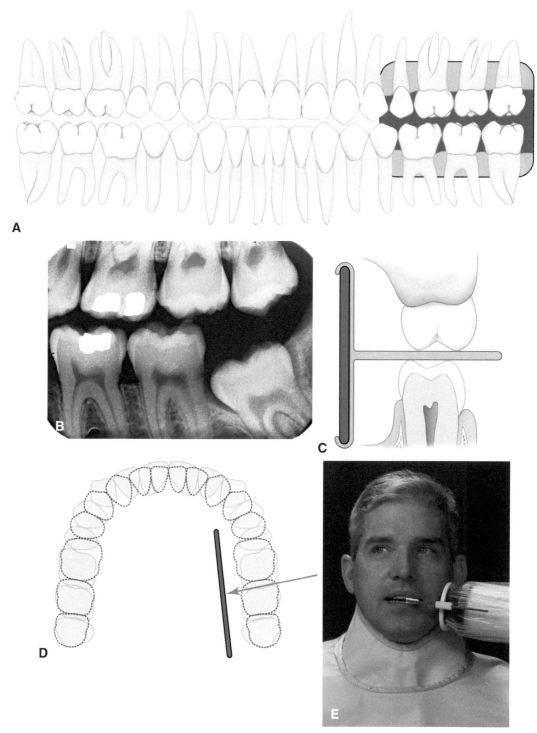

Fig. 7.22 Molar bitewing projection. (A) The shaded area outlines the image field. (B) Bitewing radiograph of the molar region. (C and D) Graphic representations of the image receptor and the x-ray beam relative to the crowns of the maxillary and mandibular molar. (E) Position of the patient with the receptor holder in place and the aiming ring aligned for exposure.

ANTERIOR MAXILLARY OCCLUSAL PROJECTION (FIG. 7.23)

Image Field: The primary field of this projection includes the anterior maxilla and its dentition and the anterior floor of the nasal fossa and teeth from canine to canine (see Fig. 7.23A and B).

Receptor Placement: Adjust the patient's head so that the sagittal plane is perpendicular and the occlusal plane horizontal to the floor (see Fig. 7.23C). Place the receptor in the mouth with the exposure side toward the maxilla, the posterior border touching the rami, and the long dimension of the receptor perpendicular to the sagittal plane. The patient stabilizes the receptor by gently closing the mouth.

Projection of Central Ray: Orient the central ray through the tip of the nose toward the middle of the receptor with approximately +45 degrees vertical angulation and 0 degrees horizontal angulation (see Fig. 7.23C).

Point of Entry: The central ray enters the patient's face approximately through the tip of the nose (see Fig. 7.23C).

TOPOGRAPHIC MAXILLARY OCCLUSAL PROJECTION (FIG. 7.24)

Image Field: This projection shows the palate, zygomatic processes of the maxilla, anteroinferior aspects of each antrum, nasolacrimal canals, teeth from second molar to second molar, and nasal septum (see Fig. 7.24A and B).

Receptor Placement: Seat the patient upright with the sagittal plane perpendicular to the floor and the occlusal plane horizontal. Place the receptor, with its long dimension perpendicular to the sagittal plane, crosswise in the mouth. Gently push the receptor in backward until it contacts the anterior border of the mandibular rami. The patient stabilizes the receptor by gently closing the mouth (see Fig. 7.24C).

Projection of Central Ray: Direct the central ray at a vertical angulation of +65 degrees and a horizontal angulation of 0 degrees to the bridge of the nose just below the nasion, toward the middle of the receptor (see Fig. 7.24C).

Point of Entry: Generally the central ray enters the patient's face through the bridge of the nose (see Fig. 7.24C).

LATERAL MAXILLARY OCCLUSAL PROJECTION (FIG. 7.25)

Image Field: This projection shows a quadrant of the alveolar ridge of the maxilla, inferolateral aspect of the antrum, tuberosity, and teeth from the lateral incisor to the contralateral third molar (see Fig. 7.25A and B). In addition, the zygomatic process of the maxilla superimposes over the roots of the molar teeth.

Receptor Placement: Place the receptor with its long axis parallel to the sagittal plane and on the side of interest, with the tube side toward the side of the maxilla in question. Push the receptor posteriorly until it touches the ramus. Position the lateral border parallel with the buccal surfaces of the posterior teeth, extending laterally approximately 1 cm past the buccal cusps. Ask the patient to close gently to hold the receptor in position (see Fig. 7.25C).

Projection of Central Ray: Orient the central ray with a vertical angulation of +60 degrees, to a point 2 cm below the lateral canthus of the eye, directed toward the center of the receptor (see Fig. 7.25C).

Point of Entry: The central ray enters at a point approximately 2 cm below the lateral canthus of the eye (see Fig. 7.25C).

ANTERIOR MANDIBULAR OCCLUSAL PROJECTION (FIG. 7.26)

Image Field: This projection includes the anterior portion of the mandible, the dentition from canine to canine, and the inferior cortical border of the mandible (see Fig. 7.26A and B).

Receptor Placement: Seat the patient tilted back so that the occlusal plane is 45 degrees above horizontal. Place the receptor in the mouth with the long axis perpendicular to the sagittal plane and push it posteriorly until it touches the rami. Center the receptor with the exposure side down and ask the patient to bite lightly to hold the receptor in position (see Fig. 7.26C).

Projection of Central Ray: Orient the central ray with −10 degrees angulation through the point of the chin toward the middle of the receptor; this gives the ray −55 degrees of angulation to the plane of the receptor (see Fig. 7.26C).

Point of Entry: The point of entry of the central ray is in the midline and through the tip of the chin (see Fig. 7.26C).

TOPOGRAPHIC MANDIBULAR OCCLUSAL PROJECTION (FIG. 7.27)

Image Field: This projection includes the soft tissue of the floor of the mouth and reveals the lingual and buccal plates of the mandible from second molar to second molar (see Fig. 7.27A and B). When this view is made to examine the floor of the mouth (e.g., for sialoliths), the exposure time should be reduced to half the time used to create an image of the mandible.

Receptor Placement: Seat the patient in a semireclining position with the head tilted back so that the ala-tragus line is almost perpendicular to the floor. Place the receptor in the mouth with its long axis perpendicular to the sagittal plane and with the tube side toward the mandible. The anterior border of the receptor should be approximately 1 cm beyond the mandibular central incisors. Ask the patient to bite gently on the receptor to hold it in position (see Fig. 7.27C).

Projection of Central Ray: Direct the central ray at the midline through the floor of the mouth approximately 3 cm below the chin, at right angles to the center of the receptor (see Fig. 7.27C).

Point of Entry: The point of entry of the central ray is in the midline through the floor of the mouth approximately 3 cm below the chin (see Fig. 7.27C).

LATERAL MANDIBULAR OCCLUSAL PROJECTION (FIG. 7.28)

Image Field: This projection covers the soft tissue of half the floor of the mouth, the buccal and lingual cortical plates of half of the mandible, and the teeth from the lateral incisor to the contralateral third molar (see Fig. 7.28A and B). When this view is used to provide an image of the floor of the mouth, the exposure time should be reduced to half that used to provide an image of the mandible.

Receptor Placement: Seat the patient in a semireclining position with the head tilted back so that the ala-tragus line is almost perpendicular to the floor (see Fig. 7.28C). Place the receptor in the mouth with its long axis initially parallel with the sagittal plane and with the exposure side down toward the mandible. Place the receptor as far posterior as possible, then shift the long axis buccally (right or left) so that the lateral border of the receptor is parallel with the buccal surfaces of the posterior teeth and extends laterally approximately 1 cm.

Projection of Central Ray: Direct the central ray perpendicular to the center of the receptor through a point beneath the chin, approximately 3 cm posterior to the point of the chin and 3 cm lateral to the midline (see Fig. 7.28C).

Point of Entry: The point of entry of the central ray is beneath the chin, approximately 3 cm posterior to the chin and approximately 3 cm lateral to the midline (see Fig. 7.28C).

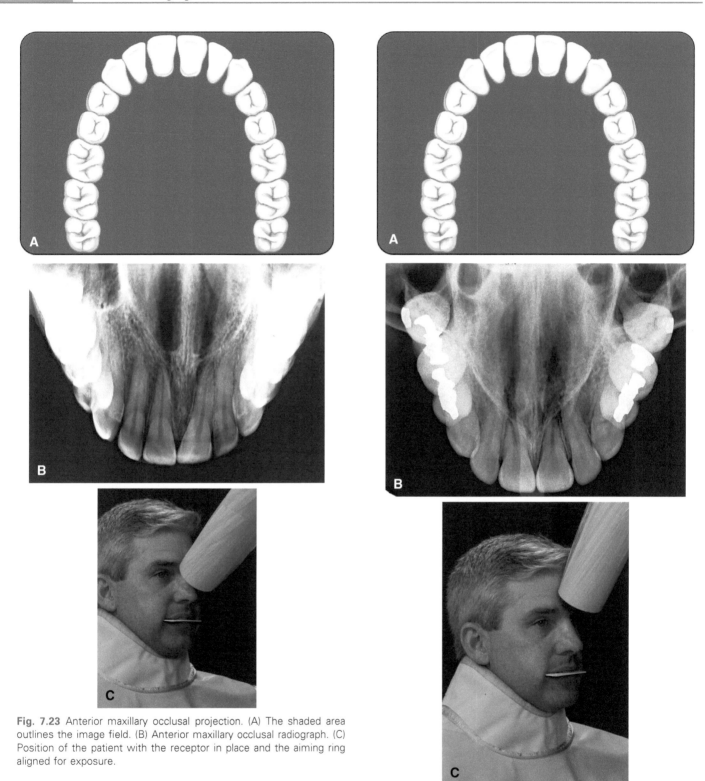

Fig. 7.23 Anterior maxillary occlusal projection. (A) The shaded area outlines the image field. (B) Anterior maxillary occlusal radiograph. (C) Position of the patient with the receptor in place and the aiming ring aligned for exposure.

Fig. 7.24 Topographic maxillary occlusal projection. (A) The shaded area outlines the image field. (B) Topographic maxillary occlusal radiograph. (C) Position of the patient with the receptor in place and the aiming ring aligned for exposure.

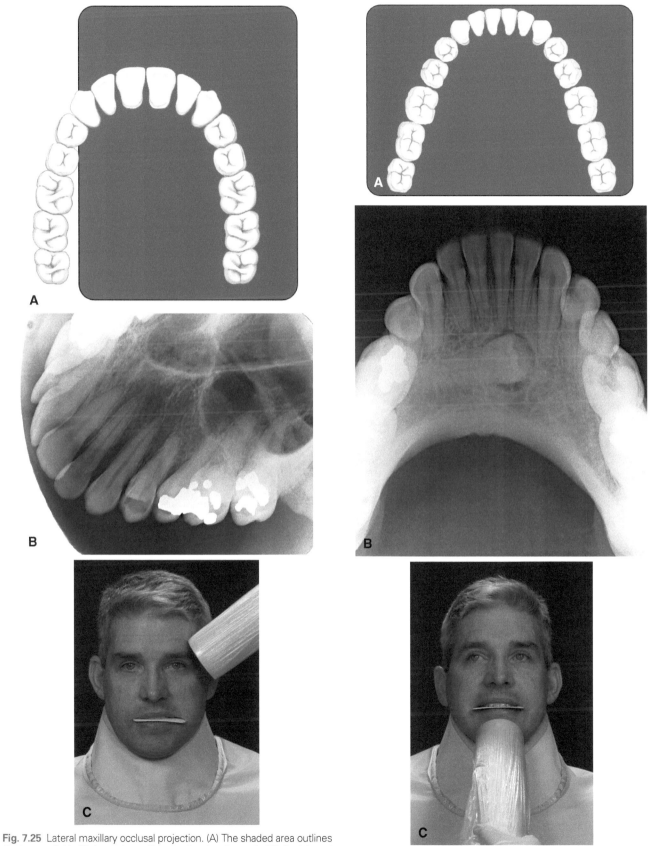

Fig. 7.25 Lateral maxillary occlusal projection. (A) The shaded area outlines the image field. (B) Lateral maxillary occlusal radiograph. (C) Position of the patient with the receptor in place and the aiming ring aligned for exposure.

Fig. 7.26 Anterior mandibular occlusal projection. (A) The shaded area outlines the image field. (B) Anterior mandibular occlusal radiograph. (C) Position of the patient with the receptor in place and the aiming ring aligned for exposure.

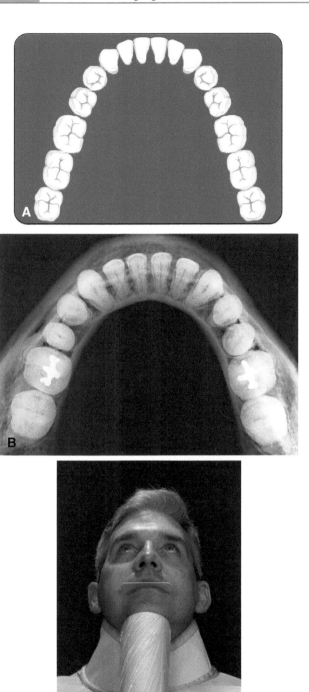

Fig. 7.27 Topographic mandibular occlusal projection. (A) The shaded area outlines the image field. (B) Topographic mandibular occlusal radiograph. (C) Position of the patient with the receptor in place and the aiming ring aligned for exposure.

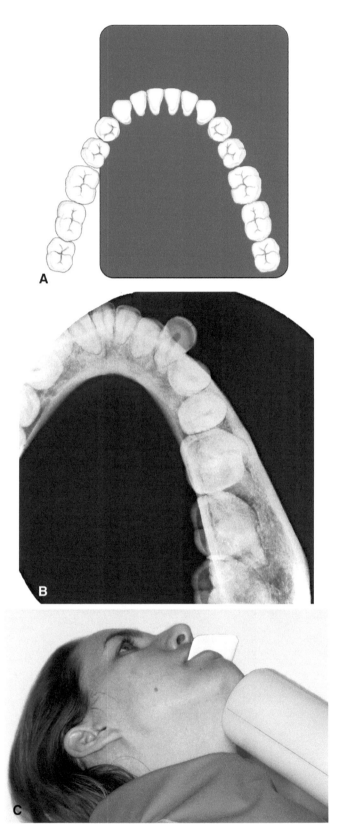

Fig. 7.28 Lateral mandibular occlusal projection. (A) The shaded area outlines the image field. (B) Lateral mandibular occlusal radiograph. (C) Position of the patient with the receptor in place and the aiming ring aligned for exposure.

IMAGING OF CHILDREN

Radiation protection is especially important for children because of their greater sensitivity to irradiation. The best way to reduce unnecessary exposure is for the dentist to make the minimal number of radiographs required for the individual patient. These judgments are based on a careful clinical examination and consideration of the patient's age, medical history, growth considerations, and general oral health as well as whether caries is present and the time elapsed since previous examinations (see Chapter 17). Bitewing examinations for caries assessment are not required when the contacts are open and the proximal surfaces can be visually examined. The frequency should be determined partly by the patient's caries rate. A periapical survey is often recommended for children early in the mixed dentition stage. Special attention should be paid to procedures that reduce exposure (see Chapter 3), including use of fast receptor, proper processing, beam-limiting devices, and protective aprons and thyroid shields.

Radiography in a child can be a challenging experience. Although the principles of periapical radiography for children are the same as for adults, in practice children present special considerations because of their small anatomic structures and possible behavioral problems. The smaller size of the arches and dentition requires the use of smaller periapical receptors. The relatively shallow palate and floor of the mouth may require further modification of receptor placement. Special radiographic examinations using an occlusal receptor for extraoral projections have been suggested.

Patient Management

Children are often apprehensive about the radiographic examination, much as they are about many other types of dental procedures. The radiographic examination usually is the first manipulative procedure performed on a young patient. If this examination is nonthreatening and comfortable, subsequent dental experiences are usually accepted with little or no apprehension. Such apprehension is best allayed by familiarizing the child with the procedure, which is done by explaining it in a manner that he or she can comprehend. It often is wise to describe the x-ray machine as a "camera used to take pictures of teeth." The child can become more comfortable with the receptor and x-ray machine by touching them before the examination. The operator should carry on a conversation with the child as a distraction and to gain his or her confidence. It may be advantageous for the child to watch an older brother or sister being radiographed or to have the parent or dental assistant serve as a model. Children who feel a gagging sensation can be asked to breathe through the nose. Techniques to distract their attention, such as asking them to curl their toes or make a fist, can be effective. However, if the procedure is postponed until the next appointment, the gag reflex may not be encountered; often it may then be much easier for the patient to control. It is especially important to explain to the patient that the procedure will be much easier the next time—plant the positive thought.

Examination Coverage

When a complete radiographic survey is necessary, it should show the periapical region of all teeth, the proximal surfaces of all posterior teeth, and the crypts of the developing permanent teeth. The number of projections required depends on the child's size. Also, an exposure appropriate to the child's size should be used. For example, a 50% reduction in the milliamperes used for an average young adult gives the proper density for patients younger than 10 years. Exposure settings (mA or s) are reduced about 25% for children 10 to 15 years old.

Primary Dentition (3 to 6 Years)

A combination of projections can be used to provide adequate coverage for the pediatric dental patient. This examination may consist of two anterior occlusal receptors, two posterior bitewing receptors, and up to four posterior periapical receptors as indicated (Fig. 7.29). For the maxillary and interproximal projections, the child is seated upright with the sagittal plane perpendicular to and the occlusal plane parallel with the floor (horizontal plane). For mandibular projections other than the occlusal, the child is seated upright with the sagittal plane perpendicular. The tragus corner of the mouth line is oriented parallel to the floor. Some dentists find that a panoramic view, rather than the four periapicals, is more informative and results in less exposure to the child (see Chapter 3).

Maxillary anterior occlusal projection. A No. 2 receptor should be placed in the mouth with its long axis perpendicular to the sagittal plane and the exposure surface toward the maxillary teeth. The receptor is centered on the midline with the anterior border extending just beyond

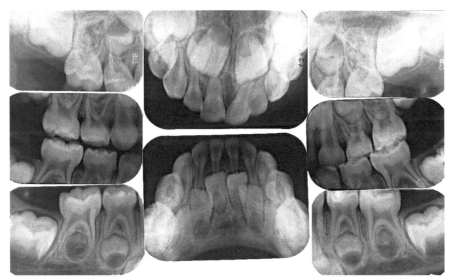

Fig. 7.29 Radiographic examination of primary dentition consists of two anterior occlusal views, four posterior periapical views, and two bitewing views. Often it is preferable to make a bitewing and panoramic examination followed by selected periapical views as indicated.

the incisal edges of the anterior teeth. The central ray is directed at a vertical angulation of +60 degrees through the tip of the nose toward the center of the receptor.

Mandibular anterior occlusal projection. The child should be seated with the head tipped back so that the occlusal plane is about 25 degrees above the plane of the floor. A No. 2 receptor is placed with the long axis perpendicular to the sagittal plane and the exposure surface toward the mandibular teeth. The central ray is oriented at −30 degrees vertical angulation and through the tip of the chin toward the receptor.

Bitewing projection. A No. 0 receptor is used with a paper loop receptor holder. The receptor is placed in the child's mouth as in the adult premolar bitewing projection. The image field should include the distal half of the canine and the deciduous molars. A positive vertical angulation of +5 to +10 degrees should be used. The horizontal angle is oriented to direct the beam through the interproximal spaces.

Deciduous maxillary molar periapical projection. A No. 0 receptor in a modified XCP or BAI (Dentsply Rinn, Elgin, IL) bite block is used, either with or without the aiming ring and indicator bar. The receptor is positioned in the midline of the palate with the anterior border extending to the maxillary primary canine. The image field of this projection should include the distal half of the primary canine and both primary molars.

Deciduous mandibular molar projection. A No. 0 receptor is positioned in a modified XCP or BAI bite block with or without the aiming ring and indicator bar between the posterior teeth and tongue. The exposed radiograph should show the distal half of the mandibular primary canine and the primary molar teeth.

Mixed Dentition (7 to 12 Years)

A complete examination of the mixed dentition, if indicated, consists of two incisor periapical views, four canine periapical views, four posterior periapical views, and two or four posterior bitewing views (Fig. 7.30). For the maxillary and interproximal projections, the child should be seated upright with the sagittal plane perpendicular and the occlusal plane parallel to the floor. For the mandibular projections, the child should be seated upright with the sagittal plane perpendicular and the ala-tragus line parallel to the floor. XCP instruments are used for larger children. Bisecting angle bite blocks may be more comfortable for smaller individuals.

Maxillary anterior periapical projection. A No. 1 receptor should be placed in the mouth behind the maxillary central and lateral incisors. The receptor should be centered on the embrasure between the central incisors.

Mandibular anterior periapical projection. A No. 1 receptor should be positioned behind the mandibular central and lateral incisors.

Canine periapical projection. A No. 1 receptor should be positioned behind each of the canines.

Deciduous and permanent molar periapical projection. A No. 1 or No. 2 receptor (if the child is large enough) should be positioned with the anterior edge behind the canine.

Posterior bitewing projection. Bitewing projections should be exposed in the premolar region with a No. 1 or No. 2 receptor as previously described, using either bitewing tabs or the Rinn bitewing instrument. Four bitewing projections should be exposed when the second permanent molars have erupted.

MOBILE INTRAORAL RADIOGRAPHY

Occasionally it is difficult to have a patient come to a conventional wall-mounted dental x-ray machine. For instance, in remote sites such as nursing homes, hospitals, or at disaster scenes, it can be highly advantageous to have a portable machine that may be taken directly to the patient. Combining such a portable x-ray generator with digital imaging provides rapid, self-contained imaging capability. Portable battery-powered x-ray generators have been approved by the U.S. Food and Drug Administration (FDA) (Fig. 7.31). Clinical trials on the Nomad handheld x-ray unit (Aribex, Inc., Orem, UT) have shown that this unit can be held stable and produce clinically acceptable images. This machine uses a high-frequency constant-potential x-ray generator (60 kV constant potential) and has a short focal spot-to-skin distance (20 cm)—both of these allow for short exposure times compared with conventional units. It has a small focus spot (0.4 mm). The operator dose is mitigated using internal shielding materials in the unit to reduce leakage exposure and a shield on the aiming cylinder to minimize backscatter from the patient. Several states in the United States have additional requirements related to training and radiation dose documentation when using these handheld units.

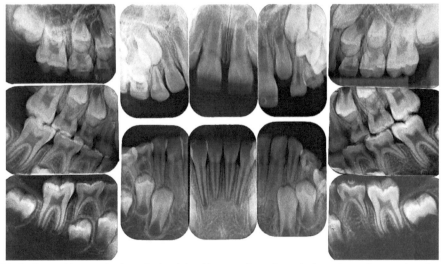

Fig. 7.30 Radiographic examination of mixed dentition consists of two incisor views, four canine views, four posterior views, and two bitewing views. Often it is preferable to make a bitewing and panoramic examination followed by selected periapical views as indicated.

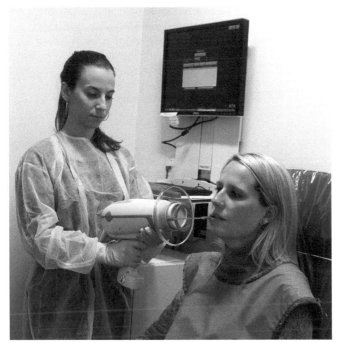

Fig. 7.31 Handheld x-ray machine for intraoral radiography. Operator dose is minimized by a shield on the aiming cylinder to reduce backscatter. (Courtesy Dr. Akrivoula Soundia and Dr. Holly Vreeburg, UCLA School of Dentistry, Los Angeles, CA.)

SPECIAL CONSIDERATIONS

The radiographic procedures described in this chapter may need to be modified for patients who have unusual difficulties or special needs. Specific modifications depend on the patient's physical and emotional characteristics. However, as with any dental procedure, the dental assistant begins the examination by showing appreciation of the patient's condition and compassionate recognition of problems that might occur. If the assistant is kind but firm, the patient's confidence increases, which helps the patient to relax and cooperate. Following are a few conditions and circumstances that may be encountered, with recommendations and suggestions that may help the clinician achieve an adequate radiographic examination.

Infection

Infection in the orofacial structures may result in edema and lead to trismus of some of the muscles of mastication. As a result, intraoral radiography may be painful to the patient and difficult for both the patient and the radiologist. Under such circumstances, panoramic or occlusal techniques may offer the only possibility of an examination. In the case of edema in an area to be examined, exposure time should be increased to compensate for the increased x-ray attenuation due to tissue swelling.

Trauma

A patient who has undergone trauma may have a dental or facial fracture. Dental fractures are well visualized on periapical or occlusal radiographs. Special care must be taken in making these views because of the condition of the patient. Skeletal fractures are usually best seen with panoramic or other extraoral views or a computed tomography examination. In some cases, patients with fractures of the facial skeleton may be non-ambulatory because of other injuries. Consequently an extraoral radiographic examination with the patient in the supine position may be necessary. However, the circumstances need not compromise the

techniques, and satisfactory intraoral images can be produced if the proper relative positions of the tube, patient, and receptor are observed.

Patients With Mental Disabilities

Patients with mental disabilities may cause some difficulty and usually is the result of the patient's lack of coordination or inability to comprehend what is expected. When the radiographic examination is performed speedily, unpredictable moves by the patient can be minimized. In some cases sedation may be required.

Patients With Physical Disabilities

Patients with physical disabilities (e.g., loss of vision, loss of hearing, loss of the use of any or all extremities, congenital defects such as cleft palate) may require special handling during a radiographic examination. These patients are usually cooperative and eager to assist. They may be accustomed to so much discomfort and inconvenience that their tolerance level is high, and they are not challenged by the relatively slight irritation represented by the x-ray procedures. Generally intraoral and extraoral radiographic examinations may be performed for these patients if a good rapport between the patient and radiology technician is established and maintained. Members of the patient's family are often helpful in assisting the patient into and out of the examination chair and in receptor positioning and holding inasmuch as they are usually familiar with the patient's condition and accustomed to coping with it.

Gag Reflex

Occasionally patients who need a radiographic examination manifest a gag reflex at the slightest provocation. These patients are usually very apprehensive and frightened by unknown procedures; others simply seem to have very sensitive tissue that precipitates a gag reflex when stimulated. This sensitivity is manifested when the receptor is placed in the oral cavity. To overcome this disability, the radiologist should try to relax and reassure the patient. The radiologist can describe and explain the procedures. Often gagging can be controlled if the operator bolsters the patient's confidence by demonstrating technical competence and showing authority tempered with compassion. The gag reflex is often worse when a patient is tired; therefore it is advisable to perform the examination in the morning, when the individual is well rested, especially in the case of children.

Stimulating the posterior dorsum of the tongue or the soft palate usually initiates the gag reflex. Consequently, during the placement of the receptor, the tongue should be very relaxed and positioned well to the floor of the mouth; this can be accomplished by asking the patient to swallow deeply just before opening the mouth for placement of the receptor. (The dentist should never mention the tongue or ask patients to relax the tongue; this usually makes them more conscious of it and precipitates involuntary movements.) The receptor is carried into the mouth parallel to the occlusal plane. When the desired area is reached, the receptor is rotated with a decisive motion, bringing it into contact with the palate or the floor of the mouth. Sliding it along the palate or tongue is likely to stimulate the gag reflex. Also, the dentist must keep in mind that the longer the receptor stays in the mouth, the greater the possibility that the patient will start to gag. The patient should be advised to breathe rapidly through the nose because mouth breathing usually aggravates this condition.

Any little exercise that can be devised which does not interfere with the x-ray examination but shifts the patient's attention from the receptor and the mouth is likely to relieve the gag reaction. Asking patients to hold their breath or to keep a foot or arm suspended during receptor placement and exposure can often create such a distraction. In extreme cases, topical anesthetic agents in mouthwashes or spray can be administered to produce temporary numbness of the tongue and palate to reduce gagging. However, in our experience, this procedure gives limited results. The most effective approach is to reduce apprehension, minimize tissue irritation, and encourage rapid breathing through the nose. If all measures fail, an extraoral

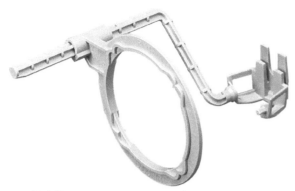

Fig. 7.32 EndoRay receptor holder used for endodontic images. This device provides room for files to be in place while making the image. (Courtesy Dentsply Rinn, Elgin, IL.)

examination may be the only means, short of administering general anesthesia, to examine the patient radiographically.

Imaging for Endodontics

Radiographs are essential for endodontic diagnosis and treatment planning. Additionally, intraoperative radiographs may be taken during the endodontic procedure to assist in confirming the working length of the endodontic instrumentation or to identify additional canals. The presence of a rubber dam, rubber dam clamp, and root canal instruments may complicate an intraoral periapical examination by impairing proper receptor positioning and aiming cylinder angulation. Despite these obstacles, certain requirements must be observed:

1. The tooth being treated must be centered in the image.
2. The receptor must be positioned as far from the tooth and apex as the region permits to ensure that the apex of the tooth and some periapical bone are apparent on the radiograph.

For maxillary projections, the patient is seated so that the sagittal plane is perpendicular and the occlusal plane is parallel to the floor. For mandibular projections, the patient is seated upright with the sagittal plane perpendicular and the tragus-to-corner of the mouth line parallel to the floor. Specially designed receptor holders for endodontic images are available (Fig. 7.32). These instruments fit over files, clamps, and the rubber dam without touching the subject tooth. The aiming cylinder is aligned to direct the central ray perpendicular to the receptor.

Often a single radiograph of a multirooted tooth made at the normal vertical and horizontal projection does not display all the roots. In these cases, when it is necessary to separate the roots on multirooted teeth, a second projection may be made. The horizontal angulation is altered 20 degrees mesially for maxillary premolars, 20 degrees mesially or distally for maxillary molars, or 20 degrees distally for an oblique projection of mandibular molar roots.

If a sinus tract is encountered, its course is tracked by threading a gutta-percha cone through the tract before the radiograph is made. It also is possible to localize and determine the depth of periodontal defects with this gutta-percha tracking technique.

A final radiograph of the treated tooth is made to demonstrate the quality of the root canal filling and the condition of the periapical tissues after removal of the clamp and rubber dam. This radiograph serves as a baseline for comparison of subsequent radiographic examination to monitor the outcome of endodontic treatment.

Pregnancy

Although a fetus is sensitive to ionizing radiation, the amount of exposure received by an embryo or fetus during dental radiography is extremely low. There have been no reports of damage to a fetus from dental radiography. Nevertheless, prudence suggests that such radiographic examinations be kept to a minimum consistent with the mother's dental needs. As with any patient, radiographic examination is limited during pregnancy to cases with a specific diagnostic indication. With the low patient dose afforded by use of optimal radiation safety techniques (see Chapter 3), an intraoral or extraoral examination can be performed whenever a reasonable diagnostic requirement exists.

Edentulous Patients

Radiographic examination of edentulous patients is important, whether the area of interest is one tooth or an entire arch. These areas may contain roots, residual infection, impacted teeth, cysts, or other pathologic entities that may adversely affect the usefulness of prosthetic appliances or the patient's health. After a determination has been made that these entities are not present, repeated examinations to detect them are not warranted in the absence of signs or symptoms.

If available, a panoramic examination of the edentulous jaws is most convenient. If abnormalities of the alveolar ridges are identified, the higher resolution of periapical receptor is used to make intraoral projections to supplement the panoramic examination.

In a completely or partly edentulous patient, a receptor-holding device is used for intraoral radiography of the alveolar ridges. Placement of the receptor-holding instrument may be complicated by its tipping into the voids normally occupied by the crowns of the missing teeth. To manage this difficulty, cotton rolls are placed between the ridge and the receptor holder, supporting the holder in a horizontal position. An orthodontic elastic band to hold cotton rolls to the bite block on the receptor holder often is useful when several such projections must be exposed. With elastics, it is simple to maneuver the cotton rolls into the areas that require support. The patient may steady the receptor-holding instrument with a hand or an opposing denture.

If panoramic equipment is unavailable, an examination consisting of 14 intraoral views provides an excellent survey. The exposure required for an edentulous ridge is approximately 25% less than that for a dentulous ridge. This examination consists of seven projections in each jaw (adult No. 2 receptor) as follows:

Central incisors (midline): one projection
Lateral canine: two projections
Premolar: two projections
Molar: two projections

BIBLIOGRAPHY

Adriaens PA, De Boever J, Vande Velde F. Comparison of intra-oral long-cone paralleling radiographic surveys and orthopantomographs with special reference to the bone height. *J Oral Rehabil*. 1982;9:355–365.

Biggerstaff RH, Phillips JR. A quantitative comparison of paralleling long-cone and bisection-of-angle periapical radiography. *Oral Surg Oral Med Oral Pathol*. 1976;62:673–677.

Dubrez B, Jacot-Descombes S, Cimasoni G. Reliability of a paralleling instrument for dental radiographs. *Oral Surg Oral Med Oral Pathol Oral Radiol Endod*. 1995;80:358–364.

Forsberg J, Halse A. Radiographic simulation of a periapical lesion comparing the paralleling and the bisecting-angle techniques. *Int Endod J*. 1994;27:133–138.

Iannucci J, Jansen Howerton L. *Dental Radiography: Principles and Techniques*. 3rd ed. St Louis: Saunders; 2006.

Scandrett FR, Tebo HG, Miller JT, et al. Radiographic examination of the edentulous patient, 1: review of the literature and preliminary report comparing three methods. *Oral Surg Oral Med Oral Pathol*. 1973;35:266–274.

Schulze RK, d'Hoedt B. A method to calculate angular disparities between object and receptor in "paralleling technique". *Dentomaxillofac Radiol*. 2002;31:32–38.

Weclew TV. Comparing the paralleling extension cone technique and the bisecting angle technique. *J Acad Gen Dent*. 1974;22:18–20.

8

Cephalometric and Skull Imaging

Sotirios Tetradis and Mel L. Kantor

In extraoral radiographic examinations, both the x-ray source and the image receptor (film or digital sensor) are placed outside the patient's mouth. This chapter describes the most common projections for extraoral radiographic examinations in which the source and sensor remain static. These include the lateral cephalometric projection of the sagittal or median plane; the submentovertex (SMV) projection of the transverse or horizontal plane; and the Waters, posteroanterior (PA), cephalometric, and reverse Towne projections of the coronal or frontal plane. Panoramic radiography is described in Chapter 9, and other more complex imaging modalities are described in Chapters 10 to 13.

SELECTION CRITERIA

Extraoral radiographs are used to examine areas not fully covered by intraoral radiographs or to evaluate the cranium, face (including the maxilla and mandible), or cervical spine for diseases, trauma, or abnormalities. Standardized extraoral (cephalometric) radiographs also assist in evaluating the relationship between various orofacial and dental structures, growth and development of the face, or treatment progression.

Before obtaining an extraoral radiograph, it is essential to evaluate the patient's complaints and clinical signs in detail. The clinician must first decide which anatomic structures need to be evaluated and then select the appropriate projection or projections. Selecting the appropriate extraoral radiographic examination for the diagnostic task at hand is the *first* step in obtaining and interpreting a radiograph. To spatially localize pathology, at least two radiographs taken at right angles to each another are obtained.

TECHNIQUE

Extraoral radiographs are produced with conventional dental x-ray machines, certain models of panoramic machines, or higher-capacity medical x-ray units. Cephalometric and skull views require at least a 20 by 25-cm (8 by 10-inch) image receptor. For film-based imaging, it is critical to label the right and left sides of the image correctly and clearly. This usually is done by placing a metal marker (an *R* or an *L*) on the outside of the cassette in a corner in which the marker does not obstruct diagnostic information.

The proper exposure parameters depend on the patient's size, anatomy, and head orientation; the speed of the image receptor; x-ray source-to-receptor distance; and whether or not grids are used. In cases of known or suspected disease, medium-speed or high-speed rare-earth screen-film combinations provide optimal balance between diagnostic information and patient exposure. For orthodontic purposes, high-speed combinations reduce patient exposure without compromising

the identification of anatomic landmarks necessary for cephalometric analysis.

Proper positioning of the x-ray source, patient, and image receptor requires patience, attention to detail, and experience. The main anatomic landmark used in patient positioning during extraoral radiography is the canthomeatal line, which joins the central point of the external auditory canal to the outer canthus of the eye. The canthomeatal line forms approximately a 10-degree angle with the Frankfort plane, the line that connects the superior border of the external auditory canal with the infraorbital rim. The image receptor and patient placement, central beam direction, and resultant image for the lateral, SMV, Waters, PA, and reverse Towne projections are summarized in Table 8.1 and described in detail in the text. Table 8.1 is organized to show the progressive head rotation in relation to the x-ray beam in the frontal views and thus clarify the resultant projected anatomy.

EVALUATION OF THE IMAGE

Extraoral images should first be evaluated for overall quality. Proper exposure and processing, when film-based, result in an image with good contrast and density. Proper patient positioning prevents unwanted superimpositions and distortions and facilitates identification of anatomic landmarks. Interpreting poor-quality images can lead to diagnostic errors and subsequent treatment errors.

The first step in the interpretation of radiographic images is the identification of anatomy. A thorough knowledge of normal radiographic anatomy and the appearance of normal variants is critical for the identification of pathology. Abnormalities cause disruptions of normal anatomy. Detecting the altered anatomy precedes classifying the type of change and developing a differential diagnosis. What is not detected cannot be interpreted.

The interpretation of extraoral radiographs should be thorough, careful, and meticulous. Images should be interpreted in a room with reduced ambient light, and peripheral light from the viewbox or monitor should be masked. A systematic, methodical approach should be used for the visual exploration or interrogation of the diagnostic image. A method for the visual interrogation of extraoral radiograph of the head and neck is illustrated for the lateral and PA cephalometric projections (see Fig. 8.3 and 8.7) but can be applied to the remaining projections as well. These methods are not the only approach to examining radiographic images. Any technique that reliably ensures that the entire image will be examined is equally appropriate.

CEPHALOMETRIC PROJECTIONS

Cephalometric projections are standardized projections that allow for reproducible imaging of the craniofacial region. All cephalometric

TABLE 8.1   Technical Aspects of Extraoral Radiographic Projections and Resultant Images

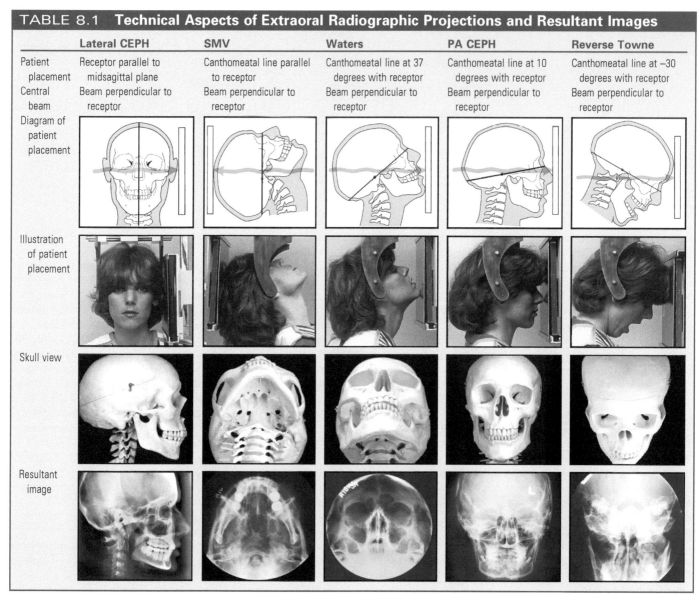

	Lateral CEPH	SMV	Waters	PA CEPH	Reverse Towne
Patient placement Central beam	Receptor parallel to midsagittal plane Beam perpendicular to receptor	Canthomeatal line parallel to receptor Beam perpendicular to receptor	Canthomeatal line at 37 degrees with receptor Beam perpendicular to receptor	Canthomeatal line at 10 degrees with receptor Beam perpendicular to receptor	Canthomeatal line at −30 degrees with receptor Beam perpendicular to receptor
Diagram of patient placement					
Illustration of patient placement					
Skull view					
Resultant image					

CEPH, Cephalometric; *PA*, posteroanterior; *SMV*, submentovertex.

radiographs, including the lateral view, are made with a cephalostat (Fig. 8.1), which helps to maintain a constant relationship between the skull, the receptor, and the x-ray beam. A cephalometric projection is made with a long source-to-object distance of 5 ft; this large distance minimizes image magnification. The object-to-receptor distance is typically 10 to 15 cm and should be maintained constant for sequential radiographs of the same patient. These projections may be made using film or digital receptors.

Skeletal, dental, and soft tissue anatomic landmarks delineate the lines, planes, angles, and distances used to generate measurements and to classify patients' craniofacial morphology. At the beginning of treatment, these measurements are often compared with an established standard or norm; during treatment, the measurements are usually compared with measurements from previous cephalometric radiographs of the same patient to monitor growth and development as well as treatment-induced changes.

Lateral Cephalometric Projection (Lateral Skull Projection)

Of the extraoral radiographs described in this chapter, the lateral cephalometric projection is the one most commonly used in dentistry.

Indications

- Evaluate the anteroposterior (AP) relationships between the maxilla, mandible, and cranial base.
- Assess skeletal and soft-tissue relationships.
- Monitor progress of treatment and treatment outcomes.
- Proceed with orthognathic surgical treatment planning.

Image Receptor and Patient Placement

The image receptor is positioned parallel to the patient's midsagittal plane. In cephalometric radiography, the patient is placed with the left side toward the image receptor (U.S. standards) and a wedge filter at

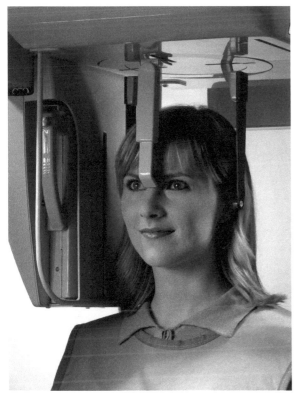

Fig. 8.1 Patient positioned for lateral cephalometric imaging in a cephalostat. The ear rods and nasion indicator help stabilize the patient's head in a standard position. (Courtesy J. Morita Mfg. Co, Kyoto, Japan.)

the tube head is positioned over the anterior aspect of the beam to absorb some of the radiation and allow visualization of soft tissues of the face. The patient is asked to occlude in his or her normal intercuspation position.

Position of the Central X-Ray Beam

The central beam is perpendicular to the midsagittal plane of the patient and the plane of the image receptor and is centered over the external auditory meatus.

Resultant Image (Fig. 8.2)

Exact superimposition of right and left sides is impossible because the structures on the side near to the image receptor are magnified less than the same structures on the side far from the image receptor. Bilateral structures close to the midsagittal plane demonstrate less discrepancy in size compared with bilateral structures farther away from the midsagittal plane. Structures close to the midsagittal plane (e.g., the clinoid processes and inferior turbinates) should be nearly superimposed.

Interpretation

Although the lateral cephalometric radiograph is obtained to evaluate the relationship of the oral and facial structures, this radiograph is still a lateral *skull* projection, providing significant diagnostic information for the anatomy of the head and neck. Therefore lateral cephalometric radiographs should first be evaluated for possible pathology and for anatomic variants that might simulate disease before cephalometric analysis. It is not sufficient to limit the interpretation to the cephalometric analysis. To ensure that all anatomic structures are assessed, a systematic

visual interrogation of lateral cephalometric radiographs should be followed. Such an approach is presented next (Fig. 8.3):

Step 1. Evaluate the base of the skull and calvaria. Identify the mastoid air cells, clivus, clinoid processes, sella turcica, sphenoid sinuses, and roof of the orbit. In the calvaria, assess vessel grooves, sutures, and diploic space. Look for intracranial calcifications (Fig 8.3B).

Step 2. Evaluate the upper and middle face. Identify the orbits, sinuses (frontal, ethmoid, and maxillary), pterygomaxillary fissures, pterygoid plates, zygomatic processes of the maxilla, anterior nasal spine, and hard palate (floor of the nose). Evaluate the soft tissues of the upper and middle face, nasal cavity (turbinates), soft palate, and dorsum of tongue (Fig 8.3C).

Step 3. Evaluate the lower face. Follow the outline of the mandible: from the condylar and coronoid processes; to the rami, angles, and bodies; and finally to the anterior mandible. Evaluate the soft tissue of the lower face (Fig 8.3D).

Step 4. Evaluate the cervical spine, airway, and area of the neck. Identify each individual vertebra, confirm that the skull-C1 and C1-C2 articulations are normal, and assess the general alignment of the vertebrae. Assess soft tissues of the neck, hyoid bone, and airway (Fig 8.3E).

Step 5. Evaluate the alveolar bone and teeth (Fig 8.3F).

Fig. 8.4 presents incidental findings identified on lateral cephalometric radiographs of asymptomatic orthodontic patients. Calcification of the intraclinoid ligament and formation of a bridged sella is a common normal variant that does not warrant any further evaluation (see Fig. 8.4A). Alternatively, expansion, irregular outlines, and destruction of the sella floor (see Fig. 8.4B) raise suspicion of an invasive lesion, such as a pituitary tumor, and require further investigation with advanced imaging and referral to a medical specialist. Multiple opacities throughout patient's calvaria are the result of superimposed hair braids (see Fig. 8.4C). Well-defined opacities at the superior aspect of the calvaria represent calcifications of arachnoid granulations and are a normal variant (see Fig. 8.4D). Enlargement of the pharyngeal adenoids and palatal tonsils (see Fig. 8.4E) is a common finding in young patients but can cause narrowing of the airway and breathing difficulties. Finally, partial agenesis of the ring of atlas (see Fig. 8.4F) is a developmental anomaly that can cause instability of the atlanto-occipital and atlanto-odontoid articulation and requires further evaluation. Fusion of the body and transverse process of the dens with the third cervical vertebra (see Fig. 8.4F), a rare normal variant, should also be noted.

After evaluation of the whole lateral skull radiograph for possible pathology, cephalometric evaluation of the patient follows. There are many cephalometric analyses based on a variety of anatomic landmarks. Steiner and Ricketts analyses are two commonly used analyses that employ the skeletal, dental, and soft tissue landmarks listed in Box 8.1. Precise identification of the various landmarks on the lateral cephalometric radiograph is necessary to generate accurate cephalometric measurements. The landmarks in Box 8.1 are shown in Fig. 8.5A, on a side view of a skull, and in Fig. 8.5B, on a 5-mm-wide midline section of an orthodontic patient imaged by cone beam computed tomography. Finally, Fig. 8.5C depicts the projected landmark position on the lateral cephalogram of an orthodontic patient.

Posteroanterior Cephalometric Projection

The second most common skull radiograph used in dentistry is the PA cephalometric projection. The PA cephalogram is mainly used for the evaluation of facial asymmetries and assessment of orthognathic surgery outcomes involving the patient's midline or mandibular-maxillary relationship.

Indications

- Evaluate craniofacial asymmetry.
- Assess jaw skeletal relationships.

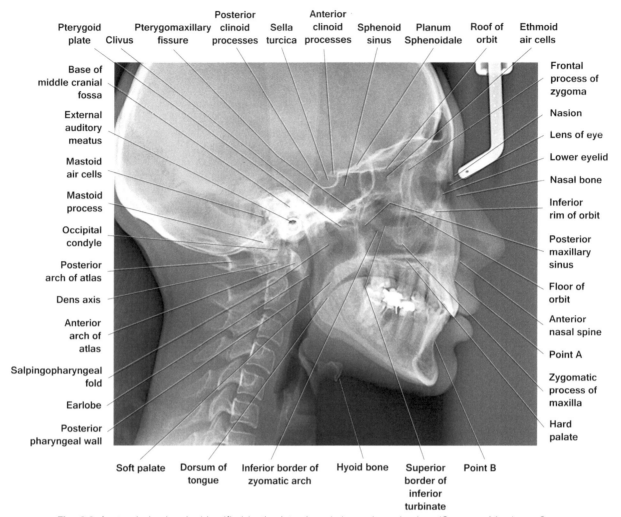

Fig. 8.2 Anatomic landmarks identified in the lateral cephalometric projection. (Courtesy Ms. Lucy Gao, University of California Los Angeles.)

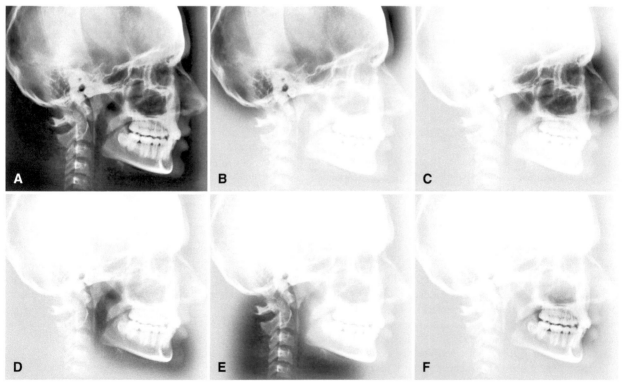

Fig. 8.3 Interrogating the lateral cephalometric projection. The radiograph in the upper left demonstrates the whole image. Subsequent radiographs correspond to the steps of interrogation.

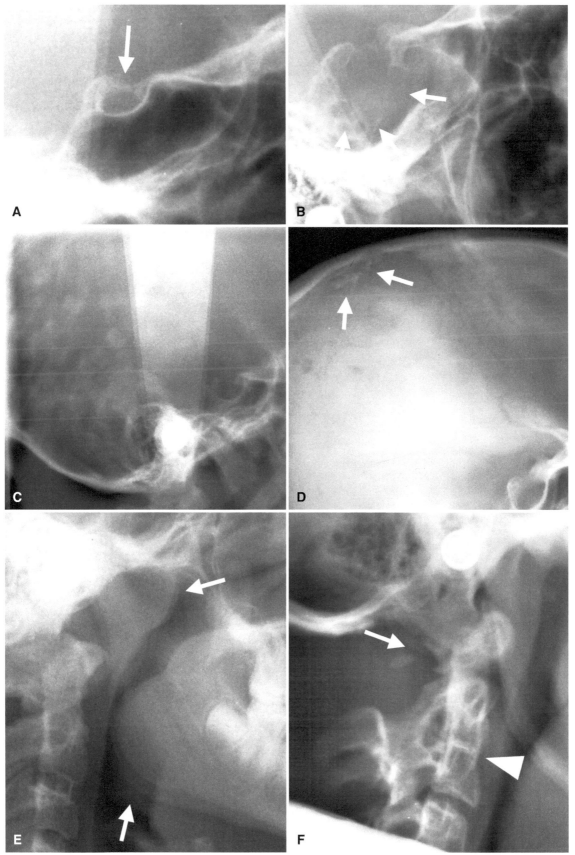

Fig. 8.4 Incidental findings on lateral cephalometric radiographs of asymptomatic orthodontic patients are indicated by *arrows*. (A) Intraclinoid ligament calcification appearing as a bridged sella. (B) Irregular and erosive expansion of the floor and anterior and posterior walls of sella turcica. (C) Hair braid shadows are superimposed over the patient's calvaria. (D) Calcification of arachnoid granulations is a normal variant. (E) Enlarged pharyngeal adenoids and palatal tonsils can be a normal finding depending on the patient's age but can compromise nasal breathing. (F) Cervical spine anomalies, such as agenesis of the posterior ring of atlas (C1) *(arrow)*, can cause spine instability, whereas vertebral fusion of dens (C2) and C3 *(arrowhead)* is a normal variant.

BOX 8.1   Definition of Cephalometric Landmarks

Skeletal Landmarks

1. Porion (P): Most superior point of the external auditory canal
2. Sella (S): Center of the hypophyseal fossa
3. Nasion (N): Frontonasal suture
4. Orbitale (O): Most inferior point of the infraorbital rim
5. PT point: Most posterior point of the pterygomaxillary fissure
6. Basion (Ba): Most anterior point of the foramen magnum
7. PNS: Tip of the posterior nasal spine
8. ANS: Tip of the anterior nasal spine
9. A point (A): Deepest point of the anterior border of the maxillary alveolar ridge concavity
10. B point (B): Deepest point in the concavity of the anterior border of the mandible
11. Pogonion (Po): Most anterior point of the symphysis
12. Gnathion: Midpoint of the symphysis outline between pogonion and menton
13. Menton (M): Most inferior point of the symphysis
14. Gonion: Most convex point along the inferior border of the mandibular ramus
15. Ramus point: Most posterior point of the posteroinferior border of the mandibular ramus
16. R1: Most inferior point of the sigmoid notch
17. R2: Arbitrary point on the lower border of the mandible below R1
18. R3: Most concave point of the anterior border of the mandibular ramus
19. R4: Most convex point of the posterior border of the mandibular ramus
20. Articulare (Ar): Point of intersection between the basisphenoid and the posterior border of the condylar head
21. Condyle top: Most superior point of the condyle
22. DC point: Center of the condylar head

Dental Landmarks

23. U6 mesial cusp: Tip of the maxillary first molar mesial buccal cusp
24. U6 mesial: Contact point on the mesial surface of the maxillary first molar
25. U6 distal: Contact point on the distal surface of the maxillary first molar
26. L6 mesial cusp: Tip of the mandibular first molar mesial buccal cusp
27. L6 mesial: Contact point on the mesial surface of the mandibular first molar
28. L6 distal: Contact point on the distal surface of the mandibular first molar
29. UI incisal: Incisal edge of maxillary central incisor
30. UI facial: Most convex point of the buccal surface of the maxillary central incisor
31. UI root: Root tip of the maxillary central incisor
32. LI incisal: Incisal edge of mandibular central incisor
33. LI facial: Most convex point of the buccal surface of the mandibular central incisor
34. LI root: Root tip of the mandibular central incisor

Soft Tissue Landmarks

35. Soft tissue glabella: Most anterior point of the soft tissue covering the frontal bone
36. Soft tissue nasion: Most concave point of soft tissue outline at the bridge of the nose
37. Tip of nose: Most anterior point of the nose
38. Subnasale: Soft tissue point where the curvature of the upper lip connects to the floor of the nose
39. Soft tissue A point: Most concave point of the upper lip between the subnasale and the upper lip point
40. Upper lip: Most anterior point of the upper lip
41. Stomion superius: Most inferior point of the upper lip
42. Stomion inferius: Most superior point of the lower lip
43. Lower lip: Most anterior point of the lower lip
44. Soft tissue B point: Most concave point of the lower lip between the chin and lower lip point
45. Soft tissue pogonion: Most anterior point of the soft tissue of the chin
46. Soft tissue gnathion: Midpoint of the chin soft tissue outline between the soft tissue pogonion and soft tissue menton
47. Soft tissue menton: Most inferior point of the soft tissue of the chin

See Fig. 8.5.

- Monitor progress of treatment and treatment outcomes.
- Proceed with orthognathic surgical treatment planning.

Image Receptor and Patient Placement

The image receptor is placed in front of the patient, perpendicular to the midsagittal plane and parallel to the coronal plane. For the PA cephalometric radiograph, the patient is placed so that the canthomeatal line forms a 10-degree angle with the horizontal plane and the Frankfurt plane and is perpendicular to the image receptor. For a standard PA skull projection, the canthomeatal line is perpendicular to the image receptor.

Position of the Central X-Ray Beam

The central beam is perpendicular to the image receptor, directed from posterior to anterior (hence the name PA), parallel to the patient's midsagittal plane, and centered at the level of the bridge of the nose.

Resultant Image (Fig. 8.6)

The midsagittal plane (represented by an imaginary line extending from the interproximal space of the central incisors through the nasal septum and the middle of the bridge of the nose) should divide the skull image into two symmetric halves. The superior border of the petrous ridge should lie in the lower third of the orbit.

Interpretation

Similar to the lateral cephalometric projection, the PA cephalogram should be viewed as a skull projection first, before any cephalometric analysis. A systematic review of the radiograph, ensuring evaluation of all structures, should be followed. Such an approach is presented next (Fig. 8.7):

Step 1. Evaluate the calvaria, sutures, and diploic space starting in the area of the left external auditory meatus, over the top of the calvaria, to the right external auditory meatus. Look for intracranial calcifications. Identify the mastoid air cells and petrous ridge of the right and left temporal bones. In this and all subsequent steps, compare the right and left sides and look for symmetry (Fig. 8.7B).

Step 2. Evaluate the upper and middle face. Identify the orbits, sinuses (frontal, ethmoid, and maxillary), and zygomatic processes of the maxilla. Assess the nasal cavity, middle and inferior turbinates, nasal septum, and hard palate (Fig. 8.7C).

Step 3. Evaluate the lower face. Follow the outline of the mandible starting from the right condylar and coronoid processes, ramus, angle, and body through the anterior mandible to the left body, angle, ramus, coronoid process, and condyle (Fig. 8.7D).

Step 4. Evaluate the cervical spine. Identify the dens, the superior border of C2, and the inferior border of C1 (Fig. 8.7E).

Step 5. Evaluate the alveolar bone and teeth (Fig. 8.7F).

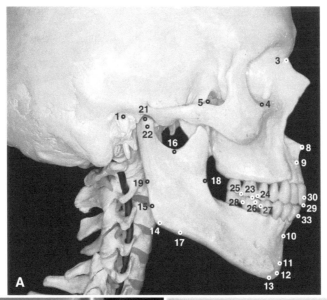

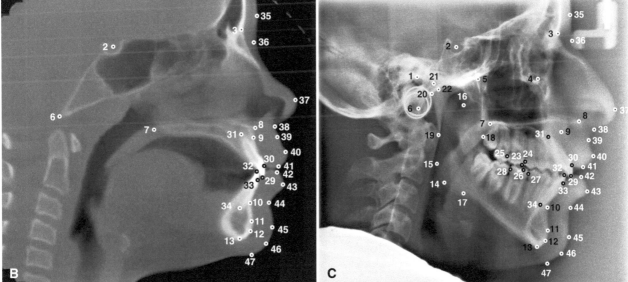

Fig. 8.5 (A) Anatomic cephalometric landmarks shown on a side view of the skull. (B) Midline anatomic cephalometric landmarks depicted on a 5-mm-wide cone beam computed tomographic section of an orthodontic patient. (C) Cephalometric landmarks used in Steiner and Ricketts cephalometric analyses *(see Box 8.1).*

CRANIOFACIAL AND SKULL PROJECTIONS

Submentovertex (Base) Projection

Indications

SMV radiographs display the base of the skull, the zygomatic arches, and the sphenoid sinuses (Fig. 8.8). These radiographs can demonstrate osseous changes from skull base tumors, fractures of the zygomatic arches, and the integrity and aeration of the sphenoid sinuses. These imaging indications are largely achieved by computed tomography (see Chapters 10, 11, and 13).

Image Receptor and Patient Placement

The image receptor is positioned parallel to the patient's transverse plane and perpendicular to the midsagittal and coronal planes. To achieve this position, the patient's neck is extended as far backward as possible, with the canthomeatal line parallel to the image receptor.

Position of the Central X-Ray Beam

The central beam is perpendicular to the image receptor, directed from below the mandible toward the vertex of the skull (hence the name SMV) and centered about 2 cm anterior to a line connecting the right and left condyles.

Resultant Image (see Fig. 8.8)

The midsagittal plane (represented by an imaginary line extending from the interproximal space of the maxillary central incisors through the nasal septum to the middle of the anterior arch of the atlas and to the dens) should divide the skull image into two symmetric halves. The buccal and lingual cortical plates of the mandible should be projected as uniform opaque lines. An underexposed view is required for the evaluation of the zygomatic arches because they will be overexposed or "burned out" on radiographs obtained with normal exposure factors.

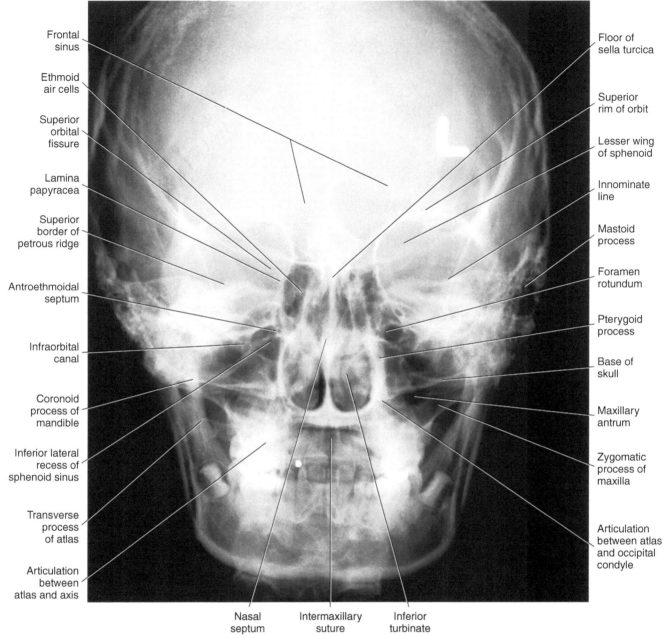

Fig. 8.6 Anatomic landmarks identified in the posteroanterior cephalometric projection.

Interpretation

As described earlier for the lateral and PA cephalometric projections, a systematic approach that ensures interrogation of the complete image and evaluation of all anatomic structures is paramount in the interpretation of the SMV projection.

Waters Projection
Indications

The Waters projection, also referred to as the occipitomental projection, displays the paranasal sinuses, predominantly the maxillary sinus and to a lesser extent the frontal sinus and ethmoid air cells. It also demonstrates the midfacial bones and orbits (Fig. 8.9). A Waters projection was used to evaluate maxillary sinusitis and midfacial fractures. Today these diagnostic objectives are accomplished by computed

tomography (see Chapters 10, 11, and 13). The American College of Radiology Appropriateness Criteria considers that this projection is usually not appropriate for the evaluation of trauma, orbits, and sinonasal disease.

Image Receptor and Patient Placement

The image receptor is placed in front of the patient and perpendicular to the midsagittal plane. The patient's head is tilted upward so that the canthomeatal line forms a 37-degree angle with the image receptor. If the patient's mouth is open, the sphenoid sinus is seen superimposed over the palate.

Position of the Central X-Ray Beam

The central beam is perpendicular to the image receptor and centered in the area of the maxillary sinuses.

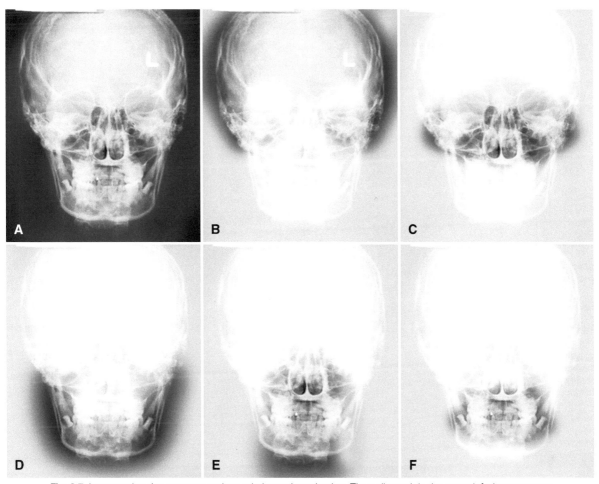

Fig. 8.7 Interrogating the posteroanterior cephalometric projection. The radiograph in the upper left demonstrates the whole image. Subsequent radiographs correspond to the steps of interrogation.

Resultant Image (see Fig. 8.9)

The midsagittal plane (represented by an imaginary line extending from the interproximal space of the maxillary central incisors through the nasal septum and the middle of the bridge of the nose) should divide the skull image into two symmetric halves. The petrous ridge of the temporal bone should be projected below the floor of the maxillary sinus.

Interpretation

As described earlier for the lateral and PA cephalometric projections, a systematic approach that ensures interrogation of the complete image and evaluation of all anatomic structures is paramount in the interpretation of the Waters projection.

Reverse Towne Projection (Open Mouth)
Indications

The reverse Towne projection was frequently used to evaluate patients with suspected fractures of the condyle and condylar neck. Today these diagnostic objectives are best achieved by computed tomography (see Chapters 10, 11, and 13).

Image Receptor and Patient Placement

The image receptor is placed in front of the patient, perpendicular to the midsagittal plane and parallel to the coronal plane. The patient's head is tilted downward so that the canthomeatal line forms a 30-degree angle with the image receptor. To improve the visualization of the condyles, the patient's mouth is opened so that the condylar heads are located inferior to the articular eminence. When requesting this image to evaluate the condyles, it is necessary to specify "open-mouth reverse Towne"; otherwise a standard Towne view of the occiput may result.

Position of Central X-Ray Beam

The central beam is perpendicular to the image receptor and parallel to the patient's midsagittal plane; it is centered at the level of the condyles.

Resultant Image (Fig. 8.10)

The midsagittal plane (represented by an imaginary line extending from the middle of the foramen magnum and the posterior arch of the atlas through the middle of the bridge of the nose and the nasal septum) should divide the skull image in two symmetric halves. The petrous ridge of the temporal bone should be superimposed at the inferior part of the occipital bone, and the condylar heads should be projected inferior to the articular eminence.

Interpretation

As described earlier for the lateral and PA cephalometric projections, a systematic approach that ensures interrogation of the complete image and evaluation of all anatomic structures is paramount in the interpretation of the reverse Towne projection.

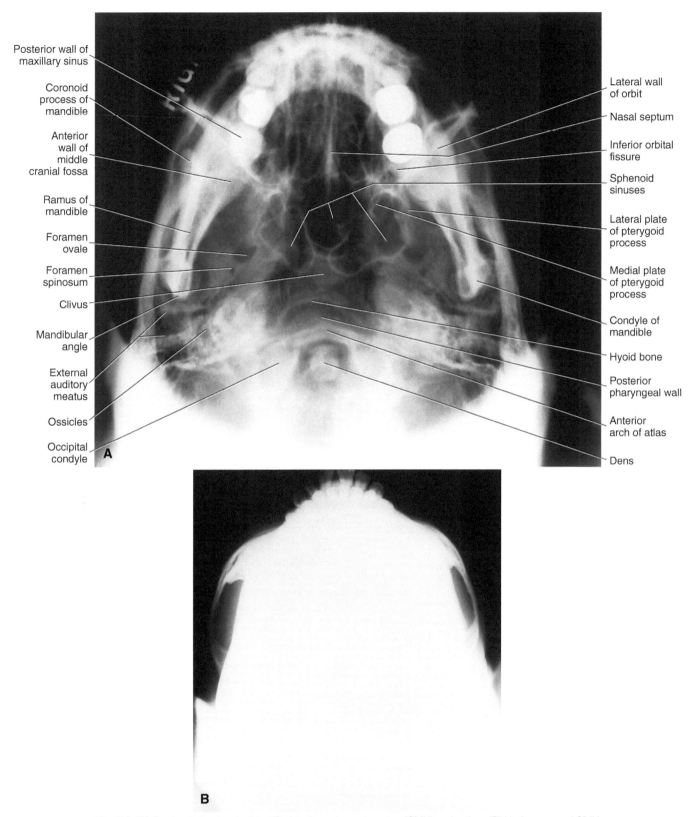

Posterior wall of maxillary sinus

Coronoid process of mandible

Anterior wall of middle cranial fossa

Ramus of mandible

Foramen ovale

Foramen spinosum

Clivus

Mandibular angle

External auditory meatus

Ossicles

Occipital condyle

Lateral wall of orbit

Nasal septum

Inferior orbital fissure

Sphenoid sinuses

Lateral plate of pterygoid process

Medial plate of pterygoid process

Condyle of mandible

Hyoid bone

Posterior pharyngeal wall

Anterior arch of atlas

Dens

A

B

Fig. 8.8 (A) Anatomic landmarks identified in the submentovertex (SMV) projection. (B) Underexposed SMV view reveals the zygomatic arches.

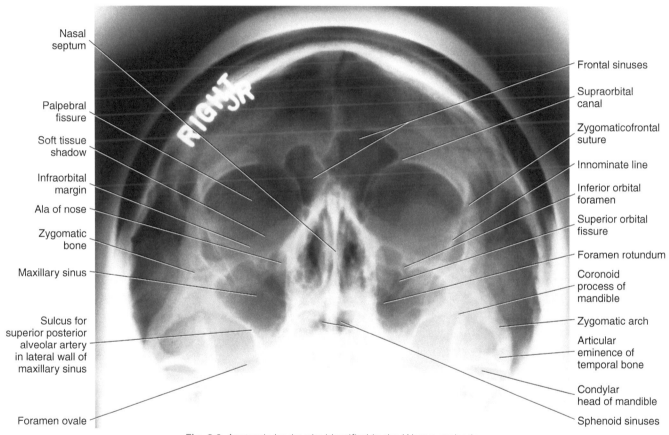

Nasal septum

Palpebral fissure

Soft tissue shadow

Infraorbital margin

Ala of nose

Zygomatic bone

Maxillary sinus

Sulcus for superior posterior alveolar artery in lateral wall of maxillary sinus

Foramen ovale

Frontal sinuses

Supraorbital canal

Zygomaticofrontal suture

Innominate line

Inferior orbital foramen

Superior orbital fissure

Foramen rotundum

Coronoid process of mandible

Zygomatic arch

Articular eminence of temporal bone

Condylar head of mandible

Sphenoid sinuses

Fig. 8.9 Anatomic landmarks identified in the Waters projection.

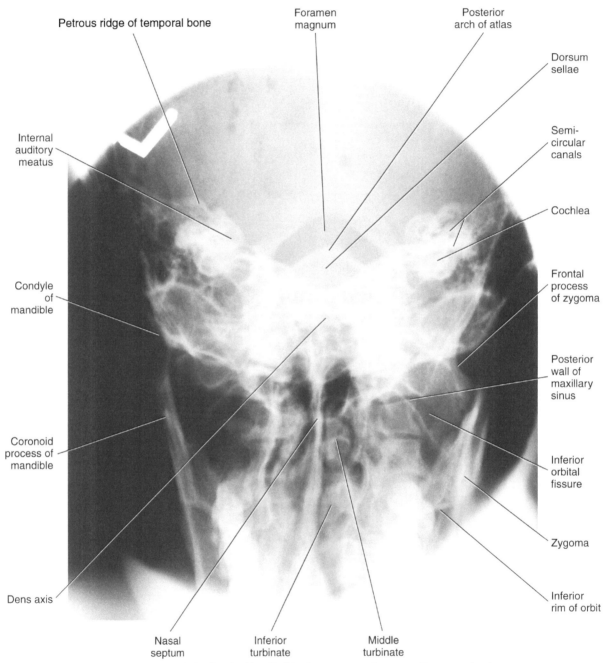

Petrous ridge of temporal bone

Foramen magnum

Posterior arch of atlas

Dorsum sellae

Semi-circular canals

Cochlea

Frontal process of zygoma

Posterior wall of maxillary sinus

Inferior orbital fissure

Zygoma

Inferior rim of orbit

Internal auditory meatus

Condyle of mandible

Coronoid process of mandible

Dens axis

Nasal septum

Inferior turbinate

Middle turbinate

Fig. 8.10 Anatomic landmarks identified in the open-mouth reverse Towne projection.

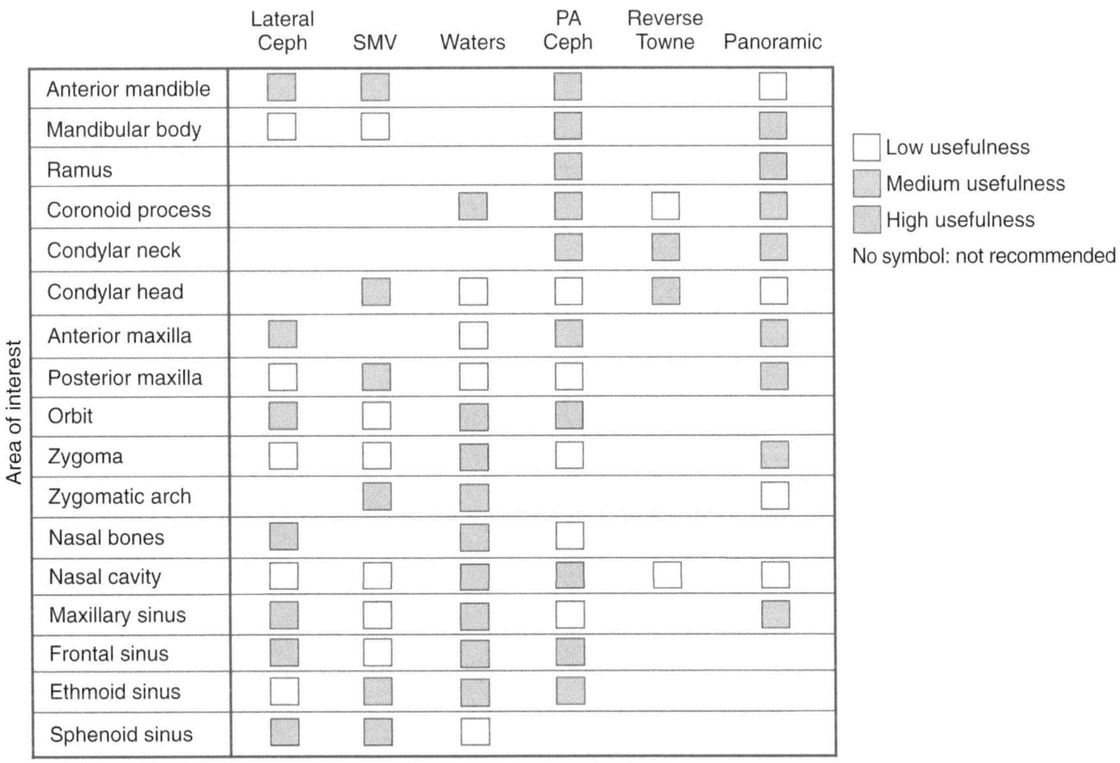

Area of interest	Lateral Ceph	SMV	Waters	PA Ceph	Reverse Towne	Panoramic
Anterior mandible	Medium	Medium		Medium		Low
Mandibular body	Low	Low		Medium		Medium
Ramus				Medium		Medium
Coronoid process			Medium	Medium	Low	Medium
Condylar neck				Medium	Medium	Medium
Condylar head		Medium	Low	Low	Medium	Low
Anterior maxilla	Medium		Low	Medium		Low
Posterior maxilla	Low	Medium	Low			Medium
Orbit	Medium	Low	Medium	Medium		
Zygoma	Low	Low	Medium	Low		Medium
Zygomatic arch		Medium	Medium			Low
Nasal bones	Medium			Low		
Nasal cavity	Low	Low	Medium	Medium	Low	Low
Maxillary sinus	Medium	Low	Medium	Low		Medium
Frontal sinus	Medium	Low	Medium	Medium		
Ethmoid sinus	Low	Medium	Medium	Medium		
Sphenoid sinus	Medium	Medium	Low			

Legend: Low usefulness / Medium usefulness / High usefulness / No symbol: not recommended

Fig. 8.11 Relative usefulness of extraoral radiographic projections to display various anatomic structures. *Ceph,* Cephalometric; *PA,* posteroanterior; *SMV,* submentovertex.

CONCLUSION

Extraoral radiography can provide valuable information for the evaluation of the dental and craniofacial complex. After assessing the patient's signs and symptoms, the clinician should choose the proper projection that provides the appropriate diagnostic information for the evaluation of the anatomic structures in question. Fig. 8.11 summarizes the use of extraoral radiographs for the evaluation of various anatomic structures. Although panoramic radiography is the subject of Chapter 9, it is included in Fig. 8.11 for comparison.

Although most extraoral radiographs in dentistry are cephalometric projections obtained for the orthodontic and orthognathic assessment of asymptomatic patients, anatomic variants that can simulate disease or affect treatment and even occult pathology can be identified. Therefore cephalometric radiographs should be viewed as skull radiographs first and interpreted following a systematic, thorough, and knowledgeable approach.

BIBLIOGRAPHY

American College of Radiology, Appropriateness Criteria. Available at https://acsearch.acr.org/list.

Kantor ML, Norton LA. Normal radiographic anatomy and common anomalies seen in cephalometric films. *Am J Orthod Dentofacial Orthop.* 1987;91:414–426.

Keats TE, Anderson MW. *Atlas of Normal Roentgen Variants That May Simulate Disease.* 9th ed. St Louis: Mosby; 2012.

Long BW, Ballinger PW, Smith BJ, et al. *Merrill's Atlas of Radiographic Positions and Radiologic Procedures.* Vol. 2. 11th ed. St Louis: Mosby; 2007.

Miyashita K. *Contemporary Cephalometric Radiography.* Tokyo: Quintessence Publishing Co; 1996.

Shapiro R. *Radiology of the Normal Skull.* Chicago: Year Book Medical Publishers; 1981.

Swischuk LE. *Imaging of the Cervical Spine in Children.* New York: Springer-Verlag; 2001.

9

Panoramic Imaging

Aruna Ramesh

Panoramic radiography (also called *pantomography*) is a body section imaging technique that results in a wide, curved image layer depicting the maxillary and mandibular dental arches and their supporting structures (Fig. 9.1). This is achieved by using a single rotation of the x-ray source and image receptor around the patient's head (Fig. 9.2). Panoramic images are most useful clinically for diagnostic challenges requiring broad coverage of the jaws (Box 9.1). Common clinical applications include evaluation of trauma including jaw fractures, location of third molars, extensive dental or osseous disease, known or suspected large lesions, tooth development and eruption (especially in the mixed dentition), impacted or unerupted teeth and root remnants (in edentulous patients), temporomandibular joint (TMJ) pain, and developmental anomalies. Panoramic imaging is often used in initial patient evaluation that can provide the required insight or assist in determining the need for other projections. Panoramic images are also useful for patients who do not tolerate intraoral procedures well.

The main disadvantage of panoramic radiography is the lack of fine anatomic detail available on intraoral periapical radiographs. Thus it is not as useful as periapical radiography for detecting small carious lesions, fine structure of the marginal periodontium, or early periapical disease. The proximal surfaces of premolars also typically overlap. The availability of a panoramic radiograph for an adult patient often does not preclude the need for intraoral films for the diagnoses of most commonly encountered dental diseases. When a full-mouth series of radiographs is available for a patient requiring only general dental care, typically little or no additional useful information is gained from a simultaneous panoramic examination. A panoramic combined with bitewings or with bitewings and selected periapical radiographs could provide diagnostic information similar to a full-mouth series. Other problems associated with panoramic radiography include unequal magnification and geometric distortion across the image. Occasionally, the presence of overlapping structures, such as the cervical spine, can hide odontogenic lesions, particularly in the incisor regions. Clinically important objects may be situated outside the focal trough and may appear distorted or not be seen at all.

PRINCIPLES OF PANORAMIC IMAGE FORMATION

The principles of panoramic radiography were first described by Paatero and Numata independently in 1948 and 1933, respectively. Fig. 9.2 shows a schematic view of the relationships between the x-ray source, the patient, the secondary collimator, and the image receptor during panoramic image formation. The following illustrations explain the formation of the *focal trough* in a panoramic machine. Imagine an assembly containing a disk with upright physical objects (represented by letters) and an image receptor (Fig. 9.3). The receptor travels upward through the beam at the same speed as objects A through C rotate

through the beam. A lead collimator in the shape of a slit located at the x-ray source limits the x-rays to a narrow vertical beam. Another collimator between the objects and the image receptor reduces scattered radiation from the objects to the image receptor. Consider first radiopaque objects A through C. As the disk rotates, their radiographic images are recorded sharply on the receptor that also moves through the beam at the same direction and speed. The spatial relationship of the shadows of these objects correctly represents the relationship of the actual objects. Because the source-receptor distance is constant and the object-receptor distance is the same for each object, all objects are magnified equally. Now consider objects D through F. They are located on the opposite side of the disk, between the x-ray source and the center of rotation of the disk. These objects move in the opposite direction of the receptor, so their shadows are reversed on the receptor. Because these objects are much closer to the x-ray source, their images are greatly magnified.

Fig. 9.4 shows that the same relationship between the rotating receptor and objects can be achieved if the disk is held stationary but the x-ray source and the receptor are rotated around the center of rotation in the disk. The x-ray beam still passes through the center of the disk and sequentially through objects A through C. Similarly, the receptor is still moved through the beam and at the same rate as the beam passes through A through C. In this situation, as before, objects A through C move through the x-ray beam in the same direction and at the same rate as the receptor. Objects D through F continue to be blurred, just as before.

Fig. 9.5 shows that a patient may replace the disk and objects A through F represent teeth and surrounding bone. The illustration demonstrates the positions of the x-ray source and the receptor early in an exposure cycle. The center of rotation is located off to the side of the arch, away from the objects being imaged. The rate of movement of the receptor is regulated to be the same as that of the x-ray beam sweeping through the dentoalveolar structures on the side of the patient nearest the receptor. Structures on the opposite side of the patient (near the x-ray tube) are distorted and appear out of focus because the x-ray beam sweeps through them in the direction opposite that in which the image receptor is moving. In addition, structures near the x-ray source are so magnified (and their borders so blurred) that they are not seen as discrete images on the resultant image. These structures appear only as diffuse phantom or ghost images. Because of both of these circumstances, only structures near the receptor are usefully captured on the resultant image.

Contemporary panoramic machines use a continuously moving center of rotation rather than multiple fixed locations (Fig. 9.6). This feature optimizes the shape of the focal trough to image best the teeth and supporting bone. This center of rotation is initially near the lingual surface of the right body of the mandible when the left TMJ region is being imaged. The rotational center moves anteriorly along an arc that

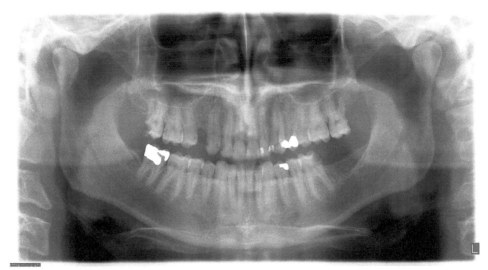

Fig. 9.1 Panoramic image demonstrating broad coverage of hard and soft tissues of adult orofacial region including maxilla, mandible, dentition, and adjacent structures. Panoramic images are made with a much lower dose than a full-mouth set and have broader coverage; however, they have lower spatial resolution.

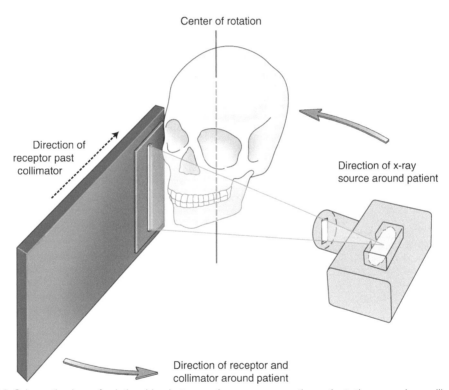

Center of rotation

Direction of
receptor past
collimator

Direction of x-ray
source around patient

Direction of receptor and
collimator around patient

Fig. 9.2 Schematic view of relationships between the x-ray source, the patient, the secondary collimator, and image receptor. As the x-ray tube head moves around one side of the patient, the receptor assembly moves toward the opposite side. The image receptor slides past the collimator, sequentially producing a latent image. With a charge-coupled device (CCD) image receptor, there is a vertical CCD linear array behind the collimator that continuously reads out the exposure to produce an image.

ends just lingual to the symphysis of the mandible when the midline is imaged. The arc is reversed as the opposite side of the jaws is imaged.

This basic principle of image formation remains the same, regardless of the type of detector used to record the image. In the case where the receptor is a charge-coupled device (CCD) array, the film is replaced by a two-dimensional CCD array. Each column of the array is read out

to construct the image. The key is to read out the columns at the same rate as an imaginary moving film would move past the array. The CCD array is read out continuously as the x-ray source and receptor travel around the patient. The resulting geometric projection characteristics are the same as in film or photostimulable phosphor (PSP) plate imaging.

Focal Trough (Image Layer)

The focal trough or image layer is a wide, three-dimensional curved zone, where the structures positioned within this zone are reasonably well defined on the panoramic image (Fig. 9.7). The anatomic structures seen on a panoramic image are primarily those positioned within the focal trough during imaging. Structures positioned in the center of the focal trough are the clearest and those that are progressively farther from the center of the focal trough become progressively less clear. Objects outside the focal trough are blurred, magnified, or reduced in size and are sometimes distorted to the extent of not being recognizable. The shape of the focal trough varies with the brand of equipment used, as well as with the imaging protocol selected within each unit. The shape and width of the focal trough is determined by the path and velocity of the receptor and x-ray tube head, alignment of the x-ray beam, and collimator width. The location of the focal trough can change with extensive machine use, so recalibration may be necessary if consistently suboptimal images are being produced.

In some panoramic machines, the shape and size of the focal trough can be adjusted to conform better to the patients' maxillomandibular anatomy allowing for better imaging of children, patients with atypical jaw morphology or specific anatomic sites of interest such as the TMJ or the maxillary sinuses. This modification is achieved by decreasing the rotational arc of the x-ray source-receptor movement to reduce the

---

BOX 9.1   Panoramic Imaging

Indications
- Overall evaluation of dentition
- Examine for intraosseous pathology, such as cysts, tumors, or infections
- Gross evaluation of temporomandibular joints
- Evaluation of position of impacted teeth
- Evaluation of eruption of permanent dentition
- Dentomaxillofacial trauma
- Developmental disturbances of maxillofacial skeleton

Advantages Compared With a Full-Mouth Examination
- Broad coverage of facial bones and teeth
- Low radiation dose
- Ease of panoramic radiographic technique
- Can be used in patients with trismus or in patients who cannot tolerate intraoral radiography
- Quick and convenient radiographic technique
- Useful visual aid in patient education and case presentation

Disadvantages
- Lower-resolution images that do not provide the fine details provided by intraoral radiographs
- Magnification across image is unequal, making linear measurements unreliable
- Image is superimposition of real, double, and ghost images and requires careful visualization to decipher anatomic and pathologic details
- Requires accurate patient positioning to avoid positioning errors and artifacts
- Difficult to image both jaws when patient has severe maxillomandibular discrepancy

---

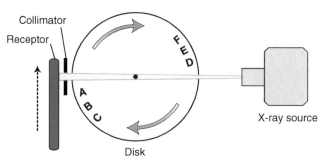

Fig. 9.3 Producing a panoramic image: In this conceptual view, the x-ray source and collimator are held stationary. The receptor moves through the beam, and the rotating disk also carries objects *A–F* through the beam. Objects *A–C* move through the beam at the same rate and direction as the image receptor and are imaged well. Objects *D–F* move through the beam at the same rate as the receptor but in the opposite direction, and so their images are blurred. The principles of panoramic image formation are the same for film-based and digital systems.

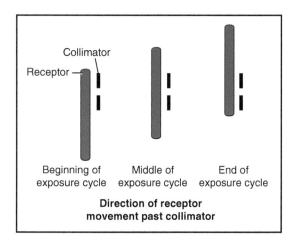

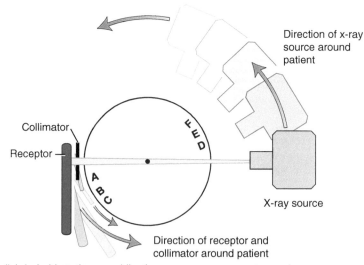

Fig. 9.4 Producing a panoramic image: The disk is held stationary while the x-ray source, receptor, and collimator rotate around the center of the disk. Nonetheless, the x-ray beam still passes through the objects to the image receptor in the same direction as in Fig. 9.3, and the same imaging results are obtained. The *inset* emphasizes how the receptor moves past the collimator during their motion around the disk.

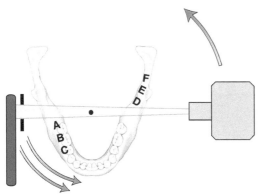

Fig. 9.5 Producing a panoramic image: The imaging geometry is the same as Figs. 9.3 and 9.4, but the disk and objects are replaced with a patient. The rate the receptor moves through the beam is the same as the rate the beam passes through objects *A–C*; thus only the dentition in the mandible near the receptor (objects *A–C*) are imaged well. Structures on the opposite side of the mandible (objects *D–F*) are blurred beyond recognition.

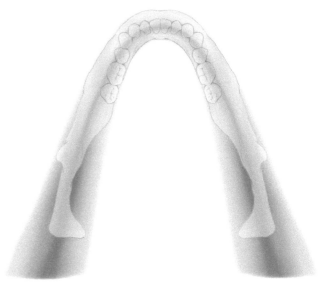

Fig. 9.7 Focal trough: The moving source and receptor generate a zone of sharpness, known as the focal trough or image layer. The closer an anatomic structure is positioned to the center of the trough, the more clearly it is imaged on the resulting radiograph. Panoramic machines typically provide laser lights to allow the operator to position the patient's dentition optimally in the focal trough.

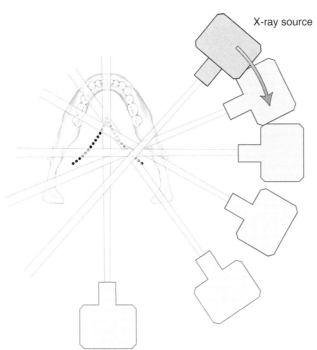

X-ray source

Fig. 9.6 Producing a panoramic image: In contrast to the preceding three schematic drawings shown in Figs. 9.3–9.5, the center of rotation of the x-ray source moves continuously as the tube and receptor rotate around the patient. Initially, the x-ray beam rotates on the end of the dotted arc on the tube side of the patient. As the x-ray source moves behind the patient, the center of rotation moves forward along the arc *(dotted line)*. The drawing shows the directions of the x-ray beam at various intervals for the first half of the exposure cycle. The x-ray source then continues to move around the patient to image the opposite side.

focal trough size to better adapt to pediatric jaws. The decreased rotational arc also results in reduced patient radiation exposure. In some panoramic units, the projection angle of the x-ray beam is modified to yield images with decreased overlap of adjacent teeth and with minimal superimposition of structures from the opposite side of the jaw.

Real, Double, and Ghost Images

Because of the rotational nature of the x-ray source and receptor, the x-ray beam intercepts some anatomic structures twice during the single

exposure cycle. Depending on their location, objects may cast three different types of images:

- *Real images:* Objects that lie between the center of rotation and the receptor form a real image. Within this zone, objects that lie within the focal trough cast relatively sharp images, whereas images of objects located outside the focal trough are blurred. Fig. 9.8A and C show the positions of the x-ray source during imaging of the left and right sides of the mandibular ramus, respectively. In Fig. 9.8A, the left ramus lies between the center of rotation and the receptor and casts a real image. Because it is within the focal trough, its image is sharp. Also demonstrated in Fig. 9.8A is the formation of the real images of the hyoid bone and cervical spine. However, because these structures are away from the center of the focal trough and closer to the x-ray source, their images are blurred and magnified. Fig. 9.8D shows in blue the anatomic region that makes real images.
- *Double images:* Objects that lie posterior to the center of rotation and that are intercepted twice by the x-ray beam form double images (green region in Fig. 9.8E). This region includes the hyoid bone, epiglottis, and cervical spine, all of which cast images on both the right and left side of the image.
- *Ghost images:* Some objects are located between the x-ray source and the center of rotation. These objects cast ghost images. On the panoramic image, ghost images appear on the opposite side of its true anatomic location and at a higher level because of the upward inclination of the x-ray beam. As the object is located outside of the focal plane and close to the x-ray source, the ghost image is blurred and significantly magnified. Several anatomic structures cast ghost images (orange region in Fig. 9.8F). For example, in Fig. 9.8A, the right mandibular ramus lies between the x-ray source and the center of rotation and its ghost image is superimposed over the left side of the image. Similarly, the ghost image of the left ramus is superimposed over the right side of the image (see Fig. 9.8C). The hyoid bone and cervical spine also form ghost images when the anterior regions of the jaws are imaged (see Fig. 9.8B). In addition, metallic accessories, such as earrings, necklaces, and hairpins, form

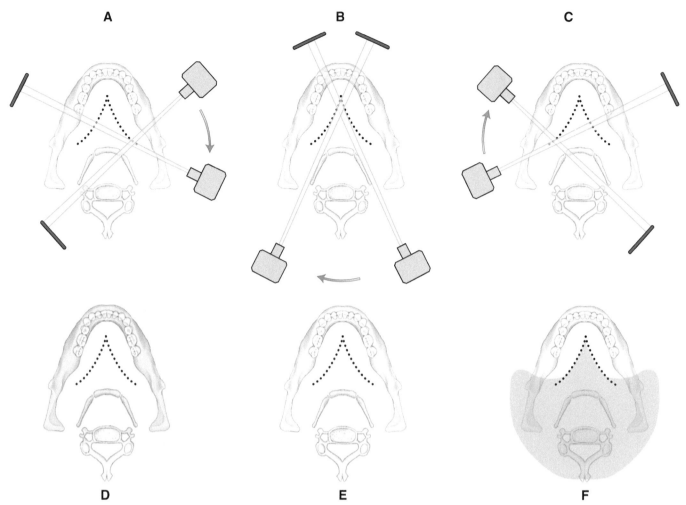

Fig. 9.8 Formation of real, double, and ghost images. (A–C) The exposure begins with the x-ray tube head on the patient's right side and continues with the tube head moving behind the patient and ending on the left side. The *dotted line* represents the path of the moving center of rotation during the exposure cycle. (D) Structures between the moving center of rotation and the receptor form real images *(blue zone)*. (E) Structures lying between the moving centers of rotation and the receptor that are imaged twice *(green zone)* cast double images. (F) Structures located between the x-ray source and moving center of rotation *(orange zone)* cast ghost images.

ghost images, which appear as blurred radiopaque images that can obscure anatomic details, mask pathologic changes, or mimic pathologic changes. The ghost images of the hard palate and mandibular body and angle are clearly visualized in a panoramic image (Fig. 9.9). Some anatomic zones form both real double and ghost images. These zones are the regions of overlap between the orange and green regions in Fig. 9.8E and F.

Image Distortion

The panoramic image necessarily produces distortion of the size and shape of the object, making it unreliable for linear or angular measurements. The image distortion is influenced by several factors, including x-ray beam angulation, x-ray source-to-object distance, path of rotational center, and position of the object within the focal trough. These parameters vary among panoramic units and among different regions of the jaws for the same unit. They are also strongly dependent on patient anatomy and positioning of the patient in the unit. These variables make it impossible to apply preset magnification factors that can be used to make reliable measurements on panoramic radiographs.

Horizontal magnification is determined by the position of the object within the focal trough. The magnitude of the horizontal distortion depends on the distance of the object from the center of the focal trough and thus is strongly influenced by patient positioning. Fig. 9.10 illustrates the influence of anterior patient positioning on image size and shape. Fig. 9.10A and B show a mandible supporting a brass ring properly aligned in the center of the focal trough. A notched positioning device (bite-block) denotes the center of the anterior aspect of the focal trough. Note the even magnification of the ring and the images of the anterior teeth in proper proportion. Fig. 9.10C–E show the same mandible positioned 5 mm posterior to the center of the focal trough and a panoramic radiograph of a patient with the same error. This position causes distortion of the ring in the horizontal dimension, with the ring appearing broader with a commensurate increase in width of the images of the teeth. Fig. 9.10F–H show the same mandible positioned 5 mm anterior to the center of the focal trough and a panoramic radiograph of a patient with the same error. The horizontal distortion results in the ring appearing narrow with a commensurate decrease in width of the projected teeth. On these images, the vertical dimension, in contrast

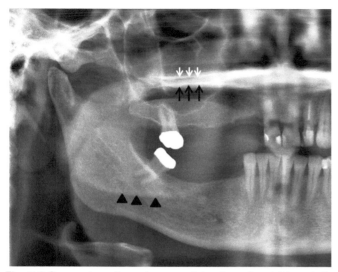

Fig. 9.9 Panoramic radiograph cropped to show the right posterior midfacial region. The hard palate appears as two radiopaque lines. The lower line *(black arrows)* represents the junction between the hard palate and lateral nasal wall on the receptor side of the patient. The upper line *(white arrows)* represents the junction between the nasal wall and hard palate on the tube side or ghost image of the opposite side. The *black arrowheads* indicate the ghost image of the opposite mandible.

to the horizontal dimension, is little altered. These distortions result from the horizontal movements of the receptor and x-ray source. Thus, as a general rule, when the structure of interest, in this case the mandible, is displaced to the lingual side of its optimal position in the focal trough, toward the x-ray source, the beam passes more slowly through it than the speed at which the receptor moves. Consequently, the images of the structures in this region are elongated horizontally on the image, and they appear wider. Alternatively, when the mandible is displaced toward the buccal aspect of the focal trough, the beam passes at a rate faster than normal through the structures. In the example shown, because the receptor is moving at the proper rate, the representations of the anterior teeth are compressed horizontally on the image, and they appear thinner.

The same principle applies to the patient's midsagittal plane being rotated in the focal trough. The posterior structures on the side to which the patient's head is rotated are magnified in the horizontal dimension because the posterior structures are positioned away from the image receptor, whereas posterior structures on the opposite side are positioned closer to the image receptor and are reduced in horizontal dimension. The resulting image has horizontally (mesiodistally) large molar teeth and mandibular ramus and severe premolar overlap on one side and horizontally (mesiodistally) smaller molar teeth and mandibular ramus on the other side (this positioning artifact is demonstrated in Fig. 9.11). This imaging appearance must not be confused with a congenital or developmental facial asymmetry.

The magnitude of horizontal distortion varies between the anterior and posterior regions of the jaws. In the anterior region, horizontal magnification increases markedly as the object moves away from the center of the focal trough. The degree of this magnification in the posterior regions is less than that in the anterior region. Two identical objects located in the anterior and posterior regions may have different horizontal magnifications. Thus overall horizontal measurements made

on panoramic radiographs are unreliable. Special attention must be paid to these considerations when following the progress of a bony lesion, especially in the anterior region. As a result of improper patient positioning, the lesion may appear relatively larger (enlarging) (see Fig. 9.10D) or smaller (healing) (see Fig. 9.10G) on successive images. The importance of careful alignment and positioning of the patient's dental arches within the focal trough is apparent.

Vertical magnification is determined by distance between the x-ray source and the object, similar to conventional radiography. In some panoramic units, this distance is maintained constant throughout the exposure cycle, resulting in a relatively constant vertical magnification in different areas of the image.

The orientation of the panoramic x-ray beam has a slight caudocranial inclination. As a result of this beam angulation, structures that are positioned closer to the source are projected higher up on the image, relative to structures that are positioned farther away from the source of radiation. Thus the spatial relationships between the objects in the vertical dimension may not accurately represent true anatomic relationships, rendering assessment of vertical relationships in panoramic radiograph unreliable. Fig. 9.12 depicts a mandibular molar and three different positions of the mandibular canal, from lingual to buccal. All three positions are in the same horizontal plane (see Fig. 9.12A). However, owing to the angulation of the x-ray beam, the image of the lingually positioned canal (orange) is projected closer to the apex of the molar, whereas the image of the buccally positioned canal (green) is projected farther away from the root apex. Thus the distance between the root apex and the mandibular canal can be misrepresented on a panoramic radiograph.

Panoramic Machines

A number of manufacturers produce high-quality film-based and digital panoramic machines. Most of these units have the versatility to allow for adjustment of focal trough shape based on patient size (adult vs. child) for panoramic image and produce tomographic cross-sectional images of selected areas of the facial skeleton. One such unit is presented in Fig. 9.13A. As mentioned previously, in addition to producing standard panoramic images of the jaws, some of these units have the capability of adjusting to patients of various sizes and making frontal and lateral images of TMJs, tomographic views through the sinuses, and cross-sectional views of the maxilla and mandible. These views are acquired by having special x-ray source and receptor movements programmed into the machine. "Extraoral bitewing" views are also offered by a few of the panoramic units that can be especially useful in patients having difficulty with intraoral receptor placement (see Fig. 9.13B). Each machine also has the capability for adding on a cephalometric attachment to allow exposure of standardized skull views. Some machines have the capability of automated exposure control; this is accomplished by measuring the amount of radiation passing through the patient's mandible during the initial part of the exposure and adjusting the imaging factors (kilovoltage peak [kVp], milliamperage [mA], and speed of imaging movements) to obtain an optimally exposed image. Finally, all of these machines are available in CCD-digital configurations, and some have cone beam imaging capability (see Chapters 11 to 13).

PATIENT POSITIONING AND HEAD ALIGNMENT

Proper patient preparation and positioning within the focal trough are essential to obtaining diagnostic panoramic radiographs. Dental appliances, earrings, necklaces, hairpins, and any other metallic objects in the head and neck region should be removed. It may also be wise to demonstrate the machine to the patient by cycling it while

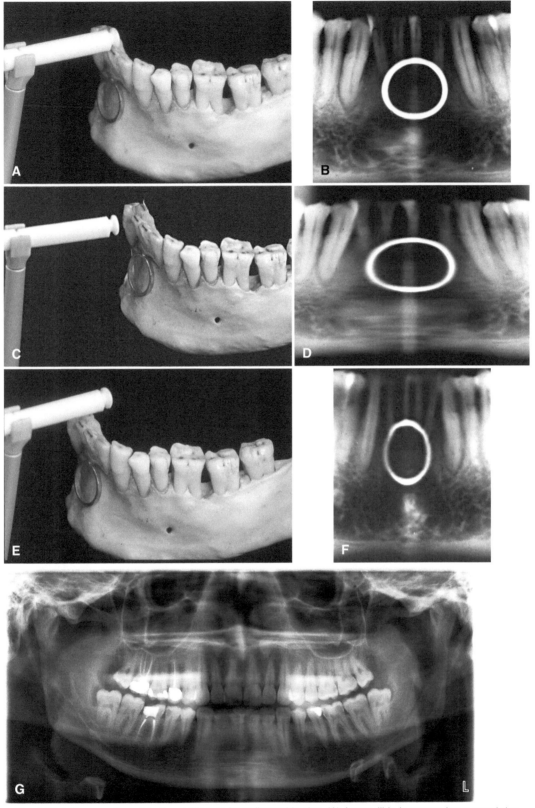

Fig. 9.10 Influence of an object's position on its radiographic size. (A) A mandible is supporting a metal ring positioned at the center of the focal trough. The mandible is positioned at the center of the focal trough by placing the incisal edges of the central incisors in a notch at the end of a bite rod-positioning device. (B) Resultant cropped panoramic radiograph shows minimal distortion of the metal ring. (C) The mandible and ring are positioned 5 mm posterior to the focal trough. (D) Resultant cropped panoramic radiograph demonstrates horizontal magnification of both the ring and the mandibular teeth. (E) The mandible and ring are positioned 5 mm anterior to the notch in the bite-block. (F) Resultant cropped panoramic radiograph demonstrates the horizontal minification of both the ring and the mandibular teeth. (G) Panoramic radiograph of a patient showing horizontal magnification in the anterior teeth due to patient positioning error as shown in *C*.

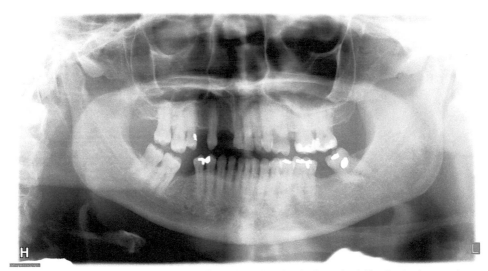

Fig. 9.10, cont'd (H) Panoramic radiograph of a patient showing horizontal minification in the anterior teeth due to patient positioning error as shown in *E*. There is also a rotation to the left present in *H*.

explaining the need to remain still during the procedure. This is particularly important for children, who may be anxious. Children should be instructed to look forward and not to follow the tube head with their eyes.

The anteroposterior head position is achieved typically by having patients place the incisal edges of their maxillary and mandibular incisors into a notched positioning device (bite-stick). Patient's midsagittal plane must be centered within the focal trough without any lateral shift in the mandible when making this protrusive movement. Most panoramic units have laser beams to facilitate alignment of the patient's midsagittal plane, Frankfort plane, and anteroposterior position within the focal trough.

Placement of the patient either too far anterior or too far posterior relative to the focal trough results in significant dimensional aberrations in the images. Too far posterior positioning results in magnified mesiodistal dimensions *("fat" teeth)* through the anterior sextants (see Fig. 9.10D). Too far anterior positioning results in reduced mesiodistal dimensions *("thin" teeth)* through the anterior sextants (see Fig. 9.10F). Failure to position the midsagittal plane in the rotational midline of the machine results in a radiograph showing right and left sides that are unequally magnified in the horizontal dimension (see Fig. 9.11). Poor midline positioning is a common error, causing horizontal distortion in the posterior regions; excessive tooth overlap in the premolar regions; and occasionally, nondiagnostic, clinically unacceptable images. A simple method for evaluating the degree of horizontal distortion of the image is to compare the apparent mesiodistal width of the mandibular first molars bilaterally. The smaller side is too close to the receptor, and the larger side is too close to the center of rotation or rotational center.

The patient's chin and occlusal plane must be properly positioned to avoid distortion. The occlusal plane is aligned so that it is slightly lower anteriorly. A general guide for chin positioning is to position the patient so that a line from the tragus of the ear to the outer canthus of the eye is parallel with the floor. If the chin is tipped too high, the occlusal plane on the radiograph appears flat or inverted, and the resultant image of the mandible is distorted (Fig. 9.14A). In addition, the radiopaque shadow of the hard palate is superimposed on the roots of the maxillary teeth. If the chin is tipped too low, the occlusal plane shows an exaggerated smile line, the teeth become severely overlapped, the

symphyseal region of the mandible may be cut off the film, and both mandibular condyles may be projected off the superior edge of the film (see Fig. 9.14B).

Patients are positioned with their backs and spines as erect as possible and their necks extended. Props such as a cushion for back support, foot support, or to straighten the spine minimize the artifact produced by vertebral shadow. Proper neck extension is best accomplished by using a gentle upward force on the mastoid eminences when positioning the head with a slight lower inclination of the chin. Allowing patients to slump their heads and necks forward causes a large opaque artifact in the midline created by the superimposition of the cervical vertebrae. This shadow obscures the entire symphyseal region of the mandible and may require that the radiograph be retaken (Fig. 9.15A). Finally, after patients are positioned in the machine, they should be instructed to swallow and hold the tongue flat against the roof of the mouth. This raises the dorsum of the tongue to the hard palate, eliminating the airspace and providing optimal visualization of the apices of the maxillary teeth. Fig. 9.15B presents improper tongue positioning with the resulting an airspace below the hard palate hindering visualization of the apices of the maxillary teeth.

IMAGE RECEPTORS

The use of digital image receptors in panoramic imaging has become very common. Both PSP and solid-state detectors (CCD or complementary metal oxide semiconductor [CMOS] device) are used in panoramic imaging (see Chapter 4). In indirect digital acquisition with the film-sized PSP plate, the image is processed by reading the latent image off of the PSP plate, yielding a digital image. Alternatively, direct digital acquisition panoramic machines use an array of solid-state detectors that transmit an electronic signal to the controlling computer, which is transmitted to the display screen, as it is being acquired. Digital modalities allow postacquisition processing to enhance the image characteristics, including contrast and density adjustments, white/black inversion, magnification, edge enhancement, and color rendering. Most units are capable of exporting the digital image in DICOM (Digital Imaging and Communications in Medicine) format or in a variety of standard image formats, such as Tagged Image File Format (tiff) or

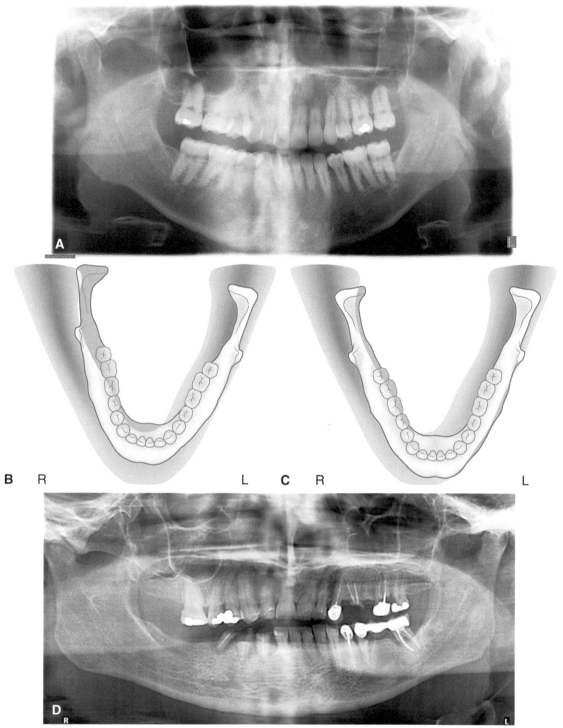

Fig. 9.11 (A) Panoramic radiographic presentation of positioning error—rotation of the sagittal plane. The patient's head was rotated to the right, placing the right jaws lingual to the focal trough and the left jaws buccal to the focal trough. As a consequence, the images of the right jaws are magnified and the images of the left jaws are minimized. Note also the interproximal overlaps of the right posterior teeth. (B) Schematic presentation of rotation of patient's head to the right side *without* a midline shift noted in Fig. 9.11A. (C and D) Schematic and radiographic presentation of shift of the patient's head to left *with* a shift in the midline, without rotation of the head. The resultant panoramic radiograph shows horizontal magnification in the anterior teeth in addition to the magnification in the right jaws.

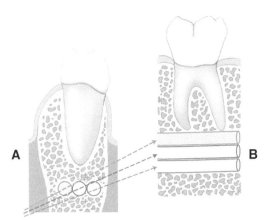

Fig. 9.12 Influence of projection geometry on spatial relationships in the vertical dimension. (A) Diagrammatic representation of a coronal cross section through the mandible. Three potential locations of the mandibular canal are shown. The locations lie in the same horizontal plane but differ in their buccolingual position. The x-ray beam *(dotted lines)* is angulated relative to the horizontal plane. (B) Apparent locations of the mandibular canals in the resultant image. When lingually positioned *(orange)*, the canal is projected more superiorly than when the canal is located buccally *(green)*.

Joint Photography Experts Group (jpeg), allowing easy exchange of radiographic images. DICOM is a standard that specifies handling, storage, printing, and transmission of medical images. The American Dental Association endorses the use of DICOM as the standard for exchange of all dental digital images and recommends that all new digital x-ray units be DICOM compliant.

Intensifying screens (see Chapter 5) are used in film-based panoramic radiography because they significantly reduce the amount of radiation required for properly exposing a radiograph. Fast films combined with high-speed (rare earth) screens are indicated for most examinations. In most cases the manufacturer provides panoramic machines with intensifying screens. The type of screen (manufacturer and model) is printed in black letters on each screen and clearly projected onto the radiograph. With rare earth screens and fast films, the patient's skin exposure from panoramic radiography is approximately equivalent to four bitewing views using F-speed film.

All panoramic radiographs must have a mechanism to indicate the patient's name, date of birth, the right and left side of the patient, date of examination and the name of the dentist, without obscuring anatomic structures. No parts of the image should be trimmed to make the film fit the patient's chart.

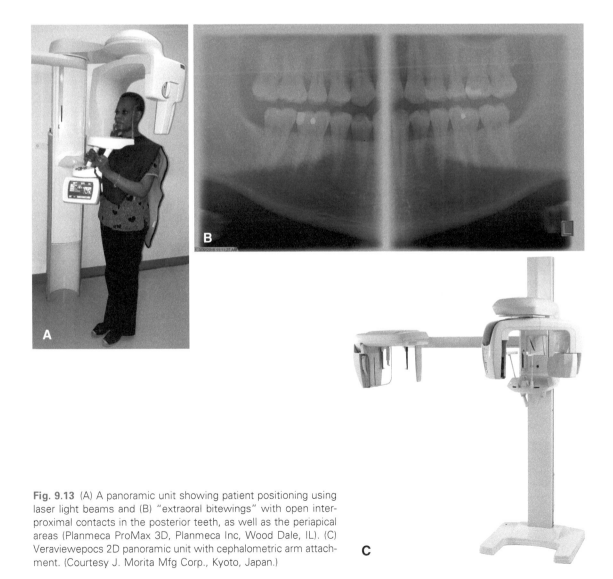

Fig. 9.13 (A) A panoramic unit showing patient positioning using laser light beams and (B) "extraoral bitewings" with open interproximal contacts in the posterior teeth, as well as the periapical areas (Planmeca ProMax 3D, Planmeca Inc, Wood Dale, IL). (C) Veraviewepocs 2D panoramic unit with cephalometric arm attachment. (Courtesy J. Morita Mfg Corp., Kyoto, Japan.)

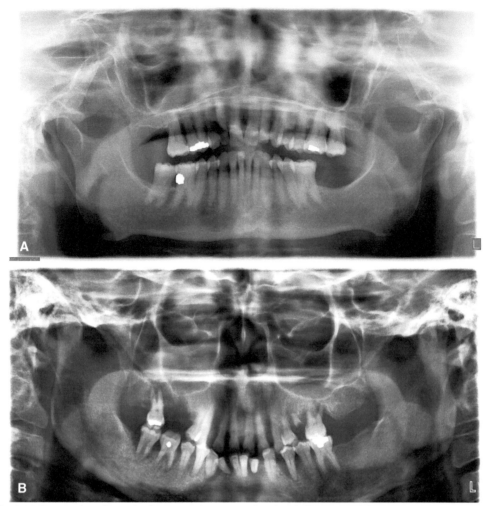

Fig. 9.14 Panoramic radiographs demonstrating poor patient head alignment. (A) The chin and occlusal plane are rotated upward, resulting in overlapping images of the teeth and an opaque shadow (the hard palate) obscuring the roots of the maxillary teeth. (B) The chin and occlusal plane are rotated downward, cutting off the symphyseal region on the radiograph and distorting the anterior teeth.

PANORAMIC FILM DARKROOM TECHNIQUES

Special darkroom procedures are needed when panoramic film is being processed. These films are far more light sensitive than intraoral films, especially after they have been exposed. A reduction in darkroom lighting from that used for conventional intraoral film is necessary. A Kodak GBX-2 (Carestream Dental LLC, Atlanta, GA) filter can be installed with a 15-watt bulb at least 4 feet from the working surface. Panoramic film should be developed either manually or in automatic film processors according to the manufacturers' recommendations in order to obtain optimal images.

INTERPRETING PANORAMIC IMAGES

The need for appropriate ambient lighting and a quiet viewing room apply equally to viewing digital images on a computer display and traditional film radiographs on a viewbox. Image interpretation starts with a systematic analysis of the image and a thorough understanding of the appearances of the normal anatomic structures and their variants on the image. Panoramic images are quite different from intraoral images and demand a disciplined and focused approach to their interpretation.

Recognizing normal anatomic structures on panoramic radiographs is challenging because of the complex anatomy of the midface, the superimposition of various hard and soft structures, and the changing projection orientation with real, double, and ghost images. The many potential artifacts associated with machine and patient movement and patient positioning must be identified and understood.

Routine imaging in dentistry is predominantly limited to two-dimensional representation of three-dimensional structures. On a posteroanterior (PA) skull film, orbital rims, nasal conchae, teeth, cervical vertebrae, and petrous ridges are all in sharp focus on the image, although they may be 8 inches apart from each other. Despite this presenting less interpretation challenge in a panoramic view, which is a curved image "slice" of the maxillomandibular complex, there is still the thickness to the tomogram that must be considered. The clinician must relate the structures on the image to their relative positions in the midfacial skeleton. An example of this three-dimensionality is the relative positioning of the external oblique and mylohyoid ridges in the mandible: On the panoramic image, they generally both appear sharp, whereas physically the external oblique ridge is on the mandibular buccal surface and the mylohyoid ridge is on the mandibular lingual surface, separated by several millimeters. When panoramic images are viewed, it is important

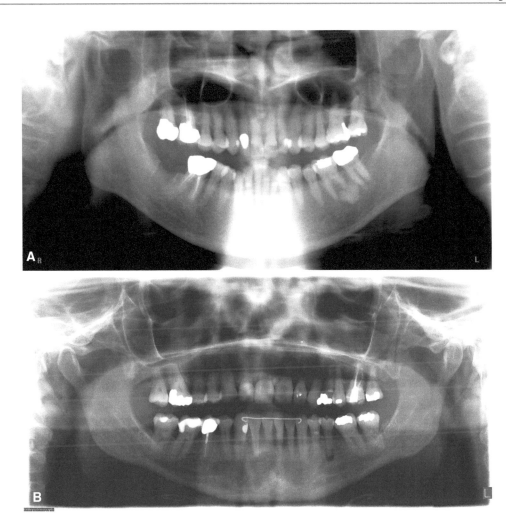

Fig. 9.15 (A) Panoramic radiograph demonstrating improper neck positioning. Note the large radiopaque region in the middle because the patient has the neck angled forward. This ghost image of the cervical spine could have been eliminated by having the patient sit straight and align or stretch the neck. (B) Panoramic radiograph showing improper tongue positioning, where the dorsum of the tongue was not positioned flat against the hard palate, resulting in the airspace below the hard palate hindering visualization of the apices of the maxillary teeth.

for the clinician to remember this principle and to attempt mental visualization of the structures three dimensionally.

It is helpful to view the image as if looking at the patient, with the structures on the patient's right side positioned on the viewer's left (Fig. 9.16), similar to the orientation of periapical and bitewing images, making the interpretation more comfortable. It is important to recognize the planes of the patient that are represented in different parts of the panoramic image. The panoramic image represents the curved jaw that is unfolded onto a flat plane. In the posterior regions, the panoramic image depicts a sagittal (lateral) view of the jaws, whereas in the anterior sextant, it represents a coronal (anteroposterior) view.

Dentition

One of the strengths of the panoramic image is the demonstration of the complete dentition. Although there is a rare situation where positioning of the patient or an ectopic tooth places the tooth out of the focal trough, all the teeth are generally seen on the image. Thus the interpretation must always include identification of all erupted and developing teeth (Fig. 9.17). The teeth should be examined for abnormalities of number, position, and anatomy. Existing dentistry, including endodontic

obturations, crowns, and other fixed restorations, should be noted. Excessively wide or narrow anterior teeth suggest malposition of the patient in the focal trough. Similarly, teeth that are wider on one side than the other suggest that the patient's sagittal plane was rotated. Gross caries and periapical and periodontal disease may be evident. However, the resolution of a panoramic radiograph is lower than that of intraoral radiographs, and additional intraoral radiographs may be needed to detect subtle disease. The proximal surfaces of the premolar teeth often overlap, which interferes with caries interpretation.

It is particularly important to examine impacted third molars closely. The orientation of the molars; the numbers and configurations of the roots; the relationships of the tooth components to critical anatomic structures, such as the mandibular canal, floor and posterior wall of the maxillary sinus, maxillary tuberosity, and adjacent teeth; and the presence of abnormalities in the pericoronal or periradicular bone must be carefully studied. However, given the two-dimensional nature of the panoramic image, such findings may need additional imaging with cone beam computed tomographic (CT) imaging to define precisely the spatial relationships of the roots of the impacted molars to the vital structures.

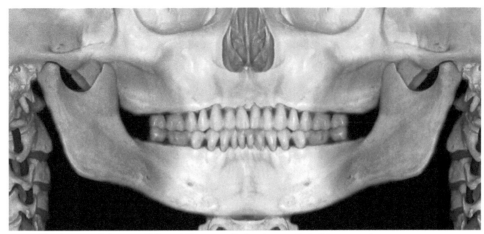

Fig. 9.16 The bones of the mandible, midface, cervical spine, and skull base as they appear on a panoramic image. The image is composed of left and right lateral views of the facial bones posterior to the canines and a coronal view anterior to the premolars.

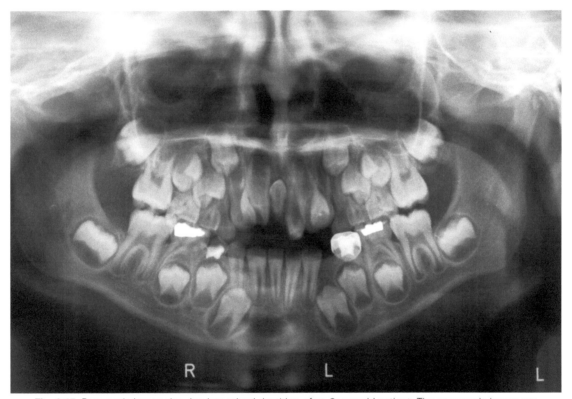

Fig. 9.17 Panoramic image showing late mixed dentition of an 8-year-old patient. The panoramic image can be useful in identifying the presence or absence of the permanent dentition, as well as assessing their developmental status. Note impacted and inverted mesiodens in the maxillary midline and malalignment of incisors.

Midfacial Region

The midface is a complex mixture of bones, air cavities, and soft tissues, all of which appear on panoramic images (Fig. 9.18). Individual bones that may appear on the panoramic image of the midface include temporal, zygoma, mandible, frontal, maxilla, sphenoid, ethmoid, vomer, nasal, nasal conchae, and palate; thus it is a misnomer to refer to the midfacial region on the panoramic image as "the maxilla." Maintaining the discipline and focus of a systematic examination of all aspects of the midfacial images is difficult and critical in the overall examination of the panoramic image.

This region can be compartmentalized into major sites for examination (see Fig. 9.18), as follows:

- Cortical boundary of the maxilla, including the posterior border and the alveolar ridge
- Pterygomaxillary fissure

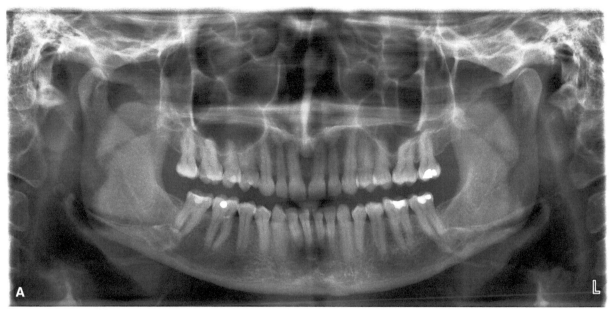

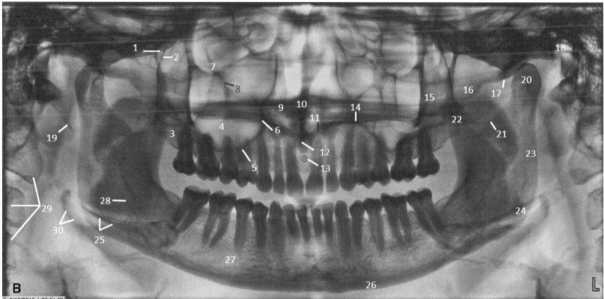

1. Pterygomaxillary fissure	11. Floor of the nasal cavity	22. Coronoid process
2. Posterior border of maxilla	12. Anterior nasal spine	23. Posterior border of the ramus
3. Maxillary tuberosity	13. Incisive foramen	24. Angle of the mandible
4. Maxillary sinus	14. Hard palate/floor of the nasal cavity	25. Hyoid bone
5. Floor of the maxillary sinus	15. Zygomatic process of maxilla	26. Inferior border of the mandible
6. Medial border of the maxillary sinus/ lateral border of the nasal cavity	16. Zygomatic arch	27. Mental foramen
7. Floor of the orbit	17. Articular eminence	28. Mandibular canal
8. Infraorbital canal	18. External auditory meatus	29. Cervical vertebrae
9. Nasal cavity	19. Styloid process	30. Epiglottis
10. Nasal septum	20. Mandibular condyle	
	21. Sigmoid notch	

Fig. 9.18 (A) Properly acquired and displayed panoramic image of an adult patient. The patient's left side is indicated on the image, and the image is oriented as if the clinician were facing the patient. This is the same orientation used with a full-mouth series. (B) Inverted image of the same panoramic radiograph identifying midfacial and mandibular anatomic structures.

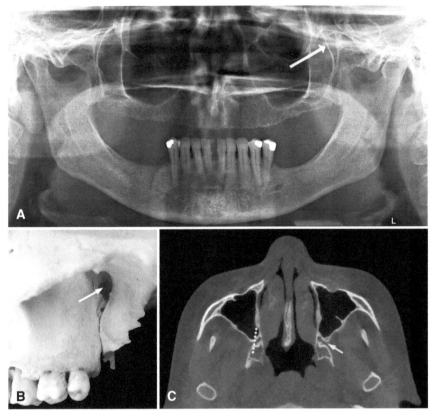

Fig. 9.19 Pterygomaxillary fissure, a space between the posterior surface of the maxilla and the anterior border of the pterygoid plates. (A) Inverted teardrop shape of the fissure on a panoramic image *(arrow)*. (B) The fissure on a dried skull *(arrow)*. (C) The approximate image section *(dotted line)* of the panoramic focal trough through the pterygomaxillary fissure *(arrow)* on an axial computed tomographic section.

- Maxillary sinuses
- Zygomatic complex, including inferior and lateral orbital rims, zygomatic process of maxilla, and anterior portion of zygomatic arch
- Nasal cavity and conchae
- TMJs (also viewed in the mandible, but visualizing important structures multiple times is always a good idea in image interpretation)
- Maxillary dentition and supporting alveolus

Examining the cortical outline of the maxilla is a good way to center the examination of the midface. The posterior border of the maxilla extends from the superior portion of the pterygomaxillary fissure down to the tuberosity region and around to the other side. The posterior border of the pterygomaxillary fissure is the pterygoid spine of the sphenoid bone (the anterior border of the pterygoid plates). Occasionally, the sphenoid sinus may extend into this structure. The pterygomaxillary fissure itself has an inverted teardrop appearance; it is very important to identify this area on both sides of the image because maxillary sinus mucoceles and carcinomas characteristically destroy the posterior maxillary border, which is manifested as loss of the anterior border of the pterygomaxillary fissure. To clarify the three-dimensional anatomy of the pterygomaxillary fissure, Fig. 9.19 shows this structure in a dried skull, in an axial CT image, and in the panoramic image.

The maxillary sinuses are usually well visualized on panoramic images. The clinician should identify each of the borders (posterior, anterior, floor, roof) and note whether they are entirely outlined with cortical bone, approximately symmetric, and comparable in radiographic density. The borders should be present and intact. The medial border of the maxillary sinus is the lateral border of the nasal cavity; however, this interface is not demonstrated on the panoramic image. The superior border, or roof, of the maxillary sinus is the floor of the orbit; this interface is demonstrated on the panoramic image in its most anterior aspect. Although it is useful to compare right and left maxillary sinuses when looking for abnormalities, it is important to remember that bilateral asymmetry in size, shape, and presence or number of septae within the maxillary sinuses is a common anatomic variation. The posterior aspect of the sinus is more opaque because of superimposition of the zygoma. Each sinus should be examined for evidence of a mucous retention cyst, mucoperiosteal thickening, and other abnormalities.

The zygomatic complex, or "buttress" of the midface, is a very complex anatomic area, with contributions from the frontal, zygomatic, and maxillary bones. It includes the lateral and inferior orbital rims, the zygomatic process of the maxilla, and the zygomatic arch. The zygomatic process of the maxilla arises over the maxillary first and second molars. The maxillary sinus can pneumatize the zygomatic process of the maxilla up to the zygomaticomaxillary suture. This can result in the appearance of an elliptical, corticated radiolucency in the maxillary sinus, possibly superimposed over the roots of a molar tooth, on a panoramic image. The inferior border of the zygomatic arch extends posteriorly from the inferior portion of the zygomatic process of the maxilla and continues posteriorly to the articular tubercle and glenoid fossa of the temporal bone. The superior border of the zygomatic arch, which curves antero-superiorly to form the lateral aspect of the lateral orbital rim, should also be noted. The zygomaticotemporal suture lies in the middle of the zygomatic arch and may simulate a fracture if visualized on the image.

In addition, the mastoid air cells occasionally pneumatize the temporal bone all the way to the zygomaticotemporal suture, giving the glenoid fossa of the TMJ the appearance of having a multilocular, or "soap-bubbly," radiolucency, which is a variant of normal.

The nasal fossa may show the nasal septum and inferior concha, including both the bone and its mucosal covering. In the anterior region, the lateral border and anterior rim of the nasal cavity are seen as a radiopaque line. The anterior nasal spine and the incisive foramen also may be seen. The floor of the nasal cavity or hard palate is seen as a horizontal radiopacity, superimposed over the maxillary sinus in the posterior regions; this is often seen as two radiopaque lines (see Fig. 9.9). The lower line is sharp and represents the junction between the lateral wall of the nasal cavity and hard palate on the tube side. The upper line is more diffuse and represents the junction on the opposite side. The conchae, composed of an internal bone, the turbinate, and covering cartilage and mucosa, are seen in a coronal manner in the anterior portion of the image and in a sagittal manner in the posterior portions of the panoramic image. They can appear as very large, homogeneous, soft tissue densities superimposed over the maxillary sinuses and occasionally the anterior nasopharynx.

Mandible

Assessment of the mandible (see Fig. 9.18) can be compartmentalized into the major anatomic areas of this curved bone, as follows:
- Condylar process and TMJ
- Coronoid process
- Ramus
- Body and angle
- Anterior sextant
- Mandibular dentition and supporting alveolus

The clinician should be able to follow a cortical border around the entire bone, with the exception of the dentate areas. This border should be smooth, without interruptions, and should have symmetric thicknesses in comparable anatomic areas (e.g., angles, inferior borders of bodies, posterior borders of rami). The trabeculation of the mandible tends to be more plentiful in the anterior regions, whereas the marrow compartment increases toward the angle and into the ramus; however, these trabecular patterns and densities should be relatively symmetric. This is especially true in children, who have very sparse trabeculation throughout the deciduous and mixed dentition stages.

The mandibular condyle is generally positioned slightly anteroinferior to its normal closed position because the patient has to open and protrude the mandible slightly to engage the positioning device in most panoramic machines. The TMJ can be assessed for gross anatomic changes of the condylar head and glenoid fossa; the soft tissues, such as the articular disc and posterior ligamentous attachment, cannot be evaluated. The glenoid fossa is part of the temporal bone, and it can be pneumatized by the mastoid air cells. This can result in the appearance of a multilocular radiolucency in the articular eminence and the roof of the glenoid fossa, which is a variant of normal. More definitive osseous assessment of the TMJ is accomplished by using cone beam computed tomography (CBCT) imaging and multidetector computed tomography (MDCT) scan. Magnetic resonance imaging is the examination of choice for evaluation of the disc and pericondylar soft tissues.

Shadows of other structures that can be superimposed over the mandibular ramal area include the following:
- Oropharyngeal and nasopharyngeal airway shadows, the former specifically when the patient is unable to expel the air and place the tongue in the palate during the exposure
- Posterior wall of the nasopharynx
- Cervical vertebrae, especially in patients with pronounced anterior lordosis, typically seen in severely osteoporotic individuals
- Earlobe
- Nasal cartilage
- Soft palate and uvula
- Dorsum of the tongue
- Ghost shadows of the opposite side of the mandible
- Real and ghost shadows of metallic jewelry or other ear, nose, tongue decorations

From the angle of the mandible, viewing should be continued anteriorly toward the symphyseal region. A fracture often manifests as a discontinuity ("step deformity") in the inferior border; a sharp change in the level of the occlusal plane indicates that the fracture passes through the tooth-bearing area, whereas a cant in the entire occlusal table without a step deformity in the occlusal plane indicates that the fracture is posterior to the tooth-bearing area. The width of the cortical bone at the inferior border of the mandible should be at least 3 mm in adults and of uniform density. There may be localized or generalized bone thinning indicating an expansile lesion such as a cyst or systemic diseases such as hyperparathyroidism and osteoporosis, respectively. The outlines of both sides of the mandible should be compared for symmetry. Asymmetry of size may result from improper patient positioning or conditions such as hemifacial hyperplasia or hypoplasia. The hyoid bone may be projected below or onto the inferior border of the mandible.

Trabeculation is most evident within the alveolar process. The mandibular canals and mental foramina are usually clearly visualized in the ramus and body regions of the mandible. Typically, the canals exhibit uniform width or gentle tapering from the mandibular foramina to the mental foramina. They may be less well demarcated in the first molar and premolar regions. When only one border of the canal is seen, it is typically the inferior border. The canals usually rise to meet the mental foramina, often looping several millimeters anterior to the mental foramina; this is termed the "anterior loop" of the mandibular canal, and its position and extent are considerations when planning dental implants in the mandibular canine regions. An expansion of the canal suggests neurovascular pathology; however, slight widening at the entry point of the canal into the body of the mandible from the ramus is a variation of normal. The mandible should be examined for radiolucencies or opacities. The midline is more opaque because of the mental protuberance, increased trabecular numbers, and attenuation of the beam as it passes through the cervical spine. Many modern panoramic machines automatically increase the exposure factors as they pass across the cervical spine region in an attempt to minimize this opacity; nevertheless, some opacity is generally seen in the anterior regions of the image. There are often depressions on the lingual surfaces of the mandible, which are occupied by the submandibular and sublingual glands. These depressions are termed the lingual salivary gland depressions, or fossae, and are often more radiolucent compared to adjacent areas. This anatomic feature is shown on a panoramic image, dry skull, coronal CT section, and periapical image in Fig. 9.20A–D.

Soft Tissues

Numerous opaque soft tissue structures may be identified on panoramic radiographs, including the tongue arching across the image under the hard palate (approximately extending from the right to the left mandibular angle), lip markings (in the middle of the image), the soft palate extending posteriorly from the hard palate over each ramus, the posterior wall of the oral and nasal pharynx, the nasal septum, the earlobes, the nose, and the nasolabial folds (Fig. 9.21A and B). Radiolucent airway shadows superimpose on normal anatomic structures and may be delineated by the borders of adjacent soft tissues. They include the nasal fossa, nasopharynx, oral cavity, and oropharynx. The epiglottis and thyroid cartilage are often seen in panoramic images (Fig. 9.22).

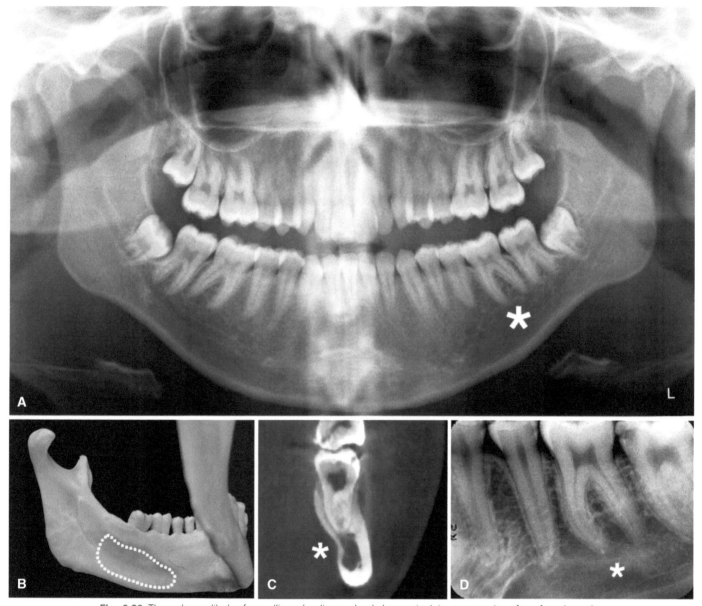

Fig. 9.20 The submandibular fossa (lingual salivary gland depression) is a concavity often found on the posterior lingual surface of the mandible. This triangularly shaped area is bounded by the mylohyoid ridge superiorly and the inferior border of the mandibular body and lies in the region of the roots of the molars and premolars. *Asterisk* indicates the area of the submandibular fossa on the various images. (A) Panoramic image. (B) Photograph of the lingual side of a dried mandible. (C) Coronal computed tomographic scan through the molar region of the mandible. (D) Mandibular molar periapical image.

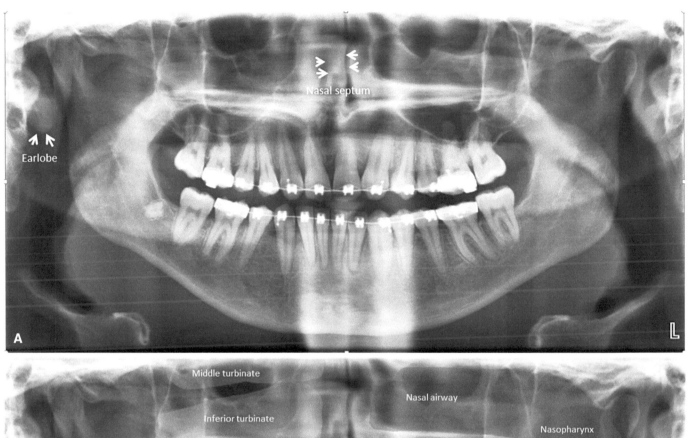

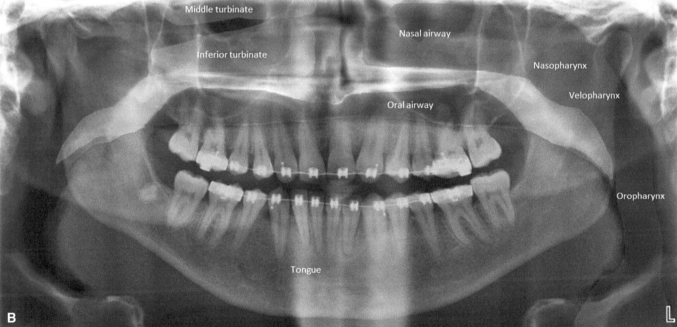

Fig. 9.21 Soft tissue images on a panoramic radiograph. (A) Properly acquired panoramic radiograph showing radiographically evident orofacial soft tissues. (B) The same panoramic image with an overlay indicating the components of the airway. The nasal airway surrounds the turbinates. The nasopharynx is posterior to the turbinates and above the level of the hard palate. The velopharynx is posterior to the soft palate. The oropharynx is below the uvula.

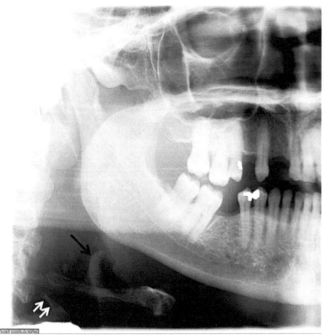

Fig. 9.22 Normal structures occasionally seen in the neck region on panoramic images. The superior aspect of the thyroid cartilage *(white arrows)* can be mistaken for a vascular calcification. The epiglottis *(black arrow)* lies posterior to the dorsum of the tongue.

BIBLIOGRAPHY

American Dental Association Council on Scientific Affairs. The use of dental radiographs: update and recommendations. *J Am Dent Assoc.* 2006;137(9):1304–1312.

Brooks SL, Brand JW, Gibbs SJ, et al. Imaging of the temporomandibular joint: a position paper of the American Academy of Oral and Maxillofacial Radiology. *Oral Surg Oral Med Oral Pathol Oral Radiol Endod.* 1997;83:609–618.

Chomenko AG. *Atlas for Maxillofacial Pantomographic Interpretation.* Chicago: Quintessence; 1985.

Farman AG, ed. *Panoramic Radiology: Seminars on Maxillofacial Imaging and Interpretation.* Berlin: Springer; 2007.

Langland OE, Langlais RP, McDavid WD, et al. *Panoramic Radiology.* 2nd ed. Philadelphia: Lea & Febiger; 1989.

McDavid WD, Dove SB, Welander U, et al. Dimensional reproduction in direct digital rotational panoramic radiography. *Oral Surg Oral Med Oral Pathol.* 1993;75:523–527.

McDavid WD, Langlais RP, Welander U, et al. Real, double and ghost images in rotational panoramic radiography. *Dentomaxillofac Radiol.* 1983;12:122–128.

Numata H. Consideration of the parabolic radiography of the dental arch. *J Shimazu Stud.* 1933;10:13.

Paatero YV. The use of a mobile source of light in radiography. *Acta Radiol.* 1948;29:221.

Paatero YV. A new tomographic method for radiographing curved outer surfaces. *Acta Radiol.* 1949;32:177.

Rushton VE, Rout J. *Panoramic radiology.* London: Quintessence Publishing Co; 2006.

Terry GL, Noujeim M, Langlais RP, et al. A clinical comparison of extraoral panoramic and intraoral radiographic modalities for detecting proximal caries and visualizing open posterior interproximal contacts. *Dentomaxillofac Radiol.* 2016;45(4):20150159.

Cone Beam Computed Tomography: Volume Acquisition

William C. Scarfe

Cone beam computed tomographic (CBCT) imaging was originally developed for angiography in the early 1980s with the first dental and maxillofacial units introduced commercially in the late 1990s and early 2000s (Fig. 10.1). Unlike other extraoral dental imaging procedures, such as panoramic and cephalometric radiography, CBCT acquires data volumetrically providing three-dimensional (3D) radiographic imaging for the assessment of the dental and maxillofacial complex facilitating dental diagnosis. With expanding availability of third party application software capable of importing data in Digital Imaging and Communications in Medicine (DICOM) file format, the role of maxillofacial CBCT has now expanded to image guidance of operative and surgical procedures and, more recently, additive manufacturing of biomodels and surgical guides.

There are three main processes in CBCT imaging: (1) image production, (2) visualization, and (3) interpretation. This chapter addresses the technical issues of image production including image data-set acquisition and "for presentation" reconstruction.

PRINCIPLES OF CONE BEAM COMPUTED TOMOGRAPHIC IMAGING

In all computed tomography (CT) techniques, a collimated x-ray source and a detector revolve around the patient (see Chapter 13, Figs. 13.1–13.3). The detector records photon attenuation by measuring the number of photons that exit the patient, registering this information at several hundred angles through the rotational arc. These recordings constitute the "raw data" that is reconstructed by a computer algorithm to create a 3D data set composed of volumetric elements (voxels) from which images are derived. The basic component of resultant grayscale images is the picture element (pixel) values. The grayscale value or intensity of each pixel is related to the intensity of the photons incident on the detector. Although providing similar images, CBCT and multidetector computed tomography (MDCT; see Chapter 13) represents separate evolutionary arms of CT imaging.

The geometric configuration and acquisition mechanics for the CBCT technique are theoretically simple (Fig. 10.2). CBCT imaging is performed using a rotating gantry or C-arm supporting an x-ray source and reciprocating area detector. A divergent x-ray source, collimated as a cone or, more commonly, as a pyramid, is directed through the region of interest (ROI) within the maxillofacial region, and the residual attenuated photons strike the detector on the opposite side. On activation, data are acquired from a series of sequential exposures as the gantry rotates around a fixed axis of rotation centered within the patient's ROI. The trajectory arc is ideally 360 degrees but can vary from 180 to 720 degrees. During the rotation, multiple sequential planar projection images are captured. These two-dimensional single-projection images constitute the raw primary data and are individually referred to as basis, frame, or raw images. Basis images appear similar to cephalometric radiographic images except that each is slightly offset from the next. There are usually several hundred basis images with the complete series known as the projection data. Because CBCT exposure incorporates the entire ROI, only one rotational scan of the gantry is necessary to acquire enough data for volumetric image construction. Software programs incorporating sophisticated algorithms including filtered back projection are applied to these projection data to generate a volumetric data set—an image volume that can be used to generate secondary reconstruction images in three orthogonal planes (axial, sagittal, and coronal). Cone beam geometry captures volumetric data with scan times ranging from less than 5 to more than 30 seconds.

COMPONENTS OF IMAGE PRODUCTION

There are three major components to CBCT image production:
- X-ray generation
- X-ray detection
- Image reconstruction

The x-ray generation and detection specifications of currently available CBCT systems (Tables 10.1 and 10.2) reflect proprietary variations in these parameters. Maxillofacial CBCT systems can be distinguished operationally according to the orientation of the patient during image acquisition (Fig. 10.3). CBCT systems can also be divided by unit functionality into dedicated CBCT or hybrid multimodality systems that combine digital panoramic and/or cephalometric radiography with a small to medium field of view (FOV) CBCT system (see Fig. 10.3).

X-Ray Generation

Although CBCT imaging is technically simple in that only a single scan of the patient is made to acquire a projection data set, numerous clinically important parameters in x-ray generation affect both image quality and patient radiation dose.

Patient Stabilization

Depending on the unit, CBCT examinations are made with the patient sitting, standing, or supine (see Fig. 10.3). Supine units are physically larger, have a greater physical footprint, and may not be accessible for patients with some physical disabilities. Standing units may not be able to be adjusted to a height low enough to accommodate wheelchair-bound patients. Although seated units are the most comfortable, they may not allow scanning of physically disabled or wheelchair-bound patients. With all systems, immobilization of the patient's head is more important than patient positioning because any head movement degrades the final image. Immobilization of the head is achieved by using some combination of a chin cup, bite fork, or other head-restraint mechanism.

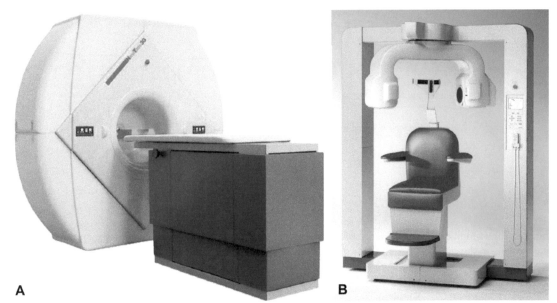

Fig. 10.1 The First Commercially Available Maxillofacial Cone Beam Computed Tomography Units in the United States. (A) The NewTom 9000 DVT (QR srl, Verona, Italy) was a supine unit with a fixed spherical field of view (FOV) of 9 inches. (B) The 3D Accuitomo XYZ Slice View Tomograph (J. Morita Corp., Kyoto, Japan) was a unit in which the patient was seated and produced a small volume, cylindrical FOV with a high resolution.

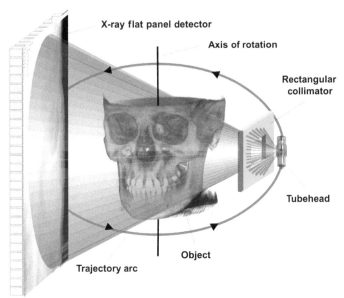

Fig. 10.2 Cone Beam Imaging Geometry. A divergent x-ray beam created at the tube head is collimated in a circle or rectangle (this example) into a three-dimensional cone or pyramid, respectively. The x-ray projection is directed through the patient onto a detector (either solid-state flat panel detector [this example] or II/charge-coupled device). After a single two-dimensional projection is acquired by the detector, the x-ray source and detector rotate a small distance around a trajectory arc. At this second angular position, another basis projection image or frame is captured. This sequence continues around the object for the entire 360 degrees (full trajectory) or along a reduced or partial trajectory capturing hundreds of individual images.

X-Ray Generator

During the scan rotation, each projection image set is made by sequential single-image capture of the remnant attenuated x-ray beam by the area detector. X-ray generation may be continuous or pulsed to coincide with the detector activation. Preferably, the x-ray production should be pulsed to coincide with the detector sampling; this means that actual exposure time can be substantially less than scanning time. This technique considerably reduces patient radiation dose.

The ALARA (*As Low As Reasonably Achievable*) principle of dose optimization necessitates that CBCT exposure factors should be adjusted on the basis of patient size and specific diagnostic task. This adjustment can be achieved by appropriate selection of tube current (milliamperes [mA]), tube voltage (kilovolt peak [kVp]), or both. In some cases, exposure time also can be adjusted to change scan time. Faster scans produce volumetric data sets from fewer basis images (see later section on scan factors). The variation in exposure parameters together with the presence of pulsed x-ray beam and size of the image field are the primary determinants of patient exposure.

Scan Volume

The dimensions of the FOV or scan volume primarily depend on the detector size and shape, the beam projection geometry, and the ability to collimate the beam. The shape of the scan volume can be either cylindrical or spherical. Collimating the primary x-ray beam limits radiation exposure to the ROI. It is desirable to limit the field size to the smallest volume that images the ROI. This field size must be selected for each patient based on individual needs. This procedure reduces unnecessary exposure to the patient and produces the best images by minimizing scattered radiation, which degrades image quality. CBCT

TABLE 10.1 Summary of Specifications for Cone Beam Computed Tomographic Systems

Specification	Variable	Parameter
Unit type	Patient position during image acquisition	Supine; standing; seated
	Functionality	CBCT only; multimodal (CBCT/pan or CBCT/pan/ceph); integrated (radiographic and simultaneous facial surface scan)
	Geometry	Fixed (full or partial) arc trajectory (degrees); variable
	Number of basis projections	Fixed; variable (number)
		Scan time (s)
X-ray generator	mA/kVp	Fixed; patient size and diagnostic task preset (settings available); variable
	X-ray source	Constant; pulsed
	AEC	Present/absent
	Focal spot size	Millimeters
Scan volume	Shape	Spherical; cylindrical; convex triangular; other
	Dimensions	Spherical (diameter); cylinder (height × diameter [cm])
Detector	Type	II/CCD; CsI/a-Si; PST; CsI/CMOS
	Voxel size	Fixed; variable (range)
	Grayscale (bit depth)	Acquired; displayed; archived (2^n)
Software	Primary reconstruction time	<1 min, 1–3 min, >3 min

AEC, Automatic exposure control; *CBCT,* cone beam computed tomography; *ceph,* cephalometric radiography; *CMOS,* complementary metal oxide semiconductor; *CsI/a-Si,* cesium iodide/amorphous silicon flat panel; *II/CCD,* area image intensifier/charge-coupled device; *kVp,* kilovolt peak; *mA,* milliamperes; *n,* bit-depth; *pan,* panoramic radiography; *PST,* proprietary Siemens Technology.

TABLE 10.2 Representative Cone Beam Computed Tomographic Imaging Systems

Products; Models	Distributor
3D Accuitomo—XYZ Slice View Tomograph[a]; FPD[a]; 3D Accuitomo 170; Veraviewepocs 3D R100; Veraviewepoc 3D F40	J Morita Mfg Corp, Kyoto, Japan
Bel-Cat; Bel-Cat PA; Bel-Cat CM	Takara Belmont Corporation, Somerset, NJ
Auge Solio; Aliloth; Alphard 3030 (PSR 9000N); Alphard 2520	Asahi Roentgen, Kyoto, Japan
I-MAX Touch 3D	Owandy Corp., Paris, France
CS 8100 3D; CS 9000 3D; CS 9300 3D; CS 9500[a]	Carestream Dental, Atlanta, GA
DaVinci D3D; Hyperion 9	My-Ray Dental Imaging, Cefla Dental Group, Imola, Italy
Comfort[a]; Compact[a]; ComfortPLUS; Orthophos XG 3D; Orthophos SL 3D	Sirona Dental Inc., Charlotte, NC
GXCB-500 HD; GXDP-700 S; KaVo 3D eXam; 3D eXam+	Gendex Dental Systems, Hatfield, PA/KaVo Dental Corp., Biberach, Germany
i-CAT Classic[a]; Next Generation (Model 17-19, Platinum)[a]; i-CAT FLX; i-CAT FLX MV	Imaging Sciences, Hatfield, PA
Picasso Series (Trio / Pro / Master)[a]; PaX-i3D; PaX-Flex 3D; PaX-Uni 3D; PaX-Duo 3D; Pax-Zenith 3D; PaX-Reve 3D	VATECH Co Ltd, Gyeonggi-Do, Republic of Korea
NewTom 9000[a]; 3G[a]; VGi; VGi-Flex; Giano; 5G	QR, Inc. Verona, Italy (a Cefla company)
OP300; OP 300 Maxio 3D	Instrumentarium Dental, Tuusula, Finland
PreXion 3D Elite	PreXion Inc, San Mateo, CA
Promax 3D; 3Ds; 3D Plus; 3D Mid; 3D Max	Planmeca Oy, Helsinki, Finland
Encompass Eagle 3D	Panoramic Corp., Fort Wayne, IN
Rayscan Alpha 3D; Alpha Plus	LED Medical Diagnostics Inc., Atlanta, GA
Scanora 3D/Cranex 3D	Soredex, Tuusula, Finland
Suni 3D; 3D HD	Suni Medical Imaging, Inc, San Jose, CA
X-Mind Trium 3D	Acteon North America, Mt. Laurel, NJ

[a]No longer manufactured/unavailable.

units are classified according to the maximum FOV incorporated from the scan or scans (Fig. 10.4).

Two approaches have been introduced to enable scanning of an ROI greater than the FOV of the detector. One method involves obtaining data from two or more separate scans and superimposing the overlapping regions of the CBCT data volumes using corresponding fiducial reference landmarks (referred to as either "bioimage registration" or "mosaicing"). Software is used to fuse adjacent image volumes ("stitching" or "blending") to create a larger volumetric data set either in the horizontal or in the vertical dimension (Fig. 10.5). The disadvantage of stitching overlapped regions is that such overlapped regions are imaged twice, resulting in double the radiation dose to such regions. A second method to increase the height or width of the FOV using a small area detector is to offset the position of the detector, collimate the beam asymmetrically, and scan only half the patient's ROI in each of the two offset scans (Fig. 10.6).

Scan Factors

The number of images that constitute the projection data from the scan is determined by the detector frame rate (number of images acquired per second), the completeness of the trajectory arc (180 to 360 degrees), and the rotation speed of the source and detector. The number of basis images of a single scan set may be fixed or variable. Higher frame rates have both desirable and undesirable effects. Higher frame rates increase the signal-to-noise ratio, producing images with less noise and reducing metallic artifacts. However, a higher frame rate is associated with a longer scan time and higher patient radiation dose. In addition, more data are obtained, and primary reconstruction time is increased. In contrast, some "quick-scan" or "fast-scan" protocols use markedly lower frame rates with considerable reduction in patient radiation dose. However, the image resolution from these scans may not be adequate for all diagnostic tasks.

CBCT units are available, providing fixed or variable rotation angles. Most CBCT units have fixed scan arcs. Fixed rotation angle units may

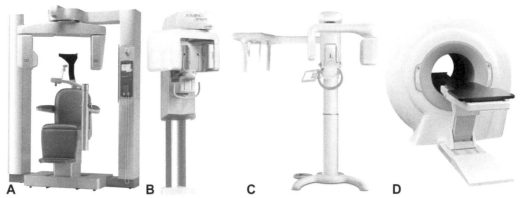

Fig. 10.3 Cone Beam Computed Tomography Units Are Distinguished Operationally by the Position of the Patient During the Scan. (A) Seated (e.g., 3D Accuitomo 170, J Morita Corp., Osaka, Japan). (B) (e.g., X-Mind trium Pan 3D, Acteon North America, Mt. Laurel, NJ) and (C) (e.g. Rayscan Alpha 3D, LED Medical Diagnostics Inc., Atlanta, GA), Standing. (D) Supine (e.g., Newtom 5G, QR srl, Verona, Italy). According to function, CBCT devices can also be categorized according to functionality and considered a dedicated unit (A and D) or a hybrid unit with panoramic (B) or panoramic and cephalometric capability (C).

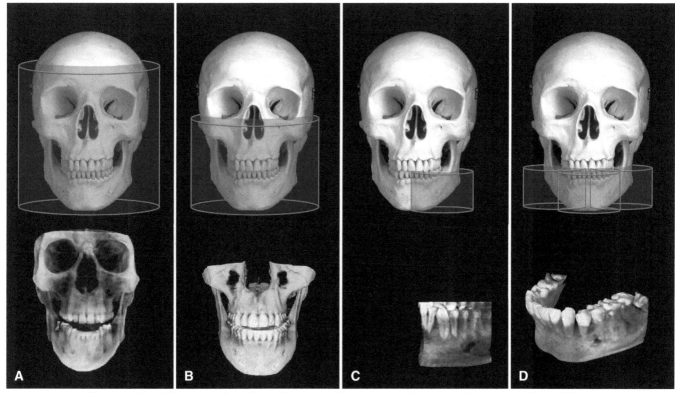

Fig. 10.4 Classification of Cone Beam Computed Tomography Units According to the Field of View (FOV). (A) Large FOV scans provide images of the entire craniofacial skeleton, enabling cephalometric analysis. (B) Medium FOV scans image the maxilla or mandible or both. (C) Focused or restricted FOV scans provide high-resolution images of limited regions. (D) Stitched scans from multiple focused FOV scans provide larger regions of interest to be imaged from superimposition of multiple scans. (Skull image courtesy and copyright of Primal Pictures, Ltd, London, UK: http://www.primalpictures.com.)

be a full 360 degrees or partial trajectory arcs. Ideally, CBCT imaging should be performed with a full scan arc to acquire adequate projection data for volumetric software reconstruction. However, many CBCT units are based on panoramic platforms, most having scan arcs less than 360 degrees. A limited scan arc potentially reduces the scan time and patient radiation dose and is mechanically easier to perform.

However, images produced by this method may have greater noise and reconstruction interpolation artifacts. Units providing variable rotation angles usually provide two options: a complete or a partial scan arc.

It is desirable to reduce CBCT scan times to as short as possible to reduce motion artifact resulting from patient movement. Patient movement can be substantial and may be a limiting factor in image resolution.

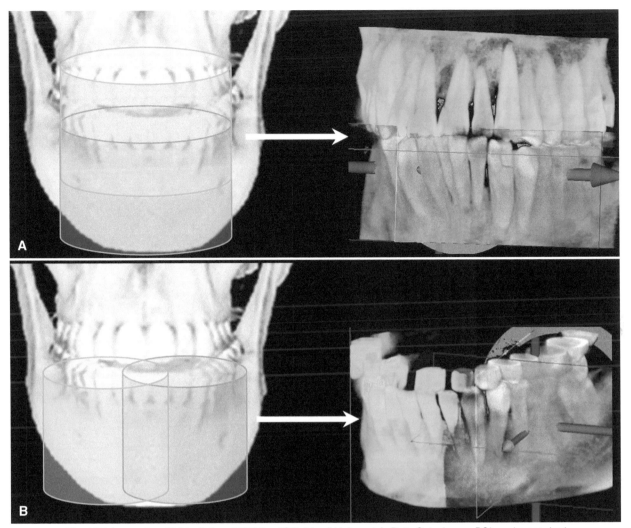

Fig. 10.5 Increasing Field of View (FOV) by "Stitching" Volumetric Data Sets. Larger ROI can be acquired by small FOV cone beam computed tomography units by "stitching" adjacent limited area volumetric data sets. This process requires acquisition of separate scans *(left)*, registration of each volume by superimposition of fiducial landmarks, and fusion to provide a larger FOV *(right)*. Units may use this technique to increase either the vertical (A) or the horizontal (B) FOV. Shown here are adjacent *(orange and blue)* volumetric data sets (KODAK CS 9000 Carestream Dental, Atlanta, GA) stitched manually using proprietary software (InVivoDental software; Anatomage, San Jose, CA).

Decreased scanning times may be achieved by increasing the detector frame rate, reducing the number of projections, or reducing the scan arc. The first method provides images of the highest quality, whereas the latter methods increase image noise.

Image Detectors

Current CBCT units can be divided into two groups based on detector type: (1) image intensifier tube/charge-coupled device (II/CCD) combination or (2) flat panel detectors (FPDs). II/CCD units are usually larger and bulkier and result in circular basis image areas (spherical volumes) rather than rectangular ones (cylindrical volumes) produced by FPDs. Most, but not all, contemporary CBCT units use FPDs. FPDs employ an "indirect" detector based on a large-area solid-state detector panel coupled to an x-ray scintillator layer (see Chapter 4). The most common flat panel configuration consists of a cesium iodide scintillator applied to a thin film transistor made of amorphous silicon. More recently, large complementary metal oxide semiconductor technology arrays have also been used.

Voxel Size

The spatial resolution—and therefore detail of a CBCT image—is determined by the dimensions of individual voxels produced in formatting the volumetric data set. CBCT units in general provide voxel resolutions that are isotropic—equal in all three dimensions. The principal determinants of nominal voxel size in a CBCT image are the matrix and pixel size of the detector. Detectors with smaller pixels capture fewer x-ray photons per voxel and result in more image noise. Consequently, CBCT imaging using higher resolutions may be designed to use higher dosages to achieve a reasonable signal-to-noise ratio for improved diagnostic image quality.

Both the focal spot size and the geometric configuration of the x-ray source are important to determine the degree of geometric unsharpness, a limiting factor in spatial resolution. The cost of x-ray tubes—and therefore of the CBCT unit—increases substantially with small focal spot size tubes. Reducing the object-to-detector distance and increasing source-to-object distance also minimizes geometric unsharpness. In

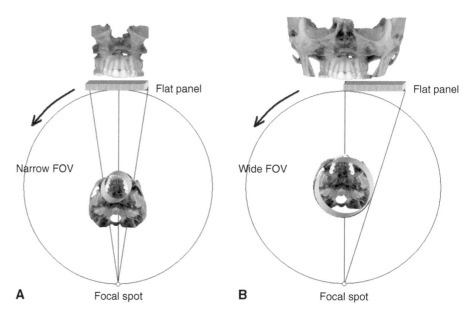

Fig. 10.6 Schematic of Asymmetric Cone Beam Computed Tomography Geometric Configuration to Increase Field of View *(FOV)* **Using a Flat Panel Detector (FPD).** (A) Conventional geometric arrangement whereby the central ray of the x-ray beam from the focal source is directed through the middle of the object to the center of the FPD. The resultant image is limited to the region of the detector (dentition in this case). (B) Alternative method increasing image size involves shifting the location of the flat panel imager and collimating the x-ray beam laterally to extend the FOV object. In this instance, the FPD is shifted to the opposite side of the midline halfway through the exposure. The resulting image doubles the horizontal ROI. (Adapted courtesy of SOREDEX, Tuusula, Finland.)

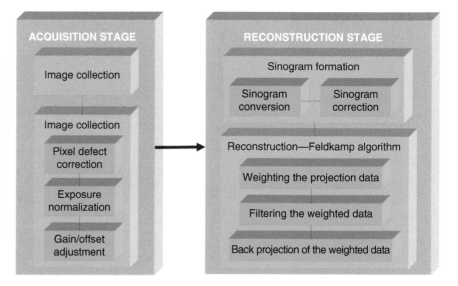

Fig. 10.7 Image Acquisition and Reconstruction. The acquisition stage involves acquisition of individual basis projections and subsequent modification of these images to correct for inconsistencies. Image correction is sequential and consists of the removal of signal voids from individual or linear pixel defects, image normalization by histogram equalization so that a full range of voxel intensity values are used, and removal of inherent electronic detector artifacts. After correction, images undergo reconstruction, which includes converting the corrected basis projection images into sinograms and application of the Feldkamp reconstruction to the corrected filters to the image and use of back-projection techniques to reconstitute the image.

maxillofacial CBCT imaging, the detector position is limited because it must be located far enough from the patient's head so that it freely rotates unobstructed by the patient's shoulders. Limitations also exist in extending the source-to-object distance because this increases the size of the CBCT unit. However, reducing source-to-object distance produces a magnified projected image on the detector, increasing potential spatial resolution. Additional factors influencing image resolution include motion of the patient's head during the exposure, the type of scintillator used in the detector, and the image reconstruction algorithms applied.

Grayscale

The ability of CBCT imaging to display differences in photon attenuation is related to the ability of the detector to reveal subtle contrast differences. This parameter is called the bit depth of the system and determines the number of shades of gray available to display the attenuation. All currently available CBCT units use detectors capable of recording grayscale differences of 12 bits or greater. A 12-bit detector provides 2^{12} or 4096 shades to display contrast. A 16-bit detector provides 2^{16} or 65,536 shades of gray. Although higher bit-depth images in CBCT

imaging are possible, this added information comes at the expense of increased computational time and substantially larger file sizes.

Reconstruction

Although a single acquisition rotation may take less than 20 seconds, it produces 100 to more than 600 individual projection frames, each with more than 1 million pixels with 12 to 16 bits of data assigned to each pixel. These data are processed to create a volumetric data set composed of cuboidal volume elements (voxels) by a sequence of software algorithms in a process called primary reconstruction. Subsequently, visual orthogonal (i.e., perpendicular) images are reformatted by sectioning the volumetric data set, referred to as secondary reconstruction. The reconstruction of these data is computationally complex. To facilitate data handling, data may be acquired by one computer (acquisition computer) and transferred by an Ethernet connection to a processing computer (workstation). In contrast to conventional CT imaging, CBCT data reconstruction is performed by personal computer–based, rather than workstation, platforms.

The reconstruction process consists of two stages, each comprising numerous steps (Fig. 10.7):

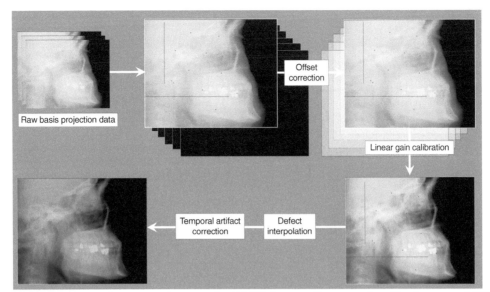

Fig. 10.8 Cone Beam Computed Tomography (CBCT) Detector Preprocessing. The first step of CBCT detector preprocessing is offset correction. This is accomplished by pixel-wise subtraction of an individual offset value computed by averaging over a series of up to 30 dark images. The second step is the linear gain calibration, consisting of dividing each pixel by its individual gain factor. The gain factors are obtained by averaging a sequence with up to 30 images of homogeneous exposures without any object between x-ray source and detector. The gain sequence is first offset corrected with its own sequence of dark images. The next procedure is the defect interpolation. Each pixel that shows unusual behavior, either in the gain image or in the average dark sequence, is marked in a defect map. The gray values of pixels classified as defective in this way are computed by linear interpolation along the least gradient descent. For flat panel detectors, there is usually an additional procedure to correct for temporal artifacts. These arise in such detectors because both the scintillator and the photodiodes exhibit residual signals.

1. Preprocessing stage (Fig. 10.8). The preprocessing stage is performed at the acquisition computer. After the multiple planar projection images are acquired, these images must be corrected for inherent pixel imperfections, variations in sensitivity across the detector, and uneven exposure. Depending on the CBCT unit, image calibration may be required routinely to remove these defects.
2. Reconstruction stage. The remaining data-processing steps are performed on the reconstruction computer. The corrected images are converted into a special representation called a sinogram, a composite image developed from multiple projection images. This process of generating a sinogram is referred to as the Radon transformation. The final image is reconstructed from the sinogram with a filtered back-projection algorithm for volumetric data acquired by CBCT imaging; the most widely used algorithm is the Feldkamp algorithm. This process is referred to as inverse Radon transformation. When all slices have been reconstructed, they are combined into a single volume for visualization.

Reconstruction times vary depending on the acquisition parameters (voxel size, size of the image field, and number of projections), hardware (processing speed, data throughput from acquisition to reconstruction computer), and software (reconstruction algorithms) used. Reconstruction should be accomplished in an acceptable time (<5 minutes) to facilitate clinical workflow.

CLINICAL CONSIDERATIONS

Operation of CBCT equipment is technically straightforward and similar, in many respects, to the performance of panoramic radiography. However, in contrast to panoramic imaging, numerous exposure and acquisition settings may be adjusted, depending on the CBCT unit used (see Table 10.1). Practitioners and operators using CBCT must have a thorough understanding of the operational parameters and the effects of these parameters on image quality and radiation safety.

Patient Selection Criteria

CBCT exposure provides a radiation dose to the patient higher than radiation doses of other dental radiographic procedures. The principal tenet of the ALARA principle must be applied: There should be justification of the exposure to the patient so that the total potential diagnostic benefits are greater than the individual detriment radiation exposure might cause. Generally, a CBCT image should be used only when a lower dose examination, such as a periapical or panoramic view, cannot provide the necessary information for patient diagnosis and treatment. Numerous consensus-derived statements providing guidelines on the clinical use of CBCT have been published. General use guidelines from the American Academy of Oral and Maxillofacial Radiology (AAOMR) and the American Dental Association (ADA) provide broad guidance to perform and interpret diagnostic CBCT images. These documents provide guidance on the appropriate use and prescription of CBCT imaging, describe the responsibilities of practitioners and licensed operators in performing the examination, outline the appropriate documentation and radiation safety considerations, and provide recommendations for quality control and patient education. In addition, specific use guidelines from the AAOMR are available for endodontics, implant dentistry, and orthodontics. Essentially, CBCT imaging should be used as an adjunctive diagnostic tool to existing dental imaging techniques for specific clinical applications, not as a screening procedure. It is advisable that the indication for the CBCT examination be documented by entry in the patient's chart or on the written request or prescriptive order for the CBCT examination.

Patient Preparation

Patients should be escorted into the scanner unit and provided with appropriate personal radiation barrier protection before head stabilization. Although the mandatory use of these devices is regulated by regional (state) or federal legislation, it is recommended that at least a leaded torso apron be applied correctly (above the collar) to the patient. Use of a leaded apron is particularly advisable for pregnant patients and for children. It is highly recommended that a lead thyroid collar also be used, provided that it would not interfere with the scan, to reduce thyroid exposure.

Immediately before the scan, the patient should be asked to remove all metallic objects from the head and neck areas, including eyeglasses, jewelry (including earrings and piercings), and metallic partial dentures. It is not necessary to remove completely removable plastic prostheses.

Each CBCT unit has a unique method of head stabilization, varying from chin cups to posterior or lateral head supports to head restraints. Patient motion can be minimized by application of one or more methods simultaneously. Image quality is severely degraded by head movement, so it is important to obtain patient compliance.

Alignment of the area of interest with the x-ray beam is critical to image the appropriate field. Often facial topographic reference planes (e.g., the midsagittal plane, Frankfort horizontal) or internal references (e.g., occlusal plane, palatal plane) are adjusted to align with external laser lights to position the patient correctly.

Unless specifically indicated otherwise (e.g., closed temporomandibular joint views or orthodontic views), it is desirable that the dentition be separated but held together firmly during the scan; this can be done with a tongue depressor or cotton rolls. Separation of the teeth is particularly useful in single arch scans where scatter from metallic restorations in the opposing arch can be reduced.

The patient should be directed to remain as still as possible before exposure, to breathe slowly through the nose, and to close the eyes. The last suggestion reduces the possibility of the patient moving as a result of following the detector as it passes in front of the face.

Imaging Protocol

An imaging protocol is a set of technical exposure parameters for CBCT imaging that depend on the specified purpose of the examination. An imaging protocol is developed to produce images of optimal quality with the least amount of radiation exposure to the patient. For specific CBCT devices, manufacturer-provided imaging protocols are usually available. Most commonly, they involve modifications in exposure settings based on patient size and acquisition settings such as imaging FOV, number of basis projections, and voxel resolution, based on diagnostic task (Fig. 10.9). Operators should be aware of the effects of all parameters on image quality and patient dose when choosing imaging protocols.

Exposure Settings

The quality and quantity of the x-ray beam depend on tube voltage (kVp) and tube current (mA). The available ranges of exposure factors in CBCT greatly depend on the manufacturer. Some CBCT manufacturers provide units with fixed, nonadjustable exposure settings, whereas others incorporate "preset" exposure settings for different-sized individuals or specific scanning protocols and allow operator "manual" adjustment of kVp or mA or both (Fig. 10.9). Operators who use CBCT units with operator-adjustable exposure settings must understand that these parameters affect both image quality (Fig. 10.10) and patient radiation dose and that careful selection is required to fulfill the ALARA principle.

A recent CBCT innovation is incorporation of automatic exposure control (AEC) as a dose reduction strategy to optimize patient doses. Used in most MDCT devices, AEC attempts to adjust and customize (i.e., modulate) tube current (mA) specifically for each patient according to the radiation intensity recorded by the detector by using a short pre-examination (scout) exposure (NewTom-FP; Quantitative Radiology s.r.l., Cefla Group, Verona, Italy) or using an exposure modulation during the rotation (SafeBeam technology, NewTom VGI evo/NewTom GiANO, Quantitative Radiology s.r.l., Cefla Group, Verona, Italy). It is anticipated that widespread implementation of AEC in CBCT will avoid the need for manual adaptation of exposure parameters based on patient size.

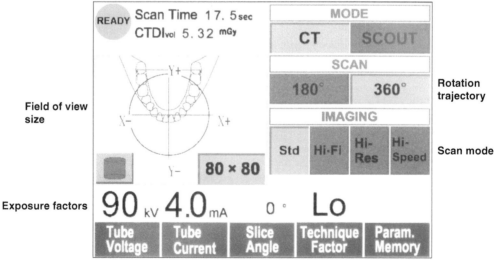

Fig. 10.9 Control panel for a cone beam computed tomography device (Accuitomo170, J. Morita Manufacturing Company, Kyoto, Japan). Icons in light green show the selected settings for a medium field of view (80 mm × 80 mm) with a rotation trajectory of 360-degrees, and a standard nominal resolution. The selected exposure factors (90 kV, 4 mA) can be adjusted to optimize for patient size. The scan time and the radiation dose (computed tomography dose index, CTDI) for these settings are displayed in the top left corner.

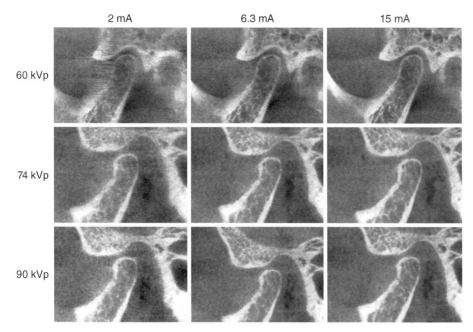

2 mA   6.3 mA   15 mA

60 kVp

74 kVp

90 kVp

Fig. 10.10 Effect of Exposure Parameters on Image Quality. Representative 0.076-mm parasagittal slices of the left temporomandibular joint of a cadaver demonstrate the effect of changing mA (columns) and kVp (rows) on image quality for high-density (cortical bone) and low-density (cancellous bone) structures. Although all images are adequate for visualization of gross morphologic changes at all values, there is increased graininess (noise) of the images made at low kVp and mA, making discernment of the fine trabecular pattern or surface irregularities of cortical plates more difficult. Little improvement in subjective image quality is achieved at settings greater than 74 kVp and 6.3 mA despite appreciable associated increases in dose.

When exposure reduction is necessary to compensate for differences in patient size, mA changes are preferable to kVp changes as the increase in noise for a given dose reduction is smaller for the former. mA adjustments affect effective dose proportionately. Similarly, a higher kVp may be considered in patients with high-density objects, such as teeth with root canal fillings or dental implants, to reduce beam-hardening artifacts from these materials. Adjustment of kV has an even greater effect on dose than does mA, with each increase in 10 kV approximately doubling the dose if all other parameters remain the same. Exposure parameters should be appropriate for both the given patient size and the diagnostic task that motivated image selection.

Spatial Resolution

Spatial resolution refers to the ability of an image to reveal fine detail. It is determined primarily by detector nominal pixel size, beam projection geometry, patient scatter, detector motion blur, fill factor (the fraction of a pixel's area capable of collecting light), focal spot size, number of basis images, and reconstruction algorithm. The voxel size with which projection images are acquired varies from manufacturer to manufacturer. In addition, CBCT units may offer a selection of voxel sizes. For these choices, the image detector collects information over a series of pixels in the horizontal and vertical directions and averages the data. This collation or pixel binning results in a substantial reduction in data processing, reducing secondary reconstruction times. Therefore voxel size should be specified as either acquisition or reconstruction. Although increased image resolution in some CBCT units does not affect changes in exposure parameters, some manufacturers incorporate reduced-dose exposure protocols for low-resolution settings.

Scan Time and Number of Projections

Adjusting the detector frame rate to increase the number of basis image projections results in reconstructed images with fewer artifacts and better image quality (Fig. 10.11). However, increasing the number of projections requires longer primary reconstruction times and increases patient radiation exposure proportionately.

Scanning Trajectory

Reconstructed images from incomplete, limited, or truncated scanning trajectories of less than 360 degrees may have limited-angle artifacts because of missing information. These include greater peripheral unidirectional streaking artifacts and more pronounced midplane cupping and photon starvation artifacts. Missing data can be compensated for with many approaches, including use of statistical knowledge of the patient's anatomy and use of numerous algorithm projection completion techniques.

Field of View

Collimation of the CBCT primary x-ray beam by adjustment of the FOV enables limitation of the x-radiation to the ROI. Reduction in the FOV usually can be accomplished mechanically or, in some instances, electronically. Mechanical reduction in the dimensions of the x-ray beam can be achieved by either preirradiation (reducing primary radiation dimensions) or postirradiation (reducing the dimensions of the transmitted radiation, before it is detected) collimation. Electronic collimation involves elimination of data recorded on the detector that are peripheral to the area of interest. Electronic collimation is undesirable because it results in greater exposure of the patient to radiation than is necessary for the imaging task.

Reduction of the FOV to the ROI improves image quality because of reduced scattered radiation (see Fig. 10.11). More importantly, a reduction in FOV is usually associated with patient dose reductions ranging from 25% to 66% depending on machine, type of collimation (vertical or horizontal), amount of mechanical collimation, and location (maxilla vs. mandible; anterior vs. posterior).

Archiving, Export, and Distribution

The process of CBCT imaging produces two data products: (1) the volumetric image data from the scan and (2) the image report generated by the operator. Both sets of data must be archived and distributed. Scan data backup is usually performed in its native or proprietary image format. However, export of image data is usually in the Digital Imaging and Communications in Medicine standard version 3 (DICOM v3) file

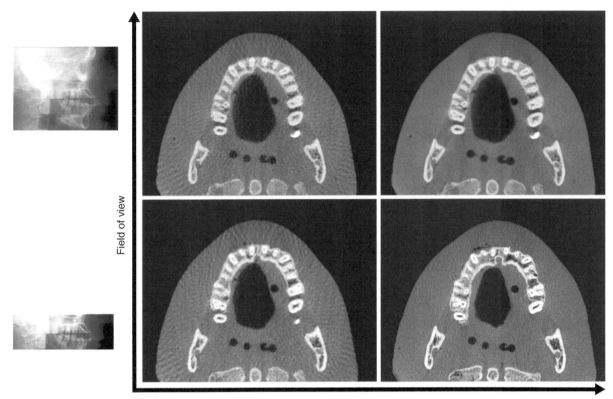

Number of basis projection images

Fig. 10.11 Pictorial Plot of the Effect of Number of Basis Projection Images and Size of Field of View (FOV) on Image Quality. Increasing number of projections in one 360-degree scan (*x*-axis) provides more data and reduces image noise; however, it increases patient dose proportionately. Reducing the number of projections creates undersampling and produces streaks. Minimizing the FOV (*y*-axis) reduces patient exposure and resultant scatter radiation and results in images with increased contrast and decreased noise.

format. This is the International Standards Organization–referenced standard for all diagnostic imaging, including medical, dental, and veterinary imaging, and includes all modalities, such as x-ray, visible light, and ultrasound. It is the dental image standard in the United States, adopted by the ADA. CBCT DICOM data can be imported into third-party application-specific software programs that provide virtual simulations that can be used to plan treatment and predict dental implant and prosthetic, surgical orthognathic, orthodontic, or prosthetic outcomes (see Chapters 11 and 14).

IMAGE ARTIFACTS

The fundamental factor that impairs CBCT image quality is image artifact (also see Chapter 13). An artifact is any distortion or error in the image that is unrelated to the subject being studied. CBCT images inherently have more artifacts than MDCT images because of the lower energy spectra used; cone beam geometry; and the introduction of additional considerations such as aliasing artifacts caused by the cone beam divergence, scatter, and a generally higher noise level. Artifacts can be classified according to their etiology.

Inherent Artifacts

Artifacts can arise from limitations in the physical processes involved in the acquisition of CBCT data. The beam projection geometry of CBCT, reduced trajectory rotational arcs, and image reconstruction methods produce the following three types of artifacts:

- Scatter
- Partial volume averaging
- Cone beam effect

Scatter results from x-ray photons that are diffracted from their original path after interaction with matter. Because CBCT uses area detectors, they capture scattered photons that contribute to overall image degradation or "quantum noise" compared with MDCT imaging (Fig. 10.12). Scatter causes streak artifacts similar to artifacts of beam hardening.

Partial volume averaging is a feature of both MDCT and CBCT imaging. It occurs when the selected voxel size of the scan is larger than the size of the object being imaged. For instance, a voxel 1 mm on one side may contain both bone and adjacent soft tissue. In this case, the displayed pixel is not representative of either bone or soft tissue but rather becomes an average of the brightness values of the different tissues. Boundaries in the resultant image may have a "step" appearance or homogeneity of pixel intensity levels. Partial volume averaging artifacts occur in regions where surfaces are rapidly changing in the *Z* direction, for example, in the temporal bone. Selection of the smallest acquisition voxel can reduce the presence of these effects.

The cone beam effect is a potential source of artifacts, especially in the peripheral portions of the scan volume. Because of the divergence of the x-ray beam as it rotates around the patient in a horizontal plane, structures at the top or bottom of the image field are exposed only when the x-ray source is on the opposite side of the patient (Fig. 10.13). The result is image distortion, streaking artifacts, and greater peripheral noise. This effect is minimized by incorporation by manufacturers of various forms of CT reconstruction. Clinically, the effect can be reduced by positioning the ROI in the horizontal plane of the x-ray beam.

Procedure-Related Artifacts

Undersampling of the object can occur when too few basis projections are provided for image reconstruction or when rotational trajectory

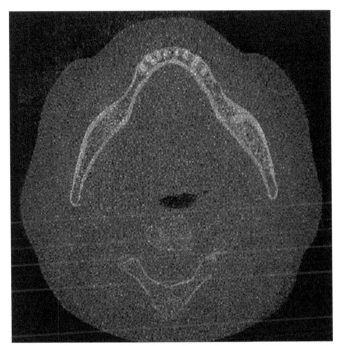

Fig. 10.12 Quantum Noise Cone Beam Computed Tomography (CBCT) Artifacts. Axial high-resolution CBCT image at default resolution (0.125 mm nominal voxel size) shows marked graininess or quantum noise caused by contamination of detector signal by scatter radiation.

arcs are incomplete. A reduced data sample leads to misregistration, sharp edges, and noisier images as a result of aliasing, which appear as fine striations in the image (Fig. 10.14). Because increasing scan time (the number of basis projections) or reducing scan arc rotation results in proportional increase or decrease to patient exposure, respectively, the importance of this artifact should be considered in relation to the diagnostic information.

Typically, scanner-related artifacts appear as circular or ring streaks resulting from imperfections in scanner detection or poor calibration (Fig. 10.15). Either of these problems results in a consistently repetitive reading at each angular position of the detector, resulting in a circular artifact.

Misalignment of the x-ray source to the detector creates a double contour artifact, similar to that created by patient motion. Repeated use of CBCT equipment over time may result in slight configuration changes, and components may need to be periodically realigned.

Introduced Artifacts

As an x-ray beam passes through an object, lower energy photons are absorbed in preference to higher energy photons. This phenomenon, called beam hardening, results in two types of artifact: (1) distortion of metallic structures as a result of differential absorption, known as a cupping artifact, and (2) streaks and dark bands, which, when present between two dense objects, create extinction or missing value artifacts (Fig. 10.16). In clinical practice, it is advised to reduce the field size, modify patient position, or separate the dental arches to avoid scanning regions susceptible to beam hardening (e.g., metallic restorations, dental implants). It is also important to remove metallic objects such as jewelry before scanning to reduce peripheral beam hardening effects superimposed on the ROI.

Patient Motion Artifacts

Patient motion can cause misregistration of data, which appear as double contours in the reconstructed image (Fig. 10.17). The smaller the voxel size (i.e., the higher the spatial resolution), the smaller the

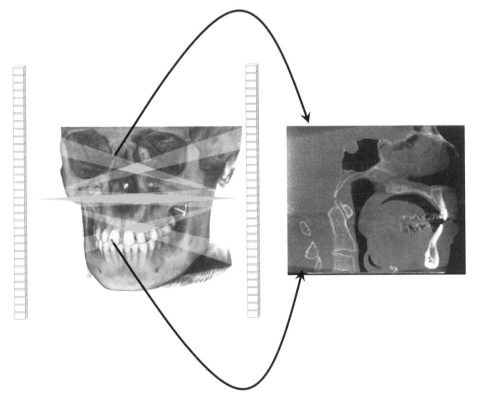

Fig. 10.13 Schematic of Cone Beam Artifact. Exaggerated projection of three representative x-ray beams (one perpendicular, one angled inferiorly, and one angled superiorly) from the focal spot point of origin is shown at two positions of the x-ray tube rotation, 180 degrees apart. The optimal amount of data collected by the detector for reconstruction corresponds to the solid blue volume between the overlapping projections. Centrally, the amount of data acquired is maximal, whereas peripherally *(transparent blue)*, the amount of data collected is appreciably less. The midsagittal section image demonstrates the visual effects of data interpolation by the reconstruction algorithm owing to inadequate data obtained at the peripheral superior and inferior extensions of the volumetric data set producing a peripheral "V" artifact of increased noise, distortion, and reduced contrast.

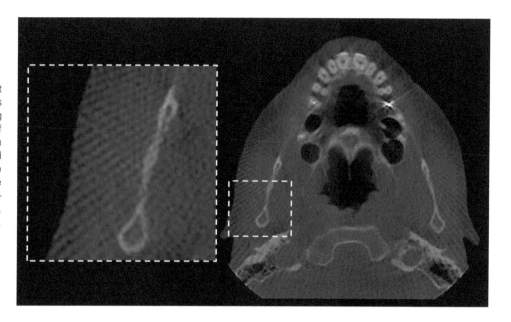

Fig. 10.14 Moiré Artifact. Too great an interval between basis projections (undersampling) or an incomplete scanning trajectory can result in misregistration of data by the reconstruction software, known as aliasing. On the cone beam computed tomographic image, particularly on the periphery *(inset)*, fine alternating hyperdense and hypodense stripes appear to be radiating from the edge of the volumetric data, resulting in a characteristic "Moiré" pattern, a type of aliasing artifact.

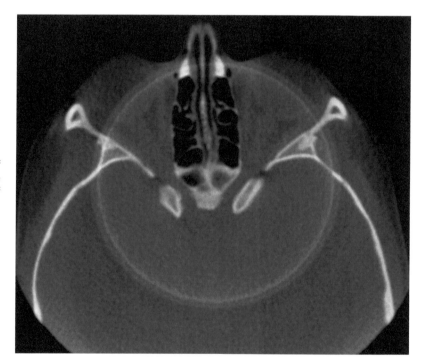

Fig. 10.15 Circular or Ring Artifacts. Visual appearance of scanner-related artifacts as circular rings on an axial image suggests imperfections in scanner detection as a result of poor calibration.

movement necessary to cause misalignment of structures. This problem can be minimized by restraining the head and using as short a scan time as possible.

STRENGTHS AND LIMITATIONS

CBCT imaging has numerous features that make it suitable for many dental applications, but it also has a number of limitations.

Strengths
Size and Cost
CBCT equipment has a greatly reduced size and physical footprint compared with conventional CT equipment, and it is approximately one-fourth to one-fifth the cost. Both of these features make it available for the dental office.

Fast Acquisition
With more recent advances in solid-state detector achievable frame rates, computer processing speed, and units incorporating reduced trajectory arcs, most CBCT scanning is performed in less than 30 seconds.

Submillimeter Resolution
All CBCT units currently use megapixel solid-state devices for x-ray detection, which provide submillimeter voxel resolution in all orthogonal planes. Some CBCT units are capable of high-resolution imaging (nominal 0.076- to 0.125-mm voxel resolution) and may be required for tasks requiring discernment of fine detail structures and disease processes, such as the periodontal space, root canal morphology, and root resorption or fracture.

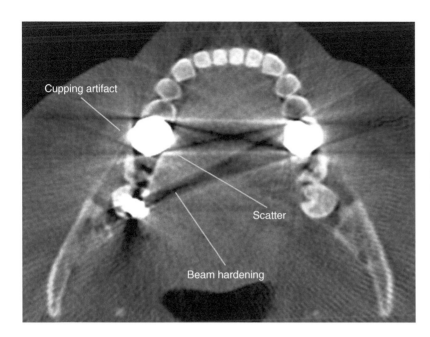

Fig. 10.16 Introduced Artifacts. Axial view demonstrating beam hardening *(dark bands)*, scatter *(white streaks)*, and cupping (image distortion) artifacts.

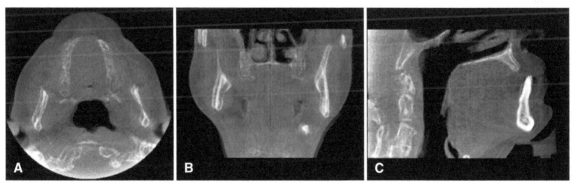

Fig. 10.17 Motion Artifacts. Patient motion during the scanning exposure can result in misregistration artifacts, which appear as double contours in the reconstructed image as demonstrated in the axial (A), coronal (B), and sagittal (C) planes.

Relatively Low Patient Radiation Dose

Published reports indicate that there is a wide range in patient effective dose (International Commission on Radiation Protection [ICRP] 2007) for maxillofacial CBCT depending on the type and model of CBCT equipment and parameters used in clinical practice, such as FOV, exposure (kVp and mA), and acquisition (e.g., rotational arc, number of basis images) settings. Reported adult effective doses for any protocol ranged from 46 to 1073 μSv for extended FOVs, 9 to 548 μSv for large FOVs, 4 to 421 μSv for medium FOVs, and 5 to 297 μSv for small FOVs. These values are approximately equivalent to 1 to 42 digital panoramic radiographs (approximately 20 μSv) or 3 to 123 days' equivalent per capita natural background radiation (approximately 3100 μSv in the United States). Patient radiation dose can be reduced by collimating the beam, elevating the chin, and using protective eyewear and thyroid and cervical spine shielding. CBCT imaging provides a range of potentially substantial dose reductions compared with conventional head MDCT imaging (range, 430 to 1160 μSv). Typical doses from standard exposure protocols from CBCT and MDCT imaging are listed in Chapter 3 (Table 3.2 and Fig. 3.4).

Interactive Analysis

CBCT data reconstruction and viewing is performed natively by use of a personal computer. In addition, some manufacturers provide software with extended functionality for specific applications, such as implant placement or orthodontic analysis (see Chapters 11, 14, and 15). Finally, the availability of cursor-driven measurement algorithms provides the practitioner with an interactive capability for real-time dimensional assessment, annotation, and measurements.

Limitations

CBCT images have limitations compared with conventional CT images.

Image Noise

The cone beam projection acquisition geometry irradiates a larger tissue volume yielding more scatter radiation from Compton interactions. Much of this scattered radiation is produced omnidirectionally and recorded by detector pixels. Consequently, the number of photons detected at each pixel does not reflect the true attenuation of an object along a specific path of the x-ray beam. This difference, referred to as noise, contributes to image degradation. The amount of scattered radiation is generally proportional to the total mass of tissue contained within the primary x-ray beam; this increases with increasing object thickness and field size. The contribution of this scattered radiation to production of the CBCT image may be greater than the primary beam. In clinical applications, the scatter-to-primary ratios are about 0.01 for single-ray CT imaging and 0.05 to 0.15 for fan-beam and spiral CT imaging and may be 0.4

to 2 in CBCT imaging. For these reasons, it is always desirable to use the smallest FOV possible when making a CBCT image.

Additional sources of image noise in CBCT are statistical variations in the homogeneity of the incident x-ray beam (quantum mottle) and added noise of the detector system (electronic). The inhomogeneity of x-ray photons depends on the number of the primary and scattered x-rays absorbed, the primary and scattered x-ray spectra incident on the detector, and the number of basis projections. Electronic noise is due to the inherent degradations of the detector system related to the x-ray absorption efficiency of energy at the detector.

In addition, because of the increased divergence of the x-ray beam over the area detector, there is a pronounced heel effect. This effect produces a large variation or nonuniformity of the incident x-ray beam on the patient and resultant nonuniformity in absorption with greater signal-to-noise ratio (noise) on the cathode side of the image relative to the anode side.

Poor Soft Tissue Contrast

Contrast resolution is the ability of an image to reveal subtle differences in image radiodensity. Variations in image intensity are a result of differential attenuation of x-rays by tissues that differ in density, atomic number, or thickness. Two principal factors limit the contrast resolution of CBCT. First, scattered radiation is a significant factor in reducing the contrast of the CBCT image. Scattered x-ray photons reduce subject contrast by adding background signals that are not representative of the anatomy, reducing image quality. CBCT units have noticeably less soft tissue contrast than MDCT units, and are inadequate for critical evaluation of soft tissue pathology.

Second, there are numerous inherent FPD-based artifacts that affect linearity or response to x-radiation. Saturation (nonlinear pixel effects above a certain exposure), dark current (charge that accumulates over time with or without exposure), and bad pixels (pixels that do not react to exposure) contribute to nonlinearity. In addition, the sensitivity of different regions of the panel to radiation (pixel-to-pixel gain variation) may not be uniform over the entire region.

CONCLUSIONS

CBCT imaging is an effective volumetric diagnostic imaging technology that produces accurate, submillimeter resolution images of diagnostic quality in formats enabling volumetric visualization of the osseous structures of the maxillofacial region at lower doses and costs compared with MDCT imaging. Although technically easy to perform, CBCT imaging should be considered an adjunctive diagnostic modality to the history and clinical examination. Imaging should be "task specific" with exposure and scan factor protocols adjusted and image formatting options tailored to optimize image display and minimize patient radiation dose.

BIBLIOGRAPHY

Principles of Cone Beam Computed Tomographic Imaging
Angelopoulos C, Scarfe WC, Farman AG. A comparison of maxillofacial CBCT and medical CT. *Atlas Oral Maxillofac Surg Clin North Am.* 2012;20:1–17.
Scarfe WC, Farman AG. What is cone-beam CT and how does it work? *Dent Clin North Am.* 2008;52:707–730.
Scarfe WC, Li Z, Aboelmaaty W, et al. Maxillofacial cone beam computed tomography: essence, elements and steps to interpretation. *Aust Dent J.* 2012;57(suppl 1):46–60.

Radiation Dose
Carrafiello G, Dizonno M, Colli V, et al. Comparative study of jaws with multislice computed tomography and cone-beam computed tomography. *Radiol Med.* 2010;115:600–611.
Ludlow JB, Timothy R, Walker C, et al. Effective dose of dental CBCT - a meta-analysis of published data and additional data for nine CBCT units. *Dentomaxillofac Radiol.* 2015;44(1):20140197.
Okano T, Harata Y, Sugihara Y, et al. Absorbed and effective doses from cone beam volumetric imaging for implant planning. *Dentomaxillofac Radiol.* 2009;38:79–85.
Pauwels R, Beinsberger J, Collaert B, et al. SEDENTEXCT Project Consortium: Effective dose range for dental cone beam computed tomography scanners. *Eur J Radiol.* 2012;81:267–271.
ICRP, Rehani MM, Gupta R, et al. Radiological protection in Cone Beam Computed Tomography (CBCT). ICRP publication 129. *Ann ICRP.* 2015;44(1):9–127.
Theodorakou C, Walker A, Horner K, et al; SEDENTEXCT Project Consortium. Estimation of paediatric organ and effective doses from dental cone beam CT using anthropomorphic phantoms. *Br J Radiol.* 2012;85:153–160.
The 2007 recommendations of the International Commission on Radiological Protection. IRCP Publication 103. *Ann ICRP.* 2007;37:1–332.

Image Reconstruction
Endo M, Tsunoo T, Nakamori N, et al. Effect of scattered radiation on image noise in cone beam CT. *Med Phys.* 2001;28:469–474.
Feldkamp LA, Davis LC, Kress JW. Practical cone-beam algorithm. *J Opt Soc Am.* 1984;1:612–619.
Siewerdsen JH, Jaffray DA. Cone-beam computed tomography with a flat-panel imager: magnitude and effects of x-ray scatter. *Med Phys.* 2001;28:220–231.

Patient Selection Criteria
American Academy of Oral and Maxillofacial Radiology. Clinical recommendations regarding use of cone beam computed tomography in orthodontics. [corrected]. Position statement by the American Academy of Oral and Maxillofacial Radiology. *Oral Surg Oral Med Oral Pathol Oral Radiol.* 2013;116:238–257.
American Association of Endodontists and American Academy of Oral and Maxillofacial Radiology. Joint position statement: use of cone beam computed tomography in endodontics 2015 update. *Oral Surg Oral Med Oral Pathol Oral Radiol.* 2015;120:508–512.
Carter L, Farman AG, Geist J, et al; American Academy of Oral and Maxillofacial Radiology. American Academy of Oral and Maxillofacial Radiology executive opinion statement on performing and interpreting diagnostic cone beam computed tomography. *Oral Surg Oral Med Oral Pathol Oral Radiol Endod.* 2008;106:561–562.
The American Dental Association Council on Scientific Affairs. The use of cone-beam computed tomography in dentistry: an advisory statement from the American Dental Association Council on Scientific Affairs. *J Am Dent Assoc.* 2012;143:899–902.
Tyndall DA, Price JB, Tetradis S, et al. Position statement of the American Academy of Oral and Maxillofacial Radiology on selection criteria for the use of radiology in dental implantology with emphasis on cone beam computed tomography. *Oral Surg Oral Med Oral Pathol Oral Radiol.* 2012;113:817–826.

Image Artifacts
Benic GI, Sancho-Puchades M, Jung RE, et al. In vitro assessment of artifacts induced by titanium dental implants in cone beam computed tomography. *Clin Oral Implants Res.* 2013;24:378–383.
Esmaeili F, Johari M, Haddadi P, et al. Beam hardening artifacts: comparison between two cone-beam computed tomography scanners. *J Dent Res Dent Clin Dent Prospects.* 2012;6:49–53.
Schulze R, Heil U, Gross D, et al. Artefacts in CBCT: a review. *Dentomaxillofac Radiol.* 2011;40:265–273.

11

Cone Beam Computed Tomography: Volume Preparation

William C. Scarfe

Cone beam computed tomographic (CBCT) imaging provides a volumetric data set that can be reformatted to present digital images in any plane. CBCT users should be familiar with software-assisted dynamic image review, and its reformatting according to task-specific protocols. Several software applications provide the ability to expand the use of this volumetric data set to facilitate digital treatment planning, image guidance of operative and surgical procedures, and additive manufacturing (AM).

Chapter 10 detailed technical aspects of CBCT image production, and optimizing conditions to produce diagnostically adequate CBCT data. This chapter focuses on the interaction and use of the subsequent volumetric data for image interpretation, and task-specific applications.

STAGES IN VOLUMETRIC DATA DISPLAY

Most software programs display the CBCT volumetric data set as secondary two-dimensional (2D) contiguous reconstructed images in three orthogonal planes (axial, sagittal, and coronal) at a default thickness (Fig. 11.1). Typically, the default view presents the three planes in individual panels in an interactive format with localizers within each orthogonal panel to spatially identify an anatomic location in all three panes. CBCT data should be considered as a volume that must be analyzed in its entirety, and from which selected images are extracted to document the findings. Technically, four stages provide an efficient and consistent systematic methodologic approach to optimize CBCT image display before image interpretation:

1. Reorient data
2. Correct data
3. Explore data
4. Format data

Reorient Data

One of the advantages of CBCT acquisition is that the resultant volumetric data set can be reoriented in relation to three orthogonal planes using imaging software. As CBCT volumetric data sets are isotropic, imaging software may align the orthogonal planes with respect to anatomic features or according to a reference plane (Fig. 11.2). The entire volume can be reoriented such that the patient's anatomic features are aligned to fixed orthogonal coordinates or alternately the volumetric data set may remain invariant and the orthogonal planes are adjusted. This stage is particularly important for aligning subsequent cross-sectional, transaxial images perpendicular to the structure of interest, such as to visualize single tooth pathology, to measure the maximal height and width of the residual alveolar ridge in an edentulous segment for implant site assessment (Fig. 11.3), to compare temporomandibular joint (TMJ) condylar morphology, or to perform a craniofacial analysis.

Optimize Displayed Images

The overall density and contrast of orthogonal images varies between CBCT units and within the same unit depending on the patient size, degree of edentulism, and scan parameters selected. Therefore to optimize image presentation and facilitate diagnosis, it is often necessary to adjust contrast (window width) and brightness (window level) parameters to favor bony structures. Although CBCT proprietary software may provide for window width and level presets, it is advisable that these parameters be adjusted for each scan. After these parameters are set, further enhancements can be performed by the application of sharpening, filtering, and edge-enhancement algorithms. The use of these functions must be weighed against the visual effects of increased noise in the image (Fig. 11.4). After these adjustments, secondary algorithms (e.g., annotation, measurement, magnification) can be applied with confidence.

Explore the Data

Because there are numerous contiguous orthogonal images in each plane, it is impractical to display all slices on one display format. Therefore each series must be reviewed dynamically by scrolling through the consecutive orthogonal image "stack." This is referred to as navigating through the volume in a "cine" or "paging" mode. It is recommended that scrolling be performed craniocaudally (i.e., from head to toe) and then in reverse, slowing down in areas of greater complexity (e.g., TMJ articulations and skull base). This scrolling process should be performed at least in two planes (e.g. coronal and axial). Viewing orthogonal projections at this stage is recommended as an overall survey for disease and to establish the presence of any asymmetry.

Format Data

All CBCT software, be it either proprietary acquisition and display original equipment manufacturer (OEM) or commercial third-party display programs, are capable of many formatting options, each directed toward visualizing specific components of the volumetric data set. Acquisition or scan protocols incorporate field of view (FOV) limitations and allow choice of specific exposure parameters. After acquisition, an image display protocol should be applied selectively on the volume to highlight anatomic features or functional characteristics for each specific diagnostic task. Overall, selection should be based on applying thin sections to show detail and thicker sections to demonstrate relationships. There are two basic format options (Fig. 11.5):

- Multiplanar reformation
- Volumetric rendering

Multiplanar Reformation

Because of the isotropic nature of acquisition, the volumetric data set can be sectioned nonorthogonally to provide 2D planar images referred

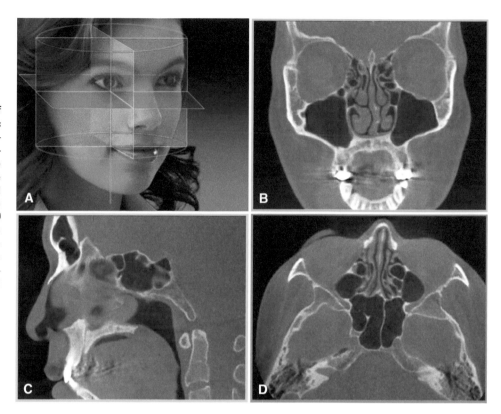

Fig. 11.1 Standard Display Modes of Cone Beam Computed Tomographic Volumetric Data. (A) Cylindrical three-dimensional volumetric data set superimposed on the head showing the three orthogonal planes in relation to the reconstructed volumetric data set: coronal *(teal)*, sagittal *(green)*, and axial *(pink)*. (B–D) Corresponding representative coronal *(teal)* (B), sagittal *(green)* (C), and axial *(pink)* (D) images. Each orthogonal plane has multiple contiguous thin-slice sections, which are interrelational. (Image of head and superimposed volumetric data set and orthogonal orientation courtesy of J. Morita Mfg Corp, Kyoto, Japan.)

to as multiplanar reformation (MPR). MPR modes include linear oblique, curved planar, and serial transaxial reformations. Several maxillofacial anatomic structures do not correspond to the standard orthogonal planes, in which case, oblique reformatting can be useful (Fig. 11.6). Linear oblique images are most often used to transect the mandibular condyle. Curved planar images are generated by manually drawing a planning line or spline by selecting multiple nodes along the centerline corresponding to the jaw arch on an appropriate axial image; this creates a "simulated" or reformatted dental panoramic image. Panoramic MPR reformatted images are useful for jaw evaluation. Such reformatted images must be thick enough to include the entire mandible to avoid missing disease. Serial sequential images perpendicular to an arbitrary linear oblique or curved planar MPR provide a dynamic representation of the anatomic structure, minimizing parallax error. These images are referred to as transaxial, tangential, or, most commonly, cross-sectional images. Cross-sectional images have two characteristics, a slice thickness and distance between adjacent cross-sectional images (interslice interval). Cross-sectional images are optimal for examining teeth and alveolar bone.

Volume Rendering

Volume rendering allows visualization of volumetric data by selective display of voxels within a data set as a 2D projection. Two specific techniques are commonly used: indirect volume rendering (IVR) and direct volume rendering (DVR).

Indirect volume rendering is a complex process requiring selection of the intensity or density of the grayscale level of the voxels to be displayed within an entire data set (called "segmentation"). This process is technically demanding and computationally difficult, requiring specific software; however, it provides a volumetric surface reconstruction with depth (Fig. 11.7). Two types of views are possible: views that are solid (surface rendering) and views that are transparent (volumetric rendering).

This volumetric procedure is optimal for visualization and analysis of craniofacial conditions and determination of relationships of various anatomic features, such as the inferior alveolar canal (IAC) to the mandibular third molar.

Direct volume rendering is a much simpler process that involves selecting an arbitrary threshold of voxel intensities, below or above which all gray values are removed. Numerous techniques are available; however, the most commonly used are ray sum and maximum intensity projection (MIP).

The slice thickness of orthogonal or MPR images can be "thickened" by increasing the number of adjacent voxels included in the display (Fig. 11.8). This creates an image slab that represents a specific volume of the patient, referred to as a ray sum. The thickness of the slab is usually determined by the thickness of the structure to be imaged. Full-thickness ray sum images in the sagittal and coronal planes can be used to generate simulated skull projections, such as lateral and posteroanterior cephalometric images (Fig. 11.9), respectively. In contrast to conventional radiographs, these ray sum images are without magnification and parallax distortion. However, this technique uses the entire volumetric data set, and interpretation is negatively affected by "anatomic noise"—the superimposition of multiple structures—also present in conventional projection radiography.

Maximum intensity projection (MIP) visualizations are achieved by evaluating each voxel value along an imaginary projection ray from the observer's eyes within a particular volume of interest and representing only the highest value as the display value. Voxel intensities that are below an arbitrary threshold are eliminated (Fig. 11.10). MIP images have great utility for demonstration of the location of impacted teeth, for TMJ evaluation, for identification of fractures, for craniofacial analysis, for surgical follow-up, for assessment of cervical spine anomalies, and for demonstration of soft tissue dystrophic calcifications.

Text continued on p. 171

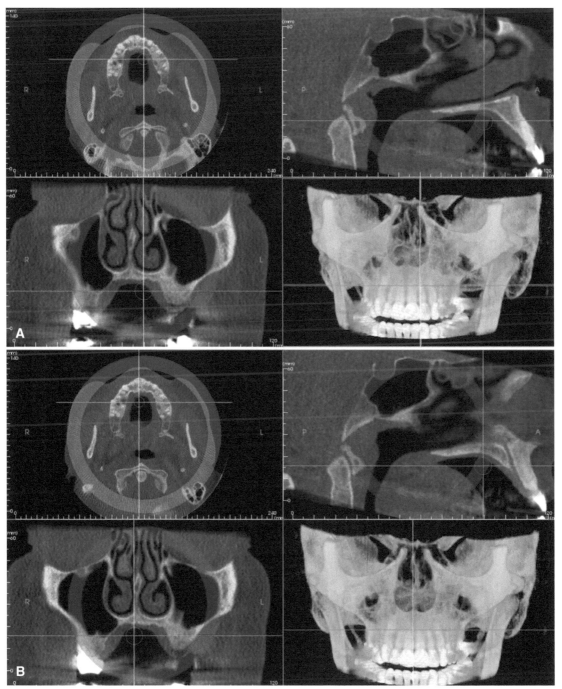

Fig. 11.2 Cone Beam Computed Tomographic (CBCT) Volumetric Data Reorientation. Axial, sagittal, and coronal orthogonal sectional images and three-dimensional volumetric rendering before (A) and after (B) reorientation of the CBCT data set to fixed orthogonal coordinates. The circular rotational tool superimposed on the respective images is selected with the cursor and adjusted to align images according to specific reference lines. In this case, axial, and sagittal orthogonal images were realigned such that the maxillary jaw was symmetrically repositioned, and the palatal plane was parallel to the floor. (Images created with InVivo Dental software, Anatomage, San Jose, CA.)

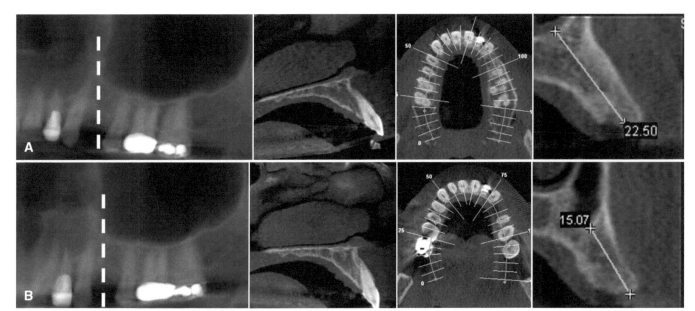

Fig. 11.3 Reorientation of Sagittal Plane to Internal Reference (Occlusal Plane). *(Left to right)* Reformatted panoramic, midsagittal, axial, and cross-sectional images of the same data set at original orientation (A) and after down-tilt of the volumetric data set in the sagittal plane such that the residual alveolar ridge is parallel to the occlusal plane (B). The lower set of images reveals the appropriate relationship of the maxillary sinus to the alveolar ridge and a substantial difference in measured height of the alveolar bone.

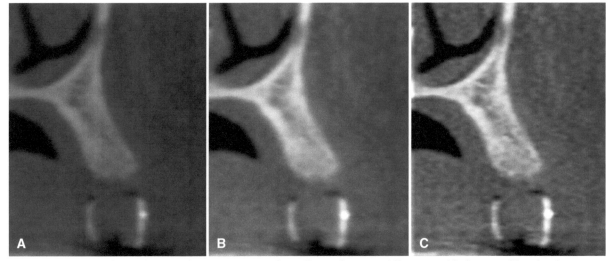

Fig. 11.4 Effect of Image Enhancement on Cone Beam Computed Tomographic Images. The visual effect of three sequential adjustments on a multiplanar reformation cross-sectional image. (A) Default image after interpolation algorithm—smoothens edges of cortical bone but adds blur to high-contrast structures. (B) Adjustment of window level and width to bone preset (W/L: 3000/500). (C) Addition of mild sharpen algorithm. (Images created with XoranCat software, Xoran Technologies, Inc., Ann Arbor, MI.)

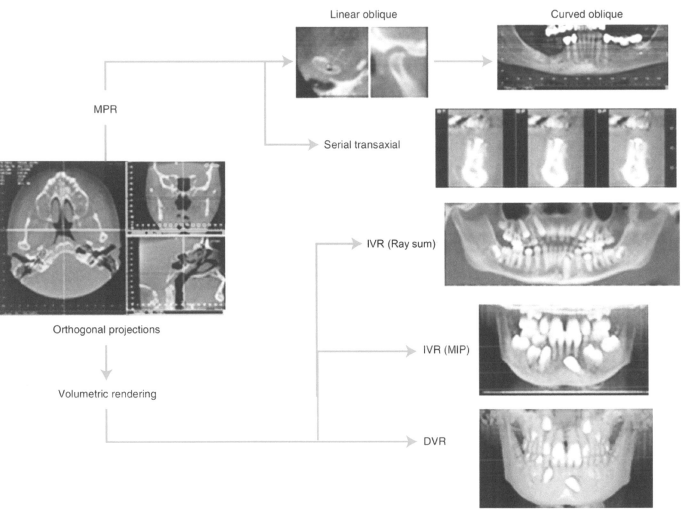

Fig. 11.5 Display Mode Options of Cone Beam Computed Tomographic Volumetric Data. Display modes can be divided into two categories: multiplanar reformation *(MPR)* consisting of linear, curved oblique, and serial transaxial images; and volumetric images including ray sum, comprising images of increased section thickness, indirect volume rendering *(IVR)*, the most common of which being maximum intensity projection *(MIP)*, and direct volume rendering *(DVR)*.

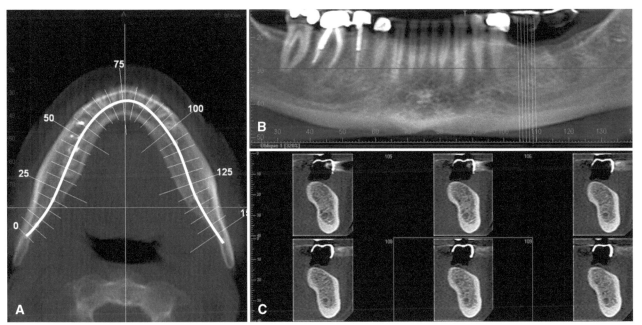

Fig. 11.6 Multiplanar Reformation (MPR). A thick axial image (A) simulating an occlusal image with an MPR oblique curved line *(white solid line)* and resultant "panoramic" image (B) and serial cross-sectional, 1-mm-thick images (C) of a potential implant site in the lower left mandible. The axial and panoramic images are used as reference images to show the location of the cross-sectional images. The cross-sectional images demonstrate the amount of lingual undercut and location of the inferior alveolar canal.

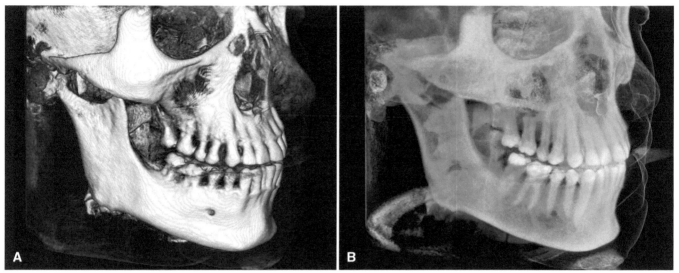

Fig. 11.7 Three-Dimensional Volumetric Surface Rendering. Manual segmentation is often accomplished by an adjustable scale determining the upper and lower limit and range of intensity values to include in the segmentation. The visual result of changes in this scale is displayed in "real time" so that the effects of incremental changes can be visualized. The segmentation may be optimized to reveal the objects of interest, including bone as a solid surface or shaded surface display (A) and bone and the dentition under the bone as a transparency (B) using volumetric imaging. (Segmentation performed with InVivo Dental software, Anatomage, San Jose, CA.)

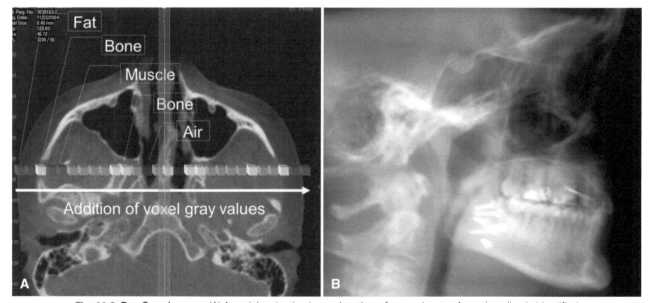

Fig. 11.8 Ray Sum Images. (A) An axial projection is used as the reference image. A section slice is identified that in this case corresponds to the midsagittal plane, and the thickness of this slice is increased to include both left and right sides of the volumetric data set. As the thickness of the "slab" increases, adjacent voxels representing elements such as air, bone, and soft tissues are added. (B) The resultant image generated from a full-thickness ray sum provides a simulated lateral cephalometric image.

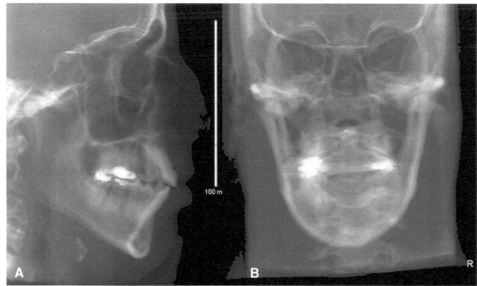

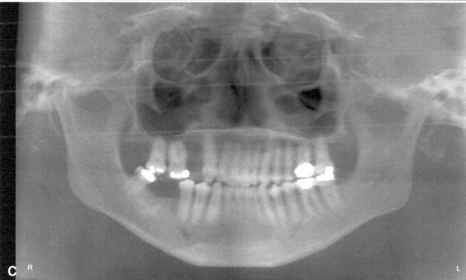

Fig. 11.9 Two-Dimensional Projections Generated With Cone Beam Data Set. This patient had an asymmetry of one side of the face. Ray sum reformation of the cone beam computed tomographic data was performed to provide multiple conventional images, such as the lateral cephalometric (A), frontal cephalometric or posteroanterior (B), and panoramic (C) projections. (Images generated with Dolphin 3D Imaging Software, Chatsworth, CA.)

INTERPRETIVE REPORT

Cone beam imaging comprises the technical component of patient exposure. It is the professional responsibility of a practitioner who operates a CBCT unit, or who requests a CBCT study, to provide a written report describing the imaging findings based on interpretation of the entire image data set. Documentation of the CBCT procedure by the inclusion of an interpretive report is an essential element of CBCT imaging and should form part of a patient's record. Patient diagnosis may often be complex, and management may involve numerous practitioners. An interpretation report serves as the optimal method of communication of interpretation findings for CBCT. Often this report includes selected images that best document significant findings.

It is imperative that all image data be systematically reviewed for disease. Competency in interpretation of both anatomic and pathologic findings on CBCT images varies depending principally on practitioner experience and the FOV of the scan. Qualified specialist oral and maxillofacial radiologists should be consulted when practitioners are not familiar with the image findings, or if they are unwilling to accept

the responsibility to review the entire CBCT volume. The essential elements of a CBCT radiologic report are outlined in Table 11.1.

TASK-SPECIFIC APPLICATIONS

CBCT technology has been applied to diagnosis in all areas of dentistry. CBCT imaging is not a replacement for panoramic or conventional projection radiographic applications but rather is best used as a complementary modality for specific applications.

Diagnosis and Preoperative Assessment
Implant Site Assessment

Perhaps the greatest impact of CBCT has been on the planning of dental implant placements (see Chapter 15). CBCT provides cross-sectional images demonstrating alveolar bone height, width, and angulation and accurately depicts vital structures, such as the inferior alveolar dental nerve canal in the mandible or the sinus in the maxilla. The most useful series of images for implant site assessment include the axial, reformatted panoramic, and cross-sectional images at the specific location

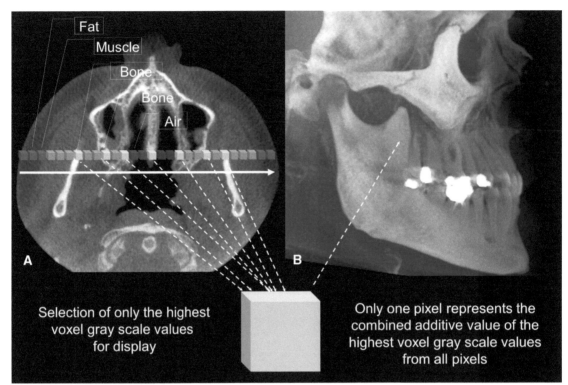

Fig. 11.10 Maximum Intensity Projection (MIP). This method produces a "pseudo"-three-dimensional image by evaluating each voxel value along an imaginary projection ray from the observer's eyes within the data set and then representing only the highest value as the display value. In this example, an axial projection (A) is used as the reference image. A projection ray is identified throughout the entire volumetric data set along which individual voxels are identified, each with varying grayscale intensity corresponding to various tissue densities, such as fat, muscle, air, and bone. The MIP algorithm selects only the values along the projection ray that have the highest values (usually corresponding to bone or metal) and represents this as only one pixel on the resultant image (B).

TABLE 11.1   Essential Elements of a Cone Beam Computed Tomographic Radiologic Report

Outline	Details
Patient information	Patient name, unique identifier code, date of birth, referring practitioner's name, rationale for procedure
Scan information	Succession number, date of procedure, date report was generated, location of facility, equipment used, scan parameters, and images provided
Image quality	Problems encountered during procedure (e.g., patient motion)
	Artifacts that compromise diagnostic evaluation
Radiologic findings	General findings should include reference to:
	• Gnathic structures: dental status including specific erupted, unerupted, impacted and missing teeth, restorative status, endodontic treatment, periapical lesions, general marginal alveolar bone status, and status of edentulous regions
	• Extragnathic structures: temporomandibular joint, paranasal sinuses, nasopharynx and oropharynx, airway, soft tissue of the neck, intracranial calcifications
	Specific findings should provide observations addressing rationale for procedure
	Significant incidental findings should be identified
Radiologic impression	Definitive or differential diagnosis, related to rationale for imaging examination or clinically significant incidental findings
	Correlation to patient presentation addressing pertinent clinical issues
	Comparison with previous imaging studies, if available
	Recommendations for follow-up or additional diagnostic or clinical studies, as appropriate, to clarify, confirm, or exclude diagnosis

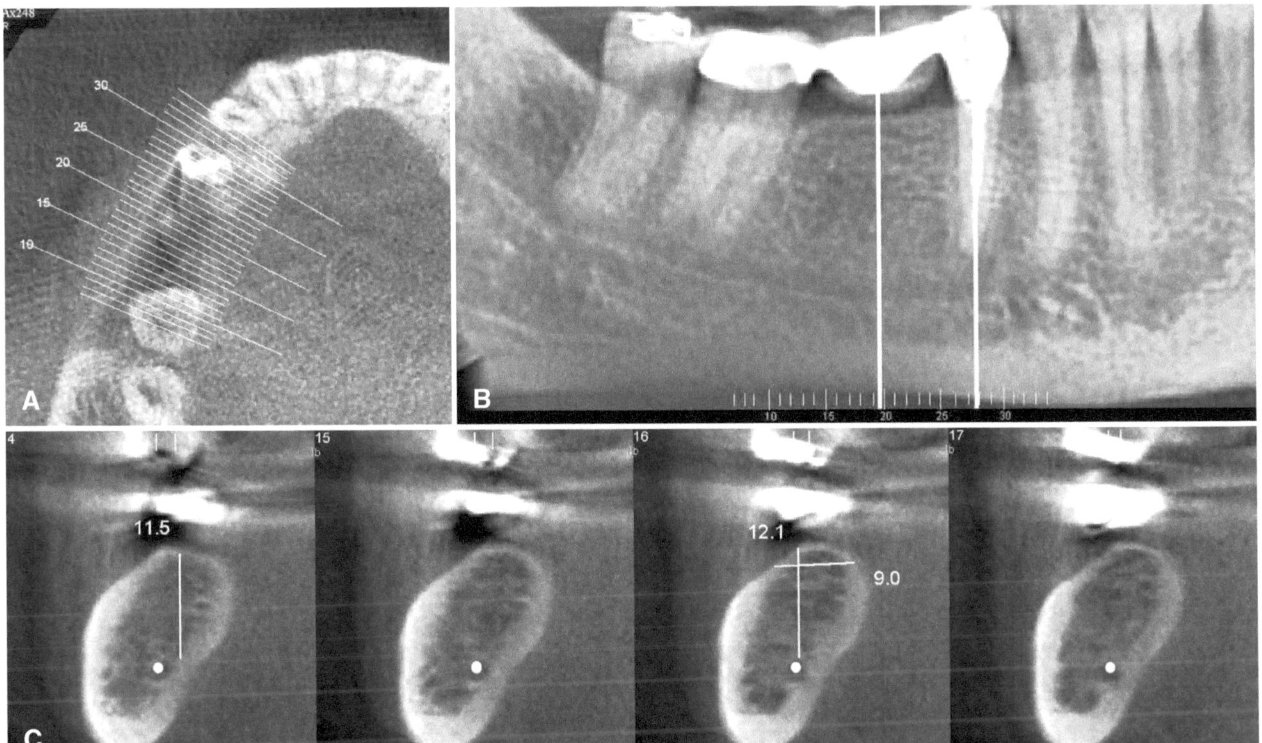

Fig. 11.11 Cone Beam Computed Tomographic Imaging for Implant Site Assessment. A curved planar multiplanar reformation (MPR) is accomplished by aligning the long axis of the imaging plane with the dental arch (A), providing a regional panorama-like thin-slice image (B). In addition, serial thin-slice transaxial images are often generated perpendicular to the curved planar MPR (C), which are useful in the assessment of specific morphologic features, such as the location of the inferior alveolar canal (shown with a *white dot*) for implant site assessment and for allowing measurement of the available alveolar bone height and width *(solid line)*. (Images created with Newtom 3G, Cefla North America, Inc., Charlotte, NC.)

(Fig. 11.11). In many instances, a radiographic template with hyperdense markers is worn by the patient during the scan (Fig. 11.12). This stent provides a precise reference of the location of the proposed implants or teeth (see Chapters 14 and 15).

Endodontics

The use of CBCT imaging in endodontics is indicated in the following clinical situations (Fig. 11.13):

- Patients who present with contradictory or nonspecific clinical signs and symptoms associated with untreated or previously endodontically treated teeth
- For the initial treatment of teeth with the potential for extra canals and suspected complex morphology, such as mandibular anterior teeth, and maxillary and mandibular premolars and molars, and dental anomalies
- For intra-appointment identification and localization of calcified canals
- If clinical examination and 2D intraoral radiography are inconclusive in the detection of vertical root fracture
- When evaluating the nonhealing of previous endodontic treatment to help determine the need for further treatment, such as nonsurgical, surgical, or extraction
- For nonsurgical retreatment to assess endodontic treatment complications, such as overextended root canal obturation material, separated endodontic instruments, and localization of perforations

- For presurgical treatment planning to localize root apex/apices and to evaluate the proximity to adjacent anatomical structures
- For the surgical placement of implants
- For diagnosis and management of limited dentoalveolar trauma, root fractures, luxation, and/or displacement of teeth, and localized alveolar fractures, in the absence of other maxillofacial or soft tissue injury that may require other advanced imaging modalities
- For the localization and differentiation of external and internal resorptive defects and the determination of appropriate treatment and prognosis

Orthodontics and Three-Dimensional Cephalometry

CBCT imaging is used in the diagnosis, assessment, and analysis of maxillofacial orthodontic and orthopedic anomalies. The most common conditions in which CBCT is useful are the identification of dental structural anomalies, such as root resorption and display of the position of impacted and supernumerary teeth and their relationships to adjacent roots or other anatomic structures. CBCT imaging facilitates surgical exposure and planning of subsequent movement. Other applications include the assessment of palatal morphologic features and dimensions, tooth inclination and torque, characterization of alveolar bone for orthodontic mini-implant placement, and determining available alveolar bone width for buccolingual movement of teeth. CBCT imaging also provides adequate visualization of the TMJ, pharyngeal airway space, and soft tissue relationships.

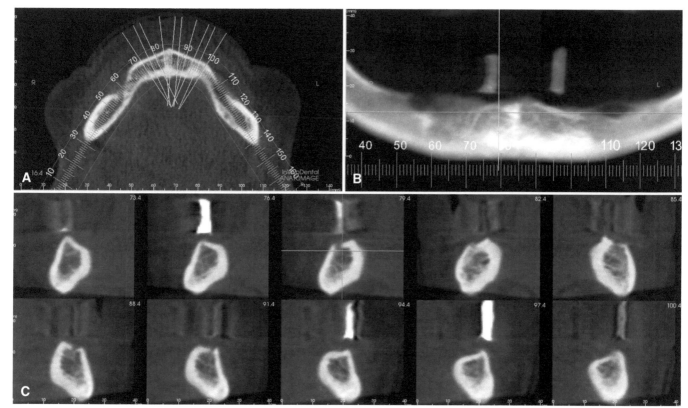

Fig. 11.12 Use of a Radiographic Template. Plastic intraoral appliances provide fiducial radiographic landmarks that can be used to correlate proposed clinical location and angulation of implants with the available alveolar bone. The axial (A) and panoramic (B) projections provide an overview of location, whereas serial cross-sectional images (C) indicate alveolar bone height. In this example of an edentulous mandible, the radiograph has two markers at proposed implant sites; the 1-mm-thick transplanar images at 3-mm intervals of the mandibular anterior region (C) indicate that although the right trajectory is optimal (*upper left* cross-sectional image), the proposed placement trajectory of the right implant *(lower left)* is too far buccal to engage the available bone. (Images generated on InVivo Dental software, Anatomage, San Jose, CA.)

CBCT imaging provides two unique contributions to orthodontic practice:
- Numerous linear images currently used in orthodontic diagnosis, cephalometric analysis, and treatment planning can be created from a single CBCT scan (see Table 8.1). This capability provides for greater clinical efficacy.
- CBCT data can be reconstructed to provide unique, previously unavailable images. Specific software provides three-dimensional (3D) visualization and analysis of the maxillofacial skeleton and soft tissue boundaries, such as the airway and facial outline. The numerous potential benefits to 3D cephalometry include demonstrating and characterizing asymmetry and anteroposterior, vertical, and transverse dentoskeletal discrepancies, incorporating the soft tissue integument, and the potential for assessment of growth and development.

Mandibular Third Molar Position

The relationship of the IAC to the roots of mandibular third molar teeth is important when considering extractions and attempting to minimize the likelihood of nerve damage that may lead to permanent loss of sensation to one side to the lower lip. Accurate assessment of the position of the IAC in relation to the impacted third molar may reduce injuries to this nerve. Panoramic imaging may be adequate when

intervening bone is present between the roots of the third molar and the IAC, but when radiographically superimposed, it is advisable to use a 3D imaging approach. Volumetric rendering with IAC annotation or "tracing" in combination with cross-sectional imaging provides useful visualization of the relationships of anatomic structures in these circumstances (Fig. 11.14).

Temporomandibular Joint

CBCT imaging provides multiplanar and potentially 3D images of the condyle and surrounding structures to facilitate analysis and diagnosis of osseous morphologic features and joint space and function, which are critical keys to providing appropriate treatment outcomes in patients with TMJ signs and symptoms. Imaging can depict the features of degenerative joint disease (Fig. 11.15) and developmental anomalies of the condyle, ankylosis, and rheumatoid arthritis. Appropriate imaging protocols should include reformatted panoramic and axial reference images; corrected parasagittal and paracoronal cross-sectional slices; and for cases in which asymmetry is suspected or surgery is contemplated, volumetric reconstructions.

Maxillofacial Pathoses

CBCT imaging can assist in the assessment of many conditions of the jaws, most notably dental conditions such as impacted canines and

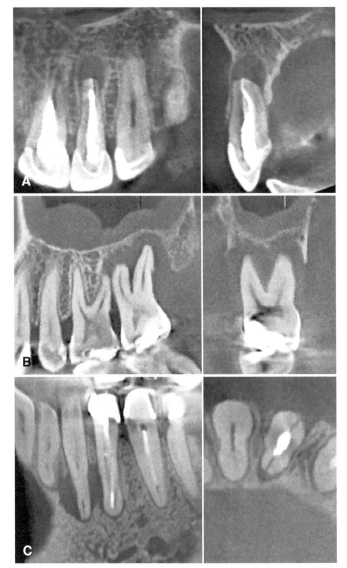

Fig. 11.13 Cone Beam Computed Tomographic (CBCT) Imaging for Endodontics. Numerous endodontically related conditions can be demonstrated in high resolution with restricted field of view CBCT imaging, including periapical conditions (A); periodontal, periapical, and sinus disease (B); and root fracture and associated alveolar bone loss (C). (Images taken created with a 3DX Accuitomo, J. Morita Mfg Corp, Kyoto, Japan.)

Treatment Planning and Virtual Simulations

The key feature of CBCT image output that makes systems interoperable is the use of image files that are conformant with the Digital Imaging and Communications in Medicine (DICOM) standard file format.

Treatment planning for a potential implant site involves an interplay of considerations of both surgical and prosthetic requirements. Implant planning software allows greater sophistication in analysis and planning, providing interactive methods of translating prosthetic planning to the surgical site (Fig. 11.18). In implant planning, software can be used to select and direct the placement of implant fixtures either directly by the use of image-guided navigation or indirectly via the construction of restrictive surgical guides.

Image fusion is the process of integration of two imaging data sets. Most commonly, CBCT volumes are fused with extraoral facial (photographic) or intraoral (impression) optical data (Fig. 11.19). After registration, numerous options allow interaction with the data sets either independently or in toto. Composite data sets provide holistic assessment of the interaction of hard tissue base with the soft tissue integument; monitoring and evaluation of changes over time; and, in combination with simulation software, predictive modeling.

Image-Guided Surgery and Additive Manufacturing

Imaged-guided surgery refers to techniques that translate software-derived virtual surgical plans developed from virtual simulations to the surgical environment. Two concepts for image-guided surgery have been developed. The first concept involves the fabrication of a plastic drilling or surgical template based on a virtual treatment plan. Numerous systems are available. Some systems are for oral and maxillofacial surgery (Fig. 11.20); however, most are for dental implant placement. The surgical templates can be a modification of a laboratory imaging stent or created directly from image data using additive manufacturing techniques. The second concept incorporates expensive navigation systems that implement the techniques of frameless stereotaxy. This real-time, in operatory, display-driven virtual guidance of surgical tools is based on the registration of the surgical instrument with the virtual patient as demonstrated by CBCT data.

Additive manufacturing (AM) is a broad term to describe a group of related processes and techniques used to fabricate physical scale models directly from 3D computer-assisted design data (see Chapter 14). 3D printing is but one of a range of AM processes in which material is extruded through fine nozzles in layers to create an object—similar to inkjet printer print heads. Prior to 2008, AM technology was only available through specific service providers such as dental laboratories and the United States military. However, desktop and in-office AM printers are now available for use in dentistry using a variety of alternate printing processes (Fig. 11.21). In maxillofacial imaging, the most obvious and widespread clinical application of the use of AM has been in the fabrication of surgical guides to assist in dental implant placement. However, biomodels, customized plastic dimensionally accurate anatomic models of the maxillofacial skeleton, can also be fabricated. DICOM data imported to proprietary software is used to compute 3D images generated by thresholding the intensity of the voxel values to be displayed and segmenting these from the background. The resulting models are used for presurgical planning of numerous complex maxillofacial surgical cases, including craniofacial reconstruction for correction of deformity caused by trauma, tumor resection, and distraction osteogenesis. Biomodels allow direct simulation of osteotomies and grafts, facilitates the measurements of segmental jaw movements, and facilitate preoperative construction of surgical templates (see Fig. 11.20) and surgical prostheses providing the practitioner with a higher level of confidence before performing a surgical procedure, reducing surgical and anesthetic time.

supernumerary teeth, fractured or split teeth, periapical lesions, and periodontal disease. Benign calcifications (e.g., tonsilloliths, lymph nodes, salivary gland stones) can also be identified by location and differentiated from potentially significant calcifications, such as may occur in carotid artery atheroma. Although CBCT imaging does not provide suitable soft tissue contrast to distinguish the contents of paranasal soft tissue attenuations, the morphologic characteristics and extent of these lesions are particularly well seen (e.g., mucous extravasation cyst). CBCT imaging is particularly useful for assessment of trauma (Fig. 11.16) and for visualizing the extent and degree of involvement of benign odontogenic (Fig. 11.17) or nonodontogenic cysts and tumors as well as osteomyelitis.

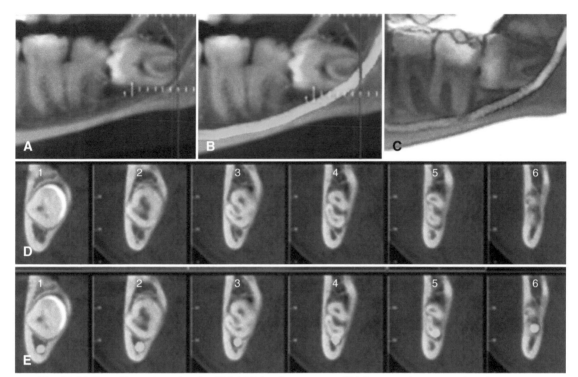

Fig. 11.14 Cone Beam Imaging for Third Molar Assessment. Third-party software used to demonstrate the location of the inferior alveolar canal (IAC) *(green)*. Nonannotated (A) and annotated (B) panoramic multiplanar reformation reformatted, volumetric transparency reconstruction (C) images with corresponding nonannotated (D) and annotated field of view (E) cross-sectional images at 1-mm intervals. Cross-sectional slices with the IAC traced *(green)*. All images demonstrate the close proximity and course of the IAC in relation to the root of the left mandibular, horizontally bony impacted and unerupted third molar. (Images created with Dolphin 3D Imaging Software, Chatsworth, CA.)

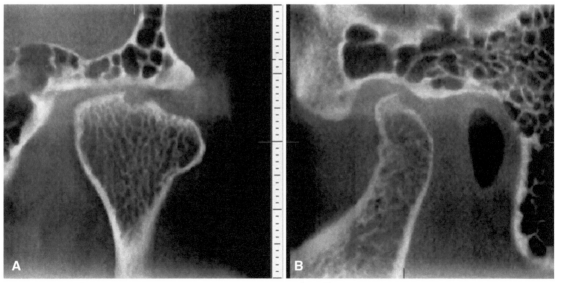

Fig. 11.15 Cone Beam Computed Tomographic Imaging of the Temporomandibular Joint (TMJ). Corrected coronal (A) and sagittal (B) images of a right TMJ with erosive defects on the superior cortical surface of the condyle associated with mild degenerative joint disease. (Images created with 3DX Accuitomo, J. Morita Mfg Corp, Kyoto, Japan.)

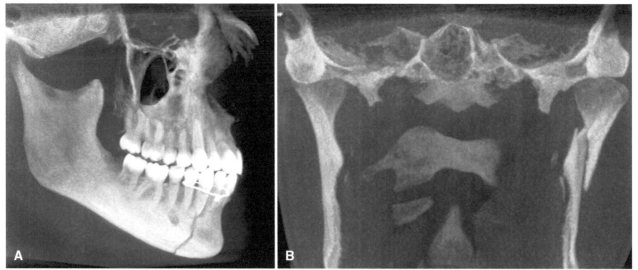

Fig. 11.16 Cone Beam Computed Tomographic Imaging of Mandibular Fractures. Use of maximum intensity projection (MIP) in the assessment of complex mandibular fractures. (A) Oblique thin slab multiplanar reformation image with MIP application demonstrates a simple, slightly displaced fracture of the right parasymphyseal region. (B) Coronal thin-slab MIP image demonstrates a comminuted displaced left subcondylar neck fracture. (Images created with i-CAT, ISI, Hatfield, PA, created using XoranCat software, Xoran Technologies, Inc, Ann Arbor, MI.)

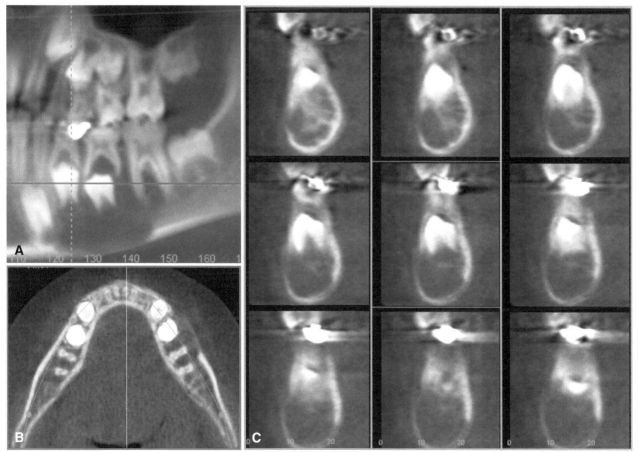

Fig. 11.17 Cone Beam Computed Tomographic Imaging of Maxillofacial Pathology. (A) Cropped reformatted ray sum panoramic view. (B) Axial slice at level of *red horizontal line* on panoramic view and outline for midportion of cross-sectional images. (C) Serial 1-mm-thick cross-sectional slices (of unilocular well-defined hypodensity) in the left premolar mandibular body of a patient in the mixed dentition phase.

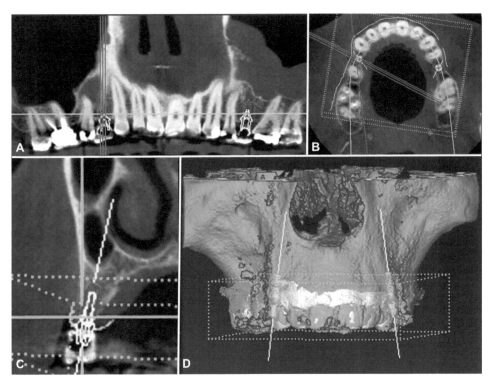

Fig. 11.18 Virtual Simulation Planning for Implant Placement. (A) Reformatted thin section panoramic of a partially dentate maxilla shows the alignment of the two virtual implant bodies *(yellow outline)* in relation to the radiographic markers providing the planned occlusal surface of the right first premolar and left second premolar teeth. (B) Axial image showing the buccopalatal position of the right implant *(yellow outline)* in the residual alveolar ridge. (D) Composite cone beam computed tomographic and optical intraoral surface scan of the teeth and mucosa *(silver)* shows the buccopalatal emergence profile *(yellow solid line)* and position (implant outline in *solid yellow*). Software also allows the use of overlay prosthetic tools, such as (1) surgical confidence marker (*dark blue outline* around each implant used to identify 0.5-mm surgical tolerance limits); (2) tapering drill confidence limit, shown on the apical portion of the implant (space between *yellow* implant and *blue outline*, C); and (3) soft tissue collar (*white outline*, C). (Images created with coDiagnostix, Dental Wings Inc., Montreal, QC, Canada.)

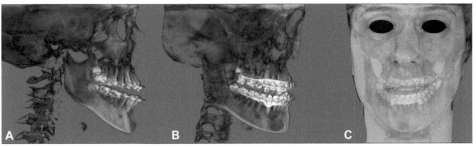

Fig. 11.19 Fusion Image. Right lateral (A), 45-degree (B), and frontal (C) three-dimensional (3D) anatomic views demonstrate image fusion possibilities. (A) Volumetric cone beam computed tomographic (CBCT) rendering. (B) CBCT data fused with high-resolution intraoral optical surface scanning of the teeth. (C) CBCT intraoral optical scan and facial digital photographs fused to form a composite 3D image set. (Images generated with Dolphin 3D Imaging Software, Chatsworth, CA; courtesy of Dr. Vinicius Dutra, Porto Alegre, Brazil.)

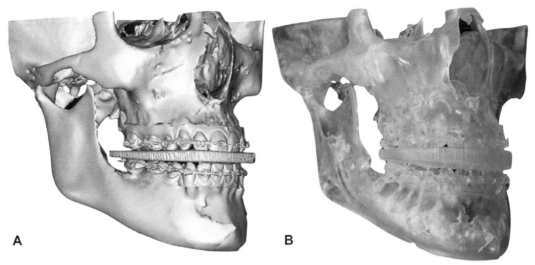

Fig. 11.20 Additive Manufacturing for Orthognathic Surgery. (A) Three-dimensional volumetric reconstruction of the maxilla and mandible after virtual surgery combining maxillofacial cone beam computed tomographic data and optical surface scans of the dentition. Note the wafer separating the maxillary and mandibular dentition that is used as a surgical guide to confirm the final relationship of the dentition. (B) Biomodel of the maxillofacial complex after virtual surgery with interposed plastic surgical stent. Modeling was performed to provide a physical model with which to confirm the actual surgery and fit of the surgical guide. (Images generated with Dolphin 3D Imaging Software, Chatsworth, CA; courtesy of Dr. Vinicius Dutra, Porto Alegre, Brazil.)

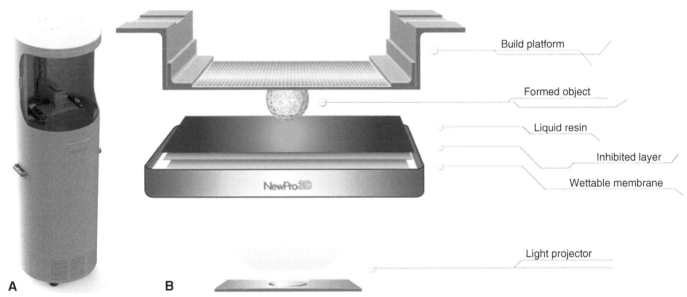

Fig. 11.21 Additive Manufacturing In-Office Printing. (A) Example of in-office three-dimensional resin based printer (NP1, NewPro3D, Burnaby, BC, Canada) using a proprietary modification of digital light processing technology (ILI Technology). (B) Schematic showing ILI technology. An accurate resin object (formed object), such as a biomodel or surgical guide, is created by projection of a light pattern (light projector) onto a wettable membrane between the photo-curing resin (liquid resin) and the light source. The object is created by sequential layering of photo-polymerized resin with upward translation of the build platform. (Images courtesy of NewPro3D, Burnaby, BC, Canada.)

CONCLUSION

CBCT technology has expanded maxillofacial CBCT imaging from diagnosis and image guidance of operative and surgical procedures into 3D printing. The use of CBCT has allowed greater predictability in the diagnosis and subsequent care of patients, especially those with complex conditions. This imaging tool brings with it an increased practitioner responsibility in the performance, optimal visualization, and interpretation of volumetric data sets.

BIBLIOGRAPHY

Radiologic Reports

American College of Radiology. ACR practice parameter for communication of diagnostic imaging findings. In: Practice guidelines and technical standards, 2014, American College of Radiology. https://www.acr.org/~/media/ACR/Documents/PGTS/guidelines/Comm_Diag_Imaging.pdf. Accessed September 12, 2017.

Carter L, Farman AG, Geist J, et al. American Academy of Oral and Maxillofacial Radiology executive opinion statement on performing and interpreting diagnostic cone beam computed tomography. *Oral Surg Oral Med Oral Pathol Oral Radiol Endod.* 2008;106:561–562.

European Society of Radiology (ESR). Good practice for radiological reporting. Guidelines from the European Society of Radiology. *Insights Imaging.* 2011;2:93–96.

Clinical Applications

Bornstein MM, Scarfe WC, Vaughn VM, et al. Cone beam computed tomography in implant dentistry: a systematic review focusing on guidelines, indications, and radiation dose risks. *Int J Oral Maxillofac Implants.* 2014;29(suppl):55–77.

Cevidanes LH, Alhadidi A, Paniagua B, et al. Three-dimensional quantification of mandibular asymmetry through cone-beam computerized tomography. *Oral Surg Oral Med Oral Pathol Oral Radiol Endod.* 2011;111:757–770.

Mitsouras D, Liacouras P, Imanzadeh A, et al. Medical 3D printing for the radiologist. *Radiographics.* 2015;35(7):1965–1988.

Scarfe WC, Azevedo B, Toghyani S, et al. Cone Beam Computed Tomographic imaging in orthodontics. *Aust Dent J.* 2017;62(suppl 1):33–50.

Scarfe WC, Farman AG, Sukovic P. Clinical applications of cone-beam computed tomography in dental practice. *J Can Dent Assoc.* 2006;72:75–80.

Scarfe WC, Levin MD, Gane D, et al. Use of cone beam computed tomography in endodontics. *Int J Dent.* 2009;2009:634567.

Special Committee to Revise the Joint American Association of Endodontists / American Academy of Oral and Maxillofacial Radiology Position Statement on use of CBCT in Endodontics. AAE and AAOMR Joint Position Statement: use of cone-beam-computed tomography in endodontics – 2015 update. *Oral Surg Oral Med Oral Pathol Oral Radiol.* 2015;120:508–512.

Swennen GR, Schutyser F. Three-dimensional cephalometry: spiral multislice vs cone-beam computed tomography. *Am J Orthod Dentofacial Orthop.* 2006;130:410–416.

The American Dental Association Council on Scientific Affairs. The use of cone-beam computed tomography in dentistry: an advisory statement from the American Dental Association Council on Scientific Affairs. *J Am Dent Assoc.* 2012;143:899–902.

Tyndall DA, Price JB, Tetradis S, et al. Position statement of the American Academy of Oral and Maxillofacial Radiology on selection criteria for the use of radiology in dental implantology with emphasis on cone beam computed tomography. *Oral Surg Oral Med Oral Pathol Oral Radiol.* 2012;113:817–826.

12

Radiographic Anatomy

Sanjay M. Mallya

Knowledge of the radiographic appearances of normal structures is the foundation of radiologic interpretation. Proficient radiologic diagnosis requires an appreciation of the wide range of variation in the appearances of normal anatomic structures. Often the ranges of normal radiographic appearance overlap with the radiographic appearance of disease. Such equivocal findings pose challenges to decision making for further investigation and management.

GENERAL PRINCIPLES OF RADIOLOGIC EVALUATION

- The radiographic appearance of structures reflects the pattern of x-ray photon attenuation. Tissues that attenuate more photons appear more radiopaque (brighter), whereas low-attenuation tissues appear radiolucent (darker). This pattern of radiodensity is the basis of all x-ray–based imaging, including intraoral, panoramic, cephalometric, and computed tomographic (CT).
- On two-dimensional projections, the anatomic structures along the path of the beam are superimposed onto the same region on the image (Fig. 12.1). In viewing these images, the clinician should combine information on the x-ray beam angulation with knowledge of anatomy, and decipher the positions and projections of individual structures.
- CT images provide visualization of the imaged anatomy in three dimensions, without superimposition. Cone beam CT (CBCT) and multidetector CT (MDCT) are typically displayed as multiplanar reconstructions of the imaged structures in three orthogonal planes (Fig. 12.2). For ease of visualization, the imaged volume is typically reoriented with tools within the CBCT software. The reorientation of the image volume is guided by the diagnostic task. For example, to examine the skull base, the axial plane is reoriented parallel to the Frankfort plane. When viewing the dentoalveolar region, the axial plane is set to be parallel to the occlusal plane. Likewise, when examining individual teeth, the image may be reoriented to along the long axis of individual roots. Sometimes it may be necessary to make additional custom reconstructions in specific planes, such as cross sections to evaluate the teeth and dentoalveolar ridges. In any single section, the plane of section may be oblique and incomplete through an anatomic site and may cause the structure to appear abnormal.
- Although the region of immediate diagnostic interest may be limited to a specific site, it is important to evaluate all structures imaged. Often, disease is an incidental finding—that is, located typically in part of the image unrelated to the reason for which the image was made. Accordingly it is critical to systematically evaluate the entire image or imaged volume.

TEETH

Hard Tissues

Teeth are composed primarily of dentin, with an enamel cap over the coronal portion and a thin layer of cementum over the root surface (see Fig. 12.1). The enamel cap characteristically appears more radiopaque than the other tissues because it is the most dense naturally occurring substance in the body. Because it is about 96% mineral, it causes the greatest attenuation of x-ray photons. Its radiographic appearance is uniformly opaque and without evidence of the fine structure. Only the occlusal surface reflects the complex gross anatomy. The dentin is about 75% mineralized, and because of its lower mineral content, its radiodensity is similar to that of bone. Dentin is homogeneous on radiographs because of its uniform morphologic features. The junction between enamel and dentin appears as a distinct interface that separates these two structures. The thin layer of cementum on the root surface has a mineral content (50% to 60%) comparable to dentin. Cementum is not usually apparent radiographically because the contrast between it and dentin is so low and the cementum layer is so thin. On periapical and bitewing radiographs, diffuse radiolucent areas with ill-defined borders may be apparent radiographically on the mesial or distal aspects of teeth in the cervical regions between the edge of the enamel cap and the crest of the alveolar ridge (see Fig. 12.2). This phenomenon, called *cervical burnout* (Box 12.1).

For most diagnostic tasks, the radiographic anatomy of teeth as displayed on intraoral radiographs is adequate to detect and evaluate dental hard tissue abnormalities. The radiographic appearance of teeth on CBCT images is similar to that on intraoral radiographs. Detailed anatomy of the teeth and the supporting periodontium is depicted better on limited field-of-view (FOV) scans than on medium- and full-FOV scans. Similar to intraoral radiographs, the teeth demonstrate a radiopaque enamel cap and a homogeneously radiopaque dentin (Fig. 12.3). As in periapical radiographs, cementum is typically not radiographically apparent because of the lack of radiographic contrast between cementum and dentin. However, unlike intraoral radiographs, CBCT also shows the buccal and lingual surfaces of the tooth. Thus morphologic variations, such as root dilacerations in the buccolingual dimension that are not apparent on periapical radiographs, are well demonstrated on CBCT examinations (Fig. 12.4).

Pulp

The pulp of normal teeth is composed of soft tissue and consequently appears radiolucent. The chambers and root canals containing the pulp extend from the interior of the crown to the apices of the roots. Although the shape of most pulp chambers is fairly uniform within tooth groups, variations exist among individuals in the size of the pulp chambers and

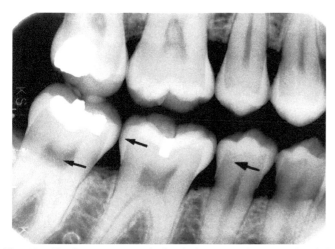

Fig. 12.1 Teeth are composed of pulp (*arrow* on the second molar), enamel (*arrow* on the first molar), dentin (*arrow* on the second premolar), and cementum (usually not visible radiographically).

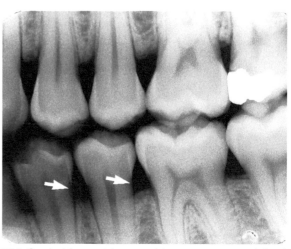

Fig. 12.2 Cervical burnout is caused by overexposure of the lateral portion of roots between the enamel and the alveolar crest and results in an ill-defined radiolucent zone *(arrows).*

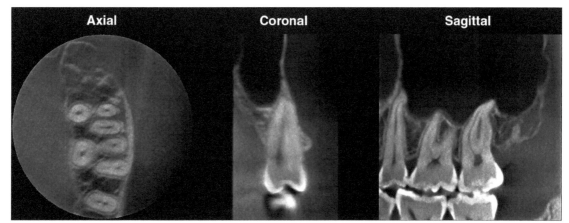

Fig. 12.3 Multiplanar reconstructions with a limited field-of-view cone beam computed tomography scan showing high-resolution axial, coronal, and sagittal sections through the dentoalveolar region of the posterior maxilla.

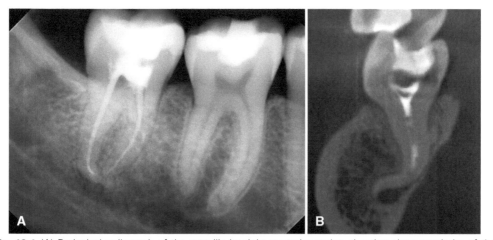

Fig. 12.4 (A) Periapical radiograph of the mandibular right posterior region showing close proximity of the root apices to the inferior alveolar canal (B) Cross section through the distal root demonstrates marked dilaceration, which was not apparent on the periapical radiograph.

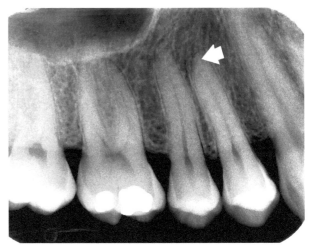

Fig. 12.6 Although the root canal is typically not radiographically visible in the apical 2 mm of a tooth, anatomically it is present and contains the vascular and neural supply to the pulp *(arrow)*.

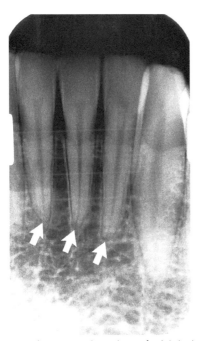

Fig. 12.5 Root canals open at the apices of adult incisors *(arrows)*.

the extent of pulp horns. Such variations must be evaluated on the radiographs, especially when planning restorative procedures.

In normal, fully formed teeth, the pulp canal may be apparent, extending from the pulp chamber to the apex of the root. An apical foramen is usually recognizable (Fig. 12.5). In other normal teeth, the canal may appear constricted in the region of the apex and not discernible in the last 1 mm or so of its length (Fig. 12.6). In this case, the canal may occasionally exit on the side of the tooth, just short of the radiographic apex. Lateral canals may occur as branches of an otherwise normal root canal. They may extend to the apex and end in a normal, discernible foramen or may exit the side of the root. In either case, two or more terminal foramina might cause endodontic treatment to fail if they are not identified.

In periapical radiographs, there may be superimposition of two pulp canals within the same root, for example, in the mesiobuccal root of the maxillary molar. Radiographs taken at different horizontal angulations may be needed to separate the images of these canals. Identification of individual pulp canals and their morphology is important for endodontic treatment planning. Despite these limitations, periapical radiographs provide adequate information for the initial evaluation of pulpal and periapical disease.

CBCT scans portray the three-dimensional morphology of the roots, pulp chambers, and pulp canals more accurately than intraoral radiographs. A pulp canal that is not evident in periapical radiographs due to

superimposition may be clearly depicted on CBCT scans. CBCT imaging is particularly useful to evaluate anatomy of multi-rooted teeth and roots with multiple pulp canals. The number and morphology of pulp canals and their course through the roots in all three planes can be examined. Reconstruction of the image volume along the long axis of each root may also be required. Individual canals are best identified on axial sections, whereas the course of the canal through the length of the root and its exit through the apex are typically assessed on coronal and sagittal sections (Fig. 12.7). When periapical radiographic findings suggest potential extra canals or complex morphology in a tooth being evaluated for endodontic treatment, limited FOV CBCT scans should be made to provide additional diagnostic information (see Chapter 17).

In a mature tooth, the shape of the pulp chamber and canal may change. A gradual deposition of secondary dentin occurs with aging. This process begins apically, proceeds coronally, and may lead to pulp obliteration. Trauma to the tooth (e.g., from caries, a blow, restorations, attrition, or erosion) also may stimulate dentin production, leading to a reduction in size of the pulp chamber and canals. Such cases usually include evidence of the source of the pathologic stimulus. However, in the case of a minor trauma to the teeth, only the patient's recollection may suggest the true reason for the reduced pulp chamber size.

Developing Teeth

At the end of a developing tooth root, the pulp canal diverges, and the walls of the root rapidly taper to a knife edge (Fig. 12.8). In the recess formed by the root walls and extending a short distance beyond is a small, rounded, radiolucent area in the trabecular bone, surrounded by a thin layer of cortical bone. This is the dental papilla bounded by its bony crypt. The papilla forms the dentin and the primordium of the pulp. When the tooth reaches maturity, the pulpal walls in the apical region begin to constrict and finally come into close apposition. Awareness of this sequence and its radiographic pattern is often useful in evaluating the stage of maturation of the developing tooth; it also helps avoid misidentifying the apical radiolucency as a periapical lesion.

SUPPORTING DENTOALVEOLAR STRUCTURES

Lamina Dura

A radiograph of sound teeth in a normal dental arch demonstrates that the tooth sockets are bounded by a thin radiopaque layer of dense bone

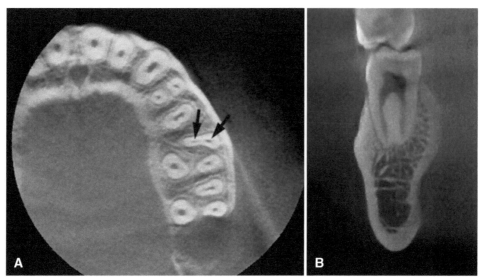

Fig. 12.7 Limited cone beam computed tomography scans demonstrates pulpal morphology. (A) Axial section through the roots of the maxillary teeth. Two pulp canals *(arrows)* are visible in the mesiobuccal root of the first molar. (B) Cross-sectional slice through the long axis of the mesial root of the mandibular first molar demonstrates the course of two pulp canals. Also, the lingual location of the inferior alveolar canal relative to the root apex is evident.

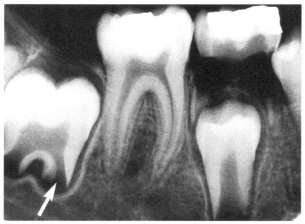

Fig. 12.8 A developing root shown by a divergent apex around the dental papilla *(arrow)*, which is enclosed by an opaque bony crypt. The apices of the first molar are still open but nearing closure.

BOX 12.2   Radiographic Projection of the Lamina Dura

The radiographic appearance of the lamina dura is determined by the angulation of the x-ray beam relative to the tooth root. When the x-ray beam is directed through a relatively long expanse of the structure, the lamina dura appears radiopaque and well defined. When the beam is directed more obliquely, the lamina dura appears more diffuse and may not be discernible. In fact, even if the supporting bone in a healthy arch is intact, identification of a lamina dura completely surrounding every root on each film is frequently difficult, although it is usually evident to some extent about the roots on each image (Fig. 12.10).

The appearance of the lamina dura is a valuable diagnostic feature. The presence of an intact lamina dura around the apex of a tooth strongly suggests a vital pulp. However, because of the variable appearance of the lamina dura, the absence of its image around an apex on a radiograph may be normal. Rarely, the lamina dura may be absent from a molar root extending into the maxillary sinus in the absence of disease. Therefore, when establishing a diagnosis and treatment, the clinician should consider other signs and symptoms as well as the integrity of the lamina dura.

(Fig. 12.9). Its name, lamina dura ("hard layer"), is derived from its radiographic appearance. This layer is continuous with the shadow of the cortical bone at the alveolar crest. It is only slightly thicker and with the same radiodensity as the trabeculae of cancellous bone in the area. Its radiographic appearance is caused by the fact that the x-ray beam passes tangentially through many times the thickness of the thin bony wall, which results in its observed attenuation (the eggshell effect). Developmentally, the lamina dura is an extension of the lining of the bony crypt that surrounds each tooth during development.

The appearance of the lamina dura on radiographs may vary, depending on the direction of the x-ray beam relative to the cortical bone thickness (Box 12.2). In addition, small variations and disruptions in the continuity of the lamina dura may result from superimpositions of cancellous bone and small nutrient canals passing from the marrow spaces to the periodontal ligament (PDL). The thickness and density of the lamina dura on the radiograph vary with the amount of occlusal stress to which the tooth is subjected. The lamina dura is thicker and more radiopaque around the roots of teeth in heavy occlusion and thinner and less dense around teeth not subjected to occlusal function.

Alveolar Crest

The gingival margin of the alveolar process that extends between the teeth is apparent on radiographs as a radiopaque line—the alveolar crest (Fig. 12.11). The level of this bony crest is considered normal when it is 0.5 to 2 mm apical to the cementoenamel junction of the adjacent teeth. The alveolar crest may recede apically with age and show marked resorption with periodontal disease. Radiographs can demonstrate only the position of the crest; determining the significance of its level is primarily a clinical decision (see Chapter 20).

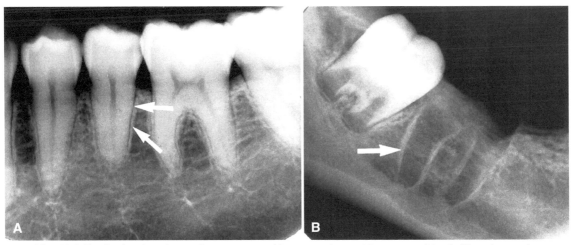

Fig. 12.9 The lamina dura *(arrows)* appears as a thin opaque layer of bone around teeth (A) and around a recent extraction socket (B).

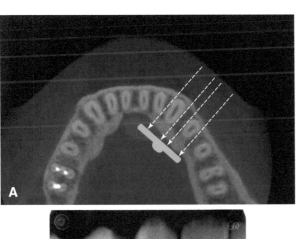

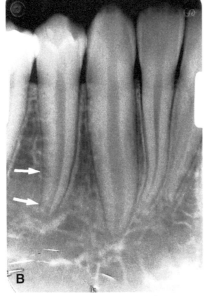

Fig. 12.10 (A) Representation of the position of the image receptor for a periapical projection of the mandibular canine and premolar. Note how the x-ray beam *(dashed arrows)* traverses through partial thicknesses of the lamina dura on the mesial surface of the canine and distal surface of the first premolar. (B) The lamina dura is poorly visualized on the distal surface of this premolar *(arrows)* but is clearly seen on the mesial surface. A broad, flat lamina dura oriented parallel to the x-ray beam produces a prominent lamina dura, whereas a curved narrow lamina dura is less visible.

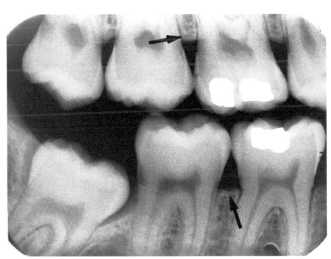

Fig. 12.11 The alveolar crests *(arrows)* are seen as cortical borders of the alveolar bone. The alveolar crest is continuous with the lamina dura.

The length of the normal alveolar crest in a particular region depends on the distance between the teeth in question. In the anterior region, the crest is reduced to only a point of bone between the close-set incisors. Posteriorly it is flat, aligned parallel with and slightly below a line connecting the cementoenamel junctions of the adjacent teeth. The crest of the bone is continuous with the lamina dura and forms a sharp angle with it. Rounding of these sharp junctions is indicative of periodontal disease.

The image of the crest varies from a dense layer of cortical bone to a smooth surface without cortical bone. In the latter case, the trabeculae at the surface are of normal size and density. In the posterior regions, this range of radiodensity of the crest is presumed to be normal if the bone is at a proper level in relation to the teeth. However, the absence of an image of cortex between the incisors is considered by many to be an indication of incipient disease, even if the level of the bone is not abnormal.

Periodontal Ligament Space

Because the PDL is composed primarily of collagen, it appears as a radiolucent space between the tooth root and the lamina dura. This space begins at the alveolar crest, extends around the portions of the tooth roots within the alveolus and returns to the alveolar crest on the opposite side of the tooth (Fig. 12.12).

The PDL width varies between individuals, from tooth to tooth in the same individual and even from location to location around one tooth (Fig. 12.13). It is usually thinner in the middle of the root and slightly wider near the alveolar crest and root apex, suggesting that the fulcrum of physiologic movement is in the region where the PDL is thinnest. The thickness of the ligament relates to the degree of function, because the PDL is thinnest around the roots of embedded teeth and teeth that have lost their antagonists. The reverse is not true, however, because an appreciably wider space is not regularly observed in persons with especially heavy occlusion or bruxism.

The shape of the tooth may create the appearance of a double PDL space. When the x-ray beam is directed so that two convexities of a root surface appear on a film, a double PDL space is seen (Fig. 12.14). A common example of this double PDL space is seen on the buccal

and lingual eminences on the mesial surface of mandibular first and second molar roots.

Cancellous Bone

The cancellous bone (also called trabecular bone or spongiosa) lies between the cortical plates in both jaws. It is composed of thin radiopaque plates and rods (trabeculae) surrounding many small radiolucent pockets of marrow. On two-dimensional radiographs, the radiographic pattern of the trabeculae comes from two anatomic sources. The first is the cancellous bone itself. The second is the endosteal surface of the outer cortical bone where the cancellous bone fuses with the cortical bone. At this surface, trabecular plates are relatively thick and make a significant contribution to the radiographic image. There is wide variation in the trabecular pattern among individuals and between different anatomic sites in the same patient. It is important to recognize the limits of this variation so that it is not confused with disease. To evaluate the trabecular pattern in a specific area, the practitioner should examine the trabecular distribution, size, and density and compare them throughout both jaws and especially with the corresponding region on the opposite side. This comparison allows the clinician to assess whether a particularly suspect region is anatomic or pathologic in nature.

The trabeculae in the anterior maxilla are typically thin and numerous, forming a fine, granular, dense pattern (Fig. 12.15), and the marrow spaces are consequently small and relatively numerous. In the posterior maxilla, the trabecular pattern is usually quite similar to the pattern in the anterior maxilla, although the marrow spaces may be slightly larger.

In the anterior mandible, the trabeculae are thicker than in the maxilla, resulting in a coarser pattern (Fig. 12.16) with trabecular plates that are oriented more horizontally. The trabecular plates are also fewer than in the maxilla, and the marrow spaces are correspondingly larger. In the posterior mandible, the periradicular trabeculae and marrow spaces may be similar to those in the anterior mandible but are usually larger (Fig. 12.17). The trabecular plates are also oriented mainly horizontally in this region. Below the apices of the mandibular molars, the number of trabeculae dwindles still more. In some cases, the area from just below the molar roots to the inferior border of the mandible may appear to be almost devoid of trabeculae. The distribution and size of the trabeculae throughout both jaws show a relationship to the thickness (and strength) of the adjacent cortical plates. It may be speculated that

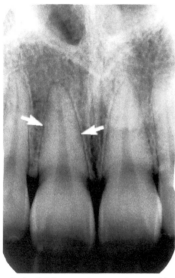

Fig. 12.12 The periodontal ligament space *(arrows)* is seen as a narrow radiolucency between the tooth root and the lamina dura.

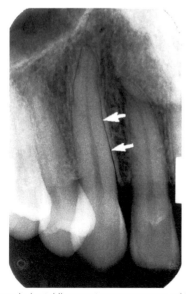

Fig. 12.13 The periodontal ligament space appears wide on the mesial surface of this canine *(arrows)* and thin on the distal surface.

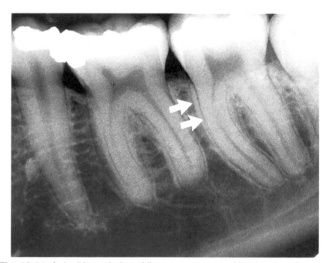

Fig. 12.14 A double periodontal ligament space and lamina dura *(arrows)* may be seen when there is a convexity of the proximal surface of the root resulting in two heights of contour. Double periodontal ligament spaces may also be seen on the mesial surfaces of both roots of the first molar.

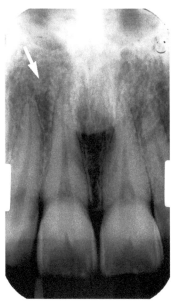

Fig. 12.15 The trabecular pattern in the anterior maxilla is characterized by fine trabecular plates and multiple small trabecular spaces *(arrow)*.

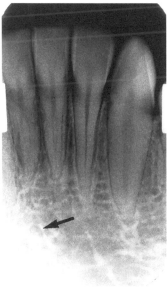

Fig. 12.16 The trabecular pattern in the anterior mandible is characterized by coarser trabecular plates *(arrow)* and larger marrow spaces than in the anterior maxilla.

where the cortical plates are thick (e.g., in the posterior region of the mandibular body), internal bracing by the trabeculae is not required, so there are relatively few except where required to support the alveoli. By contrast, in the maxilla and anterior region of the mandible, where the cortical plates are relatively thin and less rigid, trabeculae are more numerous and lend internal bolstering to the jaw. Occasionally the trabecular spaces in this region are very irregular, with some so large that they mimic pathologic lesions. This finding may be diagnostically challenging (Box 12.3).

Cortical Bone

Buccal and lingual cortical plates of the mandible and maxilla do not cast a discernible image on periapical, bitewing and panoramic radiographs. They are well depicted on CBCT images, best visualized on the

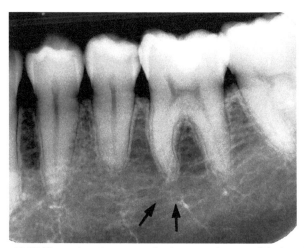

Fig. 12.17 The trabecular pattern in the posterior mandible is quite variable, generally showing large marrow spaces and sparse trabeculation, especially inferiorly *(arrows)*.

BOX 12.3 Trabecular Sparseness: Anatomic Variation Versus Disease

Sparseness or apparent absence of trabeculae may suggest the presence of disease in an otherwise asymptomatic patient.
- Considerable variation may exist in trabecular patterns among patients, so it is important to examine other regions of the jaws, preferably on the contralateral side, to assess the general trabecular pattern for that individual. Assess whether the area of trabecular sparseness deviates appreciably from that norm.
- Compare with previous radiographs of the region in question to determine whether the current appearance represents a change from a prior condition. An abnormality is more likely when the comparison indicates a change in the trabecular pattern.
- If prior films are unavailable, it is frequently useful to repeat the radiographic examination at a reduced exposure because this may demonstrate the presence of a sparse trabecular pattern that was overexposed and "burned out" in the initial projection.
- In an asymptomatic patient, it may be appropriate to expose another radiograph at a later time to monitor for interval changes.

---

axial, coronal, or cross-sectional images (see Figs. 12.7 and 12.18). Cortical bone has higher mineral content than the adjacent cancellous bone, and appears more radiopaque. The endosteal surface of the cortex is smooth and merges with the trabeculae of the cancellous bone. The thickness of the cortical bone varies with anatomic location. In particular, buccal bone adjacent to teeth is often thin and barely discerned on radiographs. CBCT images reveal the proximity of the root surface to the cortical plates of the alveolar bone and detect anatomic variations, such as fenestrations or dehiscence defects (see Fig. 12.18).

MAXILLA AND MIDFACIAL BONES

The maxilla and palatine bones form the upper jaw. The maxilla comprises a pyramidal-shaped body and four processes—alveolar, palatine, zygomatic, and frontal.

Intermaxillary Suture

The alveolar and palatine processes articulate in the midline to form the intermaxillary suture between the central incisors. On intraoral

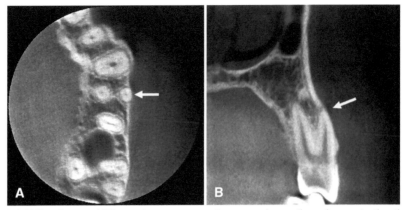

Fig. 12.18 Axial (A) and coronal (B) cone beam computed tomography sections demonstrating the proximity of the roots of the first premolar to the buccal cortical plate. Note the fenestration defect adjacent to the buccal root of the first premolar *(arrows)*.

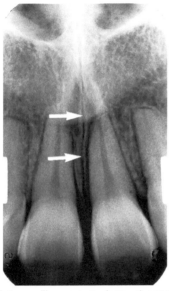

Fig. 12.19 The intermaxillary suture *(arrows)* appears as a curved radiolucency in the midline of the maxilla.

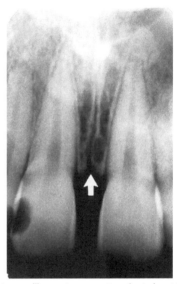

Fig. 12.20 The intermaxillary suture may terminate in a V-shaped widening *(arrow)* at the alveolar crest. This is a normal variation and should not be confused with alveolar bone loss associated with periodontal disease.

periapical radiographs this suture appears as a thin radiolucent line in the midline between the two portions of the premaxilla (Fig. 12.19). It extends from the alveolar crest between the central incisors superiorly through the anterior nasal spine and continues posteriorly between the maxillary palatine processes to the posterior aspect of the hard palate. It is not unusual for this narrow radiolucent suture to terminate at the alveolar crest in a small rounded or V-shaped enlargement (Fig. 12.20).

On CBCT images, the intermaxillary suture is best evaluated on coronal and axial sections (Plate 12.2). The suture is limited by two parallel radiopaque borders of thin cortical bone on each side of the maxilla. The radiolucent region is usually of uniform width. The adjacent cortical margins may be either smooth or slightly irregular. The appearance of the intermaxillary suture depends on both anatomic variability and, in the case of periapical radiography, on the angulation of the x-ray beam through the suture. Evaluation of the intermaxillary suture is important in planning for orthodontic expansion of the palate.

Anterior Nasal Spine

The anterior nasal spine is frequently demonstrated on periapical radiographs of the maxillary central incisors (Fig. 12.21). Located in the midline, it lies approximately 1.5 to 2 cm above the alveolar crest,

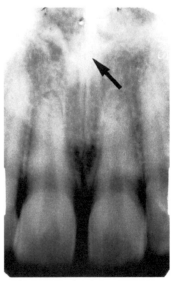

Fig. 12.21 The anterior nasal spine is seen as an opaque, irregular, or V-shaped projection from the floor of the nasal aperture in the midline *(arrow)*.

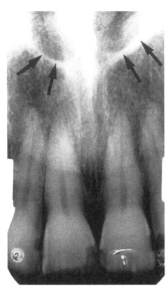

Fig. 12.22 The anterior floor of the nasal aperture *(arrows)* appears as opaque lines extending laterally from the anterior nasal spine.

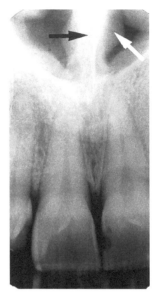

Fig. 12.23 The nasal septum *(black arrow)* arises directly above the anterior nasal spine and is covered on each side by mucosa *(white arrow)*.

usually at or just below the junction of the inferior end of the nasal septum and the inferior outline of the nasal aperture. It is radiopaque because of its bony composition and is usually V-shaped. On CBCT images, the anterior nasal spine is best observed on axial and sagittal sections as a triangular projection from the anterior surface of the maxilla at the level of the nasal floor (Plates 12.2 and 12.7).

Nasal Aperture and Nasal Cavity

Because the air-filled nasal aperture and cavity lie just above the oral cavity, its radiolucent image may be apparent on intraoral radiographs of the maxillary teeth, especially in central incisor projections. On maxillary incisor periapical views, the inferior border of the fossa aperture appears as a radiopaque line extending bilaterally away from the base of the anterior nasal spine (Fig. 12.22). Above this line is the radiolucent space of the inferior portion of the nasal cavity. The relatively radiopaque nasal septum is seen arising in the midline from the anterior nasal spine (Fig. 12.23). The shadow of the septum may appear wider than anticipated and not sharply defined because the image is a superimposition of septal cartilage and vomer bone. Also, the septum frequently deviates slightly from the midline, and its plate of bone (the vomer) is curved.

Depending on the field of view, CBCT scans may encompass the full extent of the nasal cavity. The boundaries of the nasal cavity may be evaluated in the coronal, sagittal, and axial planes. The cribriform plate of the ethmoid bone and the ethmoidal air cells form the roof of the nasal cavity. The hard palate forms the floor (see Plates 12.2, 12.4, and 12.5).

Nasal Conchae and Nasal Turbinates

The lateral walls contain thin bony projections called conchae. The conchae plus their mucosal covering are called turbinates (see Plates 12.2, 12.4, and 12.5). There are three nasal turbinates—superior, middle, and inferior—which define spaces termed superior, middle, and inferior meati (see Plate 12.4). Pneumatization of the concha is termed concha bullosa and is a common variant with a reported frequency of 14% to 53% (Fig. 12.24).

On periapical radiographs of the maxillary incisor and canine regions, the inferior nasal conchae is often visualized, extending from the right and left lateral walls for varying distances toward the septum. These

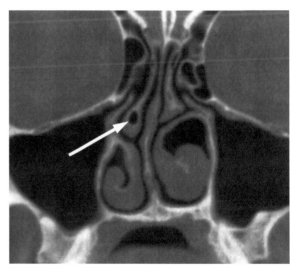

Fig. 12.24 Concha bullosa. Coronal section through the nasal turbinates showing pneumatization of the middle concha *(arrow)*, or concha bullosa.

conchae fill varying amounts of the lateral portions of the cavity (Fig. 12.25).

Nasal Floor and Hard Palate

The palatine processes are thick horizontal bony projections that form the anterior three-fourths of the hard palate and the floor of the nasal cavity. On periapical radiographs, the floor of the nasal aperture and a small segment of the nasal cavity are occasionally projected high onto a maxillary canine radiograph (Fig. 12.26). In the posterior maxillary region, the floor of the nasal cavity may be seen in the region of the maxillary sinus. It may falsely convey the impression of a septum in the sinus or a limiting superior sinus wall (Fig. 12.27).

Medium- and full-FOV CBCT scans may show the entire extent of the nasal floor (hard palate), best displayed on coronal and sagittal sections (see Plates 12.4, 12.5, and 12.7). Disruption of the hard palate suggests developmental disturbances, such as a cleft palate. Areas of bony protuberance or tori are frequently noted, especially in the midline.

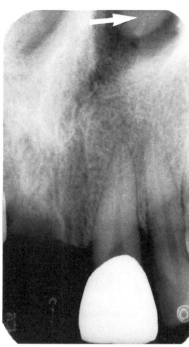

Fig. 12.25 The mucosal covering of the inferior concha *(arrow)* is occasionally visualized in the nasal cavity.

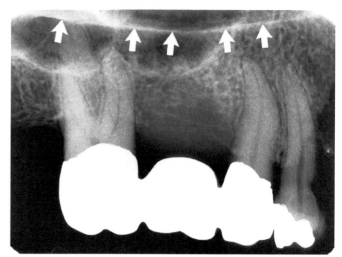

Fig. 12.27 The floor of the nasal cavity, or hard palate *(arrows)*, extends posteriorly, superimposed over the maxillary sinus.

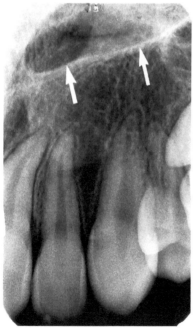

Fig. 12.26 The floor of the nasal aperture *(arrows)* often may be seen extending posteriorly from the anterior nasal spine above the maxillary lateral incisor and canine.

Numerous nutrient canals also may be observed perforating the cortical outline of the hard palate on high-resolution scans.

Nasopalatine Canal and Incisive Foramen

The nasopalatine canal originates in the anterior floor of the nasal cavity and exits on the anterior maxilla as the incisive foramen, located in the midline on the anterior aspect of the palatine process immediately palatal to the maxillary central incisors. Within this foramen are two lateral canals—the incisive canals or foramina of Stensen—that transmit the terminal branch of the descending palatine artery and the nasopalatine nerve. Occasionally there may be two additional midline canals—the foramina of Scarpa, which transmit the nasopalatine nerves.

On intraoral and panoramic radiographs, the incisive foramen is usually projected between the roots and in the region of the middle and apical thirds of the central incisors (Fig. 12.28). It appears as an ovoid radiolucency, often with diffuse borders. Occasionally the lateral walls of the nasopalatine canal are seen as a pair of radiopaque lines running vertically from the floor of the nasal aperture to the incisive foramen (Fig. 12.29A). When an exaggerated vertical angle is used, as in anterior maxillary occlusal projections, the openings of the foramina of Stensen at the nasal floor may be seen (Fig. 12.30).

There is wide variation in the appearance of the incisive foramen on periapical radiographs. The foramen varies markedly in its radiographic shape, size, and sharpness. It may appear smoothly symmetric or very irregular, and its borders may be well demarcated or ill defined. The position of the foramen's image is also variable and may be recognized at the apices of the central incisor roots, near the alveolar crest, anywhere in between, or extending over the entire distance. The great variability of its radiographic image is primarily the result of (1) the differing angles at which the x-ray beam is directed for the maxillary central incisors and (2) some variability in its anatomic size. Often, a large incisive foramen may mimic disease (Box 12.4).

CBCT images better demonstrate the anatomy of the nasopalatine canal and incisive foramen (see Fig. 12.29B and C). The shape and size of the incisive foramen is best assessed on axial sections (see Fig. 12.29B and Plates 12.2 and 12.3). The variation in the size of the nasopalatine canal is recognized on sagittal sections (Fig. 12.31 and Plate 12.7). Evaluation of the locations of the foramen and canal is important in planning implant placement in the anterior maxilla (see Chapter 15).

Lateral Fossa

The lateral fossa (also called the incisive fossa) is a gentle depression in the maxilla near the apex of the lateral incisor (Fig. 12.32A). It may appear diffusely radiolucent on periapical projections of this region, superimposed over the root of the lateral incisor (see Fig. 12.32B). An intact lamina dura around the root of the lateral incisor coupled with absence of clinical symptoms will indicate absence of periapical disease.

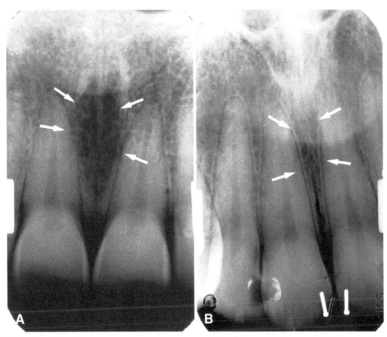

Fig. 12.28 (A) The incisive foramen appears as an ovoid radiolucency *(arrows)* between the roots of the central incisors. (B) Note its borders, which are diffuse but within normal limits.

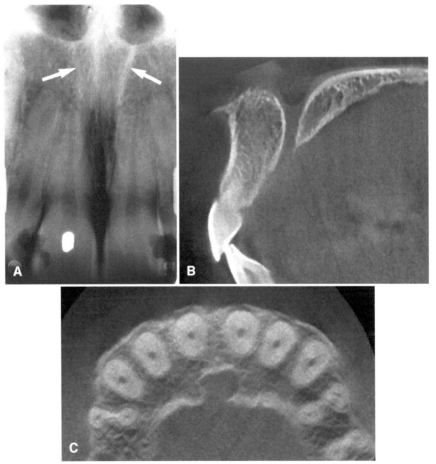

Fig. 12.29 Nasopalatine canal. (A) The lateral walls of the nasopalatine canal *(arrows)* extend from the incisive foramen to the floor of the nasal fossa. (B) Cone beam image in the sagittal plane shows superior foramina in the floor of the nasal fossa, the anterior and posterior borders of the canal, and the incisive foramen opening onto the hard palate. (C) Cone beam image in the axial plane at the level of the incisive foramen shows anterior and lateral borders of the incisive canal lying palatal to the incisor roots seen in cross section.

BOX 12.4 Nasopalatine Canal—Anatomic Variation Versus Disease

- The nasopalatine canal is a potential site of cyst formation. A nasopalatine canal cyst is radiographically discernible because it frequently causes enlargement of the foramen and canal. Often the appearance of a large incisive foramen may mimic a cyst. The presence of a cyst is presumed if the width of the foramen exceeds 1 cm or if enlargement can be demonstrated on successive radiographs.

- On a periapical radiograph, the radiolucency of the normal incisive foramen may be projected over the apex of one central incisor to mimic a periapical radiolucency. The presence of an intact lamina dura around the central incisor in question and a lack of clinical symptoms will indicate absence of periapical disease.

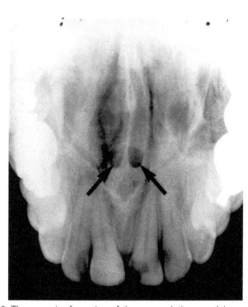

Fig. 12.30 The superior foramina of the nasopalatine canal *(arrows)* appear just lateral to the nasal septum and posterior to the anterior nasal spine.

Nose

The soft tissue of the tip of the nose is frequently seen in projections of the maxillary central and lateral incisors, superimposed over the roots of these teeth. The image of the nose has a uniform, slightly opaque appearance with a sharp border (Fig. 12.33). Occasionally the radiolucent nares can be identified, especially when a steep vertical angle is used.

Nasolacrimal Canal

The nasal and maxillary bones form the nasolacrimal canal. It runs from the medial aspect of the anteroinferior border of the orbit inferiorly to drain under the inferior concha into the nasal cavity. The anatomy of the nasolacrimal canal is distinct on CBCT and best evaluated in the axial and coronal planes (see Plates 12.2 and 12.4). Occasionally it can be visualized on periapical radiographs in the region above the apex of the canine, especially when a steep vertical angulation is used (Fig. 12.34). The nasolacrimal canals are usually seen on maxillary occlusal projections (see Chapter 7) in the region of the molars (Fig. 12.35).

Paranasal Sinuses

The paranasal sinuses consist of four pairs of air-filled cavities—the maxillary, frontal, and sphenoid sinuses and ethmoid air cells—and drain into, the nasal cavity via ostia. The sinuses are lined by mucous membrane. Only the maxillary sinuses are visualized on periapical radiographs. CBCT scans encompass the sinuses to different extents depending on the FOV and the region being imaged. Limited- and medium-FOV CBCT imaging of the posterior maxillary arch will image some portion of the maxillary sinuses, and often the ethmoid air cells. Full-FOV CBCT scans will encompass all paranasal sinuses. The intricate anatomy of the sinus boundaries and its drainage routes into the nasal cavity are the basis of radiologic sinus evaluation.

Maxillary Sinus

The maxillary sinus develops by the invagination of mucous membrane from the nasal cavity. The largest of the paranasal sinuses, it normally occupies virtually the entire body of the maxilla. Its function is unknown. The maxillary sinus may be considered as a three-sided pyramid, with

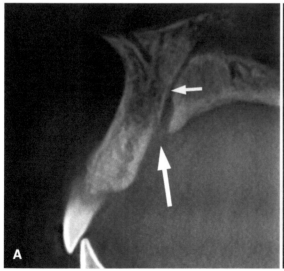
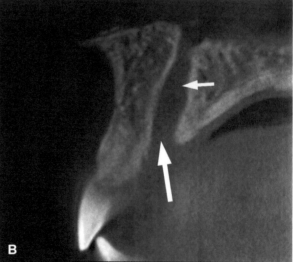

Fig. 12.31 (A) and (B) Sagittal cone beam computed tomography sections through the midsagittal plane showing the course of the nasopalatine canal *(yellow arrow)* and the opening of the incisive foramen *(white arrow)*. Note the range of normal variation in the size of these structures.

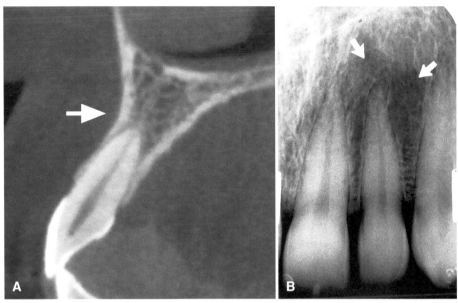

Fig. 12.32 (A) Cone beam computed tomography section through the long axis of a maxillary lateral incisor showing the lateral fossa as a depression on the buccal surface *(arrow)*. (B) The lateral fossa is a diffuse radiolucency *(arrows)* in the region of the apex of the lateral incisor.

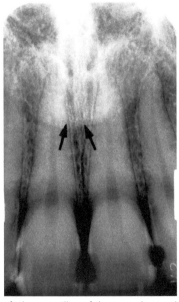

Fig. 12.33 The soft tissue outline of the nose *(arrows)* is superimposed on the anterior maxilla.

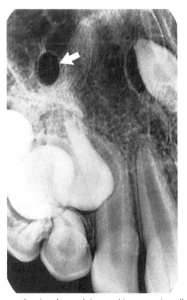

Fig. 12.34 The nasolacrimal canal *(arrow)* is occasionally seen near the apex of the canine when steep vertical angulation is used. Note the mesiodens (supernumerary tooth) in the midline superior to the central incisor.

its base the medial wall adjacent to the nasal cavity and its apex extending laterally into the zygomatic process of the maxilla. Its three sides are (1) the superior wall forming the floor of the orbit, (2) the anterior wall extending above the premolars, and (3) the posterior wall bulging above the molar teeth and maxillary tuberosity. The sinus communicates with the nasal cavity by the ostium, approximately 3 to 6 mm in diameter and positioned under the posterior aspect of the middle concha of the ethmoid bone (see Plates 12.2, 12.4, 12.5, and 12.7).

Periapical radiographs show the inferior portion of the maxillary sinus. The maxillary sinus floor is a thin layer of cortical bone and appears as a thin radiopaque line (Fig. 12.36). In adults, the sinuses are

usually seen to extend from the distal aspect of the canine to the posterior wall of the maxilla above the tuberosity. In the absence of disease, it appears continuous, but on close examination it can be seen to have small interruptions in its continuity or radiodensity. When viewed on periapical radiographs, these discontinuities are probably illusions caused by superimposition of small marrow spaces.

The maxillary sinuses show considerable variation in size. They enlarge during childhood, achieving mature size by age 15 to 18 years. They may change during adult life in response to environmental factors. The right and left sinuses usually appear similar in shape and size, although marked asymmetry is occasionally present. The floors of the

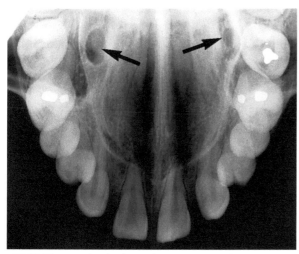

Fig. 12.35 The nasolacrimal canals are commonly seen as ovoid radiolucencies *(arrows)* on maxillary occlusal projections. They should not be confused with the greater palatine foramina, which are not apparent on maxillary occlusal projections.

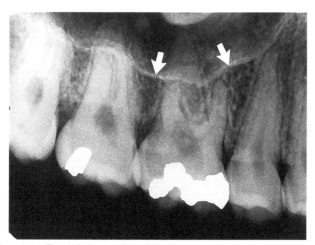

Fig. 12.36 The inferior border of the maxillary sinus *(arrows)* appears as a thin radiopaque line near the apices of the maxillary premolars and molars.

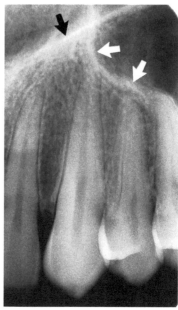

Fig. 12.37 The anterior border of the maxillary sinus *(white arrows)* crosses the floor of the nasal fossa *(black arrow)*.

BOX 12.5 Relationship Between Teeth and the Maxillary Sinus

The close relationship between the maxillary sinus and teeth leads to the possibility that clinical symptoms originating in the sinus may be perceived in the teeth and vice versa.

- Canals that carry the superior alveolar nerves traverse the anterolateral and posterolateral walls of the sinus (Fig. 12.40). The nerves are in intimate contact with the membrane lining the sinus. As a result, an acute inflammation of the sinus is frequently accompanied by pain in the maxillary teeth innervated by the portion of the nerve proximal to the area of sinus inflammation. Careful clinical evaluation of the maxillary posterior teeth to rule out dental disease is important to differentiate true odontogenic pain from sinus-related pain.
- Occasionally periapical and periodontal inflammation from the maxillary molar teeth may extend to cause inflammation of the maxillary sinus mucosa, referred to as odontogenic maxillary sinusitis (see Chapter 28). Unlike chronic rhinosinusitis, odontogenic maxillary sinusitis is usually unilateral. Approximately 10% of maxillary sinusitis is due to odontogenic causes.

---

maxillary sinus and nasal cavity are seen on periapical radiographs at approximately the same level around the age of puberty. In older individuals, the sinus may extend farther into the alveolar process; in the posterior region of the maxilla, its floor may appear considerably below the level of the floor of the nasal cavity. Anteriorly, each sinus is restricted by the canine fossa and is usually seen to sweep superiorly, crossing the level of the floor of the nasal cavity in the premolar or canine region. Consequently, on periapical radiographs of the canine, the floors of the sinus and nasal cavity are superimposed and seen crossing one another, forming an inverted "Y" in the area (Fig. 12.37).

The degree of extension of the maxillary sinus into the alveolar process is extremely variable. In some periapical projections, the floor of the sinus is well above the apices of the posterior teeth; in others, it may extend well beyond the apices toward the alveolar ridge. In response to a loss of function (associated with the loss of posterior teeth), the sinus may expand farther into the alveolar bone, occasionally extending to the alveolar ridge (Fig. 12.38). The roots of the molars usually lie in close apposition to the maxillary sinus. Root apices may project

anatomically into the floor of the sinus, causing small elevations or prominences along the maxillary sinus floor. Periapical images may convey the impression that the roots project into the sinus cavity, which is an illusion. The intimate relationship between the tooth roots and the maxillary sinus is evaluated better with CBCT (Fig. 12.39), and this is the modality of choice when critical evaluation of the maxillary sinus floor is clinically indicated. The thin layer of bone covering the root is seen as a fusion of the lamina dura and the floor of the sinus. Rarely, defects may be present in the bony covering of the root apices in the sinus floor, and the apical lamina dura may be indistinct. Due to this close relationship, manifestations of odontogenic disease and maxillary sinus disease is often diagnostically challenging (Box 12.5).

Frequently, thin radiolucent lines of uniform width are found within the periapical image of the maxillary sinus (see Fig. 12.40). These are the shadows of neurovascular canals or grooves in the lateral sinus walls

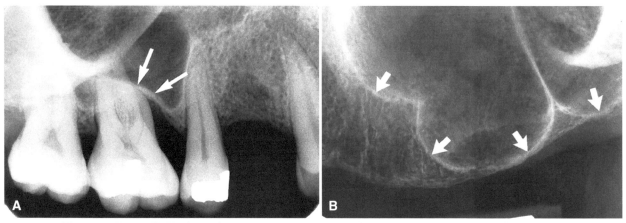

Fig. 12.38 (A) and (B) The floor of the maxillary sinus *(arrows)* often extends toward the crest of the alveolar ridge in response to missing teeth.

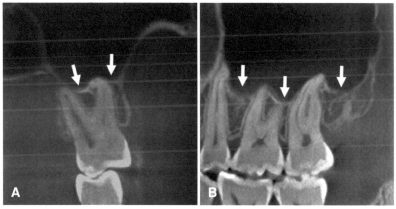

Fig. 12.39 Coronal (A) and sagittal (B) cone beam computed tomography sections through the maxillary posterior region demonstrating the relationship between the teeth and the maxillary sinus floor *(arrows)*. The corticated border of the sinus dips in between the tooth roots. Dilaceration of the mesiobuccal root of the maxillary molar is depicted on the coronal image.

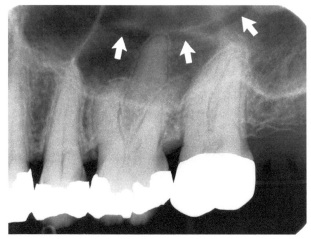

Fig. 12.40 Neurovascular canals *(arrows)* in the lateral wall of the maxillary sinus. Such vascular canals, although typically less prominent, are commonly seen in the walls of the normal maxillary sinus.

that accommodate the posterior superior alveolar vessels, their branches, and the accompanying superior alveolar nerves. Although they may be found coursing in any direction (including vertically), they are usually seen running a curved posteroanterior course that is convex toward the alveolar process.

Often one or several radiopaque lines traverse the image of the maxillary sinus (Fig. 12.41). These opaque lines are called septa. They are thin folds of cortical bone that project a few millimeters away from the floor and wall of the antrum, or they may extend across the sinus. They are usually oriented vertically and vary in number, thickness, and length. Although septa appear to separate the sinuses into distinct compartments, this is seldom the case. Rather, the septa typically extend only a few millimeters into the central volume of the sinus. Septa warrant attention because they sometimes mimic periapical disease, and the chambers they create in the alveolar recess may complicate the search for a root fragment displaced into the sinus. In these clinical situations, CBCT is the modality of choice in performing this anatomic evaluation.

The floor of the maxillary sinus occasionally shows small radiopaque projections, which are nodules of bone (Fig. 12.42). These must be differentiated from root tips, which they resemble in shape. In contrast to a root fragment, which is quite homogeneous in appearance, the bony nodules often show trabeculation; although they may be quite well defined, at certain points on their surface they blend with the trabecular pattern of adjacent bone. A root fragment may also be recognized by the presence of a root canal.

On periapical radiographs, it is common to see the floor of the nasal fossa in periapical views of the posterior teeth superimposed on the maxillary sinus (see Fig. 12.27). The floor of the nasal fossa is usually oriented more or less horizontally, depending on film placement, and

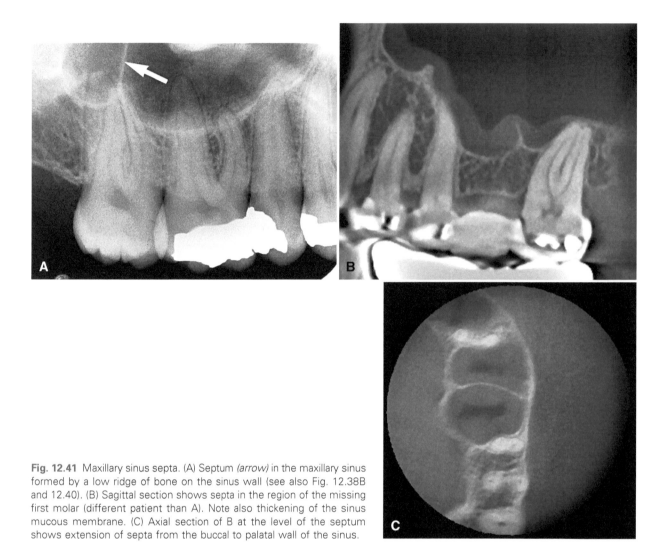

Fig. 12.41 Maxillary sinus septa. (A) Septum *(arrow)* in the maxillary sinus formed by a low ridge of bone on the sinus wall (see also Fig. 12.38B and 12.40). (B) Sagittal section shows septa in the region of the missing first molar (different patient than A). Note also thickening of the sinus mucous membrane. (C) Axial section of B at the level of the septum shows extension of septa from the buccal to palatal wall of the sinus.

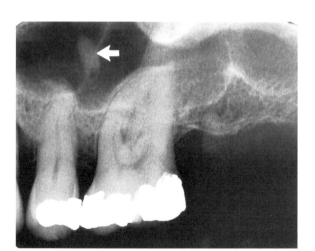

Fig. 12.42 This bony mass *(arrow)* may represent a bony nodule, a normal variant of the floor of the maxillary sinus, but is most likely a retained root fragment from a prior extraction.

is superimposed high on maxillary views. The image, a solid opaque line, frequently appears thicker than the adjacent sinus walls and septa.

Ethmoid, Sphenoid, and Frontal Sinuses

The ethmoid, sphenoid, and frontal sinuses are not in the imaging field for periapical radiography. However, these sinuses are well visualized on CBCT scans and on panoramic and cephalometric radiographs. When the paranasal sinuses are imaged on CBCT scans, the anatomic boundaries and drainage patterns of the sinus must be systematically examined (Box 12.6).

The ethmoidal sinuses are divided into the anterior and posterior ethmoidal air cells, and the number of air cells per side ranges from 3 to 18. Frequently extramural air cells—air cells outside of the ethmoid bone—can be visualized. These include agger nasi air cells, causing pneumatization of the lacrimal bone, and Haller cells, which cause pneumatization of the orbital floor. Occasionally Haller cells are seen on panoramic images (see Chapter 9).

The sphenoid sinuses are midline structures in the body of the sphenoid bone and start to develop at approximately 4 months in utero. The sinuses vary considerably in size, and the right and left sphenoid sinuses are often asymmetric and separated by a bony septum. Often multiple septa are present, giving the sinus a "locular" appearance. The sphenoid sinuses may extend inferiorly, resulting in pneumatization of

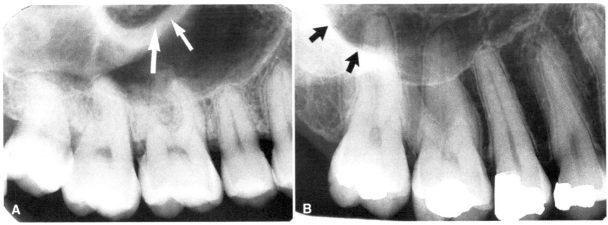

Fig. 12.43 The zygomatic process of the maxilla *(arrows)* protrudes laterally from the maxillary wall. Its size may be quite variable: small with thick borders (A) or large with thin borders (B).

BOX 12.6 Systematic Evaluation of Paranasal Sinuses on Computed Tomography Scans

In a normal paranasal sinus, the epithelial lining is relatively thin and barely visible on radiographs. Thus the sinuses appear radiolucent, with a well-corticated bony outline. Inflammatory and neoplastic changes in the sinus lining appear as a soft tissue density contrasted against the air-filled cavity. Sinuses are evaluated for the presence of soft tissue thickening, the integrity of the borders, and the patency of the drainage paths of the paranasal sinuses. Evaluation of the paranasal sinuses should include a critical examination of the following anatomic structures:

- *Osteomeatal complex:* The maxillary sinus drains via the ostium into the infundibulum—a channel between the uncinate process of the ethmoid bone and the inferomedial wall of the orbit (see Plates 12.1, 12.2, 12.4, and 12.5). The infundibulum channels drain into the hiatus semilunaris (see Plate 12.4) and then into the middle meatus. The complex of the maxillary ostium, infundibulum, uncinate process, hiatus semilunaris, ethmoidal bulla, and middle meatus is referred to as the osteomeatal complex. This region is the common drainage path for the frontal and maxillary sinuses and anterior ethmoidal air cells and thus must be carefully inspected for patency. This complex is best visualized on the coronal and axial sections.
- *Frontal recess:* This is the path for the drainage of the frontal sinus into the middle meatus. This recess is best visualized on sagittal and coronal sections (see Plate 12.4).
- *Sphenoethmoidal recess:* This is the drainage path for the sphenoid sinus and posterior ethmoidal air cells in the superior meatus at the posterior region of the nasal cavity. This recess is located between the posterior ethmoidal cells and the sphenoid sinus (see Plate 12.1). It is best appreciated in axial and sagittal sections.

the pterygoid bones. The sphenoid sinuses are not visualized on periapical images but are well demonstrated on CBCT scans and on lateral cephalometric radiographs (see Chapter 8).

The frontal sinuses are the last paranasal sinuses to develop, usually starting at approximately 6 to 7 years of age. Hypoplasia of the frontal sinus is a common normal variant, and aplasia of the frontal sinuses is noted in approximately 4% of the population. The frontal sinuses are well demonstrated on CBCT scans and on cephalometric radiographs (see Chapter 8).

Zygomatic Process and Zygoma

The zygomatic process of the maxilla is an extension of the lateral maxillary surface that arises in the region of the apices of the first and second molars and articulates with the maxillary process of the zygoma. On periapical radiographs, the zygomatic process appears as a U-shaped radiopaque line with its open end directed superiorly. The enclosed rounded end is projected in the apical region of the first and second molars (Fig. 12.43). The size, width, and definition of the zygomatic process are quite variable, and its image may be large, depending on the angle at which the beam was projected. The maxillary antrum may expand laterally into the zygomatic process of the maxilla (and into the zygomatic bone after the maxillozygomatic suture has fused), resulting in a relatively increased radiolucent region within the U-shaped image of the process.

When the sinus is recessed deep within the process, as in Fig. 12.43B (and perhaps into the zygoma), the image of the air space within the process is dark. Typically the walls of the process are thin and well defined (in contrast to the very dark radiolucent air space). When the sinus exhibits relatively little penetration of the maxillary process, as in Fig. 12.43A (usually in younger individuals or individuals who have maintained their posterior teeth and vigorous masticatory function), the image of the walls of the zygomatic process of the maxilla tends to be thicker, and the appearance of the sinus in this region is smaller and more opaque.

The inferior border of the zygoma extends posteriorly from the inferior border of the zygomatic process of the maxilla to the zygomatic process of the temporal bone. It can be identified as a uniform radiopacity over the apices of the molars (Fig. 12.44). The zygomatic process of the temporal bone and the body of the zygoma compose the zygomatic arch. The prominence of the molar apices superimposed on the shadow of the zygoma and the amount of periapical detail supplied by the radiograph depend primarily on the extent of aeration (pneumatization) of the zygoma by the maxillary sinus and on the orientation of the x-ray beam.

The zygomatic processes of the maxilla articulate posteriorly with the maxillary process of the zygoma. These two processes form the anterior segment of the zygomatic arch (see Plates 12.2 and 12.5). The zygomaticomaxillary suture is visualized as a thin, radiolucent, jagged

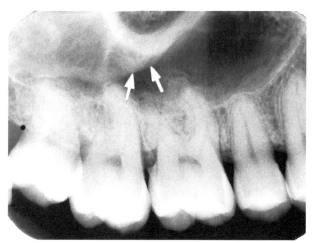

Fig. 12.44 The inferior border of the zygoma *(arrows)* extends posteriorly from the inferior portion of the zygomatic process of the maxilla.

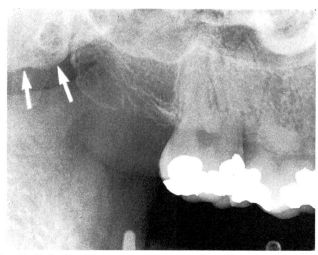

Fig. 12.46 Pterygoid plates *(arrows)* located posterior to the maxillary tuberosity.

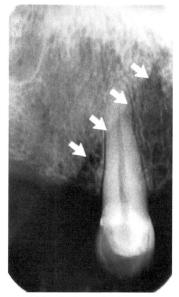

Fig. 12.45 The nasolabial soft tissue fold *(arrows)* extends across the canine-premolar region.

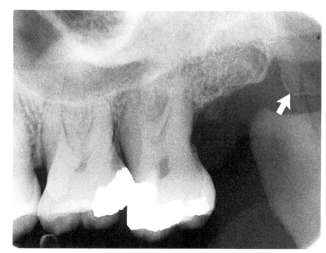

Fig. 12.47 The hamular process *(arrow)* extends inferiorly from the medial pterygoid plate.

line in this portion of the arch. Disruptions of the integrity or symmetry of the arch may be associated with craniofacial developmental abnormalities or facial trauma.

Nasolabial Fold

An oblique line demarcating a region that appears to be covered by a veil of slight radiopacity frequently traverses periapical radiographs of the premolar region (Fig. 12.45). The line of contrast is sharp, and the area of increased radiopacity is posterior to the line. The line is the nasolabial fold, and the opaque veil is the thick cheek tissue superimposed on the teeth and the alveolar process. The image of the fold becomes more evident with age, as the repeated creasing of the skin along the line (where the elevator of the lip, zygomatic head, and orbicularis all insert into the skin) and the degeneration of the elastic fibers finally lead to the formation and deepening of permanent folds. This radiographic feature frequently proves useful in identifying the side of the maxilla represented by a film of the area if it is edentulous and few other anatomic features are demonstrated.

Pterygoid Plates

The medial and lateral pterygoid plates lie immediately posterior to the maxilla. These structures are best visualized on coronal and axial CT sections (see Plates 12.2 and 12.5) and must be carefully evaluated when assessing a patient with facial trauma. Involvement of the pterygoid plates is an essential feature of Le Fort fractures (see Chapter 27). The images on these two plates are extremely variable, and they do not appear at all on many intraoral radiographs of the third molar area. When they are apparent, they almost always cast a single radiopaque homogeneous shadow without any evidence of trabeculation (Fig. 12.46). Extending inferiorly from the medial pterygoid plate is the hamular process (Fig. 12.47), which on close inspection can show trabeculae.

MANDIBLE

Symphysis

Radiographs of the region of the mandibular symphysis in infants demonstrate a radiolucent line through the midline of the jaw between the images of the forming deciduous central incisors (Fig. 12.48). This suture usually fuses by the end of the first year of life, after which it is no longer radiographically apparent. It is not frequently encountered

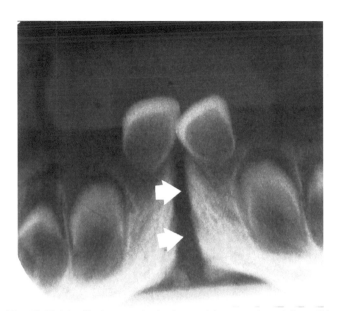

Fig. 12.48 Mandibular symphysis *(arrows)* in a newborn infant. This suture closed within the first year. Note the erupted bilateral supernumerary primary incisors.

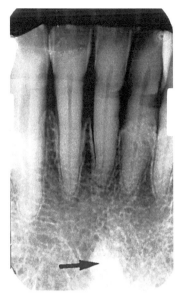

Fig. 12.50 The genial tubercles *(arrow)* appear as a radiopaque mass, in this case without evidence of the lingual foramen.

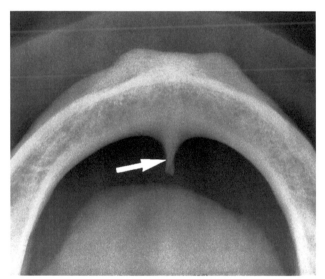

Fig. 12.49 Genial tubercle *(arrow)* on the lingual surface of the mandible in this cross-sectional mandibular occlusal view. This tubercle is unusually prominent.

on dental radiographs because few young patients have cause to be examined radiographically. If this radiolucency is found in older individuals, it is abnormal and may suggest a fracture or a cleft.

Genial Tubercles

The genial tubercles (also called the mental spine) are located on the lingual surface of the mandible slightly above the inferior border and in the midline. They are bony protuberances, more or less spine-shaped, that are often divided into a right and left prominence and a superior and inferior prominence. They attach the genioglossus muscles (at the superior tubercles) and the geniohyoid muscles (at the inferior tubercles) to the mandible. They are well visualized on mandibular occlusal radiographs as one or more small projections (Fig. 12.49). Their appearance on periapical radiographs of the mandibular incisor region is variable; often they appear as a radiopaque mass (3 to 4 mm in diameter)

in the midline below the incisor roots (Fig. 12.50). They may also not be apparent at all.

Lingual Foramen

Midline lingual foramina are present in 96% to 100% of individuals, located in the region of the genial tubercles (see Plate 12.8B). The superior foramen contains a neurovascular bundle from the lingual arteries and nerve, whereas the inferior foramen is supplied from the sublingual or submental arteries and from the mylohyoid nerve. On periapical radiographs, the lingual foramen (Fig. 12.51) is typically visualized as a single round radiolucent canal with a well-defined opaque border lying in the midline below the level of the apices of the incisors.

The anatomic location is essential in presurgical treatment planning because damage to the neurovascular bundle in the course of implant bed preparation, for example, may lead to excessive bleeding.

Mental Ridge

On periapical radiographs of the mandibular central incisors, the mental ridge (protuberance) may occasionally be seen as two radiopaque lines sweeping bilaterally forward and upward toward the midline (Fig. 12.52). They are of variable width and density and may be found to extend from low in the premolar area on each side up to the midline, where they lie just inferior to or are superimposed on the mandibular incisor tooth roots. The image of the mental ridge is most prominent when the beam is directed parallel with the surface of the mental tubercle (as in using the bisecting-angle technique).

Mental Fossa

The mental fossa is a depression on the labial aspect of the mandible extending laterally from the midline and above the mental ridge. Because of the resulting thinness of jawbone in this area, the image of this depression may be similar to that of the submandibular fossa (see later) and likewise may be mistaken for periapical disease involving the incisors (Fig. 12.53).

Mental Foramen

The mental foramen is usually the anterior limit of the inferior dental canal that is apparent on periapical radiographs (Fig. 12.54). Its image

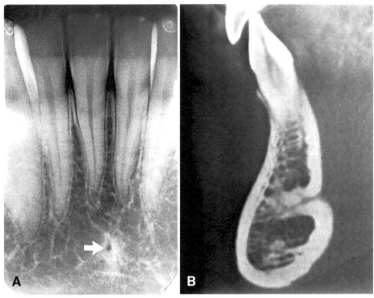

Fig. 12.51 Lingual foramen. (A) Lingual foramen on a periapical view *(arrow)*, with a sclerotic border, in the symphyseal region of the mandible. (B) Cone beam sagittal section through mandibular midline shows superior lingual foramen extending deep into the mandible from the lingual surface.

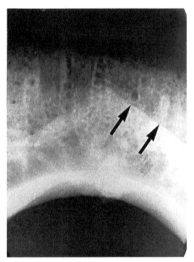

Fig. 12.52 Mental ridge *(arrows)* on the anterior surface of the mandible, seen as a radiopaque ridge. The mental ridge is most prominent when the beam is angled from well below the occlusal plane.

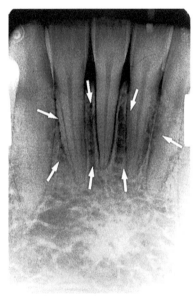

Fig. 12.53 The mental fossa is a depression on the anterior surface of the mandible and is seen as a radiolucent area with ill-defined borders *(arrows)* in the region of the incisor roots.

is quite variable, and it may be identified on periapical radiographs only about half the time because the opening of the mental canal is directed superiorly and posteriorly. As a result, the usual view of the premolars is not projected through the long axis of the canal opening. This circumstance is responsible for the variable appearance of the mental foramen. Although the wall of the foramen consists of cortical bone, the density of the image of the foramen varies, as does the shape and definition of its border. It may be round, oblong, slit-like, or very irregular and partially or completely corticated. The foramen is seen about halfway between the lower border of the mandible and the crest of the alveolar process, usually in the region of the apex of the second premolar. Also, because it lies on the surface of the mandible, the position of its image in relation to the tooth roots is influenced by projection angulation. It may be projected anywhere from just mesial of the permanent first molar roots to as far anterior as mesial of the first premolar root.

The location and size of the mental foramen is better evaluated on CT sections (Fig. 12.55 and Plate 12.3). When visualization of the mental foramen is critical to the treatment plan, as in implant placement, CBCT is the modality of choice. An important anatomic variation to detect when placing implants in the premolar region is the anterior loop, where the inferior alveolar canal extends anterior to the mental foramen before it loops posteriorly to exit through the mental foramen. The incidence of an accessory mental foramen is about 7%.

When the mental foramen is projected over one of the premolar apices, it may mimic periapical disease (Fig. 12.56). In such cases evidence of the inferior alveolar canal extending to the suspect radiolucency or a detectable lamina dura in the area would suggest the true nature of the dark shadow. However, the relative thinness of the lamina dura superimposed with the radiolucent foramen may result in considerable "burnout" of the lamina dura image, which complicates its recognition. Nevertheless, a second radiograph from another angle is likely to show the lamina dura clearly as well as some shift in position of the radiolucent foramen relative to the apex.

Inferior Alveolar Canal

The radiographic image of the inferior alveolar canal is a dark linear shadow with thin radiopaque superior and inferior borders cast by the lamella of bone that bounds the canal (Fig. 12.57). Sometimes the borders are seen only partially or not at all. The width of the canal shows some interpatient variability but is usually constant anterior to the third molar region. The canal's course may be apparent between the mandibular and mental foramina. Only rarely is the image of its anterior continuation toward the midline discernible on the radiograph.

The relationship of the inferior alveolar canal to the roots of the lower teeth may vary from one in which there is close contact with all molars and the second premolar to one in which the canal has no intimate relationship to any of the posterior teeth. In the usual picture, however, the canal is in contact with the apex of the third molar, and the distance between it and the other roots increases as it progresses anteriorly. When the apices of the molars are projected over the canal, the lamina dura may be overexposed, conveying the impression of a missing lamina or a thickened PDL space that is more radiolucent than apparently normal for the patient (Fig. 12.58). To ensure the soundness

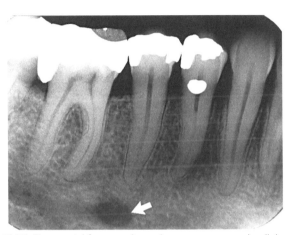

Fig. 12.54 The mental foramen *(arrow)* appears as an oval radiolucency typically near the apex of the second premolar.

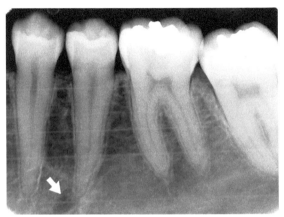

Fig. 12.56 The mental foramen *(arrow)* (over the apex of the second premolar) may simulate periapical disease. However, continuity of the lamina dura around the apex indicates the absence of periapical abnormality.

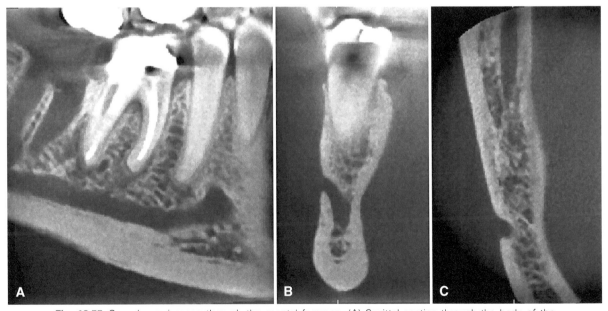

Fig. 12.55 Cone beam images through the mental foramen. (A) Sagittal section through the body of the mandible shows the inferior alveolar canal rising toward the mental foramen, which lies anterior to the apex of the second premolar. (B) Coronal section through the mental foramen shows how the inferior alveolar canal ascends to exit through the buccal cortex at the mental foramen. A clear understanding of this anatomy is important when implants are placed in this region. (C) Axial section through the mental foramen demonstrates posterior inclination of the opening of the mental foramen on the mandibular buccal surface. Note also the section of the inferior alveolar canal lying more posteriorly, inferior to the molars, and adjacent to the lingual cortex *(top of image).*

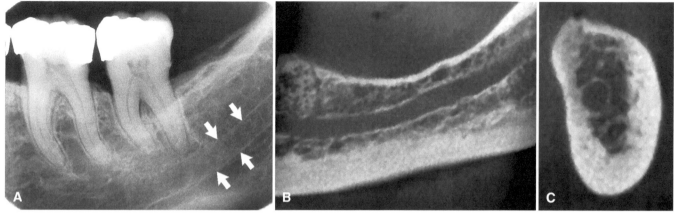

Fig. 12.57 Inferior alveolar canal. (A) On periapical view, *arrows* denote radiopaque superior and inferior cortical borders. (B) Cone beam section through the body of the mandible (different patient) shows corticated borders of the inferior alveolar canal. (C) Cone beam cross-sectional view shows the circular inferior alveolar canal with corticated borders lying adjacent to the lingual plate.

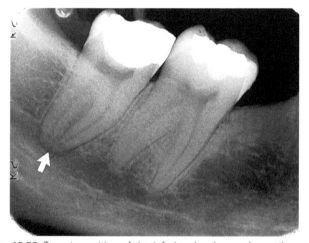

Fig. 12.58 Superimposition of the inferior alveolar canal over the apex of a molar causes the image of the periodontal ligament space to appear wider *(arrow)*. However, the presence of an intact lamina dura indicates that there is no periapical disease.

of such a tooth, other clinical testing procedures must be used (e.g., vitality testing). Because the canal is usually located just inferior to the apices of the posterior teeth, altering the vertical angle for a second periapical radiograph of the area is not likely to separate the images of the apices and canal.

The course of the inferior alveolar canal is well demonstrated on CT scans (Fig. 12.59 and Plate 12.8C and F). In cross-sectional and coronal slices, the inferior alveolar canal is typically seen as an oval or round radiolucency with corticated borders (see Fig. 12.59). Sometimes the cortication may be thin or imperceptible. The relationship of the canal to the tooth roots should be assessed. This relationship varies greatly among patients, especially in the molar region, with the inferior alveolar canal occupying a position from close to the root apices to adjacent to the inferior border of the mandible. Other variations include bifid inferior alveolar canal with a reported frequency of about 15%; these can be seen on panoramic and cone beam images (see Fig. 12.59). Patients with bifid canals are at greater risk of inadequate anesthesia or surgical complications, for example, from implant placement.

Nutrient Canals

Nutrient canals carry a neurovascular bundle and appear as radiolucent lines of fairly uniform width. They are most often seen on mandibular periapical radiographs running vertically from the inferior dental canal directly to the apex of a tooth (Fig. 12.60) or into the interdental space between the mandibular incisors (Fig. 12.61). They are visible in about 5% to 40% of all patients and are more frequent in black patients, male patients, older patients, and patients with high blood pressure, diabetes mellitus, or advanced periodontal disease. They may be accentuated in a thin ridge. Because they are anatomic spaces with walls of cortical bone, their images occasionally have hyperostotic borders. Sometimes a nutrient canal is oriented perpendicular to the cortex and appears as a small round radiolucency simulating a pathologic radiolucency.

Mylohyoid Ridge

The mylohyoid ridge (also called the internal oblique ridge) is a slightly irregular crest of bone on the lingual surface of the mandibular body. Its anterior margin lies about 10 mm inferior to the alveolar ridge lingual to the second premolar and extends posteriorly to the area of the third molar about 5 mm below the alveolar crest. This ridge serves as an attachment for the mylohyoid muscle. On a periapical radiograph, its image runs diagonally downward and forward from the area of the third molars to the premolar region at approximately the level of the apices of the posterior teeth (Fig. 12.62). This image is sometimes superimposed on the images of the molar roots. The margins of the image are not usually well defined but appear quite diffuse and of variable width. Occasionally, the ridge is relatively dense with sharply demarcated borders (Fig. 12.63). It is more evident on periapical radiographs when the beam is positioned with excessive negative angulation. Generally, as the ridge becomes less defined, its anterior and posterior limits blend gradually with the surrounding bone.

Submandibular Gland Fossa

On the lingual surface of the mandibular body, immediately below the mylohyoid ridge in the molar area, there is frequently a depression in the bone. This concavity accommodates the submandibular gland and often appears as a radiolucent area with the sparse trabecular pattern characteristic of the region (Fig. 12.64). This trabecular pattern is even less defined on periapical and panoramic radiographs of the area because it is superimposed on the relatively reduced mass of the concavity. The

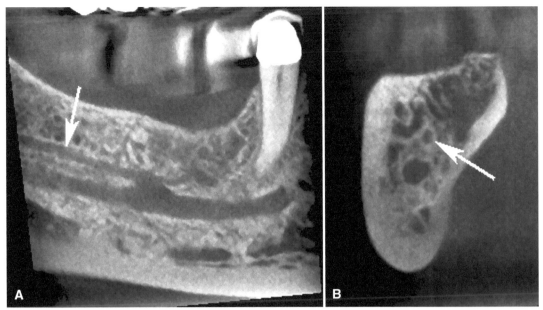

Fig. 12.59 Bifid inferior alveolar canal. (A) Cone beam sagittal section through the body of the mandible shows a bifid inferior alveolar canal. The superior branch has a smaller diameter than the primary canal *(arrow)*. (B) Cross-sectional image shows primary canal and superior secondary canal *(arrow)*.

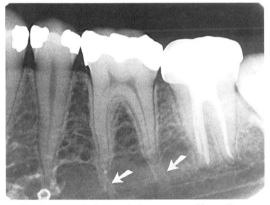

Fig. 12.60 Nutrient canals *(arrows)*, demonstrated by radiopaque cortical borders, descend from the mandibular first molar. Nutrient canals at this location are a common finding.

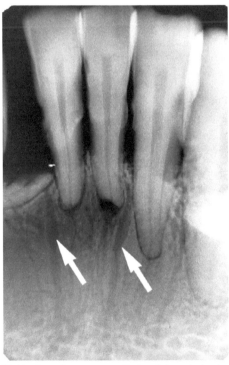

Fig. 12.61 Nutrient canals seen as vertical radiolucent structures *(arrows)* in the anterior mandible are often associated with periodontal disease as in this patient.

radiographic image of the fossa is sharply limited superiorly by the mylohyoid ridge and inferiorly by the lower border of the mandible but is poorly defined anteriorly (in the premolar region) and posteriorly (at about the ascending ramus). Although the image may appear strikingly radiolucent, accentuated as it is by the dense mylohyoid ridge and inferior border of the mandible, awareness of its possible presence should preclude its being confused with a bony lesion by inexperienced clinicians.

CBCT scans allow assessment of the submandibular fossa region in the coronal and axial planes. The extent and depth of this concavity, or undercut, varies greatly (see Plate 12.8D). The identification of this anatomic feature is crucial in examining mandibular anatomy for implant treatment planning.

External Oblique Ridge

The external oblique ridge is a continuation of the anterior border of the mandibular ramus. It follows an anteroinferior course lateral to the alveolar process and is relatively prominent in its upper part; it juts considerably on the outer surface of the mandible in the region of the

third molar (Fig. 12.65). This bony elevation gradually flattens and usually disappears at about where the alveolar process and mandible join below the first molar. The ridge is a line of attachment of the buccinator muscle. Characteristically it is projected onto posterior periapical radiographs superior to the mylohyoid ridge, with which it runs an almost parallel course. It appears as a radiopaque line of varying

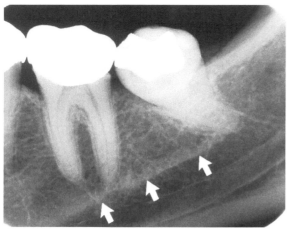

Fig. 12.62 Mylohyoid ridge *(arrows)* running at the level of the molar apices and above the inferior alveolar canal.

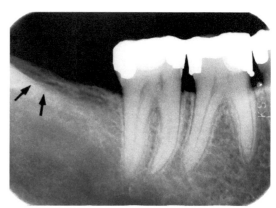

Fig. 12.65 External oblique ridge *(arrows)* on the buccal surface of the mandible, seen as a radiopaque line near the alveolar crest in the mandibular third molar region.

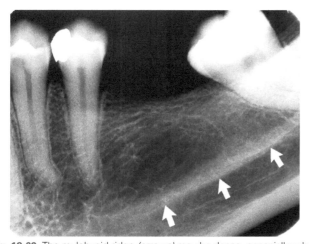

Fig. 12.63 The mylohyoid ridge *(arrows)* may be dense, especially when a radiograph is exposed with excessive negative angulation.

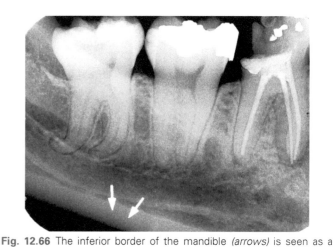

Fig. 12.66 The inferior border of the mandible *(arrows)* is seen as a dense, broad radiopaque band.

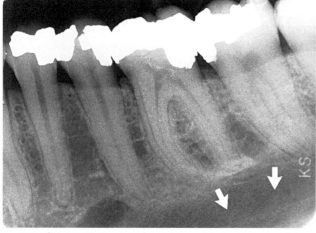

Fig. 12.64 Submandibular gland fossa *(arrows)*, indicated by a radiolucent region with ill-defined borders and sparse trabecular bone lying inferiorly to the mandibular molars.

width, density, and length, blending at its anterior end with the shadow of the alveolar bone.

Inferior Border of the Mandible

Occasionally the inferior mandibular border is seen on periapical projections (Fig. 12.66) as a characteristically dense, broad, radiopaque band of bone.

Coronoid Process

The image of the coronoid process of the mandible is frequently apparent on periapical radiographs of the maxillary molar region as a triangular radiopacity, with its apex directed superiorly and anteriorly, superimposed on the region of the third molar (Fig. 12.67). In some cases it may appear as far forward as the second molar and be projected above, over, or below these molars, depending on the position of the jaw and the projection of the x-ray beam. Usually the shadow of the coronoid process is homogeneous, although internal trabeculation can be seen in some cases. Its appearance on maxillary molar radiographs results from the downward and forward movement of the mandible when the mouth is open. Consequently, if the opacity reduces the diagnostic value of the image, the radiograph must be remade, and the second view should be acquired with the mouth minimally open. (This contingency must

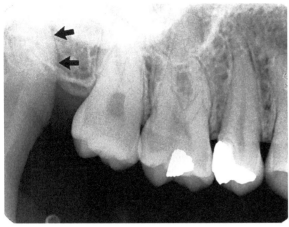

Fig. 12.67 Coronoid process of the mandible *(arrows)* superimposed on the maxillary tuberosity.

be considered whenever this area is radiographically examined.) Occasionally, especially when its shadow is dense and homogeneous, the coronoid process is mistaken for a root fragment. The true nature of the shadow can be easily demonstrated by obtaining two radiographs with the mouth in different positions and noting the change in position of the suspect shadow.

The coronoid process is viewed free of superimposition on CT images (see Plates 12.2 and 12.5). When the primary diagnostic task is evaluation of the coronoid process—for example, to assess coronoid hyperplasia—CT imaging, preferably CBCT, should be the modality of choice.

TEMPOROMANDIBULAR JOINT

The temporomandibular joint (TMJ) region is imaged on panoramic, cephalometric, and CBCT imaging. The TMJ is the articulation between the glenoid fossa of the temporal bone and the condyle of the mandible. The glenoid fossa is a concave depression located in the squamous portion of the temporal bone (see Plates 12.6 and 12.7). It is bordered anteriorly by the articular eminence and posteriorly by the squamo-tympanic and petrotympanic fissures. The articular eminence is usually described as a posterior slope, adjacent to the fossa, and the crest, which is the inferiormost tip of the eminence. The condyle is typically ellipsoid and is longer in the mediolateral dimension than in the anteroposterior dimension. The condyle is angulated with the medial pole being positioned posterior to the lateral pole, typically forming an angle of 15 to 30 degrees with the sagittal plane. When viewing sections through the TMJ, it is useful to make custom reconstructions through the axial long axis of the condylar head. The resulting oblique sections are referred to as "corrected" sagittal and frontal sections (Fig. 12.68).

- In the sagittal view, the fossa and eminence form an inverted "S" shape, characteristically seen as a smooth radiopaque line (see Fig. 12.68B). The angle of the posterior slope of the eminence can vary considerably and is typically 30 to 60 degrees to the Frankfort plane. Anatomic variation that forms a steep eminence (angle >60 degrees) is suggested to predispose to TMJ internal derangements.
- The superior surface of the condylar head is usually rounded or convex (see Fig. 12.68C), but anatomic variations, such as slight flattening or marked convexity, are frequently observed. The size and shape of the right and left condylar heads should be compared. When an asymmetry is observed, the symmetry of the entire mandible should be assessed, including the intercuspation of the teeth and any deviation of the mandible on opening.

- In adults, the articular surfaces of the condyle, glenoid fossa, and articular eminence have a corticated border. Pathologic conditions, such as osteoarthritis, often cause a thinning or loss of this normal cortication. However, this corticated border is not visualized during periods of condylar growth and thus is not seen until approximately age 18 years.
- With the teeth in maximal intercuspation, the condyle is normally seated concentrically within the glenoid fossa. Although considerable deviation from this position is observed in radiographs of asymptomatic individuals, the condyle is frequently retruded in individuals with TMJ dysfunction.

BASE OF THE SKULL

A full- and often medium-FOV CBCT scan encompasses the region of the skull base; the anatomy of this region is best evaluated on axial and coronal sections. To facilitate viewing, it is useful to orient the CBCT volume to the Frankfort plane, with the axial slices parallel to this plane and coronal slices perpendicular to it. Five bones form the skull base: ethmoid, sphenoid, occipital, frontal (paired), and temporal (paired).

The entire cranial base is evaluated for symmetry, integrity, and continuity. For example, infections or neoplasms may extend from the ethmoid air cells into the cranial fossa through the cribriform plate, disrupting this anatomic structure. Furthermore, it is important to be familiar with the various foramina and canals in the skull base.

The anterior cranial base is formed by the frontal bones (laterally), the cribriform plate and crista galli of the ethmoid bone (medially), and the lesser wing of the sphenoid bone (posteriorly). These bones also contribute to the roof of the nasal cavity, ethmoid air cells, and orbits. The anterior cranial base is best visualized on coronal and sagittal sections (see Plates 12.4, 12.5, and 12.7).

The middle cranial base is formed by the body and greater wings of the sphenoid bone and the petrous and squamous portions of the temporal bones; it overlies the sphenoid sinuses and the mastoid air cells, middle and inner ears, and infratemporal fossae (see Plates 12.5–12.7). The sella turcica is a depression in the body of the sphenoid that contains the pituitary gland. This depression, together with the anterior and posterior clinoid processes, forms a U-shaped corticated line on sagittal sections and is saddle-shaped on coronal sections. There is a broad range in the dimensions of the sella turcica, with the anteroposterior dimension ranging from 5 to 16 mm and the depth ranging from 4 to 12 mm (see Fig. 12.68). On either side of the sella turcica is the carotid groove, seen extending posteriorly to the carotid canal, which passes vertically through the petrous portion of the temporal bone (see Plate 12.2). The clivus is a triangular bone formed by the union of the basisphenoid and basiocciput bones and extends posteriorly and caudally from the sella turcica (Fig. 12.69). The union between these bones—the spheno-occipital synchondrosis—is completed by 16 to 20 years. Thus, an open synchondrosis, seen as a gap in the clivus, is a normal appearance for children younger than 16 years of age (Fig. 12.70).

There are several key communications between the middle cranial fossa and the extracranial space, as follows:

- *Superior orbital fissure* (see Plate 12.1): Located lateral to the sphenoid body and immediately below the anterior clinoid processes, it transmits cranial nerves III, IV, V, and VI and the superior ophthalmic vein.
- *Foramen rotundum:* A canal that traverses the greater wing of the sphenoid bone and transmits the maxillary division of the trigeminal nerve to the pterygopalatine fossa. The course of this canal is best visualized on coronal sections (see Plate 12.5).
- *Foramen ovale:* Located in the sphenoid body, it transmits the mandibular division of the trigeminal nerve to the infratemporal

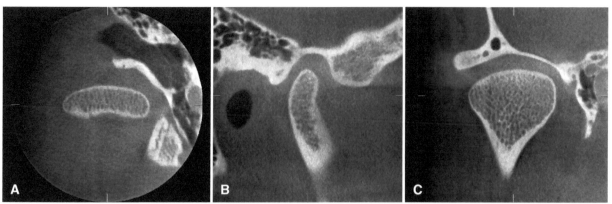

Fig. 12.68 Limited field-of-view cone beam computed tomography image of the temporomandibular joint. Axial (A), corrected sagittal (B), and frontal (C) sections. Note intact cortical borders on all articular surfaces.

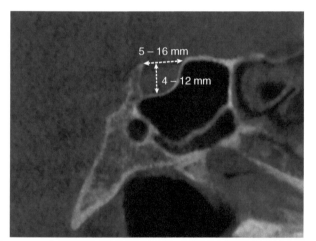

Fig. 12.69 Cone beam computed tomography section through the midsagittal plane showing the sella turcica. The range of variation in its anteroposterior and vertical dimensions is indicated.

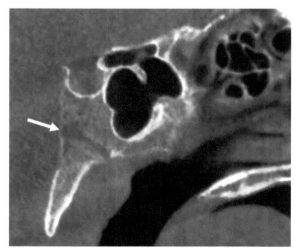

Fig. 12.70 Clivus showing incomplete spheno-occipital synchondrosis *(arrow)*. This is a normal appearance until the synchondrosis is completed, typically by 16 to 20 years. Note appearance of a completed synchondrosis in Fig. 12.69.

fossa. It is adequately visualized on axial and coronal sections (see Plates 12.2 and 12.5). There is considerable variation in the size of this foramen.

- *Foramen spinosum:* Located posterior and lateral to the foramen ovale, it is best visualized on axial sections (see Plate 12.2).

An important anatomic region to examine is the pterygopalatine fossa. This is a funnel-shaped fossa located below the skull base that has communications with the middle cranial fossa, nasal cavity, orbit, infratemporal fossa, and oral cavity (Plate 12.6). This fossa is bordered anteriorly by the posterior wall of the maxilla and posteriorly by the pterygoid process of the sphenoid bone. The opening to the pterygopalatine fossa from the lateral aspect is the pterygomaxillary fissure. On sagittal sections, the fossa is seen as an inverted pear-shaped radiolucency (see Plate 12.7); on axial and coronal sections, it appears as a rectangular area (see Plates 12.1 and 12.5).

The styloid process is noted as a bony projection from the inferior surface of the petrous temporal bone adjacent to the stylomastoid foramen. The length of this process ranges from 5 to 50 mm. The stylohyoid ligament is often calcified, with reported frequencies of up to 30%. The mastoid process is another protuberance from the inferior surface of the temporal bone. Pneumatization of this bony process by the mastoid air cells occurs starting at age 3 to 5 years. As a result of the presence of air, the mastoid air cells appear as radiolucent air spaces, and opacification of these air cells often indicates disease. Sometimes pneumatization may extend anteriorly into the articular eminence and even into the zygoma or the occipital bone adjacent to the mastoid process.

AIRWAY

Medium- to full-FOV CBCT scans often encompass the airway space from the nasal cavity to the pharynx. The pharynx is typically considered in three zones: the nasopharynx, oropharynx, and hypopharynx (Fig. 12.71 and Plate 12.7). The nasopharynx lies behind the nasal cavity and extends to the level of the hard palate. The oropharynx spans the region between the tongue and the pharyngeal wall, extending from the level of the hard palate to the base of the epiglottis. The region posterior to the soft palate from the level of the hard palate to the caudal tip of the uvula is sometimes referred to as the velopharynx. The hypopharynx is the most caudal part of the pharynx, below the epiglottis. Anatomic variations in the size of the soft palate or tongue or pathologic enlargements of the palatine tonsils can cause narrowing of the airway dimensions.

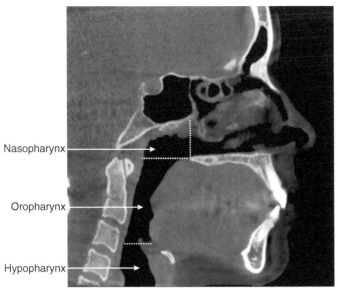

Nasopharynx

Oropharynx

Hypopharynx

Fig. 12.71 Cone beam computed tomography image through the mid-sagittal plane showing the pharyngeal airway. The *dotted lines* indicate the boundaries of the nasopharynx, oropharynx, and hypopharynx.

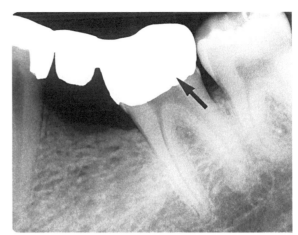

Fig. 12.73 A cast gold crown, appearing completely radiopaque *(arrow)*, serves as the terminal abutment of a bridge.

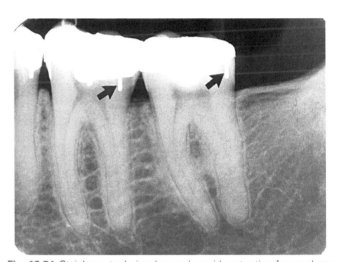

Fig. 12.74 Stainless steel pins *(arrows)* provide retention for amalgam restorations.

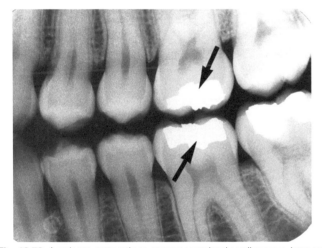

Fig. 12.72 Amalgam restorations appear completely radiopaque *(arrows)*.

RESTORATIVE MATERIALS

Restorative materials vary in their radiographic appearance, depending principally on their atomic number and also influenced by their thickness and density. A variety of restorative materials may be recognized on projection radiographs and CT scans.

- Silver amalgam is completely radiopaque (Fig. 12.72).
- Gold is equally opaque to x-rays, whether cast as a crown (Fig. 12.73) or an inlay or condensed as gold foil.
- Stainless steel pins (Fig. 12.74) and stainless steel crowns (Fig. 12.75) appear highly radiopaque.
- A calcium hydroxide base is placed in a deep cavity to protect the pulp. Such base material is typically composed to be radiopaque (Fig. 12.76) so that the development of recurrent caries (radiolucent) can be identified.
- Gutta-percha, a rubber-like substance used to fill pulp canals during endodontic therapy, is also radiopaque, but lower in radiodensity than amalgam (Fig. 12.77).

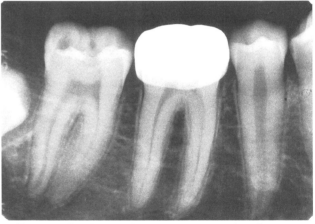

Fig. 12.75 Stainless steel crowns appear mostly radiopaque.

- Silver points, previously used to obliterate pulp canals during endodontic therapy, are highly radiopaque (Fig. 12.78).
- Composite restorations are typically partially radiopaque, as are porcelain restorations, which are usually fused to a metallic coping (Fig. 12.79).
- Orthodontic appliances around teeth (Fig. 12.80) are relatively radiopaque, although less than stainless steel crowns.

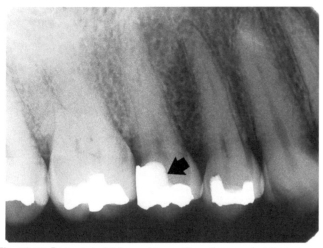

Fig. 12.76 Base material *(arrow)* is usually radiopaque but less opaque than the amalgam restoration.

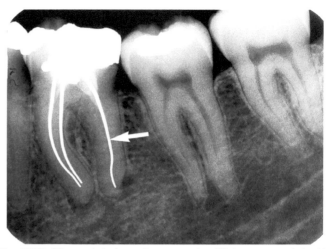

Fig. 12.78 Silver points *(arrow)* were used to fill the root canals in this patient.

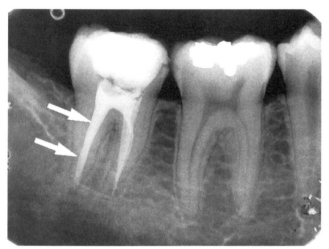

Fig. 12.77 Gutta-percha *(arrows)* is a radiopaque rubber-like material used in endodontic therapy.

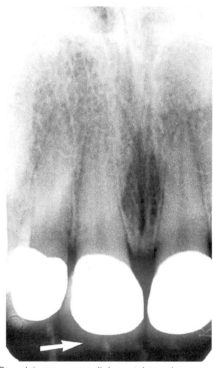

Fig. 12.79 Porcelain appears radiolucent *(arrow)* over a metal coping.

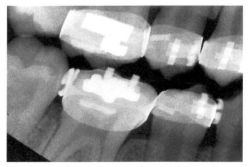

Fig. 12.80 Orthodontic appliances have a characteristic radiopaque appearance.

BIBLIOGRAPHY

Berkovitz BKB, Holland GR, Moxham BL. *Oral Anatomy, Histology and Embryology*. 4th ed. London: Mosby; 2009.

Claeys V, Waskens G. Bifid mandibular canal: literature review and case report. *Dentomaxillofac Radiol*. 2005;34:55–58.

Harnesberger HR, Osborn AG, Ross J, et al, eds. *Diagnostic and Surgical Imaging Anatomy: Brain, Head and Neck, Spine*. Salt Lake City: Amirsys; 2006.

Jacobs R, Mraiwa N, van Steenberghe D, et al. Appearance, location, course, and morphology of the mandibular incisive canal: an assessment on spiral CT scan. *Dentomaxillofac Radiol*. 2002;31:322–327.

Kasle MJ. *An Atlas of Dental Radiographic Anatomy*. 4th ed. Philadelphia: Saunders; 1994.

Liang X, Jacobs R, Lambrichts I, et al. Lingual foramina on the mandibular midline revisited: a macroanatomical study. *Clin Anat*. 2007;20:246–251.

Lusting JP, London D, Dor BL, et al. Ultrasound identification and quantitative measurement of blood supply to the anterior part of the mandible. *Oral Surg Oral Med Oral Pathol Oral Radiol Endod*. 2003;96:625–629.

Mraiwa N, Jacobs R, van Steenberghe D, et al. Clinical assessment and surgical implications of anatomic challenges in the anterior mandible. *Clin Implant Dent Relat Res*. 2003;5:219–225.

Naitoh M, Hiraiwa Y, Aimiya H, et al. Accessory mental foramen assessment using cone-beam computed tomography. *Oral Surg Oral Med Oral Pathol Oral Radiol Endod*. 2009;107:289–294.

Von Arx T, Matter D, Buser D, et al. Evaluation of the location and dimensions of lingual foramina using limited cone-beam computed tomography. *J Oral Maxillofac Surg*. 2011;69:2777–2785.

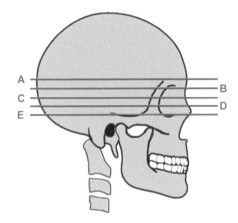

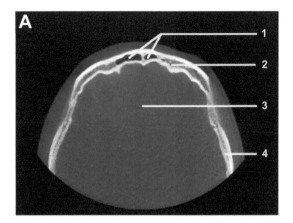

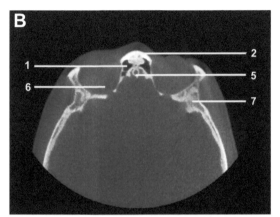

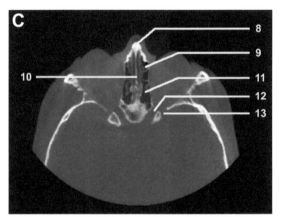

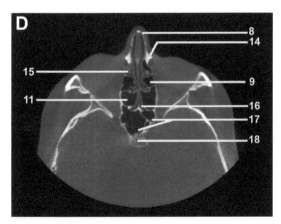

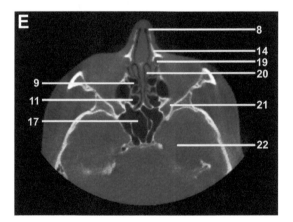

1. Frontal sinus
2. Frontal bone
3. Anterior cranial fossa
4. Squamous portion of temporal bone
5. Crista galli
6. Orbit
7. Greater wing of sphenoid bone
8. Nasal bone
9. Anterior ethmoid air cells
10. Perpendicular plate of ethmoid bone
11. Posterior ethmoid air cells

12. Optic canal
13. Superior orbital fissure
14. Nasal process of maxillary bone
15. Uncinate process
16. Sphenoethmoid recess
17. Sphenoid sinus
18. Floor of sella turcica
19. Nasolacrimal duct
20. Superior turbinate
21. Inferior orbital fissure
22. Middle cranial fossa

PLATE 12.1

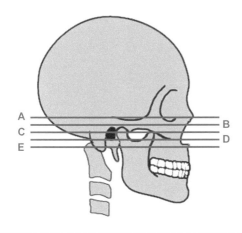

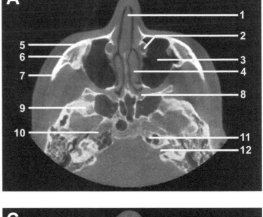

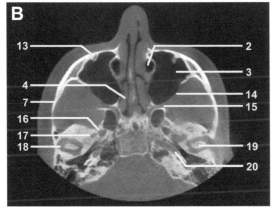

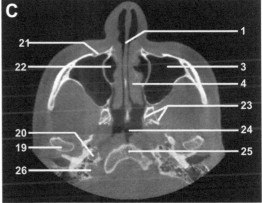

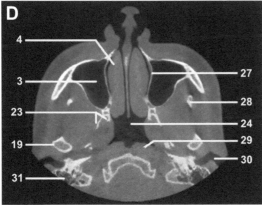

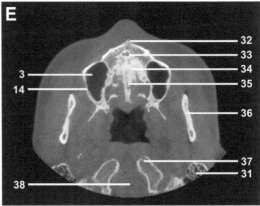

1. Nasal septum
2. Nasolacrimal duct
3. Maxillary sinus
4. Nasal turbinate
5. Zygomatic process of maxilla
6. Zygomatico-maxillary suture
7. Zygomatic arch
8. Pterygopalatine fossa
9. Greater wing of sphenoid bone
10. Carotid canal
11. Petrous portion of temporal bone
12. Internal auditory canal
13. Infraorbital canal

14. Lateral wall of maxillary sinus
15. Pterygomaxillary fissure
16. Foramen ovale
17. Foramen spinosum
18. Glenoid fossa
19. Mandibular condyle
20. Carotid canal
21. Infraorbital foramen
22. Nasal cavity
23. Pterygoid plates
24. Nasopharyngeal airway
25. Occipital bone
26. Jugular foramen

27. Medial wall of maxillary sinus
28. Coronoid process
29. Pharyngeal wall
30. External auditory meatus
31. Mastoid process
32. Anterior nasal spine
33. Nasopalatine canal
34. Hard palate
35. Intermaxillary suture
36. Ramus of mandible
37. Anterior arch of atlas (C1)
38. Foramen magnum

PLATE 12.2

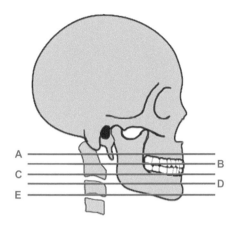

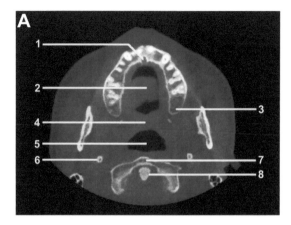

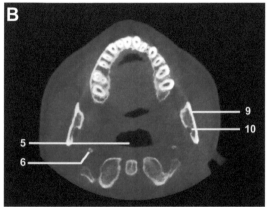

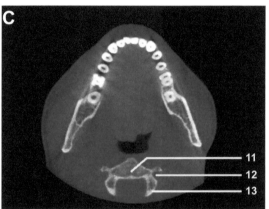

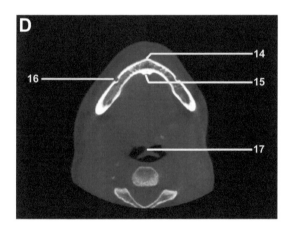

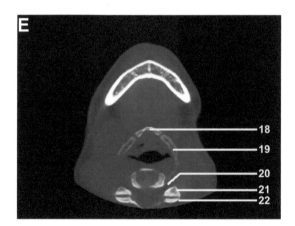

1. Incisive foramen
2. Tongue
3. Maxillary tuberosity
4. Soft palate
5. Oropharyngeal airway
6. Styloid process
7. Anterior arch of atlas (C1)
8. Odontoid process of C2
9. Ramus of mandible
10. Mandibular foramen
11. Inferior body of C2

12. Transverse foramen
13. Lamina of C2
14. Mandibular symphysis
15. Genial tubercles
16. Mental foramen
17. Epiglottis
18. Body of hyoid bone
19. Greater cornu of hyoid bone
20. C2-C3 neural foramen
21. Superior articular process of C3
22. Inferior articular process of C2

PLATE 12.3

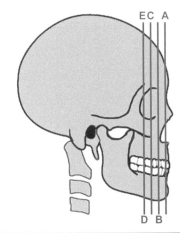

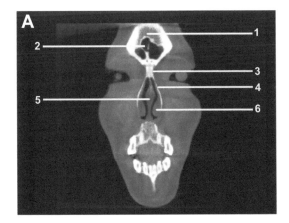

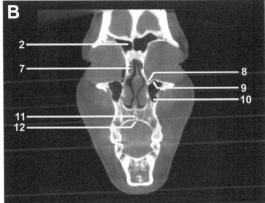

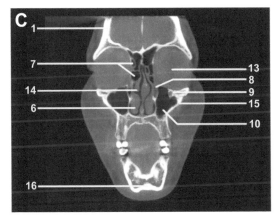

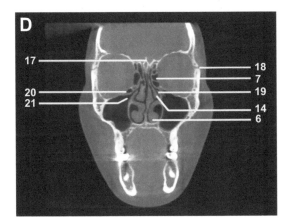

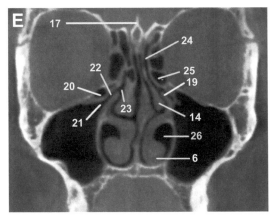

1. Frontal bone
2. Frontal sinus
3. Nasal bone
4. Maxillary bone
5. Nasal septum
6. Inferior nasal turbinate
7. Ethmoid air cells
8. Nasolacrimal duct
9. Infraorbital canal

10. Maxillary sinus
11. Nasopalatine canal
12. Incisive foramen
13. Orbit
14. Middle nasal turbinate
15. Zygomatic process of the maxilla
16. Mandible
17. Crista galli of ethmoid bone
18. Fronto-zygomatic suture

19. Uncinate process
20. Infraorbital ethmoid air cells
    (Haller cells)
21. Ostium of maxillary sinus
22. Infundibulum
23. Hiatus semilunaris
24. Frontal recess
25. Ethmoid bulla
26. Inferior meatus

PLATE 12.4

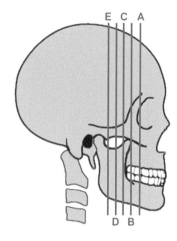

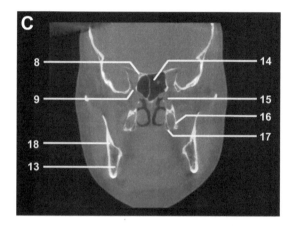

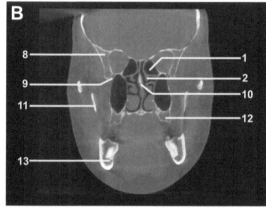

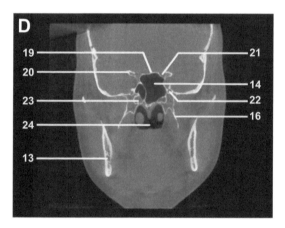

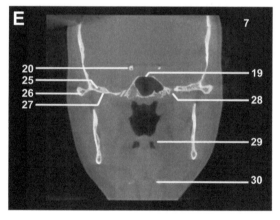

1. Ethmoid air cells
2. Superior nasal turbinate
3. Middle nasal turbinate
4. Zygomatic arch
5. Maxillary sinus
6. Inferior nasal turbinate
7. Hard palate (floor of nasal cavity)
8. Sphenoid bone
9. Inferior orbital fissure
10. Perpendicular plate of ethmoid bone

11. Coronoid process of mandible
12. Maxillary tuberosity
13. Inferior alveolar canal
14. Sphenoid sinus
15. Pterygopalatine fossa
16. Lateral pterygoid plate
17. Medial pterygoid plate
18. Mandibular ramus
19. Floor of sella turcica
20. Anterior clinoid process

21. Optic canal
22. Foramen rotundum
23. Pterygoid (vidian) canal
24. Nasopharyngeal airway
25. Squamous temporal bone
26. Zygomatic process of
    temporoal bone
27. Sphenosquamousal suture
28. Foramen ovale
29. Palatine tonsils
30. Hyoid bone

PLATE 12.5

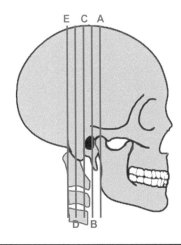

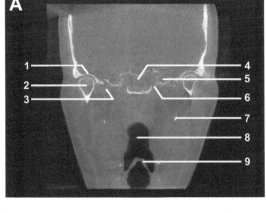

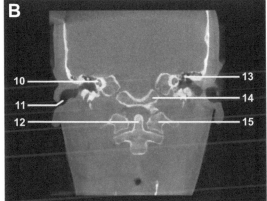

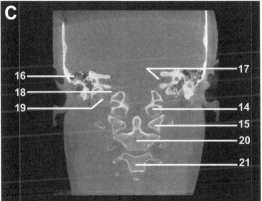

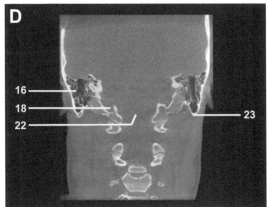

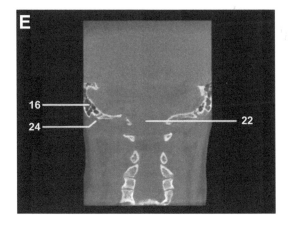

1. Glenoid fossa
2. Mandibular condyle
3. Foramen spinosum
4. Basiocciput
5. Carotid canal
6. Petrooccipital suture
7. Styloid process
8. Oropharnygeal airway
9. Epiglottis
10. Semicircular canal
11. External auditory meatus
12. Odontoid process of C2
13. Ossicles of ear
14. Occipital condyles
15. Lateral mass of C1
16. Mastoid air cells
17. Internal auditory meatus
18. Jugular foramen
19. Jugular bulb
20. Body of C2
21. Body of C3
22. Foramen magnum
23. Mastoid process
24. Occipito-mastoid suture

PLATE 12.6

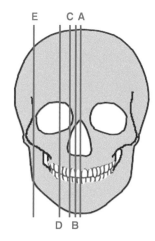

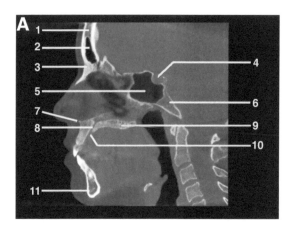

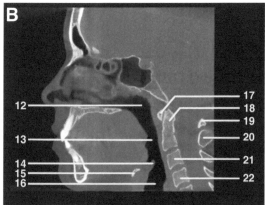

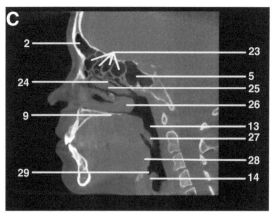

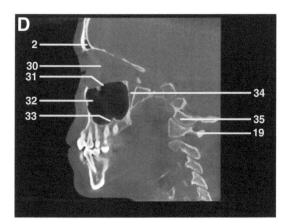

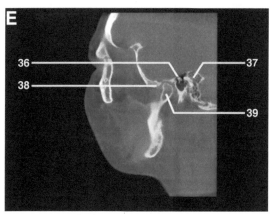

1. Frontal bone	14. Epiglottis	27. Soft palate
2. Frontal sinus	15. Hyoid bone	28. Base of tongue
3. Nasal bone	16. Hypopharynx	29. Vallecula
4. Sella turcica	17. Anterior arch of C1	30. Orbit
5. Sphenoid sinus	18. Odontoid process of C2	31. Floor of orbit/Roof of maxillary sinus
6. Clivus	19. Posterior arch of C1	32. Maxillary sinus
7. Anterior nasal spine	20. Spinous process of C2	33. Floor of maxillary sinus
8. Nasopalatine canal	21. Body of C3	34. Pterygopalatine fossa
9. Hard palate	22. Body of C4	35. Occipital condyle
10. Incisive foramen	23. Ethmoid air cells	36. Ossicle of middle ear
11. Mandibular symphysis	24. Hiatus semilunaris	37. Mastoid process
12. Nasopharyngeal airway	25. Middle turbinate	38. Articular eminence
13. Oropharyngeal airway	26. Inferior turbinate	39. Mandibular condyle

PLATE 12.7

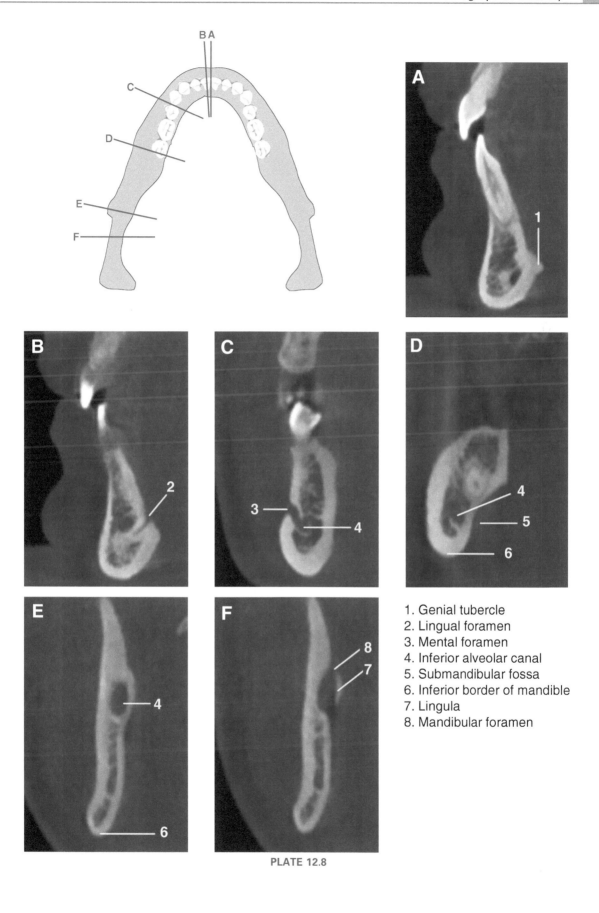

1. Genial tubercle
2. Lingual foramen
3. Mental foramen
4. Inferior alveolar canal
5. Submandibular fossa
6. Inferior border of mandible
7. Lingula
8. Mandibular foramen

PLATE 12.8

13

Other Imaging Modalities

Sanjay M. Mallya

The imaging modalities described in this chapter employ equipment and techniques that are beyond the routine needs of most general dental practitioners. Of these modalities, multidetector computed tomographic (MDCT) and magnetic resonance (MR) imaging are often prescribed by specialist dentists for diagnosis and treatment planning of maxillofacial diseases. Nuclear medicine, ultrasonography, and positron emission tomographic (PET) imaging are used for more specialized purposes, and have applications in dentistry. Thus, dentists should have a basic understanding of their operating principles and clinical applications.

MULTIDETECTOR COMPUTED TOMOGRAPHY

In 1972, Godfrey Hounsfield, an engineer, announced the invention of a revolutionary imaging technique that used image reconstruction mathematics, developed two decades before by Cormack, to produce cross-sectional images of the head. Hounsfield and Cormack shared the Nobel Prize in Physiology or Medicine in 1979 for their pioneering work that led to the invention of computed tomography (CT), considered by many to be among the top five innovations in medicine. The word "tomography" is derived from the Greek words "*tomos*" (slice) and "*graphe*" (drawing)—CT produces images of sections of the body. The basic principle of CT is the same—whether applied to *conventional single-slice CT, MDCT,* or *cone beam computed tomography (CBCT)* (see Chapters 10 and 11). In all CT techniques, a collimated x-ray source and a detector revolve around the patient (Figs. 13.1–13.3). The detector records photon attenuation by measuring the number of photons that exit the patient, registering this information at several hundred angles through the rotational arc. Complex mathematical algorithms translate this attenuation data into a three-dimensional (3D) map that spatially locates the attenuating structures.

COMPUTED TOMOGRAPHIC SCANNERS

The initial CT scanner required a 5-minute scan time. Subsequently, CT scanner design evolved through four generations and decreased this scan time to 1 to 2 seconds. In these conventional designs, the x-ray tube and detector array, mounted on a gantry assembly, revolved around the patient lying down on a table. At the end of each revolution, the table advanced through the gantry, while the x-ray tube-detector assembly returned to its original position to unwind the attached wiring that supplied power and transferred data from the detector to the computer. The first-generation scanners used a "pencil-like" beam, and recorded data with a single detector. The x-ray beam was collimated at the source and at the surface of the detector to minimize scatter radiation reaching the detector. The second- to fourth-generation scanners used an array of multiple detectors arranged in an arc or in a fixed outer ring (see Fig. 13.1A and B). The table movement through the gantry, typically 1 to 5 mm, positioned the patient for imaging of the next slice. CT scanners that use this type of "step and shoot" movement for image acquisition are called incremental scanners. The final image set consists of a series of spaced, contiguous, or overlapping images in the axial plane.

In the early 1990s, CT scanners were introduced that acquire image data in a helical fashion (see Fig. 13.2). These *helical CT scanners,* or *spiral CT scanners,* used a "slip-ring" technology that eliminated the need for directed wired connections to the moving x-ray tube and detector. The gantry, containing the attached x-ray tube and detectors, continuously revolves around the patient, while the table on which the patient is lying continuously advances through the gantry. A continuous helix of data is acquired as the x-ray beam moves down the patient. Helical CT imaging is now the prevailing scanning mode. Helical CT scanning offered several advantages. It replaced the incremental scanning process with continuous image acquisition, and markedly decreased scan times. Like incremental CT scanners, these units also used an array of detectors in a single row, allowing image capture of single slices with each gantry revolution.

Multidetector CT (MDCT), also referred to as multislice CT (MSCT), was introduced in the late 1990s and has now become the most widely used CT scanner design across the world. In MDCT, multiple rows of detectors are incorporated into the array in the *z*-axis (craniocaudal axis, patient's head to foot), allowing capture of multiple image slices during each gantry revolution (see Fig. 13.3). MDCT technology has considerably reduced scan times, limiting motion artifact from breathing, peristalsis, or heart contractions; this is important for patients who cannot hold their breath for long periods and for pediatric and trauma patients. Current detector, configurations have improved spatial resolution to submillimeter dimensions. Volumetric acquisition with isotropic imaging allows reformatting in planes different from the axial acquisition, without compromising image quality. Contemporary MDCT scanners have 64 to 128 rows of detectors, with some vendors manufacturing scanners with 320 and 640 detector rows.

X-Ray Tubes

MDCT scanners operate at high tube voltage and tube current, and thus require special x-ray tubes to meet the high demands on heat production and cooling. MDCT units use x-ray tubes with rotating anodes (see Fig. 1.9), with a high heat capacity, up to 8 million heat units (compare with dental tubes of 20,000 heat units). They typically operate at 120 kilovolt peak (kVp) (range, 80 to 140 kVp) and at high tube currents (200 to 800 mA). The high x-ray output minimizes exposure time and improves image quality by increasing the signal-to-noise ratio. The high kVp also provides a wide dynamic range by reducing bone absorption compared with soft tissue and extends tube life by reducing tube loading. The tubes operate continuously by using three-phase or high-frequency generators. To minimize patient exposure the beam is

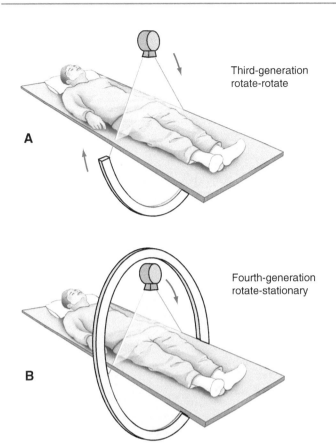

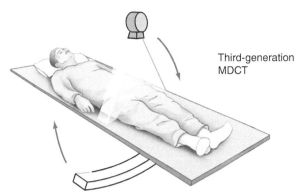

Fig. 13.3 Multidetector Computed Tomography *(MDCT)* **Scanners Use a Relatively Wide Detector Array Having 64 to 640 Rows.** In these scanners, all parts of the detector array arc are equidistant from the x-ray source. Computed tomography image formation.

Fig. 13.1 Geometry of Computed Tomography (CT) Scanners. (A) In CT scanners, the x-ray source emits a fan beam. In third-generation CT scanners, both the x-ray source and the detector array rotate around the patient in a circular path. The patient is moved incrementally between each rotation of the source. (B) In fourth-generation CT scanners, the x-ray tube rotates around the patient, and the remnant beam is detected by a fixed circular array.

collimated to a thin fan beam before it enters the patient. Some of the x-ray photons interact with the patient and are scattered. To improve image quality the residual beam is again collimated to remove the scattered photons before it reaches the detector array.

Detectors

In MDCT, the x-ray beam exiting the patient is captured by an array of solid-state detectors. These detectors are usually made of high-atomic-number scintillating materials, such as Gd_2S_2O. The detectors absorb x-ray photons and produce visible light, which is detected by photodiodes and converted into an electronic signal that forms the data to be analyzed. The scintillation detectors have a high x-ray detection efficiency and absorb almost 90% of the incident photons. This increased efficiency allows short scan times, and increases the signal-to-noise ratio. As described above, predetector collimators limit the amount of scattered radiation that strikes the detector. This decreases noise and improves image contrast.

Multidetector Computed Tomographic Image Acquisition Parameters
Field of View

The field of view (FOV) must encompass the anatomic region being imaged. For maxillofacial and mandibular CT protocols, the FOV typically ranges from 7 to 18 cm, to encompass the entire maxillofacial skeleton from the cranial base to past the mandibular inferior border. Following acquisition, the entire FOV, or a part thereof, can be reconstructed into an image data set. A scout or localizer view is first made, and is typically a lateral projection of the head. This scout view allows the technologist to define the FOV. Some automatic exposure control techniques (see later) use information from this scout view to estimate tube current based on patient size and anatomy.

Exposure Settings (kVp, mA)

Most adult CT examinations are performed at a tube voltage of 120 kVp. Lowering the kVp will decrease the radiation dose, but will increase image noise. Several pediatric MDCT protocols use a lower kVp (80 to 120 kVp) to reduce radiation dose to the patient. However, decreasing the milliampere setting (mA) is the more common method to minimize radiation dose. Notably, several units offer automatic exposure control rather than using fixed mA settings, where the mA is automatically adjusted depending on patient size and body part being examined.

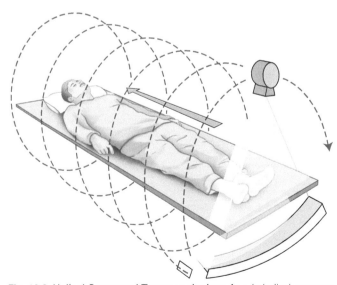

Fig. 13.2 Helical Computed Tomography Imaging. In helical scanners, the patient is moved continuously through the gantry, and the x-ray source moves continuously around the patient in a circle. The net effect is to describe a helical beam—and image—path through the patient. True axial sections are reconstructed in the software.

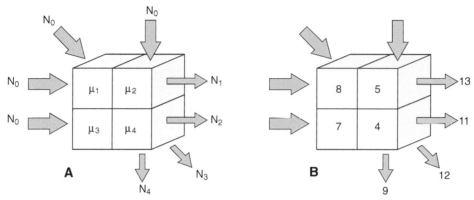

Fig. 13.4 Image Reconstruction. (A) Assume four volumes with differing linear attenuation coefficients (μ). A beam entering the object with N_0 photons is reduced in intensity by object. The intensity of the remnant beam is measured by the detector array. The value of each cell in the object can be determined by solving four (or more) independent simultaneous equations. Such a brute-force approach is computationally intensive, and in practice much faster algorithms are used to reconstruct images. (B) This task is conceptually similar to Sudoku problems in that the exposure to the detector is known, and the filtered back-projection algorithms estimate the exposure intensity at each voxel.

Slice Thickness and Detector Configurations

In conventional single-slice CT, the thickness of the imaged slice was determined by collimating the beam width. In MDCT, multiple slices are acquired in one gantry rotation, and the minimum slice thickness is dependent on the detector row width. Following acquisition, data from contiguous detector rows can be combined (binning) to reconstruct slices of different thicknesses. For example, consider a 320-slice CT scanner with detector elements that are 0.5-mm wide. The beam width would be 320 × 0.5 mm = 160 mm. The acquired volume can be reconstructed into 320 × 0.5-mm slices, 160 × 1-mm slices, 80 × 2-mm slices. The diagnostic task guides reconstructed slice thickness. For maxillofacial examinations, bone evaluation is typically accomplished with 0.5-mm– to 0.75-mm–thick slices, whereas 1-mm–thick sections are adequate for soft-tissue examination.

The *pitch* of the scan influences scan speed, overlapping of sections, and the radiation dose. For MDCT, the pitch is defined as

$$\text{Pitch} = \frac{\text{Distance moved by table per 360 degree rotation}}{\text{Beam width}}$$

When the pitch is 1, there is no overlap between slices. At a pitch less than 1, the slices overlap, yielding images with higher resolution. However, the length of tissue imaged per gantry rotation is less, resulting in longer scan times to image the same anatomic region. Importantly, the radiation dose to the patient is increased. When the pitch is greater than 1, the helical acquisitions are separated. This allows faster scan times for the same scan length, and with less radiation dose. However, the missing data between the helical rotations reduces the image resolution in the z-axis.

Computed Tomography Image Reconstruction
Reconstruction Algorithms

The photons recorded by the detectors represent a composite of the absorption characteristics of all anatomic structures in the path of the x-ray beam. Computer algorithms use these photon counts to reconstruct the sectional images. The methods used to reconstruct images are complex. Consider the object with four compartments, as shown in Fig. 13.4. The linear attenuation coefficients (densities) of each of the four cells can be computed by using four simultaneous equations to

solve for four unknowns. This method becomes computationally impracticable when there are 512^2 or 1024^2 cells. Instead, methods called filtered back-projection algorithms involving Fourier transformations are used for rapid image reconstruction. A modification of these methods, called the Feldkamp reconstruction, is used for MDCT to account for the diverging x-ray beam. This same principle is used in CBCT imaging (see Chapter 10). Additional algorithms are applied to correct for the helical motion of the scanner and to construct planar cross sections from the helical information. In recent years, an image processing technique called iterative reconstruction has been used instead of filtered back-projection to reduce noise from images. This technique allows the use of low-dose protocols yet produces images with comparable or better image quality.

Bone- and Soft-Tissue Kernels

After reconstruction, various image processing algorithms, or "filters," are applied to accentuate specific characteristics in the CT image. In clinical practice, these filters are often referred to as "bone kernels" and "soft-tissue kernels" (Fig. 13.5), and are designed to facilitate specific diagnostic objectives. For example, bone evaluation requires higher spatial resolution—application of the bone kernel will reconstruct an image with sharper detail to emphasize bone structure, although with some increase in image noise. On the other hand, evaluation of soft-tissue areas requires identification of mild differences in attenuation, and soft-tissue kernels yield images with less noise and enhanced contrast resolution.

Postprocessing of Multidetector Computed Tomographic Data Sets
Computed Tomography Numbers and Hounsfield Units

The CT image is recorded and displayed as a matrix of individual blocks called voxels (volume elements) (Fig. 13.6). Each square of the image matrix is a pixel. MDCT images are typically 512 × 512 pixels. Each pixel is assigned a CT number representing tissue density, inferred from the attenuation data by the reconstruction algorithms. This number is proportional to the degree to which the material within the voxel has attenuated the x-ray beam. CT numbers are normalized to the attenuation value of water, and expressed on a scale of arbitrary units—Hounsfield units (HU), in honor of the inventor Hounsfield.

Bone kernel   Soft-tissue kernel

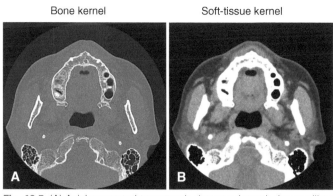

Fig. 13.5 (A) Axial computed tomography images through the maxillary dentoalveolar arch, reconstructed with bone kernel. Note details of bone trabeculation. (B) Axial slice from the same plane reconstructed with a soft-tissue kernel. Note enhanced contrast between muscles and subcutaneous fat.

In the HU scale, the CT number of water is defined as zero, and the CT number of air is defined as −1000. The mathematical derivation of CT numbers and Hounsfield units of common tissues and materials are shown in Table 13.6.

Window Width and Levels

CT images are typically 12-bit images, which means they have 4096 (2^{12}) shades of gray. Display monitors will typically display 256 to 1024 shades of gray. The human eye is capable of distinguishing approximately 32 gray levels at a fixed luminance, and thus 6- to 8-bit images are usually sufficient for CT image display. Software applications that display CT images allow the viewer to narrow the range of gray levels displayed, and this postprocessing task is known as windowing (Fig. 13.7). By setting a *window width* and *window level*, the viewer manipulates the contrast scale and brightness of the displayed image (Fig. 13.8). The window width sets the range of CT numbers that will be displayed in the grayscale. The window level is the CT number at the center of this range.

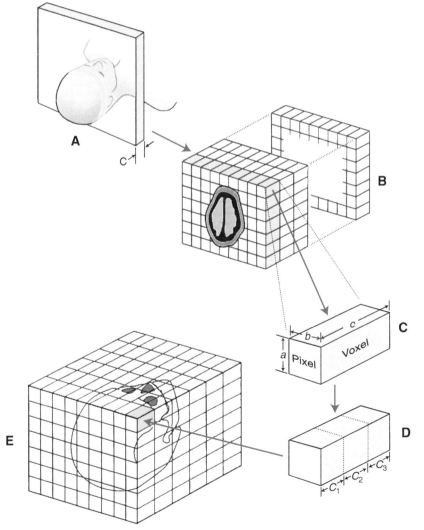

Fig. 13.6 (A) Data for a single-plane image are acquired from multiple projections made during the course of a 360-degree rotation around the patient. Slice thickness (c) is controlled by the width of the post patient collimator. (B) A single-plane image is constructed from absorption characteristics of the subject and displayed as differences in optical density, ranging from −1000 to +4000 HU. Several planes may be imaged from multiple contiguous scans. (C) The image consists of a matrix of individual pixels representing the face of a volume called a voxel. Although dimensions *a* and *b* are determined partly by the computer program used to construct the image, dimension *c* is controlled by the collimator as in A. (D) Cuboid voxels can be created from the original rectangular voxel by computer interpolation. This allows the formation of multiplanar and three-dimensional images (E).

Multiplanar and Curved Planar Reformation

Reconstructed volumetric MDCT data sets can be viewed as images in the axial, coronal, and sagittal planes or in any arbitrary plane depending on the diagnostic task. This is referred to as multiplanar reformation (MPR), and the simultaneous visualization in three orthogonal planes often facilitates radiographic interpretation (Fig. 13.9). Viewing software programs allow the user to display these images at the thickness of 1 voxel, or as thicker slices combining data from several voxels. Curved planar reformation is accomplished by creating a reformation plane along the long axis of an anatomic structure, for example, the dental arch, and can be applied to generate "panoramic" views of the jaws.

Special postprocessing techniques allow visualization of the 3D data set (Fig. 13.10). Surface rendering (or shaded surface display) provides a 3D view of a surface. These computer algorithms delineate a surface based on thresholding (identifying pixels with CT numbers within a specified range) and edge-detection (identifying pixels with sharp changes in CT numbers). The pixels are then shaded by assigning a brightness value to simulate a 3D scene. Many software programs allow the user to interact with these rendered images, such as rotation, or removal of the external surface to visualize another structure. Volume rendering is a similar but more advanced technique. Both these rendering techniques are valuable adjuncts to the primary review of the MPR images, for example, to visualize facial asymmetry and fractures (see Figs. 13.10 and 27.25).

TABLE 13.6 Typical Hounsfield Units (HU) for Air and Tissues	
Tissue	**Hounsfield Units (CT Numbers)**
Bone	+200 (trabecular) to +3000 (dense cortical)
Muscle	+40 to +80
Clotted blood	+50 to +75
Blood	+15 to +30
CSF	+15
Water	0
Fat	−60 to −100
Lung	−200 to −600
Air	−1000

$$HU = 1000 \times \frac{\mu - \mu_{water}}{\mu_{water}}$$

where μ is the linear attenuation coefficient.

CT, Computed tomography; CSF, cerebrospinal fluid.

Artifacts

Artifacts are systemic discrepancies between the CT numbers in reconstructed voxels and the true attenuation coefficients of the anatomic structures that they represent. Some commonly encountered artifacts in the maxillofacial region are described below.

Partial Volume Artifact

When a single voxel represents tissues of differing densities (e.g., bone and soft tissue), the resulting CT number for that voxel is an intermediate value that does not accurately represent either tissue. This artifact will occur when the object being imaged is smaller than the size of an individual reconstructed voxel. Practically, this artifact may appear as partial disruption of a thin layer of cortical bone, for example, the bony walls of the ethmoid air cells or the temporal bone.

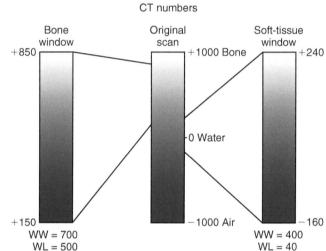

Fig. 13.7 Window Width and Level. Computed tomography (CT) numbers (HU) are scaled on cortical bone (+1000), water (0), and air (−1000). Viewing bone or soft tissue is optimized by improving the contrast of the appropriate region of the original image. Window width (WW) is the range of CT numbers used, and window level (WL) is the importation of the range. Preset parameters in the software (bone and soft-tissue window views) are used to enhance visualization of those tissues. In this example, a bone window may have a range of 700 units and a mean of 500 units, whereas a soft tissue window may have a range of 400 units and a mean of 40 units.

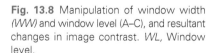

Fig. 13.8 Manipulation of window width (WW) and window level (A–C), and resultant changes in image contrast. WL, Window level.

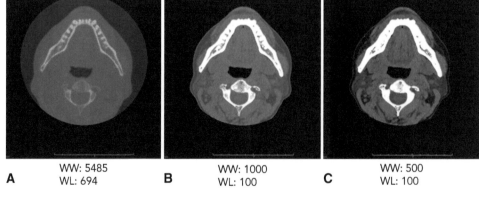

A	WW: 5485 WL: 694	B	WW: 1000 WL: 100	C	WW: 500 WL: 100

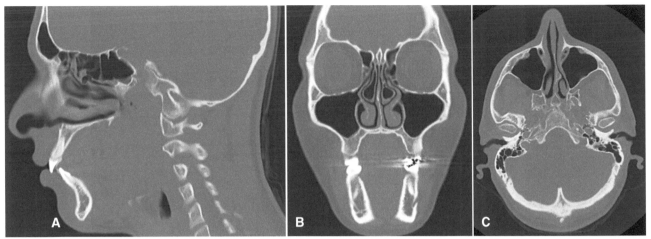

Fig. 13.9 Multiplanar Reconstruction Views Facilitate Interpretation of Complex Anatomy. (A) Computed tomography images demonstrating the sagittal plane through lateral incisors and foramen lacerum. Note the frontal, ethmoid, and sphenoid sinuses. (B) Coronal view through the ethmoid and maxillary sinuses and mental foramen in the left mandible. (C) Axial view through the level of maxillary sinuses and mandibular condyles. The patient's right side appears on the left side of the coronal and sagittal images as if the patient is lying on the back with the toes pointed toward the observer.

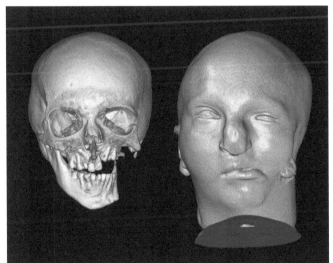

Fig. 13.10 Three-Dimensional (3D) Rendering. 3D views with the threshold setting to visualize bone *(left)* or soft tissue *(right)*, and made to appear to have depth by highlighting structures near the front and shadowing structures near the back. This patient has hemifacial microsomia and demonstrates incomplete development of the left frontal, sphenoid, temporal maxillary, zygomatic, and mandibular bones. Note also the reduced size of the left orbit, depression of the tip of the nose, missing and incompletely erupted left maxillary teeth, deviation of the right mandible to the left, sunken left midface, and malformation of the left ear. (Images courtesy Dr. P.-L. Westesson, University of Rochester, NY.)

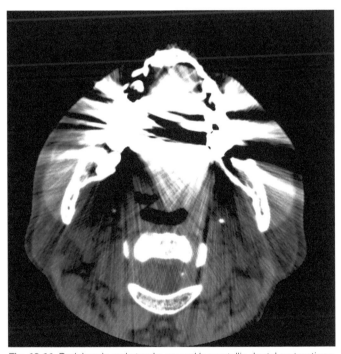

Fig. 13.11 Dark bands and streaks caused by metallic dental restorations.

Metal Streaking Artifacts

Metal streaking artifacts occur because of the near-complete absorption of x-ray photons by metallic restorations. They appear as opaque streaks in the occlusal plane (see Fig. 13.11).

Contrast Agents

Contrast agents are substances used to improve visualization of the interface between structures. CT imaging frequently uses iodine-based contrast media, administered intravenously, to enhance soft tissue and vascular image detail. The iodine in the contrast medium has a high atomic number ($Z = 53$) and efficiently absorbs x-rays (Fig. 13.12).

Beam-Hardening Artifact

X-ray tubes produce a poly-energetic x-ray beam. As it travels through the patient's tissue, the lower energy photons are preferentially attenuated, and the mean energy of the beam is increased. Beam hardening results in two types of artifacts—cupping artifacts and *streaks and dark bands* (Fig. 13.11). Beam-hardening artifacts manifest as dark streaks between two highly attenuating structures, such as compact bone, dental implants, and dental restorations.

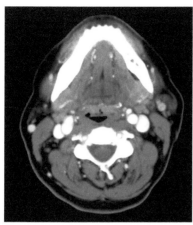

Fig. 13.12 Contrast Agents. Iodine may be administered intravenously to enhance blood vessels and structures with a rich vascular supply, including the periphery of some tumors. Computed tomography image through the mandible in the soft-tissue window and after administration of iodine. Note prominent great vessels lying just anterior and lateral to the cervical vertebrae and muscles of the floor of the mouth and neck.

Malignant facial tumors often are more vascularized than surrounding normal tissues; thus, the presence of the iodine perfusing these tissues increases their radiographic density and makes their margins more detectable. Contrast medium also helps to visualize enlarged lymph nodes containing metastatic carcinoma. However, contrast media can be nephrotoxic in elderly patients with kidney disease.

Applications

MDCT imaging has several applications in the diagnosis and treatment of dento-maxillofacial diseases. Indications for MDCT are listed in Box 13.1. For some of these clinical indications, the diagnostic objectives may be accomplished by CBCT (see Chapters 10, 11, and 17). Table 13.1 compares the spatial resolution, contrast resolution, and radiation dose of MDCT and CBCT. Compared with CBCT, MDCT has a higher radiation dose, and lesser spatial resolution.

For most intraosseous pathologies in the bone, CBCT may be adequate. However, MDCT has a high contrast resolution, and provides excellent visualization of the soft tissues. Thus, when there is evident or suspected soft-tissue involvement, MDCT is the preferred CT protocol.

MAGNETIC RESONANCE IMAGING

Magnetic resonance imaging (MRI) is an imaging technique with a revolutionary impact in diagnostic imaging, both in terms of the spectrum of tissue contrast and lack of risks associated with ionizing radiation (see Chapter 2). In 1973, Paul Lauterbur described the potential of making images based on the principles of nuclear magnetic resonance (NMR). Subsequently, Sir Peter Mansfield developed use of the magnetic field and the mathematical analysis of the signals for image reconstruction. In the 1980s, MRI was developed and refined for practical clinical application. Lauterbur and Mansfield were awarded the Nobel Prize in Physiology or Medicine in 2003.

To make an MR image, the patient is first placed inside a large magnet. This magnetic field causes the nuclei of many atoms in the body, particularly hydrogen, to align with the magnetic field. The scanner directs a radiofrequency (RF) pulse into the patient, causing some hydrogen nuclei to absorb energy (resonate). When the RF pulse is turned off, the hydrogen nuclei release the stored energy, which is detected

BOX 13.1   Indications for Maxillofacial Multidetector Computed Tomography

- Infections, including osteomyelitis and space infections
- Midfacial and mandibular trauma
- Developmental anomalies of the craniofacial skeleton
- Benign intraosseous cysts and neoplasms of the jaws
- Benign and malignant neoplasms that originate in, or extend into, the orofacial soft tissues
- Soft-tissue cysts

TABLE 13.1   Comparison of Multidetector Computed Tomography and Cone Beam Computed Tomography Parameters

Parameter	Multidetector Computed Tomography	Cone Beam Computed Tomography
Soft-tissue contrast resolution	Excellent	Poor
Typical spatial resolution, detector width	0.5 mm and above	0.08–0.4 mm
Radiation dose, maxillofacial computed tomography without contrast	Standard protocol: 0.65 mSv Low-dose protocol: 0.18 mSv	Typically, <0.1 mSv

as a signal in the scanner. This signal is used to construct the MR image—in essence, a map of the distribution of hydrogen plus local tissue properties that influence the strength of the magnetic resonance signal.

MR imaging is noninvasive and uses nonionizing radiation. It makes images with excellent soft-tissue resolution in any imaging plane. Practical limitations of MR imaging include high cost and long scan times. Additionally, metallic objects in the imaging field, such as dental restorations and orthodontic appliances, may produce image artifacts. Ferromagnetic objects, such as foreign bodies or surgical devices, may move into the strong magnetic field, injuring the patient.

Nuclear Magnetic Moment

Individual protons and neutrons (nucleons) in the nuclei of all atoms possess a spin, or angular momentum. In nuclei having equal numbers of protons and neutrons, the spin of each nucleon cancels that of another, producing a net spin of zero. However, nuclei containing an unpaired proton or neutron have a net spin. A fundamental law of physics is that a spinning, charged mass has an associated magnetic field, designated *nuclear magnetic moment*. Thus, nuclei with unpaired nucleons act as magnets with *magnetic dipoles* (north and south poles). This key property of nuclei is harvested in the making of an MR image. Table 13.2 lists abundance of biological nuclei of relevance in MRI. Of these nuclei, standard clinical MRI uses the hydrogen nucleus to produce signals for imaging.

External Magnetic Field

In clinical MR imaging, the patient is placed within a strong magnetic field. The field strengths range from 0.1 to 7 T, with 1.5 T being the most common (1.5 T is about 30,000 times the strength of the earth's magnetic field).

TABLE 13.2 **Magnetic Properties of Abundant Biological Nuclei**		
Isotope	**Abundance (%)**	**Gyromagnetic Ratio (MHz/T)**
^{1}H	99	42.6
^{12}C	98	0[a]
^{16}O	99	0[a]
^{19}F	100	40.0
^{23}Na	100	11.3
^{31}P	100	17.2

[a]Isotopes with a gyromagnetic ration of zero do not produce a magnetic resonance signal.

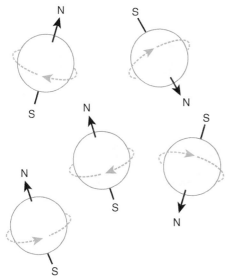

Fig. **13.13** Magnetic Dipoles. Hydrogen nuclei within a patient normally have randomly oriented dipoles and thus no net magnetic vector.

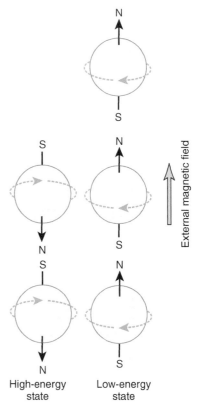

Fig. **13.14** Hydrogen Nuclei in an External Magnetic Field. In the presence of an applied strong external magnetic field, most nuclei are in the lower energy state and are aligned parallel with the magnetic field, whereas others align in the higher energy state antiparallel to the magnetic field.

A hydrogen nucleus consists of a single unpaired proton and therefore acts as a magnetic dipole. Normally, these magnetic dipoles are randomly oriented in space (Fig. 13.13). When placed within a strong external magnetic field, the magnetic moments of these individual protons align along the direction of the magnetic field (Fig. 13.14).

Two energy states are possible for the hydrogen nucleus: lower energy state (*spin-up*, magnetic moment *in the direction* of the external magnetic field), and higher energy state (*spin-down*, magnetic moment *against the direction* of the external magnetic field). Nuclei prefer to be in a lower energy state, and thus, at equilibrium more hydrogen nuclei have magnetic moments in the direction of the external magnetic field (also referred to as Z-axis). In this situation, the net magnetization (or *longitudinal magnetization, M_z*, see Fig. 13.17)—the sum of all magnetic moments from all protons—is in the direction of the magnetic field. Increasing the magnetic field strength increases the magnitude of the longitudinal magnetization.

Precession

In addition to aligning in or against the direction of the external magnetic field, the magnetic moment of the protons also precess about the external magnetic field (Fig. 13.15). This motion resembles a spinning top or gyroscope, which rotates around an upright position as it slows down. Likewise, the presence of the external magnetic field causes the axis of the spinning proton to wobble (or precess) around the axis of the

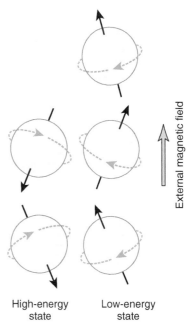

Fig. **13.15** Hydrogen Nuclei in an External Magnetic Field. The magnetic dipoles are not aligned exactly with the external magnetic field. Instead, the axes of spinning protons actually oscillate or wobble with a slight tilt from being absolutely parallel with the flux of the external magnet.

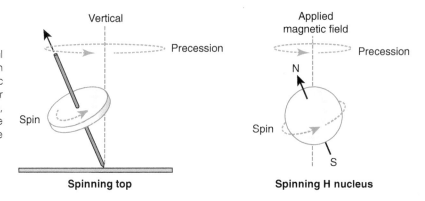

Fig. 13.16 Precession. Much as a top rotates around a vertical axis when spinning, the spin axis of a spinning hydrogen nucleus rotates around the direction of the external magnetic field. This movement is called precession, and the rate or frequency of precession is called the precessional, resonance, or Larmor frequency. The Larmor frequency depends on the strength of the external magnetic field and is specific for the nuclear species.

applied magnetic field (Fig. 13.16). The frequency of precession is called the Larmor frequency or resonance frequency and is defined by the Larmor equation. Practical applications of the Larmor equation to clinical MRI are discussed in Box 13.2.

Radiofrequency Pulse and Resonance

Hydrogen nuclei at equilibrium in the external magnetic field are in either the lower energy state or higher energy state, and switch between these energy states by absorbing or releasing energy. In MR imaging, a pulse of radiofrequency (RF, nonionizing electromagnetic radiation; see Fig. 1.3) is emitted into the patient. The RF pulse frequency matches the Larmor frequency of the hydrogen nucleus—matching the frequency of the RF pulse to the Larmor frequency causes the protons to resonate and absorb the RF energy. This energy absorbance causes some of the low-energy nuclei (spin-up) to gain energy to convert to the high-energy (spin-down) state. Consequently, the longitudinal magnetization, M_Z, is reduced (Fig. 13.17). The longer the RF pulse is applied, the less the resultant longitudinal magnetization. The RF pulse makes the protons precess in phase with each other, resulting in tissue magnetization in the transverse plane (*transverse magnetization, M_{XY}*) perpendicular to the longitudinal Z-axis (see Fig. 13.17). An RF pulse of sufficient intensity and duration can decrease the M_Z to zero (Fig. 13.18). This RF pulse is called a 90-degree RF pulse or a flip angle of 90 degrees, and maximizes the transverse magnetization M_{XY} because the magnetic moments of all nuclei are in phase.

Magnetic Resonance Signal

The precession of the transverse magnetization, M_{XY}, induces an electric current in a receiver coil (Fig. 13.19). The magnitude of this current is proportional to the overall concentration of hydrogen nuclei (proton density) in the tissue. The signal strength also depends on the degree to which hydrogen is bound within a molecule. Tightly bound hydrogen atoms, such as in hydroxyapatite in bone, do not align themselves with the external magnetic field and produce a weak signal. Loosely bound and mobile hydrogen atoms, such as those in soft tissues and liquids, react to the RF pulse and produce a detectable signal at the end of the RF pulse. The concentration of loosely bound hydrogen nuclei available to create the signal is referred to as the proton density or spin density of the tissue in question. The higher the concentration of loosely bound hydrogen atoms, the stronger the transverse magnetization, the stronger the MR signal, and the brighter the corresponding part of the MR image.

When the RF pulse is turned off, the nuclei begin to return to their original lower energy spin state, a process called relaxation. As some of the high-energy nuclei return to the low-energy state, the longitudinal magnetization, M_Z, returns to its original equilibrium state. Additionally, and independently, the individual magnetic moments of the protons

---

BOX 13.2   Practical Applications of the Larmor Equation in Clinical Magnetic Resonance Imaging

- Hydrogen nuclei are abundant and have a high gyromagnetic ratio, and thus a high Larmor frequency, which permits efficient signal production to make a magnetic resonance image.
- The gyromagnetic ratio of each nucleus is unique (see Table 13.2). Thus, for a given magnetic field strength, the Larmor frequencies of different nuclei are also unique, and this allows for the selective excitation of hydrogen nuclei during clinical imaging.
- The Larmor frequency of a nuclear species is directly proportional to the strength of the external magnetic field. In magnetic resonance imaging, a local magnetic gradient is applied across an anatomic site. This spatially separates the tissue's protons into "slices" of varying Larmor frequencies—the basis for spatially encoding magnetic resonance signals into image slices.

$$\boldsymbol{\omega} = \boldsymbol{\gamma} \times \boldsymbol{B}_0$$

where $\boldsymbol{\omega}$ is the Larmor frequency, $\boldsymbol{\gamma}$ is the gyromagnetic ratio, and $\boldsymbol{B}_0$ is the strength of the external magnetic field.

---

begin to interact with each other and dephase. This dephasing results in reduction of the magnetization in the transverse plane, M_{XY}, a condition called decay. Because of the loss of transverse magnetization and the dephasing of the hydrogen nuclei, there is a loss of intensity of the MR signal. The decreasing voltage recorded in the receiving coil is called the free induction decay signal.

T1 and T2 Relaxation

Relaxation at the end of the RF pulse results in recovery of the longitudinal magnetization; this is accomplished by transfer of energy from individual hydrogen nuclei (spin) to the surrounding molecules (lattice). This is an exponential process, and the time required for 63% of the longitudinal magnetization, M_Z, to return to equilibrium is called the T1 relaxation time or spin-lattice relaxation time. The T1 relaxation time varies with different tissues and reflects the ability of their nuclei to transfer their excess energy to surrounding molecules (Table 13.3). Tissues with a high fluid content, such as cerebrospinal fluid (CSF), tend to have long T1 times because the high inherent energy of water inhibits the transfer of energy from excited hydrogen nuclei. However, tissues with a high fat content, such as bone marrow, tend to have short T1 times reflecting the low inherent energy of fat and the relative ease by which energy is transferred from excited hydrogen nuclei.

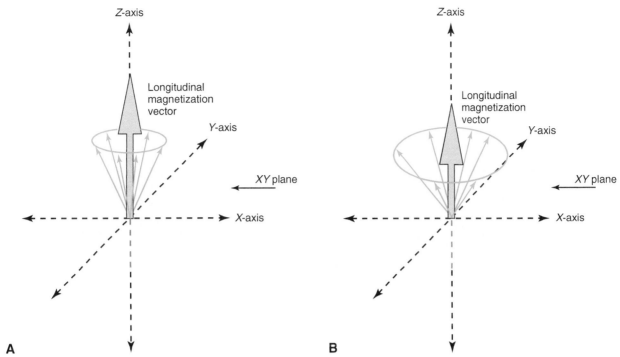

Fig. 13.17 Longitudinal Magnetization. When hydrogen nuclei are in an external magnetic field, two energy states result: spin-up, which is parallel to the direction of the field, and spin-down, which is antiparallel to the direction of the field. (A) The combined effect of these two energy states is a weak net magnetic moment, or magnetization vector parallel with the applied magnetic field. (B) When the frequency of the radiofrequency (RF) pulse matches the Larmor frequency, the protons absorb the RF energy causing some low-energy nuclei to convert to the high-energy state, reducing the net longitudinal magnetic vector (*vertical blue arrow* in Z-axis).

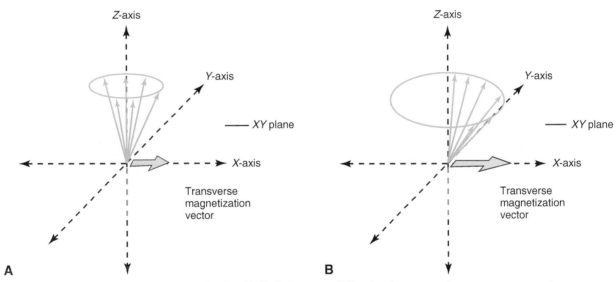

Fig. 13.18 Transverse Magnetization. (A) Radiofrequency (RF) pulse also causes the protons to precess in phase with each other, resulting in a net tissue magnetization vector in the transverse plane (*XY* plane). (B) Increasing the intensity and duration RF of the pulse increases the transverse magnetization vector because the nuclei are more nearly in phase (*horizontal blue arrow* in *X*-axis).

When the RF pulse is applied, hydrogen nuclei precess around the Z-axis in phase (or in sync with each other). After the RF pulse is stopped, the magnetic moments of adjacent hydrogen nuclei begin to interfere with one another, causing the nuclei to dephase (precess asynchronously relative to each other) with a resultant loss of the transverse magnetization, M_{XY}. The time constant that describes the exponential rate of loss of transverse magnetization is called the T2 relaxation time or the spin-spin relaxation time. As the transverse magnetization rapidly decays to zero, so does the amplitude and duration of the detected radio signal. T2 relaxation occurs more rapidly than T1 relaxation. Like T1 times, T2 times are also a feature of the tissues being examined. In fat, the molecules are closely packed, and this results in more potent dephasing interactions between adjacent hydrogen nuclei. Thus, tissues with higher fat content have short T2 relaxation times. In contrast, molecular arrangement of water is more widely spaced, and thus tissues containing more fluid have long T2 relaxation times.

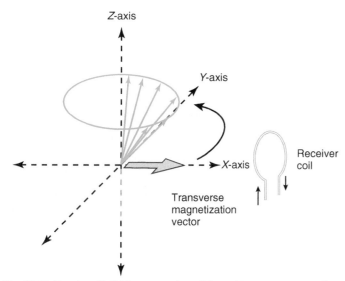

Fig. 13.19 Receiver Coil. The precession of the net transverse magnetic vector in the *XY* plane induces a current flow in a receiver coil, the magnetic resonance signal. The frequency of this induced alternating current signal matches the frequency of the radiofrequency pulse and the Larmor frequency of hydrogen nuclei.

TABLE 13.3   T1 and T2 Relaxation Times in a Main Field of 1.5 T

Tissue Type	T1 Time (ms)	T2 Time (ms)
Fat	240–250	60–80
Bone marrow	550	50
White matter of cerebrum	780	90
Gray matter of cerebrum	920	100
Muscle	860–900	50
Cerebrospinal fluid (similar to water)	2200–2400	500–1400

Clinical Magnetic Resonance Pulse Sequences and Defining Image Contrast

The MR signal produced by a single application of an RF pulse is a relatively weak signal and is inadequate to reconstruct clinically useful MR images. Clinical MR imaging protocols use repeated cycles of RF pulse application and signal detection to accumulate sufficient data to reconstruct an MR image. For example, where the MRI matrix is 256 × 256 pixels, the signal average from 256 measurements is used. Additionally, the timing and polarity of the RF pulses, and the timing of signal measurements can be modulated to generate images with different tissue contrasts. An MR *pulse sequence* describes the temporal sequence of these parameters as set by the operator to determine the appearance of the resultant image. The two fundamental MR sequences are *spin-echo (SE)* and *gradient-echo (GRE)* sequences—contemporary MR sequences are variations of these two sequences, with modulation or addition of parameters. Most maxillofacial MRI examinations are performed with modifications to the conventional spin-echo sequence, graphically depicted in Fig. 13.20.

In spin-echo MR imaging, a 90-degree RF pulse is applied to induce a transverse magnetization, M_{XY}. Following this RF pulse, the longitudinal magnetization M_Z starts to increase (T1 relaxation), and the nuclei dephase at a rate determined by tissue properties (T2 relaxation). Unrelated to tissue properties, inhomogeneity in the external magnetic field causes rapid dephasing and decrease of M_{XY} and masks differences in tissue T2 relaxation properties. To minimize this undesirable influence, a 180-degree RF pulse is applied to refocus the precession, increase the transverse magnetization M_{XY}, and produce a measurable signal that is reflective of tissue properties.

Fast spin-echo (FSE) and turbo spin-echo (TSE) are modifications of the traditional spin-echo sequence and are designed for more rapid image acquisition. Gradient-echo sequences refocus spins by applying gradient fields, rather than using a 180-degree RF pulse. Additionally, the initial RF pulse is a 90-degree or smaller RF pulse. Some modifications are designed to enhance or suppress signals from specific tissues. For example, the Short T1 Inversion Recovery (STIR), the Chemical Shift Selective (CHESS) and the Fat Saturation (FATSAT) sequences minimize the signal from fat allowing improved visualization of adjacent structures. Similarly, fluid attenuated inversion recovery (FLAIR) sequences minimize the signal from fluid, allowing for better visualization of pathology adjacent to the CSF.

The key parameters of a pulse sequence are the repetition time (TR) and echo time (TE). The TR is the duration between repeat 90-degree RF pulses (see Fig. 13.20), and determines the amount of T1 relaxation that has occurred at the time the signal is collected. The TE is the time

Fig. 13.20 Spin-Echo Pulse Sequences. The basic features of a magnetic resonance *(MR)* pulse sequence are the repetition time (*TR*, the duration between repeat 90-degree RF pulses) and the echo time (*TE*, the time after application of the 90-degree radiofrequency *(RF)* pulse when the MR signal is read). TR determines the amount of T1 relaxation that has occurred at the time the signal is collected, whereas TE controls the amount of T2 relaxation that has occurred when the signal is collected. In the spin-echo sequence, a 180-degree pulse is applied to refocus the spins. The timing of this pulse is half the TE time.

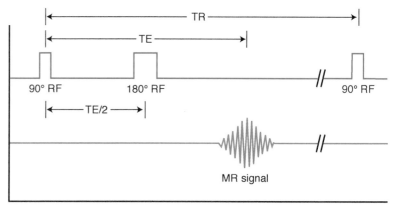

Time

between the center of the 90-degree RF pulse and the center of echo measurement, when the MR signal is read. It controls the amount of T2 relaxation that has occurred when the signal is collected. Clinical MR imaging protocols adjust the TR and TE to accentuate differences in tissues based on their T1 relaxation time, T2 relaxation time, or proton density (Table 13.4), and produce images with different spectrums of tissue contrast (Fig. 13.21).

T1-Weighted Image

A T1-weighted image emphasizes differences in T1 values of tissues (see Table 13.3); this is accomplished by use of short TR (typically 400 to 800 ms with a 1.5 T magnetic field) and short TE (20 ms). In such images, tissues with short T1 times, such as fat, appear bright, whereas tissues with long T1 times, such as CSF (water), appear dark (see Fig. 13.21). T1-weighted images are more commonly used to demonstrate anatomy.

T2-Weighted Image

A T2-weighted image emphasizes differences in T2 values of tissues (see Table 13.3); this is accomplished by use of long TR (2000 ms) and long TE (typically 80 to 150 ms). In such images, tissues with long T2

TABLE 13.4 Manipulation of Magnetic Resonance Image Contrast by Manipulation of Repetition Time and Echo Time

Image Contrast	Repetition Time	Echo Time
T1-weighted	Short (400–800 ms)	Short (≤25 ms)
T2-weighted	Long (>2000 ms)	Long (80–150 ms)
Proton density-weighted	Long (>2000 ms)	Short (≤25 ms)

Repetition and echo times (in milliseconds) for imaging in a 1.5 T magnetic field.

times, such as CSF or temporomandibular joint (TMJ) fluid, appear bright, whereas tissues with short T2 times, such as fat, appear dark (Fig. 13.22). Images with T2 weighting are used to depict pathologic changes, such as inflammation and neoplasia.

There are many pulse sequences varying the strength and timing of the RF pulses that emphasize or suppress various tissues in the resultant images.

Scanner Gradients

To generate an image, MR signals from the patient must be spatially assigned to generate an image. This is accomplished by using three gradient coils within the bore of the imaging magnet oriented in the X (left to right), Y (anterior to posterior), and Z (head to toe) planes, which modify the intensity of the magnetic field surrounding the patient. The Z-axis gradient creates a gradient magnetic field in the craniocaudal dimension. When this gradient is applied, the Larmor frequency of hydrogen nuclei varies linearly along the magnetic gradient. The RF pulse frequency is selected to match the Larmor frequency in the desired axial slice of tissue to be imaged. The slope of the gradient applied and the bandwidth (range) of the RF pulse determine the thickness of this slice. The location of the signal within the X and Y (transverse) planes is derived by switching off the Z-gradient coil followed by rapidly turning on the X-gradient and then the Y-gradient coils (termed phase encoding and frequency encoding, respectively). The resulting MR signals can now be separated based on their locations in the X, Y, and Z planes allowing for 3D reconstruction of the MR image.

Contrast Agents

Contrast agents, most commonly gadolinium, may be administered intravenously to improve tissue contrast (Figs. 13.23 and 13.24). Gadolinium is a paramagnetic substance and shortens the T1 relaxation times of tissues, making them appear brighter. Tissues that enhance include normal tissues, such as vessels with slow-flowing blood, sinus mucosa, and muscle. Pathologic tissues including neoplasms, infections, inflammations, and posttraumatic lesions often enhance allowing them to be better differentiated from surrounding normal tissue.

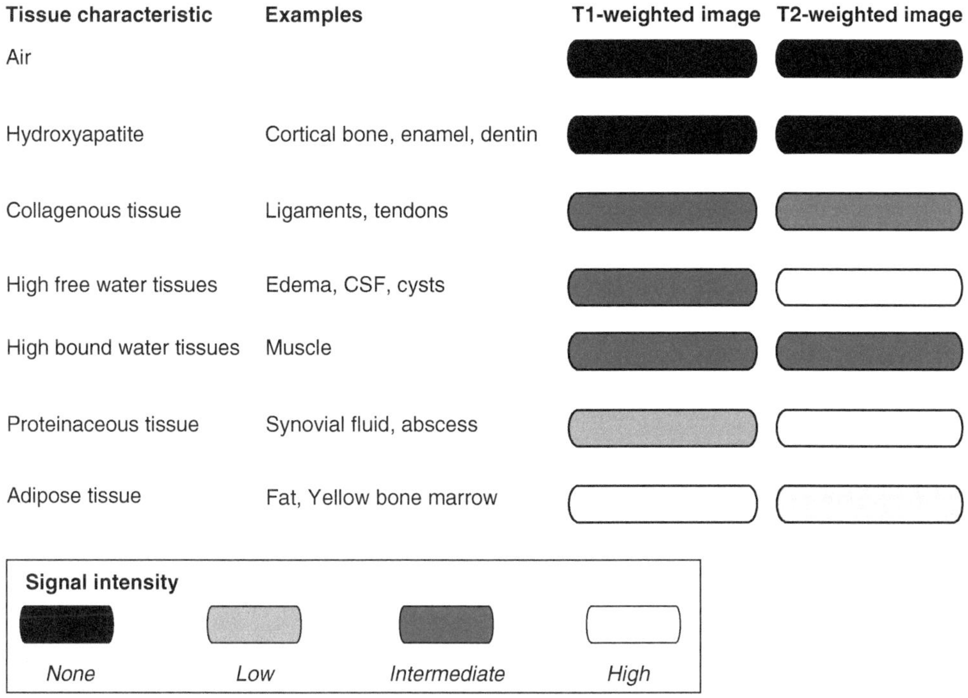

Tissue characteristic	Examples	T1-weighted image	T2-weighted image
Air			
Hydroxyapatite	Cortical bone, enamel, dentin		
Collagenous tissue	Ligaments, tendons		
High free water tissues	Edema, CSF, cysts		
High bound water tissues	Muscle		
Proteinaceous tissue	Synovial fluid, abscess		
Adipose tissue	Fat, Yellow bone marrow		

Fig. 13.21 Signal Intensity of Relevant Tissues in the Craniofacial Region on T1- and T2-Weighted Imaging. The signal intensities are characterized on a scale of no signal intensity (black) to low, intermediate, and high signal intensity (bright). CSF, Cerebrospinal fluid.

Signal intensity

| None | Low | Intermediate | High |

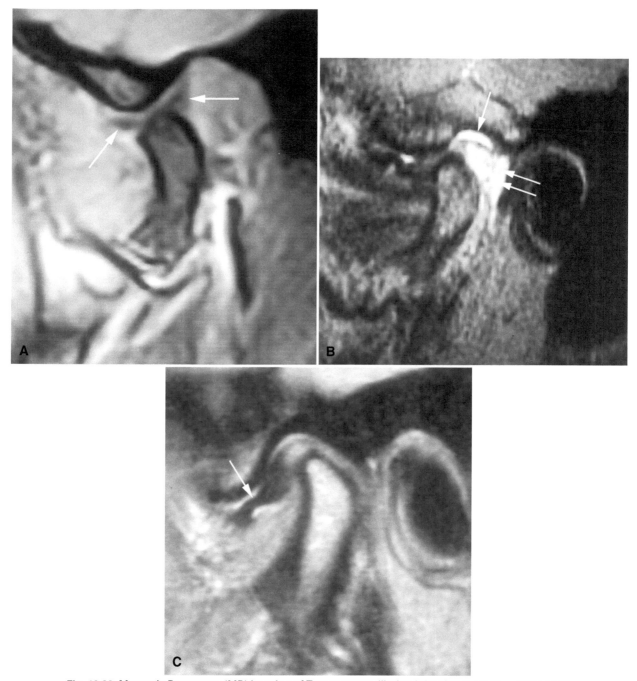

Fig. 13.22 Magnetic Resonance (MR) Imaging of Temporomandibular Joint (TMJ). (A) T1-weighted MR image of the TMJ. In this image, the jaw is partly open, as indicated by the location of the condyle relative to the articular eminence. The articular disk, which has a "bow tie" appearance *(arrows)*, is in a normal position relative to the translating condyle. (B) T2-weighted MR image of the TMJ illustrates both inflammatory effusion into the superior joint space *(arrow)* and hyperemia caused by increased vasculature in the retrodiscal tissues *(double arrows)*. (C) In this proton or spin density MR image of the TMJ, the disk is anteriorly displaced *(arrow)*, with the posterior band in the 9 o'clock position relative to the condylar head. (B and C, Courtesy Richard Harper, DDS, Dallas, TX.)

Evidence suggests an association between intravenous gadolinium administration use and nephrogenic systemic fibrosis. Primary risk factors are renal failure and a low estimated glomerular filtration rate (eGFR < 30). The American College of Radiology (ACR) recommends evaluation of serum creatinine in all patients who will receive intravenous gadolinium administration. In high-risk patients, such as patients 60 years and older, or those with a history of renal disease, the eGFR is calculated. When the eGFR is lower than 30, gadolinium administration is not recommended.

Advantages and Limitations of Magnetic Resonance Imaging

MR imaging has several advantages over other diagnostic imaging procedures.

- *Superior contrast resolution of soft tissues.* X-ray attenuation coefficients of soft tissues may vary by no more than 1%, limiting radiographic contrast. However, T1 and T2 relaxation times may vary by up to 40%.

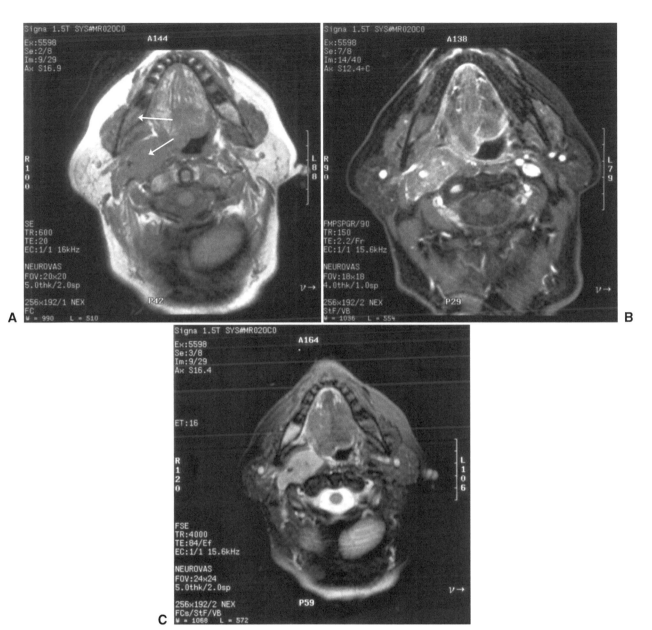

Fig. 13.23 Magnetic Resonance (MR) Images. MR imaging examination performed to evaluate a neck mass in a patient with a known diagnosis of multiple myeloma. (A) Axial T1 precontrast (no fat saturation) image through the mandible. Note abnormally dark marrow in the posterior right mandible (*upper arrow*, compare with left side) and mass in the right carotid space *(lower arrow)*. (B) Axial T1 postcontrast image with fat saturation. Note abnormal enhancement of the mass in the right carotid space. (C) Axial T2 with fat saturation demonstrating an abnormally bright signal in both the marrow in the right mandible and the mass in the right carotid space. (Courtesy Dr. Thomas Underhill, Radiology Associates, Richmond, VA.)

- No ionizing radiation associated risks.
- Direct multiplanar imaging in all three planes is possible without reorienting the patient.

Disadvantages of MR imaging include:

- Relatively long imaging times limit its use in patients who may not be able to hold still for extended periods of time.
- Patients with claustrophobia may not be able to tolerate the confined imaging space within the MRI scanner.
- The presence of ferromagnetic substances within the patient's body poses potential hazards—the strong magnetic fields can move these objects, cause excessive heating, or induce strong electrical currents, which may harm the patient. MRI is contraindicated in patients with implanted electronic medical devices such as cardiac pacemakers, some cerebral aneurysm clips, and in patients with embedded ferrous foreign bodies, such as shrapnel or bullets.
- Metals used in dental restorations do not move but often significantly distort the image in their vicinity. Titanium implants cause only minor local image degradation. Removable dental appliances must be removed prior to MRI scanning.
- *Special considerations in imaging patients undergoing orthodontic treatment:*

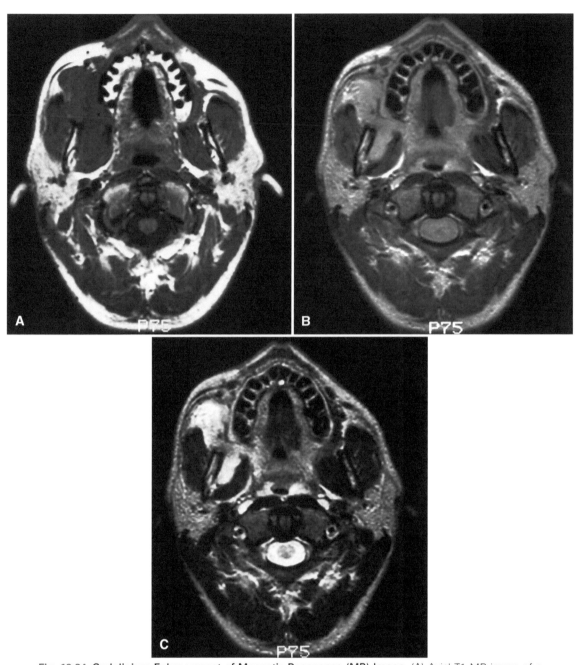

Fig. 13.24 Gadolinium Enhancement of Magnetic Resonance (MR) Image. (A) Axial T1 MR image of a rhabdomyosarcoma involving the soft tissues of the right face. The tumor cannot be distinguished from the adjacent masseter and pterygoid muscles because both have the same tissue signal. (B) Axial T1 postgadolinium MR image. The tumor now has a brighter signal (lighter) than the adjacent muscles because of its greater vascularity, enhanced by gadolinium. (C) Axial T2 MR image. The tumor has a brighter signal than adjacent muscles because of greater fluid content of the tumor.

- Steel orthodontic archwires are subject to substantially high forces and may need to be removed. Archwires made of cobalt chromium, nickel titanium, and titanium molybdenum exhibit minimal forces.
- Stainless steel brackets, bands, and fixed retainers should be checked to ensure secure attachment, and may be left in place if secure, unless they interfere with the region of the image being examined.

Applications of Magnetic Resonance Imaging in Maxillofacial Diagnosis

Because of its excellent soft-tissue contrast resolution, MR imaging is useful in evaluating soft tissue conditions. Applications of MRI in dentistry include:

- Evaluate the position and integrity of the TMJ articular disk (see Fig. 13.22).

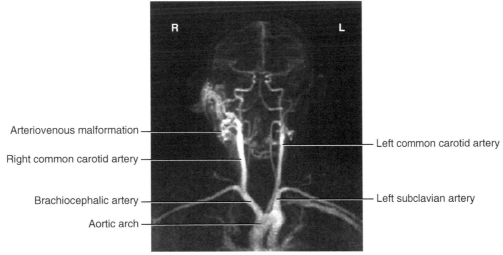

Fig. 13.25 Magnetic Resonance Angiography of the Head and Neck. This image, made with gadolinium as a contrast agent, demonstrates an arteriovenous malformation in the region of the right face. Note the widened carotid artery and rich vasculature supply in the right midfacial region. This is a maximum intensity image made from a stack of individual slices. (Image courtesy Dr. Susan White, UCLA School of Dentistry.)

- Evaluate neoplasms of oral cavity and jaws to determine soft-tissue extent, lymph node involvement, and perineural invasion (see Figs. 13.23 and 13.24).
- Evaluate salivary gland diseases, including cysts and neoplasms, infections, and obstructions.
- Evaluate vascular lesions in the orofacial region (Fig. 13.25).
- Evaluate suspected early osteomyelitis of the jaws to determine edematous changes in the fatty marrow and the surrounding soft tissue.

NUCLEAR MEDICINE

Projection radiography, CT imaging, MR imaging, and diagnostic ultrasonography are morphologic imaging techniques that record macroscopic anatomic changes in the image. In contrast, diagnostic nuclear medicine monitors incorporation of radionuclides in the tissues and provides functional information on the nature of the pathophysiologic change. Diagnostic applications of nuclear medicine relevant to maxillofacial diseases include detection and monitoring of metastatic disease, bone tumors, skeletal growth disturbances, and infection.

Radionuclide imaging uses radioactive atoms or molecules that emit γ (gamma) rays. Radionuclides allow measurement of tissue function in vivo and provide an early marker of disease through detection and measurement of biochemical change. After the radionuclides are administered, they distribute in the body according to their chemical properties, like their stable isotopes. In nuclear medicine, the patient's tissues serve as the source of radiation, and the intensity and location of the signal are the key parameters in its interpretation. In *planar scintigraphy*, a gamma camera detects γ rays and forms images to demonstrate the distribution and locations of the radionuclide in the body. *Single photon emission computed tomographic (SPECT) imaging* and *PET imaging* are advanced nuclear medicine techniques that generate tomographic views, and this functional information is often superimposed onto the morphological information from MDCT examinations.

Planar Bone Scintigraphy

Bone scintigraphy is a two-dimensional imaging technique that depicts the locations of active bone turnover. It uses the radionuclide technetium

TABLE 13.5   Three-Phase Skeletal Scintigraphy

Phase	Description	Time After Injection	Functional Information
1	Blood flow	30–60 s	Reflects vascularity
2	Blood pool	Within 10 min	Reflects soft-tissue involvement
3	Delayed	2–6 h	Reflects osteoblastic activity

99m (^{99m}Tc). ^{99m}Tc has a half-life of 6 hours and emits primarily 140 keV γ-photons. To image bone, ^{99m}Tc is bound to methylene diphosphonate (MDP), a pyrophosphate analog. The compound is stable, is not metabolized in the body, and is rapidly cleared from plasma by renal excretion, with more than 70% of the administered radioactivity cleared within 6 hours. Bone scintigraphy has a high sensitivity and can detect as low as 5% to 10% demineralization in bone. Its location to bone depends on the local vascularity and the degree of osteoblastic activity. Approximately 30% of the administered radionuclide is adsorbed onto bone, with the maximal uptake occurring within the first hour.

The three-phase bone scan is a common protocol for ^{99m}Tc-MDP imaging. A dose of 740 to 1110 megabecquerels (MBq, approximately 20 to 30 mCi) is administered by intravenous injection. Subsequently, images are acquired with a gamma camera, which uses scintillation crystals as radiation detectors, giving the technique the name scintigraphy. The effective dose from bone scintigraphy is approximately 3 to 6 mSv (see Chapter 3).

The three phases are described in Table 13.5. Both blood flow and osteoblastic activity influence uptake. Radionuclide uptake is more in trabecular bone, and in areas which have a larger mineralization surface such as the spine. In children, osteoblastic activity associated with growth in children causes increased uptake in the physes and facial bones. The low-level bone turnover associated with periodontal disease also manifests as increased uptake.

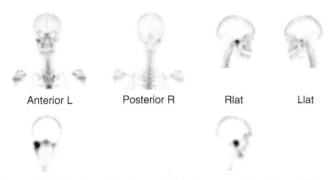

Anterior L   Posterior R   Rlat   Llat

Fig. 13.26 Radionuclide Image With Increased Uptake of ⁹⁹ᵐTc-Methylene Diphosphonate (MDP) in the Region of the Right Temporomandibular Joint. The planar images in the top row were captured with a gamma camera. The lower two tomographic images were captured with single photon emission computed tomographic (SPECT) imaging.

Single Photon Emission Computed Tomography

SPECT imaging is a tomographic nuclear medicine technique (see Fig. 13.27). In this technique, the gamma camera is rotated 360 degrees around the patient. Image acquisition takes about 30 to 45 minutes. The acquired data are processed by mathematical reconstruction algorithms into contiguous axial slices, as in CBCT and MDCT imaging. The tomographic imaging minimizes superimposition and increases the contrast and spatial resolution. SPECT images can be fused with CT images to combine the functional and morphological information (see Fig. 13.27D and E).

Applications of Bone Scintigraphy and Single Photon Emission Computed Tomography

Bone scintigraphy and SPECT have the following applications in diagnosis and treatment planning of maxillofacial disease, and capitalize on the high sensitivity of this technique.
- Primary and metastatic bone tumors
- Abnormalities of the temporomandibular joint, such as condylar hyperplasia and condylar resorption (Fig. 13.26)
- Osteomyelitis and osteonecrosis of the jaws (Figs. 13.27 and 13.28)
- Skeletal dysplasias—fibrous dysplasia and Paget disease

Positron Emission Tomographic Imaging

PET imaging is a tomographic diagnostic nuclear medicine technique. PET imaging has a sensitivity nearly 100 times that of a gamma camera, and relies on positron-emitting radionuclides. One technique uses the compound 2-[¹⁸F] fluoro-2-deoxy-D-glucose (FDG) which is incorporated into cells with a high glycolytic activity. The radiopharmaceutical emits a positron, which interacts with a free electron and mutual annihilation occurs, resulting in the production of two 551-keV photons emitted at 180 degrees to each other. The PET scanner consists of a ring of many detectors in a circle around the patient (Fig. 13.29). Electronically coupled opposing detectors simultaneously identify the pair of γ photons and this forms the basis of spatial location of the

signal origin. Contemporary PET-CT scanners sequentially acquire the PET image and the CT image and superimpose morphological and functional information (Fig. 13.30).

Applications

In maxillofacial diagnosis, FDG-PET/CT imaging is useful to detect and monitor metastatic bone disease, primary and recurrent malignancies (see Fig. 13.30), and osteomyelitis.

Ultrasonography

Sonography is a technique based on sound waves that acquires images in real time without the use of ionizing radiation. The phenomenon perceived as sound is the result of periodic changes in the pressure of air against the eardrum. The periodicity of these changes ranges from 1500 to 20,000 Hz. By definition, ultrasound has a periodicity greater than 20 kHz, which is greater than the audible range. Diagnostic ultrasonography (or sonography), the clinical application of ultrasound, uses vibratory frequencies in the range of 1 to 20 MHz.

Scanners used for sonography generate electrical impulses that are converted into ultra-high-frequency sound waves by a transducer, a device that can convert one form of energy into another—in this case, electrical energy into sonic energy. The transducer emitting ultrasound is held against the body part being examined. The ultrasonic beam passes through or interacts with tissues of different acoustic impedance. Sonic waves that reflect (echo) toward the transducer are detected by the transducer, amplified, processed, and displayed as a digital image. Current techniques permit echoes to be processed at a sufficiently rapid rate to allow perception of motion; this is referred to as real-time imaging.

The ultrasound signal transmitted into a patient is attenuated by a combination of absorption, reflection, refraction, and diffusion. The higher the frequency of the sound waves, the higher the image resolution, but the less the penetration of the sound through soft tissue. The fraction of the beam that is reflected to the transducer depends on the acoustic impedance of the tissue, which is a product of its density (and the velocity of sound through it) and the beam's angle of incidence. Because of its acoustic impedance, a tissue has a characteristic internal echo pattern. Consequently, not only can changes in echo patterns distinguish between different tissues and boundaries, but they also can be correlated with pathologic changes within a tissue. Tissues that do not produce signals, such as fluid-filled cysts, are said to be anechoic and appear black. Tissues that produce a weak signal are hypoechoic, whereas tissues that produce intense signals, such as ligaments, skin, or needles or catheters, are hyperechoic and appear bright. Thus, interpretation of sonograms relies on knowledge of both the physical properties of ultrasound and the anatomy of the tissues being scanned.

Ultrasonography is used in the head and neck region for evaluation of neoplasms in the thyroid, parathyroid, salivary glands, or lymph nodes; stones in salivary glands or ducts; Sjögren's syndrome; and the vessels of the neck, including the carotid artery for atherosclerotic plaques (see Figs. 13.30 and 13.31). Ultrasonography is also used to guide fine-needle aspiration in the neck. More recent advances include 3D imaging to allow multiplanar reformatting, surface renderings (e.g., of a fetal face), and color Doppler sonography for evaluation of blood flow (Fig. 13.32).

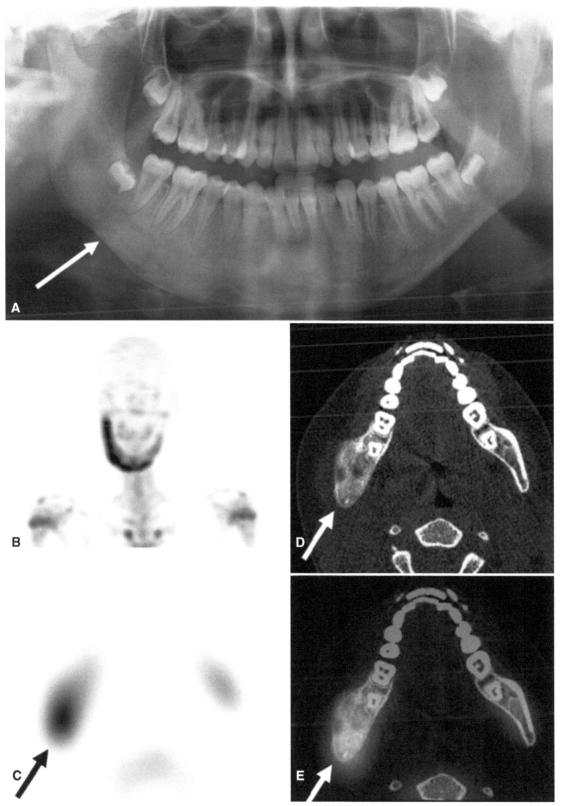

Fig. 13.27 Single Photon Emission Computed Tomographic (SPECT)/Computed Tomography (CT) Imaging of a 14-Year-Old Girl With Chronic Osteomyelitis of the Mandible. (A) Panoramic view demonstrating expansion and sclerosis of the right mandible *(arrow)*. (B) Planar radionuclide image showing uptake throughout the mandible and especially on the right side. (C) SPECT axial image showing increased activity in the posterior regions of both sides of the mandible and especially on the right side *(arrow)*. (D) CT axial image at the same level as the image in C. Note periosteal expansion and lytic areas in the right mandible *(arrow)*. (E) SPECT/ CT fusion image demonstrating the area of greatest activity in the right mandible *(arrow)*. (Modified from Strobel K, Merwald M, Huellner MW, et al: [Importance of SPECT/CT for resolving diseases of the jaw] [in German]. *Radiologe.* 2012;52:638–645.)

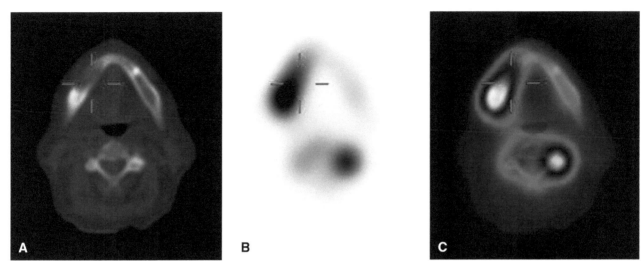

Fig. 13.28 Single Photon Emission Computed Tomographic Image of Bisphosphonate Osteonecrosis of the Jaw in a Woman With Breast Cancer Treated With Zoledronic Acid for 2 Years Because of a Metastatic Lesion to C2. (A) Axial computed tomography image demonstrating bisphosphonate-associated osteonecrosis of the jaw (BRONJ) in the left mandible that is mostly lytic but also sclerotic more posteriorly. (B) SPECT image showing extensive deposition of ^{99m}Tc pertechnetate in the left body of the mandible and region of right articular surface of C2. (C) Fusion image demonstrating isotope uptake most extensive in the sclerotic (posterior) portion of the BRONJ lesion and in the sclerotic metastatic lesion in C2. (Images courtesy Dott.ssa Franca Dore, Azienda Ospedaliero-Universitaria Trieste.)

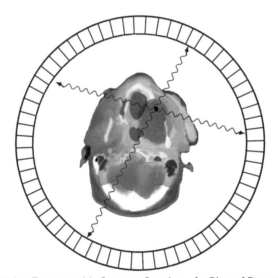

Fig. 13.29 Positron Emission Tomographic Scanner Consists of a Ring of Detectors That Measure Pairs of 511 keV γ Rays Traveling in Opposite Directions From Positron Annihilation. Each pair is recorded simultaneously; thus, the location of the radionuclide can be determined as the intersection of the pairs of detectors recording simultaneous events. The location of the common source of the radionuclide is readily determined as the intersection of the flight paths of the γ rays.

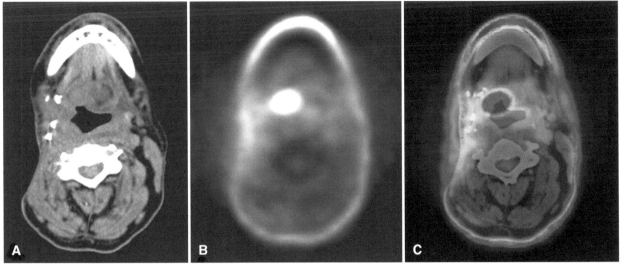

Fig. 13.30 Positron Emission Tomographic (PET) Scan and Fused Positron Emission Tomographic/Computed Tomography (CT) Scan. This patient has a known recurrent carcinoma at the base of the tongue. (A) Soft-tissue algorithm CT image at the level of the inferior border of the mandible. The four metallic objects on the patient's right side posterior to the mandible represent vascular clips from prior surgery. (B) Fluoro-2-deoxy-D-glucose (FDG)-PET scan showing an *oval-shaped* region of high metabolic activity of tumor at the right tongue base. The FDG activity in the anterior mandible is related to low-level metabolic activity in the vicinity of a reconstruction plate. (C) Fused images A and B demonstrating the region of high metabolic activity superimposed on the CT anatomy. The intensity of the FDG activity has been color-coded with red being the highest intensity and purple being the lowest. Images were acquired on a combined PET/CT scanner. (Courtesy Dr. Todd W. Stultz, Cleveland Clinic, OH.)

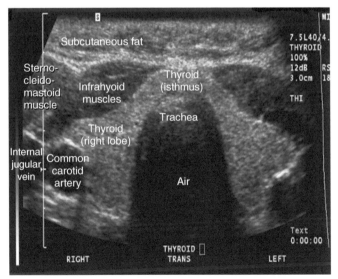

Fig. 13.31 Ultrasound Examination (Transverse Section) of a Healthy Thyroid Gland. This image shows glandular, muscular, adipose, and vascular tissues because of the different acoustic impedance of these tissues. (Courtesy Dr. Christos Angelopoulos, Columbia University, College of Dental Medicine, NY.)

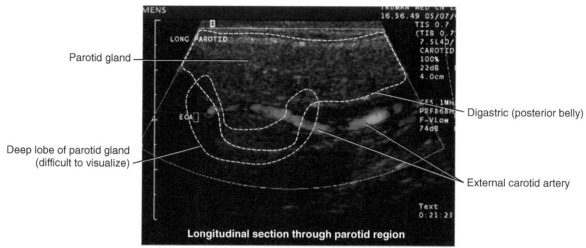

Parotid gland

Deep lobe of parotid gland
(difficult to visualize)

Digastric (posterior belly)

External carotid artery

Longitudinal section through parotid region

Fig. 13.32 Doppler Ultrasound Examination. Longitudinal section through the parotid gland, including the deep lobe, and posterior belly of digastric muscle. With Doppler ultrasound, the transducer records small changes in the direction of blood flow. In this image, the external carotid artery is coded red where blood flows toward the transducer and blue where it moves away from the transducer. (Courtesy Dr. Christos Angelopoulos, Columbia University, College of Dental Medicine, NY.)

BIBLIOGRAPHY

Computed Tomography

American College of Radiology: ACR-ASNR-SPR practice parameter for the performance of computed tomography (CT) of the extracranial head and neck. 2012; Available at: https://www.acr.org/~/media/ACR/Documents/PGTS/guidelines/CT_Head_Neck.pdf. Accessed July 30, 2017.

Bushberg JT, Seibert JA, Leidholdt EM Jr, et al. *The Essential Physics of Medical Imaging.* 3rd ed. Baltimore: Lippincott Williams & Wilkins; 2012.

Fishman EK, Jeffrey RB Jr. *Multidetector CT: Principles, Techniques, and Clinical Applications.* Philadelphia: Lippincott Williams & Wilkins; 2004.

Mahesh M. *MDCT Physics: The Basics - Technology, Image Quality and Radiation Dose.* Lippincott Williams & Wilkins; 2009.

Mahesh M. Search for isotropic resolution in CT from conventional through multiple-row detector. *Radiographics.* 2002;22(4):949–962.

Magnetic Resonance Imaging

Blink EJ. An easy introduction to basic MRI physics for anyone who does not have a degree in physics: http://mri-physics.net/.

Bushberg JT, Seibert JA, Leidholdt EM Jr, et al. *The Essential Physics of Medical Imaging.* 3rd ed. Baltimore: Lippincott Williams & Wilkins; 2012.

Bushong SC, Clarke G. *Magnetic Resonance Imaging: Physical and Biological Principles.* 4th ed. St Louis: Mosby; 2015.

Elison JM, Leggitt VL, Thomson M, et al. Influence of common orthodontic appliances on the diagnostic quality of cranial magnetic resonance images. *Am J Orthod Dentofacial Orthop.* 2008;134:563–572.

Patel A, Bhavra GS, O'Neill JR. MRI scanning and orthodontics. *J Orthod.* 2006;33:246–249.

Nuclear Medicine

Christian P, Waterstram-Rich KM. *Nuclear Medicine and PET/CT: Technology and Techniques.* 7th ed. St Louis: Mosby; 2011.

Dore F, Filippi L, Biasotto M, et al. Bone scintigraphy and SPECT/CT of bisphosphonate-induced osteonecrosis of the jaw. *J Nucl Med.* 2009;50:30–35.

Schiepers C. *Diagnostic Nuclear Medicine.* 2nd ed. Berlin: Springer; 2006.

Sharp PF, Gemmell HG, Murray AD. *Practical Nuclear Medicine.* 3rd ed. London: Springer-Verlag; 2005.

Van den Wyngaert T, Huizing MT, Fossion E, et al. Prognostic value of bone scintigraphy in cancer patients with osteonecrosis of the jaw. *Clin Nucl Med.* 2011;36:17–20.

Ultrasound

Emshoff R, Bertram S, Strobl H. Ultrasonographic cross-sectional characteristics of muscles of the head and neck. *Oral Surg Oral Med Oral Pathol Oral Radiol Endod.* 1999;87:93–106.

Kremkau FW. *Sonography: Principles and Instruments.* 8th ed. St Louis: Saunders; 2010.

Rumack CM, Wilson SR, Charboneau JW, et al. *Diagnostic Ultrasound.* 4th ed. Philadelphia: Mosby; 2011.

Shimizu M, Okamura K, Yoshiura K, et al. Sonographic diagnostic criteria for screening Sjögren's syndrome. *Oral Surg Oral Med Oral Pathol Oral Radiol Endod.* 2006;102:85–93.

Tempkin B. *Ultrasound Scanning: Principles and Protocols.* 3rd ed. St Louis: Saunders; 2009.

14

Beyond Three-Dimensional Imaging

Sanjay M. Mallya

Over the past decade, technological advances in three-dimensional (3D) imaging with computed tomography (CT) have enhanced dentomaxillofacial diagnosis and treatment planning. In parallel to the growth of cone beam CT (CBCT), there is an increasing number of digital technologies that are being applied in dentistry. Such technologies are diverse in nature with applications in electronic health record documentation and communication, computer-aided design (CAD), computer-aided manufacturing (CAM), and, more recently, machine learning and artificial intelligence. The ability to integrate digital information from different sources has yielded innovative approaches to treatment planning, fabrication of dental appliances and restorations, and monitoring of treatment. This chapter provides an overview of contemporary technologies that maximize the information provided by CBCT imaging to augment diagnosis and treatment planning.

FOUR-DIMENSIONAL IMAGING

Diagnostic imaging is often performed to assess temporal changes (e.g., to monitor disease progression or recurrence) or to evaluate outcomes of treatment. For the most part, this is typically accomplished by a subjective visual comparison of the regions of interest on two radiographic examinations that were acquired at different times. Special software applications can merge digital information from these two images to identify interval changes that are not easily perceptible by visual evaluation. These applications typically create and display a composite image to provide a visual, interactive interface to facilitate subjective and quantitative evaluation of disease- or treatment-related changes.

Previously, such comparative techniques were used to assess dental caries, periodontal disease, and healing of apical periodontal lesions on conventional two-dimensional (2D) intraoral radiographs. These techniques applied subtraction radiography, a computer-based approach, to merge information from temporally separated digital images and "subtract" the common information to portray the interval change. However, this approach is significantly limited by the 2D nature of periapical and bite-wing radiographs. Small changes in the relationships between the x-ray beam, receptor, and the patient cause perceptible changes in the projected radiographic image and yield artifacts on subtraction images, decreasing the technique's specificity. Thus subtraction radiography using intraoral images has not translated into a routine clinical practice. However, the 3D nature of CBCT images overcomes the limitations of 2D projection geometry. Several software applications have been developed for CBCT image superimposition and quantitative analysis of changes. Some commercial CBCT analysis software suites (e.g., InVivo [Anatomage, San Jose, CA] and OnDemand 3D [Cybermed Inc., Seoul, Korea]) incorporate such modules to facilitate comparison of serial imaging.

Four-dimensional (4D) CBCT imaging, also referred to as image superimposition, uses two CBCT volumes of the same patient acquired at different time points. It is imperative that these two CBCT examinations are reconstructed with the same voxel size. The first step is *image registration*—a process to spatially align the two CBCT volumes. This process establishes spatial correspondence between voxels of the two image datasets. The second step is *image transformation*—where computer algorithms identify corresponding points or regions within the two CBCT datasets and calculate the volume rotations that must be applied to maximize the alignment of corresponding points and regions. Such "rigid body" transformations change only the position and orientation of the scan volume and do not alter the shape or size of the individual CBCT volume. Image registration may be facilitated by providing external markers (e.g., placed on the patient's skin or incorporated into a custom imaging stent). However, this is seldom done in routine clinical practice. Most image registration approaches use the patient anatomy as "markers" for registration. Approaches to image registration are listed as follows.

- *Landmark-based registration.* In this procedure, corresponding anatomic landmark points are identified to serve as spatial location markers on each CBCT volume. These points are recorded via user interaction by manual selection of points on surface segmented images of the two CBCT volumes. Theoretically, three landmark points are sufficient for rigid body transformation of the maxillofacial structures. In practice, more than three points are used. The registration algorithm computes a "centroid"—an average location of the selected points on each image volume. Differences in the 3D spatial location of the two centroids are used to compute the volume rotations that must be applied until distances between corresponding point pairs are minimized.

- *Segmentation-based registration.* Surfaces of the maxillofacial skeleton or skin are identified by segmentation, and the computer algorithm transforms one image volume until the average distances between two corresponding surfaces is minimized. Segmentation is easily accomplished and is computationally less demanding, and the registration can be rapid and automated.

- *Voxel-based registration.* Spatial correspondence is achieved by matching the gray values of individual voxels. The registration algorithm may use the voxels from the entire CBCT volume or from a predefined region selected by the operator. Typically, these methods are fully automated and minimize operator-associated variations in landmark identification. For most maxillofacial applications, the base of the skull has been shown to be a reliable stable region for voxel matching. Voxel-based methods of image registration have been shown to be reliable and reproducible, with registration errors of 0.5 mm or less.

Clinical Applications

The ability to superimpose 3D CBCT volumes facilitates subjective and quantitative evaluations of temporal changes. Some commercial CBCT analysis software suites provide these features, allowing users to apply this technique to clinical practice situations. With software programs that use voxel-based registration, the process of image superimposition is typically automated, reducing operator time and variability. Several research groups have investigated the applicability and reliability of this technique to assess growth and outcomes from orthognathic surgery. Technological enhancements will likely make the process user friendly, rapid, and reliable, and facilitate its application to routine clinical care. Potential clinical applications that would benefit from 4D imaging are listed as follows.

- Evaluate skeletal and soft-tissue changes during orthodontic treatment (Fig. 14.1).
- Evaluate airway morphologic changes caused by orthognathic and orthodontic treatment manipulations and by devices used to manage obstructive sleep apnea (Fig. 14.2).
- Evaluate outcomes of orthodontic and orthognathic surgical treatment to assess stability and relapse (Fig. 14.3).
- Assess growth-associated changes in the maxillofacial skeleton.
- Monitor adaptive changes and disease patterns in the temporomandibular joint after orthodontic and maxillofacial surgical treatments.
- Evaluate osseous healing and success of bone grafts placed for ridge augmentation or surgical reconstruction.
- Monitor stability and recurrence of intraosseous pathologic lesions.

COMPUTER-GUIDED TREATMENT PLANNING

Three-dimensional CT data are valuable for presurgical assessment of the maxillofacial anatomy (e.g., to plan reconstructive maxillofacial surgery for cosmetic, functional, and prosthetic indications or to plan placement of dental implants). Several commercial software applications can use CT volumetric data for computer-aided surgical planning. Some vendors offer these advanced functions as modules that can be added to the standard CBCT analysis suite, facilitating their application to clinical practice. The application of CAD/CAM to maxillofacial surgical interventions is expected to increase. Typically, surgical planning software applications use CBCT Digital Imaging and Communication in Medicine (DICOM) data and provide 3D visualization by surface segmentation and volumetric rendering of the anatomic area imaged. The region of interest (ROI) may be a potential implant site, a pathologic lesion in the jaw, a surgical defect, a maxillofacial developmental aberration, or the site of orthognathic surgery. Via an interactive interface, the user manipulates the CT data and simulates surgical procedures (e.g., implant placement or jaw repositioning). The simulated surgical changes are then exported in digital format and a CAD/CAM-generated tangible object such as a stent or surgical guide is made to transfer the in silico plan to the patient's anatomy during surgery.

Dental implant planning: Computer-aided implant planning is widely used in standard clinical practice. The goal of dental implant treatment is functional and esthetic restoration of the patient's dentition. CT imaging provides essential diagnostic information to evaluate the morphology of the edentulous site, the bone quality at the proposed implant site, and the relationships to the adjacent vital structures and teeth. For accurate and predictable outcomes, dental implant placement should be prosthetically driven. There are several commercial software applications for computer-guided planning and placement of dental implants (see Chapters 11 and 15). Image-guided treatment applications for implant planning are described in detail in Chapter 15.

In general, proprietary implant treatment planning software programs import CBCT data in DICOM format, allowing for a relatively easy transfer of the digital CBCT data to treatment planning software application. Typically, the CBCT is acquired with a radiographic guide in place, to depict the locations of the proposed implants and preferably also the desired anatomy and position of the implant-supported restoration. The treatment planning software includes an "implant library"—customized overlays corresponding to the shape and size of individual implant types. Within the planning software the clinician can virtually place the implant overlays, with consideration to individual anatomic and functional factors, implant parallelism, and the design of the prosthetic restoration. These include the local availability of bone volume, angulation relative to the adjacent teeth, and the proximity to vital structures. The virtually placed implants can be angulated and repositioned to simulate the final desired treatment plan (Fig. 14.4A). Virtual implant treatment planning allows the clinician to assess the need for bone augmentation and whether such augmentation could be accomplished at the time of implant placement (see Fig. 14.4B).

The virtual treatment plan directs fabrication of a CAD/CAM-designed surgical guide (Fig. 14.5). The use of surgical guides allows predictable implant placement with decreased intraoperative time. These guides may be mucosa, bone, or tooth supported. Many software applications allow the user to combine data from an optical intraoral scan of the dentition for better identification of the anatomic boundaries of the teeth and edentulous site mucosa to enhance the accuracy of the surgical guide. Clinicians must be aware that computer-guided dental implant placement is not 100% accurate. Even with the use of a CAD/CAM-fabricated surgical guide, there are deviations in the positions of the final placed implants, relative to the planning. Thus the clinician should incorporate appropriate safety zones into the treatment planning process to ensure that implant placement does not compromise adjacent vital structures and teeth or other implants.

Orthognathic surgery: Conventional approaches to planning orthognathic surgery include cephalometric analysis and mock surgery on stone dental models. More recently, virtual planning has been used to plan these surgical approaches, especially in patients with complex craniofacial deformities. Virtual planning with 3D CT data provides several advantages over conventional techniques. Treatment planning software programs can integrate digital data from CT, optical scans of the dental arch, and soft tissues to provide the clinician with a combined interactive virtual model. This is especially valuable in patients with asymmetric malocclusion and facial asymmetry. Easy communication of the virtual plan facilitates collaboration between the treatment team. Importantly, this approach can decrease the operating room time and decrease surgical complications, thereby decreasing costs and improving patient outcomes. Studies have shown that computer-assisted surgical planning has high accuracy, with average errors of less than 2 mm for linear dimensions and approximately 1.2 degrees for angular measurements. Several commercial software packages are available for virtual maxillofacial surgical planning. These include Dolphin (Dolphin Imaging, Chatsworth, CA), InVivo (Anatomage, San Jose, CA), Maxilim (Mechelen, Belgium), MIMICS, and Proplan CMF (Materialise, Belgium). However, these software applications are expensive, and the process of virtual planning requires expertise and is time intensive. Many maxillofacial surgeons use third-party services for the initial planning, software manipulation, and stent construction.

Virtual orthognathic treatment planning involves several steps and starts by combining anatomic data. The skeletal anatomy is provided by CT imaging, either multidetector CT (MDCT) or CBCT. The dental anatomy is captured by optical scanning of the dentition or by digitization of conventional stone models. In addition, the natural head position and the intercuspal occlusal relationships are registered. Three-dimensional photographs provide facial soft-tissue surface information.

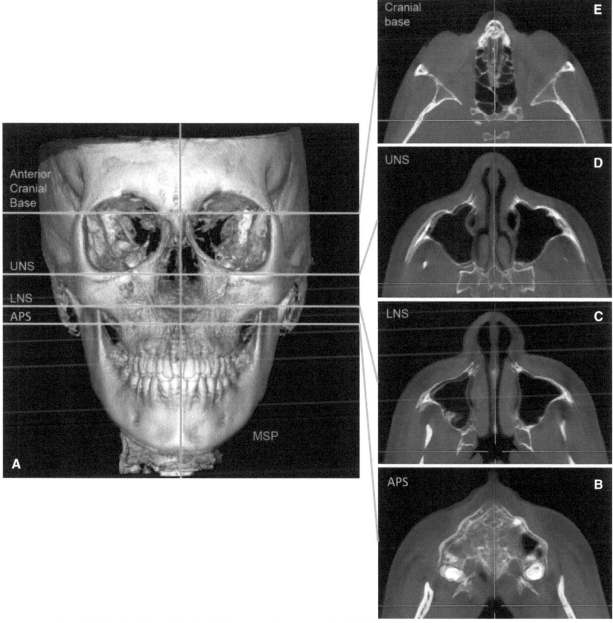

Fig. 14.1 Evaluation of Skeletal Changes Caused by Rapid Palatal Expansion. The maxillary skeletal expander is an implant-assisted device for palatal expansion. In this appliance, four microimplants provide anchorage for forces applied to expand the maxilla. The implants flank the midpalatal suture and engage the cortices of the palate and the nasal floor. Pretreatment and posttreatment cone beam computed tomography scans were registered using automated voxel-based registration (OnDemand 3D, Cybermed Inc., Seoul, Korea), using the region of the anterior cranial base for spatial correlation. Fused images were analyzed to assess treatment-induced changes in the maxilla and midfacial skeleton. Selected fused sections at axial planes through the palate (B) and the upper and lower regions of the nasal cavity (C and D) demonstrate appliance-induced changes in the maxilla, with separation of the midpalatal suture. There is excellent alignment of the osseous anatomy at the region of the anterior cranial base (E), confirming stability of this region which is unaffected by the palatal expansion device. *APS,* Axial palatal section; *LNS,* lower nasal section; *MSP,* maxillary sagittal plane; *UNS,* upper nasal section. (Image courtesy of Daniele Cantarella and Dr. Won Moon, UCLA School of Dentistry. From Cantarella D, Dominguez-Mompell R, Mallya SM, et al. Changes in the midpalatal and pterygopalatine sutures induced by micro-implant-supported skeletal expander, analyzed with a novel 3D method based on CBCT imaging. *Prog Orthod.* 2017;18:34.)

A. Superimposed volumes

B. Superimposed sections

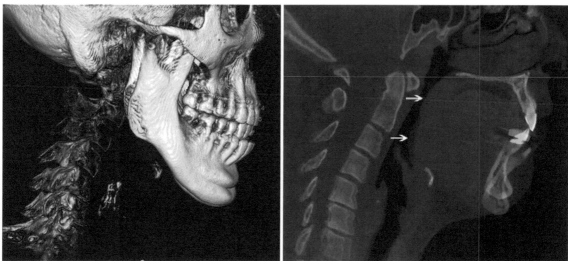

Fig. 14.2 Airway Changes Caused by a Mandibular Advancement Device for Obstructive Sleep Apnea. Obstructive sleep apnea, a chronic sleep disorder caused by upper airway collapse during sleep, is often managed with an oral appliance that advances the mandible and pulls the tongue anteriorly to increase patency of the oropharynx. Pretreatment and postappliance cone beam computed tomography scans were registered and superimposed using the InVivo software program (Anatomage, San Jose, CA). (A) Superimposed three-dimensional volumetric reconstructions showing an anterior and downward movement of the mandible when the appliance is worn. (B) Superimposed midsagittal sections showing that the appliance causes a slight anterior movement of the tongue *(white arrow)*. Note absence change in the position of the soft palate *(yellow arrow)*.

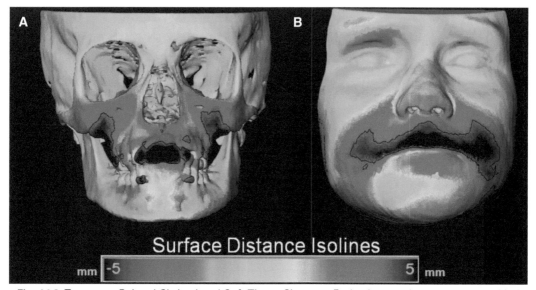

Surface Distance Isolines

mm **-5**   **5** mm

Fig. 14.3 Treatment-Related Skeletal and Soft-Tissue Changes. Fusion images demonstrate a graphical and quantitative evaluation of changes. The color scale bar at the bottom of the images depicts the magnitude and direction of the changes (*blue* = inward, *red* = outward). Three-dimensional surface model demonstrates changes in (A) the zygomatic processes of the maxilla, and (B) the soft tissue of the upper lip. (Modified from Cevidanes LH, Motta A, Proffit WR, et al. Cranial base superimposition for 3-dimensional evaluation of soft-tissue changes. *Am J Orthod Dentofacial Orthoped.* 137[4, suppl 1]: S120–S129.)

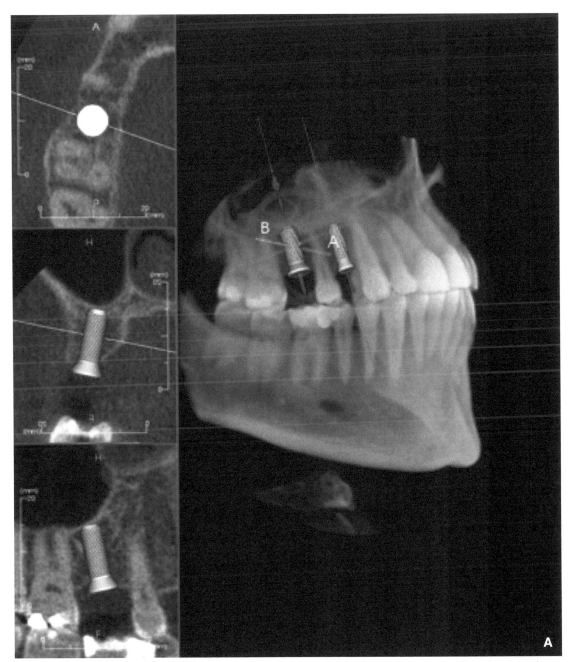

Fig. 14.4 In Silico Implant Planning. (A) Virtual implants are placed in the right maxilla. The three-dimensional volume rendered image shows virtual implants at the first premolar and first molar regions. Axial, coronal, and sagittal sections through the virtual molar implant are shown. The virtual implant is seated between the buccal and palatal cortices and engages the floor of the right maxillary sinus.

Continued

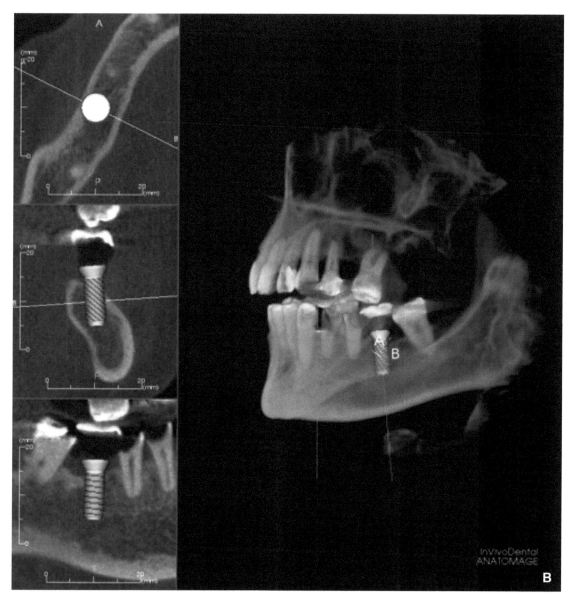

Fig. 14.4, cont'd (B) A virtual implant is positioned in the left mandibular first molar region. The location and angulation of the implant are guided by the radiopaque imaging stent. Axial, coronal, and sagittal sections through the virtual molar implant show exposure of the implant threads, indicating the need for bone augmentation.

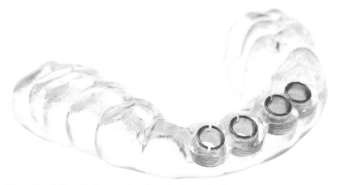

Fig. 14.5 A Tooth-Supported Surgical Guide. (Image courtesy Anatomage, San Jose, CA.)

Fiducial markers may be used to facilitate image data registration and subsequent superimposition of the these anatomic DICOM datasets. Often, these patients may have fixed orthodontic appliances, which cause considerable artifacts on the CT image. Tools in the software application allow removal of these artifactual areas. Using software tools, the surgeon then performs virtual osteotomy, mimicking surgical cuts and repositioning the virtual fragments (Fig. 14.6). The morphology of the jaws and location of vital structures guide the position of the osteotomy and the virtual placement of fixation devices. The planning software also predicts changes in the soft tissue with varying movements of the skeletal fragments. To translate the virtual plan to the operation room, a CAD/CAM fabricated interocclusal splint is fabricated to guide fragment repositioning during the actual surgery. Custom cutting plates and fixation devices can also be fabricated and printed (Fig. 14.7).

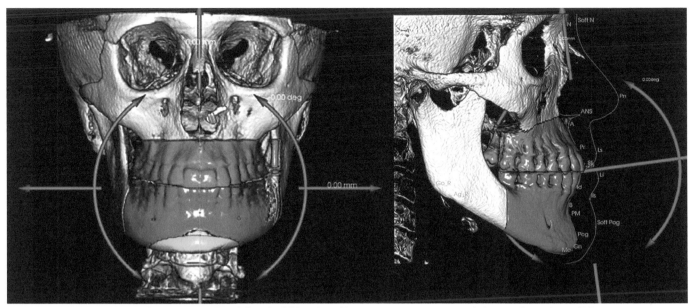

Fig. 14.6 Computer-Assisted Surgical Planning. The osteotomy segments of the maxilla and mandible can be repositioned in any plane. (Images courtesy Anatomage, San Jose, CA.)

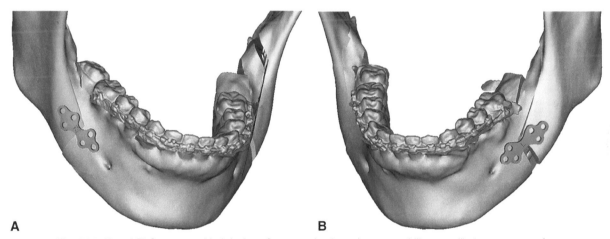

A   B

Fig. 14.7 (A and B) Computer-aided design of custom titanium plates to stabilize mandibular segments after a bilateral sagittal split osteotomy. (Modified from Li B, Shen S, Jiang W, et al. A new approach of splint-less orthognathic surgery using a personalized orthognathic surgical guide system: a preliminary study. *Int J Oral Maxillofac Surg.* 2017;46:1298–1305.)

Custom implants for facial augmentation and to restore maxillofacial defects: Proprietary software programs can design and print custom implants for facial augmentation (e.g., to augment the chin, zygomatic bones, and mandible). Similarly, maxillofacial defects from trauma or radical surgery can be restored by designing a custom implant-supported prosthesis. Custom implants provide several advantages over commercial stock implants. Custom implants have a more precise fit and are adapted to the underlying bone contours. When restoring unilateral aberrations, the unaffected side can be mirrored. Custom implants require minimal surgical alteration of the bony anatomy prior to implant placement. This reduces surgical time and cost.

THREE-DIMENSIONAL PRINTING

Three-dimensional printing, also referred to as additive manufacturing or rapid prototyping, is growing technology with increasing applications in healthcare. Initially developed to produce scale models and prototypes in the engineering industry, this technology has now grown to produce quality parts and objects in small numbers and at a lower cost. In medicine and dentistry, 3D-printed models of a patient's anatomy can be created for presurgical treatment planning, and creation of surgical templates and dental prosthesis. This technology also holds promise to print biologic tissues that may be used to print human organs and tissues.

This technology is of particular relevance to radiologic imaging, which most often provides the anatomic information that forms the basis for CAD/CAM design. In dentistry, many applications of 3D printing are based on skeletal and dental anatomy, acquired via MDCT or CBCT. Anatomic information from CT images support a wide range of 3D printing applications. CT images provide excellent contrast to differentiate between bone and soft tissue, which facilitates postprocessing. The basic steps for generation of a 3D model from CT data are described.
- *CT acquisition and reconstruction:* CT datasets should be reconstructed with isotropic voxels to maintain anatomic truth without loss of

information. MDCT examinations should be reconstructed using bone kernels (see Chapter 13). The thickness of the reconstructed sections impacts the accuracy of the printed models. For most applications, reconstruction thickness should be at least 1.25 mm. Thin sections require considerable segmentation which may be time intensive, whereas thicker sections could compromise the accuracy of the printed model. Anatomic areas such as the orbital floor, lamina papyracea, and anterior wall of the maxillary sinus consist of thin bone and require thin sections for accuracy.

- *Image segmentation:* DICOM data from the CT are imported into specialized software programs that segment the ROI. For example, if the task is to create a model of the mandible, voxels that represent the mandible have to be partitioned from the remainder of the imaged structures. On CT images, this may be accomplished initially by *thresholding,* to identify pixels in the range of bone Hounsfield units (see Chapter 13). However, thresholding will delineate pixels based on their gray values but not on spatial location. To isolate pixels that comprise an ROI, region growing segmentation algorithms can be applied. The operator initially selects one or more "seeds" within the anatomic region to be segmented. The computer algorithm compares the gray values of the neighboring pixels and, when similar, adds those pixels to expand the seed. The process is iterative and continues until no more pixels can be added. Operator input may be required to manually add in pixels, modify boundaries, or erase regions. Imperfections in the segmentation manifest as inaccuracies in the 3D-printed model.

- *Create a Standard Tessellation Language (STL) file:* The most widely used file format for 3D printing is STL. The term *tessellation* refers to tiling shapes of different geometry onto a flat surface without any overlaps or gaps. Likewise, an STL file represents the surface of the segmented region as triangular facets.

- *Creating the 3D-printed model:* The term *3D printing* or *additive manufacturing* encompasses seven categories of technologies used to create models, devices, or implants. The five technologies used in healthcare are described as follows.

  - *Vat photopolymerization:* Also referred to as *stereolithography,* this process uses a photo-curable liquid resin that solidifies on exposure to an intense light source. A laser beam is used to illuminate only the ROI cross section and cure the resin, producing a 2D cross-section layer of the model. The resin-containing vat is successively lowered (or raised for bottom-up printers) until all sections of the ROI have been printed. The model is then cured using an ultraviolet light source. The final model may require finishing to smooth edges. Small desktop devices are available for in-office use and can be used to fabricate implant guides and models of the jaws and teeth. Resins may be opaque or may be clear to demonstrate internal segmented structures such as neurovascular canals or lesions (Fig. 14.8).

  - *Material jetting:* This process is similar to inkjet printers. A nozzle moves horizontally across and jets the photopolymer onto a build platform. The layer of material is cured by ultraviolet light, and the nozzle continues to build the next layer on top of this layer, printing successive layers of the model. This process allows for multiple materials or multiple colors to be used. Materials used include polymethyl methacrylate, polystyrene, polypropylene, acrylonitrile butadiene styrene, polycarbonate, high-impact polystyrene, and high-density polyethylene. This method has been used to print dental models and implant guides.

  - *Binder jetting:* This process is similar to material jetting. The build material is a powder with a liquid binder that acts as an adhesive. The print nozzle moves horizontally to deposit layers of the powder followed by the liquid binder. The printed object

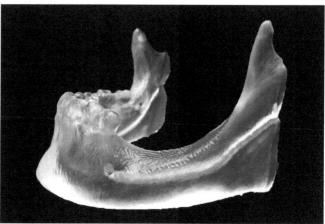

Fig. 14.8 Three-dimensional (3D)-printed model of the mandible. Mandibular anatomy from a cone beam computed tomography scan was segmented and printed using a vat polymerization 3D printer (Formlabs2). The 3D model served to perform mock surgery for a block graft from the mandibular ramus. The mandibular canal is segmented and can be seen through the clear resin. (Images courtesy Dr. Mohammed Husain, UCLA School of Dentistry, and Dr. Paul Anstey, Private Dental Practice, Beverly Hills, CA.)

is then lowered, and layers of powder and binder are deposited to successively build the model. Postprocessing includes vacuuming to remove residual powder and infiltrating the model with a resin or elastomer.

- *Material extrusion:* Also termed *fuse deposition modeling,* this process is widely used for medical and nonmedical applications due to its low cost. The build material is heated in a nozzle and deposited onto a platform, where it cools and hardens. Materials used are plastics and polymers. The resolution of this technique is lower, and the finished products are less accurate.

- *Powder bed fusion:* Technologies in this category include direct metal laser sintering, electron beam melting, selective heat sintering, selective laser melting, and selective laser sintering. A layer of powder is deposited onto a build platform, and a laser or electron beam is used to melt and fuse particles within the ROI. Successive layers of the model are built as with previous techniques. Materials used include plastics, polymers, and metals, including biocompatible materials for long-term use.

Clinical Applications of Three-Dimensional Printing

- *Craniofacial trauma and reconstruction:* Three-dimensional-printed models aid the surgeon to visualize complex trauma, in particular the location and the direction of fractures, and dislocation of the fractured segments. The models can be used to bend plates and recontour bars prior to surgery, decreasing intraoperative time. Mock surgery can be performed on the models, allowing the surgeon to anticipate potential issues that may be encountered at the time of surgery.

- *Implant surgical guides:* Following virtual implant planning, 3D-printed surgical guides may be fabricated to facilitate implant placement.

- *Maxillofacial prosthesis:* Three-dimensional printing can be used to generated CAD-designed prosthesis to restore surgical defects following radical surgery or trauma-related disfigurement.

- *Treatment planning and patient education:* Three-dimensional-printed models can be used to perform mock surgical procedures (e.g., orthognathic surgery or graft harvesting for bone augmentation).

When vital structures such as neurovascular canals are also segmented in the model, the clinician can anticipate potential intraoperative limitations and better assess the risk to these structures from the surgical procedure (see Fig. 14.8).

BIBLIOGRAPHY

Four-Dimensional Imaging

Cevidanes LH, Styner MA, Proffit WR. Image analysis and superimposition of 3-dimensional cone-beam computed tomography models. *Am J Orthod Dentofacial Orthop.* 2006;129(5):611–618.

Cevidanes LH, Hajati AK, Paniagua B, et al. Quantification of condylar resorption in temporomandibular joint osteoarthritis. *Oral Surg Oral Med Oral Pathol Oral Radiol Endod.* 2010;110(1):110–117.

Cevidanes LH, Motta A, Proffit WR, et al. Cranial base superimposition for 3-dimensional evaluation of soft-tissue changes. *Am J Orthod Dentofacial Orthop.* 2010;137(4 suppl):S120–S129.

Koerich L, Weissheimer A, de Menezes LM, et al. Rapid 3D mandibular superimposition for growing patients. *Angle Orthod.* 2017;87(3):473–479.

Nada RM, Maal TJ, Breuning KH, et al. Accuracy and reproducibility of voxel based superimposition of cone beam computed tomography models on the anterior cranial base and the zygomatic arches. *PLoS ONE.* 2011;6(2):e16520.

Ponce-Garcia C, Lagravere-Vich M, Cevidanes LHS, et al. Reliability of three-dimensional anterior cranial base superimposition methods for assessment of overall hard tissue changes: a systematic review. *Angle Orthod.* 2017.

Computer-Guided Treatment Planning

Bornstein MM, Al Nawas B, Kuchler U, et al. Consensus statements and recommended clinical procedures regarding contemporary surgical and radiographic techniques in implant dentistry. *Int J Oral Maxillofac Implants.* 2013.

Bengtsson M, Wall G, Greiff L, et al. Treatment outcome in orthognathic surgery—A prospective randomized blinded case-controlled comparison of planning accuracy in computer-assisted two- and three-dimensional planning techniques (part II). *J Craniomaxillofac Surg.* 2017;45(9):1419–1424.

De Riu G, Virdis PI, Meloni SM, et al. Accuracy of computer-assisted orthognathic surgery. *J Craniomaxillofac Surg.* 2017.

Li B, Shen S, Jiang W, et al. A new approach of splint-less orthognathic surgery using a personalized orthognathic surgical guide system: a preliminary study. *Int J Oral Maxillofac Surg.* 2017;46(10):1298–1305.

Xia JJ, Shevchenko L, Gateno J, et al. Outcome study of computer-aided surgical simulation in the treatment of patients with craniomaxillofacial deformities. *J Oral Maxillofac Surg.* 2011;69(7):2014–2024.

3D Printing

Marro A, Bandukwala T, Mak W. Three-dimensional printing and medical imaging: a review of the methods and applications. *Curr Probl Diagn Radiol.* 2016;45(1):2–9.

Mitsouras D, Liacouras P, Imanzadeh A, et al. Medical 3D printing for the radiologist. *Radiographics.* 2015;35(7):1965–1988.

15

Dental Implants

Edwin Chang

Two significant advancements have revolutionized the modern practice of dentistry: the advent and progressive refinement of dental implant rehabilitation and the widespread application of three-dimensional computed tomography imaging. Oral and maxillofacial radiology plays an increasingly crucial role in the successful planning, placement, and long-term follow-up of dental implants. This chapter provides an overview of imaging techniques used in modern dental implantology and the contribution of radiologic imaging in the preoperative, intraoperative, and postoperative phases of treatment.

IMAGING TECHNIQUES

As with all diagnostic imaging examinations, the radiographic prescription must be guided by a thorough clinical examination and the proposed imaging study must maximize diagnostic benefit while minimizing radiation risk and cost. To aid in this decision-making process, clinicians must be familiar with the indications, advantages, and limitations of imaging techniques used in oral implantology (Table 15.1 and Box 15.1).

Intraoral Radiography

Intraoral radiography is often the first-line imaging modality in the dental setting. This includes periapical, bite-wing, and occlusal images. Periapical imaging is the most commonly used examination in all phases of dental implant evaluation (Fig. 15.1). For preoperative assessment, intraoral radiography provides an evaluation of osseous healing at the edentulous site. It identifies the presence of retained roots, residual periapical pathology, and variants such as osteosclerosis, all of which complicate implant placement. Periapical radiographs allow adequate assessment of the status of the adjacent teeth and provide approximate mesiodistal and vertical distances to the adjacent anatomic boundaries and vital structures. As they are two-dimensional projection radiographs, periapical images do not provide information on the buccolingual dimension. In the past, occlusal radiographs were used to provide a basic assessment of the buccolingual contour of the mandible. However, the base of the mandibular body usually exhibits a wider buccolingual dimension than the alveolar process, resulting in overestimation of buccolingual bone width (Fig. 15.2). Anatomic limitations make occlusal radiographs ineffective in assessing edentulous sites in the maxilla. The advent and increasing accessibility of three-dimensional computed tomography (CT) in dentistry has progressively reduced the contribution of occlusal images for such purposes.

The major advantages of intraoral radiography are its relatively low cost and near-negligible radiation risk; widespread availability in dental offices; excellent spatial resolution; and, in the case of solid-state–based digital systems, the possibility of instantaneous image generation. However, intraoral imaging is limited by its relatively narrow anatomic coverage and the inability to provide accurate three-dimensional analyses.

Superimposition of contiguous structures makes it impractical to analyze the thickness of the buccal and lingual cortical plates and may obscure accurate visualization of crucial anatomic structures such as the inferior alveolar canal. Moreover, periapical imaging is subject to geometric distortion and magnification arising from elongation or foreshortening (see Chapters 6 and 7), which limits its use for linear measurements—a crucial objective of preoperative imaging for implant planning. Overall, intraoral radiography remains a valuable tool in the initial assessment of a single edentulous space or short edentulous span and should be considered as the first-line imaging modality in both intra- and postoperative phases of implant treatment.

Panoramic Imaging

Panoramic imaging is the second most commonly employed dental imaging technique because of its wide anatomic coverage, ease of acquisition, and relatively low cost. It provides a gross overview of the osseous structures of the maxillae and mandible, including the floors of the maxillary sinuses and the inferior alveolar canals—important structural considerations in posterior implant placement (Fig. 15.3). However, major limitations of panoramic imaging are image distortion and superimposition of ghost images. The degree of distortion is unpredictable—it depends on patient positioning and approximation of the patient's jaws within the standardized curvature of the focal trough. Structures located buccal to this predefined focal trough are distorted and appear narrow in the horizontal dimension, whereas structures located lingual to the focal trough will appear horizontally magnified. This nonuniform distortion precludes accurate mesiodistal measurements of the edentulous ridge and cannot be reliably corrected with software. Moreover, a vertical magnification of approximately 15% to 30% is present, and the slight negative vertical angulation of the x-ray beam projects images of lingually positioned structures more superiorly on the image. However, much like intraoral imaging, the lack of three-dimensional capabilities precludes accurate assessment of the buccolingual dimension of available bone. Moreover, the resolution of panoramic images is lower than that of intraoral radiographs. Nevertheless, panoramic imaging is of value for the initial examination of a dental implant patient, particularly when multiple implant sites are considered at once, or when intraoral images cannot be made due to difficult patient anatomy or poor patient cooperation. Guidelines from the American Academy of Oral and Maxillofacial Radiology recommend panoramic and intraoral radiography for the initial assessment of the dental implant placement.

Computed Tomography (Multidetector Computed Tomography and Cone Beam Computed Tomography)

CT is an imaging technique that generates three-dimensional cross-sectional views from multiple projections taken at several different angles

TABLE 15.1　Commonly Used Imaging Techniques for Implant Placement

Imaging Technique	Advantages	Disadvantages	Recommendation
Periapical imaging	• Readily available • High resolution • Minimal distortion • Lowest financial cost and radiation exposure	• Restricted anatomic coverage • Cannot assess buccolingual dimension • Subject to elongation and foreshortening • Anatomic superimposition • Difficult to reproduce projection geometry • May be limited by patient compliance and anatomy	• Initial assessment of single edentulous space or short edentulous span • Intraoperative imaging during implant placement • Initial postoperative radiograph and recall imaging
Panoramic imaging	• Readily available • Broad anatomic coverage • Low financial cost and radiation exposure	• Image distortion • Anatomic superimposition and ghost images • Lower resolution • Cannot assess buccolingual dimension • Technique sensitive	• Initial examination of multiple edentulous spaces • Radiographic follow-up of multiple implants
CBCT imaging	• Variable field of view: from single edentulous site to full jaws (manufacturer-dependent) • 3D tomographic imaging: no superimposition • Dimensionally accurate • Increasingly accessible • Simulate implant surgery with specialized software	• Moderate financial cost and radiation exposure • Susceptible to beam hardening artifacts • Technique-sensitive (especially to patient motion) • Special training for interpretation • Not calibrated for bone density measurements (HU) • Poor soft tissue contrast	• Following initial examination, CBCT is recommended for thorough radiologic assessment • Recommended before and after bone augmentation • Postoperatively, recommended for symptomatic implants (implant mobility, altered sensation, displaced implant) • Not appropriate for asymptomatic recall imaging

3D, Three-dimensional; *CBCT*, cone beam computed tomography; *HU*, Hounsfield units.

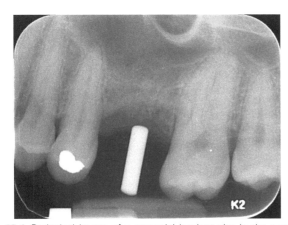

Fig. 15.1 Periapical image of a potential implant site in the posterior left maxilla. An imaging guide containing a cylindrical radiopaque marker has been inserted intraorally to depict the desired angle of implant placement.

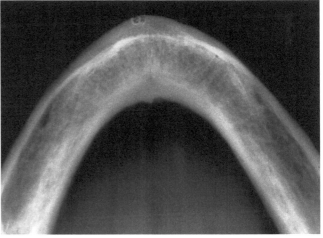

Fig. 15.2 Cross-sectional occlusal radiograph of the edentulous mandible. Note that only the widest buccolingual contours of the mandible are visualized; these are usually located inferior to the desired implant site. This could result in an overestimation of the amount of buccolingual bone available.

around the patient. Recent technologic innovations have led to the development of sophisticated multidetector CT (MDCT) systems that are widely used in medicine. MDCT images are acquired with the patient supine on a table that advances through a rotating gantry (see Chapter 13). Although MDCT has been used to evaluate several maxillofacial conditions, its higher cost, larger radiation dose, and limited accessibility to dentists have restricted its widespread adoption for the purposes of dental implant planning.

In the last two decades, cone beam CT (CBCT) has evolved to provide high-resolution three-dimensional information; it is now applied to several maxillofacial diagnostic objectives. In contrast, CBCT units acquire images with the patient in a supine, sitting, or standing position,

depending on the manufacturer and model of the unit. CBCT imaging offers the advantage of a high spatial resolution and much lower radiation doses.

Following a comprehensive patient history, clinical assessment, and initial radiographic examination with periapical and/or panoramic images, CBCT has become the imaging modality of choice for the presurgical assessment of an implant site. CBCT allows for accurate, three-dimensional analyses of the quantity of available bone, the thickness of the contiguous cortical plates, the quality and architecture of the

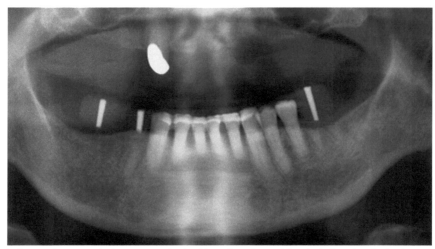

Fig. 15.3 Cropped panoramic image, acquired with an imaging guide, depicting the desired axes of three potential mandibular implants.

BOX 15.1   American Academy of Oral and Maxillofacial Radiology Recommendations for Imaging the Dental Implant Patient

Recommendation 1. Panoramic radiography should be used as the imaging modality of choice in the initial evaluation of the dental implant patient.

Recommendation 2. Use intraoral periapical radiography to supplement the preliminary information from panoramic radiography.

Recommendation 3. Do not use cross-sectional imaging, including cone beam computed tomography (CBCT), as an initial diagnostic imaging examination.

Recommendation 4. The radiographic examination of any potential implant site should include cross-sectional imaging orthogonal to the site of interest.

Recommendation 5. CBCT should be considered as the imaging modality of choice for preoperative cross-sectional imaging of potential implant sites.

Recommendation 6. CBCT should be considered when clinical conditions indicate a need for augmentation procedures or site development before placement of dental implants: (1) sinus augmentation, (2) block or particulate bone grafting, (3) ramus or symphysis grafting, (4) assessment of impacted teeth in the field of interest, and (5) evaluation of prior traumatic injury.

Recommendation 7. CBCT imaging should be considered if bone reconstruction and augmentation procedures (e.g., ridge preservation or bone grafting) have been performed to treat bone volume deficiencies before implant placement.

Recommendation 8. In the absence of clinical signs or symptoms, use intraoral periapical radiography for the postoperative assessment of implants. Panoramic radiographs may be indicated for cases requiring more extensive implant therapy.

Recommendation 9. Use cross-sectional imaging (particularly CBCT) immediately postoperatively only if the patient presents with implant mobility or altered sensation, especially if the fixture is in the posterior mandible.

Recommendation 10. Do not use CBCT imaging for periodic review of clinically asymptomatic implants.

Recommendation 11. Cross-sectional imaging, optimally CBCT, should be considered if implant retrieval is anticipated.

From Tyndall DA, Price JB, Tetradis S, et al. Position statement of the American Academy of Oral and Maxillofacial Radiology on selection criteria for the use of radiology in dental implantology with emphasis on cone beam computed tomography. *Oral Surg Oral Med Oral Pathol Oral Radiol.* 2012;113:817-826.

---

trabecular bone, and the proximity to adjacent anatomic structures and boundaries. CBCT is also the modality of choice for preoperative evaluation of the maxillary sinuses prior to sinus floor elevation, the assessment of both donor and recipient sites for autogenous bone grafting procedures, and to evaluate the outcome of these procedures. CBCT images are also used in the design and fabrication of surgical guides using computer-aided design and computer-aided manufacturing (CADCAM) technology.

As with all ionizing radiation–based imaging modalities, the use of CBCT should follow responsible and judicious image acquisition protocols. The anatomic field of view should be limited to the region of interest. Depending on the objectives of imaging, the field may be extended beyond the edentulous sites to encompass relevant adjacent anatomy, such as the maxillary sinus ostia prior to sinus lifting, the external oblique ridges for bone harvesting, or the opposing dental crowns for prosthetic planning and surgical guide fabrication. To produce a diagnostically acceptable study using the least amount of ionizing radiation, the exposure parameters should be tailored to the patient's age, size, and anatomy, and efforts should be made during image acquisition to minimize motion. Importantly, given the complexity of three-dimensional imaging volumes and the inclusion of structures beyond the dentoalveolar region, advanced training is necessary to interpret CBCT studies competently.

Image Reconstruction Techniques

Following acquisition of a CBCT volume, the imaged volume must be reconstructed in specific planes to extract the necessary information for implant planning. Owing to the curvature of the dental arch, the orthogonal anatomic planes (axial, coronal, and sagittal) are not optimal for assessing the mesiodistal and buccolingual dimensions of available bone. Therefore curved planar reformatting is applied. This is achieved through first selecting a reference axial slice of the maxillary or mandibular arch, at the midroot level of its teeth. Dedicated software tools are used to define the curve of the dental arch, tailored to the patient's anatomy (Fig. 15.4A), and subsequently to generate a series of cross-sectional images oriented perpendicular to this patient's arch in predefined, equally spaced intervals (typically 1 to 2 mm). Software tools are used to make measurements of the vertical height and buccolingual width of the edentulous site (see Fig. 15.4B). Pseudopanoramic reconstructions can also be made parallel to this customized arch, and reconstructed at various thicknesses; thinner slices allow localized anatomic visualization that is free of superimposition whereas a thicker slice will more closely resemble a panoramic radiograph (see Fig. 15.4C). Last, three-dimensional surface and volumetric renderings of the edentulous jaw can be generated to aid in visualizing the overall shape and contour of the edentulous jaw (see Fig. 15.4D). Images of CBCT reconstructions can be delivered in digital format and can be printed life size (i.e., 1:1) on high-quality photographic paper.

Other Techniques

Other radiographic imaging techniques that have been used for implant planning include the lateral oblique, lateral cephalometric, and conventional tomographic images. These techniques have been largely replaced by CBCT imaging in contemporary practice for implant treatment planning. Although magnetic resonance imaging (MRI) produces cross-sectional images of the jaws without ionizing radiation, its depiction of the hard tissue structures is inadequate for implant planning.

PREOPERATIVE ASSESSMENT AND TREATMENT PLANNING

Several functional, esthetic, and surgical considerations contribute to successful implant placement. Prior to the widespread availability of CBCT imaging, implant placement was predominantly a surgically driven approach, with the amount of available bone largely dictating the final implant position. However, with the increased accessibility and affordability of three-dimensional imaging, current trends have shifted toward a prosthetically driven approach. CBCT data can be virtually coupled with digital impression models, allowing for greater communication between the surgeon and restorative dentist. The ideal position of the putative implant is first identified based on the functional and esthetic needs of the patient as well as the state of the remaining dentition. This information is then translated into the digital environment

and, through specialized software, the implant surgery can be simulated using virtual implant libraries. Based on the amount of available bone and the shape of the residual bony ridge, the need for additional bone grafting and alveoloplasty procedures can be identified and the treatment options provided. This increased transparency and communication between the implant team and the patient allows for a more predictable outcome and keeps expectations earnest through informed decision making.

Radiologic Assessment of Bone Quantity

The principal advantage of CBCT imaging is its ability to accurately assess the quantity of available bone in all three dimensions. It is generally accepted that, ideally, the implant should be placed at least 1.5 mm from the adjacent teeth, 3 mm from an adjacent implant, and 2 mm from vital anatomic structures, such as the inferior alveolar canal. The usual anatomic boundaries are discussed further on for both the maxillae and mandible.

In the anterior maxilla, the absolute vertical limitation is the floor of the nasal fossa. However, the vertical dimension of available bone is often limited by residual ridge atrophy, which can lead to the development of a prominent buccal concavity. CBCT guides the decision for additional buccal bone grafting or restorative compromises for a shorter, more proclined implant (Fig. 15.5). In the maxillary central incisor region, proximity to the nasopalatine canal must be assessed. It is important to recognize that there are large morphologic differences in the dimensions and configuration of the nasopalatine canal; even within the same patient, the diameter of the canal can vary widely across its length (Fig. 15.6). CBCT accurately depicts the canal's topography; it is particularly valuable when there are potential space limitations, as in the case of a mesially positioned lateral incisor.

In the posterior maxilla, the floor of the maxillary sinus is the usual vertical boundary to implant placement. The pneumatization of the alveolar process is a normal physiologic process that is often accelerated by tooth loss. Although the floor of the maxillary sinus can be readily

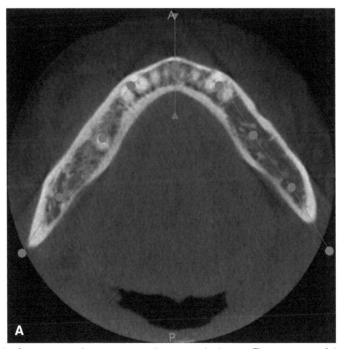

Fig. 15.4 (A) Axial reference cone beam computed tomography image. The curvature of the mandibular arch is approximated through a series of connecting dots.   *Continued*

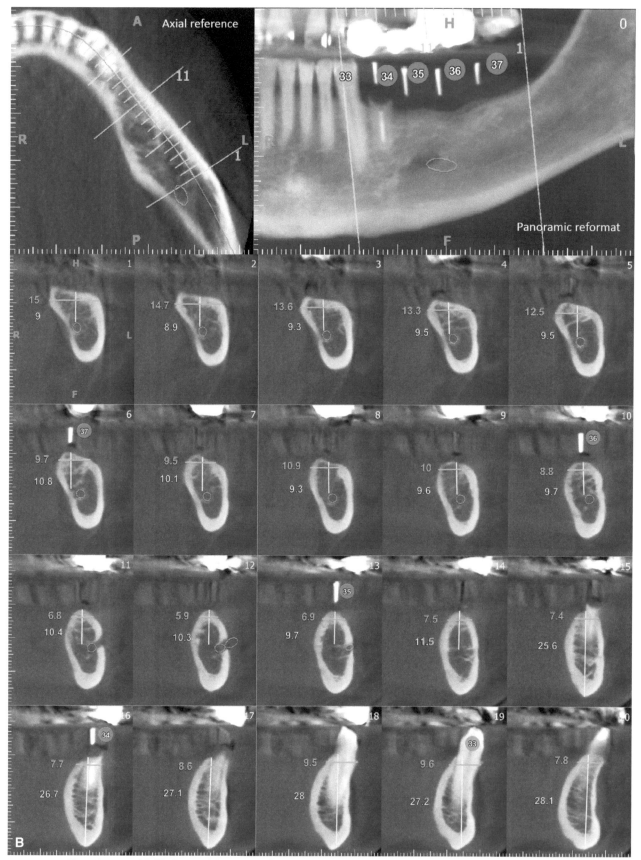

Fig. 15.4, cont'd (B) Sequential cross-sections made perpendicular to the curvature of the mandible, at 2-mm intervals. The edentulous sites are labeled (in FDI World Dental Federation notation). Vertical and buccolingual measurements are in accordance with the imaging guide. The course of the mandibular canal is outlined in *orange*.

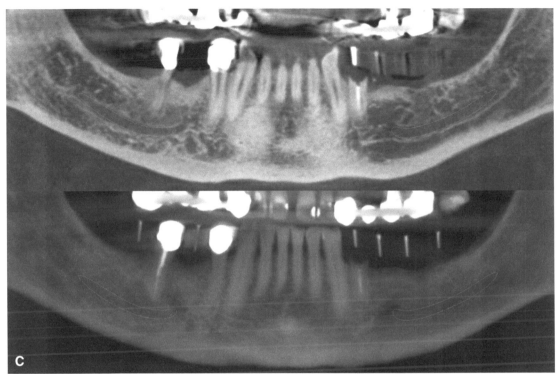

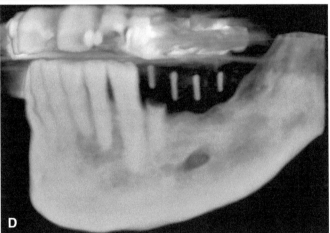

Fig. 15.4, cont'd (C) Pseudopanoramic multiplanar reformat of the mandible with a thin (0.2 mm, *top*) and thick slice thickness (40 mm, *bottom*). (D) Three-dimensional volume rendering of the edentulous posterior left mandible.

identified in two-dimensional images, the pattern of pneumatization may be variable in the transverse dimension, and the exact position of the sinus floor can be fully appreciated only with three-dimensional imaging (Fig. 15.7). If a sinus lift procedure is planned, CBCT provides crucial preoperative information, such the presence of transverse septa, inflammatory sinus disease, and prominent branches of the postero-superior alveolar artery (Fig. 15.8).

In the anterior mandible, the usual limitation to implant placement is a narrow buccolingual bone width secondary to residual ridge atrophy. Although clinical palpation of the residual ridge provides an estimate of the available buccolingual bone, only CT imaging can provide a precise assessment. Importantly, the anterior mandible contains a network of anastomosing lingual vessels that can occasionally be identified as bony canals (the median and lateral lingual foramina) (Fig. 15.9A). The mandibular incisive canal, the anterior continuation of the inferior

alveolar canal beyond the mental foramen, is another vital structure that may be radiographically apparent (see Fig. 15.9B). These structures, if breached during implant placement, have occasionally been reported to result in hemorrhage and neurosensory disturbances. CBCT depicts these canals better than two-dimensional radiographs; this may allow for a more predictable treatment outcome even within a region that is traditionally considered as a "safe zone" for implant placement.

Although the inferior alveolar canal is often assumed to be the obvious vertical limitation to implant placement in the posterior mandible, it is important to recognize that the mandibular cross-sectional morphology usually follows a sigmoid shape in the buccolingual plane (Fig. 15.10). The buccal surface of the alveolar process is often more lingually positioned than the underlying mandibular body, and a concavity is present along the lingual surface of the mandible (i.e., the submandibular

Text continued on p. 259

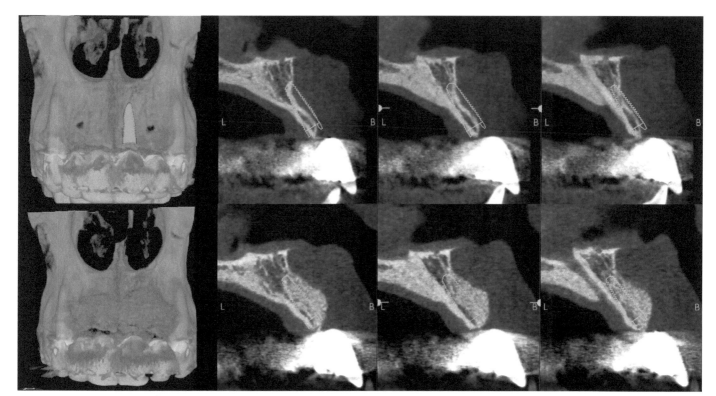

Fig. 15.5 *Top*: Three-dimensional volume rendering and buccolingual cross-sections of an edentulous maxillary left central incisor site. Note the prominent buccal concavity of the alveolar process, which prevents the desired implant to be placed without significant esthetic compromises. The virtual implant shows extensive buccal thread exposure if placed in the ideal inclination, identifying the need for buccal bone augmentation prior to implant placement. *Bottom*: Cone beam computed tomography sections following buccal bone grafting. Note how the desired implant size is now fully embedded in bone.

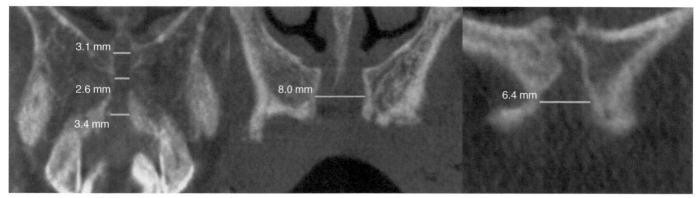

Fig. 15.6 Three examples of morphologic variation in the nasopalatine canal. Coronal slices depicting a thin, uniform canal *(left)*, two wide, converging canals *(middle)*, and a funnel-shaped canal *(right)*.

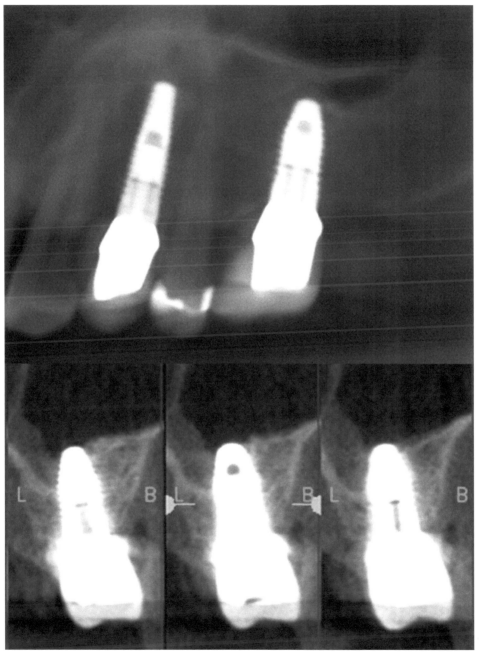

Fig. 15.7 *Top*: A simulated periapical projection reformatted from a cone beam computed tomography study. The position of the maxillary sinus floor relative to the apex of the implant placed at the maxillary left first molar site is difficult to determine due to anatomic superimposition. *Bottom*: These buccolingual cross-sections of the same implant demonstrate the irregular pneumatization of the alveolar process, which is difficult to appreciate in a projectional, two-dimensional image. The sinus floor is positioned more superiorly within the buccal aspect of the alveolar process, and more inferiorly positioned in the palatal portion of this site. The apex of this implant is more palatally oriented within the alveolar process, and has been placed beyond the sinus floor.

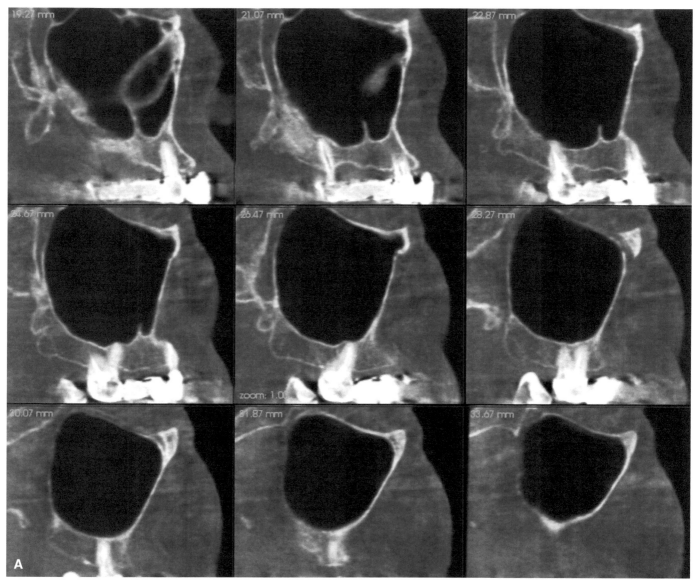

Fig. 15.8 (A) Serial sagittal cross sections of a right maxillary sinus demonstrating a transverse ridge located along the sinus floor apical to the edentulous first molar region, which may complicate a sinus lift procedure. The sinus appears otherwise normal and fully aerated.

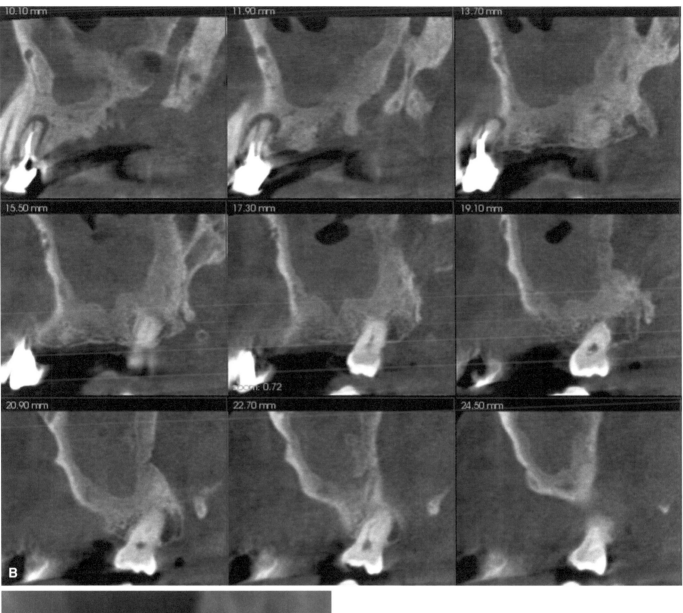

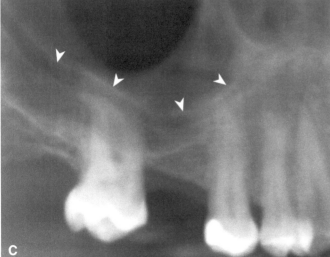

Fig. 15.8, cont'd (B) In contrast to (A), these sagittal cross sections of a left maxillary sinus show that the sinus walls are thickened and sclerotic and that most of the antral space is radiopacified. These findings could imply the possibility of sinusitis, which is a relative contraindication to a sinus lift procedure. (C) Reformatted image from a cone beam computed tomography volume of the right maxilla depicts a prominent branch of the posterior superior alveolar artery *(white arrowheads)*. The three-dimensional location of this vessel can be mapped in preparation for a sinus lift surgery.

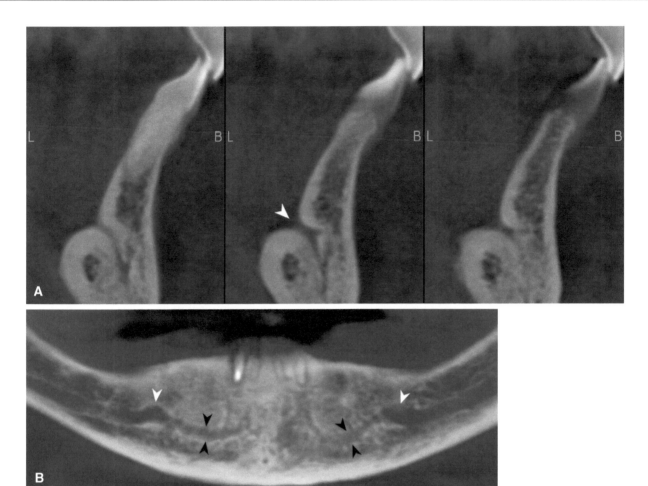

Fig. 15.9 (A) Buccolingual cross-sectional images of the mandibular midline depicting a prominent median lingual foramen *(white arrowhead)*, which could result in hemorrhage if breached during implant placement. (B) Panoramic reformatted image (3-mm slice thickness) demonstrating prominent mandibular incisive canals *(black arrowheads)* coursing anterior to the mental foramina *(white arrowheads)*.

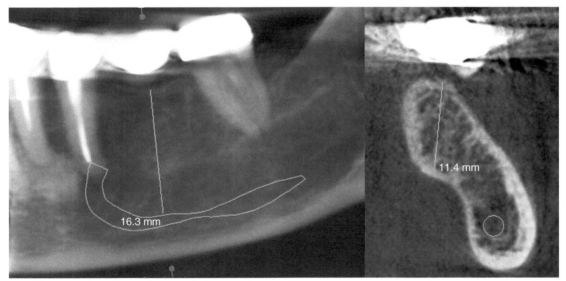

Fig. 15.10 *Left*: Cropped panoramic image reformatted from a cone beam computed tomography study of the site of the mandibular left first molar. The vertical height from the alveolar crest to the left inferior alveolar nerve canal *(outlined in orange)* measures just over 16 mm. *Right*: A cross-sectional slice at the middle of the same site (mandibular left first molar) in the buccolingual plane. A prominent lingual concavity limits implant placement at an optimal angle relative to the pontic restoration and roots of the adjacent teeth. Note that this information cannot be obtained on periapical and panoramic radiographs.

TABLE 15.2   Misch Classification of Bone Density

Classification Type	Radiographic Appearance	Typical Anatomic Location	MDCT Density Range (HU)
D1	Primarily composed of dense cortical bone Marrow spaces are hardly visible	Occasionally in anterior mandible Rarely in posterior mandible	>1250
D2	Thick outer layer of porous cortical bone Coarse trabecular bone pattern	Commonly in anterior and posterior mandible Occasionally in anterior maxilla	850–1250
D3	Thinner layer of porous cortical bone Fine trabecular bone pattern	Commonly in anterior maxilla, posterior maxilla, and posterior mandible Occasionally in anterior mandible	350–850
D4	Faint to imperceptible outline of thin cortical bone Alveolar process is primarily composed of fine trabecular bone	Commonly in posterior maxilla Rarely in anterior maxilla	150–350

HU, Hounsfield units; *MDCT*, multidetector computed tomography.
Modified from Misch CE. *Contemporary Implant Dentistry*. 3rd ed. St. Louis: Mosby; 2008.

fossa). This unique morphology is not visualized in periapical and panoramic images, which do not provide information in the buccolingual dimension, and is often undetected during clinical examination because the lingual contours of the mandibular body are difficult to palpate owing to their muscular attachments. Moreover, CBCT has been shown to be superior to panoramic images in identifying the inferior alveolar canal. This, in conjunction with the ability to objectively delineate the buccolingual contours of the mandible, can often result in changes to the size and angulation of the planned implant.

Radiologic Assessment of Bone Quality

Local bone quality is an important factor for implant success. The edentulous bone should provide primary implant stability and a pre-implant environment that is conducive to osseointegration. Currently radiologic assessment of bone quality at the edentulous site is largely a subjective evaluation of the trabecular architecture. Numerous classification systems have been proposed but few have been validated as practical clinical outcome measures. The classification system proposed by Misch et al. (Table 15.2) is most widely used and describes four categories of bone (D1 to D4) based on the thickness of cortical bone and the density and distribution of trabecular bone (Fig. 15.11). Owing to its ability to clearly visualize the thickness of cortical bone and the organization of trabecular bone, these assessments are better on cross-sectional CT images than on intraoral and panoramic images. However, the distinction between a "thick" or a "thin" cortex and "coarse" or "fine" trabecular bone relies on the subjective thresholds of the observer, which are variable among clinicians.

Objectively, bone density is formally defined as mineral mass per unit volume of bone. When applied to the diagnosis of osteoporosis and assessment of fracture risk, this assessment is typically performed using dual-energy x-ray absorptiometry (DEXA). Crude estimates of bone density obtained from the CT numbers on MDCT images (Hounsfield units, or HU) have been used to predict implant stability. HU ranges for the Misch classification of bone density have been proposed (see Table 15.2). However, owing to their wide beam geometry, increased scatter radiation, and lower contrast resolution, HU measurements from CBCT datasets are unreliable for the prediction of bone density. In general, jaw bone density in the anterior mandible is higher, whereas it is lowest in the posterior maxilla.

Radiologic imaging of proposed implant sites aids in the detection of retained root fragments and foreign bodies as well as in ruling out residual pathology. Findings that require treatment include inflammatory disease, cysts, and neoplasms, and CBCT imaging provides excellent characterization of their bony extent. Findings that do not require

treatment but may still impact implant planning are also occasionally encountered. For example, areas of osteosclerosis are common incidental findings (Fig. 15.12). Although not a direct contraindication to implant placement, the presence of osteosclerosis may cause drill deflection during implant osteotomy. Additionally, osteosclerotic areas have relatively lower vascularity, which can affect healing and osseointegration. Similarly, the presence of periapical osseous dysplasia also complicates implant placement; some case reports have shown that surgical intervention in regions of osseous dysplasia, including implant placement, can result in secondary infection of the dysplastic bone, which can lead to the development of osteomyelitis and bone sequestration (Fig. 15.13).

INTRAOPERATIVE IMAGING

During surgical implant placement, intraoperative imaging is limited to quick, in-office modalities, including digital-based periapical and panoramic radiography. These radiographs confirm appropriate pilot drill position and allow early errors to be identified so that appropriate modifications to the remaining osteotomy steps can be made. Occasionally, surgical accidents may require advanced radiologic imaging in the intraoperative phase—for example, when an implant is displaced into the maxillary sinus or placed through the inferior alveolar canal. In such situations, expedient CBCT imaging will accurately locate the implant or assess the extent of nerve canal encroachment (Fig. 15.14).

IMAGE-GUIDED APPLICATIONS

More recently, advancements in computer technology and stereolithographic prototyping have facilitated image-guided techniques for implant treatment planning and surgical placement. Several implant planning software programs use CBCT datasets to determine the optimal three-dimensional position of a proposed implant. However, the ultimate success of the procedure depends on the successful transfer of the virtual plan to the surgical suite. Various guided surgery techniques have been developed to serve as a physical conduit between the virtual and surgical environments. Such guided surgical approaches are especially helpful in cases where anatomic, functional, or esthetic requirements must be met within a relatively narrow margin of error.

Conventional stereolithographic guides are designed to be supported by one of three tissue types: teeth, mucosa, or bone. In the partially dentate patient, tooth-supported guides are usually preferred, as they allow flapless surgery to be performed while maintaining guide stability without the use of fixation pins (Fig. 15.15). This technique requires at least two or three nonmobile teeth in the arch, and the contours of these

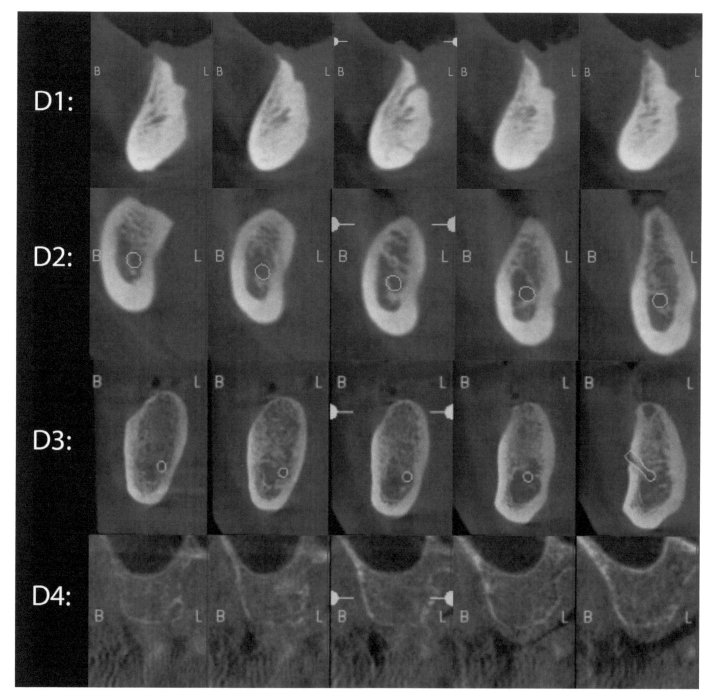

Fig. 15.11 Serial buccolingual cross-sectional images of four different edentulous sites that exemplify the Misch classifications of bone density. Mandibular nerve canals are outlined in *orange*. *First row*: The alveolar process of an edentulous anterior mandible that is primarily composed of dense cortical bone. This is suggestive of a D1 bone density classification. *Second row*: An example of a D2 classification in a posterior right mandible, with coarse trabecular bone surrounded by an outer layer of thick cortical bone. *Third row*: Thin cortical bone lining fine trabecular bone in a posterior right mandible, which is a typical example of a D3 type bone. *Fourth row*: Cross sections of a posterior right maxilla demonstrating a fine trabecular bone pattern covered by a faint lining of cortical bone. This is representative of a D4 bone density classification.

teeth can be digitally captured using three-dimensional surface optical scanning of stone models or directly via a specialized intraoral optical scanning camera. This surface model is subsequently superimposed over the CBCT dataset, which allows for accurate profiling of the tooth crowns that would otherwise be obscured by beam hardening artifacts from

restorations. Current literature suggests that tooth-supported guides are more accurate than mucosa- and bone-supported guides.

In the edentulous patient, the surgical guide can be supported only by mucosa or bone. A mucosa-supported guide will still allow a flapless surgical approach, but the accuracy of the guide depends on mucosal

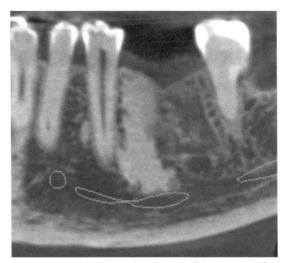

Fig. 15.12 Cone beam computed tomography section through the posterior left mandible demonstrating a large area of osteosclerosis located in the mesial aspect of an edentulous mandibular left first molar site.

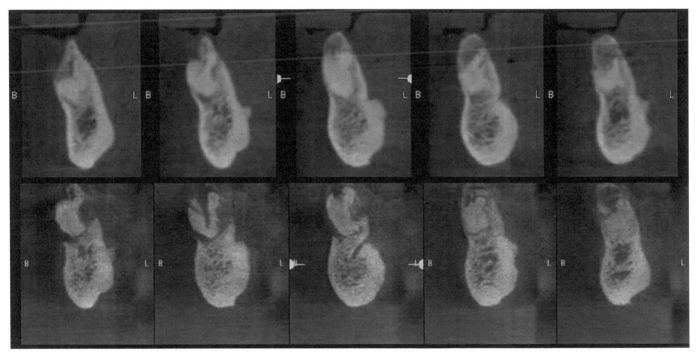

Fig. 15.13 *Top row:* Cone beam computed tomography (CBCT) images of a relatively mature focus of periapical osseous dysplasia in the anterior mandible of a patient evaluated for implant treatment planning. *Bottom row:* Following implant placement, the patient reported pain in the implant area. Two of the implants failed in the immediate postoperative period. Postoperative CBCT sections demonstrate rarefying osteitis around the foci of dysplastic bone and partial loss of the contiguous buccal and lingual cortical plates, suggestive of osteomyelitis.

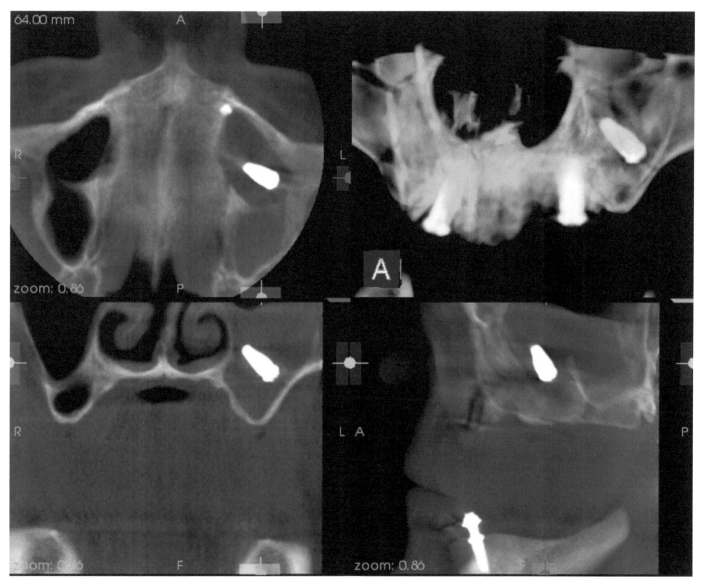

Fig. 15.14 Axial *(top left)*, coronal *(bottom left)*, sagittal *(bottom right)*, and three-dimensional volume rendering *(top right)* demonstrating a dental implant displaced into the left maxillary sinus. Note the severe mucosal thickening around the displaced implant.

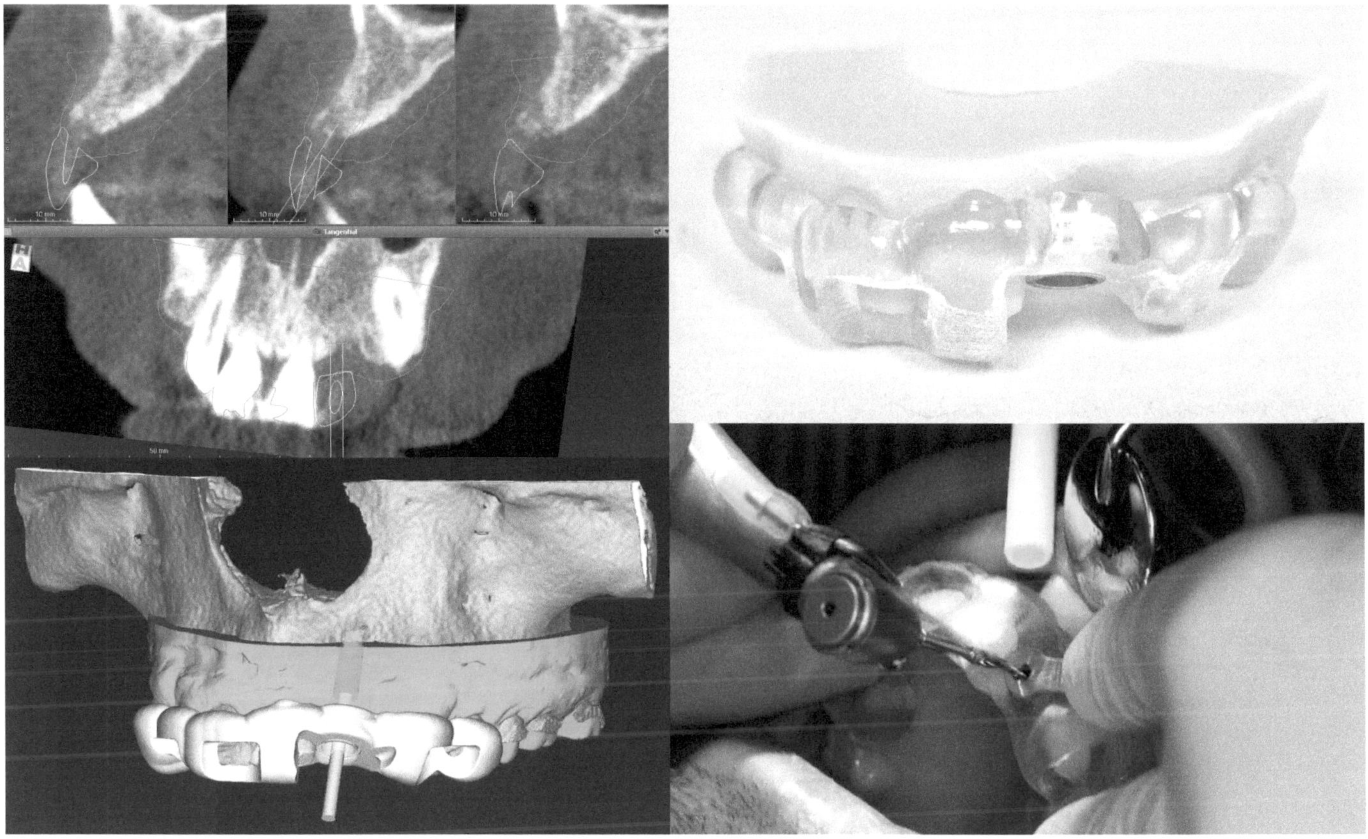

Fig. 15.15 *Top left*: Buccolingual and mesiodistal cross sections of a cone beam computed tomography (CBCT) scan acquired for implant planning at the site of an edentulous maxillary left lateral incisor. Given that the remaining teeth are present, a tooth-supported guide was planned to aid in implant placement. A stone model of the patient's arch was digitally scanned and registered with the CBCT data, which is outlined in *dark blue*. Based on the amount of available bone and the desired position of the prosthetic crown, the ideal position of the virtual implant was determined *(outlined in light blue)*. *Bottom left*: Three-dimensional surface models of the maxillae *(gray)*, the maxillary stone model *(dark blue)*, and the digitally designed surgical stent *(white)*. *Top right*: The final surgical stent printed through a rapid prototyping technique, securely seated atop a duplicate of the patient's stone model. *Bottom right*: Clinical photograph of the seated surgical stent guiding the implant osteotomy. (Courtesy Canaray: Specialists in Oral Radiology, Toronto, ON, and Dr. G. McLachlin, Calgary, AB.)

resilience and the use of fixation pins (Fig. 15.16). Alternatively, a bone-supported guide rests entirely on bone, but the surgeon must first raise an extensive flap to seat the guide (Fig. 15.17). The primary advantage of a bone-supported system is that it confers greater visualization of the surgical field, which allows early detection of positional errors through direct visualization and tactile sensation. However, the need to raise a flap increases patient discomfort and recovery time and may result in postoperative complications such as swelling and bleeding. Some studies have suggested that mucosa-supported guides confer greater clinical accuracy than bone-supported guides.

In addition to static surgical templates, more recent approaches of surgical guidance allow for a more dynamic approach. As with static planning approaches, the position and inclination of the putative implant are planned based on a preoperative CT examination. However, for implant placement in the jaw, these systems employ sophisticated intraoperative navigation technology that provides live feedback on the location and angulation of the surgical handpiece relative to the in silico planned implant position. This is typically achieved using fiducial markers registered with the CT images, positional sensors attached to the patient's stent and the handpiece, and an external digital display depicting the real-time position of the drill head in relation to the virtual planning data (Fig. 15.18). The main advantage of this approach over static surgical templates is that it allows the surgeon to make real-time modifications to the predetermined implant position while still retaining the benefits of CT guidance. However, the additional hardware and software necessary to operate these systems reduces their accessibility compared with static guides, and the added steps of tracking and displaying the surgical instrument introduce potential sources of error.

Despite its rapid evolution, surgically-guided implant placement is not used in most implant cases, and there is insufficient evidence to justify its routine use. It is important to recognize that image-guided surgical adjuncts cannot replace sound clinical skill and acumen, and it is naive to consider such a technique as a novice-friendly approach to implant placement. The surgeon must be prepared for all potential intra- and postoperative complications, including the ability to deviate from surgical guidance when unexpected situations arise, such as the need to reflect a flap and perform additional bone augmentation.

POSTOPERATIVE IMAGING AND MONITORING

Immediately following implant placement, a periapical image should be acquired to serve as a baseline image for future comparisons. If

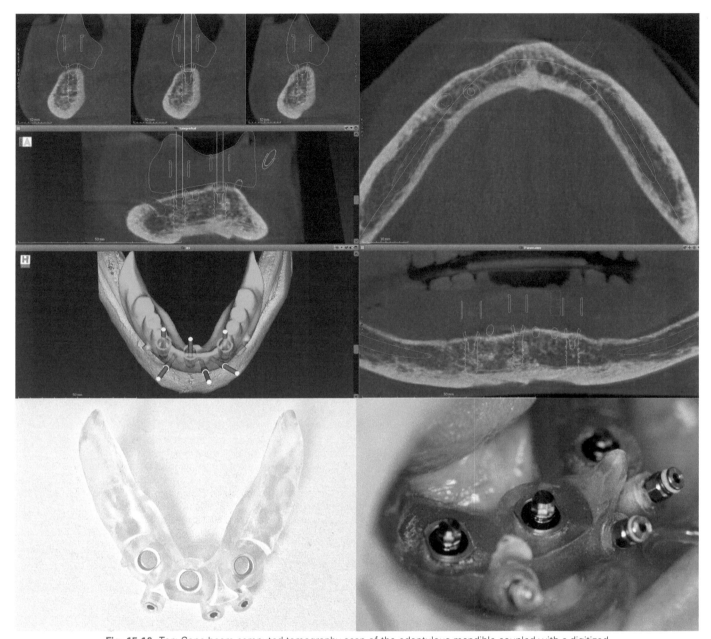

Fig. 15.16 *Top*: Cone beam computed tomography scan of the edentulous mandible coupled with a digitized model of the patient's existing complete lower denture *(dark blue)*. Three vertically oriented implants are planned in the interforaminal region of the mandible to support a fixed, implant-retained prosthesis *(light blue)*. A flapless approach was desired in this case, and a mucosa-supported guide was chosen, which was stabilized by three fixation pins positioned between these implants (also *light blue*). *Bottom left*: The final, printed mucosa-supported guide. Note the additional sleeves to allow for the insertion of fixation pins. *Bottom right*: Clinical photograph of the seated guide with the fixation pins and implants in place. (Courtesy Canaray: Specialists in Oral Radiology, Toronto, ON, Dr. J. Mahn, Paris, ON, and Ms. N. Tomkins and Ms. S. Goergen, Brantford, ON.)

multiple implants have been placed, a panoramic image may be appropriate. During the prosthetic phase of treatment, periapical or bite-wing images may be made to ensure complete seating of the implant abutment and restoration. When such images are made, it is important to position the central beam as perpendicular to the longitudinal axis of the implant fixture as possible. Small angular deviations may result in overlapping of the implant threads and allow small gaps between the fixture and prosthesis to go unnoticed (Fig. 15.19).

In the maintenance phase, annual recall imaging through the first 4 years of follow-up has been recommended for asymptomatic patients. This is particularly important in the first year of functional loading, when marginal bone loss and implant failure are most likely to occur. The most reliable indicators of implant success are clinical stability and radiographic evidence of bone adjacent to the implant body. Because of its superior resolution and ready accessibility, periapical imaging is recommended as the first-line modality to monitor implant

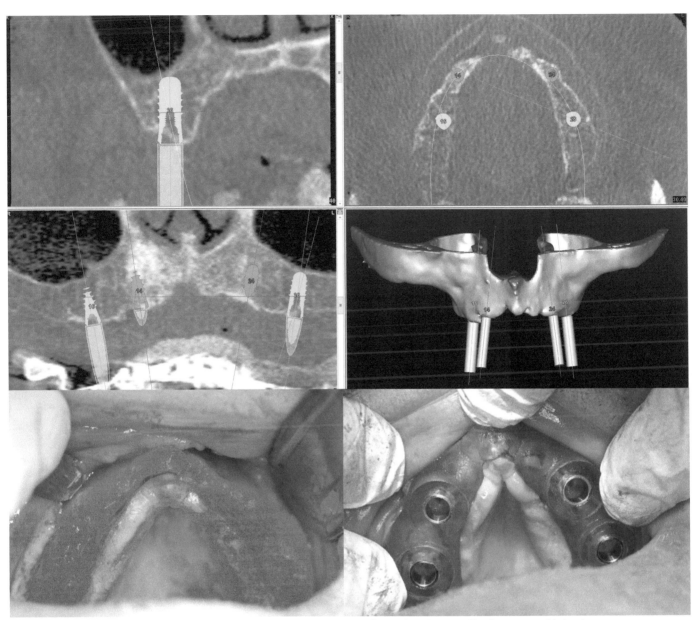

Fig. 15.17 *Top*: Cone beam computed tomography scan of the edentulous maxillae for a removable implant-supported prosthesis. Four implants were planned in the first premolar *(red)* and molar *(green)* regions, to be placed with the aid of a bone-supported guide. *Bottom*: Clinical photographs demonstrating the crestal incision made for a full mucoperiosteal flap *(left)* and the surgical guide fully seated on bone *(right)*. (Courtesy Canaray: Specialists in Oral Radiology, Toronto, ON, and Dr. J. Mahn, Paris, ON.)

osseointegration. When the instrument is ideally positioned, the image should demonstrate the apposition of normal bone around the implant threads and the reestablishment of the overlying alveolar crest (Fig. 15.20). To keep interval comparisons objective, recall images should strive to maintain the same projection geometry and exposure parameters as the immediate postoperative baseline image. Considering the radiation dose, cost, and its susceptibility to beam-hardening artifacts, CBCT imaging is not recommended for asymptomatic recall patients.

If the patient becomes symptomatic following implant placement, clinical examination and radiologic correlation are indicated. Implant mobility can arise from peri-implant bone loss subsequent to peri-implantitis, failure of the implant to osseointegrate, a loose abutment or restoration, or a fractured fixture. Similar to periodontal disease, peri-implant bone loss usually manifests as crestal bone loss with

progressive apical migration (Fig. 15.21). An implant that fails to osseointegrate will reveal a uniform radiolucent junction between the implant fixture and the surrounding bone (Fig. 15.22). In either case, implant failure may be attributed to a combination of poor plaque control, adverse loading, and systemic factors. When such a problem is identified, a CBCT examination may be prescribed to objectively characterize the extent of bone loss, particularly in the buccolingual dimension, and to assess the integrity of the adjacent cortices. These findings may be helpful in planning corrective bone augmentation procedures or the complete removal and replacement of an implant.

An implant that is placed beyond its local anatomic confines often causes symptoms. In the anterior maxilla and mandible, the presence of a prominent buccal concavity and a relatively thin buccal cortex may result in cortical perforation and thread exposure (Fig. 15.23). This can

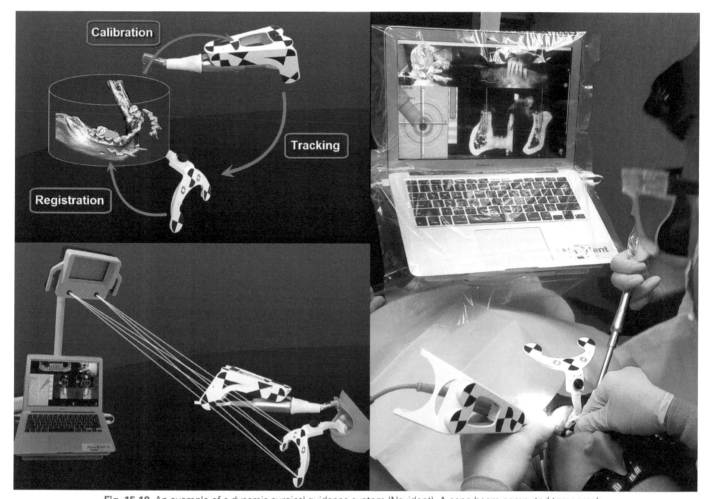

Fig. 15.18 An example of a dynamic surgical guidance system (Navident). A cone beam computed tomography (CBCT) scan is acquired with the patient wearing a specialized fiducial marker *(zig-zagging radiopaque shapes)* attached to an intraoral stent *(top left)*. A patterned optical tracking attachment is then connected to the intraoral stent during the surgery, the position of which is precisely registered to the CBCT data through the fiducial markers in the scan. Another similar tracking attachment is connected to the drill piece. Following a calibration process, the exact positions of the patient and drill head can be tracked by specialized cameras *(bottom left)* and their real-time positions relative to the CBCT volume conveyed on a laptop computer *(right)*. (Courtesy ClaroNav, Inc., Toronto, ON.)

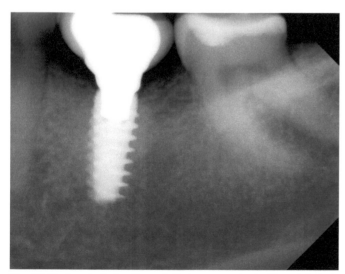

Fig. 15.19 A periapical radiograph that was acquired with an inferiorly positioned central ray, resulting in a diffuse appearance of the implant threads. The junction between the implant fixture and the restorative abutment is also poorly visualized.

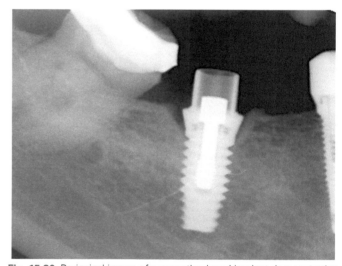

Fig. 15.20 Periapical image of a recently placed implant demonstrating the presence of normal bone adjacent to the implant threads. The overlying alveolar crest has been reestablished. These findings in conjunction with clinical immobility suggest successful implant integration.

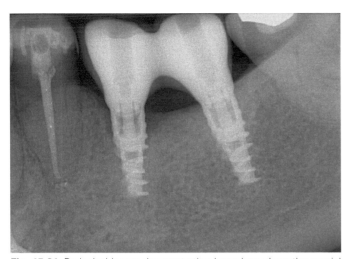

Fig. 15.21 Periapical image demonstrating bone loss along the mesial and distal surfaces of the implant placed in the region of the edentulous mandibular left second premolar.

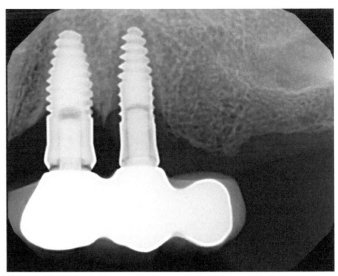

Fig. 15.22 Periapical image of the posterior left maxilla demonstrate a uniform radiolucent lining around the implant placed at the edentulous second premolar site. This could imply the presence of a soft tissue junction, indicating failed osseointegration. Mild crestal bone loss is observed around the adjacent implant at the site of the edentulous first premolar, but the remainder of this implant appears to be embedded in bone.

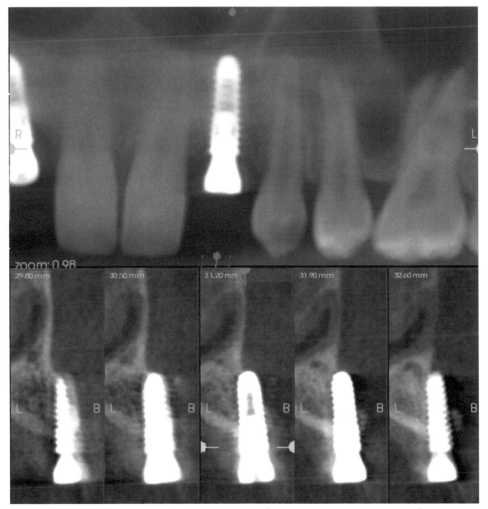

Fig. 15.23 *Top*: Cropped panoramic reformatted image of an implant placed at the site of the edentulous maxillary left lateral incisor. In this view, the implant appears to be embedded in bone. *Bottom*: Buccolingual cross-sectional images of the same implant showing that the buccal threads are exposed through a prominent buccal concavity.

lead to inflammation of the overlying soft tissue, with symptoms of pain, bleeding, and suppuration. In the posterior maxilla, implants are occasionally placed beyond the maxillary sinus floor, which may result in significant antral mucosal inflammation and the development of sinusitis (Fig. 15.24). In the posterior mandible, implants may extend into the lumen of the inferior alveolar canal, which can lead to altered sensation or numbness (Fig. 15.25). In these situations, CBCT examination may offer valuable insight in elucidating the etiology of the symptoms and in helping to guide management.

In summary, diagnostic imaging is essential for the preoperative planning of dental implants, intraoperative assessment, surgical guidance during implant placement, and the postoperative evaluation of recall and symptomatic patients. With continued scientific and technologic advancements, the practice of dental implantation will likely continue to evolve at a rapid pace. Clinicians will need to remain current with scientific literature and apply appropriate evidence-based treatment decisions that balance diagnostic efficacy, potential radiation risks, and health care costs.

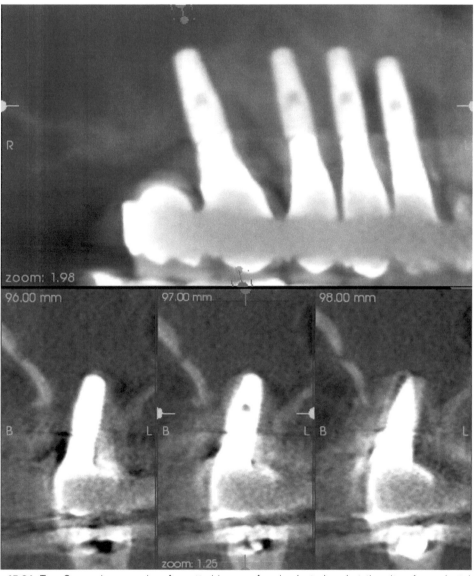

Fig. 15.24 *Top*: Cropped panoramic reformatted image of an implant placed at the site of an edentulous maxillary right first molar. *Bottom*: Buccolingual cross-sectional images of the same implant demonstrating that it has been placed through the floor of the right maxillary sinus. The right antral space is opacified and the sinus walls appear sclerotic, which could suggest the presence of sinusitis.

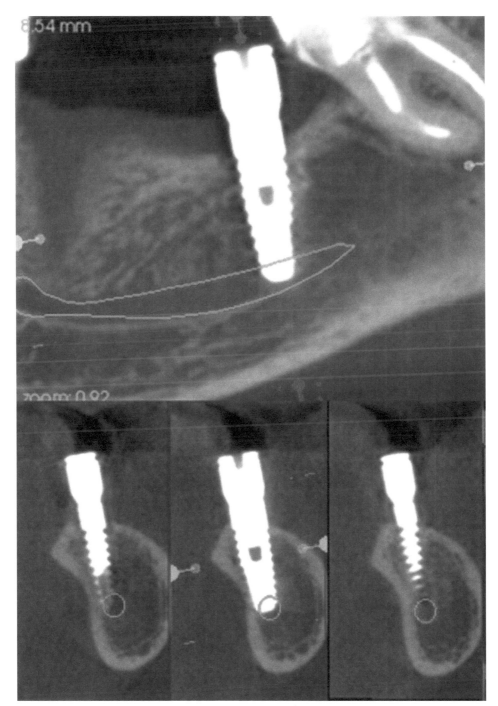

Fig. 15.25 Mesiodistal *(top)* and buccolingual *(bottom)* views of an implant that has been placed through left inferior alveolar nerve canal *(outlined in orange)* in a patient reporting numbness and altered sensation.

BIBLIOGRAPHY

Aguiar MF, Marques AP, Carvalho AC, et al. Accuracy of magnetic resonance imaging compared with computed tomography for implant planning. *Clin Oral Implants Res.* 2008;19(4):362–365.

Angelopoulos C, Thomas SL, Hechler S, et al. Comparison between digital panoramic radiography and cone-beam computed tomography for the identification of the mandibular canal as part of presurgical dental implant assessment. *J Oral Maxillofac Surg.* 2008;66(10):2130–2135.

Arisan V, Karabuda CZ, Ozdemir T. Implant surgery using bone- and mucosa-supported stereolithographic guides in totally edentulous jaws: surgical and post-operative outcomes of computer-aided vs. standard techniques. *Clin Oral Implants Res.* 2010;21(9):980–988.

Arisan V, Karabuda ZC, Ozdemir T. Accuracy of two stereolithographic guide systems for computer-aided implant placement: a computed tomography-based clinical comparative study. *J Periodontol.* 2010;81(1):43–51.

Bencharit S, Schardt-Sacco D, Zuninga JR, et al. Surgical and prosthodontic rehabilitation for patient with agressive florid cemento-osseous dysplasia. A clinical report. *J Prosthet Dent.* 2003;90:220–224.

Bornstein MM, Al-Nawas B, Kuchler U, et al. Consensus statements and recommended clinical procedures regarding contemporary surgical and radiographic techniques in implant dentistry. *Int J Oral Maxillofac Implants.* 2014;29:78–82.

Correa LR, Spin-Neto R, Stavropoulos A, et al. Planning of dental implant size with digital panoramic radiographs, CBCT-generated panoramic images, and CBCT cross-sectional images. *Clin Oral Implants Res.* 2014;25(6):690–695.

Di Giacomo GA, da Silva JV, da Silva AM, et al. Accuracy and complications of computer-designed selective laser sintering surgical guides for flapless dental implant placement and immediate definitive prosthesis installation. *J Periodontol.* 2012;83(4):410–419.

Ersoy AE, Turkyilmaz I, Ozan O, et al. Reliability of implant placement with stereolithographic surgical guides generated from computed tomography: clinical data from 94 implants. *J Periodontol.* 2008;79(8):1339–1345.

Fortin T, Bosson JL, Isidori M, et al. Effect of flapless surgery on pain experienced in implant placement using an image-guided system. *Int J Oral Maxillofac Implants.* 2006;2:298–304.

Friedrich RE, Laumann F, Zrnc T, et al. The Nasopalatine Canal in Adults on Cone Beam Computed Tomograms-A Clinical Study and Review of the Literature. *In Vivo.* 2015;29(4):467–486.

Gerlach RC, Dixon DR, Goksel T, et al. Case presentation of florid cemento-osseous dysplasia with concomitant cemento-ossifying fibroma discovered during implant explantation. *Oral Surg Oral Med Oral Pathol Oral Radiol.* 2013;115(3):e44–e52.

Gröndahl K, Lekholm U. The predictive value of radiographic diagnosis of implant instability. *Int J Oral Maxillofac Implants.* 1997;12(1):59–64.

Hämmerle CH, Stone P, Jung RE, et al. Consensus statements and recommended clinical procedures regarding computer-assisted implant dentistry. *Int J Oral Maxillofac Implants.* 2009;24(suppl):126–131.

Horner K, Islam M, Flygare L, et al. Basic principles for use of dental cone beam computed tomography: consensus guidelines of the European Academy of Dental and Maxillofacial Radiology. *Dentomaxillofac Radiol.* 2009;38:187–195.

Jung RE, Schneider D, Ganeles J, et al. Computer technology applications in surgical implant dentistry: a systematic review. *Int J Oral Maxillofac Implants.* 2009;24(suppl):92–109.

Kawai T, Hiranuma H, Kishino M, et al. Cemento-osseous dysplasia of the jaws in 54 japanese patients. A radiographic study. *Oral Surg Oral Med Oral Pathol Oral Radiol Endod.* 1999;87:107–114.

Kim YK, Park JY, Kim SG, et al. Magnification rate of digital panoramic radiographs and its effectiveness for pre-operative assessment of dental implants. *Dentomaxillofac Radiol.* 2011;40(2):76–83.

Kusum CK, Mody PV, Indrajeet, et al. Interforaminal hemorrhage during anterior mandibular implant placement: An overview. *Dent Res J (Isfahan).* 2015;12(4):291–300.

Kütük N, Demirbaş AE, Gönen ZB, et al. Anterior mandibular zone safe for implants. *J Craniofac Surg.* 2013;24(4):e405–e408.

Loubele M, Bogaerts R, Van Dijck E, et al. Comparison between effective radiation dose of CBCT and MSCT scanners for dentomaxillofacial applications. *Eur J Radiol.* 2009;71:461–468.

Ludlow JB, Timothy R, Walker C, et al. Effective dose of dental CBCT-a meta analysis of published data and additional data for nine CBCT units. *Dentomaxillofac Radiol.* 2015;44(1):20140197.

Misch CE. *Contemporary Implant Dentistry.* 3rd ed. St Louis: Mosby; 2008.

Oliveira MTF, Cardoso SV, Silva CJ, et al. Failure of dental implants in cemento-osseous dysplasia: a critical analysis of a case. *Rev Odontol UNESP.* 2014;43(3):223–227.

Ozan O, Turkyilmaz I, Ersoy AE, et al. Clinical accuracy of 3 different types of computed tomography-derived stereolithographic surgical guides in implant placement. *J Oral Maxillofac Surg.* 2009;67(2):394–401.

Pereira-Maciel P, Tavares-de-Sousa E, Oliveira-Sales MA. The mandibular incisive canal and its anatomical relationships: A cone beam computed tomography study. *Med Oral Patol Oral Cir Bucal.* 2015;20(6):e723–e728.

Raico Gallardo YN, da Silva-Olivio IR, Mukai E, et al. Accuracy comparison of guided surgery for dental implants according to the tissue of support: a systematic review and meta-analysis. *Clin Oral Implants Res.* 2016;[Epub ahead of print].

Resnik RR, Kircos LT, Misch CE. Diagnostic Imaging and Techniques. In: Misch CE, eds. *Contemporary Implant Dentistry.* 3rd ed. St. Louis: Mosby; 2008:38–67.

Ribeiro-Rotta RF, Lindh C, Pereira AC, et al. Ambiguity in bone tissue characteristics as presented in studies on dental implant planning and placement: a systematic review. *Clin Oral Implants Res.* 2011;22(8):789–801.

Rosenfeld AL, Mandelaris GA, Tardieu PB. Prosthetically directed implant placement using computer software to ensure precise placement and predictable prosthetic outcomes. Part 2: rapid-prototype medical modeling and stereolithographic drilling guides requiring bone exposure. *Int J Periodontics Restorative Dent.* 2006;26(4):347–353.

Schneider D, Marquardt P, Zwahlen M, et al. A systematic review on the accuracy and the clinical outcome of computer-guided template-based implant dentistry. *Clin Oral Implants Res.* 2009;20(suppl 4):73–86.

Sharan A, Madjar D. Maxillary sinus pneumatization following extractions: a radiographic study. *Int J Oral Maxillofac Implants.* 2008;23(1):48–56.

Tahmaseb A, Wismeijer D, Coucke W, et al. Computer technology applications in surgical implant dentistry: a systematic review. *Int J Oral Maxillofac Implants.* 2014;29(suppl):25–42.

Tyndall DA, Price JB, Tetradis S, et al. Position statement of the American Academy of Oral and Maxillofacial Radiology on selection criteria for the use of radiology in dental implantology with emphasis on cone beam computed tomography. *Oral Surg Oral Med Oral Pathol Oral Radiol.* 2012;113:817–826.

Van Assche N, Vercruyssen M, Coucke W, et al. Accuracy of computer-aided implant placement. *Clin Oral Implants Res.* 2012;23(suppl 6):112–123.

Vazquez L, Nizamaldin Y, Combescure C, et al. Accuracy of vertical height measurements on direct digital panoramic radiographs using posterior mandibular implants and metal balls as reference objects. *Dentomaxillofac Radiol.* 2013;42(2):20110429.

Yildirim YD, Güncü GN, Galindo-Moreno P, et al. Evaluation of mandibular lingual foramina related to dental implant treatment with computerized tomography: a multicenter clinical study. *Implant Dent.* 2014;23(1):57–63.

16

Quality Assurance and Infection Control

Sanjay M. Mallya

A quality assurance program in radiology is a series of procedures designed to ensure optimal and consistent operation of each component in the imaging chain. When all components function properly, the result is consistently high-quality radiographs made with optimal exposure settings, and reduced radiation dose to patients and office personnel.

The goal of an infection control program in radiology is to avoid cross-contamination among patients and between patients and the dental staff in the course of imaging.

RADIOGRAPHIC QUALITY ASSURANCE

Because radiographs are indispensable for patient diagnosis, the dentist must ensure that optimal exposure and film processing conditions are maintained. To reach this goal, a quality assurance program includes evaluation of the performance of x-ray machines, manual and automatic film processing procedures, image receptors, and viewing conditions. Optimization of all steps in the imaging chain maximizes diagnostic yield and decreases radiation dose to patients. Examples of common faults in digital sensor handling are provided in Chapter 4, and problems with film processing are presented in Chapter 5.

To effectively manage a quality assurance program, a dental office should identify one individual to assume the primary responsibility to implement the quality assurance program and to coordinate corrective action when indicated. Most quality assurance procedures are quickly accomplished and can have a significant influence on radiographic quality. The quality assurance procedures described in this section address intraoral, panoramic, cephalometric, and cone beam computed tomography (CBCT) imaging. Table 16.1 summarizes the tasks and their frequency.

Radiographic Exposures and Technique

This set of quality improvement procedures allows the office to identify a broad range of errors that impact image quality, including technical errors and x-ray source malfunction. These procedures are the same for film and digital radiography. This process helps to minimize errors in radiographic technique, including patient positioning and exposure settings. The process minimizes systematic issues that may be related to equipment calibration.

Daily Tasks

Enter findings in retake log. A simple and effective means of reducing the number of faulty radiographs is to keep a retake log. All errors for images that must be reexposed are recorded. This process quickly reveals the source of recurring problems and facilitates quick resolution.

Weekly Tasks

Review retake log. The retake record should be reviewed weekly to identify any recurring problems with film processing conditions or operator technique. This information can be used to initiate corrective actions, including staff education.

Monthly Tasks

Check exposure charts. The dental office should maintain a radiographic exposure chart next to the radiographic unit, preferably adjacent to the x-ray unit control panel where these parameters are selected. The chart should indicate the proper peak kilovoltage (kVp), milliamperes (mA), and exposure times(s) for making radiographs of each region of the oral cavity (Fig. 16.1). These tables help to ensure that all operators use the appropriate exposure factors. Typically, the mA is fixed at its highest setting; the kVp is fixed, usually at 70 kVp; and the exposure time is varied to account for patient size and location of the area of interest in the mouth.

Exposure times are initially determined empirically. In the case of photostimulable phosphor (PSP) plates and digital sensors, one should start by using the exposure times suggested by the manufacturer. Exposure times are slowly and systematically reduced to the point that image degradation is noticed. With film, careful time-temperature processing (described in Chapter 5) must be used with fresh solutions during this initial determination of exposure times.

Each month, this chart should be inspected to verify that the information is legible and accurate.

Check protective aprons and collars. Protective aprons and collars should be visually inspected for evidence of cracks. A fluoroscopic examination performed by a qualified individual can confirm any cracks in the lead shielding. These items should be replaced as necessary. Cracking is usually caused by folding the shields when not in use. It can be minimized by hanging the aprons from a hook or draping them over a handrail.

Yearly Tasks

Inspect and calibrate x-ray unit. When a new x-ray machine is purchased, it should be installed by a qualified expert, following federal and state regulations. Before its clinical use, the qualified expert performs acceptance tests. This *acceptance testing* refers to a formal group of tests that inspect the x-ray unit and confirm that the x-ray unit functions according to vendor-specific and industry standards. When in use, x-ray machines are generally quite stable, and only infrequently is a malfunction of the machine the cause of poor radiographs. The acceptance tests should be performed at periodic intervals to ensure continued

TABLE 16.1　Schedule of Radiographic Quality Assurance Procedures

	Task	Daily	Weekly	Monthly	Yearly
Monitor exposure and technique	Enter findings in retake log	•			
	Review retake log		•		
	Check exposure charts			•	
	Check protective aprons and collars			•	
	Inspect and calibrate x-ray unit				•
Film-based radiography	Replenish processing solutions	•			
	Check temperature of processing solutions	•			
	Compare film with reference film	•			
	Replace processing solutions		•		
	Clean processing equipment		•		
	Clean viewboxes		•		
	Check darkroom safelight			•	
	Clean intensifying screens			•	
	Rotate film stock			•	
Digital radiography	Calibrate image displays			•	
	Inspect PSP plates			•	
	Inspect CCD and CMOS sensors			•	
	Check digital image quality				•
	Preventive maintenance of CCD and CMOS-based panoramic and cephalometric units				•
	Preventive maintenance of PSP plate readers				•
CBCT	Detector calibration[a]	•		•	•
	Assess patient scan quality	•			
	Enter retake log	•			
	Review retake log		•		
	Preventive maintenance of CBCT unit				•
	Image quality measurement[b]			•	•

[a]Varies depending on manufacturer recommendation but should be part of annual preventive maintenance.
[b]One set of parameters is measured monthly and another set of quality parameters annually.
CBCT, Cone beam computed tomography; *CCD,* charge coupled device; *CMOS,* complementary semiconductor metal oxide; *PSP,* photostimulable phosphor.

optimal function and serves as the quality assurance program for x-ray units.

X-ray machines need to be calibrated annually, unless a specific problem is identified or substantive repair is necessary that may affect operation. A qualified expert, typically vendor service personnel, qualified medical physicists, or qualified oral and maxillofacial radiologists, should make these machine measurements because of the specialized equipment and knowledge required. The American Association of Physicists in Medicine (AAPM) Report No. 175 describes these procedures in detail and specifies the limits of tolerance for variance for the various parameters.

- *Leakage radiation:* A high-sensitivity radiation detector should be used to detect leakage radiation from the tube housing. No leakage radiation should be detected.
- *X-ray output:* A radiation dosimeter should be used to evaluate the reproducibility of radiation output (Fig. 16.2). Make at least three measurements and calculate the coefficient of variation (COV = standard deviation divided by mean). The COV should not exceed 5%.
- *Collimation and beam alignment:* The field diameter for dental intraoral x-ray machines should be no greater than 2.75 inches (7 cm). The tip of the position-indicating device (PID), or aiming cylinder, should be closely aligned with the x-ray beam.

For panoramic machines, the beam exiting the patient should not be larger than the collimator slit holding the receptor; this may be tested by taping dental films in front of and behind the collimator slit. A pin stick should be made through both films to allow subsequent realignment. Both films are exposed, processed, and realigned. The exposure to the film in front of the slit should be comparable in size to the film exposure behind the slit. Service is required if the front film exposure is larger than or not well oriented with the film exposure behind the slit.

For cephalometric radiographic units, the alignment of the x-ray beam and the cephalostat assembly should be verified. This includes adjustment of the ear rods in the vertical and horizontal planes, such that the beam is perpendicular to both ear support rods, and the receptor plane.

- *Beam energy:* The kVp of the beam should be measured to ensure accuracy and reproducibility. Measurement of kVp requires specialized equipment. Measurements should be made across the full spectrum of kVp values used for that unit, with an acceptable variation of 10% or less.
- *Beam half-value layer (HVL):* The HVL of the beam should be measured to ensure that the beam meets regulatory requirements. This is done using a dosimeter and aluminum sheets of specific thickness. The regulatory requirements of the U.S. Food and Drug Administration (FDA), 21CFR 20 are listed as follows.

X-Ray Machine: (Brand name)		
Location: (Room)		
mA: 15		
kVP: 70		
Sensor: (Brand name)		
	EXPOSURE TIME	
Projection	**Seconds**	**Impulses**
Adult periapicals		
Incisors	0.25	15
Premolars	0.30	18
Molars	0.35	21
Occlusal	0.40	24
Adult bitewings		
Premolar	0.30	18
Molar	0.35	21
Edentulous periapicals		
Incisors	0.20	12
Premolars	0.25	15
Molars	0.30	18
Occlusal	0.35	21
Children		
Anterior periapicals	0.25	15
Posterior periapicals	0.25	15
Bitewing	0.25	15
Occlusal	0.30	18

Fig. 16.1 Sample wall chart showing identification information for x-ray machine, sensor or film type, milliamperage (mA) and peak kilovoltage (kVp) settings, and appropriate exposure times for various anatomic locations and patient sizes. The optimal exposure times must be determined empirically in each office because they vary with the machine settings used, source-to-skin distance, and other factors.

Minimum Half-Value Layer (mm of aluminum)		
Peak kilovoltage (kVp)	**Intraoral Radiographic Units**	**Panoramic and Cephalometric Units**
60	1.5	1.5
70	1.5	1.8
71	2.1	2.5
80	2.3	2.9
90	2.5	3.2

- *Timer:* Electrical pulse counters count the number of pulses generated by an x-ray machine during a preset time interval. The timer should be accurate and reproducible. Deviation should not exceed 10% for timer settings greater than 10 ms.
- *mA:* The linearity of the mA control should be verified if two or more mA settings are available on the machine. Typically, an exposure using the usual adult bite-wing setting is made. The mA are then reduced to the next lower value, and the exposure time is increased to yield the same mAs (product of the mA and exposure time in seconds).

    Example: A machine has 10-mA and 15-mA settings, and 15 mA and 0.4 seconds are used for adult bite-wings

    First test exposure setting: 15 mA and 0.4 seconds (= 6 mAs)

    Second test exposure setting: 10 mA and 0.6 seconds (= 6 mAs)

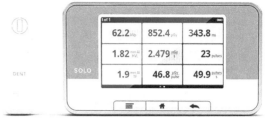

Fig. 16.2 The RaySafe X2 Solo DENT device is designed for dental offices and measures dose, dose rate, kVp, exposure time, pulses, and pulse rate. The sensor can be used for intraoral, panoramic, cephalometric and cone beam computed tomography applications. (Courtesy Fluke Biomedical, www.flukebiomedical.com.)

A discrepancy implies nonlinearity in the mA control or a fault in the timer. This variation should not exceed 10%.

- *Tube head stability:* The tube head should be stable when placed around the patient's head, and it should not drift during the exposure. When the tube head is unstable, service is necessary to adjust the suspension mechanism. The drift should be 0.5 cm or less.
- *Focal spot size:* Measure the size of the focal spot because it may become enlarged with excessive heat buildup within an x-ray machine. An enlarged focal spot contributes to geometric fuzziness in the resultant image. A specialized piece of equipment is required for this test.

Film-Based Radiography

Quality assurance tasks for film-based imaging are primarily directed to ensuring consistent and optimal conditions for film processing. These conditions, including processing chemical strength and temperature, can fluctuate rapidly; daily checks are necessary. Quality assurance tasks for film-based imaging are more frequent and typically require more time than quality assurance for digital receptors.

Daily Tasks

Replenish processing solutions. At the beginning of each work day, check the levels of the processing solutions and replenish with fresh developing solution and fresh fixing solution, as necessary. The most common cause of poor film radiographs is poor processing in the darkroom, in particular, the use of depleted solutions.

Check temperature of processing solutions. At the beginning of each work day, check the temperature of the processing solutions. The solutions must reach the optimal temperature before use—68°F (20°C) for manual processing and 82°F (28°C) for heated automatic processors. The instructions accompanying the film and processor verify the optimal temperature. Unheated automatic processors should be located away from windows or heaters that may cause their temperature to vary during the day. Proper temperature regulation is required for accurate time-temperature processing.

Compare film radiographs with reference film. A simple and effective means to routinely monitor the quality of images produced in an office is to check daily films against a reference film. A reference film provides a visual standard for optimal film processing. Comparison of daily images with the reference film may reveal problems before they interfere with the diagnostic quality of the images. When a problem is identified, it is important to determine the probable source and to take corrective action. For example, if the processing solutions have become depleted, the resultant radiographs are light and have reduced contrast. Both developer and fixer should be changed when degradation of the image quality is evident. Light images may also result from cold solutions or

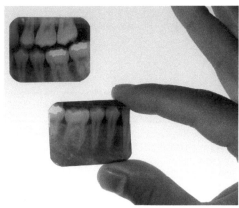

Fig. 16.3 Radiographs should be checked daily against a reference film made with fresh solutions. As processing solutions become exhausted, the daily images become increasingly light and lose contrast. When these changes are apparent, both the developer and the fixer should be changed.

insufficient developing time. Dark images may be caused by excessive developing time, developer that is too warm, or light leaks.

Reference films may be:

- *Patient images:* Soon after film processing solutions are replaced, a patient's radiograph that has been properly exposed and processed with exact time-temperature technique is mounted on a corner of the viewbox. This image, with optimal density and contrast, serves as a reference for the radiographs made in the following days and weeks (Fig. 16.3).
- *Radiographs of a standard test object:* This is the most accurate and rigorous method of testing film processing solutions but requires additional equipment and more time to perform. An aluminum step wedge serves as a test object that provides a consistent range of gray shades (see Figs. 5.22 and 5.24). A step wedge can be fabricated using few overlapping sheets of lead foils, staggered to create "steps" with multiple thicknesses of lead. The step wedge is placed on the film and exposed to make the reference image. The digital dental quality assurance (DDQA) phantom, described later, can also be used to provide a reliable test object. Daily reference images should be made with the same set of exposure settings (kVp and milliamperes-seconds [mAs]) and source-film distance. Standard images can also be made using a sensitometer to expose film to a calibrated light pattern. After processing, a densitometer is used to measure the optical density of each region of the image pattern on the film. A change in the density readings from day to day indicates a problem in film processing.

Weekly Tasks

Replace processing solutions. How frequently processing solutions are replaced depends primarily on the rate of use of the solutions and also on the size of tanks, whether a cover is used, and the temperature of the solutions. In most offices, the solutions should be changed weekly or every 2 weeks. The results of the step-wedge test help determine the proper frequency.

Clean processing equipment. Regular cleaning of the processing equipment is necessary for optimal operation. The solution tanks of manual and automatic processing equipment should be cleaned when the solutions are changed. The rollers of automatic film processors should be cleaned weekly according to the manufacturer's instructions. After cleaning, the tanks and rollers should be rinsed as the manufacturer

recommends to prevent the cleaner from interfering with the action of the film processing solutions.

Clean viewboxes. Viewboxes should be cleaned weekly to remove any particles or defects that may interfere with film interpretation.

Monthly Tasks

Check darkroom safelighting. Film becomes fogged in the darkroom because of inappropriate safelight filters, excessive exposure to safelights, and stray light from other sources. These films are dark, show low contrast, and have a muddy gray appearance. The darkroom should be inspected monthly to assess the integrity of the safelights (preferably GBX-2 filters with 15-W bulbs). The glass filter should be intact, with no cracks. To check for light leaks in a darkroom, all lights are turned off; the individual allows his or her vision to accommodate to the dark and checks for light leaks, especially around doors and vents. Light leaks should be marked with chalk or masking tape to facilitate correction. Weather stripping is useful for sealing light leaks under doors.

Clean intensifying screens. All intensifying screens in panoramic and cephalometric film cassettes should be cleaned monthly. The presence of scratches or debris results in recurring light areas on the resultant images. The foam supporting the screens must be intact and capable of holding both screens closely against the film. If close contact between the film and screens is not maintained, the image will appear unsharp.

Rotate film stock. Dental x-ray film is quite stable when it is properly handled. X-ray film should be stored in a cool, dry facility away from a radiation source. Stock should be rotated when new film is received so that old film does not accumulate in storage. The oldest film always should be used first but never after its expiration date.

Digital Radiography

An increasing number of dental offices use digital receptors for intraoral radiography. These include solid-state sensors (charge-coupled device [CCD], complementary metal oxide semiconductor [CMOS]) and PSP systems. As with film-based imaging, it is important for dental offices to periodically evaluate the components of the digital system to ensure that they maintain high-quality diagnostic imaging. Essential elements of quality assurance programs for digital dental radiography are described in the American Dental Association (ADA) Technical Report 1094 and the AAPM Report No. 175.

Monthly Tasks

Calibrate image displays. Interpretation of digital images is performed on a computer display. Such displays may be medical-grade displays designed to conform to DICOM standards or high-end consumer-grade displays—liquid crystal display (LCD) or light-emitting diode (LED) displays. Irrespective of type, displays used for radiologic diagnosis should be calibrated and checked on a monthly basis. Test pattern images, such as the Society for Motion Picture and Television Engineers (SMPTE) Medical Diagnostic Imaging Test Pattern or the AAPM TG18-QC image, should be used to assist the evaluator to adjust the brightness and contrast and to identify defects in the display. These test pattern images are publicly available via the internet and require minimal training to use, and the periodic evaluation can be completed in a few minutes.

Inspect photostimulable phosphor plates. PSP plates may become scratched in the course of use. These scratches may be seen as light streaks on processed images (see Figs. 4.22A and 4.23) and may compromise diagnostic quality and mimic pathology or foreign objects. PSP plates should be inspected monthly and removed from service when such defects are found.

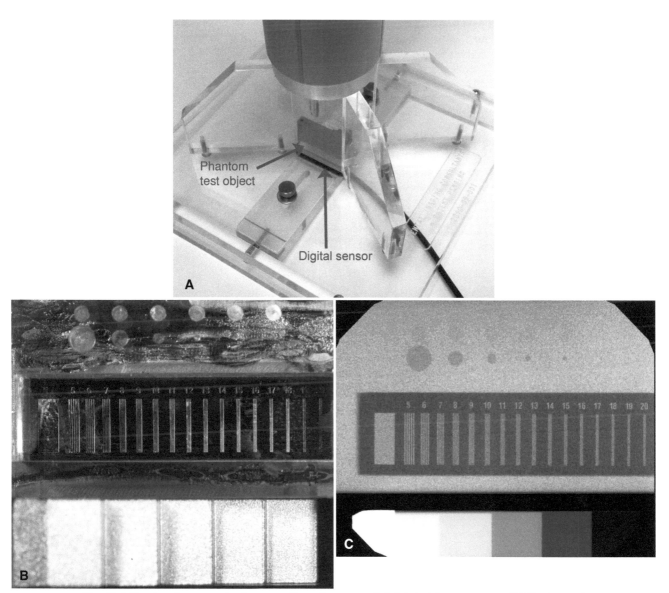

Fig. 16.4 Phantom for measuring image quality performance of digital dental x-ray systems. (A) Plastic stand allows positioning of the aiming tube of the x-ray machine over the test device, which is positioned over the digital sensor. (B) Test device contains, from the top, two rows of wells of varying diameter and depth in an acrylic background for measuring contrast detail, an etched pattern of slits in a metallic background for measuring the spatial resolution in line pairs per millimeter, and a calibrated step wedge for measuring dose response. (C) Resulting image. (Images courtesy Dr. Peter K. Mah: www.dentalimagingconsultants.com.)

Inspect CCD and CMOS sensors. CCD and CMOS sensors should be inspected monthly to confirm that the plastic housing, and cable connections to the sensor and Universal Serial Bus (USB) are intact. Although the sensor may be functional with signs of damage to these components, it may indicate an impending failure. Some of these damages may be repairable.

Yearly Tasks

Check digital image quality. The ADA Technical Report 1094 recommends that digital sensors and PSP plates be checked yearly for signs of image degradation. This is tested using phantom test objects. The DDQA phantom (Fig. 16.4) combines three components—a line pair gauge (to assess spatial resolution), a step wedge (to assess dynamic range), and variable diameter uniform depth well (to assess contrast/ detail resolution). The phantom is also designed to provide clinically relevant source-object and source-receptor distances.

Ideally, the test object images should be used to provide measurements for acceptance testing. Periodically acquired images should be compared with this initial image to assess changes in image parameters over time. It is important to recognize that the displayed image is a function of the imaging hardware (sensor or PSP plate) and the software used to display the image. Thus the effect of software upgrades or new software on displayed image quality should be tested using the test object image parameters described above.

Preventive maintenance of CCD- and CMOS-based panoramic and cephalometric units. Digital panoramic and cephalometric imaging machines should be inspected on a periodic basis, as recommended by the manufacturer. Typically, this is performed annually. In addition to the inspection and calibration of the x-ray output, as described in the section on radiographic exposure, panoramic and cephalometric CCD and CMOS detectors should be evaluated for uniformity and artifacts. The preventive maintenance schedule should calibrate and confirm proper function of the mechanical components that move the sensor during image acquisition, and the veracity of software stitching of images.

Preventive maintenance of photostimulable phosphor readers. The latent image on PSP plates are converted to a digital image in a PSP scanner. These scanners must be calibrated and tested at initial installation and at periodic intervals to ensure proper function and production of images that meet vendor system specifications and industry standards. Following the initial acceptance testing, yearly preventive maintenance should be performed to evaluate the entire PSP system. It is important to recognize that the image from a PSP system is influenced by multiple factors, including the state of the imaging plate, proper functioning of multiple mechanical and electronic components that control the laser beam and the photomultiplier tubes that collect signal, analog-to-digital processing of the signal, and eventually the calibration of the display monitor. Annual quality assurance and preventive maintenance should confirm proper functioning of these processes.

The AAPM Report No. 93 describes procedures for acceptance testing and quality control of PSP imaging systems. The measures of quality and function include dark noise and uniformity, system linearity and autoranging, image geometric uniformity, spatial resolution, and laser jitter. Notably, improper functioning of the PSP scanner components could result in dimensional inaccuracies in the image, which may impact cephalometric analysis.

Cone Beam Computed Tomography

In-office CBCT imaging has increased over the past several years. Although quality assurance protocols for image quality and radiation dose have been well established for multidetector computed tomography (MDCT), guidance for CBCT from the AAPM and ADA is under development. Broad guidelines have been published by the SEDENTEXCT consortium.

Acceptance Testing

All CBCT installations should be done by a qualified expert. Acceptance testing should include evaluation of the x-ray output parameters, mechanical and electronic controls of the equipment, and function and calibration of the detectors. The SEDENTEXCT consortium has developed guidelines for acceptance testing for dental CBCT units. The acceptance testing process includes acquiring baseline images of a test phantom to periodically monitor changes in image quality. Phantoms for CBCT image quality measurement are provided by the manufacturer or are available from third-party vendors. These include the QRM Dental CBCT phantom and the SEDENTEXCT IQ Dental CBCT-Leeds Test Object (Fig. 16.5). The phantoms should allow measurements of image uniformity, spatial resolution, contrast resolution, image noise, and geometric accuracy.

Daily Tasks

Assess patient scan quality. Dentists who acquire CBCT images in their office should include image quality assessment as part of their interpretive evaluation for every patient scan. Typically, this is accomplished within a few minutes and is an efficient means to identify hardware and software malfunction and operator errors in patient positioning and exposure. Findings that impact diagnostic quality or interpretation should be included in the radiology report.

Enter findings in retake log. As with other types of radiographic imaging, the office should maintain a log of repeat scans made. This

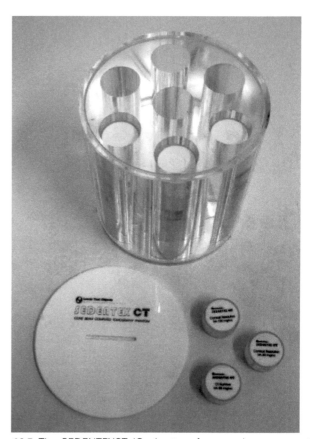

Fig. 16.5 The SEDENTEXCT IQ phantom for cone beam computed tomography image quality measurement. The insert holder is 16 cm in diameter. Attenuation in the body of the insert holder provides assessment of image uniformity and image noise. Individual inserts allow measurement of spatial resolution, contrast resolution, pixel intensity, and beam hardening artifacts. (From Pauwels R, Beinsberger J, Stamatakis H, et al. Comparison of spatial and contrast resolution for cone-beam computed tomography scanners. *Oral Surg Oral Med Oral Pathol Oral Radiol.* 2012;114(1):127–135.)

document quickly reveals the source of recurring problems and facilitates speedy resolution.

Weekly Tasks

Review retake log. The retake record should be reviewed weekly to identify any recurring problems with film processing conditions or operator technique. This information can be used to initiate corrective actions, including staff education.

Monthly Tasks

Image quality measurement. The SEDENTEXCT guidelines recommend that some parameters of image quality be evaluated on a monthly basis:

Image density: This is accomplished by measuring mean pixel intensities within a region of interest in the quality control phantom and comparing these measurements with similar baseline measurements (established during acceptance testing). The variance should not be more than 10% from baseline.

Uniformity and artifacts: Image uniformity is measured by examining pixel intensities at regions of interest in the center and periphery of the phantom. There should be no visible artifacts in the image, and the mean pixel intensities at various regions within the imaged volume should be ±10% from the mean measurement.

Annual Tasks

Preventive maintenance of cone beam computed tomography devices. Most CBCT manufacturers recommend preventive maintenance of CBCT units, typically on an annual basis. This is usually performed by a qualified service technician or a qualified expert. The maintenance tasks include evaluation of the x-ray output, beam collimation, gantry and chair mechanical components, and detector uniformity and artifacts.

Image quality measurement. In addition to the aspects of image quality evaluated on a monthly basis (described previously) the SEDENTEXCT guidelines recommend that noise, spatial resolution, contrast resolution, and geometric accuracy be measured every year.

INFECTION CONTROL

Dental personnel and patients are at increased risk for acquiring tuberculosis, herpes viruses, upper respiratory infections, and hepatitis strains A through E. After the recognition of acquired immunodeficiency syndrome (AIDS) in the 1980s, rigorous hygienic procedures were introduced in dental offices. The primary goal of infection control procedures is to prevent cross-contamination and disease transmission from patient to staff, from staff to patient, and from patient to patient. The potential for cross-contamination in dental radiography is great. In the course of making radiographs, an operator's hands become contaminated by contact with a patient's mouth and saliva-contaminated films and film holders. The operator also must adjust the x-ray tube head and x-ray machine control panel settings to make the exposure. These actions lead to the possibility of cross-contamination. Cross-contamination also may occur when an operator handles digital sensors or opens film packets to process the films in the darkroom. The procedures described in the following sections minimize or eliminate such cross-contamination (Box 16.1). Each dental office or practice should have a written policy describing its infection control practices. It is best if one individual in a practice, usually the dentist, assumes responsibility for implementing these procedures. This person also educates other members of the practice.

Standard Precautions

Standard precautions (also called universal precautions) are infection control practices designed to protect workers from exposure to diseases spread by blood and certain body fluids, including saliva. Under standard precautions, all human blood and saliva are treated as if known to be infectious for human immunodeficiency virus (HIV) and hepatitis B virus. Accordingly, the means used to protect against cross-contamination are used for all individuals. The ADA and the U.S. Centers for Disease Control and Prevention (CDC) stress the use of standard precautions because many patients are unaware that they are carriers of infectious disease or choose not to reveal this information.

BOX 16.1 Key Steps in Radiographic Infection Control

- Apply standard precautions
- Wear personal protective equipment during all radiographic procedures
- Disinfect and cover x-ray machine, working surfaces, chair, and apron
- Sterilize nondisposable instruments
- Use barrier-protected film (sensor) or disposable container
- Prevent contamination of processing equipment

Wear Personal Protective Equipment During All Radiographic Procedures

Personal protective equipment is an effective means to shield the operator from exposure to potentially infectious material, including blood and saliva.

- Hand hygiene is most important to prevent spread of infections. After the patient is seated, the practitioner should wash his or her hands using plain or antimicrobial soap, specific for health care settings. Alcohol-based hand rubs are also effective.
- Disposable gloves should be worn in sight of the patient if the operatory arrangement permits. The operator should always wear gloves when making radiographs or handling contaminated receptor barriers or associated materials such as cotton rolls and receptor-holding instruments or when removing barrier protections from surfaces and radiographic equipment.
- Operators should wear protective clothing (e.g., disposable gown or laboratory coat) that covers clothes and skin to protect against potential contamination. Eyewear, a mask, or a face shield must be worn if splash exposure to bodily fluids is anticipated.

Disinfect and Cover Clinical Contact Surfaces

Clinical contact surfaces are surfaces that might be touched by gloved hands or instruments that go into the mouth. These include the x-ray machine and control panel, chair-side computer, beam alignment device, dental chair and headrest, protective apron, thyroid collar, and surfaces on which the receptor is placed. The CDC classifies these as noncritical items. These are objects that may come in contact with saliva, blood, or intact skin but not oral mucous membranes. The goal of preventing cross-contamination is addressed by disinfecting all such surfaces and by using barriers to isolate equipment from direct contact.

Barriers made of clear plastic wrap should cover working surfaces that were previously cleaned and disinfected. Barriers protect the underlying surface from becoming contaminated and should be changed when damaged and routinely after each patient. Although barriers greatly aid infection control, they do not replace the need for effective surface cleaning and disinfection. Experience has demonstrated that failure of mechanical barriers is common during the daily activity of treatment. Whenever this happens, surfaces that become accidentally exposed must be cleaned and disinfected. Operators should avoid touching walls and other surfaces with contaminated gloves.

Any clinical contact surface that is contaminated or potentially contaminated should be disinfected. Table 16.2 lists intermediate- and low-level activity disinfectants recommended for use on clinical contact

TABLE 16.2 Disinfectants for Clinical Contact Surfaces

Activity	Disinfectant Agent	Concentration
Low	Quaternary ammonium compounds	
Low to intermediate	Phenolic compounds	0.5%–3%
	Iodophor compounds[a]	0.1%–0.2%
Intermediate	Ethyl alcohol, isopropyl alcohol	70%
	Sodium hypochlorite	1000 ppm[b]

[a]Only iodophors that are Environmental Protection Agency–registered disinfectants.
[b]5.25%–6% household bleach diluted 1:50 provides >1000 ppm available chlorine.

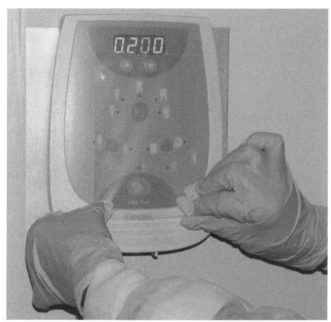

Fig. 16.6 The exposure control console should be covered with a clean barrier and changed after every patient.

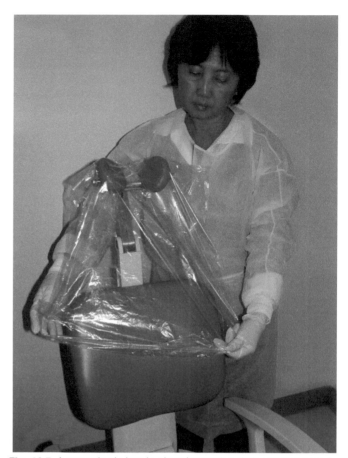

Fig. 16.7 A new plastic bag is placed over the chair and headrest for each patient.

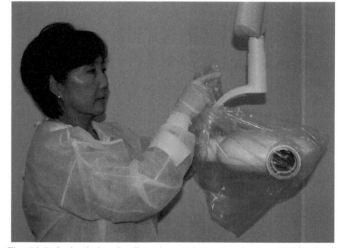

Fig. 16.8 A plastic bag is slipped over the x-ray tube head with a large rubber band just proximal to the swivel or tie ends, as shown here. The plastic is pulled tight over the position-indicating device (PID) and secured with a light rubber band slipped over the PID and placed next to the head.

surfaces. Intermediate-level disinfectants are Environmental Protection Agency (EPA)-registered agents and are tuberculocidal—an effective killer of tuberculosis—and capable of preventing other infectious diseases, including hepatitis B virus and HIV. Low-level disinfectants are EPA registered without tuberculocidal activity but inactivate hepatitis B virus and HIV. High-level disinfectants are used for chemical sterilization and should never be used on clinical contact surfaces.

- Countertops and the x-ray control console should be covered with a plastic barrier. When covering the x-ray control console, the operator should be sure to include the exposure switch and the exposure time control, if they are integral parts of the unit (Fig. 16.6). An x-ray exposure switch that is separate from the console should be covered with a plastic barrier.
- The dental chair headrest, headrest adjustments, and chair back may be easily covered with a plastic bag (Fig. 16.7). The x-ray tube head, PID, and yoke should be covered while they are still wet with disinfectant with a barrier to stop any dripping (Fig. 16.8). The bag should be secured by tying a knot in the open end or by placing a heavy rubber band over the x-ray tube head just proximal to the swivel.
- The protective apron should be cleaned, disinfected, and covered between patients because it is frequently contaminated with saliva as the result of handling (readjusting its position) during a radiographic procedure. The apron should be suspended on a heavy coat hanger to permit turning front to back. It should be sprayed with a low-level disinfectant and then wiped (Fig. 16.9).
- Exposure charts should be kept away from sources of contamination and not handled during the radiographic examination.
- Panoramic chin rest and patient handgrips should be cleaned with a low-level disinfectant. Disposable bite-blocks may be used. The head-positioning guides, control panel, and exposure switch should be carefully wiped with a paper towel that is well moistened with disinfectant. The radiographer should wear disposable gloves while positioning and exposing the patient. The gloves should be removed before the cassette is removed from the machine for processing because the cassette and film remain extraoral and should not be handled with contaminated disposable gloves.
- Cephalostat ear posts, ear post brackets, and forehead support or nasion pointer should be cleaned and disinfected. These may then also be covered with a plastic barrier.

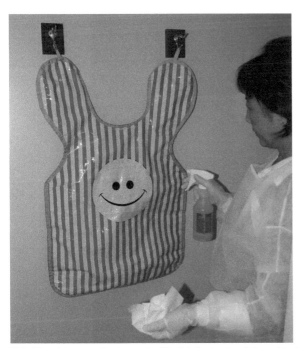

Fig. 16.9 Hanging apron is sprayed with disinfectant and then dried and covered with a garment bag.

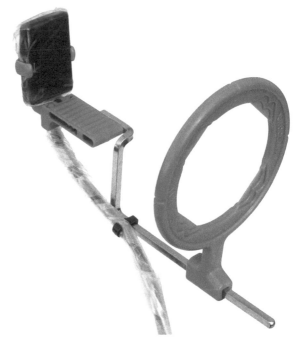

Fig. 16.10 Film-holding instrument with barrier wrapping to protect sensor and cord from saliva. (Image courtesy Dentsply Rinn: www.rinncorp.com.)

- After patient exposures are completed, the barriers should be removed, and contaminated working surfaces (including surfaces in the darkroom) and the apron should be sprayed with disinfectant and wiped as described previously. The barriers should be replaced in preparation for the next patient.

Sterilize Nondisposable Instruments

Receptor-holding instruments are classified by the CDC as semicritical items—instruments that are not used to penetrate soft tissue or bone but do come in contact with the oral mucous membrane. It is best to use receptor-holding instruments that can be sterilized, preferably by steam under pressure (autoclave). After using these instruments, disassemble the aiming ring, support arm, and bite-block. Each instrument should be cleaned with hot water and soap to remove saliva and debris. The cleaned components are then loaded into plastic or paper pouches and sterilized in an autoclave. After sterilization, the instruments should be kept in pouches for storage and subsequent transport to the radiography area. When the instruments are taken to the radiography area, it is good practice to keep them in the pouch until immediately before use. After use, instruments should be replaced in the pouch to reinforce cleanliness in the area. The same sterilization pouch should be used to transport the contaminated instruments back to the cleaning and sterilizing areas.

Use Barriers With Digital Sensors

Sensors for digital imaging cannot be sterilized by heat, so it is important to use a barrier to protect them from contamination when placed in the patient's mouth (Fig. 16.10). Typically, the manufacturers of these sensors recommend the use of plastic barrier sheaths that extend a few inches along the sensor cord. However, such barriers fail approximately 40% of the time. The supplemental use of latex finger cots provides significant added protection and is recommended for routine use when using digital sensors. Because such barriers may fail, the sensors should be cleaned and disinfected with an EPA-registered, intermediate-level hospital disinfectant after every patient. The manufacturer of such

equipment should be consulted for the proper disinfectant. Some manufacturers have designed solid-state sensors that can be immersed into a cold sterilant (a high-level EPA-registered disinfectant).

PSP sensors are placed in disposable plastic bags with a folded seal for use in the mouth. Because the entire plastic bag goes into the mouth with PSP sensors, these plates possibly can become contaminated with saliva when removed from the plastic bags for processing. This contamination could lead to cross-contamination of other plates and the processing equipment. To minimize this problem, PSP plates should be disinfected between patients, using a method recommended by the manufacturer. PSP plates may be gas sterilized with ethylene oxide.

Use Barrier-Protected Film (Sensor) or Disposable Container

To prevent contamination of bulk supplies of film, they should be dispensed in procedure quantities. The required number of films for a full-mouth or interproximal series should be prepackaged in coin envelopes or paper cups in the central preparation room. These envelopes of films should be dispensed with the film-holding instruments. For unanticipated occasions in which an unusual number of films are required, a small container of films can be on hand in the central preparation and sterilizing room. No one wearing contaminated gloves should retrieve a film from this supply. Films should be dispensed only by staff members with clean hands or wearing clean gloves.

Film packets may be prepackaged in a plastic envelope (Fig. 16.11), which protects the film from contact with saliva and blood during exposure. Barrier-protected film fits in most film-holding instruments. An attractive feature of the protective envelopes is the ease with which they may be opened and the film extracted. For best results, the packet should be immersed in a disinfectant after the films have been exposed in the patient's mouth. Then the packet should be dried and opened, allowing the film to drop out. The barrier envelopes can be conveniently opened in a lighted area, the film can be dropped onto a clean work area or into a clean paper or plastic cup, and the film can be transferred to the daylight loader or darkroom for processing.

If barrier-protected film is not used, the exposed film should be placed in a disposable container for later transport to the darkroom for processing. Paper film packets are exposed to saliva and possibly blood during exposure in the patient's mouth. To prevent saliva from seeping into a paper film packet, a paper towel should be placed beside the container for exposed films. The practitioner should use this towel to wipe each film as it is removed from the patient's mouth and before it is placed with the other exposed films. This problem may also be avoided by using film packaged in vinyl.

Prevent Contamination of Processing Equipment

After all film exposures are made, the operator should remove his or her gloves and take the container of contaminated films to the darkroom.

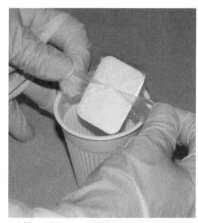

Fig. 16.11 Dental film with a plastic barrier to protect film from contact with saliva. During opening, the plastic is removed and the clean film is allowed to drop into a container.

The goal in the darkroom is to break the infection chain so that only clean films are placed into processing solutions. Two towels should be placed on the darkroom working surface. The container of contaminated films should be placed on one of these towels. After the exposed film is removed from its packet, it should be placed on the second towel. The film packaging is discarded on the first towel with the container.

The procedure to remove film from a packet without touching (contaminating) is simple. Fig. 16.12 illustrates the method for opening a contaminated film packet while wearing contaminated gloves without touching the film. The practitioner dons a clean pair of gloves, picks up the film packet by the color-coded end, and pulls the tab upward and away from the packet to reveal the black paper tab wrapped over the end of the film. Holding the film over a cup, the practitioner carefully grasps the black paper tab that wraps the film and pulls the film from the packet. When the film is pulled from the packet, it falls from the paper wrapping into the cup. The paper wrapper may need to be shaken lightly to cause the film to fall free. The packaging materials should be placed on the first paper towel. After all films are opened, the practitioner gathers the contaminated packaging and container and discards them along with the contaminated gloves. The clean films are processed in the usual manner. It is not necessary to wear gloves when handling processed films, film mounts, or patient charts.

An alternative procedure when exposing films in vinyl packaging is to place the exposed film, still in the protective plastic envelope, in an approved disinfecting solution when it is removed from the mouth and after wiping it with a paper towel. It should remain in the disinfectant after the exposure of the last film for the recommended time. Immersion for 30 seconds in a 5.25% solution of sodium hypochlorite is effective.

Automatic film processors with daylight loaders present a special problem because of the risk for contaminating the sleeves with contaminated gloves or film packets. One approach is to clean the films

Fig. 16.12 Method for removing films from packet without touching them with contaminated gloves. (A) Packet tab is opened, and lead foil and black interleaf paper are slid from wrapping. (B) Foil is rotated away from black paper and discarded. (C) Paper wrapping is opened. (D) Film is allowed to fall into a clean cup.

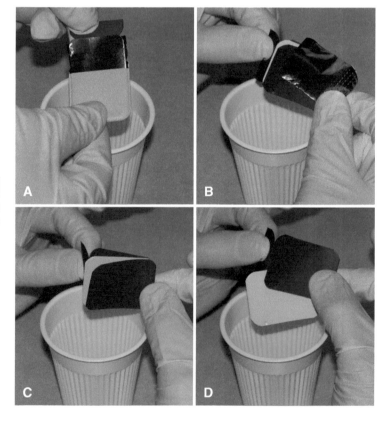

by immersion in a disinfectant, with or without a plastic envelope, as previously described. With this method, the operator cleans the films, puts on clean gloves, and takes only cleaned film packets into the daylight loader. An alternative approach is to open the top of the loader, place a clean barrier on the bottom, and insert the cup of exposed film packets into a clean cup. The operator closes the top, puts on clean gloves, pushes his or her hands through the sleeve, and opens the film packets, allowing the film to drop into the clean cup. After all film packets have been opened, the contaminated gloves are removed, the films are loaded into the developer, and hands are removed. The top of the loader may be removed, and the contaminated materials are then removed.

BIBLIOGRAPHY

Quality Assurance

American Dental Association Council on Scientific Affairs. The use of dental radiographs: update and recommendations. *J Am Dent Assoc.* 2006;137:1304–1312.

American Dental Association Council on Scientific Affairs. Dental radiographic examinations: recommendations for patient selection and limiting radiation exposure. Revised 2012. http://www.ada.org/sections/professionalResources/pdfs/Dental_Radiographic_Examinations_2012.pdf.

American Dental Association Technical Report. No. 1094. Quality assurance for digital intra-oral radiographic systems.

Buchanan A, Benton B, Carraway A, et al. Perception versus reality-findings from a phosphor plate quality assurance study. *Oral Surg Oral Med Oral Pathol Oral Radiol.* 2017;123(4):496–501.

Goren AD, Lundeen RC, Deahl ST II, et al. Updated quality assurance self-assessment exercise in intraoral and panoramic radiography, American Academy of Oral and Maxillofacial Radiology, Radiology Practice Committee. *Oral Surg Oral Med Oral Pathol Oral Radiol Endod.* 2000;89:369–374.

Carestream Dental, Dental Radiography Series: Quality assurance in dental radiography. Available at: http://www.carestreamdental.com/ImagesFileShare/.sitecore.media_library.Files.Film_and_Anesthetics.8661_US_Quality_Assurance_Brochure.pdf.

Kwan AL, Ching H, Gray JE, et al. Acceptance Testing and Quality Control of Dental Imaging Equipment. The Report of AAPM Task Group 175, 2016. Available at: http://www.aapm.org/pubs/reports/RPT_175.pdf.

Mah P, McDavid WD, Dove SB. Quality assurance phantom for digital dental imaging. *Oral Surg Oral Med Oral Pathol Oral Radiol Endod.* 2011;112:632–639.

National Council for Radiation Protection and Measurements. *Radiation Protection in Dentistry, NCRP Report No. 145.* Bethesda, MD: National Council on Radiation Protection and Measurement; 2003.

National Radiological Protection Board. Guidance notes for dental practitioners on the safe use of x-ray equipment; 2001. www.nrpb.org.uk.

Quality control recommendations for diagnostic radiography, Volume 1, Dental facilities, CRCPD Publication 01-4, July 2001.

Quality assurance in radiology and medicine. Dental Conebeam CT phantoms. http://www.qrm.de/index.htm.

Pauwels R, Beinsberger J, Stamatakis H, et al. Comparison of spatial and contrast resolution for cone-beam computed tomography scanners. *Oral Surg Oral Med Oral Pathol Oral Radiol.* 2012;114(1):127–135.

Samei E, Badano A, Chakraborty D, et al. *Assessment of Display Performance for Medical Imaging Systems, Report of the American Association of Physicists in Medicine (AAPM) Task Group 18.* Madison, WI: Medical Physics Publishing; 2005. Available at: https://www.aapm.org/pubs/reports/OR_03.pdf.

Seibert J, Bogucki T, Ciona T, et al Acceptance testing and quality control of photostimulable storage phosphor imaging systems. The report of AAPM Task Group 93, 2006. Available at: http://www.aapm.org/pubs/reports/RPT_93.pdf.

SMPTE RP-133. 1991 Specifications for medical diagnostic imaging test pattern for television monitors. Available at: https://www.smpte.org/store/product/smpte-rp-1331991-specifications-medical-diagnostic-imaging-test-pattern-television.

U.S. Department of Health and Human Services, Food and Drug Administration. Performance standards for ionizing radiation emitting products. 21 CFR 1020.30: Diagnostic x-ray systems and their major components. U.S. Food and Drug Administration, Maryland, 2014. Available at: https://www.accessdata.fda.gov/scripts/cdrh/cfdocs/cfcfr/CFRSearch.cfm?fr=1020.30.

Infection Control

American Academy of Oral and Maxillofacial Radiology infection control guidelines for dental radiographic procedures. *Oral Surg Oral Med Oral Pathol.* 1992;73:248–249.

American Dental Association Council on Scientific Affairs and American Dental Association Council on Dental Practice. Infection control recommendations for the dental office and the dental laboratory. *J Am Dent Assoc.* 1996;127:672–680.

Bartoloni JA, Chariton DG, Flint DJ. Infection control practices in dental radiology. *Gen Dent.* 2003;51:264–271.

Centers for Disease Control and Prevention. *Summary of Infection Prevention Practices in Dental Settings: Basic Expectations for Safe Care.* Atlanta, GA: US Department of Health and Human Services, Centers for Disease Control and Prevention, National Center for Chronic Disease Prevention and Health Promotion, Division of Oral Health; 2016. Available at: https://www.cdc.gov/oralhealth/infectioncontrol/pdf/safe-care.pdf.

Hubar JS, Gardiner DM. Infection control procedures used in conjunction with computed dental radiography. *Int J Comput Dent.* 2000;3:259–267.

Kalathingal S, Youngpeter A, Minton J, et al. An evaluation of microbiologic contamination on a phosphor plate system: is weekly gas sterilization enough? *Oral Surg Oral Med Oral Pathol Oral Radiol Endod.* 2010;109:457–462.

MacDonald DS, Waterfield JD. Infection control in digital intraoral radiography: evaluation of microbiological contamination of photostimulable phosphor plates in barrier envelopes. *J Can Dent Assoc.* 2011;77:b93.

Miller CH, Palenik CJ. *Infection Control and Management of Hazardous Materials for the Dental team.* 4th ed. St Louis: Mosby; 2009.

Palenik CJ. Infection control practices for dental radiography. *Dent Today.* 2004;23:52–55.

Rutala WA, Weber DJ, Healthcare Infection Control Practices Advisory Committee (HICPAC). *Guideline for Disinfection and Sterilization in Healthcare Facilities.* Atlanta, GA: Department of Health and Human Services, Centers for Disease Control and Prevention; 2008. Available at: https://www.google.com/url?sa=t&rct=j&q=&esrc=s&source=web&cd=2&ved=0ahUKEwigxM3J6P3XAhVSwWMKHTjuBNwQFgg4MAE&url=https%3A%2F%2Fwww.cdc.gov%2Finfectioncontrol%2Fpdf%2Fguidelines%2Fdisinfection-guidelines.pdf&usg=AOvVaw0LPt-NzLafoISl3DqPAAQ-.

U.S. Department of Labor, Occupational Safety and Health Administration. Occupational exposure to bloodborne pathogens, needlestick and other sharp injuries, final rule. *Fed Regist.* 2001;66:5317–5325. Available at: https://www.osha.gov/pls/oshaweb/owadisp.show_document?p_id=16265&p_table=FEDERAL_REGISTER.

17

Prescribing Diagnostic Imaging

Ernest W.N. Lam

Oral and maxillofacial imaging is a form of diagnostic testing that should be performed only when a historical finding or a clinical sign or symptom indicates that imaging is likely to contribute to the diagnosis or treatment plan. Therefore imaging should be performed only after a patient's thorough medical and dental history has been obtained and a clinical examination has been made. The specific diagnostic imaging procedure prescribed should be guided by this examination and tailored specifically to the patient's needs and the diagnostic task. Because most dentomaxillofacial imaging uses ionizing radiation, the dentist must make sure that potential diagnostic and treatment planning benefits outweigh the risks associated with radiation to the patient (Chapters 2 and 3).

RADIOLOGIC EXAMINATIONS

The design of the type and scope of the imaging examination should be guided by:
- The perceived nature or severity of an abnormality (including its size and accessibility)
- The ability of the imaging technique to accurately reveal the characteristic diagnostic features of the abnormality (sensitivity and specificity)
- The amount of image detail required (resolution)
- The radiation dose to the patient

In some instances conventional intraoral or panoramic imaging may be entirely appropriate. Other cases may require more sophisticated imaging approaches such as computed tomography (CT), magnetic resonance imaging (MRI), nuclear medicine, or ultrasound. For example, intraoral imaging provides high spatial resolution and is the best choice to critically evaluate the effects of diseases involving a tooth and its supporting structures. In contrast, panoramic imaging may allow the clinician to examine more extensive disease involving a larger area, but with lower image resolution and more image artifacts. Advanced imaging techniques such as cone beam CT (CBCT) and multidetector CT (MDCT) may be required when there is a need to evaluate the sectional anatomy of the region in three dimensions. MRI and ultrasound are better suited to demonstrate the soft tissues. When the metabolic activity of an abnormality has to be assessed, nuclear medicine may be useful. Imaging with MDCT and nuclear medicine will deliver a substantially higher radiation dose to the patient than will conventional imaging or CBCT. Thus it is important that dentists develop skills to select the most appropriate examination considering the diagnostic task, radiation dose, and cost of the imaging procedure.

Intraoral Images

Intraoral images offer the clinician the highest spatial resolution relative to other radiographic imaging modalities used in dentistry. Therefore when fine detail is important or imaging is required to investigate a possible abnormality involving a tooth or its supporting structures, intraoral imaging is the best choice.

The geometry of the incident x-ray beam and the position of the receptor relative to the x-ray beam determine the area imaged. Periapical images, where the image receptor is positioned parallel to the long axis of the teeth and the alveolar process, are optimal to demonstrate the tooth root or roots, the supporting structures (the periodontal ligament and lamina dura), and the periradicular alveolar process. A limitation of periapical imaging is geometric distortion, which occurs if the incident x-ray beam is not perpendicular to the long axis of a tooth root or the crest of the alveolar process.

Bitewing images are made with the receptor adjacent to the crowns of a sextant of the dentition and the crests of the alveolar processes of the maxilla and mandible. In the instance where the crest of the alveolar process in either or both arches has been lost, perhaps due to periodontal disease, the image receptor may be rotated so that its longer dimension is vertically oriented—the so-called vertical bitewing. A similar technique can be used to make bitewings of the anterior teeth. Bitewing images are optimal for revealing interproximal caries. These images are made with a 5- to 10- degree downward inclination of the incident x-ray beam to project the crests of the alveolar processes relative to the adjacent teeth with minimal distortion. This orientation also minimizes overlapping of the opposing cusps onto the occlusal surface and thus improves the probability of detecting early occlusal lesions at the dentine-enamel junction.

Occlusal images are made with the image receptor located between the occlusal surfaces of the teeth. These images can be made in children who may have small or shallow mouths in lieu of periapical images or in adults to supplement periapical and bitewing images. In adults, occlusal images are often made with larger receptors (American National Standards Institute [ANSI]) number 4), so that larger areas of the jaws can be imaged without compromising image resolution; in children, smaller (ANSI number 2) receptors are typically used.

Extraoral Images

Extraoral images allow the clinician to visualize a larger region of anatomy than intraoral images, but with much lower image resolution. As the term implies, extraoral images are made with the image receptor located outside the mouth. Depending on the positions of the incident x-ray beam and receptor, numerous views of the face and jaws can be made to specifically depict various anatomic structures. The most commonly used extraoral imaging techniques in dentistry are panoramic imaging (Chapter 9), and cephalometric imaging (Chapter 8). Less commonly, conventional projection images of the skull, midface, and jaw may be made using the lateral oblique, Caldwell, occipitomental (Waters), frontooccipital (Towne) or submentovertex (basal) projections (Chapter 8).

Panoramic imaging is a form of thin-section imaging or tomography that creates a broad view of the midface and jaws as well as adjacent structures utilizing a moving x-ray beam and image receptor. However, panoramic images have lower spatial resolution than intraoral images, and x-ray beam angulation and projection geometry result in image distortion. Furthermore, panoramic imaging is susceptible to patient movement during acquisition, and the complex pattern of superimposition of anatomic structures complicate its interpretation. Thus, although a broad view of the anatomy is advantageous, the disadvantages of lower resolution, anatomical superimposition, image distortion, and potential patient movement during image acquisition do not allow evaluation of the fine anatomic detail provided by intraoral imaging.

Advanced Imaging

For most dentomaxillofacial pathology, the decision to use three-dimensional advanced imaging modalities—including CBCT, MDCT, and MRI—should be made if intraoral, panoramic, or cephalometric imaging does not provide the necessary diagnostic and treatment planning information. Importantly, the dentist should recognize that these advanced imaging techniques typically produce images with lower spatial resolution than intraoral and panoramic images and that CBCT and MDCT deliver substantially greater radiation doses. Advanced imaging techniques are discussed in Chapters 10, 11, and 13. Although the use of these modalities has increased, it is important to recognize that the decision to employ them should be guided by the historical findings and clinical examination. When conventional two-dimensional imaging is considered inappropriate or inadequate, prescribing advanced imaging may be appropriate. Dentists who choose to operate their own advanced imaging systems must be well versed in all aspects of that imaging technology, including imaging physics, image artifact generation, image reconstruction, and interpretation of disease on advanced imaging modalities. In general these topics require specialized knowledge and training; hence dentists should consider referring their patients to a specialist in oral and maxillofacial radiology for these procedures.

GUIDELINES FOR ORDERING IMAGING

Guidelines form a framework for the image ordering practices of dentists. Guidelines are not hard and fast rules but rather principles upon which decisions may be made. This includes appropriateness of the imaging examination to provide the needed diagnostic information and radiation-associated risks. Nevertheless the dentist must apply guidelines only after a detailed review of the patient's medical and dental histories has been completed along with a thorough clinical examination to identify signs or symptoms of possible disease. Importantly, the imaging findings should potentially help to direct the patient's diagnosis and/or treatment plan.

Previous Diagnostic Images

Many patients may have already been seen by another dentist and images may have already been made. Such images may be helpful, regardless of when they were made. Even when these previous images do not reflect the current clinical condition of the patient, they may be of value to demonstrate whether a condition (e.g., caries, periodontal disease) has remained unchanged, worsened, or shown resolution or healing. Images made relatively more recently may be adequate for the current diagnostic task, thus precluding the need to make images during the current visit. For all new patients, the dentist must review the patient's prior imaging history as part of the initial visit and attempt to obtain these images from the prior dental office.

Administrative Images

Administrative images are those made for reasons other than diagnosis; these may include images made for an insurance company to approve a treatment or for a dental examining board beyond what might be required for diagnosis. Images made for administrative purposes typically do not benefit the patient, be it the patient's diagnosis or treatment plan; therefore making such images should be avoided. The National Council on Radiation Protection and Measurements Report No. 145 provides specific guidance: "*Administrative use of radiation to provide information not related to health of the patient shall not be permitted. Students shall not be permitted to perform radiographic exposures of patients, other students, or volunteers solely for purposes of their education or licensure.*"

Guidelines for Ordering Dental Radiographic Examinations

The following general categories of situations dictate a need for imaging:
- Where there is clinical evidence of an abnormality that cannot be fully assessed by physical examination alone
- Where there is a high probability of disease that is not clinically evident

In the first category, a patient may have a hard swelling in the premolar region of the mandible with expansion of the buccal and lingual surfaces. Such clinical evidence alerts the dentist to the need for a diagnostic image to determine the nature of the swelling. In the second category, a patient may seek general dental care after not having seen a dentist for many years and clinical examination shows no evidence of caries. Nevertheless bitewing images may be indicated. Because this patient has not had interproximal radiographs for many years, it is reasonable to assume that the bitewing images will be of potential benefit by detecting interproximal caries that is not clinically evident. In the absence of clinical indicators of early caries, the dentist must rely on knowledge of the prevalence of caries and the risk factors for this disease to decide whether bitewing imaging may yield potential diagnostic benefit in this particular patient.

In the mid-1980s, a panel of general and specialist dentists and scientists was convened by the US Food and Drug Administration (FDA) to develop practice parameters for prescribing dental imaging. The guidelines were developed as a radiation protection measure to reduce x-ray exposure to patients without compromising the quality of care for new or recall patients seeking general dental care. The guidelines were revised in 2004 and again in 2012 in collaboration with the American Dental Association (ADA) (Box 17.1 and Table 17.1) It is important to appreciate that in the interval since the first document of 1987, there has been no change in the philosophy underpinning the original guidelines.

The selection criteria that are a part of the FDA/ADA guidelines describe circumstances that suggest a need for diagnostic imaging. These circumstances, referred to as selection criteria, include patient age, the identification of a medical or dental historical finding, or a sign or symptom. The 2012 revised guidelines recognize 6 positive historical findings and 23 positive clinical signs or symptoms for which imaging may be warranted (Box 17.1). In many instances, the selection criteria can become known to the dentist only after an interview and/or clinical examination of the patient. The identification of selection criteria suggests the type of imaging examination most likely to benefit the patient by yielding reliable diagnostic information. Although guidelines provide the dentist with the principles underlying the ordering of diagnostic imaging, their application relies heavily on the dentists' clinical judgment. Therefore the practitioner, who may be the only individual who knows the patient's medical and dental histories and susceptibility to oral disease, must make the ultimate decision on whether to order images by using the guidelines as a resource rather than a regulation. The ADA was an equal partner with the government agencies in the revision of the guidelines and recommends their use. These guidelines therefore form the basis of the recommendations in this chapter.

BOX 17.1   American Dental Association Selection Criteria for Prescribing Dental Radiographs

Positive Historical Findings	Positive Clinical Signs or Symptoms
1. Previous periodontal or endodontic treatment	1. Clinical evidence of periodontal disease
2. History of pain or trauma	2. Large or deep restorations
3. Familial history of dental anomalies	3. Deep carious lesions
4. Post-operative evaluation of healing	4. Malposed or clinically impacted teeth
5. Remineralization monitoring	5. Swelling
6. Presence of implants or evaluation for implant placement	6. Evidence of dental/facial trauma
	7. Mobility of teeth
	8. Sinus tract ("fistula")
	9. Clinically suspected sinus pathology
	10. Growth abnormalities
	11. Oral involvement in known or suspected systemic disease
	12. Positive neurologic findings in the head and neck
	13. Evidence of foreign objects
	14. Pain and/or dysfunction of the temporomandibular joint
	15. Facial asymmetry
	16. Abutment teeth for fixed or removable partial prosthesis
	17. Unexplained bleeding
	18. Unexplained sensitivity of teeth
	19. Unusual eruption, spacing or migration of teeth
	20. Unusual tooth morphology, calcification or color
	21. Unexplained absence of teeth
	22. Clinical tooth erosion
	23. Peri-implantitis

From Dental Radiographic Examinations: Recommendations for patient selection and limiting radiation exposure. 2012.

The guidelines underscore the importance of balancing diagnostic benefit with patient risk. Therefore dentists should expose patients to radiation only when there is a reasonable expectation that the diagnostic image will benefit patient care. The selection criteria relate to a finding or a sign or symptom found in the patient's medical or dental history or, on a clinical examination, and suggest that a radiologic examination would yield clinically useful information. A key concept in the use of the selection criteria and the application of the guidelines is recognition of the need to consider each patient as an individual. In other words, the images that a dentist chooses to make are a prescription based on individual need just as a medication is prescribed on the basis of individual need. In some jurisdictions, therefore, this practice is called prescription radiology. Without some specific indication, it is inappropriate to irradiate the patient "just to see if there is something there." The major exception to this rule is the example we used earlier; that of bitewing images for the detection of interproximal caries when no clinical signs exist of even early carious lesions. The probability of finding occult disease in a patient with all permanent teeth erupted and no clinical or historical evidence of abnormality or risk factors is so low that making any image just to look for such disease is not indicated. The decision to prescribe imaging to a patient without having obtained a dental or medical history or having completed a clinical examination is not considered responsible.

Applying these guidelines to the specific circumstances with each patient requires both discipline and clinical judgment, bringing together the dentist's knowledge, experience, and concern for the well-being of the patient. Clinical judgment is also required to recognize situations that are not described by the guidelines but in which patients would need diagnostic images nonetheless.

Initial Visit

For a child in the primary dentition who is cooperative and has closed posterior contacts, only bitewing images are required to detect interproximal caries. Additional imaging is recommended only when the medical or dental history or the clinical examination reveals cause. Children without evidence of abnormality and with open proximal contacts may not require a radiologic examination at this time.

For a child in the mixed dentition following the eruption of a permanent first molar tooth, the guidelines recommend bitewing images to detect interproximal caries and a panoramic image or selected periapical or occlusal images to detect abnormalities that may arise during growth and development.

For partially or fully dentate adolescents and adults, the guidelines recommend individualized radiologic examinations based on the patient's medical or dental history or if the clinical examination reveals cause for additional imaging. The presence of widespread disease (e.g., generalized caries or periodontal disease) may indicate a need for a full-mouth series of bitewing and periapical images. Alternatively, if disease is localized, a more limited examination consisting of a subset of these images may be completed. In a circumstance with no evidence of past or current dental disease, only bitewing images may be made to investigate the patient for interproximal caries.

For an edentulous patient requesting prosthodontic care, the guidelines recommend an individualized examination that is based on the patient's medical or dental history or if the clinical examination reveals cause for additional imaging. This may include selected periapical, occlusal, or panoramic images and CBCT if dental implants are being considered.

Recall Visit

Patients who return after their initial treatment is completed will require careful examination before determining the need for additional diagnostic images. As with the initial examination, images should be obtained if the patient's medical or dental history, or if the clinical examination reveals cause for further imaging or evaluation.

The guidelines recommend bitewing images for recall patients to detect interproximal caries. The optimal frequency for these views depends on the age of the patient and the probability of finding this disease as it relates to disease risk. If the patient has high risk factors for dental caries (e.g., poor diet, poor oral hygiene, etc.) or clinically demonstrable caries, bitewing images may be made at intervals as short as 6 to 12 months for children and adolescents and 6 to 18 months for adults until no carious lesions are clinically evident. The recommended intervals are longer for patients not at a high risk for caries: 12 to 24 months for a child, 18 to 36 months for an adolescent, and 24 to 36 months for an adult. Because an individual's risk category can change, the interval between imaging can also change. Besides screening for interproximal caries with bitewing imaging, the guidelines discourage imaging at predetermined, regular time intervals without clinical indication.

TABLE 17.1   American Dental Association Guidelines for Prescribing Dental Radiographs

Type of Encounter	PATIENT AGE AND DENTAL DEVELOPMENTAL STAGE	
	Child With Primary Dentition (Before Eruption of First Permanent Tooth)	Child With Transitional Dentition (After Eruption of First Permanent Tooth)
New patient[a] being evaluated for oral diseases	Individualized radiographic exam consisting of selected periapical/occlusal views and/or posterior bitewings if proximal surfaces cannot be visualized or probed. Patients without evidence of disease and with open proximal contacts may not require a radiographic examination at this time	Individualized radiographic exam consisting of posterior bitewings with panoramic exam or posterior bitewings and selected periapical images
Recall patient[a] with clinical caries or at increased risk for caries[b]	Posterior bitewing exam at 6- to 12-month intervals if proximal surfaces cannot be examined visually or with a probe	
Recall patient[a] with no clinical caries and not at increased risk of developing caries[b]	Posterior bitewing examination at 12- to 24-month intervals if proximal surfaces cannot be examined visually or with a probe	
Recall patient[a] with periodontal disease	Clinical judgment as to the need for and type of radiographic images for the evaluation of periodontal disease. Imaging may consist of but is not limited to selected bitewing and/or periapical images of areas in which periodontal disease (other than nonspecific gingivitis) can be demonstrated clinically	
Patient (new and recall) for monitoring of dentofacial growth and development and/or assessment of dental/skeletal relationships	Clinical judgment as to need for and type of radiographic images for evaluation and/or monitoring of dentofacial growth and development or assessment of dental and skeletal relationships	
Patient with other circumstances, including but not limited to proposed or existing implants, other dental and craniofacial pathosis, restorative/endodontic needs, treated periodontal disease, and caries remineralization	Clinical judgment as to need for and type of radiographic images for evaluation and/or monitoring of these conditions	

PATIENT AGE AND DENTAL DEVELOPMENTAL STAGE

Adolescent With Permanent Dentition (Before Eruption of Third Molars)	Adult, Dentate or Partially Edentulous	Adult, Edentulous
Individualized radiographic exam consisting of posterior bitewings with panoramic exam or posterior bitewings and selected periapical images; full-mouth intraoral radiographic exam is preferred when patient has clinical evidence of generalized dental disease or a history of extensive dental treatment		Individualized radiographic exam based on clinical signs and symptoms
Posterior bitewing exam at 6- to 12-month intervals if proximal surfaces cannot be examined visually or with a probe	Posterior bitewing examination at 6- to 18-month intervals	Not applicable
Posterior bitewing exam at 18- to 36-month intervals	Posterior bitewing exam at 24- to 36-month intervals	Not applicable
Clinical judgment as to the need for and type of radiographic images for the evaluation of periodontal disease. Imaging may consist of, but is not limited to, selected bitewing and/or periapical images of areas in which periodontal disease (other than nonspecific gingivitis) can be demonstrated clinically		Not applicable
Clinical judgment as to need for and type of radiographic images for evaluation and/or monitoring of dentofacial growth and development or assessment of dental and skeletal relationships. Panoramic or periapical exam to assess developing third molars	Usually not indicated for monitoring of growth and development. Clinical judgment as to the need for and type of radiographic images for evaluation of dental and skeletal relationships	
Clinical judgment as to need for and type of radiographic images for evaluation and/or monitoring of these conditions		

[a]Refer to Box 17.1.
[b]Factors increasing risk for caries may be assessed using the American Dental Association Caries Risk Assessment forms (0 to 6 years of age) and (greater than 6 years of age), available at http://www.ada.org.
Note. The recommendations in this table are subject to clinical judgment and may not apply to every patient. They are to be used by dentists only after reviewing the patient's medical and dental histories, and completing a clinical examination. Because every precaution should be taken to minimize radiation exposure, protective thyroid collars and aprons should be used whenever possible.
From Dental Radiographic Examinations: Recommendations for patient selection and limiting radiation exposure. 2012.

The 2012 FDA/ADA guidelines also include a new section related to evaluation and monitoring of bone loss due to periodontal disease. Some form of periodontal disease may affect older adults, and this disease is responsible for a substantial portion of tooth loss. Radiologic imaging plays an important role in the evaluation of patients with periodontal disease after the disease is initially detected on clinical examination and for monitoring of disease progression. Imaging may assist in the demonstration of bone support for the dentition; also, imaging may also help to demonstrate local irritation factors that may contribute to the disease, including the presence of calculus and faulty restorations. Occasionally the length and morphologic features of the tooth roots, visible on periapical images, may also be crucial factors in the prognosis of the disease. These observations suggest that when clinical evidence of periodontal disease exists, it is appropriate to make intraoral images, generally a combination of periapical and bite-wing images, to help establish and monitor the severity of the periodontal bone loss.

Guidelines for Ordering Cone Beam Computed Tomography Examinations

Unlike the guidelines for dental imaging, guidelines for ordering CBCT imaging are relatively new, and their selection criteria are largely untested. SEDENTEXCT, a European consortium of researchers and clinical oral and maxillofacial radiologists, has published a comprehensive document that addresses selection criteria, quality assurance, and approaches to minimize patient radiation dose. The SEDENTEXCT consortium extensively reviewed the literature for evidence for CBCT use in a wide range of clinical scenarios in dentistry. Among the broad topics addressed is imaging of the developing dentition (e.g., impacted teeth), imaging requirements for assisting in the restoration of the dentition (e.g., the assessment of periapical disease, endodontics, trauma), and oral and maxillofacial surgical applications (e.g., tooth extraction, dental implant placement, orthognathic surgery, treatment of the temporomandibular joint). The document is a comprehensive resource that guides practitioners in the CBCT decision-making process. The approach taken by this group is appropriately conservative in the use of ionizing radiation.

Along the same lines as the guidelines for ordering dental radiographic examinations, the SEDENTEXCT consortium recommends that CBCT examinations

- Must not be prescribed unless a history and clinical examination have been performed
- Must be justified for each patient to ensure that the benefits outweigh the risks
- Should potentially add new information to aid the patient's management.

Of the many applications discussed in the SEDENTEXCT document, two general themes emerge as best practices for CBCT imaging examinations. First, if, in the past, MDCT has been the imaging modality of choice for a particular investigation of hard tissues, CBCT should now be used. This statement recognizes that radiation doses from CBCT are generally lower than doses from MDCT for similar examinations. Second, the size of the imaging field should be limited to only the area of interest and not go beyond. In keeping with the first theme, smaller field sizes deliver smaller radiation doses than do larger fields of view.

Guidelines for CBCT use in specific clinical disciplines have been developed by several professional organizations. The American Academy of Oral and Maxillofacial Radiology (AAOMR) and the American Association of Endodontists jointly developed a position statement to guide clinicians on the use of CBCT for specific diagnostic tasks in endodontics. These evidence-based guidelines considered diagnostic efficacy of CBCT and its impact on guiding appropriate endodontic treatment; they provide 11 recommendations that address CBCT use in nonsurgical and surgical endodontic management (Box 17.2).

To provide guidance on the use of CBCT in orthodontic diagnosis and treatment planning, the AAOMR convened a panel of oral and maxillofacial radiologists and orthodontists to develop clinical recommendations. The panel identified several specific clinical situations that could potentially benefit from CBCT imaging beyond that provided by two-dimensional imaging with panoramic and cephalometric radiography (Box 17.3).

Several professional organizations throughout the world have developed guidelines for CBCT use in dental implantology. The AAOMR position statement provides active recommendations to guide presurgical evaluation of potential implant sites and postsurgical assessment of implant placement and related complications (see Box 15.1). These recommendations are discussed in more detail in Chapter 15.

BOX 17.2 Recommendations for the Use of Cone Beam Computed Tomography in Endodontic Diagnosis and Treatment Planning

1. Intraoral radiographs should be considered the imaging modality of choice in the evaluation of the endodontic patient.
2. Limited field-of-view (FOV) cone beam computed tomography (CBCT) should be considered the imaging modality of choice for diagnosis in patients who present with contradictory or nonspecific clinical signs and symptoms associated with untreated or previously endodontically treated teeth.
3. Limited FOV CBCT should be considered the imaging modality of choice for initial treatment of teeth with the potential for extra canals and suspected complex morphology, such as mandibular anterior teeth, maxillary and mandibular premolars and molars, and dental anomalies.
4. If a preoperative CBCT has not been taken, limited FOV CBCT should be considered as the imaging modality of choice for intra-appointment identification and localization of calcified canals.
5. Intraoral radiographs should be considered the imaging modality of choice for immediate postoperative imaging.
6. Limited FOV CBCT should be considered the imaging modality of choice if clinical examination and two-dimensional intraoral radiography are inconclusive in the detection of vertical root fracture (VRF).
7. Limited FOV CBCT should be the imaging modality of choice in evaluating the nonhealing of previous endodontic treatment to help determine the need for further treatment, such as nonsurgical or surgical treatment or extraction.
8. Limited FOV CBCT should be the imaging modality of choice for nonsurgical retreatment to assess endodontic treatment complications, such as overextended root canal obturation material, separated endodontic instruments, and localization of perforations.
9. Limited FOV CBCT should be considered as the imaging modality of choice for presurgical treatment planning to localize root apex/apices and to evaluate the proximity to adjacent anatomic structures.
10. Limited FOV CBCT should be considered as the imaging modality of choice for surgical placement of implants.
11. Limited FOV CBCT should be considered the imaging modality of choice for diagnosis and management of limited dentoalveolar trauma, root fractures, luxation, and/or displacement of teeth and localized alveolar fractures in the absence of other maxillofacial or soft tissue injury that may require other advanced imaging modalities.
12. Limited FOV CBCT is the imaging modality of choice in the localization and differentiation of external and internal resorptive defects and the determination of appropriate treatment and prognosis.

From AAE-AAOMR Joint Position Statement. Use of cone beam computed tomography in endodontics. *Oral Surg Oral Med Oral Pathol Oral Radiol Endod.* 2015;120:508-512.

IMAGING CONSIDERATIONS IN THE ABSENCE OF A POSITIVE FINDING

In the absence of a historical finding or a clinical sign or symptom, the dentist must consider four factors before ordering imaging: the prevalence of an abnormality in the jaws, the probability that such an abnormality would not produce a clinically detectable sign or symptom, the ability of the imaging modality to detect the disease, and whether the detection of such an abnormality would influence the management of the patient.

There is, unfortunately, little prevalence data for abnormalities of the jaws. Most of the information is biased toward data reported by academic oral and maxillofacial pathology services that archive data

From AAOMR. Clinical recommendations regarding use of cone beam computed tomography in orthodontic treatment. *Oral Surg Oral Med Oral Pathol Oral Radiol.* 2013;116(2):238-257.

BOX 17.3 Clinical Indications for the Use of Cone Beam Computed Tomography in Orthodontic Diagnosis and Treatment Planning

1. To assess anomalies in the structure and eruption of teeth
2. To evaluate dental-alveolar boundaries
3. To assess craniofacial skeletal asymmetry
4. To assess maxillomandibular discrepancies
5. To evaluate the temporomandibular joints
6. To assess airway morphology
7. To plan for combined orthodontic and orthognathic surgical management
8. To identify optimal locations for temporary anchorage devices
9. To assess skeletal and dental changes produced by maxillary expanders

from biopsy submissions. However, because a majority of abnormalities are never biopsied and only noted in the records of patients, it is difficult to obtain reliable information. Abnormalities developing centrally within the jaw bones have an approximately 85% likelihood of occurring in the periapical areas of the teeth and are primarily odontogenic in origin. Approximately 7% are reported to be developmental in origin; the remaining 8% are said to form the basis of the decision-making process. That is, do we order imaging to look for these? As a group, odontogenic tumors are rare. Data from various oral and maxillofacial pathology biopsy services report tumor incidences ranging from approximately 0.7% to 2.7% of all accessions—a very small number. Odontogenic cysts are, however, more common, with an incidence of approximately 17%, with the largest percentage of cysts being interpreted by oral and maxillofacial pathologists as being radicular cysts. Nonodontogenic cysts, by comparison, are even rarer, representing approximately 1% of accessions, with the incisive canal or nasopalatine cyst being the most common nonodontogenic cyst found.

In the United States, a review of approximately 30 million health insurance records determined that the detection of quiescent disease (disease without any clinical sign or symptom) is not justified on the basis of economic and radiobiologic costs and the morbidity and mortality to the patients. In patient-based studies, where selection criteria have been carefully applied, only a small number of entities are missed—resorbed roots, retained primary tooth roots, hypercementoses, and osteosclerosis. Typically these entities require no management.

Some dentists establish procedures in their practices so that new or recall patients are seen by a dental assistant or hygienist who makes a predetermined set of diagnostic images at the beginning of the appointment, even before the dentist has had a chance to examine the patient. Although this may be perceived as making more efficient use of the dentist's time, it is contrary to best clinical practices whereby the selection of images is based on the findings of the medical or dental history or the clinical examination. Conducting a thorough patient interview and examination before ordering images should be the standard protocol in any dental practice.

Radiation doses from diagnostic oral and maxillofacial imaging are typically very low, and there is negligible risk of harm for any individual patient from one set of images. However, there is a large societal cost, both in terms of health care costs and radiation risk, if millions of dental patients receive examinations without a diagnostic yield, as would happen if widespread routine or screening examinations were conducted. Furthermore, there is now a growing concern among the public and

the health professions about the increasing use of ionizing radiation in health care in general and the risks it poses to the public. In dentistry, this concern has come to the fore most recently with the application of large field-of-view CBCT systems.

In summary, there is insufficient evidence to justify imaging, periodic or otherwise, solely to detect quiescent jaw pathology. Often, dentists use such "defensive" approaches and perform imaging to reduce their exposure to malpractice liability. Although lawsuits can be filed for many reasons, it is unlikely that they will be successful if it can be shown that the practitioner performed within the parameters of care—documenting a thorough medical and dental history and clinical examination and carefully considered the guidelines to order diagnostic imaging when clinically indicated.

SPECIAL CONSIDERATIONS

Pregnancy

Occasionally it is necessary to obtain diagnostic images of a pregnant patient. Although imaging is not contraindicated in a pregnant patient, many dentists and expectant mothers have concerns about the irradiation of a developing fetus. When radiation protection practices are followed (see Chapter 3), including collimation, fast or digital receptors, and protective shielding, the doses from diagnostic dentomaxillofacial radiology are negligible (see Table 3.2, and Fig. 3.4). Indeed, fetal doses from dentomaxillofacial radiography are approximately 42,000-fold lower than the threshold dose for deterministic effects on the embryo and fetus (see Chapter 2). Because radiologic imaging in all patients is predicated on there being a diagnostic need, the guidelines apply equally to pregnant patients as well as to those who are not pregnant. It is, however, recommended that when imaging is performed in all patients, including those who may be pregnant, a protective thyroid collar be used when it does not obstruct an essential anatomic region of the image.

Radiation Therapy

Patients with a diagnosed malignancy in the oral or perioral regions may receive radiation therapy for their disease. During treatment, oral tissues may receive 50 Gy or more, and although such patients are often apprehensive about receiving diagnostic imaging, radiation doses from dental imaging procedures are relatively insignificant compared with the therapeutic doses they have already received. Patients who have received radiation therapy may have radiation-induced xerostomia and are at a high risk for the development of caries, which may produce serious consequences if extractions are needed in the future. Patients who have undergone radiation therapy including the oral cavity should be carefully monitored because they are at special risk for dental disease.

EXAMPLES OF USE OF THE GUIDELINES

In the following examples, consider the ways in which the guidelines can be applied to different clinical situations:
- The first visit of a 5-year-old boy to a dental office. The patient's parent reports no known medical conditions, and the patient is cooperative. Clinical examination of the child reveals that there are open contacts between all the primary teeth and there is no evidence of caries. Because the child has grown up in a community that has a fluoridated water supply, a reasonably good diet is being observed, and the parent seems well motivated to promote good oral hygiene, no radiologic examination is required at this time. Images for the detection of developmental abnormalities are not in order at this age because a complete appraisal cannot be made at age 5 years.

Even if it could be made, it may be too early to initiate treatment for such abnormalities.

- The first visit of a 10-year-old girl in the mixed dentition to the dental office. The patient's first visit to the dentist occurred when she was 6, and her family has recently moved to your community from one that does not have water fluoridation. Unfortunately you were unable to obtain previous images of the patient. The parent reports no known medical conditions, and the patient is cooperative. The patient has stainless steel crowns on the two remaining deciduous molar teeth and some conservatively placed two-surface amalgams on a single deciduous maxillary molar. Clinical examination of the child reveals that there is no evidence of decay, and where adjacent teeth are present, there are contacts between them. At this time it may be reasonable to image the posterior teeth for interproximal decay with two bitewing images. In addition, it may be useful to make a panoramic image of this patient to evaluate the developing dentition, which will also allow the dentist to identify the presence of any developing dental anomalies.
- The recall visit of a 17-year-old adolescent male to a dental office. You have seen this patient since he was 4 years old. When the patient was a child, he was allowed to drink juice before bedtime, so you were able to bring a stop to this practice by the patient's parents but not before extensive treatment of the patient's deciduous dentition was performed. Fortunately your efforts to enforce good oral hygiene practices have worked out well and the 17-year old has a caries-free permanent dentition. In the past, you placed fissure sealants in all of the permanent premolar and molar teeth. The patient's last bitewing images were made approximately 26 months ago. At this time it may be reasonable to image the posterior teeth for interproximal decay with two bitewing images. In addition, it may be useful to make a panoramic image of this patient to evaluate the presence of developing third molars.
- A 25-year-old woman receiving a 6-month checkup after her last treatment for a fractured incisor. The patient does not have high-risk factors for caries, there are no clinical signs of caries, and no caries is evident on bitewing images made 6 months ago. In addition, the patient shows no evidence exists of periodontal disease or other remarkable signs or symptoms in general or associated with the recently fractured tooth. As long as the fractured incisor shows normal vitality testing, no radiographs are recommended for this patient. If the pulp of the tooth becomes nonvital, a periapical view of this tooth should be made.
- A 45-year-old man returning to the dentist's office after 1 year. At his last visit, two three-surface amalgam restorations were placed on the maxillary right first and second premolars, and root canal therapy was performed on the mandibular right first molar. Also at this time, the patient is found to have a 5-mm pocket in the buccal furcation of the maxillary left first molar but no other evidence of chronic periodontitis. The guidelines recommend that this patient receive bitewing images to determine if he still has active caries and periapical images of the maxillary right premolars and the mandibular right first molar to evaluate the extent of the periodontal disease and periapical inflammatory disease, respectively.
- A 65-year-old woman coming to the office for the first time. No previous radiologic images are available. The patient has a history of root canal therapy in two teeth, although she does not know which teeth were treated. Clinical examination reveals multiple carious teeth, multiple missing teeth, and periodontal pockets of between 3 and 7 mm involving most of the remaining teeth. The guidelines recommend a full-mouth series examination including bitewing images for this patient because of the high probability of finding caries, periodontal disease, and periapical inflammatory disease.

BIBLIOGRAPHY

Guidelines for Ordering Imaging

American Association of Endodontists, American Academy of Oral and Maxillofacial Radiology Joint Position Statement. Use of cone beam computed tomography in endodontics. *Oral Surg Oral Med Oral Pathol Oral Radiol Endod.* 2015;120:508–512.

American Academy of Oral and Maxillofacial Radiology. Clinical recommendations regarding use of cone beam computed tomography in orthodontic treatment. *Oral Surg Oral Med Oral Pathol Oral Radiol.* 2013;116(2):238–257.

American Academy of Oral and Maxillofacial Radiology Position Statement. Selection criteria for the use of radiology in dental implantology with emphasis on cone beam computed tomography. *Oral Surg Oral Med Oral Pathol Oral Radiol.* 2012;1113:817–826.

American Dental Association Council on Scientific Affairs. The use of dental radiographs. *JADA.* 2006;137:1304–1312.

American Dental Association Council on Scientific Affairs. Dental radiographic examinations: recommendations for patient selection and limiting radiation exposure. Revised 2012: http://www.ada.org/sections/professionalResources/pdfs/Dental_Radiographic_Examinations_2012.pdf.

American Dental Association Council on Scientific Affairs. The use of cone-beam computed tomography in dentistry. An advisory statement from the American Dental Association Council on Scientific Affairs. *J Am Dent Assoc.* 2012;143:899–902.

Atchison KA, Luke LS, White SC. An algorithm for ordering pretreatment orthodontic radiographs. *Am J Orthod Dentofac Orthop.* 1992;102:29–44.

Bohay RN, Stephens RG, Kogon SL. A study of the impact of screening or selective radiography on the treatment and post delivery outcome for edentulous patients. *Oral Surg Oral Med Oral Pathol Oral Radiol Endod.* 1998;86:353–359.

Brooks SL. A study of selection criteria for intraoral dental radiography. *Oral Surg Oral Med Oral Pathol.* 1986;62:234–239.

Brooks SL, Brand JW, Gibbs SI, et al. Imaging of the temporomandibular joint: a position paper of the American Academy of Oral and Maxillofacial Radiology. *Oral Surg Oral Med Oral Pathol Oral Radiol Endod.* 1997;83:609–618.

Flack VF, Atchison KA, Hewlett ER, et al. Relationships between clinician variability and radiographic guidelines. *J Dent Res.* 1996;75:775–782.

Kantor ML. Trends in the prescription of radiographs for comprehensive care patients in U.S. and Canadian dental schools. *J Dent Educ.* 1993;57:794–797.

Kantor ML. Use of radiology practice guidelines and compliance with accreditation standards in US and Canadian dental schools. *J Dent Educ.* 2000;79:1532–1536.

McClean PM, Miller JW. Recommendations on administratively required radiographs. *JADA.* 1983;107:61–63.

National Council on Radiation Protection and Measurements. Dental x-ray protection, NCRP Report 145, Bethesda, MD, 2003, National Council on Radiation Protection and Measurements.

Rushton VE, Horner K, Worthington HV. Routine panoramic radiography of new adult patients in general dental practice: relevance of diagnostic yield to treatment and identification of radiographic selection criteria. *Oral Surg Oral Med Oral Pathol Oral Radiol Endod.* 2002;93:488–495.

SEDENTEXCT. Radiation Protection Number 172, Cone beam CT for dental and maxillofacial radiology (Evidence-based guidelines) http://www.sedentexct.eu/files/radiation_protection_172.pdf. Accessed January 12, 2017.

Tyndall DA, Price JB, Tetradis S, et al. Position statement of the American Academy of Oral and Maxillofacial Radiology on selection criteria for the use of radiology in dental implantology with emphasis on cone beam computed tomography. *Oral Surg Oral Med Oral Pathol Oral Radiol.* 2012;113:817–826.

U.S. Department of Health and Human Services, Public Health Service, Food and Drug Administration, and American Dental Association, Council on Dental Benefit Programs, Council on Scientific Affairs. The selection of patients for dental radiographic examinations, revised (2012):

http://www.fda.gov/Radiation-EmittingProducts/
RadiationEmittingProductsandProcedures/MedicalImaging/
MedicalX-Rays/ucm116504.htm.

White SC, Heslop EW, Hollender LG, et al. Parameters of radiologic care: an official report of the American Academy of Oral and Maxillofacial Radiology. *Oral Surg Oral Med Oral Pathol Oral Radiol Endod.* 2001;91:498–511.

Disease Detection

Atchison KA, White SC, Flack VF, et al. Efficacy of the FDA selection criteria for radiographic assessment of the periodontium. *J Dent Res.* 1995;74:1424–1432.

Atchison KA, White SC, Flack VF, et al. Assessing the FDA guidelines for ordering dental radiographs. *J Am Dent Assoc.* 1995;126:1372–1383.

Atieh MA. Diagnostic accuracy of panoramic radiographs in determining the relationship between the inferior alveolar nerve and mandibular third molar. *J Oral Maxillofac Surg.* 2010;68:74–82.

Corbet EF, Ho DK, Lai SM. Radiographs in periodontal disease and management. *Austral Dent J.* 2009;54(suppl 1):S27–S43.

Daley TD, Wysocki GP, Pringle GA. Relative incidence of odontogenic tumors and oral and jaw cysts in a Canadian population. *Oral Surg Oral Med Oral Pathol.* 1994;77:276–280.

Devereux L, Moles D, Cunningham SJ, et al. How important are lateral cephalometric radiographs in orthodontic treatment planning? *Am J Orthod Dentofac Orthop.* 2011;139:e175–e181.

Jindal SK, Sheikh S, Kulkarni S, et al. Significance of pre-treatment panoramic radiographic assessment of edentulous patients - a survey. *Med Oral Pathol Oral Cir Buccal.* 2011;16:e600–e606.

Jing W, Xuan M, Lin Y, et al. Odontogenic tumours: a retrospective study of 1642 cases in a Chinese population. *Int J Oral Maxillofac Surg.* 2007;36:20–25.

Madden RP, Hodges JS, Salmen CW, et al. Utility of panoramic radiographs in detecting cervical calcified carotid atheroma. *Oral Surg Oral Med Oral Pathol Oral Radiol Endod.* 2007;103:543–548.

Masood F, Robinson W, Beavers KS, et al. Findings from panoramic radiographs of the edentulous population and review of the literature. *Quintessence Int.* 2007;38:e298–e305.

Moles DR, Downer MC. Optimum bitewing examination recall intervals assessed by computer simulation. *Commun Dent Health.* 2000;17:14–19.

Mupparapu M, Kim IH. Calcified carotid artery atheroma and stroke: a systematic review. *J Am Dent Assoc.* 2007;138:483–492.

Osterne RLV, de Matos Brito RG, Nues Alves APV, et al. Odontogenic tumors: a 5-year retrospective study in a Brazilian population and analysis of 3406 cases reported in the literature. *Oral Surg Oral Med Oral Pathol Oral Radiol Endod.* 2011;111:474–481.

Reddy MS, Geurs NC, Jeffcoat RL, et al. Periodontal disease progression. *J Periodontol.* 2000;71:1583–1590.

Schiffman E, Ohrbach R, Truelove E, et al. Diagnostic criteria for temporomandibular disorders (DC/TMD) for clinical and research applications. Recommendations of the International RDC/TMD Consortium Network and the Orofacial Pain Special Interest Group. *J Orofac Pain Headache.* 2014;28:6–27.

Senel B, Kamburoglu K, Ucok O, et al. Diagnostic accuracy of different imaging modalities in detection of proximal caries. *Dentomaxillofac Radiol.* 2010;39:501–511.

Tawfik MA, Zyada MM. Odontogenic tumors in Dakahlia, Egypt: analysis of 82 cases. *Oral Surg Oral Med Oral Pathol Oral Radiol Endod.* 2010;198:e67–e73.

White SC, Atchison KA, Hewlett ER, et al. Efficacy of FDA guidelines for ordering radiographs for caries detection. *Oral Surg Oral Med Oral Pathol.* 1994;77:531–540.

White SC, Atchison KA, Hewlett ER, et al. Clinical and historical predictors of dental caries on radiographs. *Dentomaxillofac Radiol.* 1995;24:121–127.

Yoon SJ, Yoon W, Kim OS, et al. Diagnostic accuracy of panoramic radiographs in the detection of calcified carotid arteries. *Dentomaxillofac Radiol.* 2008;37:104–108.

Zeichner SJ, Ruttimann UE, Webber RL. Dental radiography: Efficacy in the assessment of intraosseous lesions of the face and jaws in asymptomatic patients. *Radiol.* 1987;162:691–695.

Radiation Dose and Effects

Falk A, Lindhe JE, Rohlin M, et al. Effects of collimator size of a dental X-ray unit on image contrast. *Dentomaxillofac Radiol.* 1999;28:261–266.

Goske MJ, Applegate KE, Boylan J, et al. The "Image Gently" campaign: increasing CT radiation dose awareness through a national education and awareness program. *Pediatr Radiol.* 2008;38:265–269.

Ludlow JB, Timothy R, Walker C, et al. Effective dose of dental CBCT - a meta analysis of published data and additional data for nine CBCT units. *Dentomaxillofac Radiol.* 2015;44:20140197.

Ludlow JB, Davies-Ludloe LE, White SC. Patient risk to common dental radiographic exams: the impact of 2007 ICRP recommendations regarding dose calculation. *JADA.* 2008;139:1237–1243.

Ludlow JB, Ivanovic M. Comparative dosimetry of dental CBCT devices and 64 row CT for oral and maxillofacial radiology. *Oral Surg Oral Med Oral Pathol Oral Radiol Endod.* 2008;106:930–938.

Rohlin M, White SC. Comparative means of dose reduction in dental radiography. *Curr Opin Dent.* 1992;2:1–9.

Sikorski PA, Taylor KW. The effectiveness of the thyroid shield in dental radiology. *Oral Surg Oral Med Oral Pathol.* 1984;58:225–236.

Velders XL, van Aken J, van der Stelt PF. Absorbed dose to organs in the head and neck from bitewing radiography. *Dentomaxillofac Radiol.* 1991;20:161–165.

White SC, Mallya SM. Update on the biological effects of ionizing radiation, relative dose factors, and radiation hygiene. *Aust Dent J.* 2012;57(suppl 1):2–8.

Wood RE, Harris AMP, van der Merwe EJ, et al. The lead apron revisited: Does it reduce gonadal radiation dose in dental radiology? *Oral Surg Oral Med Oral Pathol.* 1991;171:642–646.

18

Principles of Radiographic Interpretation

Mariam T. Baghdady

Dentists are expected to have basic skills in interpreting the radiologic images that they make in their dental practices. This ability requires the mastery of two identifiable and nonseparable components of visual diagnosis: perception, the ability to recognize abnormal patterns in the image, and cognition, the ability to interpret these abnormal patterns to arrive at an interpretation or diagnosis. This chapter provides an overview of diagnostic reasoning in oral radiology and an analytic framework to aid in the interpretation of diagnostic images. This framework will equip the reader with a systematic strategy for image analysis.

ADEQUATE DIAGNOSTIC IMAGES

Any method of image analysis is limited by the information contained in the available diagnostic images. An essential first step is making sure that there are an adequate number of images of diagnostic quality that display the region of interest in its entirety. When plain or projection images are being used, multiple images at slightly different projection angles as well as images made at right angles to one another often provide significant additional information. When appropriate, the use of advanced forms of diagnostic imaging can also provide valuable information (see Chapters 11 and 14).

VISUAL SEARCH STRATEGIES

The ability to find and identify abnormal patterns in the diagnostic image first involves a visual search of the entire image. The ability to recognize an abnormal pattern requires both an appreciation and an in-depth knowledge of the variations of appearances of normal anatomy. This is especially true in searching panoramic images. Recent research has shown that the employment of a systematic search strategy by novice clinicians improves their ability to detect abnormalities in panoramic images.

A systematic search strategy involves the identification of a list of normal anatomic structures that would be contained within the image. In a periapical image, the list might include the crown, root structure, pulp chamber and root canal system, periodontal ligament space, and lamina dura. In a panoramic image, this strategy might involve identifying the posterior border of the maxilla, the floor of the maxillary sinus, the zygomatic process of the maxilla, and the orbital rim. In a data set of cone beam computed tomography (CBCT) images, normal anatomy

would be reviewed through the entire image volume in the axial, coronal, and sagittal imaging planes. In the face of a complex assortment of anatomic structures, the use of a systematic search strategy will enable the novice clinician to search the complete image in a more meaningful manner. A thorough appreciation of normal anatomy and its variants is a vital first step in image interpretation. When an abnormality is detected in an image, the clinician must then focus on formulating an interpretation or diagnosis of the abnormality.

DIAGNOSTIC REASONING IN ORAL RADIOLOGY

Clinical reasoning in diagnostic oral and maxillofacial radiology can be considered unique in that the initial task requires the dentist to engage in a complex perceptual phase that involves differentiating normal and abnormal anatomic structures on two-dimensional images of three-dimensional structures. After the search process, if a finding is deemed abnormal, the clinician forms a mental three-dimensional representation of the abnormality that includes the precise location, size, internal structure, and how the abnormality affects the surrounding normal structures. This complex perceptual step is a method of identifying those features of the abnormality that will serve to arrive at a plausible interpretation or diagnosis.

Commonly the novice clinician may memorize specific features associated with each type of abnormality and then attempt to use this information to interpret images. This approach has been shown to be ineffective in the correct interpretation of radiographic abnormalities. Alternatively, it has been found that understanding the basic disease mechanism underlying the changes that each type of abnormality can produce in the diagnostic image is more effective in enhancing a novice clinician's diagnostic accuracy.

Worth, a pioneer in diagnostic oral and maxillofacial radiology, stated, "Radiographic appearances are governed by anatomic and physiologic changes in the presence of disease processes. Radiologic diagnosis is founded on knowledge of these alterations, the prerequisite being awareness of disease mechanisms." The terms *disease mechanism* and "basic science" are used interchangeably to describe the pathophysiology of abnormalities at the biochemical, cellular, tissue, and organ levels. More recent research suggests that an understanding of disease mechanisms plays an essential role in enhancing diagnostic accuracy in novice clinicians. This approach may assist the novice in creating a truer understanding of diagnostic entities and their features by creating

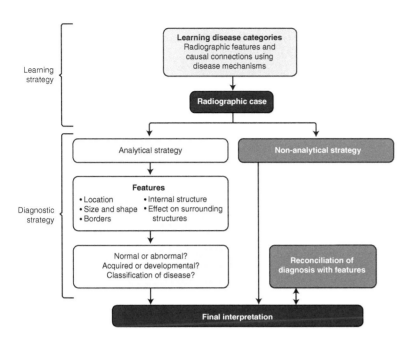

Fig. 18.1 Diagram illustrating the diagnostic process in oral radiology. The learning strategy phase represents the stage at which a novice learns about disease categories. The diagnostic strategy phase demonstrates the diagnostic techniques used by the clinician when faced with an abnormality.

coherent mental representations of different disease categories. Hence, when the dentist understands why certain features occur, he or she is better able to make the interpretation or diagnosis that makes sense, rather than simply focusing on radiologic feature counting and rote memory. Furthermore, the teaching of disease mechanisms and radiographic feature identification in a more integrated fashion produces a higher level of diagnostic accuracy in the novice clinician than when these subjects are covered in a more segregated manner.

ANALYSIS OF ABNORMAL FINDINGS

There are two main forms of diagnostic processing in radiology; the first is the analytic or systematic strategy, which we have already mentioned. This approach relies on a step-by-step analysis of all the imaging features of an abnormal finding so that an interpretation or diagnosis can be made based on these findings (Fig. 18.1). This analytic process is believed to reduce bias and premature closure of the decision-making process.

The second form, which is a nonanalytic strategy, assumes that viewing an abnormality in its entirety on a more global level can automatically lead to a more holistic diagnostic hypothesis. This hypothesis is then tested by initiating a deliberate search for features that support the hypothesis. This nonanalytic approach suggests that the clinician can make a more automatic decision regarding the diagnosis without a thorough feature analysis of the image. The expert oral and maxillofacial radiologist may rely on "pattern recognition" as a nonanalytic diagnostic strategy. There is, however, some empiric evidence that nonanalytic reasoning can be successfully employed by novice clinicians. Critics of teaching novices to rely on nonanalytic processing argue that the success of this diagnostic strategy is limited by the novice's minimal experience and the varied appearances of both normal anatomy and pathologic disorders in images. Although nonanalytic and analytic reasoning may be viewed as separate and distinct processes, research has demonstrated that they may be complementary. Students learning oral radiology could potentially benefit from specific training in the use of combining analytic and nonanalytic diagnostic strategies.

An analytic tool for the identification of abnormal findings is presented in the next section. The main function of this tool is to collect all the available imaging characteristics of the abnormal finding. Once the information is assembled, it is useful in the diagnostic process. As the imaging characteristics are being collected, it is important to integrate the disease mechanism underlying these characteristics when possible. For instance, Fig. 18.2 depicts the maturation of cemento-osseous dysplasia. In the early stage (see Fig. 18.2A), the periapical bone is resorbed and replaced with fibrous connective tissue; therefore, it appears radiolucent in the image. In a later more mature stage, this abnormality produces immature bone in the center (see Fig. 18.2B), resulting in the appearance of a radiopaque focus located at the center of the radiolucency. Knowledge of the disease mechanism underlying the development of cemento-osseous dysplasia allows the dentist to make the correct diagnosis even though the lesion is in an unusual location (the maxilla) and after the associated tooth has been extracted (see Fig. 18.2C).

ANALYTIC OR SYSTEMATIC STRATEGY

Step 1: Localize the Abnormality
Localized or Generalized
The anatomic location of the abnormality and its extent should be described. If an abnormal appearance affects all the osseous structures of the maxillofacial region uniformly, generalized disease processes, such as metabolic or endocrine abnormalities of bone, should be considered. If the abnormality is localized, is the abnormality unilateral or bilateral? Abnormal conditions such as fibrous dysplasia are more commonly unilateral, whereas Paget disease of bone and cherubism are always seen bilaterally in the jaws (Fig. 18.3).

Position in the Jaws

Identification of the geometric center or epicenter of a lesion may assist in determining the cell or tissue types contained within the abnormality in question. The epicenter can be estimated by identifying the midpoint of the mesial-distal, superior-inferior, and buccal-lingual extensions of the abnormality. This estimation may become less accurate with very

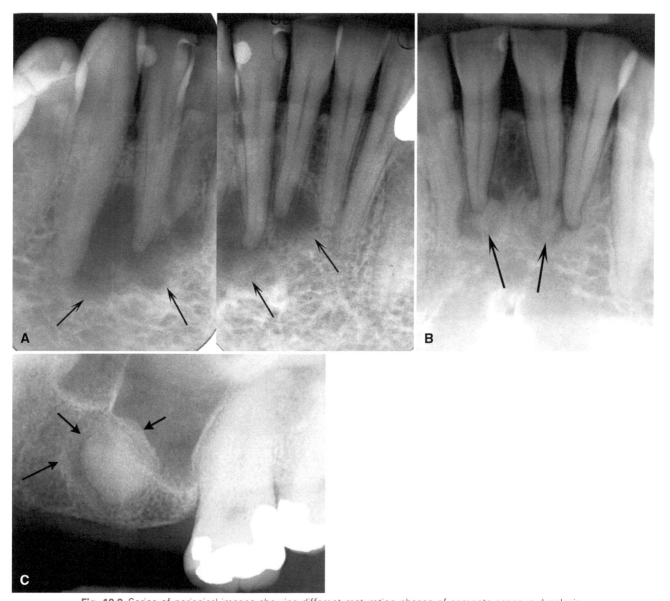

Fig. 18.2 Series of periapical images showing different maturation phases of cemento-osseous dysplasia. (A) Early radiolucent phase after periapical bone has been resorbed and replaced with connective tissue. (B) Late maturation phase *(arrows)* showing central amorphous bone (radiopaque) surrounded by a radiolucent internal border. (C) Mature phase *(arrows)* of cemento-osseous dysplasia in an unusual location and after the associated tooth has been extracted.

large lesions or lesions with poorly defined borders. The following are a few examples of relating the epicenter of the lesion to the tissue of origin:

- If the epicenter is located coronal to a tooth, the lesion probably is likely to be odontogenic in origin (Fig. 18.4).
- If the epicenter is located superior to the inferior alveolar canal (IAC), the likelihood is greater that it is of odontogenic origin (Fig. 18.5).
- If the epicenter is located inferior to the IAC, it is unlikely to be odontogenic in origin (Fig. 18.6); rather, it is more likely to have arisen from nonodontogenic cell sources.
- If the epicenter is located within the IAC, the lesion is likely neural or vascular in nature (Fig. 18.7).
- The probability of lesions arising from cartilaginous sources is greater in the condylar head region.

- If the epicenter is within the maxillary antrum, the lesion is not of odontogenic origin, as opposed to a lesion that has displaced the antral floor from the alveolar process of the maxilla (Fig. 18.8).

The other reason to establish the exact location of the lesion is that some abnormalities may be found in very specific locations within the jaws, although location in and of itself should never be used as the sole characteristic feature when abnormalities are being interpreted. The following are a few examples of this observation:

- The epicenters of central giant cell lesions are commonly located mesial to the first molar teeth in the mandible and mesial to the canine teeth in the maxilla in young patients.
- Osteomyelitis occurs more commonly in the mandible and rarely in the maxilla.
- Periapical osseous dysplasia occurs in the periapical regions of teeth (see Fig. 18.2).

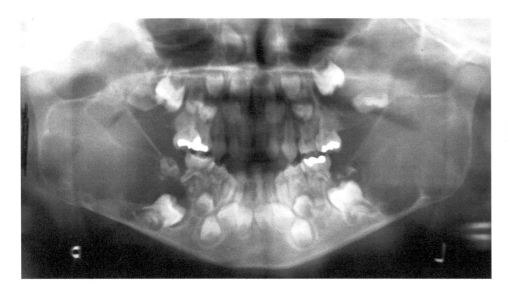

Fig. 18.3 This lesion, called *cherubism*, is bilateral, manifesting in both the left and the right mandibular rami. Because the origin of the lesion is in the midramus region, the mandibular molars have been displaced mesially on both sides.

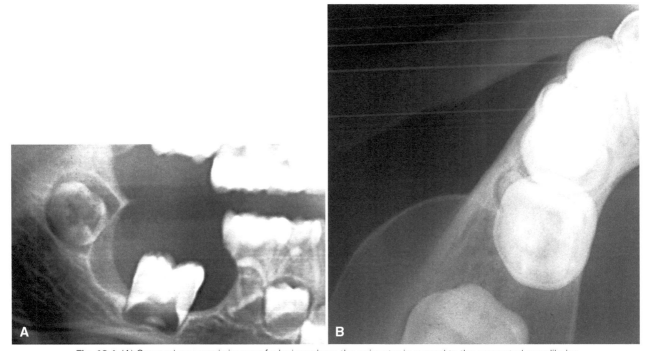

Fig. 18.4 (A) Cropped panoramic image of a lesion where the epicenter is coronal to the unerupted mandibular first molar. (B) Occlusal projection providing a right-angle view of the same lesion.

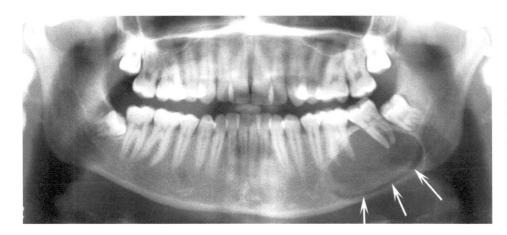

Fig. 18.5 Panoramic image revealing an ameloblastoma within the body of the left mandible. The inferior alveolar nerve canal has been displaced inferiorly to the inferior cortex *(arrows)*, indicating that the lesion started superior to the canal.

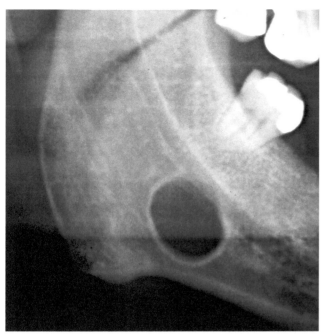

Fig. 18.6 Cropped panoramic image displaying a lesion (a submandibular salivary gland or Stafne defect) located inferior to the inferior alveolar canal and thus unlikely to be of odontogenic origin.

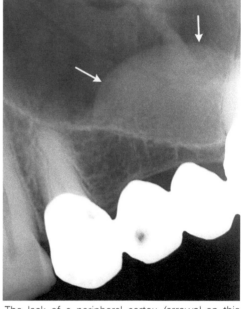

Fig. 18.8 The lack of a peripheral cortex *(arrows)* on this retention pseudocyst indicates that it originated in the sinus and not in the alveolar process. Therefore it is unlikely to be of odontogenic origin.

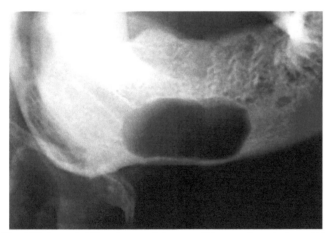

Fig. 18.7 Lateral oblique image of the mandible revealing a lesion within the inferior alveolar canal. The smooth fusiform expansion of the canal indicates a neural lesion.

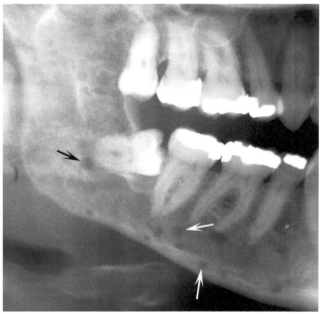

Fig. 18.9 Cropped panoramic image revealing several small punched-out lesions of multiple myeloma (a few are indicated by *arrows*) involving the body and ramus of the mandible.

Single or Multiple

Establishing whether an abnormality is solitary or multiple aids in understanding the disease mechanism of the abnormality. Additionally, the list of possible multiple, similarly appearing abnormalities in the jaws is relatively short. Examples of lesions that can be multifocal in the jaws are cemento-osseous dysplasia, odontogenic keratocysts, metastatic malignant lesions, multiple myeloma (Fig. 18.9), and leukemic infiltrates. Exceptions, of course, may occur, but these general criteria serve as a guide to an accurate interpretation or diagnosis.

Step 2: Assess the Periphery and Shape of the Abnormality

Is the periphery well or poorly defined? If an imaginary pencil can be used to reproducibly and confidently trace the border of the lesion, the border is likely well defined (Fig. 18.10). The clinician should not become overly concerned if some areas are poorly defined; this may be due to the shape of the lesion or direction of the x-ray beam at that particular location. A well-defined lesion is one in which most of the periphery is well defined. In contrast, it is difficult to exactly and reproducibly delineate a poorly defined periphery (Fig. 18.11).

The transition between a lesion and the normal adjacent bone is another important feature of the periphery to consider. The periphery of a lesion can display a zone of transition between the abnormal and

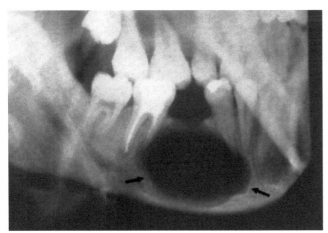

Fig. 18.10 Lateral oblique image of the mandible showing the well-defined border *(arrows)* of a residual cyst.

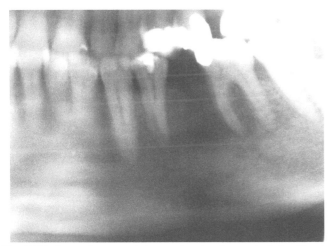

Fig. 18.11 Cropped panoramic image showing the poorly defined border of a malignant neoplasm that has destroyed bone between the first molar and the first bicuspid.

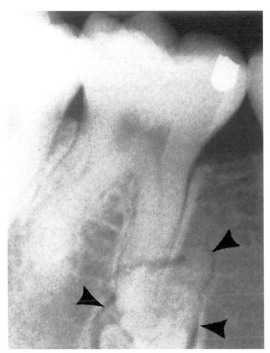

Fig. 18.12 Thin, radiolucent periphery indicates a connective tissue capsule positioned between the internal radiopaque structure of this odontoma and the radiopaque outer cortical boundary *(arrows)*.

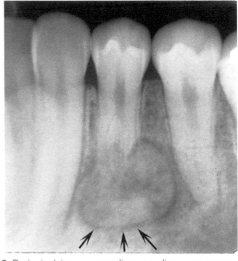

Fig. 18.13 Periapical image revealing a radiopaque mass associated with the root of the first premolar. The prominent radiolucent periphery *(arrows)* is characteristic of a connective tissue capsule of this cementoblastoma.

normal bone patterns. For example, a lesion with a thin radiopaque cortex at its periphery displays a narrow zone of transition; that is, the transition of the abnormal lesion to the normal adjacent bone across the cortex is narrow. Lesions with a sclerotic border exhibit a relatively wide zone of transition. Further analysis of these two types of peripheries or borders can help define the nature of the lesion.

Well-Defined Borders

Punched-out border. A punched-out border is one that has a sharp and very narrow zone of transition; there is no bone reaction immediately adjacent to the abnormality. The term *punched out* points to something similar to punching a hole in a piece of film or paper with a hole punch. The border of the resulting hole is well defined and the adjacent bone has a normal appearance up to the edge of the hole. This type of border is sometimes seen in multiple myeloma (see Fig. 18.9).

Corticated border. A corticated border is one that displays a thin, uniform, radiopaque line of bone at the periphery of a lesion. This is commonly seen with cysts and benign neoplasms or tumors (see Fig. 18.4).

Sclerotic border. A sclerotic border is one that shows a wider, more diffuse zone of transition between the lesion and the normal surrounding bone. The radiopaque border represents reactive bone that is usually

not uniform in width. This border may be seen in periapical osseous dysplasia and may indicate the ability of the lesion to stimulate the production of surrounding bone (see Fig. 18.2).

Internal radiolucent "soft tissue" periphery. A centrally located radiopaque lesion may be surrounded by a radiolucent rim of variable width. These lesions are described as having a mixed radiolucent and radiopaque internal structure. Histologically, the radiolucent rim represents nonmineralized connective tissue and is sometimes referred to as a "soft tissue capsule." This radiolucent rim may be seen in conjunction with a corticated periphery, as is observed with odontomas and cementoblastomas (Figs. 18.12 and 18.13).

Poorly Defined Borders

Blending border. A poorly defined border is one that is difficult to resolve. The zone of transition is often gradual and wide between the adjacent normal bone trabeculae and the abnormal-appearing trabeculae of the lesion. The focus of this observation is on the trabeculae rather than the radiolucent marrow spaces. Examples of conditions with this type of margin are sclerosing osteitis (Fig. 18.14) and fibrous dysplasia.

Invasive border. An invasive border is one in which there are few or no trabeculae between the periphery of the lesion and the normal bone. Furthermore, the zone of transition is typically wide (Fig. 18.15). In contrast to the blending border described earlier, the focus of this observation is on the enlarging radiolucency at the expense of normal adjacent bone trabeculae. These borders have also been described as permeative because the lesion grows around existing trabeculae, producing radiolucent, finger-like, or bay-type extensions at the periphery. This growth may result in enlargement of the marrow spaces at the periphery (Fig. 18.16). Invasive borders are usually associated with rapid growth and can be seen with malignant lesions.

Shape

The lesion may have a particular shape, or it may be irregular. Two examples follow:
- A circular or "hydraulic" shape, similar to an inflated or water-filled balloon, is characteristic of a cyst (see Fig. 18.4).

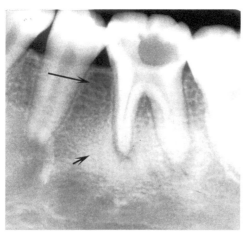

Fig. 18.14 Periapical image shows a gradual transition from the dense trabeculae of sclerosing osteitis *(short arrow)* to the normal trabecular pattern near the crest of the alveolar process *(long arrow)*. This is an example of a poorly defined blending border.

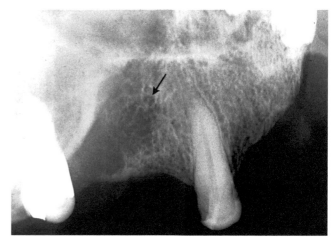

Fig. 18.16 Lateral occlusal image of a lesion revealing an ill-defined periphery with enlargement of the small marrow spaces at the margin *(arrow)*. This is characteristic of a malignant neoplasm—in this case a lymphoma.

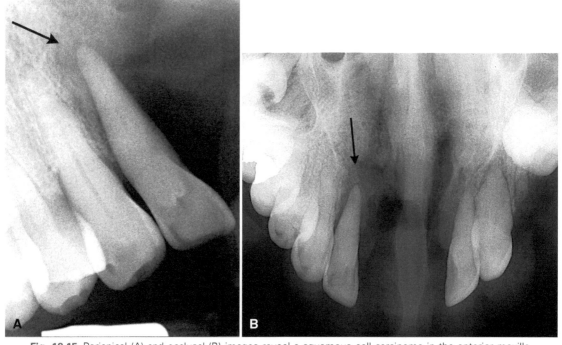

Fig. 18.15 Periapical (A) and occlusal (B) images reveal a squamous cell carcinoma in the anterior maxilla. The invasive margin extends beyond the lateral incisor *(arrow)*, and the radiolucent region with no apparent trabeculae represents bone destruction behind this margin.

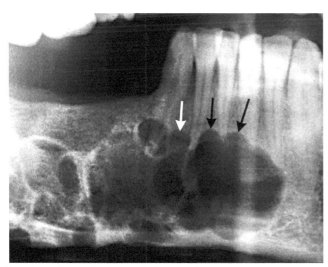

Fig. 18.17 Cropped panoramic image of an odontogenic keratocyst displaying a scalloped border, especially around the apex of the associated teeth *(arrows)*.

- Scalloping describes a series of contiguous arcs or semicircles that may develop around the roots of teeth or within adjacent bone or bone cortices. Scalloping may reflect the mechanism of a lesion's growth (Fig. 18.17). This shape may be seen in cysts (e.g., odontogenic keratocyst), cyst-like lesions (e.g., simple bone cysts), and some benign neoplasms. Occasionally a lesion with a scalloped periphery is referred to as multilocular; however, the term *multilocular* is reserved for the description of the internal structure in this text.

Step 3: Assess the Internal Structure

The internal appearance of a lesion can be classified into one of three basic categories: totally radiolucent, totally radiopaque, or mixed radiolucent and radiopaque ("mixed density"). Total radiolucency is characteristic of a lesion where the normal bone has been completely resorbed. This is commonly seen in cysts (see Fig. 18.4A). In contrast, total radiopacity implies that the lesion is filled with some sort of mineralized matrix; this is observed in osteomas. Mixed radiolucent and radiopaque lesions are those in which calcified material (radiopaque) is deposited against a radiolucent background. A challenging part of this analysis may be deciding whether the perceived calcified material is located within the lesion itself or is located buccal or lingual to the lesion; this difficulty is inherent to using two-dimensional images to represent three-dimensional structures. The shape, size, pattern, and density of the calcified material should be examined. For example, bone can be identified by the presence of a trabecular pattern. Also, the degree of radiopacity may help. For instance, enamel is more radiopaque than bone. The following is a list of most radiolucent to most radiopaque material seen in plain radiographs:
- Air, fat, and gas
- Fluid
- Soft tissue
- Bone marrow
- Trabecular bone
- Cortical bone and dentin
- Enamel
- Metal

This list is useful, but the amount of the tissue or material in the area can affect the degree of radiolucency or radiopacity. For example, a large amount of cortical bone may be as radiopaque as enamel.

The following section describes possible internal structures that may be seen in mixed radiolucent and radiopaque lesions.

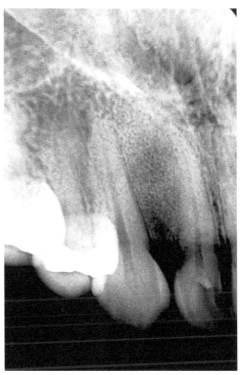

Fig. 18.18 Periapical image of a small lesion of fibrous dysplasia between the lateral incisor and canine demonstrates a change in bone pattern. A greater number of trabeculae per unit area are present; they are small and thin and randomly oriented in an orange peel-like pattern.

Abnormal Trabecular Patterns

Abnormal bone may exhibit various trabecular patterns that are different from those that are seen in normal bone. These variations result from a difference in the numbers, lengths, widths, and orientations of the trabeculae. For instance, in fibrous dysplasia, the trabeculae are usually greater in number, shorter, and not aligned in response to applied forces to the bone. Rather, they are randomly oriented, resulting in patterns described as having orange peel– or ground glass–like appearances (Fig. 18.18). Another example is the stimulation of new bone formation on existing trabeculae in response to inflammation. The result is thick trabeculae, giving an area a more radiopaque appearance (see Fig. 18.14).

Internal Septation

Septations represent striations of bone found within a lesion that appear to divide the lesion into two or more compartments. The term *multilocular* is used to describe the resultant compartments. The origin of this internal bone may be trapped normal bone, such as in ameloblastomas. In other lesions such as central giant cell lesions, cells within the tumor can manufacture bone in a recognizable linear pattern. The length, thickness, and orientation of a septum should be assessed. The appearance of the septa can inform the clinician about the nature and pathogenesis of the lesion. For instance, septa that are curved and coarse may be seen in ameloblastoma, giving rise to an internal pattern that is multilocular or "soap bubble" in appearance. This pattern reflects small nests of tumor cells or cyst-like formations within the tumor at the histopathologic level within the ameloblastoma. The small tumor nests or cyst-like areas entrap and remodel the bone around them as they increase in size (Fig. 18.19A and B). This pattern may also sometimes be observed in odontogenic keratocysts. Odontogenic myxomas also exhibit internal septation. In some cases this tumor contains a few straight, thin septa. In central giant cell lesions, reactive bone in the

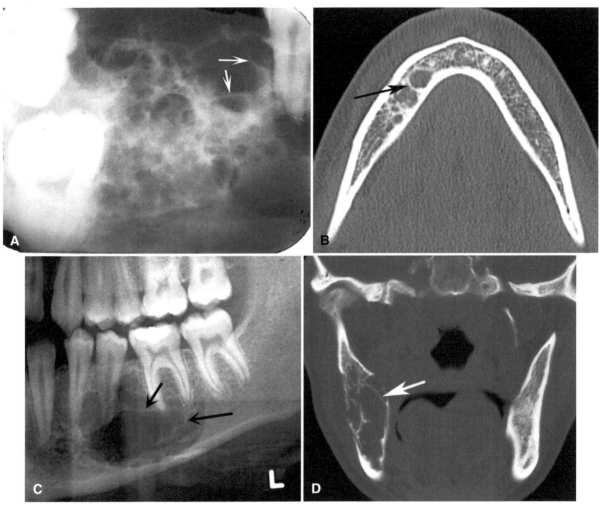

Fig. 18.19 (A) Periapical image of an ameloblastoma. The multilocular pattern created by septa *(arrows)* divides the internal structure into smaller, soap bubble–like compartments. (B) Axial multidetector computed tomography image of an ameloblastoma has typically curved septa *(arrow)*. (C) A cropped panoramic image of a central giant cell lesion with faint septations *(arrows)*. (D) Coronal computed tomography image of an odontogenic myxoma with typically straight septa *(arrow)*.

form of poorly calcified osteoid may develop, and appear as low-density and wispy or granular septations in the image.

Dystrophic Calcification

Dystrophic calcification is mineralization that occurs in damaged soft tissue. It is most commonly seen in calcified lymph nodes that appear as dense, cauliflower-like masses in the soft tissue. In chronically inflamed cysts, the calcification may have a very delicate, particulate appearance without a recognizable pattern.

Amorphous Bone

This type of dystrophic bone has a homogeneous, dense, poorly organized structure and is sometimes organized into round or oval shapes or clumps (see Fig. 18.2).

Tooth Structure

Tooth structure can usually be identified by organization into enamel, dentin, and pulp chambers. Also, the density of this material is equivalent to the normal density of tooth structure and is of greater density than the surrounding bone (see Fig. 18.12).

Step 4: Assess the Effects of the Lesion on Adjacent Structures

Evaluating the effects of a lesion on adjacent structures allows the dentist to infer biologic behavior, and this behavior may aid in identification of the disease. However, having knowledge of disease mechanisms is required. For instance, periapical inflammatory disease can stimulate bone resorption (rarefaction) or formation (sclerosis). Bone formation may occur on the surface of existing trabeculae, resulting in thickened trabeculae, and this may be reflected in an overall increase in the radiopacity of the bone (see Fig. 18.14). A space-occupying lesion, such as a cyst or a benign neoplasm or tumor, slowly creates its own space by displacing teeth and other surrounding structures (see Fig. 18.4). The following sections give examples of effects on surrounding structures and the conclusions that may be inferred from the behavior of the lesions.

Teeth, Lamina Dura, and Periodontal Ligament Space

Displacement of teeth is seen more commonly with benign slower-growing space-occupying lesions. The direction of tooth displacement is significant. Lesions with an epicenter above the crown of a tooth

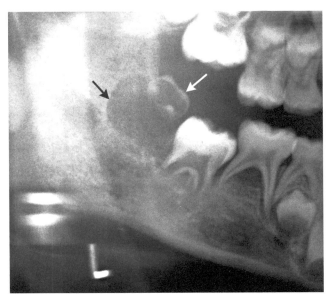

Fig. 18.20 Leukemic infiltration of the mandible shows coronal displacement of the developing second molar *(white arrow)* from the remnants of its crypt *(black arrow)*. There is a lack of a lamina dura around the apex of the first molar and widening of the periodontal ligament space around the second deciduous molar.

(i.e., dentigerous cysts and occasionally odontomas) will displace the tooth apically (see Fig. 18.4A). The central giant cell lesions arising in cherubism have a propensity to displace teeth in a mesial (anterior) direction given the epicenters of these lesions (see Fig. 18.3). Some lesions (e.g., lymphoma, leukemia, Langerhans cell histiocytosis) grow in the papillae of developing teeth and may push a developing tooth in a coronal direction (Fig. 18.20).

Resorption of teeth usually occurs with a more chronic or slowly growing process (see Fig. 18.4A). It may also result from chronic inflammation. Although tooth resorption is more commonly related to benign processes, some malignant tumors, particularly sarcomas, can occasionally resorb teeth.

Widening of the periodontal ligament space may be seen with a number of abnormalities. It is important to observe whether the widening is localized or generalized, irregular or uniform. As well, the adjacent lamina dura should be assessed to determine its condition. For instance, orthodontic movement of teeth results in generalized widening of the periodontal ligament space around tooth roots, but the lamina dura remains intact. Malignant lesions can rapidly grow down and invade the ligament space, resulting in irregular widening, and destruction of the lamina dura (Fig. 18.21).

Surrounding Bone Reaction

Some abnormalities can stimulate a bone reaction at the periphery. An example is the cortex of a cyst or the often sclerotic border seen in cemento-osseous dysplasia as previously described. The corticated border of a cyst is not actually part of the cyst but is a bone reaction that develops in response to the cyst as it enlarges. Identification of peripheral bone formation provides a behavioral characteristic suggesting that the abnormality has the ability to stimulate an osteoblastic reaction. Periapical rarefying osteitis can also stimulate a sclerotic bone reaction (see Fig. 18.14), as can some metastatic prostate and breast lesions.

Inferior Alveolar Canal and Mental Foramen

Changes to the IAC can be characteristic of specific disease processes. Superior displacement of the IAC is strongly associated with fibrous dysplasia when the epicenter occurs inferior to the canal. Widening of the IAC with the maintenance of a cortical boundary may indicate the presence of a benign lesion of vascular or neural origin within the canal (see Fig. 18.7). Irregular widening with cortical destruction may indicate the presence of a malignant neoplasm growing down the length of the canal.

Cortical Bone and Periosteal Reactions

The cortical boundaries of bone may remodel in response to the growth of a lesion within the maxilla or mandible. A slowly growing lesion may allow time for the surface periosteum to manufacture new bone, so that the resulting expanded bone surface appears to have maintained an outer cortex (see Fig. 18.4B). In contrast, a rapidly growing lesion outstrips the ability of the periosteum to respond, and the cortex may be lost (Fig. 18.22). The remodeled external shape of the mandible or maxilla can provide information on the growth pattern of the entity. For instance, a tumor such as ossifying fibroma often has a concentric growth pattern with a clear epicenter. Whereas a bone dysplasia such as fibrous dysplasia, will enlarge the bone with a growth pattern that is along the bone without an obvious epicenter (Fig. 18.23).

Exudate from an inflammatory lesion can stimulate the periosteum to lay down new bone (Fig. 18.24). When this process occurs more than once, an onionskin type of pattern can be seen. This pattern is most commonly seen in inflammatory lesions and more rarely in tumors such as leukemia and Langerhans cell histiocytosis. Other examples of patterns of reactive periosteal bone formation include a spiculated new bone formed at right angles to the surface cortex, which is seen with metastatic lesions of the prostate gland or in a radiating pattern of spiculated bone seen in osteosarcoma (Fig. 18.25) or a hemangioma.

Step 5: Formulate an Interpretation

The preceding steps enable the dentist to collect a series of radiologic findings in an organized and systematic fashion. (Box 18.1 presents the process in abbreviated form.) Now the significance of each observation must be determined and weighted. The ability to give more significance to some observations over others comes with experience.

After an initial working interpretation has been reached, ambiguities are resolved either by searching for more features or by putting more weight on one feature or the other. For instance, in the analysis of a hypothetical lesion, observations of tooth movement, tooth resorption, and an invasive destructive border are made. The effects on the teeth in this example may indicate a benign process; however, the invasive border and bone destruction are more important characteristics and indicate a malignant process. In the analytic approach (see Fig. 18.1), all these accumulated characteristics are used to make a diagnostic decision. A diagnostic algorithm such as that shown in Fig. 18.26 can aid in this decision-making process. Following this algorithm, the observer makes decisions regarding which general disease category the entity fits into and then proceeds to smaller, more specific categories. This is not an infallible method because any algorithm may occasionally fail, since lesions sometimes do not behave as expected.

Decision 1: Normal or Abnormal

The clinician should determine whether the entity of interest is a variation of normal or an abnormality. This is a crucial decision because variations of normal do not require treatment or further investigation. Therefore the clinician must develop an in-depth knowledge and appreciation

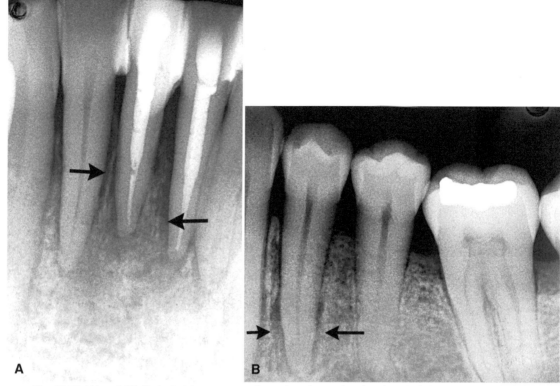

Fig. 18.21 (A) and (B) Periapical images revealing a lymphoma that has invaded the mandible. There is irregular widening of the periodontal ligament spaces *(arrows)*.

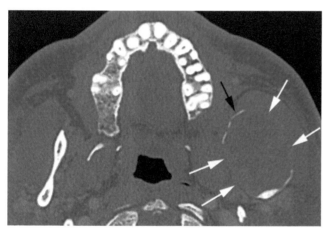

Fig. 18.22 Axial computed tomography image of an ameloblastoma involving the left mandibular ramus shows significant expansion of the ramus with displacement of the bone border *(black arrow)*. In some areas *(white arrows)* the speed of growth of the tumor has exceeded the ability of the bone to keep it confined.

for the variations in the appearances of normal anatomy. The importance of this cannot be overstated.

Decision 2: Developmental or Acquired

If the area of interest is abnormal, the next step is to decide whether the radiographic characteristics represent a developmental abnormality or an acquired change. For example, the observation that a tooth has an abnormally short root leads to the pertinent question, "Did the tooth develop a short root, or did the root develop to a normal length and then become shorter?" If the answer is the latter, the process must be

external root resorption (an acquired abnormality). If the tooth merely developed a short root, the pulp canal should not be visible to the very end of the root because of normal apex development. In contrast, external root resorption may shorten the root, but the canal remains visible to the end of the root (Fig. 18.27).

Decision 3: Disease Classification

If the abnormality is acquired, the next step is to select the most likely disease category for the acquired abnormality. The disease category can be established by observing the features and how they reflect a particular disease mechanism. The categories may include inflammation, cysts, benign neoplasia, malignant neoplasia, bone dysplasia, vascular abnormalities, metabolic diseases, or physical changes such as fractures (i.e., trauma). The following chapters describe the characteristic radiologic features of diseases in these categories based on the mechanisms that give rise to these abnormalities. The analysis should strive to narrow the interpretation to one of these disease categories; this directs the next course of action for continued investigation, referral, and treatment. This may also be a good time to bring the clinical information—such as patient history and clinical signs and symptoms—into the decision-making process. This additional information may help the clinician to refine the interpretation to a short list (a differential interpretation) of diseases within the category. When possible, considering this information at the end helps avoid the problem of doing an incomplete search of the images or trying to make the radiographic characteristics fit a preconceived diagnosis.

Decision 4: Ways to Proceed

After a disease category or a differential interpretation of diseases is determined, the clinician must decide how to proceed. This decision may require further imaging, biopsy, observation (watchful waiting),

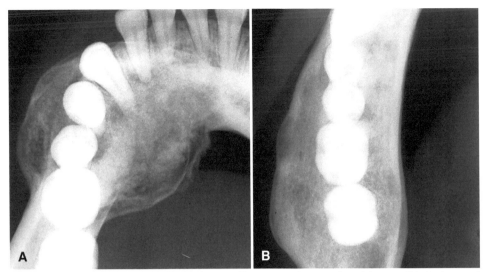

Fig. 18.23 (A) Occlusal image of an ossifying fibroma. The concentric expansion of the mandible is characteristic of a benign tumor. (B) Occlusal image of fibrous dysplasia with mild fusiform expansion of the mandible but without an obvious epicenter.

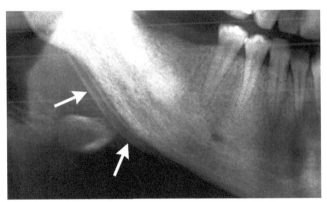

Fig. 18.24 Panoramic image of osteomyelitis revealing at least two layers of new bone *(arrows)* produced by the periosteum at the inferior aspect of the mandible.

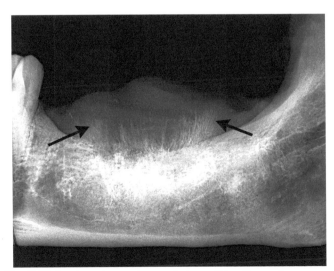

Fig. 18.25 Specimen image of a resected mandible with an osteosarcoma. Note the fine linear spicules of bone at the superior margin of the alveolar process *(arrows)*.

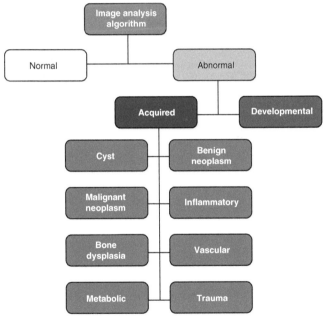

Fig. 18.26 Algorithm representing the diagnostic process that follows evaluation of the radiographic features of an abnormality.

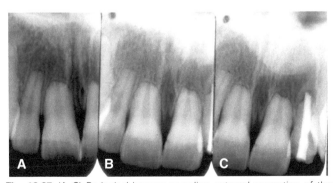

Fig. 18.27 (A–C) Periapical images revealing external resorption of the maxillary incisors, which is an acquired abnormality because of the presence of the wide pulp chambers at the apex of the roots of the teeth.

BOX 18.1   Analysis of Intraosseous Lesions

Step 1: Localize the Abnormality
- Anatomic position (epicenter)
- Localized or generalized
- Unilateral or bilateral
- Single or multifocal

Step 2: Assess Periphery and Shape of the Abnormality
Periphery
- Well defined
- Punched out
- Corticated
- Sclerotic
- Soft tissue capsule
- Poorly defined
- Blending
- Invasive

Shape
- Circular
- Scalloped
- Irregular

Step 3: Analyze the Internal Structure
- Totally radiolucent
- Totally radiopaque
- Mixed radiolucent and radiopaque (describe pattern)

Step 4: Assess the Effects of Lesion on Surrounding Structures
- Teeth, lamina dura, periodontal ligament space
- Inferior alveolar nerve canal and mental foramen
- Maxillary antrum
- Surrounding bone density and trabecular pattern
- Outer cortical bone and periosteal reactions

Step 5: Formulate an Interpretation

or definitive treatment. For example, if a lesion fits into the category of malignant neoplasia, the patient first should be referred to an oral and maxillofacial radiologist for possible advanced imaging to further characterize and stage the lesion. Advanced imaging may also help to determine an optimal site for biopsy and treatment. Periapical osseous dysplasia may not require any further investigation or treatment. In other cases, a period of watchful waiting followed by reexamination in a few months may be indicated if the abnormality appears benign and there is no clear need for immediate treatment.

With advanced training or experience in diagnostic imaging, the dentist may be better able to name one specific abnormality or at least make a short list of abnormalities from one or two of the disease categories. It is important to recognize, however, that imaging is but one diagnostic test available to the dentist, and it is not infallible. It is therefore important for the dentist to understand the limitations of imaging and recognize its value alongside other clinical information and diagnostic testing that may be ordered.

WRITING A DIAGNOSTIC IMAGING REPORT

When analyzing diagnostic images, it is advisable to create a formal report for the purposes of documentation and communication with other clinicians. The radiographic report can be subdivided into the following subsections.

General Patient Information

This section appears at the beginning of the report, and includes the patient's name, age, sex, and any alphanumeric identification such as a clinic or medical registration number. Also, the name of the referring clinician (if applicable) and the date of the report are also included.

Imaging Procedure

This section summarizes the imaging procedures provided along with the date of the examination. Specific information should be provided regarding CBCT. For example, field of view, slice thickness, and distance between slices. An example for reporting imaging procedure could be the following: "The imaging examination consists of panoramic and intraoral maxillary standard occlusal images, and contrast enhanced axial and coronal MDCT images of the mandible conducted on February 20, 2017."

Clinical Information

This is an optional section that includes pertinent clinical information regarding the patient's condition provided by the referring clinician or by the clinician dictating the report if a clinical examination was made before the radiologic examination. The clinical information should be brief and should summarize the information pertaining to the abnormality in question. For example, "Clinicial examination revealed a mass in the floor of mouth, possibly a ranula. The patient has a history of lymphoma."

Findings

This section comprises an objective detailed list of observations made from the diagnostic images. This can follow the previously presented step-by-step analysis of the anatomic location, extent of the lesion, periphery and shape, internal structure, and effects on surrounding structures. This section does not include a radiologic interpretation.

Interpretation

The collected observations from the radiologic image or images allow the dentist to elucidate their meaning, and this is called an interpretation. If additional information from the patient history is available or if clinical or other diagnostic information is available together with the radiologic interpretation results, a diagnosis can be made. In some instances, however, the radiologic features can be pathognomonic of a disease, in which case the interpretation is the diagnosis.

When possible, the clinician should endeavor to provide a definitive interpretation of the abnormality that has been imaged. When this is not possible, a short list of abnormalities or a differential interpretation (listed in order of likelihood) is acceptable. This list should not, however, be exhaustive; ideally it should be limited to diseases within one or perhaps two disease categories at most. In some situations, advice regarding additional studies, when required, and treatment may be included. Last, the name and signature of the clinician composing the report is included.

SELF-TEST

To practice the analytic technique presented, the reader should examine Fig. 18.4A and B and write down all observations and the results of the diagnostic algorithm before reading the following section.

Description
Location

The abnormality is singular and unilateral, and the epicenter lies coronal to the mandibular first molar.

Periphery and Shape

The lesion has a well-defined cortical periphery that attaches to the cementoenamel junction and the shape is round.

Internal Structure

The internal structure is completely radiolucent.

Effects on Adjacent Structures

The occlusal radiograph reveals that the buccal cortical plate has expanded in a smooth, curved shape, and a thin cortical boundary still exists.

Effects on Adjacent Teeth

This lesion has displaced the first molar in an apical direction, which reinforces the decision that the origin was coronal to this tooth. Also, the lesion has displaced the second molar distally and the second premolar in a mesial direction. Apical resorption of the distal root of the second deciduous molar has occurred.

Analysis

Making all the observations is an important first step in the interpretation process. To accomplish this next step, further knowledge of the pathologic condition and a certain amount of experience are required. The first objective is to select the correct category of diseases (e.g., inflammation, benign neoplasia, cyst); at this point, the clinician should try not to let all the names of specific diseases be overwhelming.

These images reveal an abnormal appearance. The coronal location of the lesion suggests that the tissue making up this abnormality is probably derived from a component of the dental follicle. The effects on the surrounding structures indicate that this abnormality is acquired.

The displacement and resorption of teeth, intact peripheral cortex, curved shape, and radiolucent internal structure all indicate a slow-growing, benign, space-occupying lesion, most likely in the cyst category. Odontogenic tumors, such as an ameloblastic fibroma, may be considered but are less likely because of the shape. The most common type of cyst in a follicular location is a dentigerous cyst. Odontogenic keratocysts are occasionally seen in this location, but the tooth resorption and degree of expansion are not characteristic of that pathologic condition. Therefore, the final interpretation is a dentigerous cyst, with odontogenic keratocyst and ameloblastic fibroma as possibilities in the differential interpretation, although less likely. Treatment usually is indicated for dentigerous cysts, and such a patient should be referred for consultation with an oral and maxillofacial surgeon.

BIBLIOGRAPHY

Baghdady M, Carnahan H, Lam EW, et al. The integration of basic sciences and clinical sciences in oral radiology. *J Dent Educ.* 2013;77: 757–763.

Baghdady M, Carnahan H, Lam EW, et al. Dental and dental hygiene students' diagnostic strategy and instructional method. *J Dent Ed.* 2014;8:1279–1285.

Baghdady M, Pharoah M, Regehr G, et al. The role of basic sciences in diagnostic oral radiology. *J Dent Educ.* 2009;73:1187–1193.

Eva KW, Hatala RM, LeBlanc VR, et al. Teaching from the clinical reasoning literature: combined reasoning strategies help novice diagnosticians overcome misleading information. *Med Educ.* 2007;41:1152–1158.

Woods N. Science is fundamental: the role of biomedical knowledge in clinical reasoning. *Med Educ.* 2007;41:1173–1177.

Worth HM. *Principles and Practice of Oral Radiologic Interpretation.* Chicago: Year Book Medical Publishers; 1972.

19

Dental Caries

Daniel P. Turgeon

DISEASE MECHANISM

Dental caries is a multifactorial disease that develops as a result of the interaction of three factors: the tooth, the plaque and the diet. In addition, other factors may also contribute to the process; for example, saliva, the application of fluoride, the immune system, the duration of exposure to microorganisms, and the patient's socioeconomic status. *Streptococcus mutans* in plaque plays a pivotal role in the process of demineralization. The number of *S. mutans* present is both responsive and directly proportional to the amount of sugar consumed from the diet.

Lactic acid is produced by the fermentation of fructose by *S. mutans* in the bacterial biofilm; this, in turn, causes a reduction in the local pH and demineralization of the tooth structure. The demineralization process in early carious lesions begins beneath the enamel surface, leaving behind a thin, mineralized, intact surface layer of precipitated calcium and phosphate that may persist for some time. The caries process itself does not progress in a manner that is temporally linear. Rather, it is a continuous cycle of demineralization and remineralization in which the demineralization process eventually dominates. The process can be modified and tipped in favor of remineralization by influencing factors that have been previously mentioned: reducing sugar intake, removing the plaque-containing *S. mutans*, and applying topical fluoride to strengthen the tooth surface. Should this be successful, an arrested lesion results. An arrested lesion may, however, become active again if there is renewed activity in the plaque.

Demineralization of tooth structure, called the carious lesion, represents the effect of the disease rather than the disease itself. Clinically, the appearance of caries will vary with time; an early, active lesion will appear as a white, chalky spot, whereas an older, arrested lesion will appear darker (black or brown). The rate of demineralization will vary based on the factors previously mentioned, but will also vary depending on the crystalline structure of the tooth. Enamel is composed mostly of closely packed mineralized acellular hydroxyapatite crystals. In comparison, dentin is composed approximately of 45% inorganic apatite crystals, 30% organic matrix, and 25% water. These differences result in a greater rate of demineralization within the dentin. Destruction of the outer enamel surface (cavitation) usually occurs after dentin involvement, and demineralization can progress to the pulp, causing necrosis and/or destruction of the tooth (Fig. 19.1).

ROLE OF IMAGING IN THE DETECTION OF CARIOUS LESIONS

A thorough clinical examination that includes imaging is needed to diagnose carious lesions. A clinical examination may be able to identify carious lesions on the occlusal and exposed smooth surfaces of the teeth. However, it is nearly impossible to clinically identify caries occurring on the proximal surfaces of teeth (i.e., interproximal caries), unless there has been cavitation. When this occurs, it usually means that the carious lesion has become large enough to be identified clinically. Unfortunately, when a caries lesion reaches this stage, the affected tooth may require endodontic treatment or, if the tooth is determined to be unrestorable, it may require extraction.

The intraoral bitewing image is the preferred image to detect interproximal caries in posterior teeth. As long as the operator can position the image receptor (sensor or film) correctly, the proximal surfaces should be clearly visible (Fig. 19.2). Since a caries lesion causes a demineralization of the enamel and the dentin, more x-ray photons will penetrate a demineralized region of the tooth, creating a radiolucent (dark) region on the images. Caries are sometimes visible on a panoramic image, but in these cases the caries are usually large enough to be clinically apparent. Since panoramic images have comparatively poor resolution compared with intraoral receptors, they should not be relied on to detect caries (see Chapter 9).

Even when demineralization is detected on an image, this does not mean that it represents an active carious lesion. This could simply represent an older, inactive (arrested) lesion that can be described as a "scar" in the enamel. This is possible because the minerals from the saliva are in the contact with the outermost surface of the tooth and can remineralize it but cannot reach into deeper tissues. No single image can differentiate active caries from arrested caries; to do so requires a second image, made at another time point, for comparison (Fig. 19.3).

The recommended interval between imaging examinations can vary substantially; between 6 months for patients at higher risk to 36 months for patients at low risk. The decision to obtain images must therefore be tailored for each patient. Those factors that increase risk are summarized in Table 19.1.

Recently some panoramic image systems have incorporated an "extraoral bitewing image" application (Fig. 19.4). Even though some manufacturers claim that this may be more effective than intraoral bitewing images in detecting caries, studies have shown equivocal results. We therefore continue to be of the opinion that intraoral images are still the preferred method with which to diagnose interproximal caries. Extraoral bitewing images can be used when it is impossible to obtain intraoral images—for example, with uncooperative patients, patients with a severe gag reflex, or those with anatomic constraints such as large mandibular tori.

Despite our best clinical monitoring practices, some carious lesions are not diagnosed because they may not be visible on an image. Because caries lesions progress slowly, especially in enamel, it is important for dentists to take an approach that is individualized to each patient, to understand the factors that contribute to disease, and to incorporate imaging examinations as necessary.

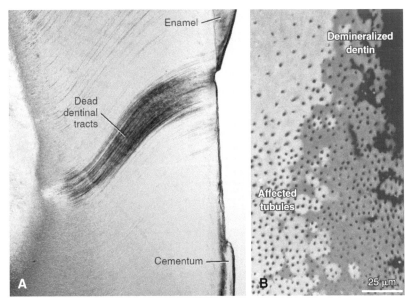

Fig. 19.1 (A) Light micrograph showing dead tracts on the radicular carious lesion that appear dark under transmitted light. (B) Scanning electron micrograph showing empty tubules under a carious lesion. (From Nanci A. *Ten Cate's Oral histology: Development, Structure, and Function.* St. Louis: Mosby Elsevier; 2013. Courtesy Dr. A. Nanci, Montréal, QC.)

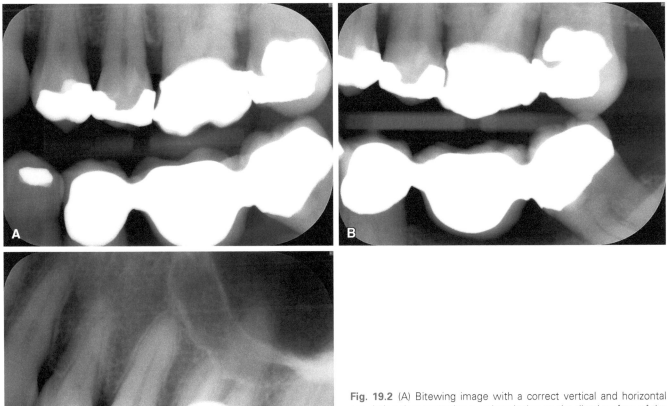

Fig. 19.2 (A) Bitewing image with a correct vertical and horizontal angulation demonstrating a carious lesion on the distal surface of the maxillary left first molar. (B) Bitewing image of the same patient with incorrect horizontal angulation, causing an overlap of the interproximal regions hiding the carious lesion. (C) Periapical image of the same patient with an incorrect vertical angulation, causing an overlap of the coronal restoration with a portion of the root and hiding the carious lesion.

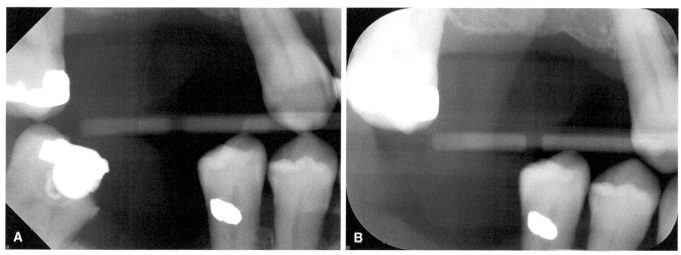

Fig. 19.3 (A) Bitewing image showing a carious lesion on the distal surface of the mandibular right first premolar. (B) Bitewing image of the same patient, obtained 5 years later. Note the absence of growth from the carious lesion.

TABLE 19.1   Factors Increasing the Risk for Caries
1. Multiple previous caries
2. Recurrent caries
3. Existing restorations of inadequate quality
4. Poor oral hygiene
5. Insufficient fluoride exposure
6. Frequent consumption of sugary drinks (including prolonged nursing)
7. Family history of poor dental health
8. Enamel defects
9. Xerostomia
10. Inability to have proper dental hygiene (possibly from a disability)
11. Head and neck radiation therapy
12. Eating disorders (bulimia)
13. Alcohol and drug abuse
14. Irregular dental care

EXAMINATION WITH DIGITAL INTRAORAL SENSORS

Digital sensors are rapidly replacing film in clinical dentistry. As we saw in Chapter 4, two different sensor types are available: solid-state sensors and photostimulable phosphor plates (PSPs). For some patients, solid-state sensors may be more difficult to place because of their size (mostly their thickness), causing patient discomfort. Furthermore, this may create more positioning difficulties for the dentist or his or her staff. That said, manufacturers are developing newer sensors that are thinner with characteristics that make them more comfortable for patients, including rounded corners. Unfortunately the active surface area of solid-state sensors is smaller than that of their film equivalents, sometimes leading to the necessity for a second image to complete the examination (Fig. 19.5). Although PSPs are slightly thicker and more rigid than film, they are similar in size and may therefore be as easy as film to position.

Holder devices for sensors are available on the market for both solid-state and PSP sensors. These position-indicating devices (PIDs) facilitate the positioning of the sensors and x-ray beam to avoid the overlap of adjacent proximal surfaces. Multiple studies have shown digital images to be equivalent to conventional films with respect to the sensitivity of caries detection. An exception is enamel caries detection, where film images have a reported higher sensitivity. For adolescents and adults, larger American National Standards Institute (ANSI) sensors (no. 2) are used to acquire bitewing images. Smaller ANSI sized sensors (no. 0 or no. 1) can be used in children. In adults with their second or third molars, there is nearly always the need for two images per side. And as is the case with film images, digital images should also be viewed on a high-quality monitor with an appropriate gray scale and in a room with subdued light.

EXAMINATION WITH CONVENTIONAL INTRAORAL FILM

As with digital sensors, ANSI no. 2 film is used for bitewing examinations in adolescents and adults, but it can also be used in younger patients when first molar teeth have erupted. In these cases, only one image may be necessary. In smaller children, ANSI no. 0 or no. 1 film can be used. Before being analyzed, the films should be mounted in frames with dark borders, and they should then be viewed in a darkened room with a light box and a magnifying glass to optimize the resolution of the film. The use of ANSI no. 3 film should be discouraged. The size (length) of the film is such that when placed in the mouth, the plane of the film bends, thus distorting the images of the teeth and bone crests.

DETECTION OF CARIOUS LESIONS

Proximal Surfaces

Typical Appearance

As the enamel rods are oriented at 90 degrees to the surface of the enamel, the penetration of acid and therefore demineralization occurs along the long axes of the enamel rods. Thus the classic shape of an enamel caries lesion is a triangle with its broad base on the proximal surface of the tooth and its tip pointing toward the dentinoenamel junction (DEJ) (Fig. 19.6). Other shapes may also be seen; these can include a band, a rectangle, or simply a notch (Fig. 19.7). When the leading edge of a caries lesion reaches the DEJ, it spreads along the enamel-dentin interface and penetrates the dentin, where a second triangle forms. Here, the broad base is located at the DEJ and its tip is pointed toward the pulp chamber. One can expect the demineralization in the dentin to be more aggressive because of the lower mineralized

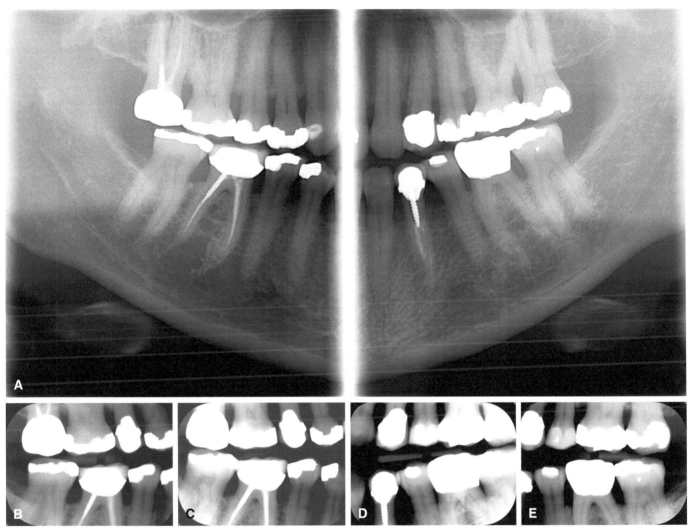

Fig. 19.4 (A) Extraoral bitewing image. (B–E) Intraoral bitewing images of the same patient. Note the higher resolution of the intraoral images. (Courtesy Dr. M. Michaud, Montréal, QC.)

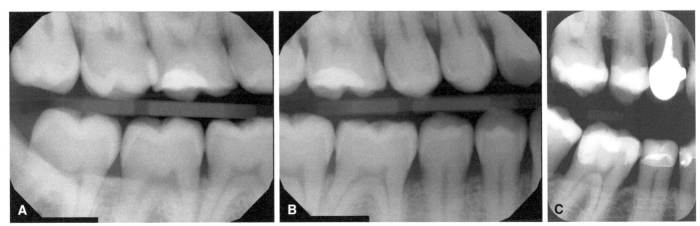

Fig. 19.5 (A) and (B) Two bitewing images from the patient's left side to cover the interproximal surfaces from the distal part of the canines to the distal part of the most posterior teeth. Note the carious lesion on the distal surface of the mandibular left second premolar. Vertical bitewing images (C) can also be obtained and are often used when the patient presents with periodontal bone loss.

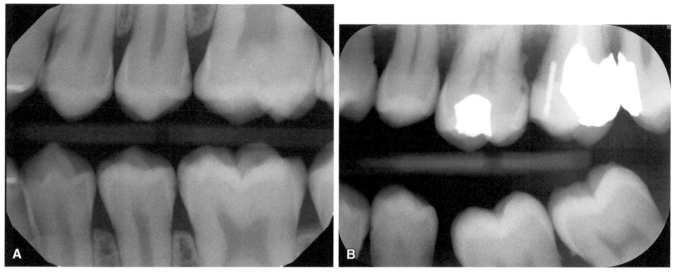

Fig. 19.6 Two bitewing images showing the triangular shape of carious lesions on the distal surface of the maxillary and mandibular left second premolars (A) and on the distal surface of the mandibular left first premolar and mesial surface of the mandibular left second premolar (B). (A, Courtesy Dr. T. N. Ly, Montréal, QC.)

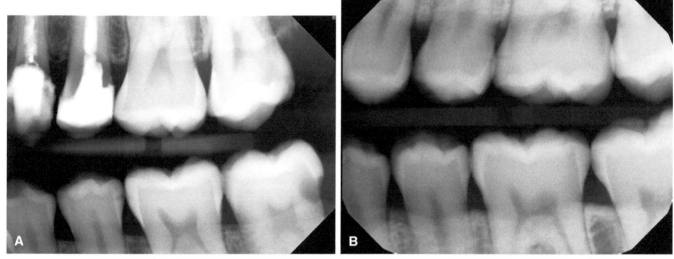

Fig. 19.7 (A) Bitewing image showing a carious lesion with a band-like appearance on the distal surface of the mandibular left second premolar. (B) Bitewing image showing a carious lesion with a rectangular shape on the mesial surface of the mandibular left second molar. Multiple other interproximal carious lesions are visible. ([B] Courtesy Dr. T. N. Ly, Montréal, QC.)

content, creating a triangle with a wider base than in the enamel. The caries lesion then progresses through the dentinal tubules toward the pulp chamber. Compared with enamel demineralization, once a dentinal lesion has reached a certain size, it may lose its triangular shape, especially if cavitation has occurred.

Interproximal carious lesions are most commonly found in a region that extends between the contact points of teeth apically to near the free gingival margin. The inferiormost point of this area may be most relevant in patients with periodontal bone loss (Fig. 19.8). The localization of caries in this very defined region of the tooth is of great help in differentiating caries from a common artifact of intraoral imaging: cervical burnout. There is a higher risk of caries on an interproximal surface that is in contact with either a carious lesion or a restoration. Special attention must therefore be given to the investigation of these seemingly intact surfaces.

Because of the buccal/lingual thickness of the proximal surfaces of posterior teeth, a small amount of demineralization in the middle of

the proximal surface may not be visible radiographically. There must be demineralization of approximately 35% of the enamel before these lesions can be observed on an image. This is one of the reasons why the true depth of a lesion (verified histologically) is most often greater than what can be seen on an image. Other studies have also shown that operator experience plays an important role in this diagnosis.

False-Positive Interpretations

Every published study on this subject has shown that there is not 100% agreement on caries diagnosis between different observers. This is especially true with enamel caries but can also sometimes occur with dentin caries. As mentioned earlier, the experience of the observer also plays a pivotal role in the interpretation process. When a carious lesion is thought to be detected on an image but the tooth structure is in fact intact, it is called a false-positive finding. Although this can be caused by a variation in the morphology of the tooth, the most common source of error is the misinterpretation of cervical burnout as dental caries.

Cervical burnout produces an artifact that mimics a carious lesion near the cementoenamel junction (CEJ) area of the tooth. As the x-ray beam meets the convex proximal surface of the tooth, those x-ray photons that pass almost tangentially through the tooth surface "see" less tooth structure than those photons that pass deeper through the tooth. This area of convexity is commonly located apical to the CEJ, near the normal height of the alveolar crest. The thinner tooth structure here absorbs fewer x-rays; consequently the area appears relatively more radiolucent on an image. Cervical burnout can also be seen in multirooted teeth when roots that are more buccally positioned do not overlap perfectly with a lingual or palatal root in a mesiodistal direction (Fig. 19.9). The presence of a shallow furcation on either the mesial or distal surface of the tooth can make the area appear more radiolucent. However, the presence of two overlapping roots can be confirmed by identifying the periodontal ligament spaces of each root.

The presence of demineralization that cannot be seen (or cannot yet be seen) is called a false-negative finding. Lack of training or experience is often the cause of this error, but it can be made worse when the images used do not provide an accurate representation of the proximal surfaces of a tooth. The most common technical error in this instance is overlap between the proximal surfaces of adjacent teeth. However, this can easily be corrected by modifying the position of the sensor or the horizontal angulation of the x-ray beam (see Fig. 19.2).

Staging and Cavitation

Multiple classification or scoring systems have been used over the years to categorize caries size and depth. One of the most recent is the International Caries Classification and Management System (ICCMS). This system separates caries progression into four stages: sound (0), initial (RA), moderate (RB), and extensive (RC) enamel and subcategories therein. In the initial stage (RA), demineralization is scored as appearing as a radiolucency within the outer half of the enamel (RA1), the inner half of the enamel without or with involvement of the DEJ (RA2) and the outer third of the dentin (RA3). The moderate stage (RB) is scored as a radiolucency reaching the middle third of the dentin (RB4). Finally, when the radiolucency reaches the inner third of the dentin or the pulp, it is scored as RC5 and RC6, respectively (Fig. 19.10). A study has shown that on average 32% of carious lesions extending into the outer third of the dentin also present with clinical cavitation. This value climbs to 72% for lesions in the middle third of the dentin or deeper. The ability to identify or at least suspect cavitation is important, because once this occurs, the bacteria in the lesion will maintain the activity of the carious lesion unless it is managed surgically.

When there are no metallic restorations in the vicinity, some reports have maintained that a cone beam computed tomography (CBCT) examination (see Chapter 11) will be extremely accurate in determining both the depth and cavitation status of a proximal surface. However, the use of CBCT for this sole purpose is not only discouraged but not evidence based. Moreover, the higher radiation dose imparted by this examination should prohibit its use for this purpose. When a CBCT is obtained for another reason, the entire volume should be evaluated for other anomalies and pathologies, including caries (Fig. 19.11).

Treatment Considerations

The decision to treat a carious lesion surgically is based on several factors. The dentist must take into account the caries risk status of the patient, the depth of the lesion, and whether there is cavitation. Generally speaking, conservative interventions like oral hygiene instruction and topical fluoride application can be put in place for caries in the ICCMS RA categories (enamel or outer third of the dentin), whereas surgical

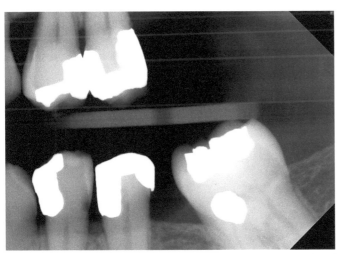

Fig. 19.8 Bitewing image of a patient with moderate horizontal periodontal bone loss and a carious lesion with an epicenter at the CEJ on the distal surface of the mandibular left first premolar.

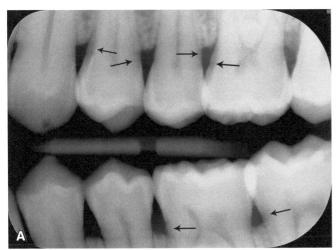
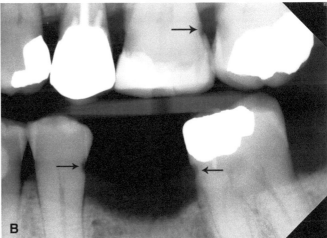

Fig. 19.9 (A) Bitewing image showing cervical burnout *(arrows)*, which can mimic a carious lesion. (B) Bitewing image with carious lesions *(arrows)*, which, compared with burnout, demonstrate an irregular border and a discontinuity of the tooth surface; they are often present in patients with periodontal bone loss.

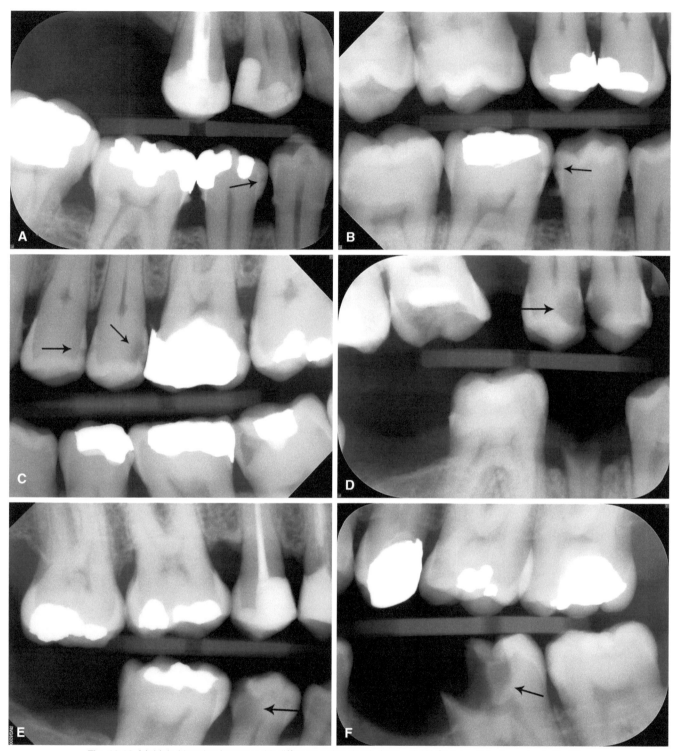

Fig. 19.10 Multiple bitewing images with different caries depth *(arrows)*. (A) Caries within the outer half of the enamel (RA1). (B) Caries within the inner half of the enamel (RA2). (C) Caries within the outer third of the dentin (RA3). (D) Caries within the middle third of the dentin (RB4). (E) Caries within the inner third of the dentin (RC5). (F) Caries in contact with the pulp (RC6).

management is needed when there is cavitation or the carious lesion has reached the middle third of the dentin (RB). The differences in management strategies between patients will mostly be based on caries risk status; a patient with a higher risk for caries would benefit from a more proactive approach versus a patient with a low risk for caries (see Table 19.1). When the decision is made not to manage a carious lesion

surgically, a follow-up imaging schedule should be put into place to monitor the carious lesion. The follow-up period should be based on the patient's risk for caries. Ideally, when new images are made, they should be as similar as possible to the originals so that any comparison will be as accurate as possible. The follow-up image can be compared with the original image to see if the lesion has grown (active) or not (arrested). If the lesion has progressed, the decision regarding surgical treatment may be revised.

Occlusal Surfaces
Typical Appearance
Caries can occur on the occlusal surfaces of premolar and molar teeth, most often in children and adolescents. Development and penetration of the enamel and dentin occurs in a similar way as it does on proximal surfaces. The difference lies in the radiographic appearance of occlusal caries. It is nearly impossible to detect occlusal caries limited to the enamel in a radiograph. The enamel is simply too thick for a carious lesion to be detectable. Once the lesion reaches the dentin, instead of creating a triangular shape, it will create a more semicircular shape, with the broad base of the semicircle at the DEJ.

Compared with proximal caries, clinical detection of occlusal caries is often more reliable, in particular for identifying small carious lesions. Clinically, new lesions may appear chalky white, whereas older lesions, possibly inactive, will have a darker coloration (brown or black). Once there is suspicion of occlusal caries, an image should be obtained to assess the depth of the lesion.

False-Positive Interpretations
Occlusal lesions can easily be missed, particularly those small caries that are limited to the enamel. Since these lesions are located at the bottom of occlusal pits and fissures, there is often a superposition from the surrounding sound enamel, which leads to these false-negative results. This is one of the reasons why a clinical examination is vital to detect occlusal caries. Multiple studies have shown that a clinical examination is more accurate than a radiograph in detecting these small lesions.

In the same way that a caries lesion progresses through proximal enamel, occlusal caries penetrating enamel will spread along the DEJ first, before entering the dentin proper. Within dentin, the caries lesion will often take on a circular shape, centered on the occlusal pit (Fig. 19.12). With occlusal caries, the dentist may see a radiolucent line along the DEJ; this can be confused with wider spreading of the carious lesion. Although this appearance can also be seen with proximal surface caries, it is often more pronounced in this location. This artifact, which is caused by the differential contrast between the more radiopaque

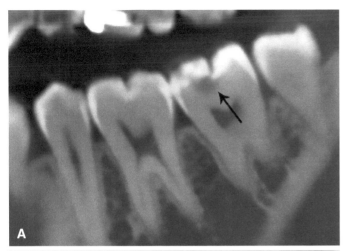
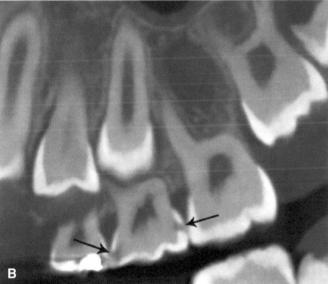

Fig. 19.11 Cone beam computed tomography images revealing carious lesions *(arrows)*. (A) A carious lesion on the occlusal surface of the second molar. (B) Carious lesions on both interproximal surfaces of the deciduous second molar.

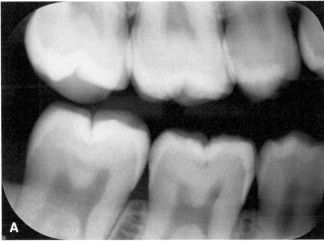
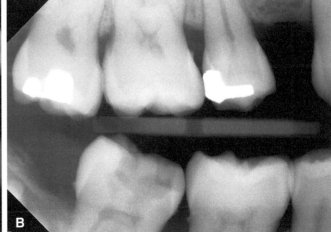

Fig. 19.12 Bitewing images with the classical appearance of occlusal caries; a small radiolucency is centered on an occlusal pit on both mandibular molars (A). If left untreated, these could cavitate and grow larger (B).

enamel and the less radiopaque dentin, is called the *Mach-band effect* (Fig. 19.13). First described by Ernst Mach in 1865, this visual and perceptual artifact arises as a result of the differential stimulation and inhibition of neighboring receptors in the retina. When a set of retinal receptors in the eye is "overstimulated" by the perception of the very radiopaque density of enamel, adjacent receptors that perceive the more radiolucent dentin are inhibited. The result of this differential response of retinal receptors results in the perception of a radiolucent band that runs in the superficial dentin just adjacent to the DEJ. To overcome the Mach-band effect, the dentist can mask the more radiopaque enamel; then the Mach band should disappear if caries are not present. If, however, the Mach band does not disappear, its presence indicates caries involvement of the DEJ. When a lesion is perceived in this way and is visible only on the image and there is no clinical evidence of disease, it would be reasonable to observe and monitor the area so as to avoid unnecessary treatment.

Cavitation and Treatment Considerations

As the occlusal lesion spreads to involve more dentin, there may not be enough dentin remaining to support masticatory forces; this may

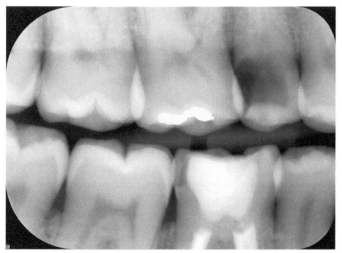

Fig. 19.13 A radiolucent line is visible at the occlusal dentin-enamel junction. This is caused by the contrast difference between the two tissues and is called the Mach band.

lead to cavitation of the surface. When that happens, it becomes easy to identify the carious lesion clinically. Even in these instances, it is still important to obtain images of the tooth—possibly both a bitewing image to assess the depth and a periapical image to assess the apical region (Fig. 19.14). This will allow the dentist to know beforehand the approximate depth of the carious lesion and if the pulp chamber may be involved.

If discoloration is noted in a fissure without cavitation, a bitewing image may be needed to evaluate the possibility of caries and the depth of the lesion. Even without clinical cavitation, occlusal caries reaching into the dentin will most likely require operative treatment.

Buccal and Lingual Surfaces

Caries arising on the buccal and lingual surfaces of the teeth can occur in the pits and fissures of these surfaces or on the smooth surfaces near the gingiva. In viewing these lesions on a single image, it is impossible to localize the lesion as being on the buccal or lingual surface. A second image incorporating a different horizontal angulation can be made to help make this determination (see the tube-shift technique or the buccal object rule in Chapter 6). Caries developing in these areas usually have a circular or oval shape and are well defined. Furthermore, the surrounding tooth structure is intact (Fig. 19.15). When a buccal or lingual carious lesion is near the occlusal surface, it can be confused with an occlusal lesion due to image superimposition. However, occlusal lesions are usually more extensive, are not as well defined, and will present a radiolucent line in the occlusal enamel. In either case, a clinical examination will confirm the diagnosis.

Root Surfaces

Caries involving the roots can be detected in patients with gingival recession or periodontal bone loss. The cementum is softer and thinner than the enamel (approximately 20 to 50 μm near the CEJ), causing the caries to progress more rapidly. The difficulty with a root caries lesion is to differentiate it from cervical burnout (see Fig. 19.9). Some radiographic signs can prove helpful to the practitioner. First, when there is no bone loss around a tooth, it is very likely that the radiolucency at the edge of the root is simply cervical burnout. Furthermore, with caries, clinical examination would demonstrate an irregularity or a depression. With cervical burnout, the root surface would be intact. Finally, the shape of the radiolucency from burnout can often be explained by the anatomy of the tooth (see Fig. 19.9A). Fortunately most root lesions

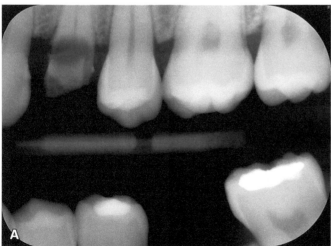
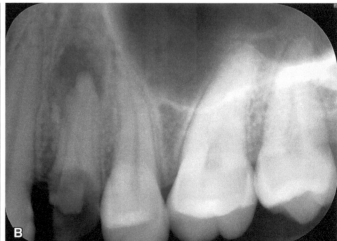

Fig. 19.14 (A) Near-complete coronal destruction from caries on the maxillary left first premolar. Once a lesion is large enough that it reaches or is near the pulp, a periapical image should be obtained to evaluate the apical region for an inflammatory lesion (osteitis), which is the case here (B).

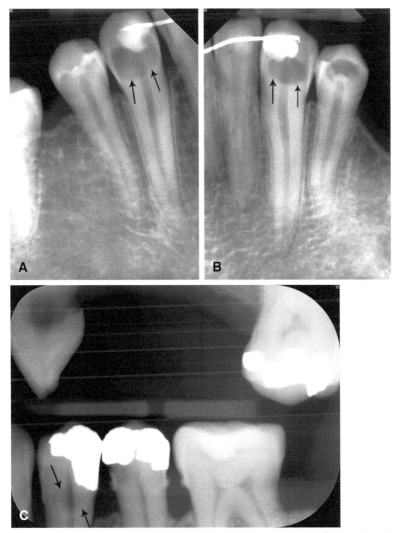

Fig. 19.15 (A–C) Buccal caries *(arrows)* usually have a circular shape, are well defined, and are in the cervical area.

can and should be detected clinically, whether they are buccal, lingual, or interproximal.

Rampant Caries

Rampant caries is the term used to describe rapid progression with severe and widespread involvement. This is most often seen in young children who have poor oral hygiene habits coupled with poor dietary habits (e.g., going to sleep with a bottle of milk or juice) (Fig. 19.16). Indeed, the increased availability of fluoride in drinking water and the use of topical fluoride delivery systems have helped to control the development of caries in these patients. Multiple carious lesions can also be seen in adult patients with xerostomia. This is often seen following radiotherapy for head and neck cancers. Imaging examinations of these patients can demonstrate advanced, generalized caries, involving smooth surfaces and teeth that usually do not present carious lesions (Fig. 19.17). These lesions, often referred to as "radiation caries," are mostly smooth-surface caries located near the cervical areas of the teeth. Impeccable hygiene along with topical fluoride and saliva substitutes can help negate the effects of the xerostomia and limit the impact on the teeth.

Associated With Dental Restorations

Some carious lesions will develop at the margin of an existing restoration. These are called recurrent (or secondary) caries and represent

new demineralization (Fig. 19.18). These new carious lesions can be caused by either a defective restoration and/or ineffective dental hygiene. Such lesions will appear as radiolucencies in the tooth structure at the junction between the restoration and the tooth. Another type of carious lesion associated with a restoration is called residual caries. These are different from recurrent caries in the sense that residual caries represent areas of demineralization that remain when the original lesion is incompletely removed. Although this can be involuntary, most often it can be purposeful when a large carious lesion encroaches on the pulp. A temporary restoration is put in place that can stimulate the development of tertiary dentin (indirect pulp capping). A few months later, the remainder of the carious lesion is removed and a final restoration can be placed.

One of the difficulties in detecting interproximal recurrent caries is to obtain an image that shows the radiolucency. Unfortunately, if the image obtained has been made at an improper vertical angulation, the restoration can hide the recurrent carious lesion. Therefore it is vital to examine the area thoroughly and to obtain high-quality images where the x-ray beam is optimally oriented to allow visualization of the interface between the tooth and the restoration. This is best obtained with a bitewing image (see Figs. 19.2 and 19.19). When in doubt, a second image with a different angulation can be acquired.

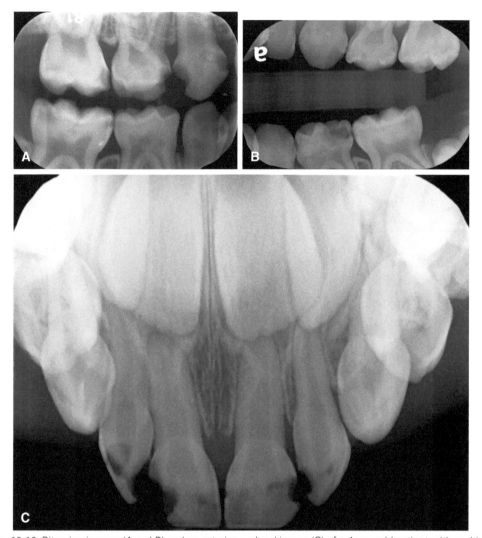

Fig. 19.16 Bitewing images (A and B) and an anterior occlusal image (C) of a 4-year-old patient with multiple carious lesions (rampant caries). (Courtesy Dr. C. Quach, Montréal, QC.)

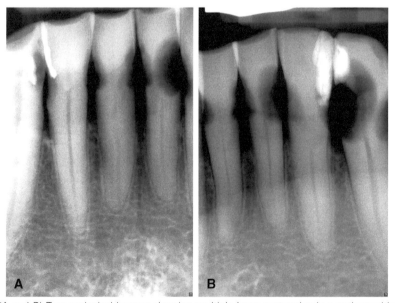

Fig. 19.17 (A and B) Two periapical images showing multiple large root caries in a patient with xerostomia following radiation therapy of the head and neck.

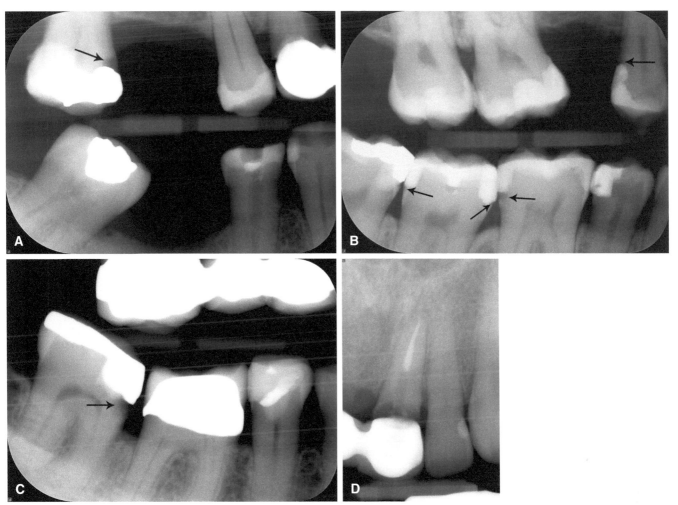

Fig. 19.18 (A) Bitewing image showing a recurrent carious lesion on the mesial surface of the maxillary right second molar *(arrow)*. (B) Bitewing image revealing multiple recurrent caries *(arrows)*. (C) Bitewing image showing a recurrent caries on the mesial surface of the mandibular right second molar *(arrow)*. (D) Anterior periapical image showing a large recurrent carious lesion on this central incisor supporting a bridge.

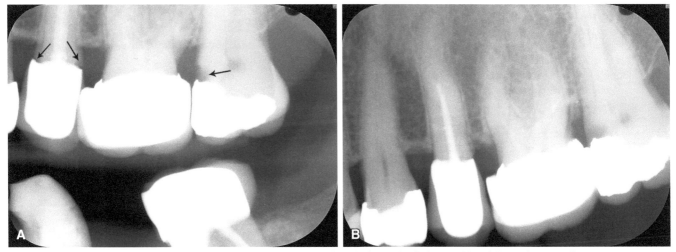

Fig. 19.19 (A) Bitewing image showing recurrent carious lesion on both the mesial and distal of the maxillary left second premolar and on the mesial of the second molar *(arrows)*. (B) Periapical image of the same region where the carious lesions around the premolar are not visible because of the increased vertical angulation. The carious lesion on the second molar is still visible, but it is not as well defined as on the bitewing.

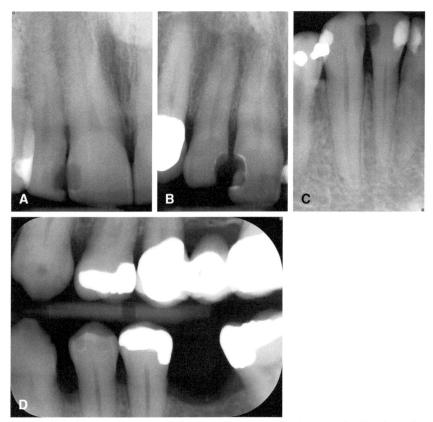

Fig. 19.20 (A) Periapical image showing radiolucent restorations placed on the distal surface of the central incisor and mesial surface of the lateral incisor. They have a well-defined shape compared with a carious lesion. (B) Periapical image showing radiolucent restorations with a radiopaque liner placed beneath the composite. This helps to confirm the diagnosis and rule out caries. (C) Periapical image with radiolucent restorations, again with a radiopaque liner on the distal surface of the lateral incisor and mesial surface of the canine. (D) Bitewing image showing two occlusal radiolucent restorations with radiopaque liner on the mandibular left first premolar. These restorations are not common on posterior teeth.

Some materials used in operative dentistry have a radiolucent appearance and may be confused with recurrent or residual caries. These materials are usually used as a base placed beneath a restoration. The shape of the radiolucency can help the dentist differentiate between a radiolucent dental material and residual caries. The clinical history of the operative procedure should also confirm this. Since liner and base materials should not extend to the periphery of a restoration (i.e., the cavity-surface margin), they should not be confused with recurrent caries. Other types of restorative materials, including older composite materials, can also mimic carious lesions. These materials were often used for interproximal restorations in the anterior maxilla and can be differentiated from caries because of their well-defined borders, their shapes, and sometimes the radiopaque base or liner at their periphery (Fig. 19.20).

ALTERNATIVE DIAGNOSTIC TOOLS TO DETECT DENTAL CARIES

Besides imaging, other methods have been developed to identify carious lesions. These have included light-induced fluorescence, lasers, transillumination and electrical conductance. The light-induced fluorescence systems can be used to identify demineralization on smooth surfaces. The other systems are more commonly used on occlusal and interproximal surfaces. Such systems work by giving the dentist a number or value indicating the presence or absence of demineralization. Some of these systems may, however, have difficulty identifying carious lesions beneath and around dental restorations. For the time being, they should be used to complement imaging examinations.

TREATMENT CONSIDERATIONS

The decision to treat or not to treat a carious lesion depends on a multitude of factors, including the patient's oral hygiene, his or her dental history, caries risk factors, and the depth and number of carious lesions. Demineralization limited to the enamel often does not require operative treatment. Rather, these lesions should be addressed noninvasively with topical fluoride application, better oral hygiene, and by reducing the frequency and amount of sugar intake. Furthermore, such lesions should be followed up to confirm that they have arrested. This is also true when a lesion has just reached the dentin. In these cases operative treatment may or may not be needed. When a carious lesion involves the deeper dentin or causes cavitation, it must be mechanically removed and a put in its place.

BIBLIOGRAPHY

Abesi F, Mirshekar A, Moudi E, et al. Diagnostic accuracy of digital and conventional imagery in the detection of non-cavitated approximal dental caries. *Iran J Radiol.* 2012;9(1):17–21.

American Dental Association Council on Scientific Affairs, US Food and Drug Administration. Dental imaging examinations: Recommendations for patient selection and limiting radiation exposure. Revised 2012. http://www.ada.org/sections/professionalResources/pdfs/Dental_Imageic_Examinations_2012.pdf.

Atchison KA, White SC, Flack VF, et al. Assessing the FDA guidelines for ordering dental images. *J Am Dent Assoc.* 1995;126(10):1372–1383.

Bahrami G, Hagstrøm C, Wenzel A. Bitewing examination with four digital receptors. *Dentomaxillofac Radiol.* 2003;32(5):317–321.

Berry HM Jr. Cervical burnout and Mach band: two shadows of doubt in radiologic interpretation of carious lesions. *J Am Dent Assoc.* 1983;106(5):622–625.

Haiter-Neto F, Wenzel A, Gotfredsen E. Diagnostic accuracy of cone beam computed tomography scans compared with intraoral image modalities for detection of caries lesions. *Dentomaxillofac Radiol.* 2008;37(1):18–22.

Hilton TJ, Ferracane JL, Broome JC. Caries management: diagnosis and treatment strategies. In: *Summit's Fundamentals of Operative Dentistry: A Contemporary Approach.* Hanover Park: Quintessence; 2013:93–130.

Kamburoglu K, Kolsuz E, Murat S, et al. Proximal caries detection accuracy using intraoral bitewing image, extraoral bitewing imagery and panoramic imagery. *Dentomaxillofac Radiol.* 2012;41(6):450–459.

Nanci A. Dentin-pulp complex and repair and regeneration of oral tissues. In: *Ten Cate's Oral Histology: Development, Structure, and Function.* St. Louis: Mosby Elsevier; 2013:165–204, 337–354.

NIH Consensus Development Conference on Diagnosis and Management of Dental Caries Throughout Life. Bethesda, MD, March 26–28, 2001. Conference papers. *J Dent Educ.* 2001;65(10):935–1179.

Pitts NB, Ismail AI, Martignon S, et al. ICCMS guide for practitioners and educators, ICCMS implementation workshop; 2014.

Selwitz RH, Ismail AI, Pitts NB. Dental caries. *Lancet.* 2007;369(9555):51–59.

SUGGESTED READINGS

Caries Detection

Abdinian M, Razavi SM, Faghihian R, et al. Accuracy of digital bitewing imagery versus different view of digital panoramic imagery for detection of proximal caries. *J Dent Tehran UMS.* 2015;12(4):290–297.

Akdeniz BG, Grondahl HG, Magnusson B. Accuracy of proximal caries depth measurements: comparison between limited cone beam computed tomography, storage phosphor and film imagery. *Caries Res.* 2006;40(3):202–207.

Hellén-Halme K, Petersson A, Nilsson M. Effect of ambient light and monitor brightness and contrast settings on the detection of approximal caries in digital images: an in vitro study. *Dentomaxillofac Radiol.* 2008;37(7):380–384.

Hintze H, Wenzel A, Danielsen B. Behaviour of approximal carious lesions assessed by clinical examination after tooth separation and imagery: a 2.5-year longitudinal study in young adults. *Caries Res.* 1999;33(6):415–422.

Isidor S, Faaborg-Andersen M, Hintze H, et al. Effect of monitor display on detection of approximal caries lesions in digital images. *Dentomaxillofac Radiol.* 2009;38(8):537–541.

Jacobsen JH, Hansen B, Wenzel A, et al. Relationship between histological and imageic caries lesion depth measured in images from four digital imagery systems. *Caries Res.* 2004;38(1):34–38.

Jørgensen PM, Wenzel A. Patient discomfort in bitewing examination with film and four digital receptors. *Dentomaxillofac Radiol.* 2012;41(4):323–327.

Mejáre I. Bitewing examination to detect caries in children and adolescents—when and how often? *Dent Update.* 2005;32(10):588–590, 593–594, 596–597.

Mejáre I, Stenlund H, Zelezny-Holmlund C. Caries incidence and lesions progression from adolescence to young adulthood: a prospective 15-year cohort study in Sweden. *Caries Res.* 2004;38(2):130–141.

Mjör IA, Toffenetti F. Secondary caries: a literature review with case reports. *Quintessence Int.* 2000;31(3):165–179.

Poorterman JHG, Weerheijm KL, Groen HJ, et al. Clinical and imageic judgement of occlusal caries in adolescents. *Eur J Oral Sci.* 2000;108(2):93–98.

Qvist V, Johannesen L, Bruun M. Progression of approximal caries in relation to iatrogenic preparation damage. *J Dent Res.* 1992;71(7):1370–1373.

Ratledge DK, Kidd EA, Beighton D. A clinical and microbiological study of approximal carious lesions, 1: the relationship between cavitation, imageic lesion depth, the site specific gingival index and the level of infection of the dentine. *Caries Res.* 2001;35(1):3–7.

Simon JC, Lucas S, Lee R, et al. Near-infrared imaging of secondary caries lesions around composite restorations at wavelengths from 1300-1700 nm. *Dent Mater.* 2016;32(4):587–595.

Wenzel A. A review of dentists' use of digital imagery and caries diagnosis with digital systems. *Dentomaxillofac Radiol.* 2006;35(5):307–314.

Wenzel A, Anthonisen PN, Juul MB. Reproducibility in the assessment of caries lesion behaviour: a comparison between conventional film and subtraction imagery. *Caries Res.* 2000;34(3):214–218.

Wenzel A, Haiter-Neto F, Gotfredsen E. Risk factors for a false positive test outcome in diagnosis of caries in approximal surfaces: impact of imageic modality and observer characteristics. *Caries Res.* 2007;41(3):170–176.

Wenzel A, Hirsch E, Christensen JH, et al. Detection of cavitated approximal surfaces using cone beam CT and intraoral receptors. *Dentomaxillofac Radiol.* 2013;42(1):39458105.

Young SM, Lee JT, Hodges RJ, et al. A comparative study of high-resolution cone beam computed tomography and charge-coupled device sensors for detecting caries. *Dentomaxillofac Radiol.* 2009;38(7):445–451.

Treatment Decision

Bader JD, Shugars DA. The evidence supporting alternative management strategies for early occlusal caries and suspected occlusal dentinal caries. *J Evid Based Dent Pract.* 2006;6(1):91–100.

Bjørndal L, Kidd EA. The treatment of deep dentine caries lesions. *Dent Update.* 2005;32(7):402–404, 407–410, 413.

Evans RW, Pakdaman A, Dennison PJ, et al. The caries management system: an evidence-based preventive strategy for dental practitioners. Application for adults. *Aust Dent J.* 2008;53(1):83–92.

Evans RW, Dennison PJ. The caries management system: an evidence-based preventive strategy for dental practitioners. Application for children and adolescents. *Aust Dent J.* 2009;54(4):381–389.

Gordan VV, Garvan CW, Heft MW, et al. Restorative treatment thresholds for interproximal primary caries based on imageic images: findings from the dental practice-based research network. *Gen Dent.* 2009;57(6):654–663.

Kakudate N, Sumida F, Matsumoto Y, et al. Restorative treatment thresholds for proximal caries in dental PBRN. *J Dent Res.* 2012;91(12):1202–1208.

Pitts NB. Are we ready to move from operative to non-operative/preventive treatment of dental caries in clinical practice? *Caries Res.* 2004;38(3):294–304.

Ricketts DN, Kidd EA, Innés N, et al. Complete or ultraconservative removal of decayed tissue in unfilled teeth. *Cochrane Database Syst Rev.* 2006;(3):CD003808.

20

Periodontal Diseases

Susanne E. Perschbacher

The periodontium supports the teeth in the jaws, and is composed of the gingiva, the periodontal ligament (PDL), cementum, and the alveolar processes of the jawbones. The periodontal diseases are a heterogeneous collection of conditions affecting these structures and are characterized by an inflammatory host response in the periodontal tissues that may lead to localized or generalized alterations in the supporting bone and soft tissues around the teeth. Left untreated, these changes may ultimately result in the loss of teeth.

In recent years, the health burden of the periodontal diseases has been increasing in the population, particularly among those in lower socioeconomic groups. The reported prevalence of periodontal disease in the U.S. population can vary between studies, and depends on the method of assessment and the threshold used. For example, when the criteria of clinical attachment loss measuring greater than 4 mm is used, the prevalence is about 23%. A recent large-scale study in the United States found that 46% of adults over the age of 30 years had periodontitis. In this study, periodontitis was defined by both clinical attachment loss (3 mm or greater) and periodontal probing depths (4 mm or greater). The identification, management, and follow-up of the periodontal diseases are an important responsibility of dental professionals, and imaging plays an important role in the successful diagnosis, treatment planning, and monitoring of these conditions.

DISEASE MECHANISM

Dental plaque biofilm plays a primary role in the initiation of the periodontal diseases. Periodontal disease-implicated bacteria, predominantly gram-negative rods and spirochetes, colonize the tooth and root surfaces between the root and the gingival margin, and in some cases invade the surrounding tissue. While these bacteria can directly damage host tissues through the release of toxins, more significantly, they may also indirectly stimulate a host inflammatory reaction. The release of inflammatory mediators as part of this response is responsible for much of the damage to the surrounding soft tissues and stimulation of osteoclastic bone resorption. Furthermore, the inflammatory response causes loss of and apical migration of the junctional epithelium, and this in turn leads to the development of periodontal pocket formation, which further facilitates bacterial colonization.

Periodontal disease often progresses in bursts, with manifestations of the process being mild or slight, moderate, or severe. As with all inflammatory processes, there are cyclic periods of active inflammation and tissue destruction, followed by times of quiescence with no appreciable changes. The relative duration of the destructive and quiescent phases depends on the form of periodontal disease, the nature of the bacterial pathogens, and the host response. Oral hygiene practices disrupt local dental plaque biofilm, and they are a primary factor determining the development and progression of periodontal disease. The onset of disease and its progression may be modified by systemic factors that alter the host immune response, and may include age, stress, smoking, or systemic disease. Hormonal changes that arise during puberty, pregnancy, and menopause may also contribute to the onset and progression of periodontal disease. Greater rates of periodontal disease are also seen in lower socioeconomic populations, and those in whom dental care is neglected.

The clinical indicators of the periodontal diseases reflect the host tissue response to oral bacterial biofilm, and these are manifest as signs of inflammation. Inflammation of the gingival tissues, gingivitis, is seen as gingival swelling, edema, and erythema. Progression to periodontitis is manifested with progressive clinical attachment and bone loss that is characterized by pocket formation and/or gingival recession. Other clinical signs include bleeding on probing, purulent exudates, and tooth mobility. The disease usually is painless, and most patients are unaware of its presence until tooth mobility becomes advanced and there is tooth loss.

ASSESSMENT OF PERIODONTAL DISEASE

Contributions of Diagnostic Imaging

In the diagnosis of the periodontal diseases, the clinical and radiologic examinations are complementary. In the assessment of the periodontal status of a patient, the clinical examination is completed first in order to determine what further testing, including acquisition of diagnostic images, is required.

The clinical examination may include taking the gingival index, performing periodontal probing, identifying bleeding sites, measuring gingival recession, determining clinical attachment loss, tooth mobility, and evaluating of the amount of attached gingiva. Radiologic images are an adjunct to this examination, and the prescription of imaging is indicated when the clinical examination suggests periodontitis.

Once it has been determined that the further investigation is warranted with diagnostic imaging, such images may contribute important information about the status of the periodontium which cannot be derived from the clinical examination. Images also provide a permanent record of the condition of the bone at any point in the course of the disease. Diagnostic images aid the clinician in identifying the extent of destruction of the alveolar processes, local predisposing factors, and features of the periodontium that may influence prognosis. Radiologic images also help the dentist assess the clinical crown-to-root ratio, a factor that can influence the prognosis of the tooth and any planned prosthesis. A summary of important radiologic features related to periodontal status that may be identified in diagnostic images are listed in Box 20.1.

BOX 20.1 Radiographic Assessment of Periodontal Conditions

Radiographs are especially helpful in the evaluation of the following features:

- Amount of bone present
- Condition of the alveolar crests
- Bone loss in the furcation areas
- Width of the periodontal ligament space
- Local irritating factors that increase the risk of periodontal disease
- Calculus
- Poorly contoured or overextended restorations
- Root length and morphology and crown-to-root ratio
- Open interproximal contacts, which may be sites for food impaction
- Anatomic considerations
- Position of the maxillary sinus in relation to a periodontal deformity
- Missing, supernumerary, impacted, and tipped teeth
- Pathologic considerations
- Caries
- Periapical lesions
- Root resorption

In summary, a complete diagnosis of periodontal disease requires a thorough clinical examination of the patient, combined with evidence identified on diagnostic images.

The dentist must also determine the optimal frequency of imaging examinations for patients being managed for periodontal disease. The extent of continued disease activity, which can be determined clinically, should dictate the frequency of subsequent imaging examinations.

IMAGING MODALITIES FOR THE ASSESSMENT OF PERIODONTAL DISEASE

Intraoral Imaging

Intraoral images provide the highest spatial resolution of any imaging modality, which allows the dentist to detect fine details of the periodontium. Image detail is essential since the structures being assessed are often submillimeter in size, and many of the radiologic signs of periodontal disease are subtle, including early loss of bone, and changes to the PDL space and lamina dura. Intraoral imaging modalities used for the assessment of periodontal disease include bitewing (interproximal) and periapical images.

Bitewing images should be considered the primary imaging choice for characterizing the periodontal diseases. These images most accurately depict the distance between the cementoenamel junction (CEJ) and the crest of the interradicular alveolar process because the incident x-ray beam is oriented at almost right angles to the long axes of the teeth. Periapical images have the benefit of demonstrating the full length of the tooth, which allows for the evaluation of the percentage of root affected by bone loss. However, periapical images may provide a distorted view of the relationship between the teeth and the location of the alveolar crest because of greater variations in the obliquity of the primary x-ray beam. This occurs most commonly in the maxilla because of anatomical limitations placed on receptor positioning by the height of the palatal vault. In such circumstances, the level of the buccal alveolar crest may be projected near or above the level of the palatal CEJ, making the bone height appear greater than it actually is.

The usefulness of intraoral images in the evaluation of the periodontal diseases can be optimized by making images of high technical quality. The technique for obtaining bitewing and periapical images is covered in greater detail in the chapters on projection geometry and intraoral projections (see Chapters 6 and 7), but the features that are particularly important for imaging the relationship between the teeth and the alveolar processes are emphasized here. The plane of the image receptor should be placed parallel to the long axis of the tooth or tooth row, or as near to this ideal position as the anatomical limitations of the mouth permit. The x-ray beam is directed along an axis that is perpendicular to the long axis of the tooth and the plane of the image receptor; this orientation minimizes distortion of the images of the teeth and periodontal tissues. In doing this, the teeth are depicted in their correct positions relative to the alveolar process when there is (1) no overlapping of the interproximal contacts between the tooth crowns; (2) no overlapping of the roots of adjacent teeth; and (3) the buccal and lingual cusps of molars are superimposed over one another.

In patients with moderate to severe clinical attachment loss that has been identified on the clinical examination, standard (i.e., horizontal) bitewing images may not depict the alveolar crest because of the extent of bone loss. In this instance, the dentist must decide before the images are made, to reorient the receptor 90 degrees so that a vertical bitewing image can be made. The vertical bitewing method uses the same American National Standards Institute (ANSI) size 2 image receptors, but oriented in such a way that the long axis of the receptor is in a vertical orientation. Although the image geometry is unchanged compared with the standard horizontal method, the additional receptor area made available by reorienting it allows the dentist to visualize the alveolar process when there has been significant clinical attachment loss (Fig. 20.1).

Limitations of Intraoral Images

Intraoral bitewing and periapical images may not, however, provide a complete representation of the status of the periodontium because of the limitations inherent to these techniques. First, bitewing and periapical images are two-dimensional representations of three-dimensional anatomic structures. Because the image cannot reveal the three-dimensional nature of this anatomy, interproximal bony defects may not be effectively visualized, as the buccal and/or lingual walls may superimpose themselves over the defect itself or the other wall. In addition, in some cases, overlapping tooth structure may superimpose over the interproximal bone, masking it from being clearly seen. However, the subtle decrease in the apparent density of the root structure (i.e., where the root may appear more radiolucent) may indicate bone loss on the buccal or lingual surface of the root. Making use of multiple images acquired at different angulations (e.g., in a full-mouth series) may allow the dentist to use the buccal object rule to obtain three-dimensional information. As an example of this, two intraoral images made in adjacent locations may allow the dentist to determine whether a cortical plate has been lost on the buccal or lingual surface of the tooth root. Second, intraoral images typically show less severe bone loss than is actually present. The earliest (Stage I) destructive lesions in bone do not cause a sufficient change to be detectable. Third, intraoral images do not demonstrate soft tissue-to-hard tissue relationships, and thus provide no information about the depth of soft tissue pockets (which is why a complementary clinical examination is necessary). And, finally, bone level is often measured relative to the position of the CEJ; however, this reference point is not valid in situations where there is supraeruption of teeth, or where there is passive eruption in patients with severe attrition. For these reasons, although intraoral images play an invaluable role in the diagnosis and treatment planning of patients with periodontal disease, their use must be adjunctive to careful clinical examination.

Panoramic Imaging

The panoramic image has many features that are attractive for the dentist. Panoramic images are relatively quick and comfortable to acquire,

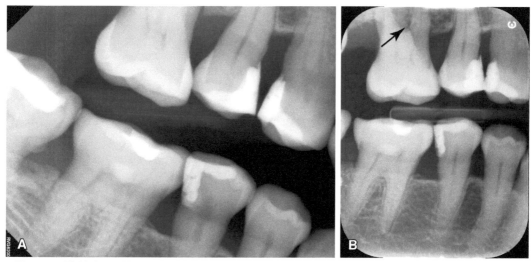

Fig. 20.1 (A) Horizontal bitewing projection, which does not demonstrate the periodontal bone levels at the distal surface of the maxillary first molar nor the mesial surface of the mandibular first premolar. (B) Vertical bitewing projection in the same site captures these surfaces as well as revealing furcation involvement of the first molar *(arrow)*.

and provide an overview of the teeth and jaws in a single image. However, panoramic images are inherently limited by the method in which they are produced. This extraoral imaging procedure creates images with superimpositions and distortions that do not arise in intraoral images, and their lower resolution relative to intraoral images makes detailed investigations difficult, particularly in the anterior areas of the jaws. Furthermore, the limitations that have already been discussed with regard to intraoral imaging are not overcome with panoramic images. And, finally, the acquisition of panoramic images can be technically challenging, resulting in additional patient positioning errors that only add to many compromises of this technique.

High-quality panoramic images can demonstrate changes to the periodontal structures, and some studies have shown that they can provide comparable diagnostic information to intraoral images. Some authors suggest that a panoramic image supplemented with selected intraoral images may be adequate for periodontal assessment. However, unless a panoramic system is already available or prescribed for another diagnostic query, the use of panoramic imaging as a primary imaging tool for characterizing periodontal disease is discouraged. The selection of imaging modalities must always be based on optimizing patient benefit for diagnosis, while minimizing risk. And, certainly, carefully selected intraoral images best achieve these goals.

Cone Beam Computed Tomography

Cone beam computed tomography (CBCT) has, as one powerful advantage, the ability to visualize the osseous supporting structures of the teeth from any angle, without anatomical superimpositions. This feature overcomes many of the limitations associated with intraoral and panoramic imaging techniques. CBCT imaging allows better visualization of some periodontal defects that are not well depicted on conventional two-dimensional images. For example, CBCT imaging may permit a more complete assessment of the architecture of complex vertical defects and craters, furcations, and buccal and lingual cortical plate loss (Fig. 20.2). In addition, anatomic features, such as root morphology or cortical fenestration, and coexistent periapical pathosis, which may be pertinent to diagnosis, treatment planning, and prognosis, may also be better visualized. The use of CBCT imaging can, however, be limited by imaging artifacts caused by metallic restorations, and these may obscure the details of the bony architecture being examined.

Compromised signal-to-noise ratios and low contrast resolution may also limit the visibility of lower density osseous structures on CBCT images present in some patients. Current evidence does not support the routine use of CBCT imaging for imaging of the periodontium because it does not offer a significant advantage over intraoral imaging techniques, particularly when the additional cost and radiation dose are considered. However, CBCT imaging, particularly small-volume and high-resolution systems, may be indicated in guiding the management of selected bony lesions, especially when surgery is being considered.

Special Techniques

Computer software and image processing techniques have been used to enhance images to achieve the improved detection of bone loss associated with periodontal disease. The most widely used of these techniques is digital subtraction radiography (see Chapter 4). The advantage of this method is that it allows better detection of small amounts of bone loss between images made at different times than can be achieved by visual inspection alone. However, image subtraction is difficult to use because the subtraction technique relies on making two images where the incident x-ray beam, the location of the bone and teeth on the image and image receptor are identical, which is difficult to accomplish in general practice. The more recent introduction of software programs that can correct for some discrepancies in positioning and alignment in sequential digital images makes subtraction techniques more forgiving. Nonetheless, this diagnostic technique remains primarily a research tool.

Another modality that is under development is called *tuned aperture computed tomography* (TACT). TACT can create image slices through the alveolar processes, and aims to allow better visualization of osseous defects, without an increase in dose over intraoral imaging. This technique is not yet commercially available.

APPEARANCE OF NORMAL ANATOMY

The appearance of the normal alveolar processes that supports the dentition has a characteristic appearance. A thin layer of radiopaque cortical bone often overlies the crest of the alveolar process, and the height of the crest lies at a level that is approximately 0.5 to 2.0 mm apical to the levels of the CEJs of adjacent teeth. Between posterior

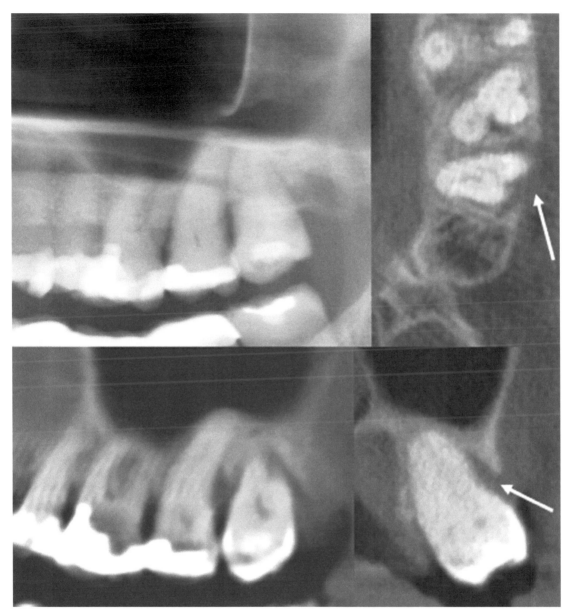

Fig. 20.2 Cropped panoramic image *(top left)* demonstrates moderate bone loss between the second and third molars. Axial *(top right)*, coronal *(bottom right)*, and parasagittal *(bottom left)* cone beam computed tomography images demonstrate the bone defects in this region more clearly. Periodontal bone loss around the buccal surface of the third molar is well visualized *(arrows)*, which could not be appreciated on the panoramic image.

teeth, the alveolar crest is oriented parallel to an imaginary line connecting adjacent CEJs (Fig. 20.3). In contrast, between anterior teeth, the alveolar crest is a point between the teeth that may have a well-defined cortex (Fig. 20.4). A well-mineralized cortical surface to the alveolar crest indicates the absence of periodontitis. However, a lack of a well-mineralized alveolar crest may be found in patients both without and with periodontitis.

The alveolar crest is continuous with the lamina dura of adjacent teeth. In the absence of disease, the junction between the alveolar crest and lamina dura of posterior teeth forms a sharp angle adjacent to the tooth root. The PDL space is a thin, even, radiolucent space that encircles the entire root surface that is located between the thin radiopaque lamina dura and the tooth root surface. The PDL space is often slightly wider around the cervical portions of tooth roots, particularly the premolar teeth, and in adolescents with erupting teeth. In this situation,

if the lamina dura still forms a sharp, well-defined angle with the alveolar crest, the condition should be considered a variant of normal and not an indication of disease. The buccal/lingual thickness of the alveolar crest varies widely, and it may be very thin coronally. This may appear in a two-dimensional image as an increase in bone radiolucency toward the crest. These sorts of variations in density alone are not an indication of disease. Rather, they may be a variation of normal.

IMAGING FEATURES OF PERIODONTAL DISEASES

Because gingivitis is an inflammatory condition confined to the gingiva, there are no changes to the underlying bone. Therefore the appearance of the bone in a diagnostic image is normal.

For all types of periodontal disease, the changes seen in diagnostic images reflect changes seen with any inflammatory condition of bone.

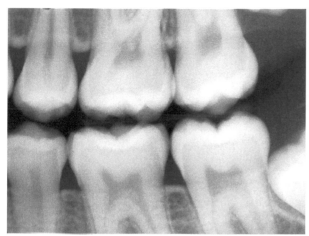

Fig. 20.3 The normal alveolar crest lies 0.5 to 2.0 mm apical to the adjacent cementoenamel junctions and forms a sharp angle with the lamina dura of the adjacent tooth. The crests may not always appear with a well-defined outer cortex.

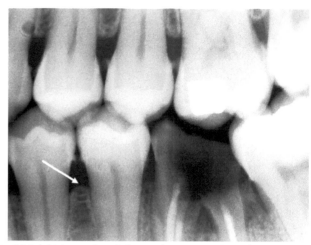

Fig. 20.5 Initial periodontal disease is seen as a loss of cortical density and a rounding of the junction between the alveolar crest and the lamina dura *(arrow)*. Note also the more pronounced bone loss around the mandibular first molar and the generalized interproximal calculus.

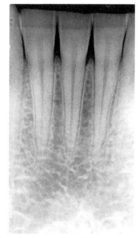

Fig. 20.4 Between the anterior teeth, the normal alveolar crest is pointed and well corticated, and is located within 0.5 to 2.0 mm of the adjacent cementoenamel junctions.

These changes can be divided into changes in the morphology of the supporting bone, and changes to the trabecular density and pattern.

Changes in morphology become apparent by observing a loss of the interproximal crestal bone, and the bone overlapping the buccal or lingual surfaces of the tooth roots. Alterations to the trabecular pattern of the alveolar processes reflect either a reduction or an increase in bone structure, or a combination of both. A reduction is seen as an increase in radiolucency (rarefaction) because of a decrease in either the number or density of existing trabeculae, or both. An increase in bone is seen as an increase in radiopacity (sclerosis) as the result of an increase in the thickness and/or density of trabecula, and/or their number. As with all inflammatory lesions of bone, periodontal disease usually involves a combination of both bone loss and bone formation. However, acute early lesions predominantly display bone loss, whereas chronic lesions have a greater component of bone sclerosis. The following patterns of bone loss may be seen in the diagnostic image as the result of periodontitis.

Changes in Morphology of Alveolar Processes
Early Bone Changes

The early bone changes that occur in periodontitis appear as areas of localized erosion of the interproximal alveolar crest (Fig. 20.5). In the anterior regions of the jaws, there is blunting of the alveolar crests and slight loss of alveolar crestal bone height. In the posterior regions of the jaws, there may be loss of the normally acute angle between the lamina dura and alveolar crest. In early stages of periodontal disease, this angle may lose its normal cortical surface (margin) and appear "rounded off," with an irregular and diffuse border. Even if only slight changes are apparent, the onset of the disease process may not be recent, because there is a delay before evidence of bone loss is visible in an image. As well, variations in the projection angle of the incident x-ray beam can cause a slight change in the apparent height of the alveolar crest. Small regions of bone loss on the buccal or lingual aspects of the teeth are also much more difficult to detect.

A Stage I or II lesion does not always develop into a more severe lesion later; however, if there is progression of the periodontal disease, bone changes can extend beyond the early changes to the alveolar crest. Defects in the morphology of the alveolar process and crest may be described as being horizontal or vertical (angular) in nature, as interdental craters and furcation defects, and as a loss of the buccal or lingual cortical plate loss. The presence and severity of these bone defects may, of course, vary regionally within a patient, and certainly among different patients.

Horizontal Bone Loss

Horizontal bone loss describes the appearance of a loss in height of the alveolar process where the crest is still horizontal (i.e., parallel to an imaginary line joining the CEJs of adjacent teeth). The bone crest is positioned more apically than the 0.5 mm to 2.0 mm from the CEJ that is considered to be the range of normal. In horizontal bone loss, the crest of the buccal and lingual cortical plates and the intervening interdental bone have been resorbed (Fig. 20.6).

Early stage (I) bone loss may be defined as loss of up to 15% of the tooth root length, or a probing depth of 4 mm or less. Stage II periodontitis is defined as bone loss between 15% and 33% of the root length, and probing depths of up to 5 mm. More severe Stages III and IV periodontal disease are defined as bone loss extending to the

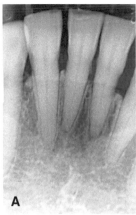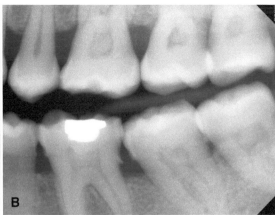

Fig. 20.6 Horizontal bone loss is seen in the anterior region (A) and the posterior region (B) as a loss of the buccal and lingual cortical plates and interdental alveolar bone.

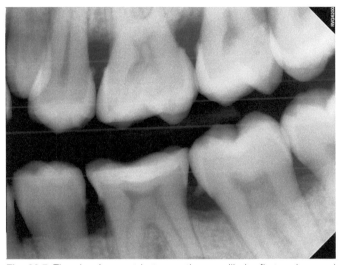

Fig. 20.7 The alveolar crest between the mandibular first and second molars appears angled but is approximately parallel to the imaginary plane created by the adjacent cementoenamel junctions, differentiating it from a vertical (angular) bone defect. There is an interproximal crater and reactive bone sclerosis present at this site.

disease and subsequent successful therapy will show reduced bone height (i.e., reduced periodontium), but the bone level may remain stable. Reestablishment of the cortication of the alveolar crest is a good indicator of stabilization of the periodontium.

Vertical Bone Defects

A vertical (or angular, infrabony) defect describes the appearance of bone loss that is localized at one or both root surfaces of a single tooth, although an individual may have multiple vertical osseous defects. These defects are associated with Stages III and IV periodontitis, and develop when bone loss progresses down the root of the tooth, resulting in a deepening of the periodontal pocket. This manifests as a V- or triangular-shaped defect within the bone that extends apically along the root of the affected tooth from the alveolar crest. Radiologically, the outline of the remaining alveolar process typically displays an angulation that is oblique to an imaginary line connecting the CEJ of the affected tooth to the adjacent tooth. In its early form, a vertical defect appears as abnormal widening of the PDL space at the alveolar crest (Fig. 20.9A).

The vertical defect is described as three-walled (surrounded by three bony walls) when both the buccal and lingual cortical plates remain intact. It is described as two-walled when one of these plates has been resorbed, and as one-walled when both plates have been lost (see Fig. 20.9B). Depending on the amount of bone loss, vertical bitewing images may be required to show the entire extent of the loss (Fig. 20.10). The distinctions among these groups are important in designing the treatment plan. The number of walls associated with a vertical defect is difficult or impossible to recognize on intraoral images, because one or both of the cortical bony plates may remain superimposed over the defect. Visualization of the depth of pockets may be aided by inserting a gutta-percha point before making the intraoral image. The point appears to follow the defect, because gutta-percha is relatively inflexible and radiopaque (Fig. 20.11). Clinical and surgical inspections are the best means of determining the number of remaining bony walls. CBCT imaging can also help characterize a defect more clearly, although this should not be routinely used for this purpose (Fig. 20.12).

Interdental Craters

The interproximal crater is a two-walled, trough-like depression that develops in the crest of the alveolar process between adjacent teeth. The buccal and lingual outer cortical walls of the interproximal bone extend further coronally than the cancellous bone between them, which has been resorbed. In an image, this appears as a band-like or irregular region of bone with less density at the crest, immediately adjacent to the more dense normal bone apical to the base of the crater (Fig. 20.13). These defects are more common in the posterior segments of the jaws

middle-third of the tooth root and beyond, with probing depths of 6 mm or more. The normal crest of the alveolar process can be up to as much as 2 mm apical to the CEJ, and therefore assessment of the quantity of bone loss must be considered from this point and not from the CEJ itself.

When the CEJs of adjacent teeth are at different horizontal levels, the alveolar crest may have an angled appearance. Careful assessment of the imaginary line connecting the adjacent CEJs, as well as the sharp angle made by the bone crest to the lamina dura, should not be confused with a true vertical (angular) bone defect (Fig. 20.7). Care must also be taken in using the CEJ as a reference point in cases of tooth supraeruption and severe attrition (Fig. 20.8). With supraeruption, the alveolar process will not necessarily remodel so that a normal relationship is maintained to the CEJ. The situation is similar in passive eruption, which may accompany severe attrition, although in this case, bone loss is not due to periodontitis. Even so, there may still be loss of attachment, which could be of clinical significance.

It is important to recognize that the extent of bone loss evident at a single examination does not indicate the current activity of the disease. For example, a patient who previously had generalized periodontal

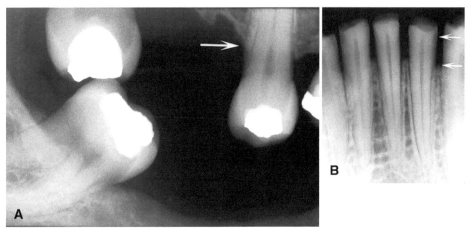

Fig. 20.8 (A) This maxillary second premolar is supraerupted; the etiology of the low bone level *(arrow)* relative to the cementoenamel junction (CEJ) is not necessarily the result of periodontal disease. (B) An example of passive eruption related to severe attrition resulting in the apparent increase in the distance from the CEJ to the bone height *(arrows)* cannot be attributed to periodontal disease. However, the resultant change in bone level relative to the CEJ still may be clinically significant.

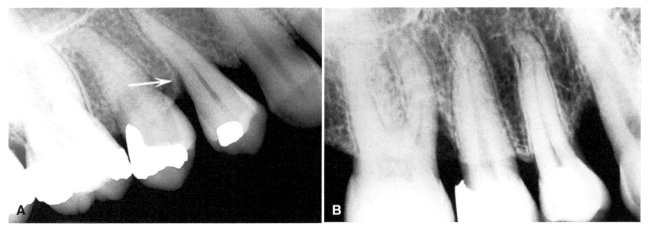

Fig. 20.9 (A) A developing vertical defect. Note the abnormal widening of the periodontal ligament space close to the crest *(arrow)*. (B) Maxillary periapical image reveals two examples of more severe vertical defects affecting the mesial surface of the first molar and the distal surface of the canine.

as a result of the broader buccal-lingual dimension of the alveolar crest in these regions.

Buccal or Lingual Cortical Plate Loss

The buccal or lingual cortical plate adjacent to the teeth may resorb. Loss of a cortical plate may occur alone or with another type of bone loss, such as horizontal bone loss. This type of bone loss is seen as an increase in the radiolucency of the tooth root near the alveolar crest. The shape seen is usually semicircular, with the depth of the radiolucency directed apically in relation to the tooth (Fig. 20.14). Lack of bone loss at the interproximal region of the tooth may make this kind of defect difficult to detect on conventional images.

Osseous Deformities in the Furcations of Multirooted Teeth

Progressive periodontal disease and the associated bone loss may extend into the furcations of multirooted teeth. As bone loss extends apically along the surface of a multirooted tooth, the bone covering the root can reach the level of the furcation or beyond. Widening of the PDL space at the apex of the interradicular bony crest of the furcation is strong evidence that the periodontal disease process involves the furcation (Fig. 20.15A). If there has been sufficient loss of bone on either the lingual and buccal surfaces of a mandibular molar furcation, the radiolucent image of the furcation defect becomes prominent (see Fig. 20.15B). The furcation defect may also involve only the buccal or lingual cortical plate, and extend into and apical to the roof of the furcation. In such a case, if the defect does not extend through to the opposing cortical plate, involvement of the furcation may appear more irregular and radiolucent than the adjacent normal bone. Use of the buccal object rule with images made at different angulations may enable the dentist to determine whether the buccal or the lingual cortical plate has been lost.

If the bone crest is located apical to the furcation but the disease process has not extended into the interradicular bone, the width of the periodontal ligament space appears normal. In addition, the septal bone may appear more radiolucent but otherwise be normal. In the mandible, the external oblique ridge may mask furcation involvement of the third molars (see Fig. 20.15C). Convergent roots may also obscure furcation defects in maxillary and mandibular second and third molars.

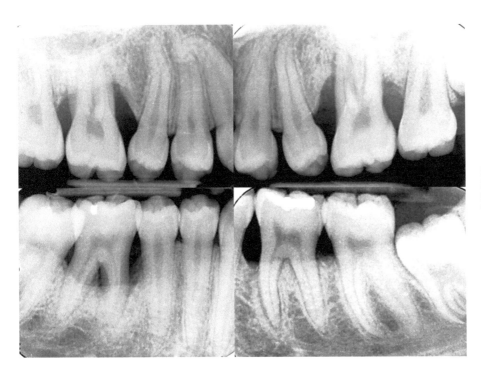

Fig. 20.10 Typical Vertical Bone Loss in Stage IV Periodontitis. Note the bone loss is confined to the region of the first molars. (Courtesy Dr. T. Charbeneau, Dallas, TX.)

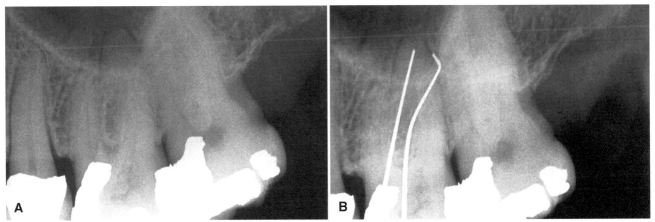

Fig. 20.11 Gutta-Percha May Be Used to Visualize the Depth of Infrabony Defects. (A) The image fails to show the osseous defect without the use of the gutta-percha points. (B) The image reveals an osseous defect extending to the region of the apex. (Courtesy Dr. H. Takei, Los Angeles, California.)

The loss of interradicular bone in the furcation of a maxillary molar may originate from the buccal, mesial, or distal surfaces of the tooth. The most common route for furcation involvement of the maxillary permanent first molar is from the mesial surface of the tooth. The image of furcation involvement is not as sharply defined around maxillary molars as it is around mandibular molars, because the palatal root is superimposed over the defect (see Fig. 20.15D). However, this pattern of bone destruction is occasionally prominent and appears as an inverted "J-shape" radiolucency, with the hook of the "J" extending into the trifurcation (see Fig. 20.15E) or as a radiolucent triangle superimposed over the roots of the involved tooth with its apex pointing toward the furcation (see Fig. 20.10).

A definitive diagnosis of complex furcation deformities requires careful clinical examination and sometimes surgical exploration. Intraoral images are an important tool in identifying potentially involved sites as well as providing information about root morphology and length,

which is of significance to treatment planning and prognosis. CBCT imaging can also be used to confirm involvement of a tooth and allow more detailed characterization of osseous furcation defects in cases where this information is necessary for treatment planning purposes.

Changes to the Internal Density and Trabecular Pattern of Bone

As with all other inflammatory lesions, the periodontal diseases may stimulate a reaction in the adjacent surrounding bone. The peripheral bone may appear more radiolucent or radiopaque, or more commonly, display a mixture of these patterns. Very rarely, no apparent change is seen in the surrounding bone. A radiolucent change reflects a loss of density and number of trabeculae. The trabeculae appear very faint, which is more commonly seen in early or acute lesions (Fig. 20.16A). If the trabeculae are sufficiently decalcified, they may not clearly appear in the image, even though they are still present; this accounts for the

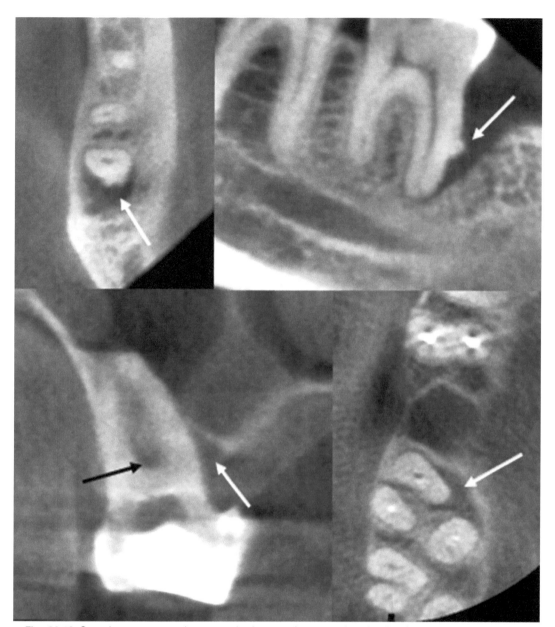

Fig. 20.12 Cone beam computed tomography images demonstrating details of the architecture of two three-walled vertical defects *(white arrows)*. Axial *(upper left)* and parasagittal *(upper right)* reconstructions show a deep vertical defect on the distal surface of the mandibular left second molar. Calculus is seen on the root surface. Coronal *(lower left)* and axial *(lower right)* images of another case show a three-walled defect on the palatal aspect of the mesiobuccal root of a maxillary molar. Early furcation involvement is also detected on this tooth *(black arrow)*.

apparent redevelopment of bone in some cases where acute inflammation resolves with successful treatment and the trabeculae remineralize. The radiopaque or sclerotic bone reaction appears because of the deposition of bone on existing trabeculae at the expense of the marrow, resulting in thicker trabeculae that may eventually be so dense so as to appear as an amorphous radiopaque mass (see Fig. 20.16B). This sclerotic reaction may extend some distance from the periodontal lesion, sometimes to the inferior cortex of the mandible. Usually the surrounding bone reaction is a mixture of both bone loss (rarefaction) and sclerosis. Furthermore, inflammatory products from a periodontal lesion may diffuse through the cortex of the floor of the maxillary sinus to cause

a regional mucositis (Fig. 20.17). In rare cases, a periosteal reaction might be seen in the adjacent alveolar process.

CLASSIFICATION OF THE PERIODONTAL DISEASES

The periodontal diseases are classified based on the tissues affected (i.e., gingiva only or with involvement of the alveolar process), stage (i.e., disease severity and complexity of management), grade (i.e., historical rate of progression and future risk of progression), or association with other conditions (i.e., systemic involvement, genetic conditions, or combined endodontic-periodontic lesions). A simplified overview

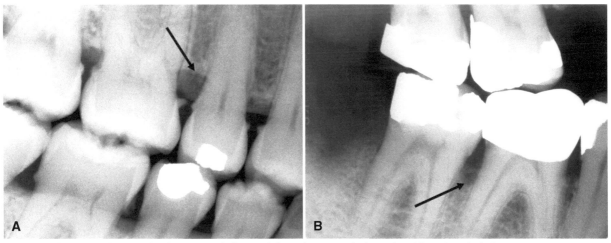

Fig. 20.13 Interproximal craters, existing as defects between the buccal and lingual cortical plates, seen as a radiolucent band (A) or trough (B) apical to the level of the crestal edges. The *arrows* indicate the base of the craters.

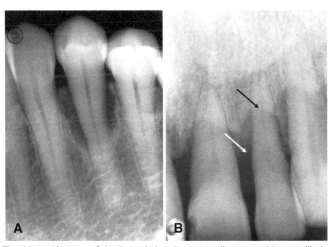

Fig. 20.14 (A) Loss of the lingual alveolar crest adjacent to this mandibular first premolar without associated interproximal bone loss. (B) Loss of the buccal cortical bone adjacent to the maxillary central and lateral incisors. The *black arrow* indicates the level of the buccal alveolar crest, which demonstrates more profound loss relative to the lingual alveolar crest *(white arrow)*.

of the classification of periodontal diseases is shown in Box 20.2 and Table 20.1.

Gingival diseases may be dental-biofilm-induced or non-biofilm. Dental biofilm-induced gingivitis is much more common than non-dental biofilm-induced inflammatory diseases affecting the gingiva. Non dental biofilm-induced gingivitis may be caused by viral or fungal infections, mucocutaneous and allergic conditions, and traumatic injuries. Gingivitis, as an inflammatory condition of the soft tissue surrounding the teeth, may manifest as gingival swelling, edema, and erythema. Periodontitis is distinguished from gingivitis by the clinically detectable destruction of host tissues, manifest as the loss of clinical soft tissue attachment and supporting bone of the involved teeth. Although periodontitis is always preceded by gingivitis, gingivitis does not always progress to periodontitis.

All the types of changes in bone morphology or trabecular pattern described above may be present to varying degrees in any patient with periodontitis. The same bone changes can also present in necrotizing periodontitis and periodontitis as a manifestation of systemic disease.

Necrotizing Periodontal Diseases

Necrotizing periodontal disease (NPD) includes necrotizing gingivitis and necrotizing periodontitis. Conditions predisposing to NPD include HIV infection, malnutrition, stress, and smoking. The clinical and gingival changes are common to both NPD conditions and include severe pain, fever and malaise with gingival erythema, bleeding, ulceration, and necrosis. Necrotizing periodontitis further presents with rapid loss of attachment. The diagnosis of necrotizing periodontal disease is made by clinical examination, but imaging aids in characterizing the extent of the bone loss.

Periodontitis as a Manifestation of Systemic Disease

This disease category includes diseases in which periodontal destruction is a manifestation of a systemic condition. Examples of such diseases include hematologic diseases (e.g., acquired neutropenia and leukemia) and genetic diseases (e.g., familial or cyclic neutropenia, Down syndrome, leukocyte adhesion deficiency syndrome, Papillon-Lefèvre syndrome, and Chédiak-Higashi syndrome). The oral changes in these conditions are the result of an impaired immune response to periodontal pathogens or a connective tissue abnormality in the periodontium that results in greater destruction. Periodontitis as a manifestation of systemic diseases may present with severe gingival and/or bone changes. Papillon-Lefèvre syndrome might be considered if there is a history of premature loss of deciduous teeth, and the permanent teeth are rapidly lost soon after erupting. This syndrome is usually seen with an associated hyperkeratosis of palmar and plantar surfaces.

OTHER CONDITIONS AFFECTING THE PERIODONTIUM

Periodontal Abscess

A periodontal abscess is a rapidly progressing, destructive lesion that usually originates in a deep soft tissue periodontal pocket. It occurs when the coronal portion of the pocket becomes occluded or when foreign material becomes lodged between a tooth and the gingiva. Clinically, pain and swelling, and sometimes a draining fistula, are present in the

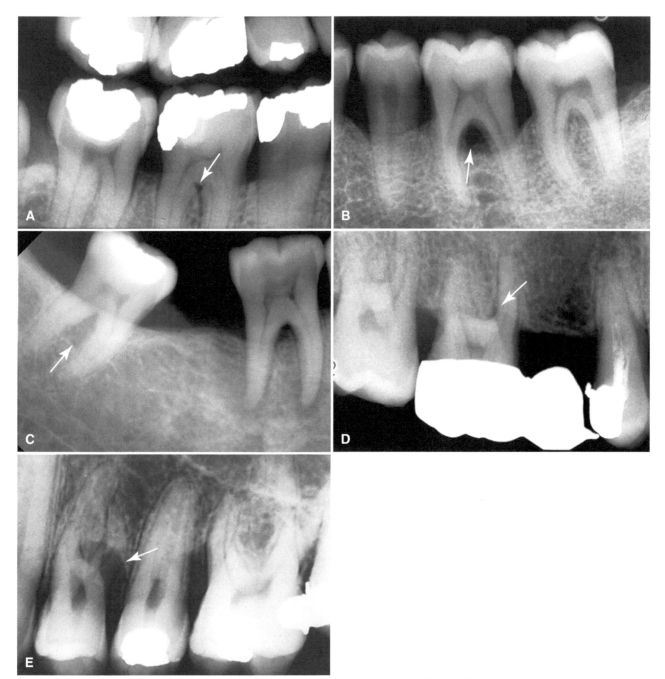

Fig. 20.15 (A) Periapical image revealing very early furcation involvement of a mandibular molar characterized by slight widening of the periodontal ligament (PDL) space in the furcation region *(arrow)*. (B) Periapical image revealing a profound radiolucent lesion within the furcation region *(arrow)* resulting from loss of bone in the furcation region and the buccal and lingual cortical plates. (C) Large furcation defect associated with the mandibular right third molar, which is less easily visualized due to superimposition by the external oblique ridge. There is also a combined periodontic-endodontic lesion of the first molar *(arrow)*. (D) Angulation of this periapical view of a maxillary first molar projected the palatal root away from the trifurcation region revealing early widening of the furcation PDL space *(arrow)*. (E) Example of an inverted "J-shape" radiolucent lesion *(arrow)* resulting from bone destruction extending into the trifurcation region of a three-rooted maxillary first bicuspid.

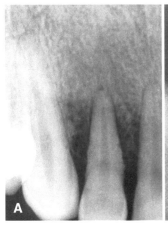
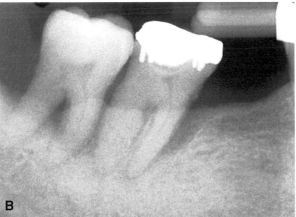

Fig. 20.16 (A) Example of a primarily radiolucent reaction around this maxillary lateral incisor. The trabeculae toward the alveolar crest on the mesial and distal aspect of the tooth are barely perceptible, and the marrow spaces are enlarged. (B) Periapical image revealing a predominantly sclerotic bone reaction resulting from the periodontal disease involving the mandibular molars. The trabeculae are thickened, and the marrow spaces are barely perceptible.

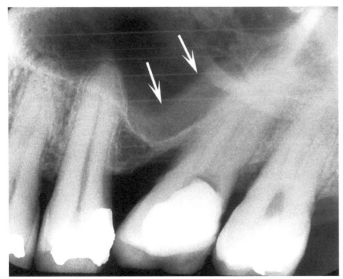

Fig. 20.17 Periapical image revealing a localized mucositis within the maxillary sinus (arrows) immediately adjacent to a vertical periodontal defect.

region. If the lesion is acute, there may be no visible changes in the image. If the lesion persists, a radiolucent region appears, often superimposed over the root of a tooth. The radiolucency may be a focal, round area of rarefaction, with loss of the lamina dura on the involved root surface, and a bridge of bone may be present over the coronal aspect of the lesion, separating it from the crest of the alveolar ridge (Fig. 20.18). After treatment, some of the lost bone may regenerate.

Endodontic-Periodontic Lesions

Inflammatory lesions from either a periodontal or pulpal origin may develop independently and merge with one another, or one lesion may induce the other. A periodontal lesion may extend to the apex of a tooth root causing secondary pulpitis, or periapical inflammatory disease may extend coronally to the crestal bone, causing a retrograde periodontitis. A combined periodontic-endodontic lesion appears as a deep angular bone defect on imaging, extending to the apex of a tooth and communicating with a concomitant focus of periapical rarefying osteitis (Fig. 20.19). The bone defect usually has a relatively uniform width or

---

BOX 20.2 Periodontal Disease Classification

I. Periodontal health, gingival diseases and conditions
   a. Periodontal health and gingival health
   b. Gingivitis: dental biofilm-induced
   c. Gingival diseases: non-dental biofilm induced
II. Periodontitis
   a. Necrotizing periodontal diseases
     i. Necrotizing gingivitis
     ii. Necrotizing periodontitis
     iii. Necrotizing stomatitis
   b. Periodontitis
     i. Stages
       1. Stage I: Initial periodontitis
       2. Stage II: Moderate periodontitis
       3. Stage III: Severe periodontitis with potential for additional tooth loss
       4. Stage IV: Severe periodontitis with potential for loss of the dentition
     ii. Extent and distribution: localized; generalized; molar-incisor distribution
     iii. Grades: Evidence or risk of rapid progression, anticipated treatment response
       1. Grade A: Slow rate of progression
       2. Grade B: Moderate rate of progression
       3. Grade C: Rapid rate of progression
   c. Periodontitis as a manifestation of systemic disease
III. Other conditions affecting the periodontium
   a. Systemic diseases or conditions affecting the periodontal support system
   b. Periodontal abscesses and endodontic-periodontic lesions
   c. Mucogingival deformities and conditions
   d. Traumatic occlusal forces
   e. Tooth and prosthesis related factors

Modified from Canton JG, Armitage G, Berglundh T, et al. A new classification scheme for periodontal and peri-implant diseases and conditions—Introduction and key changes from the 1999 classification. *J Periodontol* 2018;89(1):S1-S8.

TABLE 20.1	Periodontitis Classification			
Periodontitis Stage		I	II	III	IV
Severity	Radiographic Bone Loss	Coronal third of root (<15%)	Coronal third of root (15% to 33%)	Extending to the middle third of root and beyond	Extending to the middle third of root and beyond
Complexity	Local	Maximum probing depth ≤4 mm that is mostly horizontal bone loss	Maximum probing depth ≤5 mm that is mostly horizontal bone loss	Stage II complexity and: Probing depth ≥6 mm; vertical bone loss ≥3 mm; Class II or III furcation; moderate ridge defect	Stage III complexity and: severe ridge defect and <20 remaining teeth (10 opposing pairs)

Modified from Papapanou PN, Sanz M Buduneli N, et al. Periodontitis: Consensus report of workgroup 2 of the 2017 World Workshop on the Classification of Periodontal and Peri-Implant Diseases and Conditions. *J Periodontol* 2018; 89(1):S173-S182.

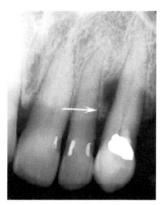

Fig. 20.18 Example of a periodontal abscess related to the maxillary canine; note the well-defined area of bone loss over the midroot region of the tooth and extending in a mesial direction toward the lateral incisor. There appears to be a layer of bone *(arrow)* separating the area of bone destruction from the crest of the alveolar process.

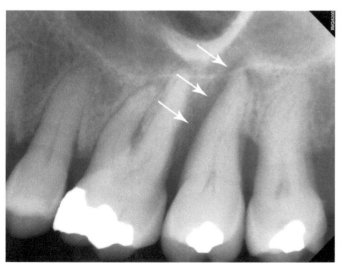

Fig. 20.19 Combined Endodontic-Periodontic Lesion. There is an angular bone defect extending the whole length of the mesial surface of the second molar, from the crest to the apex *(arrows)*.

widens slightly at the alveolar crest, creating a funnel-like shape (see Fig. 20.14C). Periodontic-endodontic lesions may affect one or multiple surfaces of the tooth, or they may be circumferential around the entire root. Treatment of these defects is complicated and involves both endodontic and periodontal therapy.

Occlusal Trauma

Traumatic occlusion causes degenerative changes in bone in response to occlusal forces that are greater than the physiologic tolerances of the tooth's supporting tissues. These changes occur either as a result of maladaptation in response to excessive occlusal forces on teeth or by normal occlusal forces on a periodontium already compromised by bone loss. In addition to clinical signs and symptoms such as increased mobility, wear facets, unusual response to percussion, and a history of contributing habits, there are associated findings in the images, including widening of the PDL space, thickening of the lamina dura, bone loss, and an increase in the number and size of trabeculae. Other sequelae of traumatic occlusion may include hypercementosis and root fractures. Traumatic occlusion alone does not cause gingivitis or periodontitis, affect the epithelial attachment, or lead to pocket formation. However, in the presence of preexisting periodontitis, bone loss may be accelerated. Traumatic occlusion can be definitively diagnosed only by clinical evaluation and not by the imaging findings alone.

Tooth Mobility

Widening of the PDL space suggests tooth mobility, which may result from occlusal trauma or a lack of bone support arising from advanced bone loss. If the affected tooth has a single root, the socket may develop an hourglass shape. If the tooth is multirooted, it may show widening of the PDL space at the apices and in the region of the furcation. These changes can develop when the tooth moves about an axis of rotation at some midpoint on the roots. In addition, the image of the lamina dura may appear broad and hazy, and show increased density.

Open Contacts

When the mesial and distal surfaces of adjacent teeth are not in contact, the patient has an open contact. Open contacts are associated with sites of periodontal disease more than closed contacts. An open contact may be dangerous to the periodontium because of the potential for food debris to become impacted in the opening. Trapped food particles may damage the soft tissue and induce an inflammatory response, and contribute to the development of localized chronic periodontal disease. Similar potential situations in which periodontal disease may develop are discrepancies in the height of two adjacent marginal ridges or tipped teeth (Fig. 20.20). Abnormal tooth alignment does not cause periodontal disease but, again, provides an environment where disease may develop as a result of difficulty in maintaining adequate oral hygiene.

Local Irritating and Factors

Other local factors that are apparent in an image may provide an environment where periodontal disease may develop or may aggravate existing periodontal disease. For example, deposits of calculus (Fig. 20.21) can prevent effective cleansing of a sulcus and lead to enhanced plaque formation and the progression of periodontal disease. Calculus is most commonly seen in association with the mandibular incisors but may be localized to any surface or generalized throughout the dentition. Other local tooth-related factors include enamel pearls and cervical enamel projections, which are aberrant enamel formations most commonly found in the furcation regions of multirooted teeth. These anomalies alter the periodontal attachment to the tooth and create sites prone to biofilm accumulation and periodontal breakdown. Defective restorations with overhanging or poorly contoured margins can also lead to the accumulation of plaque owing to difficulty in cleaning around them, thus providing an environment where periodontal disease may develop (Fig. 20.22).

OTHER MODIFIERS OF PERIODONTAL DISEASE

Diabetes mellitus is a common disease and known risk factor for periodontitis, and glycemic control in diabetes is impaired by periodontal inflammation. There is thus is a two-way systemic relationship between these diseases. Uncontrolled diabetes may result in protein breakdown, degenerative vascular changes, lowered resistance to infection, and increased severity of infections. Consequently, patients with uncontrolled diabetes are more disposed to the development of periodontal disease than individuals with normal glucose metabolism. Patients with uncontrolled diabetes and periodontal disease also show more severe and rapid resorption of the alveolar processes, and are more prone to the development of periodontal abscesses. In patients whose diabetes is under control, periodontal disease responds normally to traditional treatment.

HIV infection and acquired immunodeficiency syndrome (AIDS) is another modifier of periodontal disease. The incidence and severity of periodontal disease is high in patients with HIV/AIDS. In these individuals, the disease process is characterized by a rapid progression that leads to bone sequestration and loss of several teeth. These patients may not respond to standard periodontal therapy.

High-dose irradiation to the oral tissues as a treatment for malignant conditions in the head and neck may have a detrimental effect on the

Fig. 20.20 The second molar has tipped mesially after loss of the first molar, creating an abnormal tooth alignment that was difficult for the patient to maintain, leading to localized periodontal disease. Note the calculus on the mesial surface of the second molar. The crown on the second premolar was constructed with an enlarged distal contour to stop further tipping of the molar.

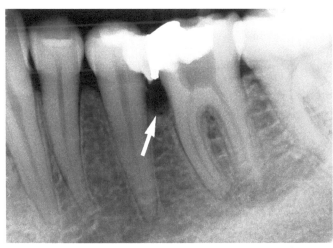

Fig. 20.22 These overhanging restorations provided an environment suitable for plaque accumulation and subsequent localized periodontal bone loss *(arrow).*

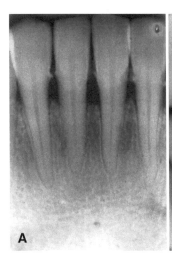
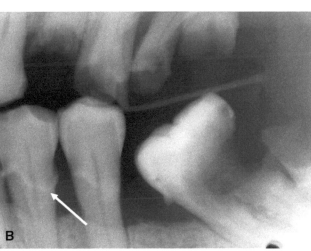

Fig. 20.21 Calculus may be seen as small angular radiopaque deposits projecting between interproximal surfaces of the teeth (A) or as radiopaque bands across the roots representing circumferential accumulation *(arrow* in B).

periodontium. Radiation therapy to the jaws results in bone that is hypovascular, hypocellular, and hypoxic. This bone may be less able to remodel and be more susceptible to infections, resulting in rapid bone loss that is indistinguishable from the characteristics of periodontal disease seen on imaging. Teeth that have been exposed to high-dose radiation fields have been shown to demonstrate greater recession, attachment loss, and mobility than teeth in the same mouth that were not within the field.

EVALUATION OF PERIODONTAL THERAPY

Occasionally, signs of successful treatment of periodontal disease are visible in the posttreatment images. Reestablishment of the interproximal crestal cortex (Fig. 20.23) and the sharp line angle between the cortex and lamina dura are good indicators of stabilization of the disease, although these signs are not seen in all patients. The relatively radiolucent margins of bone that were undergoing active resorption before treatment may become more sclerotic (radiopaque) after successful therapy. In some cases, there may have been considerable mineral loss of the cancellous bone (appearing radiolucent), so that the bone is not apparent in

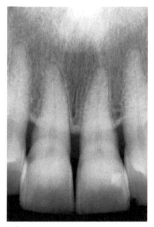

Fig. 20.23 Example of a case in which the interproximal cortex of the alveolar crest has re-formed after successful periodontal therapy.

the image. Successful treatment may result in remineralization, causing the bone to become visible in the image, giving the false impression that bone has actually grown into periodontal defects. Clinicians must be conscious of the fact that beam angulation and x-ray exposure settings may affect the visibility of the alveolar crests. Sequential images made with different beam angulations may give the false impression that bone has "grown into" the periodontal defects. Too high an x-ray exposure increases the density of the image (more black), and thin bone such as the alveolar crest may not be apparent, giving the false impression that the bone has been resorbed. Alternatively, light images may give the false impression of bone growth. In many cases, there are no apparent changes in the images after successful treatment. Also, intraoral images do not disclose the therapeutic elimination of soft tissue periodontal pockets; therefore, healing is best assessed clinically.

DIFFERENTIAL INTEPRETATION

Most cases of bone loss around teeth are caused by the periodontal diseases. This fact can make the clinician less sensitive to other diseases with similar manifestations that should always be considered in the differential diagnosis. Occasionally, more serious diseases are missed or recognized late. The most likely clinical sign of disease other than periodontal disease is the presence of one or a few adjacent loose teeth when the rest of the mouth shows no signs of periodontal disease. Suspicion should be heightened if the bone destruction does not have the pattern or morphology normally associated with periodontal disease.

Periodontal disease originates in the gingival sulcus at the alveolar crest, and progresses along the periodontium, against the affected tooth. Thus bone loss caused by periodontal disease, such as vertical defects, should appear larger at the coronal aspect and less severe at the leading edge apically. This appearance differs from other diseases, which may destroy the supporting bone in a more widespread or invasive pattern.

Malignant neoplasms—in particular, squamous cell carcinoma—involving the alveolar process may mimic the appearance of periodontal disease. And occasionally malignant neoplasia is treated as periodontal disease, resulting in a delay in diagnosis and treatment (Fig. 20.24A). This malignancy may display characteristics in the image that suggest its true nature, such as extensive bone destruction of a localized region beyond the periodontium, or invasive characteristics (see Chapter 26).

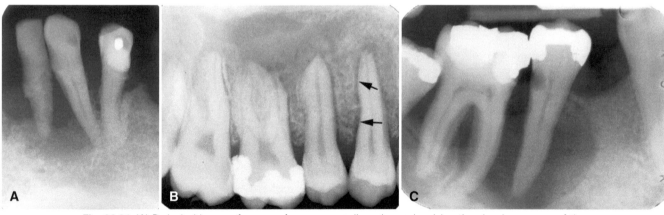

Fig. 20.24 (A) Periapical image of a case of squamous cell carcinoma involving the alveolar process of the mandible; note the irregular bone destruction. (B) Periapical image of a malignant tumor extending from the maxillary sinus into the alveolar process and invading the periodontal ligament space of the adjacent teeth. Note the irregular widening *(arrows)*. (C) Periapical image of Langerhan cell histiocytosis demonstrating a lesion with destruction of the alveolar process. Note the epicenter in the midroot region instead of the alveolar crest, as seen in periodontal disease.

Irregular widening of the PDL space along its entire length, with a ragged or irregular periphery, and destruction of the lamina dura are suggestive of infiltration by a malignancy rather than periodontal disease. In some cases, squamous cell carcinoma may mimic periodontal disease, and only the clinical characteristics of the lesion and the failure to respond to treatment indicate the presence of malignancy.

Any lesion resulting in bone destruction that has ill-defined borders and lacks a peripheral bone response (sclerosis) should be viewed with suspicion. Another disease to be considered is Langerhan cell histiocytosis (see Fig. 20.24B). Often this disease may manifest as single or multiple regions of bone destruction around the roots of teeth, similar to periodontal disease. The appearance of "teeth floating in space" may appear similar to severe periodontitis. Also, in histiocytosis, the epicenter of the bone destruction is in the midroot level of the tooth rather than at the crest, which may give early lesions an "ice cream scoop" appearance, with the alveolar crest less resorbed or even intact (see Chapter 26).

BIBLIOGRAPHY

Classification
Canton JG, Armitage G, Berglundh T, et al. A new classification scheme for periodontal and peri-implant diseases and conditions—Introduction and key changes from the 1999 classification. *J Periodontol*. 2018;89(suppl 1):S1–S8.
Papapanou PN, Sanz M, Buduneli N, et al. Periodontitis: Consensus report of workgroup 2 of the 2017 World Workshop on the Classification of Periodontal and Peri-Implant Diseases and Conditions. *J Periodontol*. 2018;89(1):S173–S182.

Clinical Characteristics of Periodontal Diseases
Herrera C, González I, Sanz M. The periodontal abscess (I): clinical and microbiological findings. *J Clin Periodontol*. 2000;27:387–394.
Newman MG, Takei HH, Klokkevold PR, et al. *Carranza's Clinical Periodontology*. Philadelphia: Saunders; 2006.
Walsh TF, al-Kohail OS, Fosam EB. The relationship of bone loss observed on panoramic radiographs with clinical periodontal screening. *J Clin Periodontol*. 1997;24:153–157.

Epidemiology
Eke PI, Dye BA, Wei L, et al. Update on prevalence of periodontitis in adults in the United States: NHANES 2009 to 2012. *J Periodontol*. 2015;86(5):611–622.
Melvin WL, Sandifer JB, Gray JL. The prevalence and sex ratio of juvenile periodontitis in a young racially mixed population. *J Periodontol*. 1991;62:330–334.
Papapanou PN. Periodontal diseases: epidemiology. *Ann Periodontol*. 1996;1:1–36.
Position paper: epidemiology of periodontal diseases. American Academy of Periodontology. *J Periodontol*. 1996;67:935–945.

Etiology
Bimstein E, Garcia-Godoy F. The significance of age, proximal caries, gingival inflammation, probing depths, and the loss of lamina dura in the diagnosis of alveolar bone loss in the primary molars. *ASDC J Dent Child*. 1994;61:125–128.
Page RC, Offenbacher S, Schroeder HE, et al. Advances in the pathogenesis of periodontitis: summary of developments, clinical implications and future directions. *Periodontol 2000*. 1997;14:216–248.
Salvi GE, Lawrence HP, Offenbacher S, et al. Influence of risk factors on the pathogenesis of periodontitis. *Periodontol 2000*. 1997;14:173.
Schwartz Z, Goultschin J, Dean DD, et al. Mechanisms of alveolar bone destruction in periodontitis. *Periodontol 2000*. 1997;14:158.
Van Dyke TE, Serhan CN. Resolution of inflammation: a new paradigm for the pathogenesis of periodontal diseases. *J Dent Res*. 2003;82:82–90.

Radiographic Manifestations
Gutteridge DL. The use of radiographic techniques in the diagnosis and management of periodontal diseases. *Dentomaxillofac Radiol*. 1995;24:107–113.
Jeffcoat MK, Wang IC, Reddy MS. Radiographic diagnosis in periodontics. *Periodontol 2000*. 1995;7:54–68.
Khocht A, Zohn H, Deasy M, et al. Screening for periodontal disease: radiographs vs PSR. *J Am Dent Assoc*. 1996;127:749–756.
Koral SM, Howell TH, Jeffcoat MK. Alveolar bone loss due to open interproximal contacts in periodontal disease. *J Periodontol*. 1981;52:447–450.
Mann J, Pettigrew J, Beideman R, et al. Investigation of the relationship between clinically detected loss of attachment and radiographic changes in early periodontal disease. *J Clin Periodontol*. 1985;12:247–253.
Nielsen IM, Glavind L, Karring T. Interproximal periodontal intrabony defects: prevalence, localization, and etiological factors. *J Clin Periodontol*. 1980;7:187–198.
Rams TE, Listgarten MA, Slots J. Utility of radiographic crestal lamina dura for predicting periodontitis disease activity. *J Clin Periodontol*. 1994;21:571–576.
Waite IM, Furniss JS, Wong WM. Relationship between clinical periodontal condition and the radiological appearance at first molar sites in adolescents: a 3-year study. *J Clin Periodontol*. 1994;21:155–160.

Radiographic Technique
Scarfe WC, Azevedo B, Pinheiro LR, et al. The emerging role of maxillofacial radiology in the diagnosis and management of patients with complex periodontitis. *Periodontol 2000*. 2017;74:116–139.
Bragger I. Radiographic diagnosis of periodontal disease progression. *Curr Opin Periodontol*. 1996;3:59–67.
Gröndahl K, Gröndahl HG, Webber RL, et al. Influence of variations in projection geometry on the detectability of periodontal bone lesions: a comparison between subtraction radiography and conventional radiographic technique. *J Clin Periodontol*. 1984;11:411–420.
Pepelassi EA, Diamanti-Kipioti A. Selection of the most accurate method of conventional radiography for the assessment of periodontal osseous destruction. *J Clin Periodontol*. 1997;24:557–567.
Reed B, Polson A. Relationships between bitewing and periapical radiographs in assessing crestal alveolar bone levels. *J Periodontol*. 1984;55:22–27.
Zaki HA, Hoffmann KR, Hausmann E, et al. Is radiologic assessment of alveolar crest height useful to monitor periodontal disease activity? *Dent Clin North Am*. 2015;59:859–872.

Subtraction Radiography
Eickholz P, Hausmann E. Evidence for healing of periodontal defects 5 years after conventional and regenerative therapy: digital subtraction and bone level measurements. *J Clin Periodontol*. 2002;29:922–928.

Cone Beam Computed Tomographic Imaging
Mol A, Balasundaram A. In vitro cone beam computed tomography imaging of periodontal bone. *Dentomaxillofac Radiol*. 2008;37:319–324.
Vandenberghe B, Jacobs R, Yang J. Detection of periodontal bone loss using digital intraoral and cone beam computed tomography images: an in vitro assessment of bony and/or infrabony defects. *Dentomaxillofac Radiol*. 2008;37:252–260.
Walter C, Weiger R, Zitzmann NU. Accuracy of three-dimensional imaging in assessing maxillary molar furcation involvement. *J Clin Periodontol*. 2010;37:436–441.

Occlusal Trauma
Burgett FG. Trauma from occlusion: periodontal concerns. *Dent Clin North Am*. 1995;39:301–311.
Wank GS, Kroll YJ. Occlusal trauma: an evaluation of its relationship to periodontal prostheses. *Dent Clin North Am*. 1981;25:511–532.

Systemic Disease
Knight ET, Liu J, Seymour GJ, et al. Risk factors that may modify the innate and adaptive immune responses in periodontal diseases. *Periodontol 2000*. 2016;71:22–51.

Emrich LJ, Shlossman M, Genco RJ. Periodontal disease in non-insulin-dependent diabetes mellitus. *J Periodontol*. 1991;62:123–131.

Epstein JB, Lunn R, Le N, et al. Periodontal attachment loss in patients after head and neck radiation therapy. *Oral Surg Oral Med Oral Pathol Oral Radiol Endod*. 1998;86:673–677.

Farzim I, Edalat M. Periodontosis with hyperkeratosis palmaris and plantaris (the Papillon-Lefèvre syndrome): a case report. *J Periodontol*. 1974;45:316–318.

Nelson RG, Schlossman M, Budding LM, et al. Periodontal diseases and NIDDM in Pima Indians. *Diabetes Care*. 1990;13:836–840.

Rateitschak-Plüss EM, Schroeder HE. History of periodontitis in a child with Papillon-Lefèvre syndrome: a case report. *J Periodontol*. 1984;55:35–46.

Winkler JR, Grassi M, Murray PA. Clinical description and etiology of HIV-associated periodontal disease. In: Robinson PB, Greenspan JS, eds. *Prospectus on Oral Manifestations of AIDS*. Littleton, MA: PSG Publishing; 1988.

21

Dental Anomalies

Aditya Tadinada and Anitha Potluri

Dental anomalies can develop in a variety of ways, and are broadly classified as being congenital, developmental, or acquired. Congenital abnormalities are typically genetically inherited, and developmental anomalies occur during the formation of a tooth or teeth. These anomalies may include variations in the normal number, size, morphology, or eruptive pattern of the teeth. Acquired abnormalities result from changes to teeth after normal formation. Teeth that form abnormally short roots may represent congenital or developmental anomalies, whereas the shortening of normal tooth roots by external resorption represents an acquired change.

DEVELOPMENTAL ABNORMALITIES

Number of Teeth

Supernumerary Teeth

Disease mechanism. Teeth that develop in addition to the normal complement as a result of excess dental lamina in the jaws are referred to as supernumerary or supplemental teeth, or parateeth. These additional teeth may be morphologically normal or abnormal. When supernumerary teeth have normal morphologic features, the term supplemental is sometimes used. Supernumerary teeth that occur in the anterior maxilla are termed mesiodens. Those that occur in the premolar area are termed peridens, and those that occur in the molar area are termed distodens or, sometimes, paramolars. Recent studies in animals have suggested a genetic etiology to the development of supernumerary teeth—specifically, the roles signaling molecules such as bone morphogenetic protein (BMP) and fibroblast growth factor (FGF), and signaling pathways, that include the wingless-related (Wnt) and sonic hedgehog (SHH) pathways. The exact mechanisms through which these molecules act (e.g., up- or downregulation of pathways), however, still remain unclear.

Clinical features. Supernumerary teeth occur in 1% to 4% of the population, and are easily identified by counting and recording all the teeth in the jaws. Supernumerary teeth may have a greater incidence in Asian and Indigenous populations, and occur twice as often in males. Although supernumerary teeth can arise in either the deciduous or the permanent dentitions, they are more common in the permanent dentition and can arise anywhere in the jaws.

Single supernumerary teeth are most common in the anterior maxilla, where they are referred to as mesiodens (Figs. 21.1 to 21.3), and in the maxillary molar region (Fig. 21.4), whereas multiple supernumerary teeth occur most frequently in the premolar regions, usually in the mandible, and are often positioned in the lingual aspect of the alveolar process (Figs. 21.5 and 21.6).

Supernumerary teeth are usually discovered on images because they interfere with normal tooth eruption (Fig. 21.7). When a supernumerary tooth does erupt, it commonly erupts outside the normal archform because of space restrictions.

Imaging features. The imaging features of supernumerary teeth are variable. They may appear entirely normal in both size and shape, but they may also be smaller in size compared with the adjacent normal dentition or have a conical shape with the appearance of a canine tooth. In extreme cases, the supernumerary teeth may appear grossly deformed.

Images may reveal supernumerary teeth in the deciduous dentition (Fig. 21.8) after 3 or 4 years of age when the deciduous teeth have formed, or in the permanent dentitions of children between 9 and 12 years of age. Although supernumerary teeth may be identified initially on two-dimensional images such as periapical, panoramic, or occlusal images, three-dimensional cone beam computed tomography (CBCT) may aid in determining the location and number of unerupted supernumerary teeth, associated pathosis, and any effects they may have on adjacent teeth and anatomical structures. In particular, care should be taken to review panoramic images for supernumerary teeth, because these may be obscured in the anterior maxilla by the image of the cervical spine, or they may appear distorted if they lie outside the focal trough.

Differential interpretation. Multiple supernumerary teeth have been associated with genetic syndromes, including cleidocranial dysplasia (see Chapter 29), familial adenomatous polyposis, Gardner syndrome (see Chapter 24), and pyknodysostosis.

Management. The management of supernumerary teeth depends on many factors, including their potential effect on the developing normal dentition, their position and number, and the potential complications that may result from surgical intervention. If supernumerary teeth erupt, they can cause malalignment of the normal dentition. Supernumerary teeth that remain in the jaws may cause root resorption of adjacent teeth and their follicles, may develop dentigerous cysts, or may interfere with the normal eruption sequence. All the preceding factors influence the decision to either remove a supernumerary tooth or keep it under observation.

Missing Teeth

Disease mechanism. The expression of developmentally missing teeth includes the absence of one or a few teeth (hypodontia), the absence of numerous teeth (oligodontia), and the failure of all teeth to develop (anodontia). Developmentally missing teeth may also be the result of numerous independent pathologic mechanisms that can affect the orderly formation of the dental lamina (e.g., orofaciodigital syndrome), failure of a tooth germ to develop at the optimal time, lack of necessary space imposed by a malformed jaw, or disproportion between tooth mass and jaw size.

Clinical features. Hypodontia in the permanent dentition, excluding third molars, is found in 3% to 10% of the population, and is more frequently found in Asian and Indigenous populations. Although missing primary teeth are relatively uncommon, when one tooth is missing, it

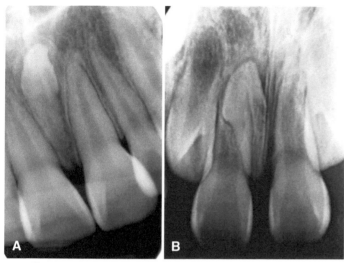

Fig. 21.1 (A and B) Periapical images of inverted mesiodens.

is usually a maxillary incisor. The most commonly missing teeth are third molars, followed by mandibular second premolars (Fig. 21.9) and maxillary lateral and mandibular central incisors. The absence may be either unilateral or bilateral. Children who have developmentally missing teeth tend to have more than one absent and more than one morphologic group (incisors, premolars, and molars) involved.

Imaging features. The development of teeth may vary markedly among individuals. Missing teeth may be recognized by identifying and counting the teeth present. For some individuals, the eruption of some teeth may be delayed by a number of years after the normally established eruption time (especially mandibular second premolars), whereas others may erupt up to 1 year after the contralateral tooth.

Differential interpretation. A tooth may be considered to be developmentally missing when it cannot be discerned clinically or through imaging, and no history exists of its extraction. Oligodontia or anodontia may occur in patients with several conditions like cleft lip and palate, and syndromes including ectodermal dysplasia (Fig. 21.10), trisomy 21, Rieger syndrome, and Book syndrome.

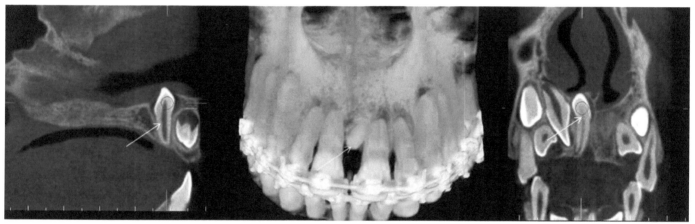

Fig. 21.2 Cone beam computed tomography reconstructions showing a supernumerary tooth between the two maxillary central incisors *(arrow)*.

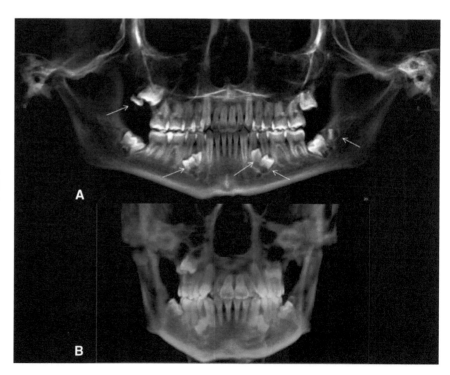

Fig. 21.3 Multiple Supernumerary Teeth. (A) Panoramic reconstruction of a cone beam computed tomography (CBCT) volume *(arrows)*. (B) Three-dimensional reconstruction from a CBCT volume.

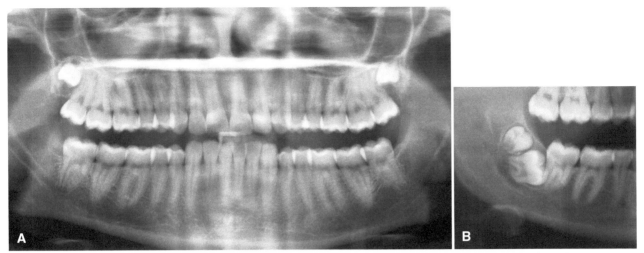

Fig. 21.4 (A) Example of two supernumerary teeth in the maxillary third molar area (distodens). (B) Example in the mandibular third molar region. ([A] Courtesy Dr. H. Grubisa, Oakville, Ontario.)

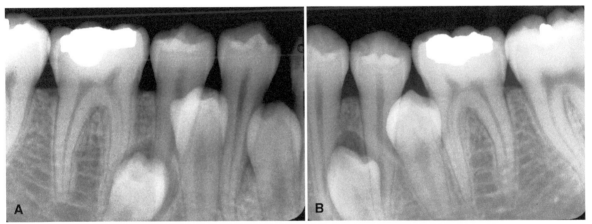

Fig. 21.5 (A and B) Periapical images show bilateral supplemental premolar teeth (peridens).

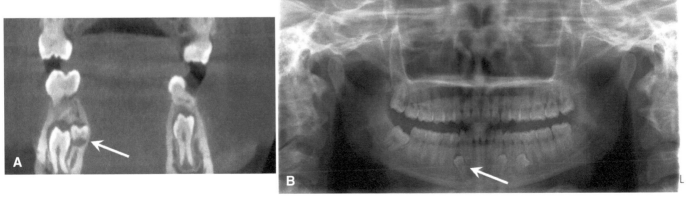

Fig. 21.6 (A) Left cross-sectional and (B) panoramic, cone beam computed tomography, and panoramic views of peridens *(arrows)* developing to the lingual of the adjacent mandibular first premolar.

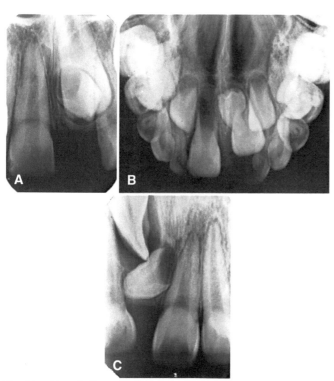

Fig. 21.7 (A to C) Examples of mesiodens interfering with eruption of adjacent permanent teeth.

Fig. 21.8 Supernumerary deciduous molar *(arrow).*

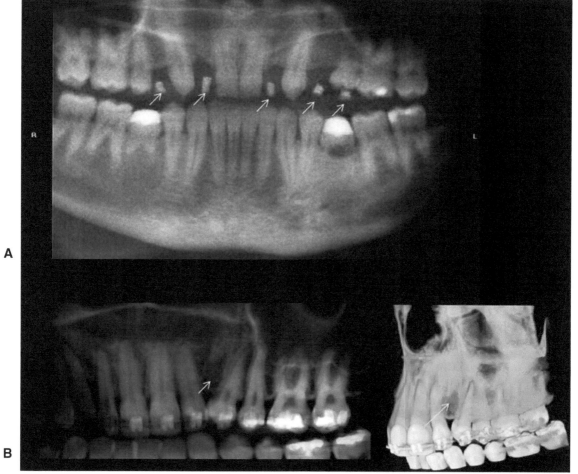

Fig. 21.9 (A) Multiple missing teeth in a patient with oligodontia. *White arrows* show radiographic markers for planning dental implants. (B) Panoramic reconstruction of a cone beam computed tomography volume. *White arrow* shows a developmentally absent maxillary left canine.

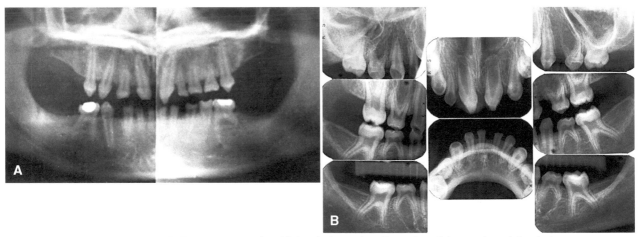

Fig. 21.10 (A and B) Two examples of multiple missing and malformed teeth in ectodermal dysplasia.

The ectodermal dysplasias are a genetically diverse group of abnormalities that include 186 distinct diseases that involve 64 gene mutations. In addition to missing teeth, phenotypically, these individuals may also lack sweat glands; have thin, fine hair; thin, delicate skin; and malformed nails. When the teeth are involved, the condition may manifest with multiple missing or malformed teeth that often have a conical or canine shape, or a notable decrease in tooth size. The ectodermal dysplasias have been subdivided into two groups. Group A ectodermal dysplasia includes entities with abnormalities involving two or more of the classically involved structures previously mentioned, and group B includes abnormalities of one of these structures, and another abnormality of ectodermal origin that may include the mammary glands, thyroid gland, thymus, anterior pituitary gland, cornea, conjunctiva, lacrimal gland, lacrimal duct, or meibomian glands.

Management. Missing teeth, abnormal occlusion, or altered facial appearance may cause some patients psychological distress. If the extent of hypodontia is mild, the associated changes likewise may be slight and can be managed by orthodontic intervention. In more severe cases, restorative, implant, and prosthetic procedures may be considered.

Size of Teeth

A positive correlation exists between tooth size (mesiodistal or buccolingual dimension) and body height. Males also have larger primary and permanent teeth than females. Beyond these normal variations, individuals may occasionally have unusually large or small teeth.

Macrodontia

Disease mechanism. In macrodontia, the teeth are larger than normal; however, macrodontia rarely affects the entire dentition. Often a single tooth, individual contralateral teeth, or a group of teeth may be involved (Fig. 21.11). Macrodontia may occur sporadically, and its cause is unknown. Vascular abnormalities such as a hemangioma (arising from within the bone or the adjacent soft tissues) can result in an increase in the size and accelerate the development of adjacent teeth. Macrodontia can also occur in hemihypertrophy of the face or in pituitary gigantism.

Clinical features. Clinically, macrodont teeth appear large and may be associated with crowding, malocclusion, or impaction.

Imaging features. Images reveal the increased size of both unerupted and erupted macrodont teeth. The shape of the tooth is usually normal, but some cases may exhibit mildly distorted morphology. Crowding may cause impaction of adjacent teeth. Periapical or panoramic imaging is most commonly used to identify this condition.

Differential interpretation. The differential interpretation of a sporadic macrodont tooth includes gemination and fusion. When fusion occurs, a count of the teeth present reveals a missing tooth. In gemination, all the teeth may be present, and often evidence exists of a division or cleft of the crown or root of the tooth. The differentiation between these three conditions may not influence the management provided.

Management. In most cases, macrodontia does not require treatment. Orthodontic treatment may be necessary if a malocclusion is present.

Microdontia

Disease mechanism. In microdontia, the teeth are smaller than normal. As with macrodontia, microdontia may involve all the teeth or be limited to a single tooth or group of teeth. Often the lateral incisors and third molars may be small. Generalized microdontia is extremely rare, although it does occur in some patients with pituitary dwarfism. Supernumerary teeth may also be microdont teeth.

Clinical features. The involved teeth are noticeably small and may have altered morphology. Microdont molars may have an altered shape. For example, mandibular molars may have four cusps rather than five, and maxillary molars may have four cusps rather than three (Fig. 21.12). Microdont lateral incisors may be peg-shaped (Fig. 21.13).

Imaging features. These small teeth are frequently malformed.

Differential interpretation. The recognition of small teeth indicates the diagnosis. The number and distribution of microdont teeth may also suggest consideration of associated abnormalities (e.g., congenital heart disease, progeria).

Management. Restorative or prosthetic treatment may be considered to create a more normal-appearing tooth, especially when considering esthetic concerns in the anterior dentition.

Eruption of Teeth
Transposition

Disease mechanism. Transposition is the condition in which two typically adjacent teeth have exchanged positions in the dental arch.

Clinical features. The most frequently transposed teeth are the permanent canine and the first premolar. Second premolars infrequently lie between the first and second molars. The transposition of central and lateral incisors is rare. Transposition can occur with hypodontia, supernumerary teeth, or the persistence of a deciduous predecessor. Transposition in the primary dentition has not been reported.

Imaging features. Images reveal transposition when the teeth are not in their usual sequence in the dental arch (Fig. 21.14). Panoramic

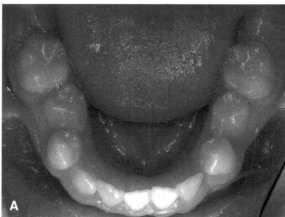

Fig. 21.11 (A) Clinical photograph of mandibular second premolar macrodontia. (B) Panoramic image shows the greater mesial/distal widths of the tooth crowns compared with their respective first premolars. (Courtesy Dr. H. Grubisa, Oakville, Ontario, Canada.)

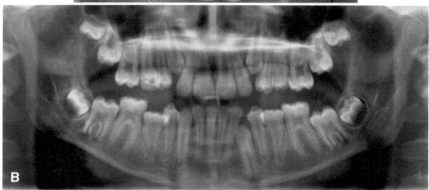

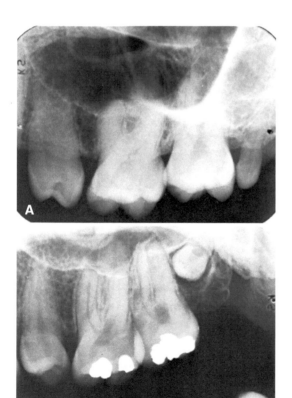

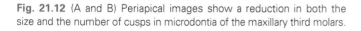

Fig. 21.12 (A and B) Periapical images show a reduction in both the size and the number of cusps in microdontia of the maxillary third molars.

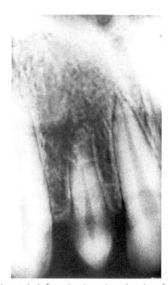

Fig. 21.13 Peg-shaped deformity in microdontia of a maxillary lateral incisor.

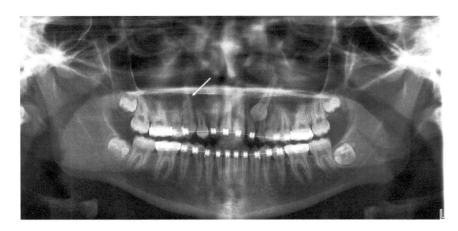

Fig. 21.14 Panoramic image demonstrating transposition of the right maxillary canine *(arrow)* and first premolar.

and CBCT imaging can aid in determining the positions and locations of these teeth.

Differential interpretation. Transposed teeth are usually easily recognized by examining the individual morphologies of the involved teeth.

Management. Transposed teeth are frequently altered prosthetically for function or esthetics, or both.

Altered Morphology of Teeth
Fusion

Disease mechanism. Fusion of teeth results from the union of adjacent tooth germs of developing teeth. Some authors believe that fusion results when two tooth germs develop so close together that, as they grow, they contact and fuse before calcification is complete. Other authors contend that a physical force or pressure produced during development causes contact of adjacent tooth buds. Males and females experience fusion in equal numbers, and the incidence is higher in Asian and Indigenous populations.

Clinical features. Fusion results in a reduced number of teeth in the arch. Although fusion is more common in the deciduous dentition, it may also occur in the permanent dentition. When a deciduous canine and lateral incisor fuse, the corresponding permanent lateral incisor may be absent. Fusion is more common in anterior teeth of both the deciduous and permanent dentitions (Fig. 21.15). Fusion may be total or partial, depending on the stage of odontogenesis and the proximity of the developing teeth. The result can vary from a single tooth of about normal size to a tooth of nearly twice the normal size. The crowns of fused teeth usually appear to be large and single, although incisal clefts of varying depth or a bifid crown can sometimes occur.

Imaging features. Periapical images, or small or limited field of view (FOV) CBCT, will be helpful in disclosing the unusual shapes or sizes of the fused teeth. The true nature and extent of the union are frequently more evident on an image than can be determined by clinical examination. Fused teeth may also show an unusual configuration of the pulp chamber or root canal.

Differential interpretation. The differential interpretation for fused teeth includes gemination and macrodontia. Fusion may be differentiated from gemination when the number of teeth is reduced by one, except in the unusual case in which a normal tooth and a supernumerary tooth have fused. The differentiation is usually academic because little difference exists in the treatment provided.

Management. The management of a case of fusion depends on which teeth are involved, the degree of fusion, and the morphologic result. If the affected teeth are deciduous, they may be retained as they are. If the clinician contemplates extraction, it is important first to

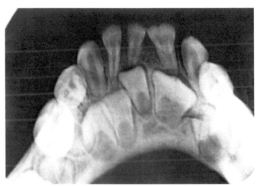

Fig. 21.15 Fusion of the central and lateral incisors in both the primary and the permanent dentitions. Note the reduction in number of teeth and the increased width of the fused tooth mass.

determine whether the permanent teeth are present. In the case of fused permanent teeth, the fused crowns may be reshaped with a restoration that mimics two independent crowns. The morphology of fused teeth requires radiologic examination before the teeth are reshaped. Endodontic therapy may be necessary and perhaps may be difficult or impossible if the root canals are of unusual shape. In some cases, it is most prudent to leave the teeth as they are.

Concrescence

Disease mechanism. Concrescence occurs when the roots of two or more primary or permanent teeth are fused through cementum. Although the cause is unknown, many authorities suspect that space restriction during development, local trauma, excessive occlusal force, or local infection after development plays an important role. If the condition occurs during development, it is sometimes referred to as true concrescence. If the condition occurs later, it is referred to as acquired concrescence.

Clinical features. Maxillary molars are the teeth most frequently involved, especially a third molar and a supernumerary tooth. Involved teeth may fail to erupt or may erupt incompletely. The sexes are equally affected.

Imaging features. An imaging examination may not always reveal concrescence; teeth may be in close contact or are simply superimposed (Fig. 21.16). When the condition is suspected on an image and extraction of one of the teeth is being considered, additional intraoral images made at different angles, or small FOV CBCT may be obtained to delineate the condition better.

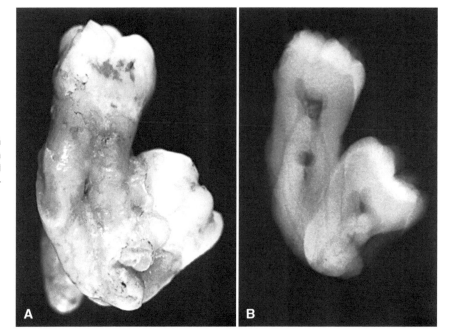

Fig. 21.16 (A) Concrescence occurs when two teeth are joined by cementum. (B) Extraction of one tooth may result in the unintended removal of the second because the cementum bridge may not be well visualized. (Courtesy Dr. R. Kienholz, Dallas, TX.)

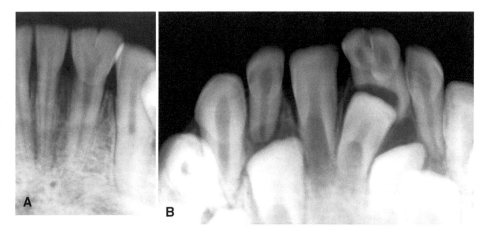

Fig. 21.17 (A) Gemination of a mandibular lateral incisor showing bifurcation of the crown and pulp chamber. (B) Almost complete gemination of a deciduous lateral incisor.

Differential interpretation. It is usually impossible to determine with certainty whether the images of teeth whose roots appear to be superimposed are actually joined. If the roots are joined, it may be impossible to tell whether the union is by cementum or by dentin (fusion). In this regard, the absence of a periodontal ligament (PDL) space between the roots may be helpful.

Management. Concrescence affects treatment only when the decision is made to remove one or both of the involved teeth because this condition complicates the extraction. The clinician should warn the patient that an effort to remove one might result in the unintended and simultaneous removal of the other.

Gemination

Disease mechanism. Gemination or twinning is a rare anomaly that arises when a single tooth bud attempts to divide. The result may be an invagination of the crown with partial clefting or, in rare cases, complete division through the crown and root, producing identical structures. Complete twinning results in a normal tooth plus a supernumerary tooth in the arch. The cause of gemination is unknown, but some evidence suggests that it may have a genetic basis.

Clinical features. Although gemination may occur in both the deciduous and the permanent dentitions, the primary teeth are more often affected, usually in the incisor region. It can be detected clinically after the anomalous tooth erupts. The occurrence in males and females is about equal. The enamel or dentin of geminated teeth may be hypoplastic or hypocalcified.

Imaging features. Images reveal the altered shape of the hard tissue and pulp chamber of the geminated tooth. Multiple periapical images made from different angles, panoramic, or CBCT images can aid in the diagnosis. Radiopaque enamel outlines the clefts in the crowns and invaginations, and accentuates them. The pulp chamber is usually single and enlarged, and may be partially divided (Figs. 21.17 and 21.18). In the rare case of premolar gemination, the tooth image suggests a molar with an enlarged crown and two roots.

Differential interpretation. The differential interpretation of gemination includes fusion. If the malformed tooth is counted as one, individuals with gemination have a normal tooth count, whereas individuals with fusion are seen to be missing a tooth.

Management. A geminated tooth in the incisor area may compromise arch esthetics and arch length. Areas of hypoplasia, invagination lines,

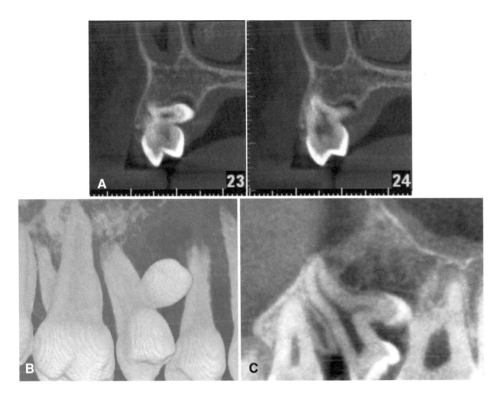

Fig. 21.18 (A) Gemination of a maxillary left second premolar on cross-sectional slices. (B) Three-dimensional surface rendering demonstrating the geminating tooth and its association with the premolar. (C) Coronal cone beam computed tomography image of another case of gemination of a second premolar. Note the common root canal. ([A and B] Courtesy Dr. B. Friedland, Cambridge, MA.)

or areas of coronal separation represent caries-susceptible sites that may in time result in pulpal inflammation. Affected teeth can cause malocclusion and lead to the development of periodontal disease. Consequently, the affected tooth may be removed (especially if it is deciduous), the crown may be restored or reshaped, or the tooth may be left untreated and periodically examined to preclude the development of complications. Before treatment is initiated on a primary tooth, the status of the permanent tooth and configuration of its root canals should be determined by imaging.

Taurodontism

Disease mechanism. The bodies of taurodont teeth appear elongated, and the roots are short. The pulp chamber extends from a normal position in the crown throughout the length of the elongated body, resulting in a more apically positioned pulpal floor.

Taurodontism may affect any tooth in either the primary or permanent dentitions, and is usually fully expressed in the molars and less often in the premolars. Single or multiple teeth may show taurodont features.

Clinical features. The distinguishing features of taurodont teeth are not recognizable clinically, because the body and roots of taurodont teeth are within the bone.

Imaging features. The distinctive morphology of taurodont teeth is quite apparent on images. The peculiar feature is the elongated pulp chamber and the more apically positioned furcation (Fig. 21.19). The shortened roots and root canals are a function of the long body and normal length of the tooth. The dimensions of the crown are normal. Periapical and panoramic images help with the diagnosis of this condition.

Differential interpretation. The image of the taurodont tooth is characteristic and easily recognized on imaging. The developing molar may appear similar; however, identification of the wide apical foramina and incompletely formed roots aids in the differential interpretation. Taurodontism has been reported in hypophosphatemia and with greater frequency in patients with trisomy 21.

Management. Taurodont teeth do not require treatment.

Dilaceration

Disease mechanism. Dilaceration is a disturbance in tooth formation that produces a sharp bend or curve in the tooth anywhere in the crown or the root. Although this anomaly is likely developmental in nature, one of the oldest hypotheses is that dilaceration is the result of mechanical trauma to the calcified portion of a partially formed tooth.

Clinical features. Most cases of radicular dilaceration are not recognized clinically. If the dilaceration is so pronounced that the tooth does not erupt, the only clinical indication of the defect is a missing tooth. If the defect is in the crown of an erupted tooth, it may be readily recognized as an angular distortion (Fig. 21.20).

Imaging features. Imaging provides the best means of detecting a radicular dilaceration. One or more teeth may be affected, and the condition occurs most often in maxillary premolars. If the roots dilacerate mesially or distally, the condition is clearly apparent on a periapical image (Fig. 21.21). However, when the roots are dilacerated buccally (labially) or lingually, the central x-ray passes approximately parallel to the deflected portion of the root, and the apical end of the root may have the appearance of a circular or oval radiopaque area with a central radiolucency (the apical foramen and root canal), giving the appearance of a "bull's-eye". The periodontal ligament space around this dilacerated portion may be seen as a radiolucent halo encircling the radiopaque area (Fig. 21.22). In some cases, especially in the maxilla, the geometry of the projections may preclude the recognition of a dilaceration.

Differential interpretation. Occasionally, dilacerated roots may be difficult to differentiate from fused roots, sclerosing osteitis, or a dense bone island. However, these usually can be discerned by making a second image at a different angle.

Management. A dilacerated root generally does not require treatment because it provides adequate support. If the tooth is to be extracted for some other reason, the removal can be complicated, especially if the clinician is not prepared with a preoperative image. In contrast, dilacerated crowns are frequently restored with a prosthetic crown to improve esthetics and function.

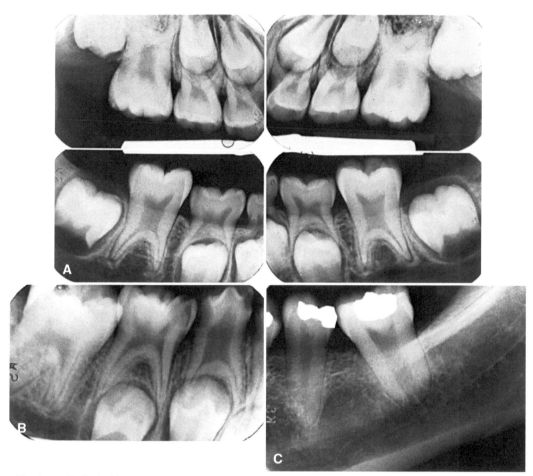

Fig. 21.19 Periapical images reveal enlarged pulp chambers and apically positioned furcations in permanent first molars (A), a primary first molar (B), and a permanent molar (C).

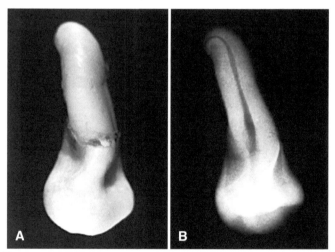

Fig. 21.20 (A) Dilaceration of the crown may be recognized clinically. (B) Image of the specimen in A. (Courtesy Dr. R. Kienholz, Dallas, Texas.)

Dens Invaginatus, Dens in Dente, and Dilated Odontome

Disease mechanism. Dens invaginatus, dens in dente, and dilated odontome represent varying degrees of invagination or infolding of the enamel surface into the interior of a tooth. The least severe form of this infolding is dens invaginatus, and the most severe form is dilated

odontome. The invagination can occur in the crown or the root during tooth development. It may also involve the pulp chamber or root canal system; this may result in a deformity of either the crown or the root, although these anomalies are seen most often in tooth crowns.

Based on the severity of the invagination, Oehler classified them into three types. In type I, the invagination is confined to the crown and does not extend apical to the cementoenamel junction. In type II, the invagination extends to the pulp chamber but remains within the root canal with no communication to the periodontal ligament space. In type IIIA, the invagination extends through the root and communicates to the periodontal ligament space. And in type IIIB, the invagination extends through the root and communicates with the periodontal ligament space at the apical foramen.

Coronal invaginations usually originate from an anomalous infolding of the enamel organ into the dental papilla. In a mature tooth, the result is a fold of hard tissue within the tooth characterized by enamel lining the fold (Fig. 21.23). When the abnormality involves the root, it may be the result of an invagination of the Hertwig epithelial root sheath and produce an accentuation of the normal longitudinal root groove.

In contrast to the coronal type, which is lined with enamel, the radicular type of defect is lined with cementum. If the invagination retracts and is cut off, it leaves a longitudinal structure of cementum, bone, and remnants of the periodontal ligament within the root canal. The structure often extends for most of the root length. In other cases, the root sheath may bud off a sac-like invagination that produces a circumscribed cementum defect in the root. Mandibular first premolars

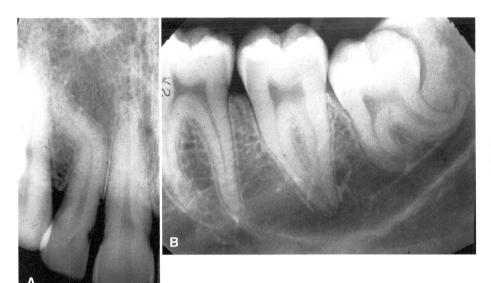

Fig. 21.21 Dilaceration of the root of a maxillary lateral incisor (A) and mandibular third molar (B).

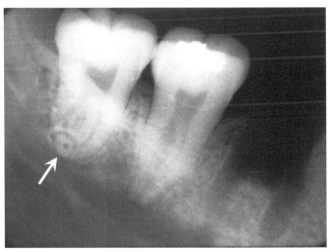

Fig. 21.22 The most apical portion of this third molar root is dilacerated in the buccal-lingual direction so that its long axis lies along the path of the x-ray beam. Note the "bull's-eye" appearance of the root apex produced by the root canal, tooth root, and periodontal ligament space *(arrow).*

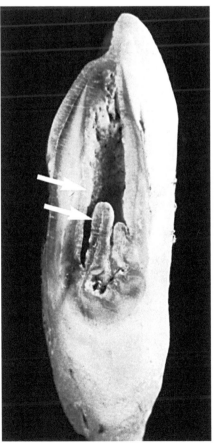

Fig. 21.23 Dens in Dente Is Characterized by an Infolding of Enamel Into the Tooth. This sectioned canine with a dens in dente shows enamel *(arrows)* folded into the tooth's interior.

and second molars are especially prone to develop the radicular variety of this invagination anomaly.

Among Caucasians and Asians, there is little difference in frequency of occurrence. If all types of expression of invagination are included, the condition is found in approximately 5% of these two population groups. The condition appears to be rare in individuals of African descent. No sexual predilection exists. Although no specific mode of inheritance seems to fit all the data, a high degree of inheritability seems to exist.

Clinical features. Dens invaginatus may appear as nothing more than a small pit between the cingulum and the lingual surface of an incisor tooth (Fig. 21.24). In dens in dente, the pit is located at the incisal edge of the tooth, and crown morphology may appear abnormal, having the appearance of a peg-shaped microdont tooth (Fig. 21.25). A dilated odontome is the most extreme form of tooth invagination, and has roughly the shape of a doughnut with a central radiolucent soft tissue region surrounded by radiopaque dental hard tissue.

Dens invaginatus and dens in dente occur most frequently in the permanent maxillary lateral incisors, followed by (in decreasing frequency) the maxillary central incisors, premolars, and canines, and less often the posterior teeth. Invagination is rare in the crowns of mandibular teeth and in deciduous teeth. The abnormality occurs symmetrically

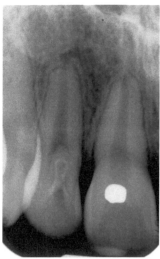

Fig. 21.24 Radiopaque, inverted teardrop outline of dens invaginatus in a maxillary lateral incisor. Note the position of the invagination in the cingulum area of the tooth crown.

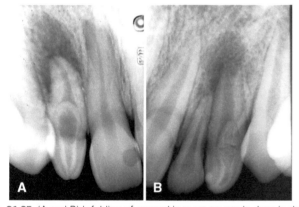

Fig. 21.25 (A and B) Infolding of enamel is more severe in dens in dente as seen in these two periapical images. The invagination begins near the incisal edge of these abnormally peg-shaped lateral incisors.

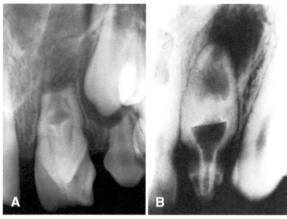

Fig. 21.26 (A and B) Severe forms of dens in dente usually result in necrosis of the pulp, open apices, and rarefying osteitis at the tooth apices.

in about half the cases, and involvement of both the central and lateral incisors may occur.

The clinical importance of dens invaginatus and dens in dente is the risk of pulpal inflammation and necrosis. The base of the invagination is usually separated from the pulp chamber by a relatively thin wall of enamel and dentin that line the base of the invagination. Here, the enamel is frequently thin, often of poor quality, and even missing in some areas. The opening of the invagination communicates with the oral cavity through a narrow constriction. The pit that is seen clinically is often difficult, if not impossible to keep clean, and consequently it offers conditions favorable for the colonization of bacteria, and the development of caries. Carious lesions are difficult to detect clinically, and rapidly involve the pulp. In addition, sometimes fine canals extend between the invagination and the pulp chamber, resulting in pulpal disease even in the absence of caries.

Imaging features. Most cases of dens invaginatus or dens in dente are discovered with imaging, and can be identified in the image even before the tooth erupts. The infolding of the enamel lining is more radiopaque than the surrounding tooth structure and can be identified easily as an inverted teardrop-shaped radiolucency with a radiopaque border (see Figs. 21.24 and 21.25). Less frequently, the radicular invaginations appear as poorly defined, slightly radiolucent structures running longitudinally within the root. The defects, especially the coronal variety, may vary in size and shape from small and superficial to large and deep. If a coronal invagination is extensive, then the crown is typically malformed, and the apical foramen is usually wide (Fig. 21.26). A frequent cause of an open apical foramen is the cessation of root development that occurs as a result of death of the pulpal tissue. In the most severe form (dilated odontome), the tooth is severely deformed, having a circular or oval shape with a radiolucent interior (Fig. 21.27). Severe forms of invagination may require CBCT to further evaluate the classification and plan appropriate treatment.

Differential interpretation. The appearance and usual occurrence in incisors are so characteristic that, once recognized, little probability exists that the anomaly will be confused with another condition.

Management. Although it is important to evaluate every case individually, the placement of a prophylactic restoration in the defect is typically the treatment of choice and should ensure a normal life span for the tooth. Failure of early identification and treatment may result in premature tooth loss or the need for root canal therapy.

Dens Evaginatus

Disease mechanism. In contrast to dens invaginatus or dens in dente, dens evaginatus (or Leong premolar) is the result of an evagination or outpouching of the enamel organ. The resultant enamel-covered tubercle usually occurs in or near the middle of the occlusal surface of premolar or occasionally molar teeth (Fig. 21.28). Lateral incisors are most commonly involved, whereas canines are rarely affected. The frequency of occurrence of dens evaginatus is highest in Asian and Indigenous populations.

Clinical features. Clinically, dens evaginatus appears as a tubercle of enamel on the occlusal surface of the affected tooth. A hard, polyp-like protuberance predominantly exists in the central groove or lingual ridge of a buccal cusp of posterior teeth and in the cingulum fossa of anterior teeth. Dens evaginatus may occur bilaterally and usually in the mandible. The tubercle often has a dentin core, and a very slender pulp horn frequently extends into the evagination. After the tubercle is worn down by the opposing dentition, it appears as a small circular facet with a small black pit in the center (Fig. 21.29). Wear, fracture, or indiscriminate surgical removal of this tubercle may precipitate exposure of the pulp and an inflammatory response. In rare cases, a microscopic direct communication may occur between the pulp and the oral cavity through

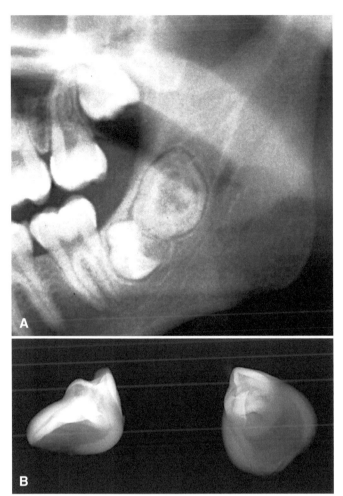

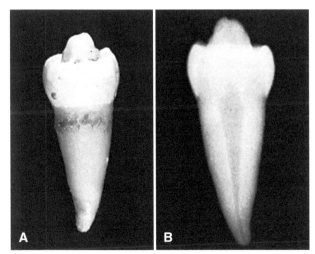

Fig. 21.27 (A) Dilated odontome, the most severe enamel invagination, is positioned just posterior to the developing mandibular third molar in this panoramic image. (B) Images of the extracted dilated odontome from two different angulations.

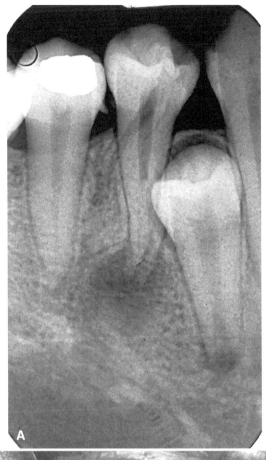

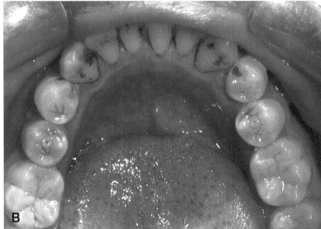

Fig. 21.29 (A) Periapical image of a mandibular first premolar with a dens evaginatus and apical rarefying osteitis. (B) Clinical photograph of another case of dens evaginatus involving the mandibular second premolar teeth, bilaterally.

Fig. 21.28 (A) Occlusal tubercle of dens evaginatus as seen in a mandibular premolar. (B) Periapical image of the specimen. (Courtesy Dr. R. Kienholz, Dallas, TX.)

this tubercle. In these instances, the pulp may become infected shortly after eruption.

Imaging features. Imaging shows an extension of a dentin tubercle on the occlusal surface unless the tubercle is already worn down. The dentin core is usually covered with radiopaque enamel. A fine pulp horn may extend into the tubercle, but this may not be visible in the image. If the tubercle has been worn to the point of pulpal exposure or has fractured, pulpal necrosis may result (see Fig. 21.29). Necrosis is indicated by an open apical foramen and periapical radiolucency. Multiple root formation is often associated with dens evaginatus, especially in mandibular premolars.

Differential interpretation. The clinical and imaging appearances may be characteristic or may be difficult to visualize if the tubercle has been worn down to the occlusal surface.

Management. If the tubercle causes any occlusal interference or shows evidence of marked abrasion, it probably should be removed under aseptic conditions, and the pulp should be capped, if necessary. Such a precaution may preclude pulpal exposure and infection as the result of accidental fracture or advanced abrasion.

Molar-Incisor Malformation

Disease mechanism. Molar-incisor malformation (MIM) is a rare developmental dental anomaly seen in the primary second molars and permanent first molars, and sometimes the permanent maxillary central incisors. The etiology of MIM is not fully understood at this time, although it is believed to be the result of an epigenetic factor linked to a systemic condition affecting the central nervous system when the patient is 1 to 2 years of age. Parents may report a history of neurological medical complications at birth or in the first 2 years of life.

Clinical features. Clinical features may include poor incisor esthetics, impactions of teeth, early exfoliation, space loss, periapical inflammatory disease, and spontaneous pain. The major manifestations are severe coronal cervical constriction of the affected molars and significant underdevelopment of one or more roots. MIM may also present with ectopic eruption of teeth.

Imaging features. The imaging features include constriction of the crowns at the cervical region, and some patients may show an abnormal notch-like defect at the cervical enamel of the permanent maxillary central incisors. The roots of all permanent first molars may appear hypoplastic with compromised bone support, and there may also be furcation involvement.

Management. As there is often a stronger expression in the molars, identifying spontaneous ectopic eruption of permanent first molars and cervical constriction is important for management. Maintaining good periodontal health and circumferential bone is vital for adequate support to the tooth and, potentially, future implant placement. Careful planning using a team-based approach with the patient's pediatric dentist and orthodontist will be the key to manage this condition.

Amelogenesis Imperfecta

Disease mechanism. Amelogenesis imperfecta is a genetic anomaly arising from mutations that may have occurred in one or more of four candidate genes that play some role in enamel formation: amelogenin (*AMELX*), enamelin (*ENAM*), enamelysin (*MMP20*), and kallikrein 4 (*KLK4*). The mutation may be inherited in an autosomal dominant or recessive manner, or it may be inherited in an X-linked pattern. These mutations lead to changes in the enamel of teeth in both dentitions, and are not related to any time or period of enamel development or any clinically demonstrable alteration (disease or dietary abnormality) in other tissues. In the hypoplastic and hypomineralized types of AI, the enamel may lack the normal prismatic structure and be laminated throughout its thickness or at the periphery. In these cases, the teeth have been reported to be more resistant to decay. The dentin and root form are usually normal. Eruption of the affected teeth is often delayed, and a tendency for tooth impaction exists. Although at least 14 variants of the condition have been described, four general types have been delineated on the basis of their clinical or imaging appearances: a hypoplastic type, a hypomaturation type, a hypocalcified type, and a hypomaturation-hypoplastic type associated with taurodontism.

Clinical features

Hypoplastic type. The enamel of the affected teeth fails to develop to its normal thickness. Consequently, the color of the underlying dentin

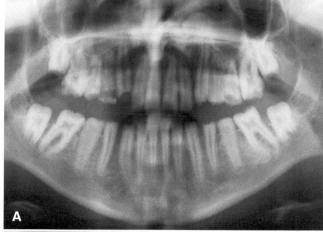
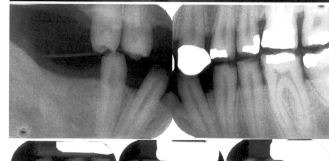
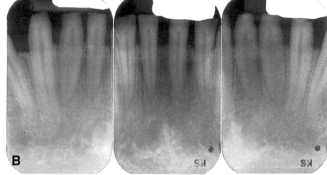

Fig. 21.30 (A) Cropped panoramic image of hypoplastic amelogenesis imperfecta. Note the absence of interproximal contacts and the "picket fence"–like appearance of the teeth. (B) Intraoral images of another case of amelogenesis imperfecta. Note the very thin enamel layer. ([A] Courtesy Dr. S. Roth, Halifax, Nova Scotia, Canada.)

imparts a yellow-brown color to the tooth. In addition, the enamel may be abnormal; the surface may be rough, pitted, smooth, or glossy. The crowns of the teeth may appear undersized with a roughly square shape. The reduced enamel thickness also causes a generalized loss of interproximal contacts between adjacent teeth (Fig. 21.30). The occlusal surfaces of the posterior teeth are relatively flat with low cusps. This is a result of the attrition of cusp tips that were initially low and not fully formed. Hypoplastic amelogenesis imperfecta is the type that is most easily identifiable on imaging.

Hypomaturation. In the hypomaturation form of amelogenesis imperfecta, the enamel has a mottled appearance but is of normal thickness. The enamel is softer than normal, its density comparable to dentin, and it may break away from the crown. Its color may range from clear to cloudy white, yellow, or brown. In one form of hypomaturation amelogenesis imperfecta, the teeth may be capped with white, opaque enamel. This appearance has been referred to as "snow-capped" teeth.

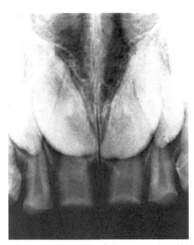

Fig. 21.31 The reduced radiopacity of the enamel and the rapid abrasion of the crowns of the primary teeth are features of hypomineralized amelogenesis imperfecta.

Hypocalcification. The hypocalcific form of amelogenesis imperfecta is more common than the hypoplastic variety. The crowns of the teeth are normal in size and shape when they erupt because the enamel is of regular thickness (Fig. 21.31). However, because the enamel is poorly mineralized (it is less dense than dentin), it starts to fracture shortly after it comes into function, and this creates clinically recognizable defects. The soft enamel abrades rapidly, and the softer dentin also wears down rapidly, resulting in a grossly worn tooth, sometimes to the level of the gingiva. An explorer point under pressure can penetrate the soft enamel, yet caries in these worn teeth is unusual. The hypocalcified enamel has increased permeability and becomes stained and darkened. The teeth of a young person with generalized hypomineralization of the enamel are frequently dark brown from food stains.

Hypomaturation-hypoplastic with taurodontism. This classification indicates a combination of hypomaturation and hypoplastic with taurodontism.

Imaging features. Amelogenesis imperfecta is identified primarily by its clinical features, although imaging can help substantiate the clinical impression. The imaging features of hypoplastic amelogenesis imperfecta include a square crown, a relatively thin radiopaque layer of enamel, low or absent cusps, and multiple open contacts between the teeth. The anterior teeth on images are said to have a "picket fence"—type appearance. The density of the enamel is normal. When the enamel is pitted, the appearance is that of sharply localized areas of mottled density, quite different from the image cast by a tooth that is normal in shape and density. The hypomaturation form exhibits a normal thickness of the enamel, but the normal density between enamel and dentin is lost. In such cases, the enamel may be very similar in density to dentin. In the hypocalcified forms, the enamel thickness is normal, but its density is even less (i.e., more radiolucent) than that of dentin. With advanced abrasion, obliteration of the pulp chambers may complicate recognition of the image.

Differential interpretation. If advanced abrasion is present and secondary dentin obliterates the pulp chambers, the imaging features of amelogenesis imperfecta may appear similar to that of dentinogenesis imperfecta. However, the presence of bulbous crowns and narrow roots, the relatively normal density of any remaining enamel, and the obliteration of pulp chambers and root canals, in the absence of marked attrition, are characteristic features of dentinogenesis imperfecta (see the following section), and should distinguish it from amelogenesis imperfecta.

Management. Appropriate treatment for amelogenesis imperfecta is restoration of the esthetics and function of the affected teeth.

Dentinogenesis Imperfecta

Disease mechanism. Dentinogenesis imperfecta or hereditary opalescent dentin is a genetic anomaly involving primarily the dentin, although the enamel may be thinner than normal in this condition. Dentinogenesis imperfecta occurs with equal frequency in both sexes. Both the deciduous and the permanent dentition may have this defect. Three forms of dentinogenesis imperfecta have been described, and each has been associated with a particular gene. Type I dentinogenesis imperfecta, which is associated with osteogenesis imperfecta, is caused by mutations of one of two genes involved in collagen synthesis: the collagen type I alpha 1 (*COL1A1*) and collagen type I alpha 2 (*COL1A2*) genes. Types II and III dentinogenesis imperfecta are caused by mutations of the dentin sialoprotein (*DSP*) and dentin sialophosphoprotein (*DSPP*) genes.

The tooth roots and pulp chambers of type I teeth are generally small and underdeveloped, and the primary dentition may be more severely affected than the permanent dentition. Type II dentinogenesis imperfecta is similar to type I but affects the dentin only without any skeletal defects. The expression of type II dentinogenesis imperfecta is variable, and occasionally individuals exhibit enlarged pulp chambers in the primary teeth. Type III dentinogenesis imperfecta, or the so-called Brandywine isolate, was described in a population of less than 200 persons in the Brandywine region of Maryland. There is some controversy regarding the differentiation between types II and III; however, type III teeth are said to exhibit enlarged pulp chambers, making them more susceptible to pulp exposure.

Dentinogenesis imperfecta is found in association with approximately 25% of cases of osteogenesis imperfecta, a hereditary disorder characterized by an inborn error in the synthesis of type I collagen. The abnormality is usually transmitted as an autosomal dominant trait. Osteogenesis imperfecta results in brittle bones, but in addition, patients may have blue sclerae, wormian bones (bones in skull sutures), skeletal deformities, and progressive osteopenia. Oral findings may also include class III malocclusions and an increased incidence of impacted first and second molars.

Clinical features. The appearance of teeth with dentinogenesis imperfecta is characteristic. The crowns exhibit a high degree of amber-like translucency and various colors from yellow to blue-gray. The colors change according to whether the teeth are observed with transmitted or reflected light. The enamel easily fractures from the teeth, and the crowns wear readily. In adults, the teeth frequently may wear down to the gingiva. The exposed dentin becomes stained. The color of the abraded teeth may change to dark brown or black. Some patients demonstrate an anterior open bite.

Imaging features. The crowns in patients with dentinogenesis imperfecta are usually normal in size, but there is a marked constriction of the tooth crown in the cervical region of the tooth that gives the crown a bulbous appearance. Images may reveal attrition of the occlusal surface. The roots are usually thin and slender, and there may be partial or complete obliteration of the pulp chambers. Early in development, the teeth may appear to have large pulp chambers, but these are quickly obliterated by the formation of dentin. Ultimately, the root canals may be narrow and threadlike, or obliterated (Fig. 21.32). Occasionally areas of rarefying osteitis may be seen in association with what appear to be sound teeth without evidence of pulpal involvement. These changes may occur as a result of microscopic communications between the residual pulp and the oral cavity. These lesions do not occur as frequently as in dentin dysplasia. The architecture of the bone in the maxilla and mandible is normal.

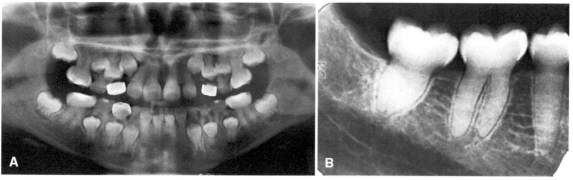

Fig. 21.32 (A and B) Dentinogenesis imperfecta characteristically shows bulbous crowns, constriction of tooth at the cementoenamel junction, short roots, and a reduced size of the pulp chamber and root canals.

Differential interpretation. Dentin dysplasia (see the following section) is the differential interpretation.

Management. The placement of prosthetic crowns on the affected teeth is usually unsuccessful unless the teeth have good root support. The teeth should not be extracted from patients 5 to 15 years old. It is generally preferable to place full overdentures on the teeth to prevent alveolar resorption. In adults, extraction of the teeth and their replacement can be recommended.

Dentin Dysplasia

Disease mechanism. Dentin dysplasia is a genetically inherited autosomal dominant abnormality that affects dentin. In type I or radicular dentin dysplasia, the most marked changes are found in the appearances of the tooth roots. In type II or coronal dentin dysplasia, changes to the crowns are most clearly seen in the altered shape of the pulp chambers. Mutations of the *DSPP* gene, the same gene that has been implicated in dentinogenesis imperfecta types II and III, have also been implicated in type II dentin dysplasia. Dentin dysplasia occurs less frequently than dentinogenesis imperfecta (1 : 100,000 vs. 1 : 8000).

Clinical features. Clinically, teeth with type I radicular dentin dysplasia have mostly normal color and shape in the primary and adult dentitions. Occasionally, a slight bluish brown translucency is apparent. The teeth are often misaligned in the arch, and patients may describe drifting and spontaneous exfoliation with little or no trauma. In type II coronal dentin dysplasia, the crowns of the primary teeth appear to be of the same color, size, and contour as teeth with dentinogenesis imperfecta—an interesting coincidence in light of the purported close genetic linkage between the two dentin abnormalities. Although not universally accepted, reports exist that primary teeth rapidly abrade. The permanent teeth have clinically normal-appearing crowns.

Imaging features. In type I dentin dysplasia, the roots of both the primary and the permanent teeth are either short or abnormally shaped (Fig. 21.33). The molar roots have been described as having a shallow W-shape. The roots of primary teeth may be only thin spicules. The pulp chambers and root canals become completely obliterated before eruption; however, this is variable. In addition, about 20% of teeth with type I dentin dysplasia are associated with rarefying osteitis—likely the result of microscopic communications between the residual pulp and the oral cavity. Association of periapical inflammatory disease with noncarious teeth is an important feature for recognition of this particular entity. In type II dentin dysplasia, obliteration of the pulp chamber (Fig. 21.34) and reduction in the calibers of the root canals occur after eruption (at least by 5 or 6 years), in contrast with type I dentin dysplasia. As the pulp chambers of the molars are filled with hypertrophic dentin, the pulp chambers may become flame- or thistle-shaped, and there may be multiple pulp stones. Occasionally, the anterior teeth and

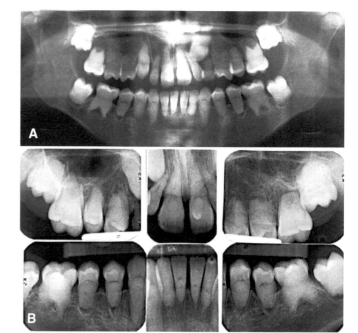

Fig. 21.33 Panoramic (A) and periapical (B) images of the same case show the short, poorly developed roots; obliterated pulp chambers and root canals; and periapical rarefying osteitis associated with type I (radicular) dentin dysplasia. Note the half-moon or "demilune" shape of the pulp chambers.

premolars develop a pulp chamber that is thistle tube in shape because of its extension into the root. The roots of the coronal variety are normal in shape and proportions.

Differential interpretation. The differential interpretation for dentin dysplasia includes only dentinogenesis imperfecta because both abnormalities can appear clinically similar. Both entities can produce crowns with altered color and obliterated pulp chambers. The finding of a thistle tube–shaped pulp chamber in a single-rooted tooth strengthens the probability of dentin dysplasia. However, in type II dentin dysplasia, the pulp chambers become obliterated after eruption.

Sometimes crown size can help distinguish between the two. The teeth in dentinogenesis imperfecta typically have bulbous-shaped crowns with a constriction in the cervical region, whereas the crowns in dentin dysplasia are usually of normal shape, size, and proportion. If the roots are short and narrow, the condition is likely to be dentinogenesis imperfecta. Normal-appearing roots or practically no roots at all should

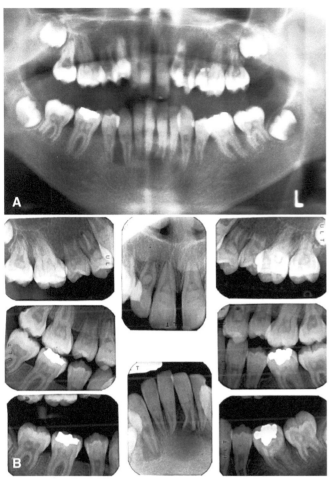

Fig. 21.34 Panoramic (A) and periapical (B) images of the same case show obliteration of the pulp chamber, reduction in the caliber of root canals, and pulp stones obscuring the flame-shaped or thistle-shaped pulp chambers associated with type II (coronal) dentin dysplasia. Note the areas of rarefying osteitis associated with some of the mandibular anterior teeth.

suggest dentin dysplasia. Periapical rarefying osteitis in association with noncarious teeth is more commonly seen in dentin dysplasia.

Management. Teeth with type I dentin dysplasia have such poor root support that prosthetic replacement is about the only practical treatment. Teeth that are of normal shape, size, and support (type II) can have coronal coverage with fixed prosthodontic treatment, if they seem to be rapidly abrading. The esthetics of discolored anterior teeth can be improved by prosthetic treatment.

Regional Odontodysplasia

Disease mechanism. Regional odontodysplasia, or "ghost teeth," is a rare condition in which both enamel and dentin are hypoplastic and hypocalcified. This localized arrest in tooth development typically affects only a few adjacent teeth in a quadrant—ergo "regional." These teeth may be either primary or permanent. If the primary teeth are affected, their successors are usually also involved. Although many theories exist regarding the etiology of this condition, including a vascular etiology, its cause is unknown.

Clinical features. Teeth affected with regional odontodysplasia are small and mottled brown as a result of staining of the hypocalcified and hypoplastic enamel. They are especially susceptible to caries, brittle,

and subject to fracture and pulpal infection. Central incisors are most often affected, with lateral incisors and canines also occasionally exhibiting the defect (most often in the maxilla). Eruption of the defective teeth is often delayed, and in severe cases they may not erupt.

Imaging features. Because these teeth are very poorly mineralized, the images of teeth with regional odontodysplasia have been described as having a "ghost-like" appearance. The pulp chambers are large and the root canals are wide because the hypoplastic dentin is thin, serving just to outline the image of the root (Fig. 21.35). Also, the poorly outlined roots are short. The enamel likewise is thin and less dense than usual— sometimes so thin and poorly mineralized that it may not be evident on the image. The tooth is little more than a thin shell of hypoplastic enamel and dentin. Teeth that do not erupt are so hypomineralized and hypoplastic that they appear to be resorbing.

Differential interpretation. The malformed teeth occasionally seen in one of the expressions of dentinogenesis imperfecta occasionally may be confused with teeth in regional odontodysplasia. Only a few teeth of either dentition in an isolated segment of the arch are affected in regional odontodysplasia, whereas dentinogenesis imperfecta that resembles regional odontodysplasia is generalized. In addition, the enamel in regional odontodysplasia is hypoplastic, which is not the case in dentinogenesis imperfecta. Finally, the fact that the dentinogenesis imperfecta trait usually carries a history of familial involvement, in contrast to regional odontodysplasia (which is not hereditary), is another important distinguishing feature.

Management. With the advent of newer restorative materials, it is recommended to retain and restore the affected teeth as much as possible. Unerupted teeth should be retained during the period of skeletal growth. Severely damaged permanent teeth with pulpal involvement may require extraction and replacement.

Enamel Pearl

Disease mechanism. The enamel pearl or enameloma is a small formation of enamel 1 to 3 mm in diameter that occurs on the roots of molars (Fig. 21.36). It is found in about 3% of the population, probably formed by cells in the Hertwig epithelial root sheath before the epithelium loses its enamel-forming potential. Usually only one pearl develops, but occasionally more may develop. Enamel pearls may have a core of dentin and rarely a pulp horn extending from the chamber of the host tooth.

Clinical features. Most enamel pearls form apical to the gingival crest, and are not detected during a clinical examination. They typically develop in the furcal areas of molar teeth, often lying at or just apical to the cementoenamel junction. Enamel pearls that form on the maxillary molars are usually in the mesial or distal furca, and pearls that develop in mandibular molars are located in the buccal or lingual furca. Usually no clinical symptoms are associated with their presence, although they may predispose to formation of a periodontal pocket and subsequent periodontal disease.

Imaging features. The enamel pearl appears smooth, round, and comparable in degree of radiopacity to the enamel covering the crown (Fig. 21.37). Occasionally the dentin casts a small, round, radiolucent shadow in the center of the radiopaque sphere of enamel. If projected over the crown, it may be obscured.

Differential interpretation. It is possible to mistake an enamel pearl for an isolated piece of calculus or a pulp stone. The differentiation between a pulp stone and an enamel pearl can be made by increasing the vertical angle of projection to move the image of the enamel pearl away from the pulp chamber. If the opacity is a calculus, it is usually clinically detectable. Occasionally, oblique views of maxillary or mandibular molars may cause superimposition of a portion of the roots in the region of the furcation, producing a density that appears similar

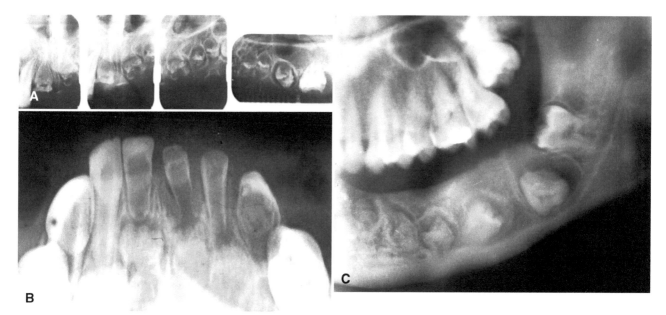

Fig. 21.35 Periapical Images Reveal Poor Mineralization of All of the Dental Hard Tissues in Regional Odontodysplasia. Note in the images how only one portion of the arch is involved. (A) Involvement of the maxillary left dentition. (B) Involvement of the primary incisors and canines. (C) Involvement of the left mandibular premolars and first and second molars. Note the lack of eruption and hypoplasia of enamel and dentin expressed mainly as short roots.

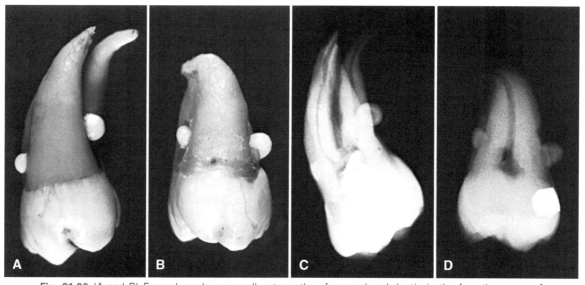

Fig. 21.36 (A and B) Enamel pearls are small outgrowths of enamel and dentin in the furcation areas of teeth. (C and D) Images of the teeth in A and B. (Courtesy Dr. R. Kienholz, Dallas, Texas.)

to that of an enamel pearl. In this case, producing another image at a slightly different horizontal angle eliminates this radiopaque region.

Management. As a rule, the recognition that a radiopaque mass superimposed on the tooth is an enamel pearl precludes the necessity for treatment. The clinician can remove the mass if its location at the cementoenamel junction predisposes to periodontal disease. The possibility must always be considered that it may contain a pulp horn.

Talon Cusp

Disease mechanism. The talon cusp is an anomalous hyperplasia of the cingulum of a maxillary or mandibular incisor. It results in the formation of a supernumerary cusp. Normal enamel covers the cusp

and fuses with the lingual aspect of the tooth. Any developmental grooves that are present may become caries-susceptible areas. The cusp may or may not contain an extension (horn) of the pulp. No apparent ethnic predilection exists.

Clinical features. The talon cusp is infrequently encountered. It may be found in either sex, and on both primary and permanent incisors. It varies in size from that of a prominent cingulum to a cusp-like structure extending to the level of the incisal edge. When viewed from its incisal edge, an incisor bearing the cusp is T-shaped with the top of the incisal edge. Although it usually occurs as an isolated entity, its incidence has been reported to be increased in teeth related to cleft palate syndromes and in association with other anomalies.

Imaging features. The radiopaque image of a talon cusp is superimposed on that of the crown of the involved incisor (Fig. 21.38). The cuspal outline is smooth, and a layer of normal-appearing enamel is generally distinguishable. The image may not reveal a pulp horn. The cusp is often apparent before eruption and may simulate the presence of a supernumerary tooth.

Differential interpretation. The appearance of a talon cusp is quite distinctive. Although it may not be distinguishable from a supernumerary tooth with a single image, a second image with either the parallax or the buccal object technique can demonstrate continuity with the tooth.

Management. If developmental grooves are present where the cusp fuses with the lingual surface of the incisor, treatment may be required to prevent the development of decay. If the cusp is large, it may pose an esthetic or occlusal problem. Slowly removing the cusp over a long period may stimulate the formation of secondary dentin and prevent exposure of a pulp horn.

Turner Hypoplasia

Disease mechanism. Turner hypoplasia, or Turner tooth, is a term used to describe a permanent tooth with a local hypoplastic enamel defect. This defect may have been caused by the extension of periapical inflammatory disease from its deciduous predecessor, by mechanical trauma transmitted through the deciduous tooth or a protracted systemic illness affecting tooth mineralization. If the insult occurs while the crown is forming, it may adversely affect the ameloblasts of the developing tooth, and result in some degree of enamel hypoplasia or hypomineralization.

Clinical features. Turner hypoplasia most often affects the mandibular premolars, generally because of the relative susceptibility of the deciduous molars to caries, their proximity to the developing premolars, and their relative time of mineralization. The severity of the defect depends on the severity of the infection or mechanical trauma and on the stage of development of the permanent tooth. It may disturb matrix formation or calcification, in which case the result varies from a hypoplastic defect to a region of hypomineralization in the enamel. The hypomineralized area may become stained, and the tooth usually shows a brownish spot on the crown. If the insult is severe enough to cause hypoplasia, the crown may show pitting or a more pronounced defect.

Imaging features. The enamel irregularities associated with Turner hypoplasia alter the normal contours of the affected tooth and are often apparent on an image (Fig. 21.39). The involved region of the crown may appear as an ill-defined radiolucent region. A stained hypomineralized spot may not be apparent because of an insufficient difference in the degree of radiopacity between the spot and the crown of the tooth. Also, the hypomineralized areas may become remineralized by continued contact with saliva.

Differential interpretation. Other conditions that result in deformation of the tooth crown, such as the delivery of high-dose therapeutic

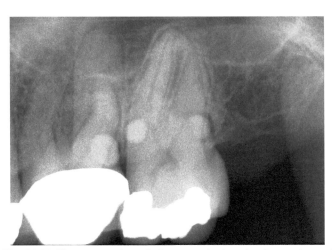
Fig. 21.37 Three enamel pearls (one attached to the first molar and two on the second molar) are apparent in this periapical image.

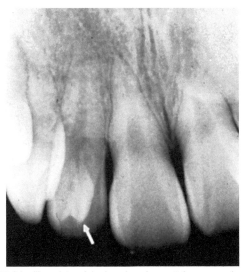
Fig. 21.38 Maxillary lateral incisor bearing a talon cusp *(arrow)*. The tooth also has two enamel invaginations, one near the incisal edge and a second in the cingulum area. (Courtesy Dr. R. A. Cederberg, Dallas, TX.)

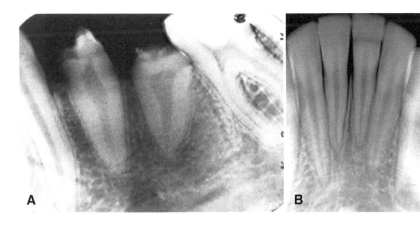

Fig. 21.39 (A) Turner hypoplasia shown as an extensive malformation and hypomineralization of the crowns of both premolars. (B) Band of hypoplasia extending across the crown of the mandibular left central incisor.

radiation during tooth development should be considered, although usually several adjacent teeth are involved. Small defects may simulate the appearance of carious lesions but can be easily differentiated by clinical inspection.

Management. If an image of a tooth affected by Turner hypoplasia shows that the tooth has good root support, the esthetics and function of the deformed crown can be restored.

Congenital Syphilis

Disease mechanism. Approximately 30% of individuals with congenital syphilis have dental hypoplasia that involves the permanent incisors and first molars. Development of primary teeth is seldom disturbed. The affected incisors are called Hutchinson incisors and the molars are called "mulberry molars." The changes characteristic of the condition seem to result from a direct infection of the developing tooth because the syphilitic spirochete has been identified in the tooth germ.

Clinical features. The affected incisor has a characteristic screwdriver-shaped crown, with the mesial and distal surfaces tapering from the middle of the crown to the incisal edge (Fig. 21.40). The effect is that the crown may be no wider mesio-distally than the cervical area of the tooth. The incisal edge is also frequently notched. Although maxillary central incisors usually demonstrate these syphilitic changes, the maxillary lateral and mandibular central incisors may also be involved.

As with incisor crowns, the crowns of affected first molars are quite characteristic, usually smaller than normal, and may be even smaller than second molar crowns. The most distinctive feature is the constricted occlusal third of the crown, with the occlusal surface no wider than the cervical portion of the tooth. The cusps of these molars are also reduced in size and poorly formed. The enamel over the occlusal surface is hypoplastic, unevenly formed in irregular globules, similar to the surface of a mulberry, a small berry having an appearance similar to a blackberry.

Imaging features. The characteristic shapes of the affected incisor and molar crowns can be identified in the image. Because the crowns of these teeth form at about 1 year of age, images may reveal the dental features of congenital syphilis 4 to 5 years before the teeth erupt.

Management. Hutchinson teeth and mulberry molars often do not require dental treatment. Esthetic restorations may be used to correct the hypoplastic defects as indicated clinically.

ACQUIRED ABNORMALITIES

Acquired changes of the dentition—that is, changes that are initiated after development of the tooth range in severity from changes that have no clinical significance to changes that cause tooth loss. In the latter case, early detection and treatment are required to preserve the tooth.

Attrition
Disease Mechanism

Attrition is physiologic wearing of the dentition resulting from occlusal contacts between the maxillary and mandibular teeth. It occurs on the incisal, occlusal, and interproximal surfaces. Interproximal wear causes the contact points to become broad and flat. Attrition occurs in more than 90% of young adults, and is generally more severe in men than women. The extent of attrition depends on the abrasiveness of the diet, salivary factors, mineralization of the teeth, and emotional tension. Physiologic attrition is also a component of the aging process. When the loss of dental tissue becomes excessive such as from bruxism, the attrition becomes pathologic.

Clinical Features

The tooth wear patterns from attrition are characteristic. Wear facets first appear on cusps, and marginal, oblique, and transverse ridges. The incisal edges of the maxillary and mandibular incisors show evidence of broadening. The wear facets on the occlusal surfaces of molars become more pronounced, with the lingual cusps of maxillary teeth and the buccal cusps of mandibular posteriors showing the most wear. When the dentin is exposed, it usually becomes stained, and the color contrast between stained dentin and enamel highlights the areas of attrition. The incisal edges of mandibular incisors tend to become pitted or "dished out" because the dentin wears more rapidly than its surrounding enamel. In the case of pathologic attrition, the patterns of wear are generally not as uniformly progressive as the patterns described for physiologic attrition. The wear facets develop at a faster rate. Moreover, attrition can be related to different cultural customs (dietary and otherwise) of a population.

Imaging Features

The imaging appearance of attrition results in a change in the normal outline of the tooth structure, altering the normal curved surfaces into flat planes. The crown is shortened coronal-apically, and is bereft of the incisal or occlusal surface enamel (Fig. 21.41). Often many adjacent

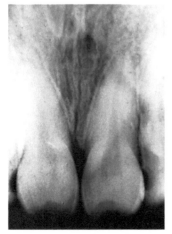

Fig. 21.40 Congenital syphilis may induce a developmental malformation of the maxillary central incisors referred to as "Hutchinson incisors." The abnormal morphology is characterized by tapering of the mesial and distal surfaces toward the incisal edge with notching of the incisal edge.

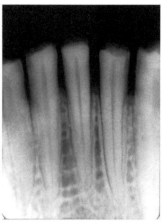

Fig. 21.41 Physiologic wear or attrition is demonstrated on this periapical image of the mandibular incisors.

teeth in each arch show this wear pattern. Reduction in the size of the pulp chambers and canals may occur because attrition stimulates the deposition of secondary dentin. This secondary dentin may result in complete obliteration of the pulp chamber and canals. A simultaneous widening of the PDL space frequently occurs if the tooth is mobile. Occasionally, evidence of hypercementosis is present.

Differential Interpretation

Recognition of physiologic attrition is usually not difficult given the characteristic history, location, and extent of wear. The general pattern is predictable and familiar.

Management

Physiologic attrition does not generally require treatment unless the teeth become symptomatic or there is some cosmetic concern.

Abrasion

Abrasion is the nonphysiologic wearing of teeth as a result of increased friction produced when the tooth is in contact with a foreign material. A history or clinical examination usually reveals the cause. Although many causes exist, two occur with moderate frequency and can usually be eliminated: toothbrush and dental floss injury. Other causes include pipe smoking, opening hairpins with the teeth, improper use of toothpicks, denture clasps, and cutting thread with the teeth.

Toothbrush Injury

Clinical features. Toothbrush abrasion is probably the most frequently observed type of injury to the dental hard tissues. The use of toothbrushes with hard bristles, or the improper horizontal "back-and-forth" movements of the toothbrush with heavy pressure, can cause the bristles to create a V-shaped wedge defect into the cervical area of the tooth, usually involving enamel and the softer root surface.

Abraded teeth may become sensitive as the dentin is exposed. The abraded areas are usually most severe at the cementoenamel junction on the labial and buccal surfaces of maxillary premolars, canines, and incisors, in approximately that order. The enamel generally limits the coronal extension of abrasion. The lesions are also more common and more pronounced on the left side for a right-handed person, and vice versa. The deposition of secondary dentin opposite the abraded areas usually keeps pace with the destruction at the surface, so pulpal exposure is rarely a complication.

Imaging features. The imaging appearance of toothbrush abrasion involves radiolucent defects at the cervical level of teeth. These defects have well-defined semicircular or semilunar shapes with borders of increasing radiopacity. The pulp chambers of the more seriously involved teeth are frequently partially or completely obliterated. The most common location of this injury is the premolar areas, usually in the upper arch.

Dental Floss Injury

Clinical features. Excessive and improper use of dental floss, particularly in conjunction with toothpaste, may result in abrasion of the dentition (Fig. 21.42). The most frequent site is the cervical portion of the proximal surfaces, just above the gingiva.

Imaging features. The imaging appearance of dental floss abrasion is narrow semilunar radiolucency in the interproximal surfaces of the cervical area. Most often the radiolucent grooves on the distal surfaces of the teeth are deeper than the grooves on the mesial surfaces, probably because it is easier to exert more pressure in a forward direction by pulling than by pushing the floss backward into the mouth.

Differential interpretation. Dental floss abrasion is readily identified by its clinical and imaging appearances. Its location provides some

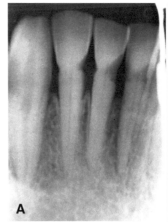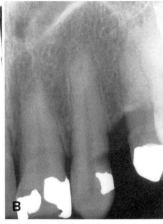

Fig. 21.42 (A) Abrasion of the cervical areas of these incisor teeth is evident from excessive (and improper) use of dental floss. Note the obliteration of the pulp chambers and reduction in size of the root canals. (B) Abrasion on the distal aspect of the maxillary canine from a denture clasp.

evidence regarding the nature of the cause. This can be verified by the patient history. Occasionally, the radiolucencies simulate carious lesions located at the cervical region of the tooth. The diagnosis can be confirmed by clinical inspection.

Management. The primary treatment recommended for abrasion is elimination of the causative agents or habits. Extensively abraded areas can be restored.

Erosion
Disease Mechanism

Erosion of teeth results from a chemical action not involving bacteria. Although in many cases the cause is not apparent, in others it is obviously the contact of acid with teeth. The source of the acid may be from chronic vomiting or acid reflux from gastrointestinal disorders, or from a diet rich in acidic foods, citrus fruits, or carbonated beverages. Regurgitated acids demineralize lingual or palatal tooth surfaces, and dietary acids primarily demineralize labial surfaces. Some occupations involve contact with acids that can induce dental erosion. The location of the erosion, the pattern of eroded areas, and the appearance of the lesion usually provide clues regarding the origin of the decalcifying agent.

Clinical Features

Dental erosion usually affects incisors, often involving multiple teeth. The lesions are generally smooth, glistening depressions in the enamel surface, frequently near the gingiva. Erosion may result in so much loss of enamel that a pink spot shows through the remaining enamel.

Imaging Features

Areas of erosion appear as radiolucent defects on the crown. Their margins may be either well defined or diffuse. A clinical examination usually resolves any questionable lesions.

Differential Interpretation

The diagnosis of erosion is based on the clinical recognition of dished-out or V-shaped defects in the buccal and labial enamel and the dentinal surfaces. The margins of a restoration may project above the remaining tooth surface. The edges of lesions caused by erosion are usually more rounded off compared with lesions caused by abrasion.

Management

As with abrasion, erosion is managed with identification and removal of the causative agent. If the cause is chronic vomiting from an eating disorder, a daily fluoride rinse should be prescribed during counseling therapy. If the cause is unknown, management depends solely on restoration of the defect. Restoration prevents additional damage, possible pulp exposure, and objectionable esthetic appearance.

Resorption

Resorption is the removal of tooth structure by osteoclast-like cells, referred to as odontoclasts when they resorb tooth structure. Resorption is classified as internal or external on the basis of the surface of the tooth being resorbed. External resorption affects the outer surface of the tooth, and internal resorption affects the pulp chamber and root canal walls. These two types differ in their imaging appearance and treatment. The resorption discussed here is not that associated with the normal physiologic process that affects deciduous teeth. Although the etiology of most resorptive lesions is unknown, at least presumptive evidence exists that some lesions are the sequelae of chronic inflammation, excessive pressure and function, or adjacent tumors and cysts.

Internal Resorption

Disease mechanism. Internal resorption occurs within the pulp chamber or root canal system, and involves resorption of the adjacent dentin wall. This form of resorption results in a focal enlargement of the size of the pulp space at the expense of tooth structure, and may be transient and self-limiting, or progressive. The etiology of the recruitment and activation of odontoclasts is unknown but may be related to inflammation within the pulp. Internal resorption has been reported to be initiated by acute trauma to the tooth, direct and indirect pulp capping, pulpotomy, and enamel invagination.

Clinical features. Internal resorption may affect any tooth in either the primary or the secondary dentitions. It occurs most frequently in permanent teeth, usually in central incisors, and first and second molars. The resorptive process most commonly begins during the fourth and fifth decades, and is more common in men. When the lesion originates in the pulp chamber of the crown, a radiolucent area may appear within the crown. If the enlarging pulp perforates the dentin and the enamel becomes involved, the area may appear clinically as a pink spot. If the condition is not intercepted, it may perforate the crown, with hemorrhagic tissue projecting from the perforation, and lead to pulpitis. When the lesion occurs in the root of a tooth, it is, for the most part, clinically silent. If resorption is extensive, it may weaken the tooth and result in fracture. It is also possible that the pulp may expand into the PDL and communicate with a deep periodontal pocket or the gingival sulcus, leading to pulpal inflammation.

Imaging features. Images can reveal symptomless early lesions of internal resorption. The lesions are localized; radiolucent; and round, oval, or elongated within the root or crown and are continuous with the image of the pulp chamber or root canal. These changes are now easily demonstrated using high-resolution, small FOV CBCT. The outline is usually sharply defined and smooth or slightly scalloped. The result is an irregular widening of the pulp chamber or canal (Fig. 21.43). It is characteristically homogeneously radiolucent, without bony trabeculation or pulp stones. However, the internal structure may seem to be apparent if the surface of the resorbed tooth structure is very irregular and has a scalloped texture. In some cases, virtually the entire pulp may enlarge within a tooth, although more commonly the lesion remains localized.

Differential interpretation. The most common lesions that can be confused with internal root resorption are dental caries on the buccal or lingual surface of a tooth and external root resorption. Carious lesions have more diffuse borders than lesions caused by internal root resorption. Clinical inspection quickly reveals caries on the buccal or lingual surface of a tooth. In addition, the mesial and distal surfaces of the pulp chamber and canal can usually be separated from the borders of the carious lesion. However, with internal root resorption, the image of the resorption cannot be separated from the pulp chamber or canal by altering the horizontal angulation of the x-ray beam.

Management. The management of internal resorption depends on the condition of the tooth. If the process has not led to a serious weakening defect in the structure, endodontic treatment halts the resorption. If the expanding pulp has not structurally compromised the tooth but a perforation of the root has occurred, the perforated surface may be surgically exposed and retrofilled. If the tooth has been badly resorbed and weakened by the resorption, extraction may be the only alternative.

External Resorption

Disease mechanism. In external resorption, odontoclasts resorb the outer surface of the tooth. This resorption most commonly involves the root surface but may also involve the crown of an unerupted tooth. The resorption may involve the dentin and cementum, and in some cases gradually extends to the pulp. Because the recruitment of odontoclasts requires an intact blood supply, only sections of the tooth with soft tissue coverage are susceptible to this resorption. This resorption may occur to a single tooth, multiple teeth, or in rare cases, all of the dentition. In many cases, the etiology is unknown, but causes can be attributed in other cases to localized inflammatory lesions, reimplanted teeth, tumors and cysts, excessive mechanical and occlusal forces, and impacted teeth.

Clinical features. External resorption is usually not recognized because often no characteristic signs or symptoms exist. Even when considerable loss of tooth structure occurs, the tooth in question is frequently firm and immobile in the dental arch. In advanced resorption, some nonspecific pain or fracture of the resorbed root occurs.

External resorption may appear at the apex of the tooth or on the lateral root surface, although it most commonly occurs in the apical and cervical regions. It is slightly more prevalent in mandibular teeth than in maxillary teeth and involves primarily the central incisors, canines, and premolars. External root resorption is common. One study of men and women 18 to 25 years old found that all patients exhibited some degree of external root resorption in four or more teeth.

Imaging features. Common sites for external root resorption are the apical and cervical regions. When the resorptive event begins at the apex, it generally causes a smooth loss of tooth structure, resulting in blunting of the root apex (Fig. 21.44). Almost always, the bone and lamina dura follow the resorbing root and exhibit a normal appearance around this shortened structure—that is, the lamina dura and periodontal ligament space are preserved. When external root resorption occurs as the result of a periapical inflammatory lesion, the lamina dura and periodontal ligament space are lost around the apex. After normal apexification (constriction of the walls of the pulp canal at the apex) of the pulp canal, it is very difficult or impossible to see the canal exit at the apex of the tooth. However, if resorption of the apical region has occurred, the pulp canal is visible and is abnormally wide at the apex (Fig. 21.45).

Occasionally, external root resorption can involve the lateral surfaces of roots (Fig. 21.46). Such lesions tend to be irregular, may involve one side more than the other, and occur in any tooth. A common cause of external resorption on the side of a root is the presence of an unerupted adjacent tooth. Examples of external root resorption include resorption

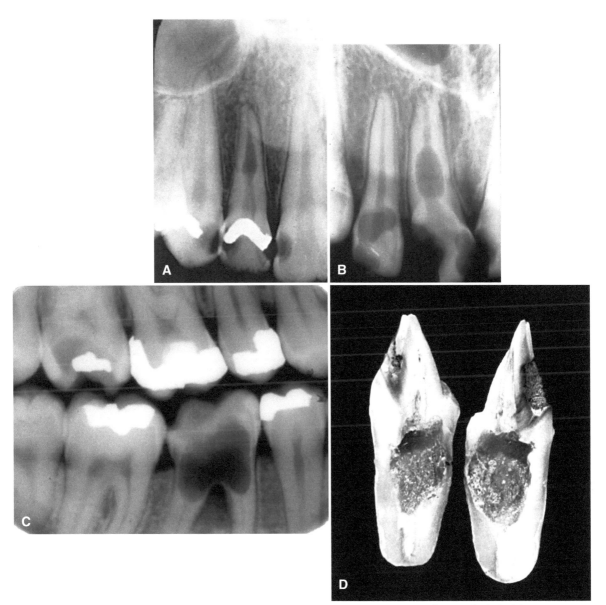

Fig. 21.43 Internal root resorption may occur in either the crown or the root of teeth. Periapical images show internal resorption centered in the root canal system (A and B) and in both the crown and the roots (C and D) in a sectioned incisor (after crown reduction).

of the distal surfaces of the roots of a maxillary second molar by the crown of the adjacent third molar, and resorption of the root of a permanent central or lateral incisor, or both, by an unerupted maxillary canine. External resorption of an entire tooth can occur when the tooth is unerupted and completely embedded in bone (Fig. 21.47), usually involving the maxillary canine or third molar. In such instances, the entire tooth, including the root and crown, may undergo resorption. Mandibular molar tooth roots can also become externally resorbed in the presence of an adjacent dense bone island; however, the resorption is self-limiting.

Differential interpretation. External root resorption on the apex or lateral surface of a root is easily visualized with imaging. When the lesion lies on the buccal or lingual surface of a root, and coronal to the adjacent bone, the differential interpretation includes caries and internal resorption. Internal resorption characteristically appears as a focal enlargement of the pulp chamber or root canal. In the case of external resorption, the image of the normal intact pulp chamber or canal may

be traced through the radiolucent area of external resorption. Also, images made at different angles can be compared. The location of the radiolucency caused by external root resorption moves with respect to the pulp canal, whereas the image of internal resorption remains fixed to the canal.

Management. When the cause of external root resorption is known, the treatment is usually to remove the etiologic factors. Treatment may involve cessation of excessive mechanical forces, surgical management of an adjacent impacted tooth, cyst, tumor, or source of inflammation. If the area of resorption is broad and on an accessible surface of the root (e.g., in the cervical location), curettage of the defect and the placement of a restoration usually stops the process.

Secondary Dentin
Mechanism
Secondary dentin is dentin deposited in the pulp chamber after the formation of primary dentin has been completed. Secondary dentin

Fig. 21.44 (A) Cone beam computed tomography cross sections demonstrate an area of external resorption affecting the palatal surface of the crown of a maxillary central incisor at the cementoenamel junction and proceeding internally into the tooth crown. (B) Three-dimensional surface rendering of the maxillary central incisor shows the resorptive defect on the palatal aspect of the tooth.

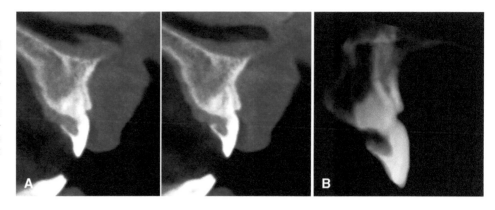

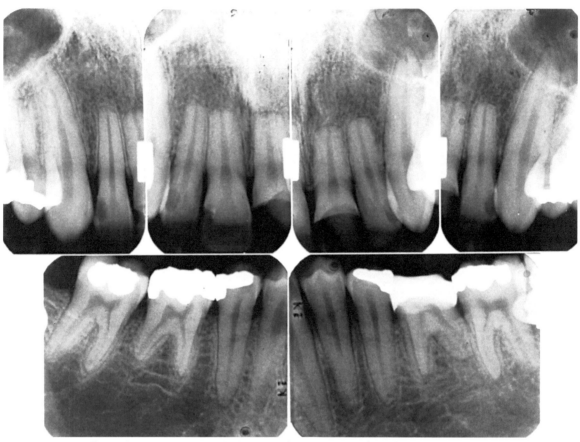

Fig. 21.45 External root resorption results in a loss of tooth structure from the apex. Note the blunted root apices, the widened pulp root canals, and the intact lamina dura.

Fig. 21.46 (A) External root resorption of the lateral surface of the root of the mandibular central incisors. These are sharply defined radiolucencies confined to the root surfaces. (B) The root has been replaced by an ingrowth of bone. This is sometimes referred to as inostosis. (C) Sagittal cone beam computed tomography image of external resorption of the palatal surface of the root of a central incisor with bone ingrowth into the defect.

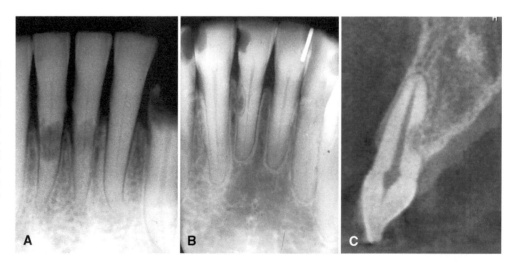

deposition may be part of physiologic aging, or it may result from such innocuous stimuli as chewing or minor trauma. Secondary dentin can also develop after long-term trauma from pathologic conditions such as moderately progressive caries, trauma, erosion, attrition, abrasion, or a dental restorative procedure. This specific stimulus promotes a more rapid and localized coronal response than that seen during normal aging. The term tertiary dentin has been suggested to identify dentin specifically initiated by nonphysiologic stimuli—that is, stimuli other than the normal aging response or normal biologic function.

Clinical Features

The response of odontoblasts in producing secondary dentin reduces the sensitivity of teeth to stimuli from the external environment. In elderly individuals with extensive secondary dentin formation, this reduced sensitivity may be especially pronounced. Similarly, the formation of an additional layer of dentin between the pulp and a region of insult reduces the sensitivity often felt by individuals with recent dental restorations or coronal fractures.

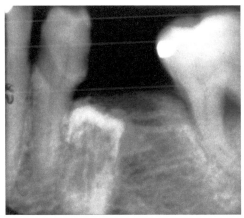

Fig. 21.47 External resorption of an impacted second premolar. Although both enamel and dentin have been resorbed, the residual enamel of the crown can still be seen as well as a hint of a pulp chamber.

Imaging Features

Secondary dentin is indistinguishable from primary dentin on imaging. Its presence is manifested as a reduction in size of the normal pulp chamber and root canal (Fig. 21.48). When secondary dentin arises from the normal aging process, the result is a generalized reduction in pulp chamber area and root canal caliber, maintaining a relatively normal shape. Often there remains only a thin, narrow pulp chamber and canal. The pulp horns usually disappear relatively early, followed by a reduction in size of the pulp chamber and narrowing of the canals. When more specific stimuli initiate secondary dentin formation, it begins in the region adjacent to the source of stimuli and alters the normal shape of the pulp chamber. Although formation of secondary dentin may continue until the pulp appears to be completely obliterated, histologic studies show that even in these extreme cases, a small thread of viable pulp tissue remains.

Differential Interpretation

Secondary dentin is recognized indirectly by the reduction in size of the pulp chamber. This appearance differs from that of the pulp stone. The pulp stone (see the following description) simply occupies some pulp chamber or canal space, but it has a round-to-oval shape (conforming to the chamber).

Management

Secondary dentin deposition per se does not require treatment. The precipitating cause is removed if possible, and the tooth is restored when appropriate.

Pulp Stones
Mechanism

Pulp stones are foci of calcification in the dental pulp. They are probably apparent microscopically in more than half of teeth from young people, and in almost all teeth from people older than 50 years. Although most are microscopic, they vary in size, with some 2 or 3 mm in diameter, almost filling the pulp chamber. Only larger pulp stones can be visualized on imaging. Although the larger stones represent only 15% to 25% of pulpal calcification, they are a common imaging finding and may appear in a single tooth or several teeth. Their cause is unknown, and no firm evidence exists that they are associated with any systemic or pulpal disturbance.

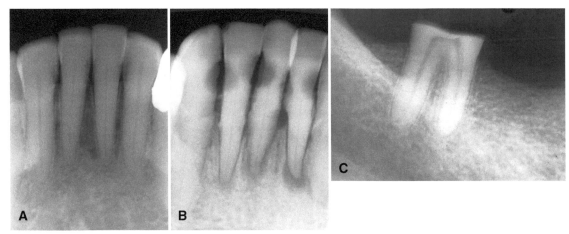

Fig. 21.48 (A) Normal formation of secondary dentin causes recession of the pulp chamber and narrowing of the root canals. (B) Secondary dentin has obliterated the pulp chambers and narrowed the root canals. This is likely a result of the carious lesions. (C) Secondary dentin formation has obliterated the pulp chamber stimulated by the severe attrition of the coronal aspect of this molar.

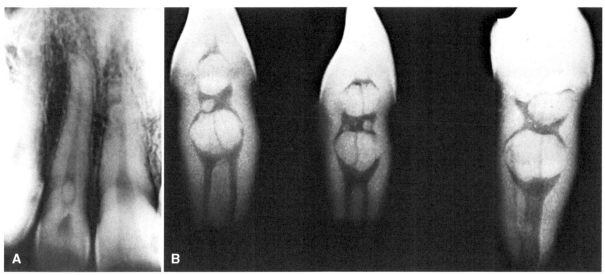

Fig. 21.49 (A) Pulp stones may be found as isolated calcifications in the pulp. (B) When large, they may cause deformation of the pulp chamber and root canals.

Clinical Features

Pulp stones are not clinically discernible.

Imaging Features

The imaging appearance of pulp stones is quite variable. They may be seen as radiopaque structures within pulp chambers or root canals, or they may extend from the pulp chamber into the root canals (Fig. 21.49). No uniform shape or number exists. They may occur as a single dense mass or as several small radiopacities. They may be round or oval, and some pulp stones that potentially occupy most of the pulp chamber conform to its shape. Their outline likewise varies from sharply defined to a more diffuse margin. They occur in all tooth types but are most common in molars. In rare instances, the canal remodels and increases its girth to accommodate a large stone.

Differential Interpretation

Although pulp stones are variable in size and form, their recognition is usually not difficult. However, in some cases, differentiation from pulpal sclerosis is difficult.

Management

Pulp stones do not require treatment; however, when endodontic treatment is being considered for a tooth with pulp stones, careful planning to understand the location and extent is important for successful endodontic therapy. Small FOV CBCT is being used increasingly to preoperatively evaluate teeth with pulp stones undergoing endodontic treatment.

Pulpal Sclerosis
Mechanism

Pulpal sclerosis is another form of calcification in the pulp chamber and canals of teeth. In contrast to pulp stones, pulpal sclerosis is a diffuse process. Its specific cause is unknown, although its appearance correlates strongly with age. About 66% of all teeth in individuals 10 to 20 years old and 90% of all teeth in individuals 50 to 70 years old show histologic evidence of pulpal sclerosis. Histologically, the pattern of calcification is amorphous and unorganized, being evident as linear strands or columns of calcified material paralleling blood vessels and nerves in the pulp.

Clinical Features

Pulpal sclerosis is a clinically silent process without clinical manifestations.

Imaging Features

Early pulpal sclerosis, a degenerative process, is not demonstrable on imaging. Diffuse pulpal sclerosis produces a generalized, ill-defined collection of fine radiopacities throughout large areas of the pulp chamber and pulp canals (Fig. 21.50).

Differential Interpretation

The differential diagnosis includes small pulp stones, but this differentiation is academic because neither pulpal sclerosis nor pulp stones require treatment.

Management

Pulpal sclerosis does not require treatment. Pulp stones and pulpal sclerosis become important when endodontic therapy is indicated for other reasons.

Hypercementosis
Disease Mechanism

Hypercementosis is excessive deposition of cementum on the tooth roots. In most cases, its cause is unknown. Occasionally, it appears on a supraerupted tooth after the loss of an opposing tooth. Another cause of hypercementosis is inflammation, usually resulting from rarefying or sclerosing osteitis. In the context of inflammation, cementum is deposited on the root surface adjacent to the apex. Hypercementosis occasionally has been associated with teeth that are in hyperocclusion or that have been fractured. Finally, hypercementosis occurs in patients with Paget disease of bone (see Chapter 25) and with hyperpituitarism (gigantism and acromegaly).

Clinical Features

Hypercementosis does not cause any clinical signs or symptoms.

Imaging Features

Hypercementosis is evident on images as an excessive buildup of cementum around all or part of a root (Fig. 21.51). The root outline is usually smooth but occasionally may be seen as an irregular but

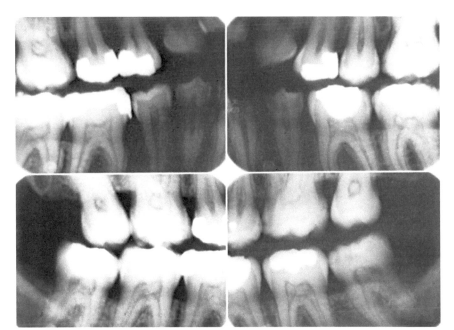

Fig. 21.50 Pulpal sclerosis is seen as diffuse calcification of the pulp chamber and canals.

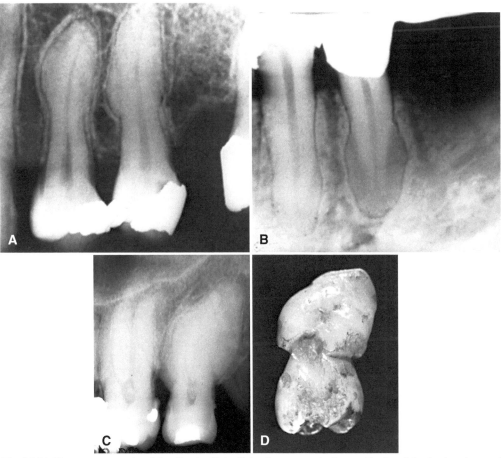

Fig. 21.51 Hypercementosis of the Roots. (A to C) In all cases, note the continuity of the lamina dura and the periodontal ligament space that encompasses the extra cementum. (D) An extracted molar exhibits extensive hypercementosis. (Courtesy Dr. R. Kienholz, Dallas, TX.)

bulbous enlargement of the root. It is most evident in the apical thirds of tooth roots, and is usually seen as a mildly irregular accumulation of cementum. This cementum is slightly more radiolucent than dentin. Of importance is the fact that the lamina dura and PDL space encompass the enlarged root. In the case of Paget disease of bone, the hypercementosis is usually very exuberant and irregular in outline.

Differential Interpretation

The differential interpretation may include any radiopaque structure that is seen within the vicinity of the root, such as a dense bone island or mature periapical osseous dysplasia. The differentiating characteristic is the presence of the periodontal ligament space around the hypercementosis. There may be a resemblance to a small cementoblastoma. Occasionally, a severely dilacerated root may have the appearance of hypercementosis.

Management

Hypercementosis requires no treatment. If a related condition, such as a periapical inflammatory disease, exists, treatment is necessary. The primary significance of hypercementosis may relate to the difficulty that the root configuration can pose if extraction is indicated.

BIBLIOGRAPHY

Developmental Abnormalities

Bergsma D, ed. *Birth Defects Compendium.* 2nd ed. New York: Alan R Liss; 1979.

Dixon GH, Stewart RE. Genetic aspects of anomalous tooth development. In: Stewart RE, Prescott GH, eds. *Oral Facial Genetics.* St Louis: Mosby; 1976.

MacDougall M, Dong J, Acevedo AC. Molecular basis of human dentin diseases. *Am J Med Genet A.* 2006;140A:2536–2546.

Pindborg JJ. *Pathology of the Dental Hard Tissues.* Copenhagen: Munksgaard; 1970.

Schulze C. Developmental abnormalities of the teeth and jaws. In: Gorlin RJ, Goldman HM, eds. *Thoma's Oral Pathology.* Vol. 1. 6th ed. St Louis: Mosby; 1970.

Witkop CJ Jr. Amelogenesis imperfecta, dentinogenesis imperfecta and dentin dysplasia revisited: problems with classification. *J Oral Pathol.* 1989;17:547–553.

Witkop CJ Jr, Rao S. Inherited defects in tooth structure. In: Bergsma D, eds. *Birth Defects, XI: Orofacial Structures.* Vol. 7, no 7. Baltimore: Williams & Wilkins; 1971.

Worth HM. *Principles and Practice of Oral Radiologic Interpretation.* Chicago: Year Book Medical; 1963.

Wright JT. The molecular etiologies and associated phenotypes of amelogenesis imperfecta. *Am J Med Genet A.* 2006;140A:2547ures.

Supernumerary Teeth

Grahnen H, Lindahl B. Supernumerary teeth in the permanent dentition: a frequency study. *Odontol Rev.* 1961;12:290–294.

Grimanis GA, Kyriakides AT, Spyropoulos ND. A survey on supernumerary molars. *Quintessence Int.* 1991;22:989–995.

Lu X, Yu F, et al. The epidemiology of supernumerary teeth and the associated molecular mechanism. *Organogenesis.* 2017;13(3):71–82. do i:10.1080/15476278.2017.1332554.

Niswander JD. Effects of heredity and environment on development of the dentition. *J Dent Res.* 1963;42:1288–1296.

Rao SR. Supernumerary teeth. In: Bergsma D, eds. *Birth Defects Compendium.* 2nd ed. New York: Alan R Liss; 1979.

Yusof WZ. Non-syndrome multiple supernumerary teeth: literature review. *J Can Dent Assoc.* 1990;56:147–149.

Developmentally Missing Teeth

al-Emran S. Prevalence of hypodontia and developmental malformation of permanent teeth in Saudi Arabian school children. *Br J Orthod.* 1990;17:115–118.

Garn SM, Lewis AB. The relationship between third molar agenesis and reduction in tooth number. *Angle Orthod.* 1962;32:14–18.

Keene HJ. The relationship between third molar agenesis and the morphologic variability of the molar teeth. *Angle Orthod.* 1965;35:289–298.

Levin LS. Dental and oral abnormalities in selected ectodermal dysplasia syndromes. *Birth Defects Orig Artic Ser.* 1988;24:205–227.

O'Dowling IB, McNamara TG. Congenital absence of permanent teeth among Irish school-children. *J Ir Dent Assoc.* 1990;36:136–138.

Visioni AF, Lisboa-Costa TN, Pagnan NAB, et al. Ectodermal dysplasias: clinical and molecular review. *Am J Med Genet.* 2009;149A:1980–2002.

Macrodontia

Garn SM, Lewis AB, Kerewsky BS. The magnitude and implications of the relationship between tooth size and body size. *Arch Oral Biol.* 1968;13:129–131.

Transposition

Schacter H. A treated case of transposed upper canine. *Dent Rec (London).* 1951;71:105–108.

Fusion

Hagman FT. Anomalies of form and number, fused primary teeth, a correlation of the dentitions. *ASDC J Dent Child.* 1988;55:359–361.

Sperber GH. Genetic mechanisms and anomalies in odontogenesis. *J Can Dent Assoc (Tor).* 1967;33:433–442.

Gemination

Ferrazzano GF, Festa P, Cantile T, et al. Multidisciplinary approach to the treatment of double bilateral upper permanent incisors in a young boy. *Eur J Paediatr Dent.* 2017;18(2):94–98. doi:10.23804/ejpd.2017.18.02.02. PMID: 28598178.

Tannenbaum KA, Alling EE. Anomalous tooth development: case report of gemination and twinning. *Oral Surg Oral Med Oral Pathol.* 1963;16:883–887.

Taurodontism

Bixler D. Heritable disorders affecting dentin. In: Steward RE, Prescott GA, eds. *Oral Facial Genetics.* St Louis: Mosby; 1976.

Dens in Dente

Oehlers FA. The radicular variety of dens invaginatus. *Oral Surg Oral Med Oral Pathol.* 1958;11:1251–1260.

Rushton MA. A collection of dilated composite odontomes. *Br Dent J.* 1937;63:65–86.

Soames JV, Kuyebi TA. A radicular dens invaginatus. *Br Dent J.* 1982;152:308–309.

Dens Invaginatus

Oehlers FA, Lee KW, Lee EC. Dens invaginatus (invaginated odontome): its structure and responses to external stimuli. *Dent Pract Dent Rec.* 1967;17:239–244.

Sykaras SN. Occlusal anomalous tubercle on premolars of a Greek girl. *Oral Surg Oral Med Oral Pathol.* 1974;38:88–91.

Yip WK. The prevalence of dens invaginatus. *Oral Surg Oral Med Oral Pathol.* 1974;38:80–87.

Gallacher A, Ali R, Bhakta S. Dens invaginatus: diagnosis and management strategies. *Br Dent J.* 2016;221:383–387. Published online: 7 October 2016. doi:10.1038/sj.bdj.2016.724.

Molar-Incisor Malformation

Brusevold IJ, Bie TMG, Baumgartner CS, et al. Molar incisor malformation in six cases: description and diagnostic protocol. *Oral Surg Oral Med Oral Pathol Oral Radiol.* 2017;124(1):52–61. doi:10.1016/j.oooo.2017.03.050. [Epub 2017 Apr 4].

Lee HS, Kim SH, et al. A new type of dental anomaly: molar-incisor malformation (MIM). *Oral Surg Oral Med Oral Pathol Oral Radiol.* 2014;118(1):101–109.e3. doi:10.1016/j.oooo.2014.03.014. [Epub 2014 Apr 5].

McCreedy C, Robbins H, Newell A, et al. Molar-incisor malformation: two cases of a newly described dental anomaly. *J Dent Child (Chic)*. 2016;83(1):33–37.

Amelogenesis Imperfecta

Bailleul-Forestier I, Molla M, Verloes A, et al. The genetic basis of inherited anomalies of the teeth. Part 1: clinical and molecular aspects of non-syndromic dental disorders. *Eur J Med Genet*. 2008;51:273–291.

Gasse B, Prasad M, Delgado S, et al. Evolutionary analysis predicts sensitive positions of MMP20 and validates newly- and previously-identified MMP20 mutations causing amelogenesis imperfecta. *Front Physiol*. 2017;8:398. doi:10.3389/fphys.2017.00398. eCollection 2017. PMID:28659819.

Seymen F, Kim YJ, et al. Recessive mutations in ACPT, encoding testicular acid phosphatase, cause hypoplastic amelogenesis imperfecta. *Am J Hum Genet*. 2016;99(5):1199–1205. doi:10.1016/j.ajhg.2016.09.018. [Epub 2016 Oct 27]; PMID:27843125.

Wright JT. The molecular etiologies and associated phenotypes of amelogenesis imperfecta. *Am J Med Genet A*. 2006;140:2547–2555.

Dentinogenesis Imperfecta and Dentin Dysplasia

Kim JW, Simmer JP. Hereditary dentin defects. *J Dent Res*. 2007;86:292–299.

MacDougall M, Dong J, Acevedo AC. Molecular basis of human dentin diseases. *Am J Med Genet A*. 2006;140:2536–2546.

O Carroll MK, Duncan WK, Perkins TM. Dentin dysplasia: review of the literature and a proposed subclassification based on imaging findings. *Oral Surg Oral Med Oral Pathol*. 1991;72:119–125.

Regional Odontodysplasia

Crawford PJ, Aldred MJ. Regional odontodysplasia: a bibliography. *J Oral Pathol Med*. 1989;18:251–263.

Enamel Pearl

Moskow BS, Canut PM. Studies on root enamel, II: enamel pearls: a review of their morphology, localization, nomenclature, occurrence, classification, histogenesis, and incidence. *J Clin Periodontol*. 1990;17:275–281.

Talon Cusp

Meskin LH, Gorlin RJ. Agenesis and peg-shaped permanent lateral incisors. *J Dent Res*. 1963;42:1476–1479.

Natkin E, Pitts DL, Worthington P. A case of talon cusp associated with other odontogenic abnormalities. *J Endod*. 1983;9:491–495.

Turner Hypoplasia

Via WF Jr. Enamel defects induced by trauma during tooth formation. *Oral Surg Oral Med Oral Pathol*. 1968;25:49–54.

Congenital Syphilis

Bradlaw RV. The dental stigmata of prenatal syphilis. *Oral Surg Oral Med Oral Pathol*. 1953;6:147–158.

Putkonen T. Dental changes in congenital syphilis: relationship to other syphilitic stigmata. *Acta Derm Venereol*. 1962;42–62.

Sarnat BG, Shaw NG. Dental development in congenital syphilis. *Am J Orthod*. 1943;29:270.

Acquired Abnormalities

Baden E. Environmental pathology of the teeth. In: Gorlin RJ, Goodman HM, eds. *Thoma's Oral Pathology*. Vol. 1. 6th ed. St Louis: Mosby; 1970.

Mitchell DF, Standish SM, Fast TB. *Oral Diagnosis/Oral Medicine*. Philadelphia: Lea & Febiger; 1978.

Pindborg JJ. *Pathology of the Dental Hard Tissues*. Philadelphia: Saunders; 1970.

Shafer WG, Hine MK, Levy BM. *Oral Pathology*. 4th ed. Philadelphia: Saunders; 1983.

Attrition

Johnson GK, Sivers JE. Attrition, abrasion, and erosion: diagnosis and therapy. *Clin Prev Dent*. 1987;9:12–16.

Murphy TR. Reduction of the dental arch by approximal attrition: quantitative assessment. *Br Dent J*. 1964;116:483–488.

Russell MD. The distinction between physiological and pathological attrition: a review. *J Ir Dent Assoc*. 1987;33:23–31.

Seligman DA, Pullinger AG, Solberg WK. The prevalence of dental attrition and its association with factors of age, gender, occlusion, and TMJ symptomatology. *J Dent Res*. 1988;67:1323–1333.

Abrasion

Bull WH, Callender RM, Pugh BR, et al. The abrasion and cleaning properties of dentifrices. *Br Dent J*. 1968;125:331.

Corica A, Caprioglio A. Meta-analysis of the prevalence of tooth wear in primary dentition. *Eur J Paediatr Dent*. 2014;15(4):385–388.

Erwin JC, Buchner CM. Prevalence of tooth wear in primary dentition. *Eur J Paediatr Dent*. 2014;15(4):385–388. Review.

Erosion

Bruggen Cate HJ. Dental erosion in industry. *Br J Ind Med*. 1968;25:249.

Carvalho TS, Colon P, et al. Consensus Report of the European Federation of Conservative Dentistry: erosive tooth wear diagnosis and management. *Swiss Dent J*. 2016;126(4):342–346. PMID:27142130.

Kisely S, Sawyer E, et al. The oral health of people with anxiety and depressive disorders - a systematic review and meta-analysis. *J Affect Disord*. 2016;200:119–132. doi:10.1016/j.jad.2016.04.040. [Epub 2016 Apr 21]. Review. PMID:27130961.

Stafne EC, Lovestedt SA. Dissolution of tooth substance by lemon juice, acid beverages, and acid from some other sources. *J Am Dent Assoc*. 1947;34:586–592.

Resorption

Bakland LK. Root resorption. *Dent Clin North Am*. 1992;36:91–507.

Bennett CG, Poleway SA. Internal resorption, postpulpotomy type. *Oral Surg Oral Med Oral Pathol*. 1964;17:228–234.

Goldman HM. Spontaneous intermittent resorption of teeth. *J Am Dent Assoc*. 1954;49:522–532.

Massler M, Perreault JG. Root resorption in the permanent teeth of young adults. *J Dent Child*. 1954;21:158–164.

Phillips JR. Apical root resorption under orthodontic therapy. *Angle Orthod*. 1955;20:1–22.

Simpson HE. Internal resorption. *J Can Dent Assoc*. 1964;30:355.

Solomon CS, Notaro PJ, Kellert M. External root resorption: fact or fancy. *J Endod*. 1989;15(5):219–223.

Stafne EC, Austin LT. Resorption of embedded teeth. *J Am Dent Assoc*. 1945;32:1003–1009.

Tronstad L. Root resorption: etiology, terminology, and clinical manifestations. *Endod Dent Traumatol*. 1988;4:241–252.

Wang J, Feng JQ. Signaling pathways critical for tooth root formation. *J Dent Res*. 2017;96(11):1221–1228. 22034517717478. doi:10.1177/0022034517717478.

Secondary Dentin

Kuttler Y. Classification of dentin into primary, secondary and tertiary. *Oral Surg Oral Med Oral Pathol*. 1959;12:966–969.

Pulp Stones

Moss-Salentijn L, Hendricks-Klyvert M. Calcified structures in human dental pulps. *J Endod*. 1988;14:184–189.

Da Silva EJ, Prado MC, et al. Assessing pulp stones by cone-beam computed tomography. *Clin Oral Investig*. 2016 Dec 9. PMID:27942985.

22

Inflammatory Conditions of the Jaws

Ernest W.N. Lam

Inflammation is the most common pathologic condition arising in the jaws. Unlike the other bones in the skeleton, the jaws are unique in the sense that teeth create a direct pathway for agents or processes, be they pathogenic microorganisms, or chemical or physical agents, to enter bone. Consequently, the inflammatory response that is mounted by the body attempts to destroy or isolate the injurious stimulus so that an environment can be created for the repair of the damaged tissue.

Under normal conditions, bone metabolism is a balance of osteoblastic bone production and osteoclastic bone resorption. And in this very complex, interdependent relationship, osteoblasts mediate the resorptive activity of osteoclasts. The pathogenicity of bacterial microorganisms, the host immune response, tissue vascularity, and time can all alter this balance to favor of either bone formation or resorption. For the purposes of this chapter, all inflammatory conditions of bone, regardless of specific etiology, are considered as part of a spectrum or continuum of conditions with different clinical features and radiologic appearances.

The four cardinal signs of inflammation (**redness**, **swelling**, **heat**, and **pain**) may be observed to varying degrees in the jaws. Acute lesions tend to have a typically rapid onset, causing pronounced pain. Also, acute inflammatory lesions are often accompanied by fever and swelling. In contrast, chronic lesions are generally less severe with a more prolonged course, and the pain is generally less intense. Furthermore, fever may be intermittent and low grade, and swelling may develop gradually. Indeed, low-grade inflammatory lesions may not produce any significant clinical symptoms at all.

When the initial source of the inflammatory response is a pathogenic microorganism and a necrotic tooth pulp, the bony lesion that develops is restricted to the tooth root apex. This condition is referred to as periapical inflammatory disease. When the dissemination occurs through the gingival tissues, the inflammatory response is referred to as periodontal disease if it involves the supporting structures of the teeth or pericoronitis if it involves the crown of a partially erupted tooth. Wider dissemination of microorganisms and the inflammatory response through the bone marrow may be augmented by tissue vascularity and the host immune response.

However, in some patients, a pathogenic microorganism or a source of the infection cannot be identified, and hematogenous spread from a distant source is presumed to be the origin. In other cases, the inability to culture a microorganism may be due to prior antibiotic therapy, or the method of bone sampling may be inadequate to reveal small, isolated pockets of infected bone. When the inflammatory response spreads through the bone via the Haversian system and Volkmann's canals to an adjacent tissue space so that it is no longer localized to the vicinity of the tooth root apex, and there is death or necrosis of bone, it is called osteomyelitis. The names of the various inflammatory conditions tend to describe their clinical and imaging presentations and behavior; however, all have the same underlying disease mechanism, including a common response of the bone to the injury.

PERIAPICAL INFLAMMATORY DISEASE

Terminology

Apical periodontitis (acute and chronic), (periapical, radicular, or periradicular) abscess, (periapical, radicular, or periradicular) granuloma, and (periapical, radicular, or periradicular) cyst are some of the many terms that have been used synonymously to refer to periapical inflammatory disease. Some of the terms that have been used refer to histopathologic interpretations of disease processes that are associated with characteristic microscopic features that cannot be identified by radiologic imaging. In contrast, the term apical periodontitis is used to describe a disease process that involves the inflammation and destruction of the apical periodontium of pulpal origin (an etiologic link that sometimes cannot be made by simply viewing an image).

"Rarefying osteitis" is the preferred radiologic term when referring to an inflammatory process in bone associated with bone destruction at the apex around a tooth root. In this context, the term "rarefying," which is derived from the word "rarefaction," refers to a loss of bone mineralization and the term "osteitis" refers to inflammation of bone. The net result of this process is an appearance of increased radiolucency. In contrast, the term "sclerosing osteitis" is used to refer to an inflammatory process in bone associated with bone deposition around a tooth root. "Sclerosis" is a term that refers to a "hardening" of the bone and radiologically, this appears as an increase in the radiopacity of bone. Focal sclerosing osteitis and "condensing osteitis" have both been used synonymously to refer to this latter condition, although the use of the term "condensing" as an adjective that describes the biologic response of bone to inflammation should be discouraged.

Disease Mechanism

The local response of the bone around a tooth as a result of pulp necrosis is the most common cause of periapical inflammatory disease (Fig. 22.1). Necrosis of the pulp commonly occurs as a result of bacterial invasion into the dental pulp through dental caries or tooth trauma. Metabolites derived from the necrotic pulp exit the tooth root apex, inciting an inflammatory response in the periapical periodontal ligament space and surrounding bone (apical periodontitis). This reaction is characterized histopathologically by an inflammatory infiltrate consisting of multinucleated cells, such as neutrophils in the more acute stages, followed by monocytes/macrophages and lymphocytes in the more chronic stages of disease.

Depending on the severity of the response, the neutrophils may collect, and pus may form, resulting in an abscess. This series of

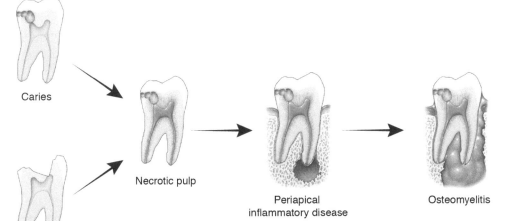

Caries

Trauma

Necrotic pulp

Periapical
inflammatory disease

Osteomyelitis

Fig. 22.1 The development of periapical inflammatory disease at the tooth root apex and dissemination into the adjacent bone.

events is often thought of as the more acute inflammatory response. Alternatively, in an attempt to heal the apical inflammatory response, the body may signal the formation of granulation tissue mixed with a chronic inflammatory cell infiltrate composed predominantly of lymphocytes, plasma cells, and histiocytes, giving rise to a granuloma. Entrapped epithelium from the epithelial cell rests of Malassez may be stimulated to proliferate, developing a lining within the area of apical bone destruction forming a cyst. Should the adjacent surrounding bone and bone marrow become more involved in the inflammatory response, a compensatory response of the bone may be to isolate the inflammatory lesion by depositing bone at the periphery of the radiolucent lesion—the process of sclerosis. As the inflammatory reaction becomes more widely disseminated, pathogenic microorganisms as well as inflammatory mediators may reach the surface of the bone and the overlying periosteum.

The periosteum is a dense and irregularly thick layer of connective tissue that lines the floors of air cavities and covers the surfaces of the jawbones. Extensions of collagen from the bone, called Sharpey's fibers, anchor the periosteum to the bone surface. The periosteum consists of two discrete cell layers: an inner osteogenic layer that harbors mesenchymal pluripotential stem cells and an outer fibrous layer that contains fibroblasts and collagen. Under the right conditions, the stem cells within the osteogenic layer can differentiate into osteoblasts, and these cells can produce bone. Pathogenic microorganisms and inflammatory mediators can travel through the Haversian system and Volkmann's canals from the focus of inflammation to the outer bone surface and the inner surface of the periosteum. Here, the pathogenic agents may broadly distend or lift the adherent periosteum from the bone surface so that the periosteum becomes elevated. However, as Sharpey's fibers attach the periosteum to the bone surface, the amount of distension may be limited. Inflammatory mediators also stimulate the stem cells in the osteogenic layer of the periosteum, and these can differentiate into osteoblasts, and new bone may be laid down in a response called periosteal new bone formation. Should the blood supply to bone become compromised, the bone may undergo necrosis, giving rise to sequestra (dying or dead bone).

Clinical Features

The symptoms of periapical inflammatory disease can range from being asymptomatic to an occasional toothache to severe pain without or with facial swelling, fever, and lymphadenopathy. In the more acute stages of disease, an abscess can be associated with severe pain, swelling, and pain of the overlying tissues to palpation. As well, a tooth may become mobile and tender to percussion, and sometimes elevated in the tooth socket. Spontaneous drainage of the abscess into the oral cavity through a fistula (parulis) may result in pain relief. The acute lesion may evolve into one that is more chronic (i.e., granuloma or cyst), which may be asymptomatic except for intermittent flare-ups of tooth pain, which may be acute exacerbations of the chronic lesion. In such instances, patients may give a history of intermittent pain. The associated tooth may be asymptomatic, or it may be mobile or sensitive to percussion. More often, however, the periapical lesion arises in a chronic form de novo, and in this case, it may be completely asymptomatic. It is important for the dentist to recognize that the clinical presentation of periapical inflammatory disease does not necessarily correlate with the histologic or imaging findings.

Imaging Examination

An initial imaging examination consisting of intraoral periapical and occlusal, and panoramic images may be useful to characterize the extent of the lesion and the teeth involved. While rarefaction and sclerosis may be visible on panoramic imaging, occlusal images can be useful for depicting periosteal new bone formation. Depending on the exuberance of the bone response, multidetector computed tomography (MDCT) or cone beam computed tomography (CBCT) are the imaging modalities of choice for detecting periosteal new bone formation and sequestration of bone. Additionally, magnetic resonance imaging (MRI) may be useful to visualize changes to the bone marrow and a nuclear medicine examination with technetium (^{99m}Tc) and gallium (^{67}Ga) may help to confirm the diagnosis. With inflammatory lesions, a positive ^{99m}Tc result depicting increased bone metabolic activity and a positive ^{67}Ga scan in the same location reflecting an inflammatory cell infiltrate can confirm the MDCT, CBCT, or MRI results.

Imaging Features

The imaging features of periapical inflammatory disease may vary depending on the stage of the disease. Very early lesions may show very subtle changes, if any, to the periapical tissues on images, and diagnosis may rely solely on the patient's clinical signs and symptoms (Fig. 22.2). More longstanding lesions may show a radiolucent region at the root apex of a tooth, and a more diffuse, surrounding area of radiopacity.

Location

In most cases, lesions of periapical inflammatory disease develop within the apical portion of the periodontal ligament space. Less commonly, such lesions are centered about another region of the tooth root, arising from accessory root canals, perforations of the root from root canal instrumentation of the pulp canal, or root fracture. The epicenter of a periapical inflammatory lesion is located subjacent or apical to the apex of the involved tooth root (Fig. 22.3). However, as the lesion enlarges, the epicenter begins to move in a more apical direction, away from the tooth root apex.

Periphery

In most instances, the periphery of periapical inflammatory lesions is poorly defined, showing a zone of bone transition that varies from one that is narrow to one that is broad, depending on the amount of peripheral sclerosis and the chronicity of the disease process (Fig. 22.4). Rarely, the periphery may be well-defined with a narrow zone between the lesion and normal bone. In such instances, a corticated periphery may sometimes be seen.

Internal Structure

Early periapical inflammatory disease may show no apparent change to the normal bone pattern at the apex of a tooth root. The inability to perceive a change may be due, in part, to the amount of bone turnover necessary to visualize the change. Indeed, the percentage range in bone turnover may be broad, with some authors reporting a visual change in bone radiolucency with as little as a 12% to 15% turnover of the bone matrix to as much as a change of two-thirds of the matrix.

The earliest radiologic change of bone structure at the apex of a tooth root may involve loss of definition of the periapical lamina dura, and this may be accompanied by a focal widening of the apical periodontal ligament space (see Fig. 22.3). As the lesion enlarges beyond the apical periodontal ligament space, the area of bone resorption is usually centered on, or just apical to, the apex of the tooth root. This radiolucent region may lack most, if not all internal bone structure.

Effects on Surrounding Structures

In the early stages of periapical inflammatory disease there may be little effect on the adjacent bone. As the disease evolves, bone deposition may be seen around the focus of rarefaction, altering the normal morphology of the trabecular bone pattern and marrow spaces (see Fig. 22.4 and 22.5). The degree to which the appearance of periapical inflammatory disease is radiolucent (rarefying osteitis) or radiopaque (sclerosing osteitis) is variable. Closer inspection of the peripheral sclerotic regions reveals thicker than normal trabeculae and sometimes an increase in the number of trabeculae per unit area. With time, the new bone formation may result in a very dense sclerotic region of bone, obscuring individual trabeculae and reducing the size of the marrow spaces. Occasionally, the lesion may appear to be composed entirely of sclerotic bone (sclerosing osteitis), but usually some evidence exists of apical periodontal ligament space widening that may persist (Fig. 22.6). In some instances, the sclerotic reaction of the bone may be localized to a small region around the tooth root apex. However, given the aggressiveness of the pathogenic microorganism and the exuberance of host immune response, as well as tissue vascularity and chronicity, the sclerotic response may extend to adjacent teeth or to a bone border. Should the inflammatory response extend to a bone border, whether the floor of an airspace, such as the maxillary sinus or the cortex of the mandible, the inflammatory response may stimulate the surface

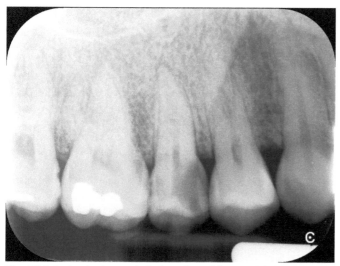

Fig. 22.2 A developing early lesion of rarefying osteitis involving the root apex of the maxillary right second premolar without significant change to the adjacent bone. Note the loss of the apical lamina dura and subtle increase in the apical width of the periodontal ligament space.

Fig. 22.3 Rarefying osteitis associated with a mandibular right first molar (A) and a maxillary lateral incisor (B). In both cases, the epicenter of the inflammatory response is located apical to the root apex. Also, note the gradual widening of the periodontal ligament space characteristic of an inflammatory lesion and the loss of definition of the lamina dura.

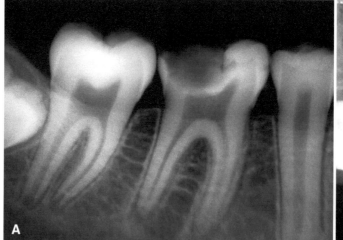

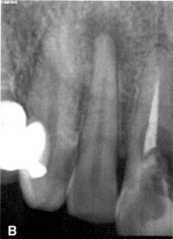

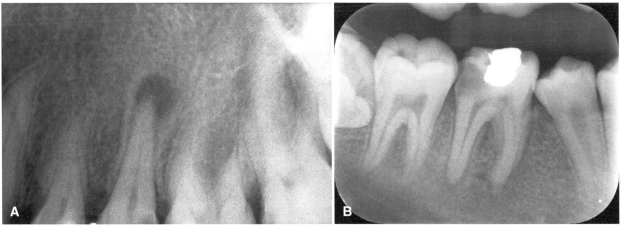

Fig. 22.4 Examples of both rarefying and sclerosing osteitis affecting a maxillary left second premolar (A) and the roots of a mandibular right first molar (B). Note the similarity of the pattern, comprising a radiolucent region at the apex of the tooth surrounded by a diffuse radiopaque reaction of sclerotic bone extending into the adjacent bone from the area of rarefaction.

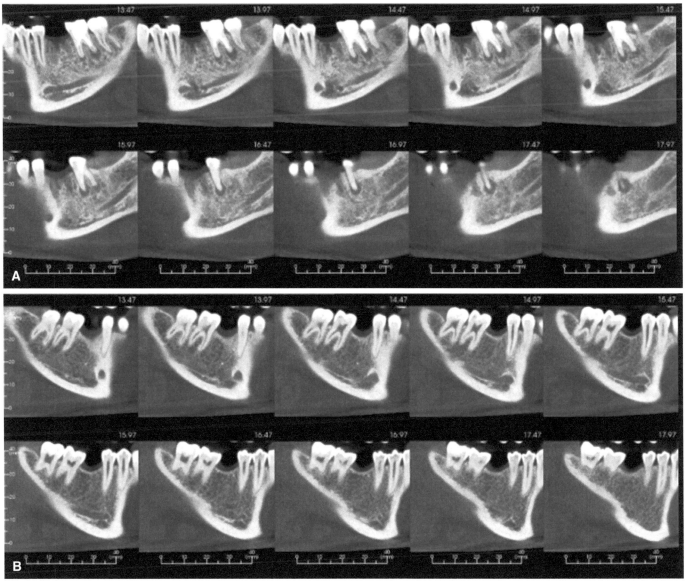

Fig. 22.5 Corrected sagittal cone beam computed tomography images of rarefying and sclerosing osteitis affecting the roots of a mandibular left second molar. Note the loss of normal trabecular bone pattern (A) compared with the unaffected side (B). The sclerotic response extends to the inferior cortex of the mandible. This change gives a particular prominence to the inferior alveolar canal.

periosteum resulting in periosteal new bone formation. Alternatively, depending on the exuberance of the inflammatory response, the bone border may be perforated and lost.

The symptoms of inflammation are often described by patients as being cyclical in nature. That is, patients commonly experience times of quiescence and relief, and times of exacerbation. In times of quiescence, the osteoblasts deposit new bone on the inner fibrous layer of the elevated periosteum, and radiologically, a radiopaque line is visible paralleling the cortex of the bone surface with an intervening radiolucent line.

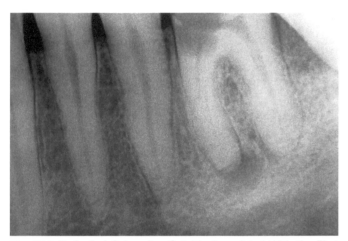

Fig. 22.6 Periapical Sclerosing Osteitis Associated With the First Molar. This is called a sclerosing lesion because most of the lesion is bone forming, resulting in a very radiopaque density. Note, however, the small region of rarefaction at the root apex and the widening of the periodontal ligament space.

However, in times of exacerbation, the periosteum is again distended from the newly formed surface cortex stimulating the differentiation of additional pleuripotential cells into osteoblasts. During the next period of quiescence, another new layer of radiopaque new bone is deposited on the underlying radiolucent fibrous layer of periosteum. The result of this process is one or more thin paired layers of connective tissue and new bone being created adjacent to the bone surface. When this process occurs around the root apex adjacent to the floor of an airspace, such as the maxillary sinus, the appearance is referred to as a "halo pattern." When the process occurs at the surface of the bone, it is referred to as an "onion skin" pattern (Fig. 22.7). Periosteal reactions may also occur on the buccal or lingual surfaces of the alveolar processes, and in rare cases involve the inferior surface of the mandible.

Should periapical inflammatory disease involve the floor of the nasal fossa or maxillary sinus, inflammatory mediators may also stimulate the adjacent mucosal lining of the air cavity producing a regional mucositis within the adjacent floor of the airspace (Fig. 22.8).

Effects on Adjacent Teeth

In many regards, the response of a tooth to periapical inflammatory disease, irrespective of whether or not the tooth is the reason for the inflammatory response or an adjacent tooth, closely mirrors the response of the bone to inflammation. In some instances, tooth roots can undergo external resorption and this may be seen on an image as a change in the normally smooth, tapering surface contour of the root. Alternatively, tooth roots may undergo hypercementosis, and this may be visualized as bulbous-shaped roots. The response of the tooth root, whether external resorption or hypercementosis, may be asymmetric and not uniform around the circumference of the root. When rarefying osteitis involves deciduous teeth, eruption of the underlying permanent dentition may be disrupted (Fig. 22.9).

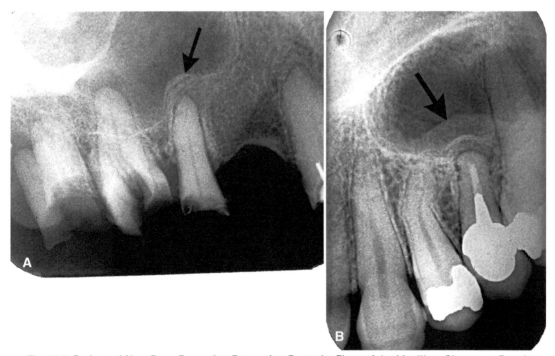

Fig. 22.7 Periosteal New Bone Formation Emanating From the Floor of the Maxillary Sinus as a Result of the Adjacent Areas of Rarefying Osteitis. (A) Laminated type of periosteal bone formation *(arrow)*. (B) Periostitis and sinus mucosal floor thickening (mucositis). Mucositis is characterized by a slight radiopaque band *(arrow)* next to periosteal bone formation.

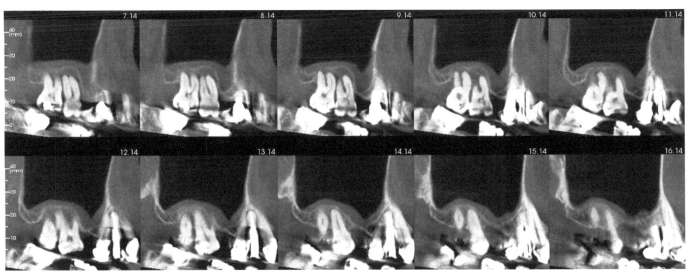

Fig. 22.8 Corrected sagittal cone beam computed tomography images demonstrating maxillary sinus floor periostitis and mucositis.

Differential Interpretation

The two types of lesions that most commonly must be differentiated from periapical inflammatory disease are periapical cemento-osseous dysplasia (PCOD) and a dense bone island (DBI) located at the apex of a tooth root. In the early radiolucent phase of PCOD, the imaging characteristics cannot be used to reliably differentiate this lesion from one of periapical inflammatory disease (Fig. 22.10). The diagnosis may rely solely on the clinical examination, which often includes a test of tooth pulp vitality. Depending on the age of the patient and the chronicity of the periapical inflammatory disease, the pulp chamber of the involved tooth may be larger than the adjacent teeth. More mature PCOD lesions may show the development of a radiopaque focus centrally within the radiolucent area, which helps in the differential interpretation since the radiopacity seen with periapical inflammatory disease occurs at the periphery of the radiolucent focus. External root resorption is also more commonly identified in inflammation than in PCOD.

When a DBI is centered on the root apex, it may mimic a focus of sclerosing osteitis. In these instances, the DBI does not alter the width of the periodontal ligament space around the apex of the tooth (Fig. 22.11). Some DBIs, particularly when they arise adjacent to mandibular molar root apices, may cause external resorption of a tooth root. Although the amount of resorption seen is limited, the root apex of such a tooth may be blunted and nontapering. However, even in such instances, a retained, thin periodontal ligament space can be visualized between the resorbed root apex and the DBI. Moreover, the zone of transition between the DBI and the normal adjacent bone is narrow, unlike in sclerosing osteitis.

If a patient has undergone successful orthograde endodontic treatment or retrograde treatment with apical surgery, a radiolucent area may persist at the root apex, which can appear to be periapical rarefying osteitis. In such cases, the bone may be undergoing healing or it may be healed, and the central radiolucent area may not yet be fully mineralized. Because the healing of such defects is by secondary intention, the central radiolucent focus consists of dense connective tissue. Often, some osseous healing may be visible around the periphery of the radiolucent area and adjacent to the normal cancellous bone. The periphery of the radiolucent area may display a granular type of bone pattern or a series of radiating trabeculae extending from the border of the central radiolucent focus

to the normal adjacent bone. This periphery is sometimes described as having a "rolled border," and the "doughnut pattern" of this entity is called a "fibrous scar" (Fig. 22.12). If the radiologic interpretation is uncertain, the patient's treatment history as well as the clinical signs and symptoms must be considered.

In rare cases, metastatic lesions and blood-borne malignancies, such as leukemia, may develop within the periapical portion of the periodontal ligament space. Close inspection of the surrounding bone may reveal other bone changes, which may include small regions of cancellous bone destruction.

Persistent Periapical Inflammatory Disease

Persistent and recurrent periapical inflammatory disease following endodontic treatment can occur. Possible etiologies can include inadequate orthograde root canal treatment, the perforation of an outer root surface with a rotary instrument, unusual morphology of the root canal, an untreated accessory canal, and root fracture. The application of high-resolution, limited field-of-view CBCT may be useful in determining the etiology of persistent or recurrent disease.

OSTEOMYELITIS

The root "myel" in the term osteomyelitis refers to bone marrow, and therefore the disease process osteomyelitis is used to describe inflammation of the bone marrow. It is noteworthy that rarefying osteitis can also involve the bone marrow, so most authors use the term osteomyelitis to refer to a more widespread response of the bone to inflammation that includes not only the marrow, but also the cortical and cancellous bone as well as the periosteum. However, even this description may be inadequate. As we have seen in the previous section, even lesions of rarefying osteitis can extend to a bone periphery to involve the cortex and periosteum. Where a localized focus of rarefying osteitis becomes more widely disseminated involves some subjectivity. A hallmark feature of osteomyelitis is the identification of a sequestrum (pl. sequestra)—one or more fragments of diseased bone that are losing or have lost their blood supply, and have undergone necrosis as a consequence of this ischemic injury.

Osteomyelitis may resolve spontaneously or with appropriate antibiotic therapy. However, if the condition is not effectively managed,

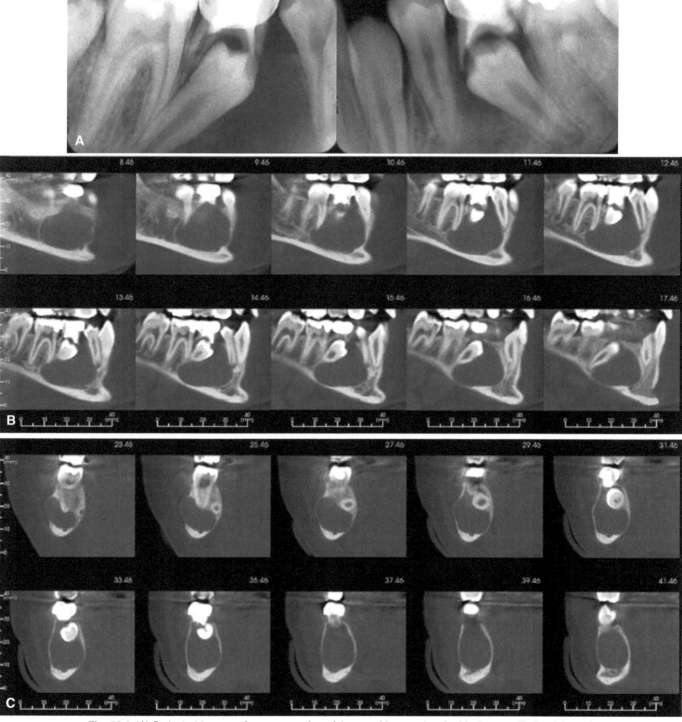

Fig. 22.9 (A) Periapical images of two areas of rarefying osteitis associated with the mandibular right and left second deciduous molars that have undergone pulpectomy procedures. Corrected sagittal (B) and buccal-lingual cross-sectional (C) images of the area of rarefying osteitis associated with the mandibular right second deciduous molar from Fig. 22.8. Note the curved, hydraulic characteristics of the border contours, and the buccal and lingual expansion of the mandible.

the infection agent may persist and continue to spread in some patients; particularly those with preexisting chronic systemic diseases, immunosuppressive states, and disorders of decreased vascularity (e.g., osteopetrosis, sickle cell disease, and HIV/AIDS).

Terminology

Numerous forms of osteomyelitis have been described and many synonyms have been used for the disease process. Consequently, confusion

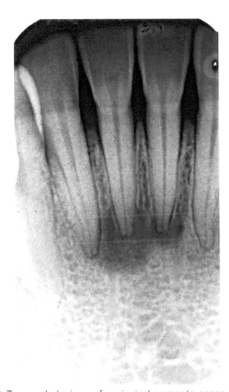

Fig. 22.10 Two early lesions of periapical cemento-osseous dysplasia located at the apical region of the mandibular central incisors. Note the similarities to rarefying osteitis.

has arisen because some forms or synonyms describe clinical progression (acute or chronic), while others make reference to an infectious agent (pyogenic), a clinical finding (suppuration), or a radiologic feature (proliferative periostitis, diffuse sclerosis). And some forms make use of multiple descriptors (Garrè's chronic nonsuppurative sclerosing osteitis). For the sake of simplicity, we will describe osteomyelitis and its associated imaging features with respect to its progression (acute and chronic) along a time continuum.

Disease Mechanism

The acute phase of osteomyelitis is caused by infection that has spread to the bone marrow, and in the jaws, the most common source of infection arises from periapical inflammatory disease from a tooth with a nonvital pulp. Infection may also occur as a result of local spread from the gingiva or by hematogenous spread from a distant site through the bone to the bone surface and periosteum. With this condition, the medullary spaces of the bone contain an inflammatory infiltrate consisting predominantly of neutrophils and, to a lesser extent, mononuclear cells.

Clinical Features

The acute phase of osteomyelitis can affect people of all ages, and it has a strong male predilection. It is much more common in the mandible than in the maxillae, possibly a consequence of the vascular supply to the mandible which tends to be more poor. The typical signs and symptoms of the acute phase are rapid onset, pain, swelling of the adjacent soft tissues, fever, lymphadenopathy, and leukocytosis. The involved teeth may be mobile and sensitive to percussion, and purulent drainage also may be present. Paresthesia of the lower lip in the third division of the trigeminal nerve distribution has also been reported.

The chronic phase of osteomyelitis may be a sequela of inadequately treated acute phase osteomyelitis, or it may arise de novo. The symptoms associated with the chronic phase are generally less severe, and symptom history may involve a greater period of time than the acute form. In comparison with the acute phase, the signs and symptoms associated with the chronic phase include intermittent, recurrent episodes of swelling, pain, fever, and lymphadenopathy. As with the acute form,

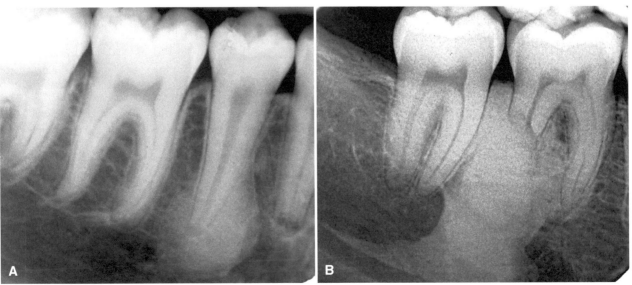

Fig. 22.11 Dense bone islands associated with mandibular molar (A) and premolar (B) teeth. In comparison to sclerosing osteitis, the periodontal ligament space is uniform in width with dense bone islands.

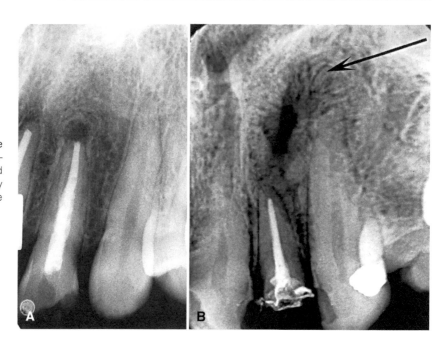

Fig. 22.12 Fibrous Scars After Successful Orthograde Endodontic Treatment. An alternating pattern of concentric radiolucent and radiopaque rings extends inward from the periphery of the healed periapical inflammatory lesion (A). A pattern of internally radiating or spoke-like radiopaque lines also can be seen (B).

paresthesia and drainage with fistula formation also may occur. In some cases, the patient may have little or no pain, or the pain may be limited to times of disease exacerbation. Histopathologically, sparse involvement of the medullary spaces may be seen with marrow fibrosis and chronic inflammatory cell infiltrates with scattered regions of inflammation. At this stage of the disease, culture results usually are negative and the pathogenic microorganism rarely found. If left untreated, osteomyelitis can spread throughout the jaw. In the mandible, this can include the temporomandibular joint, and cause septic arthritis. Ear infections and infection of the mastoid air cells may also develop.

Chronic osteomyelitis as described here is similar to the bone lesions described in chronic recurrent multifocal osteomyelitis (CRMO) and SAPHO syndrome; Synovitis (inflammatory arthritis), Acne (pustulosa), Pustulosis (psoriasis, palmoplantar pustulosis), Hyperostosis (acquired), and Osteitis (osteomyelitis) with respect to the imaging findings, negative microbiologic cultures, and clinical features such as intermittent recurrent pain and swelling of the involved bone. These forms of osteomyelitis arise de novo without going through an acute phase of osteomyelitis where a pathogenic microorganism can be identified. Therefore, some authors have used the term "primary chronic osteomyelitis" to describe this group of diseases and "secondary chronic osteomyelitis" to describe the entity that evolves from the acute phase of osteomyelitis where a pathogenic microorganism can be identified.

CRMO is a condition that often occurs symmetrically in the long bones in children, and is characterized by pain of the affected bone without or with swelling. CRMO has been described as a nonpurulent osteomyelitis with negative microbiologic cultures. The imaging features are identical to chronic osteomyelitis, which will be described here. Treatment has consisted of systemic steroids, nonsteroidal antiinflammatory drugs (NSAIDs), and bisphosphonates because antibiotic and surgical therapy have not been effective treatments. Chronic osteomyelitis of the jaw in children not having a clear etiology may be a unifocal variant of CRMO.

Imaging Examination

An initial imaging examination consisting of panoramic, as well as intraoral periapical and occlusal images may be useful to characterize the extent of the lesion and the teeth involved. While rarefaction and

sclerosis may be visible on panoramic imaging, occlusal images can be useful for depicting periosteal new bone formation. Depending on the exuberance of the bone response, MDCT or CBCT are the imaging modalities of choice for detecting periosteal new bone formation and sequestra. Additionally, MRI may be useful to visualize changes to the bone marrow and a nuclear medicine examination with technetium (^{99m}Tc) and gallium (^{67}Ga) may help to confirm the diagnosis. With acute inflammatory lesions, a positive ^{99m}Tc result depicting increased bone metabolic activity and a positive ^{67}Ga scan in the same location reflecting an inflammatory cell infiltrate can confirm the MDCT, CBCT, or MRI results during the acute phase. As the disease progresses into the chronic phase, a ^{67}Ga examination is not particularly useful because there may be no inflammatory cell population to detect.

Imaging Features

As with periapical inflammatory disease, the imaging features of osteomyelitis may vary depending on the stage of the disease, and while inflammatory cells and exudate may be found in the bone, no changes may be apparent on the diagnostic images in the early acute phase of the disease.

Location. In general terms, the posterior body of the mandible is the most common site of disease, which is, purportedly, the result of the relatively poor blood supply to the bone in this region. Osteomyelitis involving the maxilla is rare.

Periphery. The acute phase of osteomyelitis most often presents with a poorly defined, noncorticated periphery. With time, the periphery may become better defined, but disease extension may still be difficult to visualize. With increasing chronicity, a wide zone of transition may become more visible as the abnormal dense bone transitions to normal trabeculae.

Internal structure. In the acute phase of osteomyelitis, there may be a slight decrease in the density of the involved bone, with a loss of sharpness of the existing trabeculae. As the disease process begins to spread, bone resorption becomes more profound with time, resulting in an area of radiolucency in one or more focal areas scattered regions throughout the involved bone (Fig. 22.13). With time, the appearance of sclerotic regions of bone becomes apparent, and internal bone density may increase to the point where the cancellous bone is uniformly

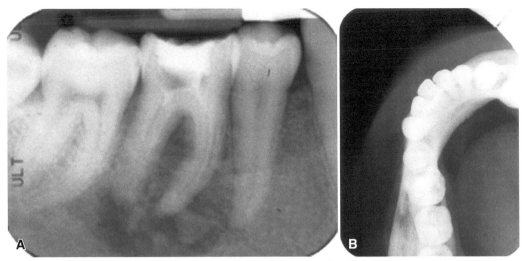

Fig. 22.13 Periapical image (A) showing a mixed radiolucent and radiopaque pattern at the apices of a mandibular right first molar. The cross-sectional occlusal image shows periosteal new bone formation on both the buccal and lingual surfaces of the mandible (B).

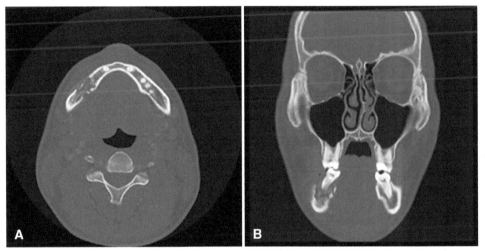

Fig. 22.14 Axial (A) and coronal (B) bone window multidetector computed tomography images of the same patient shown in Fig. 22.10 shows sequestration of the lingual cortex.

radiopaque with a density similar to cortical bone. Sequestra may then develop (see Fig. 22.13), and these can be identified by closely inspecting a region of bone resorption (radiolucency) for an island of radiopaque bone internally. Sequestra may vary in size from a small dot (smaller sequestra usually are seen in young patients) to larger islands of radiopaque bone (Fig. 22.14). Detection may require bright illumination of the radiolucent regions of the film image with an intense light source. Computed tomography (CT) is superior for revealing the internal structure of the abnormal bone, and sequestra, especially in cases where the bone is very densely sclerotic (Figs. 22.15 and 22.16). The bone pattern usually is very granular, obscuring individual bone trabeculae. A similar appearance can be seen in cases of SAPHO syndrome (Fig. 22.17).

Effects on surrounding structures. Acute osteomyelitis can stimulate either bone resorption or bone formation. Portions of cortical bone may be resorbed, and there may be new bone formation on the bone surface as a result of periosteal stimulation described earlier. On the diagnostic image, the "onion skin" pattern of periosteal new bone formation can appear as a series of one or more pairs of alternating radiolucent and radiopaque bands or lines oriented parallel or slightly convex to the surface of the bone (Fig. 22.18). The first radiopaque line of new bone is separated from the surface of the bone by a radiolucent line that represents the fibrous connective tissue inner layer of the periosteum. In some instances, the new bone may be very faint depending on its degree of mineralization. As the lesion develops into a more chronic phase, new bone (bone arcades) may continue to extend into the adjacent underlying connective tissue to support the new surface. The cyclic and periodic acute exacerbations may lift the periosteum again, stimulating the outer osteogenic layer to form a second layer of bone. This second layer can be detected in the image as a second radiopaque line almost parallel to the first and separated from it by a radiolucent band. This process may continue and may result in several lines (the "onion-skin" appearance), and eventually a massive amount of new bone may be formed adjacent to the native bone surface (Fig. 22.19). This condition is referred to as proliferative periostitis and is seen more often in children. The exuberance of the periosteal response in children reflects a thicker and more loosely attached periosteum than in adults, and the higher osteogenic potential of periosteum in younger people.

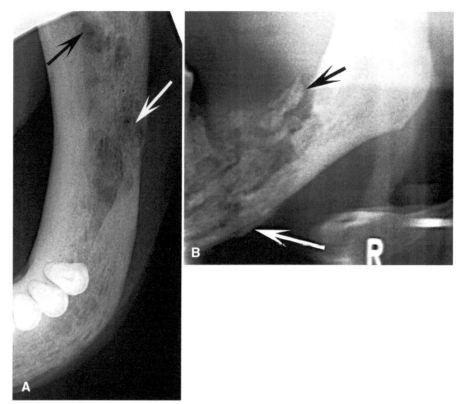

Fig. 22.15 Examples of Sequestra. Cross-sectional occlusal image (A) demonstrates small sequestra as radiopaque islands of bone on a radiolucent background in osteomyelitis *(arrows)*. Panoramic image (B) reveals a large sequestrum *(black arrow)* and a periosteal reaction at the inferior border of the mandible in osteomyelitis *(white arrow)*.

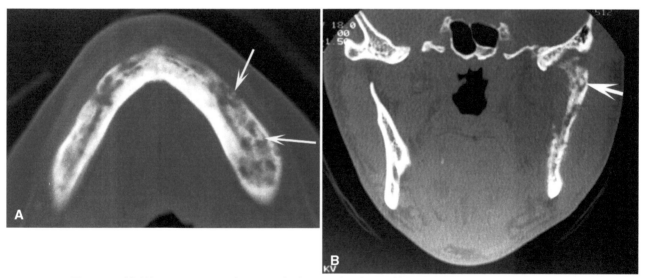

Fig. 22.16 Multidetector computed tomography images showing multiple sequestra within the body of the mandible (A) and in the condylar head (B).

With time and disease chronicity, the radiolucent lines that separate the layers of periosteal new bone from one another may begin to fill in with a granular or sclerotic bone pattern as the intervening bone arcades increase in thickness, increasing radiopacity (Fig. 22.20). When this occurs, it may be impossible to identify the original cortex or the individual layers of periosteal new bone, and this may make it difficult to determine whether the new bone is derived from the periosteum. After a considerable amount of time, a bony hard asymmetry may be seen clinically on the affected side with an altered outer contour and abnormal shape. In patients with extensive chronic osteomyelitis, the disease may slowly spread to the mandibular condyle and the temporomandibular joint resulting in septic arthritis. Further spread may involve

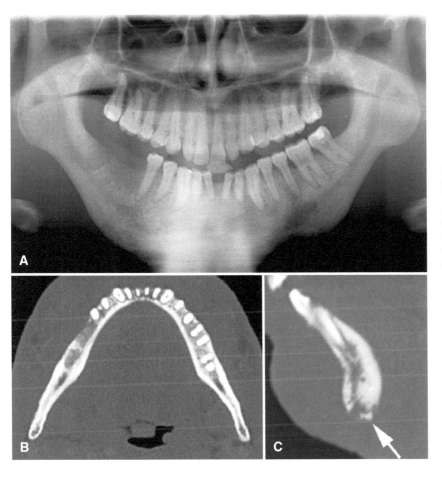

Fig. 22.17 A Case of SAPHO Syndrome in Which Both the Wrist and the Mandible Were Involved. The panoramic image (A) shows a diffuse sclerotic bone reaction, bone resorption of the inferior border of the mandibular body, and widening of the periodontal ligament spaces around many teeth. The axial multidetector computed tomography (MDCT) image shows the mostly sclerotic bone reaction with some regions of bone resorption, while the sagittal MDCT image of the anterior mandible (C) shows resorption of the inferior cortex and a sequestrum *(arrow)*.

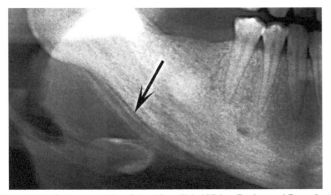

Fig. 22.18 Osteomyelitis of the Mandible With a Periosteal Reaction Located at the Inferior Cortex. Note the radiolucent line *(arrow)* between the inferior cortex of the mandible and the first layer of periosteal new bone. A second radiolucent line separates the second layer of new bone from the first layer.

the inner ear and mastoid air cells. Chronic lesions may also develop a fistula, which may appear as a well-defined break in the outer cortex or in the periosteal new bone (Fig. 22.21).

Effects on adjacent teeth. The effects on the teeth and lamina dura may be the same as the effects described for periapical inflammatory disease in the acute phase of osteomyelitis. The roots of teeth may undergo external resorption or hypercementosis, and the lamina dura may become less apparent as it blends with the surrounding sclerotic bone. If the tooth pulp is nonvital, the widened periodontal ligament

space at the root apex will be enlarged and prominent against the highly sclerotic bone.

Differential Interpretation

Clinically, the differential diagnosis of a unilateral facial or jaw swelling may include osteomyelitis and fibrous dysplasia in children, or malignancy in an adult. Therefore the clinical signs of acute inflammation may be helpful in guiding the imaging examination, and in the identification of key radiologic features. Radiographically, the presence of sequestra is a hallmark of osteomyelitis.

In the acute phase of osteomyelitis in children, the appearance of a unilateral jaw swelling may require an inflammatory lesion to be differentiated from fibrous dysplasia. A useful radiographic feature in this instance may be the way in which the bone enlarges in response to the two diseases. In fibrous dysplasia, the new bone is manufactured from within, and the outer cortex may be thinned by the changes; the location of the surface cortex does not change. Also, bone sequestration is not seen in fibrous dysplasia. In contrast, the new bone that enlarges the jaws in osteomyelitis is laid down on the bone surface by periosteal new bone deposition and is superficial to the bone cortex. In the chronic phase of osteomyelitis, the native bone cortex may be indistinct or difficult to see. In these cases, inspection of the most peripheral surface of the bone may reveal subtle evidence of periosteal new bone formation that has not yet mineralized. These points of differentiation are important because the histopathologic appearance of a biopsy specimen of new periosteal bone in osteomyelitis may be similar to that of fibrous dysplasia, and the condition may be reported erroneously should a radiologic image not be made available to the oral and maxillofacial pathologist.

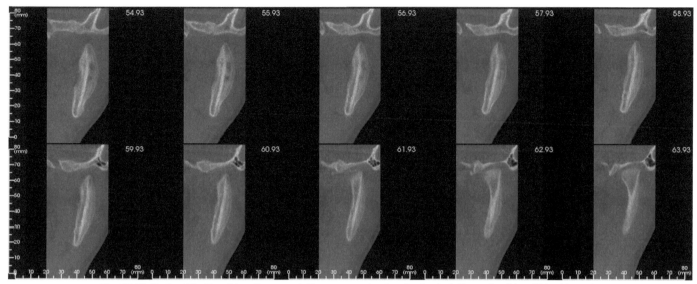

Fig. 22.19 Periostitis Resulting From an Inflammatory Lesion in the Left Posterior Mandible. Note the multiple, alternating layers of both high-attenuation (new bone) and low-attenuation (connective tissue) signal resulting in an onion-skin appearance.

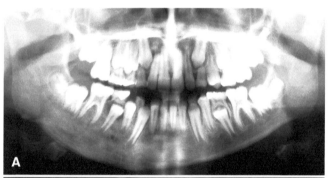

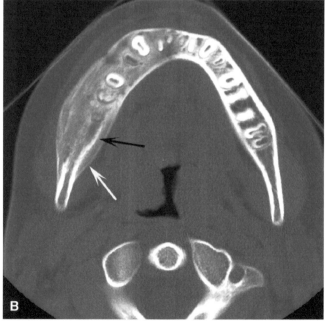

Fig. 22.20 Chronic Osteomyelitis. The panoramic image (A) demonstrates increased density and size of the right mandible compared with the left side. Note the increase in width of the mandible, periosteal new bone *(white arrow)* and evidence of the original cortex *(black arrow)*. There is a general increase in bone density on the right side (B) as well as a loss of definition of the more low-attenuation (radiolucent) component of the response as the disease process becomes chronic.

Malignant neoplasia, whether invading the jawbones from an adjacent soft tissue space or growing within the bone may, at times, be difficult to differentiate from the acute phase of osteomyelitis. This may be the case, particularly if the malignant neoplasm has become secondarily infected via an oral ulcer, and may result in an overlap of inflammatory and malignant radiographic characteristics. It is notable that some malignant neoplasms can also stimulate periosteum and create the "onion-skin" type of appearance seen radiologically in osteomyelitis, namely Langerhans cell histiocytosis, leukemia, lymphoma, and Ewing sarcoma. Should there be destruction of adjacent structures, or of the periosteal bone itself, the possibility of a malignant neoplasm should be considered. For example, Langerhans cell histiocytosis causes ill-defined, noncorticated, radiolucent regions of bone destruction, but the lesion rarely stimulates the sclerotic bone reaction seen in osteomyelitis. Ewing sarcomas will be accompanied by an often rapidly growing and exuberant soft tissue enlargement. In such instances, these lesions usually produce bone destruction, which is characteristic of malignancies.

Malignant neoplasms such as osteosarcoma and chondrosarcoma have the capability of creating new bone within the lesion itself, but this may be accompanied by adjacent areas of bone destruction. Intralesional mineralization may be sporadic and irregular, or dense and granular bone, depending on the maturation of the cells.

Paget disease of bone may affect the mandible bilaterally, which is rare in osteomyelitis; periosteal new bone formation and sequestra are not seen in Paget disease.

The imaging strategy in these instances is either CBCT or MDCT imaging because of its ability to reveal sequestra and periosteal new bone. Furthermore, if soft tissue changes need to be seen, MDCT is the imaging modality of choice.

Management

As with all inflammatory lesions of the jaws, removal of the source of inflammation is the primary goal of therapy. Removal of a tooth, or root canal therapy, may be indicated. Antimicrobial treatment is the mainstay of treatment of acute osteomyelitis, along with surgical incision and drainage.

Chronic osteomyelitis may be more difficult to manage than the acute form. In cases involving an extreme osteoblastic response where the bone may become very sclerotic, the subsequent decrease of blood

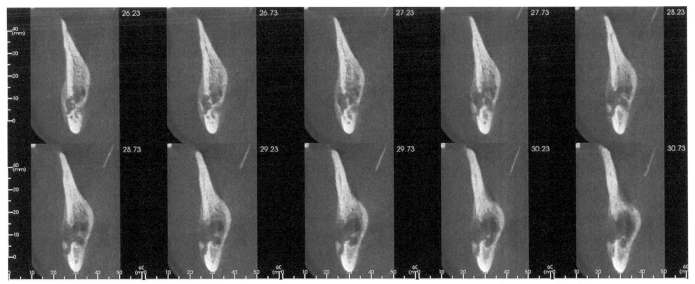

Fig. 22.21 Coronal cone beam computed tomography image showing an increase of bone density. Also, note the thick new buccal cortex of the mandible as the connective tissue layers between the periosteal new bone fill in with more sclerotic bone. A fistula can also be seen perforating the native buccal cortex from the developing mandibular ramal lesion.

supply into the bone may work against healing. Hyperbaric oxygen therapy and creative modes of long-term antibiotic delivery have been used with limited success. Surgical intervention, which may include sequestrectomy, decortication, or resection, often is necessary. The probability of successful treatment, especially when using long-term antibiotic therapy with decortication is greater in the first 2 decades of life. If microbiological cultures are negative, antibiotic therapy is not effective. It may be that the inflammatory response has become the main disease process, and antiinflammatory agents, such as steroids and NSAIDs, may be more effective. More recently, the use of bisphosphonate therapy has provided some therapeutic success.

RADIATION-INDUCED CHANGES TO THE JAWS

Disease Mechanism

Many of the imaging features identified in osteomyelitis can overlap with changes to bone as a consequence of physical or chemical insult. And without a clinical history, it may be difficult, if not impossible, to differentiate the imaging features of these diseases from one another. Therapeutic radiation is an example of a physical insult, prescribed for the treatment of a malignancy in the head and neck. Radiation damages the cellular elements of bone as well as those structures contained within the bone. At the macromolecular level, this damage may involve DNA, or protein or lipid molecules, and these changes could impair DNA replication, enzyme function, or cell membrane permeability. Moreover, such changes could result in the misrepair of radiation-induced damage, arrested cell division, or cell death. The stage of differentiation of cells within and of the bone as well as the dose, dose rate, and fraction of radiation are factors that affect how the bone responds to this injury.

At very low radiation doses in the order of 1 to 4 Gy, radiation has been reported to have a stimulatory effect on osteoblasts, and this may be seen radiographically as new bone formation. Above this dose range, however, therapeutic doses of 10 Gy can result in chondroblast and osteoblast cell death. Macroscopically, a 20-Gy single dose of radiation to the long bones in a young child can result in irreversible growth retardation and short stature. In contrast, the tolerance of mature bone to radiation is higher. Radiation damage to mature, intact bone, a more

radioresistant tissue, has been reported to occur at higher doses, generally between 60 and 70 Gy.

It is important to recognize that bone contains a number of other tissues that may be affected by radiation. One such tissue system is the vasculature. Indeed, many of the late effects of radiation injury that are seen involving bone may arise as a consequence of damage to the vasculature. Although vascular endothelial cells in large vessels are generally radioresistant, the thinner vessel walls of smaller vessels may have greater sensitivity. However, the damage of this population of cells lining the walls of small vessels may compromise their ability to proliferate, and the bone may become hypocellular and hypovascular as a result. The lack of sufficient vascularity results in a hypoxic environment in which adequate healing of bone is compromised. Should the dose, dose rate, or fractionation scheme of radiation delivery exceed the tolerance of the bone to repair, the bone may undergo cell death or necrosis, otherwise referred to as osteoradionecrosis. Therapeutic radiation exposure can cause bone damage and changes without necrosis, although it is possible that such changes may make the bone more susceptible to necrosis, especially after surgical intervention.

Radiation-induced necrosis or osteoradionecrosis is characterized by the presence of exposed bone after the delivery of radiation therapy. The exposed bone may completely sequestrate, often leading to the exposure of more bone. Although bone located anywhere within the jaws is susceptible, the posterior mandible is affected more often than other areas because it is frequently in the radiation field, particularly when lymph nodes are included in the treatment. Intense pain may occur with intermittent swelling and drainage extra-orally. However, many patients feel no pain with bone exposure. The loss of normal structure may compromise the integrity of the bone, and in some cases, the bone can fracture.

Histopathologically, bone necrosis is defined by the absence of osteocytes within lacunae. The overlying mucosal covering can be lost, and the necrotic bone becomes exposed to the oral environment where it can become secondarily infected. It is also possible that irradiated bone becomes more susceptible to necrosis from an odontogenic infection, dental extraction, or denture trauma. Also, depending on the extensiveness of the necrosis, the bone may be susceptible to fracture.

Imaging Examination

An initial imaging examination consisting of panoramic, as well as intraoral periapical and occlusal images may be useful to image the teeth and periodontal structures. Also, as many of the imaging features overlap with the features seen in osteomyelitis, a CBCT or MDCT examination should be completed for the identification of sequestra.

Imaging Features

Immediately following radiation therapy, there may be no visible changes on imaging. The earliest changes may be seen in the posterior mandible because of the generally less vascularized nature of the mandible compared with the maxilla. The abnormal bone may have a poorly defined, noncorticated periphery, and there may be irregular and ill-defined regions of bone resorption and sclerosis. In the maxilla, parts of the cortical borders of the sinus, for example, may be lost (Fig. 22.22). An early change seen in the outer cortical plate of the mandible is a sharply defined region of bone resorption. Should the normal architecture of the bone be sufficiently disrupted, jaw fractures may also be seen.

In the alveolar processes of the jaws, the most frequently occurring change is an irregular but uniform widening of the periodontal ligament space around the teeth. Furthermore, the widening that is seen lacks a discrete epicenter and there is no bone loss (Fig. 22.23). A recent study

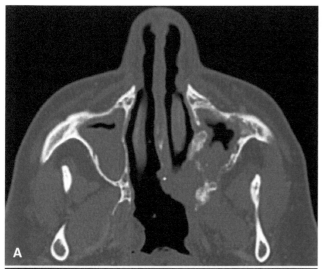

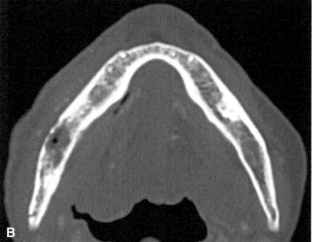

Fig. 22.22 Postradiation Changes. (A) The axial multidetector computed tomography image shows significant resorption of the posterior maxilla. In the mandible (B) there is both resorption and sclerosis.

has shown the cumulative incidence of periodontal ligament space widening to range from 12% in the first 12 months following radiation therapy to 34% in the second year, and finally 55% in the third year with widening more significant with mandibular doses greater than 45 Gy. Other changes that may also be seen include periodontal disease-like bone loss and sclerosis.

The radiologic interpretation of osteoradionecrosis relies on the identification of sequestra in addition to the patient history (Fig. 22.24). Although fractures of the bone can develop (Fig. 22.25), the appearance of a fracture is not necessarily diagnostic. Bone sequestra are seen more commonly in the mandible, and often the sequestra are fragments of detached cortical bone. The presence of osteoradionecrosis cannot always be diagnosed from the diagnostic image, and often clinically obvious signs of exposed necrotic bone (see Fig. 22.24) may not have significant changes in the panoramic image. In these cases, CT imaging is required.

Differential Interpretation

Radiation-induced widening of the periodontal ligament space must be distinguished from periapical inflammatory lesions of the teeth to avoid unnecessary endodontic or tooth extraction. In periapical inflammatory disease, the widest part of the periodontal ligament space is at the apex of the tooth root, and an epicenter is visible. In periodontal disease, the change in the width of the periodontal ligament space is seen at the alveolar crest. Vitality testing of the tooth pulp, and a thorough patient history and clinical examination are important to avoid unnecessary endodontic treatment. Radiation-induced periodontal bone-like loss is difficult to differentiate from conventional periodontal disease as the regions of bone resorption and sclerosis may be very similar.

Bone resorption secondary to radiation therapy may simulate bone destruction from a malignant neoplasm, especially in the maxilla. For this reason, the detection of a recurrence of the malignant neoplasm in the presence of osteoradionecrosis may be very difficult. If the recurrence of a malignancy is suspected, MDCT or MRI may be used to detect an associated soft tissue mass. Differentiating radiation-induced changes from osteomyelitis is less difficult because of the history of radiation therapy.

Management

Treatment of radiation-induced necrosis at the present time is unsatisfactory. Decortication with sequestrectomy and hyperbaric oxygen with antibiotics have been used with limited success because of poor healing following surgery. More conservative approaches, which aim to maintain the integrity of the mandible by keeping the site free of infection and the patient free of pain, may prove more successful in the long term. The incidence of osteoradionecrosis has declined because of the use of intensity-modulated radiotherapy (IMRT) and preventive therapies that can include the removal of teeth with a poor periodontal or pulpal prognosis before radiation treatment, and excellent oral and denture hygiene are the mainstays of preventive regimens.

MEDICATION-RELATED OSTEONECROSIS OF THE JAWS

Some medications can cause chemical insult to bone, altering the balance of osteoblastic and osteoclastic activity, creating a disease state. As with therapeutic radiation, many of the imaging features identified in medication-related osteonecrosis of the jaws overlap with osteomyelitis.

Disease Mechanism

Bisphosphonates and RANK ligand inhibitors are drugs that act to inhibit osteoclast function and bone resorption. Although these drugs

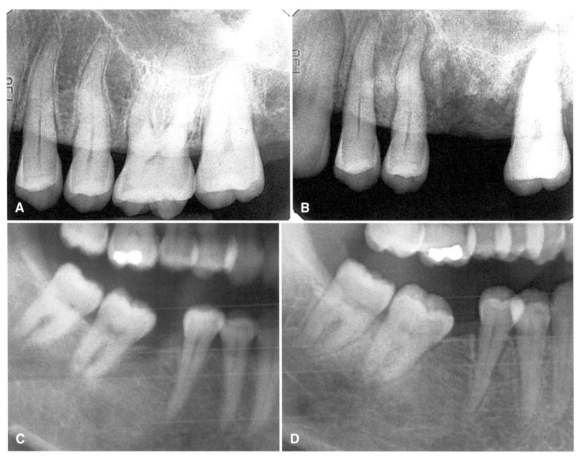

Fig. 22.23 Changes in the Maxillary Dentition After Therapeutic Radiation Exposure. Periapical images were made prior to (A) and within 6 months of receiving the radiation (B). Note the combination of bone destruction and sclerosis, and the nonconcentric widening of the periodontal ligament space. In another case, the cropped panoramic image (C) shows the condition of the bone and teeth prior to radiation and the nonconcentric widening of the ligament space after radiation (D).

have become important treatment modalities of the bone lesions of multiple myeloma, hypercalcemia of malignancy, metastatic disease, and osteoporosis, the intraoral exposure of necrotic bone in patients undertaking this pharmacologic treatment is now a well-known complication. The bone exposure occurs more commonly in patients receiving the more potent aminobisphosphonates intravenously, and after an invasive procedure, such as tooth extraction, periodontal or endodontic surgery, or implant placement. More recently, this has become a more common finding in patients who use oral bisphosphonates.

Clinical Features

Clinically, patients typically develop an area of exposed bone after an invasive dental surgical procedure, although cases related to denture trauma and spontaneous cases have also occurred (Fig. 22.26). Ulceration of palatal tori, for example, resulting in bone exposure, is most likely the result of trauma. The most common areas affected are the posterior mandible (60%) and the maxilla (40%), although both jaws (9%) may be affected. The incidence of bone exposure is difficult to determine, but more recent studies suggest that approximately 3% of patients receiving these drugs have exposed bone. The patients may be asymptomatic, or patients may present with pain and swelling.

Imaging Features

A spectrum of radiographic findings may or may not correlate well with the clinical symptoms. More often than not, there are no specific imaging findings with the clinically exposed bone; however, imaging may demonstrate the detachment. In other cases, the radiographic changes may be indistinguishable from the more chronic phase of osteomyelitis (Fig. 22.27) with increased bone sclerosis and sequestra (Fig. 22.28). Other reported findings include widening of the periodontal membrane space seen with radiation, and thickening of the lamina dura (Fig. 22.29).

Management

Treatment of medication-related bone exposure is unsatisfactory as surgical intervention and hyperbaric oxygen therapy have not been consistently successful. The mainstay of therapy is preventive in nature. Patients who are scheduled to be administered the drugs intravenously should have a dental examination to remove potential and real sources of infection to obviate the need for invasive dental procedures in the future. The situation is further complicated by the fact that the half-life of some of these drugs in bone can be very long—as much as 12 years. Once bone is exposed, management is aimed at controlling the symptoms

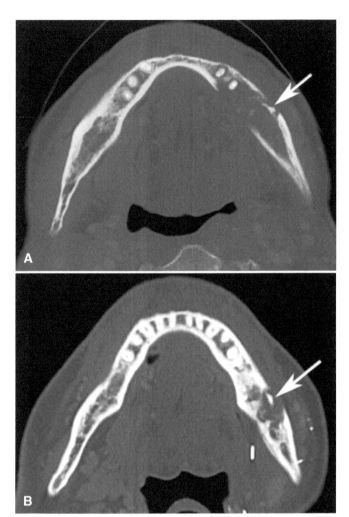

Fig. 22.24 Examples of Radiation Induced Necrosis (Osteoradionecrosis). Axial multidetector computed tomography images showing extensive bone resorption and sequestra *(arrow)* (A). The sclerotic response is more prominent in (B) as is the periosteal response on the lingual surface of the left mandible.

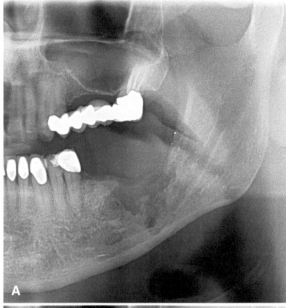

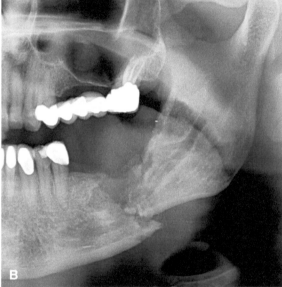

Fig. 22.25 Cropped panoramic image of a patient with bone resorption secondary to therapeutic radiation exposure (A) and the development of a fracture secondary to the loss of bone integrity in the same patient 3 months later (B).

of pain and infection with antibiotic mouth rinses and systemic antibiotic therapy.

DIAGNOSTIC IMAGING OF SOFT TISSUE INVOLVEMENT

Diagnostic imaging may be used to confirm the presence and extent of soft tissue involvement. MDCT and MRI may be used to differentiate soft tissue neoplasia from inflammatory lesions that extend to the bone surface and into the adjacent soft tissues. MDCT is usually used with an intravenous contrast agent, and the imaging features that suggest the presence of soft tissue extension of the inflammatory response include an increase in the attenuation (or radiopacity) of the normally low-attenuation (i.e., radiolucent) appearance of fat that underlies the skin. In these cases, one may observe a series of fine high-attenuation lines extending through the fat to the skin surface, with the lines being oriented perpendicular to the overlying skin surface. This is referred to as "fat streaking" (Fig. 22.30).In addition, one may see enlargement of the adjacent muscle and skin as well as abnormal collections of gas in the soft tissue. Over time, the contrast between soft tissue planes may disappear, and the presence of an abscess may become evident as a well-defined

region of low-attenuation surrounded by a wide border of contrast-enhanced (i.e., more highly attenuated or radiopaque) tissue. T_1- or T_2-weighted MRI can be used with gadolinium enhancement and fat suppression to detect the presence of adjacent soft tissue involvement, including edema. Lymphadenopathy arising from infections also may be visualized on MDCT and MR images within the fascial spaces of the head and neck (Fig. 22.31).

PERICORONITIS

Disease Mechanism

The term pericoronitis refers to inflammation of the soft tissues (i.e., the operculum) surrounding the crown of a partially erupted tooth. This condition, also referred to as operculitis, is seen most often in

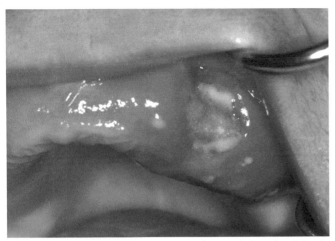

Fig. 22.26 Bisphosphonate-related exposed necrotic bone involving the buccal aspect of a maxillary edentulous ridge in the premolar region.

association with mandibular third molars in young adults. The gingiva surrounding the erupted portion of the crown becomes inflamed when food or microbial debris become trapped under the soft tissue. The gingiva subsequently becomes swollen and may become secondarily traumatized by the opposing occlusion. This inflammation may also extend into the bone surrounding the crown of the tooth.

Clinical Features

Pericoronitis can affect patients of any age or sex, but it is most commonly seen during the time of eruption of the third molars in young adults. Patients with pericoronitis typically complain of pain and swelling, with trismus being a common presentation. When the partially erupted tooth is a mandibular third molar, pain is often felt on occlusion with an ulcerated operculum usually the source of the pain.

Imaging Features

The imaging features of pericoronitis can range from no changes when the inflammatory lesion is confined to the soft tissues to localized

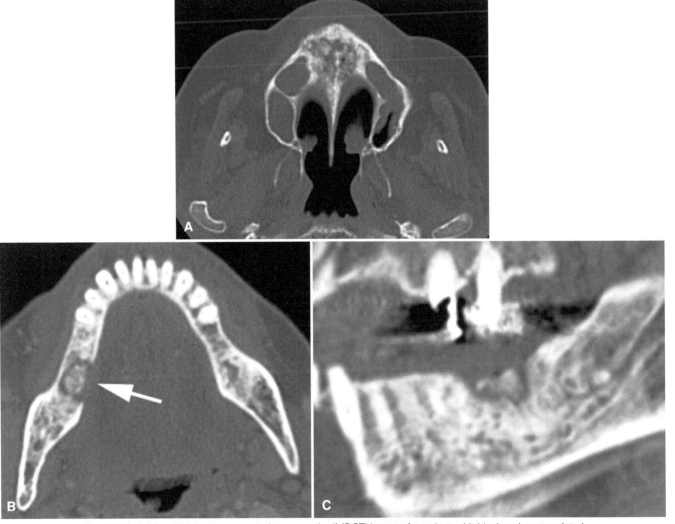

Fig. 22.27 Axial multidetector computed tomography (MDCT) image of a patient with bisphosphonate-related osteonecrosis. Note several sequestra in the anterior palate (A). Axial (B) and sagittal (C) MDCT images show a single large sequestrum in the right posterior mandible.

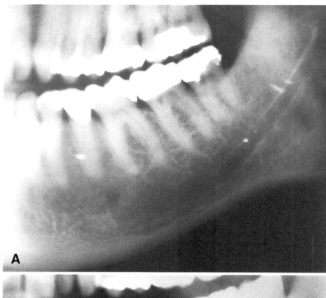

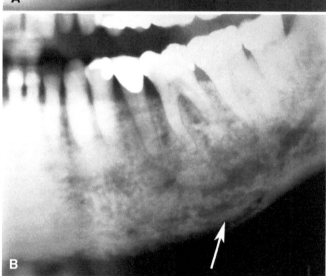

Fig. 22.28 Two cropped panoramic images (A and B) of the same patient taken 1 year apart show the changes to the normal bone pattern following bisphosphonate therapy. Note the developing sclerotic bone pattern and the sequestrum *(arrow)* of the inferior cortex.

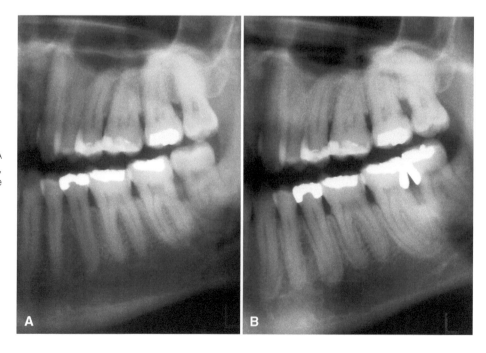

Fig. 22.29 Two cropped panoramic images (A and B) of the same patient shown in Fig. 22.27, made 7 years apart, reveals thickening of the lamina dura around the teeth.

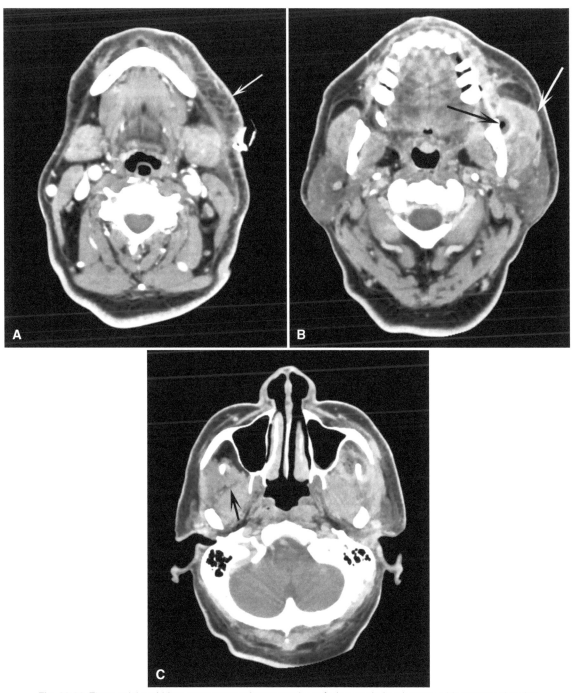

Fig. 22.30 Three axial multidetector computed tomography soft tissue window images with contrast showing an infection involving the soft tissues overlying the left mandibular ramus. There are changes to the fat underlying the adjacent skin (fat streaking or reticulation) and thickening of the skin *(arrow)*. Also, there is thickening of the masseter muscle *(white arrow)* and a radiolucent pocket of gas *(black arrow)* adjacent to the bone (B). There is also a loss of distinctive fat tissue planes between the soft tissues (C). Note that the individual muscles defined by fat planes (the lateral border of the normal lateral pterygoid muscle *[arrow]* is not apparent on the opposite affected side). (Courtesy Stuart White, DDS, Los Angeles, CA.)

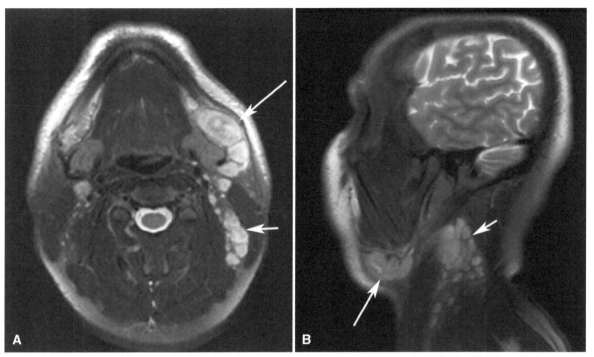

Fig. 22.31 Axial (A) and sagittal (B) T2-weighted magnetic resonance images of a patient with tuberculosis. Note the significant lymphadenopathy involving the submandibular lymph nodes *(long arrows)* and level II nodes *(short arrows)*.

rarefaction around the tooth crown and root to sclerosis of the adjacent bone. Should the inflammatory response become more exuberant, the changes can extend to the bone surface, producing periosteal new bone formation and osteomyelitis in the most severe cases.

Location

The mandibular third molar region is the most common location. When bone changes are associated with pericoronitis, they are centered on the follicular space or the portion of the crown still embedded in bone or in close proximity to bone.

Periphery

The periphery of the bone changes are poorly defined with a gradual transition of the normal trabecular pattern to sclerosis.

Internal Structure

The internal structure of bone adjacent to the area of pericoronitis is most often sclerotic with thickened trabeculae (Fig. 22.32). An area of bone loss or radiolucency immediately adjacent to the crown that enlarges the follicular space may be seen. If this lesion spreads considerably, the internal pattern appears identical to the imaging features of osteomyelitis.

Effects on Surrounding Structures

As with periapical inflammatory disease, pericoronitis may cause rarefaction and/or sclerosis of the surrounding bone. With more extensive involvement, evidence of periosteal new bone formation may be seen along an adjacent bone surface, and this may extend superiorly as high as the sigmoid notch of the mandible (Fig. 22.33).

Differential Interpretation

The diagnosis of pericoronitis is made clinically rather than radiographically. The differential interpretation of pericoronitis includes other mixed

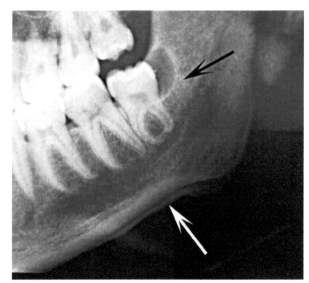

Fig. 22.32 Cropped panoramic image of a case of pericoronitis related to a partially erupted third molar. Note the sclerotic bone reaction adjacent to the follicular cortex *(black arrow)* and the periosteal reaction *(white arrow)*.

radiolucent and radiopaque, or sclerotic, entities that can exist adjacent to the crown of a partially erupted third molar. These may include a DBI and fibrous dysplasia. The clinical symptoms, which are indicative of an inflammatory lesion, usually exclude these conditions. Neoplasms to be considered include squamous cell carcinoma (in older patients) and the sclerotic form of osteosarcoma. The occurrence of squamous cell carcinoma in the midst of a preexisting inflammatory lesion may be difficult to identify. Features characteristic of malignant neoplasia,

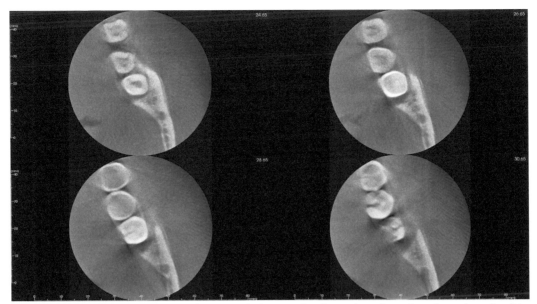

Fig. 22.33 Axial cone beam computed tomography images showing periosteal new bone formation adjacent to the lateral surface of the ramus in a patient with pericoronitis.

such as profound cortical bone destruction and invasion, may assist with the diagnosis.

Management

The treatment aim of pericoronitis is removal of the partially erupted tooth. However, in the acute phase, when trismus may prevent adequate access, antibiotic therapy and reduction of the occlusion of the opposing tooth should relieve symptoms until definitive treatment can be provided.

BIBLIOGRAPHY

Periapical Inflammatory Lesions
Bender IB, Seltzer S. Roentgenographic and direct observation of experimental lesions in bone: I. 1961. *J Endod.* 2003;29:702–706.
Bender IB, Seltzer S. Roentgenographic and direct observation of experimental lesions in bone: II. 1961. *J Endod.* 2003;29:707–712.
Worth HM. *Infections of the Jaws in Principles and Practice of Oral Radiologic Interpretation.* Chicago: Year Book Medical Publishers; 1963.

Pericoronitis
Blakey GH, White RP Jr, Offenbacher S, et al. Clinical/biological outcomes of treatment for pericoronitis. *J Oral Maxillofac Surg.* 1996;54:1150–1160.

Osteomyelitis
An CH, An SY, Choi BR, et al. Hard and soft tissue changes of osteomyelitis of the jaws on CT images. *Oral Surg Oral Med Oral Pathol Oral Radiol.* 2012;114:118–126.
Ledermann HP, Kaim A, Bongartz G, et al. Pitfalls and limitations of magnetic resonance imaging in chronic posttraumatic osteomyelitis. *Eur Radiol.* 2000;10:1815–1823.
Monsour PAK, Dalton JB. Chronic recurrent multifocal osteomyelitis involving the mandible: case reports and review of the literature. *Dentomaxillofac Radiol.* 2010;39:184–190.
Morrison WB, Schweitzer ME, Batte WG, et al. Osteomyelitis of the foot: relative importance of primary and secondary MR imaging signs. *Radiology.* 1998;207:625–632.
Nordin U, Wannfors K, Colque-Navarro P, et al. Antibody response in patients with osteomyelitis of the mandible. *Oral Surg Oral Med Oral Pathol Oral Radiol Endod.* 1995;79:429.

Orpe EC, Lee L, Pharoah MJ. A radiological analysis of chronic sclerosing osteomyelitis of the mandible. *Dentomaxillofac Radiol.* 1996;25:125–129.
Petrikowski CG, Pharoah MJ, Lee L, et al. Radiographic differentiation of osteogenic sarcoma, osteomyelitis, and fibrous dysplasia of the jaws. *Oral Surg Oral Med Oral Pathol Oral Radiol Endod.* 1995;80:744–750.
Suei Y, Taguchi A, Tanimoto K. Diagnostic points and possible origin of osteomyelitis in synovitis, acne, pustulosis, hyperostosis and osteitis (SAPHO) syndrome: a radiographic study of 77 mandibular osteomyelitis cases. *Rheumatology.* 2003;42:1398–1403.
Suei Y, Tanimoto K, Taguchi A, et al. Possible identity of diffuse sclerosing osteomyelitis and chronic recurrent multifocal osteomyelitis: one entity or two? *Oral Surg Oral Med Oral Pathol Oral Radiol Endod.* 1995;80:401–408.
Van Merkesteyn JP, Groot RH, Bras J, et al. Diffuse sclerosing osteomyelitis of the mandible: clinical radiographic and histologic findings in twenty seven patients. *J Oral Maxillofac Surg.* 1988;46:825–829.
Wannfors K, Hammarström L. Infectious foci in chronic osteomyelitis of the jaws. *Int J Oral Surg.* 1985;14:493–503.
Wood RE, Nortjé CJ, Grotepass F, et al. Periostitis ossificans versus Garré's osteomyelitis, Part I: what did Garré really say? *Oral Surg Oral Med Oral Pathol.* 1988;65:773–777.

Radiation-Induced Changes to Bone
Becker M, Schroth G, Zbären P, et al. Long-term changes induced by high dose irradiation of the head and neck region: imaging findings. *Radiographics.* 1997;17:5–26.
Hall EJ, Giaccia AJ. *Radiobiology for the Radiologist.* 7th ed. Philadelphia: Lippincott Williams & Wilkins; 2012.
Williams HJ, Davies AM. The effect of x-rays on bone: a pictorial review. *Eur Radiol.* 2006;16:619–633.

Osteoradionecrosis
Chan KC, Perschbacher SE, Lam EW, et al. Mandibular changes on panoramic imaging after head and neck radiotherapy. *Oral Surg Oral Med Oral Pathol Oral Radiol.* 2016;121:666–672.
Curi MM, Dib LL. Osteoradionecrosis of the jaws: a retrospective study of the background factors and treatment in 104 cases. *J Oral Maxillofac Surg.* 1997;55:540–544.
Hermans R, Fossion E, Ioannides C, et al. CT findings in osteoradionecrosis of the mandible. *Skeletal Radiol.* 1996;25:31–36.
Marx RE. Osteoradionecrosis: a new concept of its pathophysiology. *J Oral Maxillofac Surg.* 1983;41:283–288.

Wong JK, Wood RE, McLean M. Conservative management of osteoradionecrosis. *Oral Surg Oral Med Oral Pathol Oral Radiol Endod.* 1997;84:16–21.

Medication-Related Osteonecrosis

Jadu F, Lee L, Pharoah M, et al. A retrospective study assessing the incidence, risk factors and comorbidities of pamidronate-related necrosis of the jaws in multiple myeloma patients. *Ann Oncol.* 2007;18:2015–2019.

Subramanian G, Kalyoussef E, Blitz-Goldstein M, et al. Identifying MRONJ-affected bone with digital fusion of functional imaging (FI) and cone-beam computed tomography (CBCT): case reports and hypothesis. *Oral Surg Oral Med Oral Pathol Oral Radiol.* 2017;123:e106–e116.

Woo SB, Hellstein J, Kalmar JR. Narrative [corrected] review: bisphosphonates and osteonecrosis of the jaws. *Ann Intern Med.* 2006;144:753–761.

23

Cysts

Ernest W.N. Lam

A true cyst is a pathologic cavity in bone; it is lined by epithelium and may contain a small amount of fluid drawn from adjacent cells and tissues. The epithelium may be derived from odontogenic or nonodontogenic sources. Odontogenic sources include the dental lamina, the reduced enamel epithelium, and the epithelial rests of Malassez, or remnants of Hertwig epithelial root sheath; nonodontogenic sources may include respiratory epithelium or remnant epithelial rests within areas of tissue fusion. A thin connective tissue layer separates the base of the epithelium from the adjacent bone. Pseudocysts are a group of cysts that may not be lined by epithelium or they may not be cavities in the bone at all. Rather, pseudocysts may have some but not all of the radiologic features of a true cyst.

DISEASE MECHANISM

The proliferation of remnant epithelial cells within the bone is the initiating event in the pathogenesis of a true cyst. Epithelial proliferation may be the result of a genetic mutation or due to the release of a signaling molecule or mediator from an adjacent cell or tissue that stimulates proliferation. As the cells proliferate, they begin to displace the adjacent bone, so that space is made available for their increasing numbers (Fig. 23.1). Cells closer to the center of the developing mass become more distant from the periphery as the population proliferates and differentiates, and there is a reduction in the nutrient supply they receive from the adjacent vasculature and tissues. With time, intraluminal epithelial cell debris accumulates at the center of the cavity, and the increasing osmotic gradient that develops across the developing cyst draws fluid in from adjacent cells and tissues. With time, the developing cavity increases in size as more fluid is drawn in and more debris accumulates centrally. In addition, a thin connective tissue layer develops between the basal epithelial cells and the adjacent bone, and osteoclasts are recruited to accommodate the growing cyst within the bone. The result is a cavity within bone that expands much as a balloon would expand as it filled with water.

CLINICAL FEATURES

The most common clinical feature is a firm to bony-hard swelling that may be accompanied by pain if the cyst is related to a tooth with a nonvital pulp or has become secondarily infected.

APPLIED DIAGNOSTIC IMAGING

Diagnostic imaging has many important roles in the assessment and management of a cyst. First, imaging may aid in the initial diagnosis of a cyst and may describe its extent within bone. Radiologic investigations

may also help to determine the extent of extraosseous involvement and assist in determining the best site for biopsy.

Intraoral images may reveal subtle changes occurring around the teeth, including the effects of the cyst on the periodontal ligament space and lamina dura. Panoramic imaging can provide an overall assessment of the osseous structures of the jaws and reveal relevant changes such as alterations to the borders of the maxillary sinus. Both cone beam computed tomography (CBCT) or multidetector computed tomography (MDCT) may be useful to demonstrate the three-dimensional involvement of bone, whereas MDCT and magnetic resonance imaging (MRI) may show the involvement of adjacent tissues.

IMAGING FEATURES

Location

Cysts may occur anywhere centrally within the maxilla or mandible but are rare in the condylar and coronoid processes of the mandible. Odontogenic cysts are most commonly found in the tooth-bearing areas of the jaws; in the mandible, they develop superior to the inferior alveolar canal. Some nonodontogenic cysts can originate within the antrum, whereas others can develop in the soft tissues around the face and neck.

Periphery

Cysts that arise centrally from within bone have a well-defined periphery and a cortex characterized by a fairly uniform, thin, radiopaque line. When a cyst becomes secondarily infected, the cortex may become less discrete and take on a thicker, somewhat sclerotic and less radiopaque appearance. In addition, some cysts may insinuate themselves around the roots of teeth or against a bone cortex, creating a series of contiguous arcs; this is referred to as *scalloping*.

Shape

Cysts have curved borders that may give them an overall round or oval shape. Sometimes resembling a fluid-filled balloon, a cyst is often described as having a hydraulic shape or hydraulic pattern of expansion within the bone.

Internal Structure

Cysts are most often totally radiolucent; however, long-standing cysts may contain cellular debris, including cholesterol granules or dystrophic calcification, both of which can give them a sparse, particulate radiopaque appearance. In some cysts, the epithelium can proliferate differentially, with some areas showing slower or faster proliferation. This type of differential proliferation may give the cyst a multilocular appearance and result in the development of bony walls or septa between the loculations. Occasionally scalloping of an adjacent bone by the cyst can produce ridges within the endosteal surface of the bone cortex, which may give the false impression that these are septa.

Effects on Surrounding Structures

Cysts develop and increase in size slowly, and when the periphery encounters an adjacent bone border, the bone border thins where it engages the cyst's periphery. With time, bone will expand to accommodate the cyst, and the pattern of expansion produces a smooth, curved surface. Cysts may displace the inferior alveolar nerve canal in an inferior direction or displace the floor of the maxillary sinus, maintaining a thin layer of bone separating the cyst cavity from the antrum.

Effects on Adjacent Teeth

The slowly growing nature of cysts can cause displacement of adjacent teeth as well as external resorption of a tooth's roots, producing an often sharp, curved border that mirrors the curvature of the cyst's border. This is referred to as "directional external resorption." Also, the lamina dura and the periodontal ligament space may be lost.

ODONTOGENIC CYSTS

Radicular Cyst

The radicular cyst is discussed in Chapter 22 in the context of periapical inflammatory disease. As the radiologic features of an abscess, granuloma, or cyst that arises in the radicular or periradicular areas cannot be used to differentiate one of these lesions from any of the others, the "umbrella term" *rarefying osteitis* is used in oral and maxillofacial radiology to describe a localized inflammatory condition arising within the jaws. It is only after a focus of rarefying osteitis has undergone biopsy that the oral and maxillofacial pathologist can identify the lesion as a radicular cyst. In this situation, the epithelial lining that is identified is derived from the epithelial cell rests of Malassez, and these cells are stimulated to proliferate by inflammatory mediators and signals derived from a tooth with a nonvital pulp.

Dentigerous Cyst
Disease Mechanism

The dentigerous or follicular cyst develops from the proliferation of the reduced enamel epithelium. Consequently the cyst is associated with the crown of an unerupted tooth or supernumerary tooth. The eruption cyst is the soft tissue counterpart of a dentigerous cyst.

Clinical Features

Dentigerous cysts are the second most common type of cyst in the jaws. Clinical examination may reveal a missing tooth or teeth and possibly a hard swelling that can manifest as facial asymmetry.

Imaging Features

Location. The epicenter of a dentigerous cyst is located coronal to the crown of the involved tooth, most commonly a third molar or a maxillary canine (Fig. 23.2). An important diagnostic point is that the cyst's periphery engages the tooth at its cementoenamel junction. Dentigerous cysts developing in association with maxillary third molar teeth will enlarge into the maxilla and displace the floor of the maxillary sinus as they enlarge. Cysts developing in association with mandibular third molars may extend a considerable distance into the ramus.

Periphery. Dentigerous cysts have a well-defined and corticated periphery. If the periphery of the cyst perforates an adjacent bone surface, a portion of the cortex may be lost (Fig. 23.3). Moreover, if the cyst cavity has become secondarily infected by oral microorganisms, both the periphery and the cortex may not be as clearly seen.

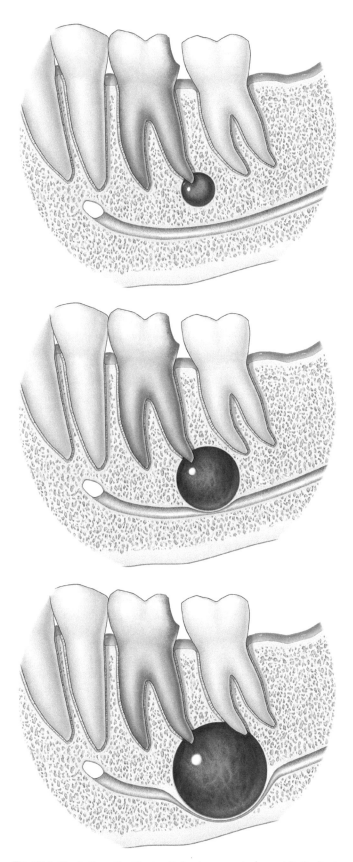

Fig. 23.1 The balloon-like "hydraulic" enlargement of a cyst in the jaws, and displacement of the adjacent inferior alveolar canal as it increases in size.

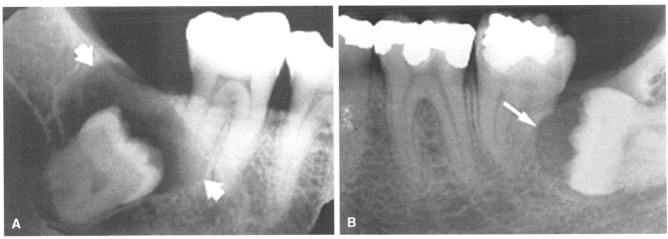

Fig. 23.2 (A) A dentigerous cyst surrounds the crown of the mandibular right third molar *(arrows)*. Note the association of the cyst with the distal cementoenamel junction. (B) A dentigerous cyst has caused resorption of the distal root of the mandibular left second molar *(arrow)*.

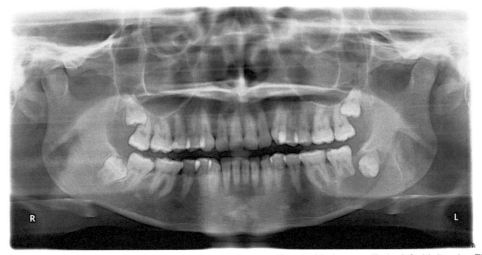

Fig. 23.3 A panoramic image shows a dentigerous cyst associated with the mandibular left third molar. The cortical boundary is not continuous around the entire cyst. The third molar has been displaced into the mandibular ramus, and there has been external resorption of the second molar roots.

Internal structure. Internally, a dentigerous cyst is completely radiolucent except for the crown of the involved tooth.

Effects on surrounding structures. As dentigerous cysts are slow-growing lesions, adjacent bone borders—whether the floor of the maxillary sinus or an adjacent cortex of bone—may be displaced as the cyst enlarges. Furthermore, adjacent anatomic structures such as the inferior alveolar canal can be displaced apically, away from the cyst (Fig. 23.4). In cases where the dentigerous cyst has broached the crest of the alveolar process in either the maxilla or mandible and the intraluminal osmotic pressure has been relieved, the cyst may be in a state of decompression, obviating its ability to expand and affect adjacent structures.

Effects on adjacent teeth. A dentigerous cyst has a propensity to displace and resorb adjacent teeth (see Figs. 23.2B, 23.3, and 23.4). In addition, a dentigerous cyst can displace the associated tooth in an apical direction, away from the cyst's epicenter, and this may be considerable. For instance, maxillary third molars (Fig. 23.5) or canine (Fig. 23.6) teeth may be displaced to the floor of the orbit, and mandibular third molars may be displaced into the condylar or coronoid processes or to the inferior cortex of the mandible.

Differential Interpretation

The histopathologic appearance of the lining epithelium of a dentigerous cyst is not specific. Therefore the diagnosis relies on both the radiographic interpretation and surgical observation of the attachment of the cyst to the cementoenamel junction. However, histopathologic examination must always be done to eliminate other similar-looking lesions that could mimic a dentigerous cyst.

One of the most difficult differential interpretations to make is between a hyperplastic follicle developing around a tooth crown and a dentigerous cyst. A cyst should be considered with any evidence of tooth displacement or expansion of the bone or with asymmetric enlargement of the follicle. If uncertainty remains, the region should be reexamined in 4 to 6 months to detect any increase in shape or influence on surrounding structures characteristic of cysts.

The differential interpretation of a dentigerous cyst may also include an odontogenic keratocyst (OKC), an ameloblastic fibroma, and a unicystic or cystic ameloblastoma. An OKC does not expand the bone to the same degree as a dentigerous cyst, is less likely to resorb teeth, and may attach further apically on the root or coronally on the crown

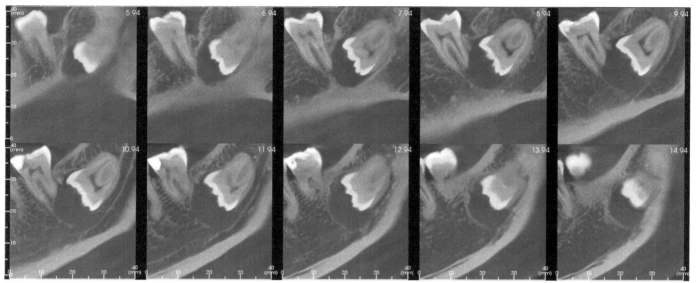

Fig. 23.4 Corrected sagittal cone beam computed tomographic images of a dentigerous cyst associated with the mandibular left third molar. Note the displacement of the inferior alveolar canal and the external resorption of the adjacent second molar distal root.

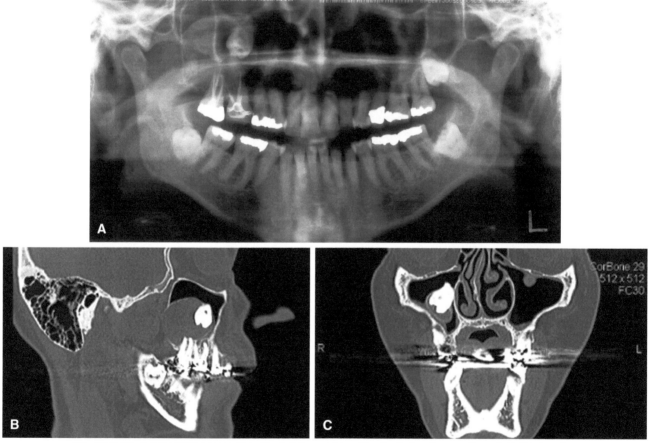

Fig. 23.5 (A) A panoramic image showing a large cystic entity displacing the maxillary right third molar. Sagittal (B) and coronal (C) multidetector computed tomography images show the cystic entity associated with the cementoenamel junction of the displaced molar.

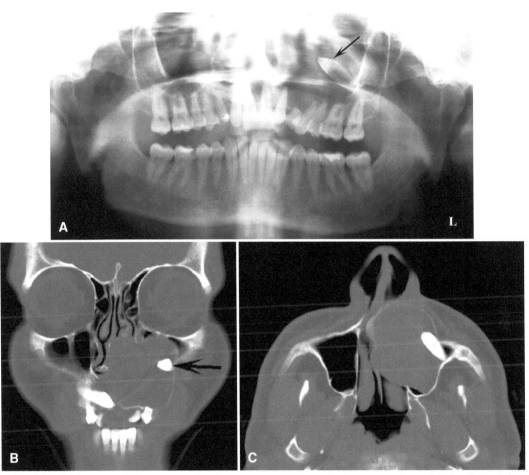

Fig. 23.6 (A) A panoramic image revealing the presence of a large dentigerous cyst associated with the left maxillary canine *(arrow)*, which has been displaced. Note the displacement and resorption of other teeth in the left maxilla. Coronal (B) and axial (C) multidetector computed tomography images of the same case show superolateral displacement of the canine, expansion of the anterior wall of the maxilla, and expansion of the cyst into the nasal fossa.

instead of at the cementoenamel junction. It may be impossible to differentiate a small ameloblastic fibroma or cystic or unicystic ameloblastoma from a dentigerous cyst if there is no internal structure. Other less common lesions that may have a pericoronal relationship to an impacted tooth include the adenomatoid odontogenic tumor, the calcifying epithelial odontogenic tumor, and calcifying odontogenic cysts (COCs), all of which can surround the crown and root of the involved tooth. Evidence of a radiopaque internal structure is sometimes found in these lesions. Occasionally rarefying osteitis developing at the apex of a primary tooth may appear to envelop the crown of an adjacent developing permanent tooth positioned apical to it, giving the false impression of a dentigerous cyst associated with the permanent tooth. This occurs most often with the mandibular deciduous molar and the developing premolar teeth. In these cases, the clinician should look for extensive caries or large restorations in a primary tooth—an etiology that would support an interpretation of a rarefying osteitis.

Management

Dentigerous cysts are treated by surgical removal, which usually includes the tooth as well. Large cysts may be treated by marsupialization before removal. The cyst lining should be submitted for histopathologic examination because other lesions have been reported to arise from the dentigerous cyst epithelium—namely ameloblastoma, squamous cell carcinoma, and mucoepidermoid carcinoma, although this occurs rarely.

Odontogenic Keratocyst
Disease Mechanism

The epithelial lining of OKCs is derived from the dental lamina and is distinctive for its thin, keratinized epithelium (four to eight cells thick). When the keratin sloughs from the surface of the epithelium, a collection of viscous or cheesy material can be found in the cyst's lumen. In contrast to most cysts, which are thought to enlarge solely by intraluminal osmotic pressure, the epithelium in the OKC appears to have some innate growth potential. Occasionally budlike proliferations of epithelium grow from the basal layer of the epithelium into the underlying connective tissue. Also, islands of epithelium in the wall may give rise to satellite microcysts, which can enlarge independently. These differences in the mechanism of growth give the OKC a different radiographic appearance from other cysts. The ability of the basal epithelial cells to undergo "budding" can sometimes create a multilocular appearance on an image, and mutations have been identified involving the human homolog of the *Drosophila PTCH* gene, which may contribute to its non–cystlike behavior.

Clinical Features

OKCs can develop in association with an unerupted tooth or as solitary entities in bone. OKCs usually cause no symptoms, although mild swelling may occur. Pain may occur with secondary infection. Aspiration of the cavity may reveal a thick, yellow, cheesy material (keratin). In contrast to other odontogenic cysts, OKCs have a great propensity for recurrence, possibly because of small satellite cysts or fragments of epithelium left behind after surgical removal.

Imaging Features

Location. Although odonotogenic keratocysts can occur anywhere in the jaws, they most commonly arise in the posterior body of the mandible (90% occur distal to the canine teeth) and mandibular ramus (>50%). The epicenter is located superior to the inferior alveolar canal. Occasionally OKCs may develop in association with the crown of an unerupted or impacted tooth and may be difficult to distinguish from dentigerous cysts. A change to the contour of the follicle coronal to the cementoenamel junction in an OKC, where the follicle enlarges smoothly and uniformly from the cementoenamel junction, is one way to distinguish this lesion from a dentigerous cyst (Fig. 23.7).

Periphery. OKCs have a well-defined and corticated periphery. The periphery is smooth, but its border may scallop a thick bone cortex (Fig. 23.8).

Internal structure. The internal structure is most commonly radiolucent. The presence of internal keratin does not increase the radiopacity. In some cases, curved internal septa may be present, giving the lesion a multilocular appearance.

Effects on surrounding structures. An important characteristic of the OKC is its propensity to grow through the bone without significant bone expansion (Fig. 23.9). This "tunneling" type of growth pattern with minimal expansion occurs throughout the body of the mandible except for the ramus and coronoid process, where considerable expansion may be seen due to the very thin nature of the bone in these locations. This tunneling effect can also be seen within the alveolar process of the maxilla (Fig. 23.10A). Adjacent to an airspace such as the nasal fossa or maxillary sinus, OKCs expand in a concentric and hydraulic manner (see Fig. 23.10B) that is more classical for a cyst; as the cyst enlarges, it can reduce the volume of the adjacent airspace.

Occasionally the bone expansion created by large lesions may exceed the ability of the periosteum to form new bone to accommodate the OKC, and the epithelium may contact soft tissue adjacent to the outer surface of the mandible. The relatively slight expansion common to these lesions potentially contributes to their late detection, which occasionally allows them to reach a large size. The inferior alveolar nerve canal may be displaced inferiorly.

Effects on adjacent teeth. OKCs occasionally displace teeth and resorb tooth roots, but to a lesser degree than dentigerous cysts.

Differential Interpretation

When an OKC develops in a pericoronal position, it may be indistinguishable from a dentigerous cyst. The lesion is likely to be an OKC if the cyst periphery is associated with the tooth at a point apical or coronal to the cementoenamel junction or if little or no expansion of the bone has occurred. The scalloped margin or a multilocular appearance of an OKC may resemble an ameloblastoma, but the latter has a greater propensity to expand bone. Occasionally large lateral periodontal cysts, especially in the maxilla, have a growth pattern similar to that of an OKC, with minimal bone expansion. The mild expansion and multilocular appearance of the odontogenic myxoma may make it indistinguishable from an OKC. A simple bone cyst (SBC) often has a scalloped border and minimal bone expansion, similar to an OKC; however, the margins of an SBC usually are more delicate and often difficult to detect, and there is little or no effect on the teeth or the supporting structures.

Management

If an OKC is suspected, referral to an oral and maxillofacial radiologist for a complete radiologic examination is advisable. If, on plain imaging, a cortical perforation is detected, MDCT should be used to investigate the possibility of soft tissue extension. Otherwise CBCT can be ordered. Because this entity has a propensity to recur, an accurate determination of the extent and location of any cortical perforations with soft tissue extension is best achieved with MDCT.

Surgical treatment may vary and can include resection, curettage, or marsupialization to reduce the size of large lesions before surgical excision. More attention is usually devoted to complete removal of the cystic walls so as to reduce the chance of recurrence. After surgical treatment, it is important to reexamine the patient at regular intervals to detect any recurrence. Recurrent lesions usually develop within the first 5 years but may occur as much as 10 years later.

Nevoid Basal Cell Carcinoma Syndrome
Disease Mechanism

Nevoid basal cell carcinoma, or Gorlin-Goltz syndrome, is an autosomal dominant disorder related to mutations of the human homolog of the *Drosophila PTCH* gene.

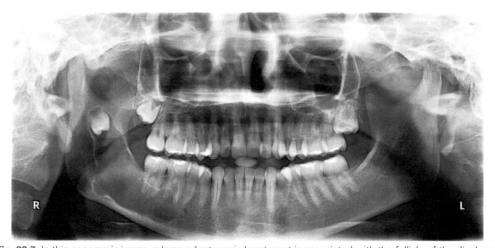

Fig. 23.7 In this panoramic image, a large odontogenic keratocyst is associated with the follicle of the displaced mandibular right third molar. Note the change to the contour of the third molar follicle. The contour of the follicle and the change in its size occur coronal to the cementoenamel junction of the third molar.

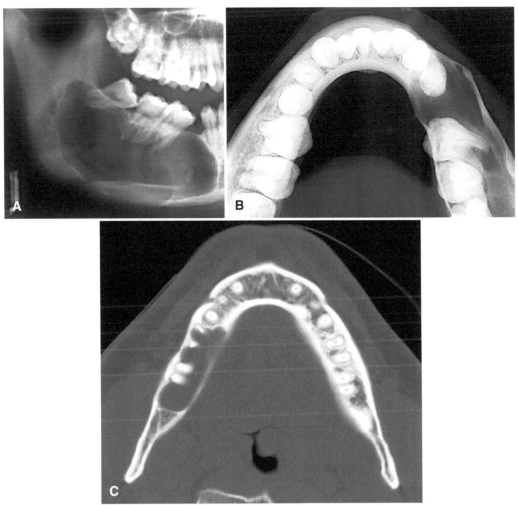

Fig. 23.8 A large odontogenic keratocyst occupying most of the right body and ramus of the mandible (A). Despite the cyst's large size, the buccal and lingual surfaces of the mandible have been expanded only slightly, as can be seen in the occlusal image (B). The multidetector computed tomography image shows a lack of expansion of the mandible and the cyst scalloping between the roots of the teeth (C).

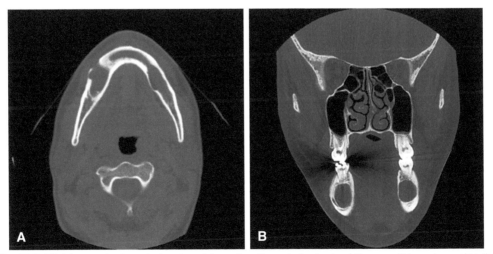

Fig. 23.9 (A) A large odontogenic keratocyst tunneling through the body of the mandible and crossing the midline to involve both the right and left sides. (B) Despite the cyst's very large size, there has been little, if any, buccal or lingual expansion of the bone.

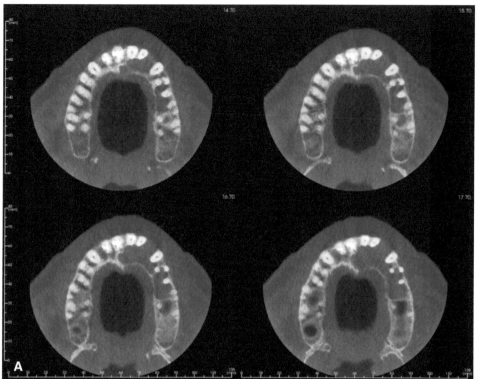

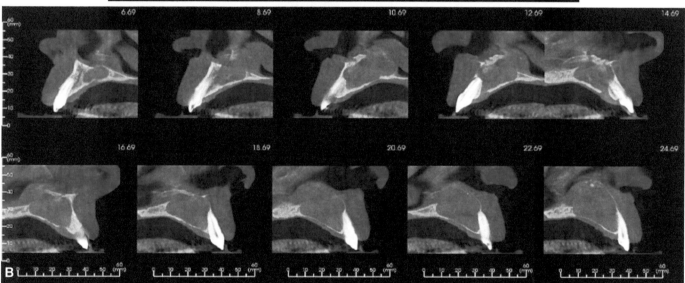

Fig. 23.10 Axial (A) and buccal palatal (B) cone beam computed tomographic images of a maxillary odontogenic keratocyst (OKC). Note that the OKC is generally confined to the borders of the bone except superiorly, where there has been hydraulic expansion of the nasal floor.

The expressivity of the phenotypes is variable, although they may include multiple basal cell carcinomas of the skin, palmar and plantar pitting, skeletal abnormalities such as bifid ribs, vertebral fusion, polydactyly, shortening of the metacarpals, temporal and temporoparietal bossing, minor hypertelorism, mild prognathism, calcification of the falx cerebri and other parts of the dura, medulloblastoma, and multiple OKCs.

Clinical Features

Nevoid basal cell carcinoma syndrome may be detected early in life, usually in the second or third decade, with the development of OKCs within the jaws and skin basal cell carcinomas. Although genetic testing of relatives is a useful diagnostic tool, approximately 20% of new diagnoses represent spontaneous mutations of the *PTCH* gene. Typically multiple OKCs develop in multiple quadrants earlier in life (Fig. 23.11). A thorough radiologic examination including MDCT or CBCT imaging is required to detect all the jaw lesions, and regular follow-up of patients diagnosed with the syndrome is important to identify new and recurrent OKCs early, particularly because the recurrence rate of OKCs associated with the syndrome is higher than of solitary OKCs.

Imaging Features

The imaging features of OKCs that arise in nevoid basal cell carcinoma syndrome are identical to those associated with solitary OKCs.

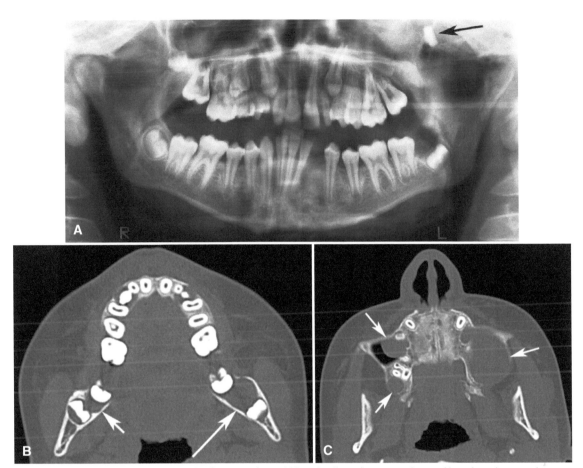

Fig. 23.11 A panoramic image (A) of a case of nevoid basal cell carcinoma syndrome. Note the odontogenic keratocyst (OKC) related to the developing mandibular left third molar and a large OKC within the left maxilla that has displaced the left maxillary third molar *(arrow)*. Axial multidetector computed tomography (MDCT) image of the same case (B) showing the OKC associated with the mandibular left third molar *(long arrow)*, also seen in the panoramic image, and another very small OKC *(short arrow)* in the right posterior mandible, which is not visible in the panoramic image. Another axial MDCT image (C) from the same case reveals the large OKC in the left maxilla and two other OKCs *(arrows)* not readily apparent in the panoramic image.

Differential Interpretation

The presence of a corticated periphery and the hydraulic cystic features of the lesions differentiates nevoid basal cell carcinoma syndrome from other abnormalities characterized by multiple radiolucencies (e.g., multiple myeloma). Cherubism presents with bilateral multilocular, radiolucent lesions with internal septations, but these usually produce significant jaw expansion—features that are not characteristic of nevoid basal cell carcinoma syndrome. In addition, the lesions of cherubism displace teeth anteriorly or mesially, which is a distinctive characteristic. Occasionally, patients with multiple dentigerous cysts may show some similarities, but dentigerous cysts are more expansile.

Management

OKCs in nevoid basal cell carcinoma syndrome are treated more aggressively than solitary OKCs because they appear to have an even greater propensity for recurrence. It is reasonable to examine the patient annually for new and recurrent cysts with panoramic and intraoral imaging. Should these images reveal areas that are suspicious for new or recurrent OKCs, MDCT or CBCT should be ordered. A referral to a medical geneticist should also be made.

Buccal Bifurcation Cyst
Disease Mechanism

The epithelial lining of the buccal bifurcation cyst (BBC) is probably derived from the epithelial cell rests of Malassez in bifurcation of multirooted teeth. The histopathologic characteristics of the lining are not distinctive and overlap with other odontogenic cysts. Therefore both histopathologic and radiologic examinations are necessary to make the appropriate diagnosis.

The etiology of the BBC is not known. One hypothesis identifies inflammation as the stimulus for epithelial proliferation, but inflammation is not always present.

It is possible that the paradental cyst of the third molar and the BBC are the same entity. An associated enamel extension into the furcation of third molars with paradental cysts has not been documented with molars with BBC. In addition, the inflammatory component associated with paradental cysts is not always present with BBCs.

Clinical Features

Commonly the BBC is associated with mandibular molars; they can also arise in association with maxillary molar teeth. On clinical examination, the molar may be unerupted or the tooth may be partially erupted with its lingual cusp tips abnormally protruding through the mucosa, higher than the position of the buccal cusps. The first molar is involved more frequently than the second molar, and the pulps of these teeth are vital.

A hard swelling may be palpable buccal to the involved molar, and if it is secondarily infected, the patient has pain. The age of detection is younger, within the first two decades of life rather than in the third decade, with a paradental cyst of the third molar.

Imaging Features

Location. The BBC is associated with multirooted molar teeth with the mandibular first molar being the most commonly associated tooth followed by the second molar (Fig. 23.12). Occasionally BBCs can occur bilaterally (Fig. 23.13), and they can involve maxillary molars as well. The epicenter of the cyst is always in the buccal furcation of the affected molar. On panoramic or periapical images, the lesion may appear to

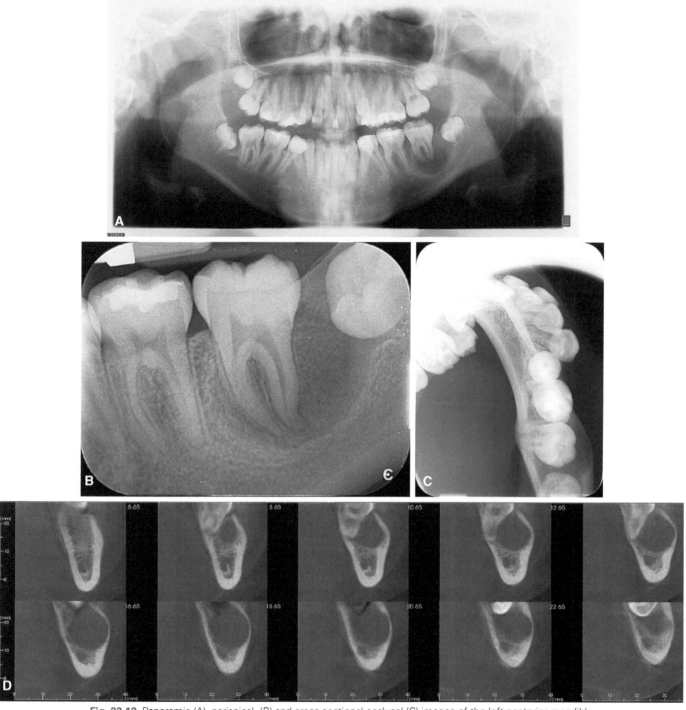

Fig. 23.12 Panoramic (A), periapical, (B) and cross-sectional occlusal (C) images of the left posterior mandible show a buccal bifurcation cyst associated with a tipped mandibular left second molar. Note the tipping of the tooth crown in (A) and the displacement of the roots of the second molar into the lingual cortex of the mandible (C). The buccal epicenter of the cyst is seen in the buccal lingual cross-sectional cone beam computed tomographic images, as is the compression of the inferior alveolar canal (D).

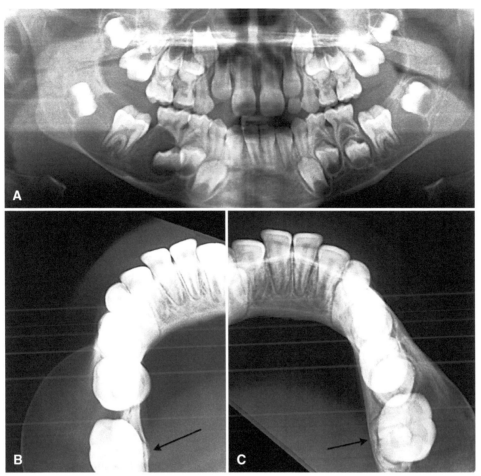

Fig. 23.13 Bilateral Buccal Bifurcation Cysts. A panoramic image (A) shows cysts related to the mandibular first molars. The occlusal surface of each tooth has been tipped in relation to the other teeth, and adjacent teeth have been displaced. Occlusal images of the same case (B) and (C). Note the smooth curved expansion of the buccal cortex and the displacement of the roots of the first molars into the lingual cortical plate *(arrows)*.

be centered slightly distal to the furcation of the involved tooth because of x-ray beam obliquity.

Periphery. In some cases, the periphery is not always readily apparent, and the lesion may have a very subtle radiolucent appearance superimposed over the roots of the molar. In other cases, the lesion may have a well-defined and corticated border.

Internal structure. The internal structure is radiolucent.

Effects on surrounding structures. As the cyst begins to enlarge and engage the buccal surface of the bone, expansion of the surface is seen. Owing to the cyst's very slow growth rate, the surface of the bone will remodel to accommodate the cyst. With the expansion of the bone surface, the cortex remains intact but is often significantly thinned. If the cyst is secondarily infected, periosteal new bone formation is seen on the buccal cortex adjacent to the involved tooth (Fig. 23.14).

Effects on adjacent teeth. The most striking diagnostic characteristic of the BBC is the tipping of the involved molar so that the root tips are displaced into the lingual cortex of the bone and the occlusal surface is tipped toward the buccal surface (see Fig. 23.12). This accounts for the lingual cusp tips being positioned higher than the buccal tips. This tipping may be detected in a periapical or panoramic image if the image of the occlusal surface of the affected tooth is apparent and the unaffected teeth are not. The best diagnostic image is the cross-sectional (standard)

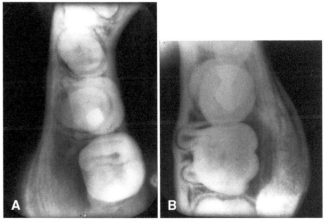

Fig. 23.14 Occlusal views (A and B) of buccal bifurcation cysts that have been secondarily infected. Note the laminated periosteal new bone formation on the buccal aspect of the first molars and the abnormal position of the roots of the first molar in (B). (Courtesy Dr. Doug Stoneman, University of Toronto.)

mandibular occlusal image, which demonstrates the abnormal position of the tooth roots adjacent to or within the lingual cortex.

Differential Interpretation

The major differential interpretations of the BBC include rarefying osteitis and dentigerous cyst. Rarefying osteitis can easily be excluded because the epicenter of periapical inflammatory disease is located apical to the root apex of the involved tooth, whereas the epicenter of the BBC is located within the furcation. Although obliquity of the x-ray beam may superimpose the cyst near the crown of an unerupted, developing molar, the occlusal image will readily show the expansile nature of the bone to be adjacent to the molar furcation. Should the BBC become secondarily infected and periosteal new bone formation or sclerosis can be visualized, the cyst could be confused with a periodontal abscess or Langerhans cell histiocytosis. The fact that only a BBC tilts the molar as described helps to differentiate it from other lesions.

Management

A BBC is managed by conservative curettage, although some cases have resolved without intervention. The involved molar need not be removed, and BBCs do not recur.

Residual Cyst

Disease Mechanism

A residual cyst is a cyst that develops after incomplete removal of epithelium associated with a previous cyst. The most common sources of this epithelium include an inflammatory cyst (i.e., rarefying osteitis) and a dentigerous cyst.

Clinical Features

A residual cyst is usually asymptomatic and is often identified in a radiologic examination of an edentulous area. If not identified, the cyst can enlarge, resulting in a painless swelling of the jaw. If it is secondarily infected, a residual cyst may be identified by the pain it elicits.

Imaging Features

Location. Residual cysts can occur in both jaws, although they are found slightly more often in the mandible than the maxilla. The epicenter of a residual cyst is located in the former periapical region of the involved and/or missing tooth and in the mandible; it is always superior to the inferior alveolar canal (Fig. 23.15).

Periphery. A residual cyst has a well-defined and corticated border unless it has become secondarily infected.

Internal structure. The internal aspect of a residual cyst typically is radiolucent, although dystrophic calcifications may be present in long-standing cysts.

Effects on surrounding structures. Residual cysts may cause expansion of an adjacent bone surface and thinning of the overlying cortex. In the maxilla, a residual cyst may displace the floor of the maxillary sinus or course of the inferior alveolar canal.

Effects on adjacent teeth. Residual cysts can displace teeth or resorb tooth roots.

Differential Interpretation

Without a patient history and/or previous images, clinicians may have difficulty determining whether a solitary cyst in the jaws is a residual cyst. Other examples of common solitary cysts include OKCs. A residual cyst has, however, greater potential for expansion of bone than an OKC. The Stafne defect is located more inferiorly in the mandible, away from the tooth-bearing areas of the jaws, and the cortex of the Stafne defect is usually very thick.

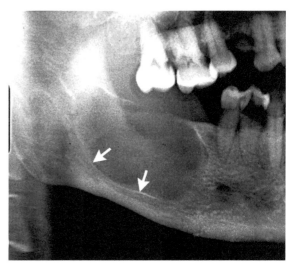

Fig. 23.15 The epicenter of this residual cyst is located superior to the inferior alveolar canal; it has displaced the canal in an inferior direction *(arrows)*. The cortical boundary is not continuous around the entire cyst.

Management

The treatment of residual cysts is surgical removal, marsupialization, or both if the cyst is large.

Lateral Periodontal Cyst

Disease Mechanism

The lateral periodontal cyst is thought to arise from remnants of the epithelial cell rests of Malassez in the periodontal ligament space adjacent to the surface of the tooth root. This lesion is usually is unicystic, but it may appear as a cluster of small cystic cavities—a condition referred to as a botryoid odontogenic cyst. It has been postulated that a lateral periodontal cyst is the intrabony counterpart of the gingival cyst in an adult.

Clinical Features

The lateral periodontal cyst is often small and usually asymptomatic (Fig. 23.16A). If these cysts become secondarily infected, they can mimic a lateral periodontal abscess.

Imaging Features

Location. The lateral periodontal cyst usually develops in the incisor and premolar areas of the mandible. In the maxilla, it usually develops in the lateral incisor and the canine area.

Periphery. A lateral periodontal cyst has a well-defined and corticated border. Although it is most often round to oval in shape, a larger cyst can take on a more irregular appearance.

Internal structure. Internally, the lateral periodontal cyst is radiolucent. The botryoid variety may have a multilocular appearance, although this description is related more to its histopathologic appearance.

Effects on surrounding structures. Occasionally large lateral periodontal cysts have a growth pattern similar to that of OKCs, with minimal expansion of the involved bone (see Fig. 23.16B and C).

Effects on adjacent teeth. The lateral periodontal cyst may efface the lamina dura of the adjacent root, and larger cysts can displace adjacent teeth.

Differential Interpretation

The lateral periodontal cyst is sometimes said to be an interpretation of exclusion. Because the radiographic appearance of a lateral

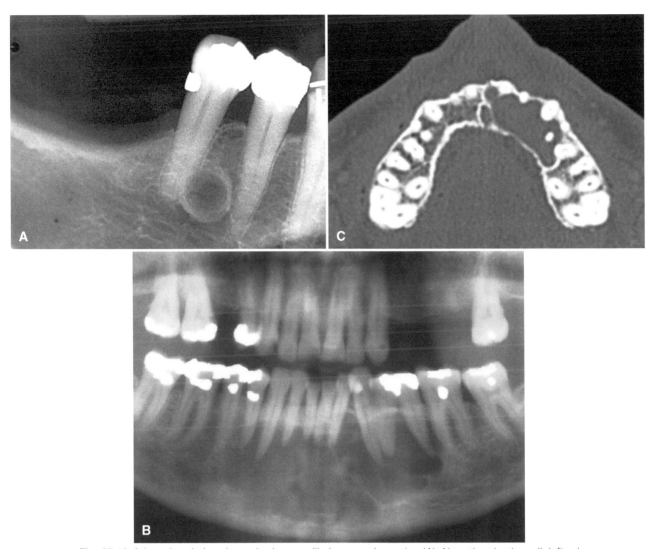

Fig. 23.16 A lateral periodontal cyst in the mandibular premolar region (A). Note the classic well-defined cortical border. Cropped panoramic image with a large lateral periodontal cyst crossing the midline of the mandible (B). Axial multidetector computed tomography image of a large lateral periodontal cyst causing minimal expansion of the maxilla (C).

periodontal cyst is similar to that of many other solitary cysts, the following lesions should be included in the differential interpretation: a small OKC, neurofibroma, ameloblastoma, and a focus of rarefying osteitis located at the foramen of a lateral (accessory) root canal. If the lateral periodontal cyst has a botryoid appearance, it may also resemble a small ameloblastoma.

Management

Lateral periodontal cysts usually do not require sophisticated imaging beyond intraoral or panoramic images because of their small size. Excisional biopsy or simple enucleation is the treatment of choice because these cysts do not tend to recur.

Glandular Odontogenic Cyst
Disease Mechanism

The glandular or sialoodontogenic cyst is a rare cyst derived from odontogenic epithelium with a spectrum of characteristics including salivary gland features such as mucous-producing cells. Some

authors hypothesize a relationship to the central mucoepidermoid carcinoma.

Clinical Features

There is a slight female predilection with a mean age in the fifth decade of life. This cyst shows aggressive behavior and a tendency to recur after surgery.

Imaging Features

Location. The glandular odontogenic cyst occurs more commonly in the mandible and most often in the anterior mandible and the maxilla.

Periphery. There is usually a cortical border that may be smooth or scalloped.

Internal structure. The glandular odontogenic cyst may be radiolucent, although multilocular lesions have been reported (Fig. 23.17).

Effects on surrounding structures. Expansion of an adjacent bone border has been reported, with perforation through the cortex.

Effects on adjacent teeth. Displacement of adjacent teeth has been reported.

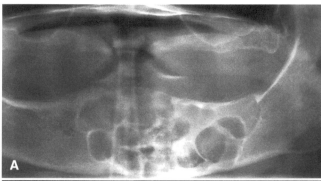
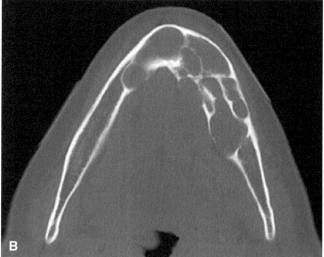

Fig. 23.17 A cropped panoramic image (A) of a glandular odontogenic cyst with a multilocular appearance very similar to an ameloblastoma. Axial multidetector computed tomography image (B) detailing the multilocular internal cystic structure.

Differential Interpretation

This cyst can appear similar to any unilocular or multilocular radiolucent entity, including odontogenic keratocyst, ameloblastoma, and central mucoepidermoid carcinoma.

Treatment

Because of the high rate of recurrence with conservative treatments such as enucleation, more aggressive management, including resection, may be considered. Treated cases should be followed with periodic radiographic examinations to assess for recurrence.

Calcifying Odontogenic Cyst
Disease Mechanism

The COC is known by a number of other names, including calcifying epithelial odontogenic cyst, dentinogenic ghost cell tumor, and Gorlin cyst.

COCs are uncommon, slow-growing, benign lesions. They have a spectrum of appearances with the characteristics of a cyst and in some instances a solid neoplasm. These cells within this lesion can produce a calcified matrix identified as dysplastic dentin; in some instances, the lesion is associated with an odontoma. This lesion also sometimes contains a more solid component that gives it an appearance resembling that of an ameloblastoma, although it does not behave like one.

Clinical Features

The COC has a wide age distribution. Clinically the lesion usually presents as a slow-growing, painless swelling in the jaw. Occasionally the patient may complain of pain. Aspiration often yields a viscous granular yellow fluid.

Imaging Features

Location. Most COCs occur centrally in bone, with a nearly equal distribution between the jaws. Most (75%) occur mesial to the first molar, especially in the incisor and canine areas, where the tumor can sometimes manifest as a pericoronal radiolucency.

Periphery. The periphery can vary from being well defined and corticated with a curved, cyst-like shape to being poorly defined and irregular.

Internal structure. The internal structure can vary. The lesion may be completely radiolucent or may show evidence of small foci of calcified material that appear as white flecks or small smooth pebbles. Also, larger, more solid amorphous radiopaque masses can be seen (Fig. 23.18). In rare cases the lesion may appear multilocular.

Effects on surrounding structures. The lesion may expand the bone and perforate an adjacent cortex when it is large enough to extend to the bone surface.

Effects on adjacent teeth. In 20% to 50% of cases the COC is associated with an unerupted or impacted tooth (most commonly a canine) that impedes its eruption. Displacement of adjacent teeth and resorption of roots may also occur.

Differential Interpretation

When there is no evidence of internal calcifications, the COC may be indistinguishable from a dentigerous cyst or an OKC. Other lesions to be considered that have internal calcifications include an adenomatoid odontogenic tumor as well as the ameloblastic fibro-odontoma and calcifying epithelial odontogenic tumor. It is not, however, common for the COC to occur in locations where the ameloblastic fibro-odontoma or the calcifying epithelial odontogenic tumor commonly arises. Finally, some long-standing cysts may display internal dystrophic calcification, giving a similar appearance to the COC.

Management

The COC is treated with enucleation and curettage. Because clinicians generally have little experience with the more solid neoplastic variants, it is wise to follow treatment with periodic imaging examinations for recurrence.

NONODONTOGENIC CYSTS

Nasopalatine Cyst
Disease Mechanism

The nasopalatine (duct) or incisive canal usually contains remnants of the nasopalatine duct, a primitive organ of smell, and the nasopalatine vessels and nerves. The nasopalatine (duct) or incisive canal cyst forms in the nasopalatine canal when these embryonic epithelial remnants within the canal undergo proliferation and cystic degeneration.

Clinical Features

Nasopalatine cysts account for about 10% of jaw cysts. The age distribution is broad, with most cases being discovered in the fourth through sixth decades, and the incidence is three times higher in males than in females.

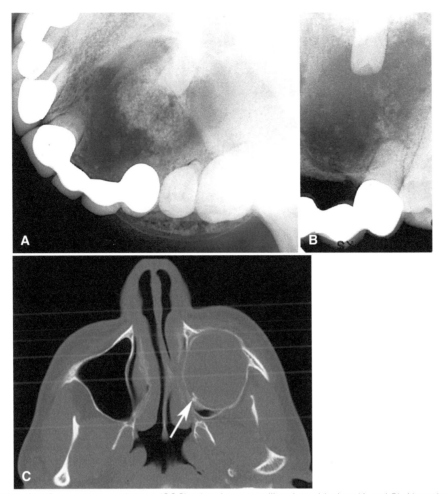

Fig. 23.18 Calcifying odontogenic cyst (COC) related to a maxillary lateral incisor (A and B). Note the well-defined corticated border, internal calcifications, and resorption of part of the root of the central incisor. Axial multidetector computed tomography image (C) of a large COC invaginating into the maxillary sinus. Note the small calcifications along the posterior border *(arrow)*.

Most cysts are asymptomatic; however, as they increase in size, the most frequent chief complaint is a swelling just posterior to the palatine papilla. This swelling usually is fluctuant and blue in color if the cyst is near the surface. A less superficial nasopalatine cyst is covered by normal-appearing mucosa unless it is ulcerated from masticatory trauma. As the cyst expands, it may penetrate the labial cortex and produce a swelling below the maxillary labial frenulum or to one side of it. The lesion may also bulge into the nasal cavity and distort the nasal septum. Pressure from the cyst on the adjacent nasopalatine nerves that occupy the same canal may cause a burning sensation or change in sensation over the palatal mucosa. In some cases cystic fluid may drain into the oral cavity through a sinus tract or a remnant of the nasopalatine duct, and the patient may report a salty taste.

Imaging Features

Location. Most nasopalatine cysts are centered in the midline in the nasopalatine foramen or canal. However, this cyst can also expand asymmetrically, extending posteriorly into the hard palate or laterally into the lateral incisor area.

Periphery. The nasopalatine cyst has a well-defined and corticated periphery, and it is round or oval in shape (Fig. 23.19). Sometimes the image of the anterior nasal spine may be superimposed over the cyst, giving it a heart shape.

Internal structure. Most nasopalatine duct cysts are radiolucent. Rarely, nasopalatine cysts may develop internal dystrophic calcifications; these may appear as ill-defined, amorphous, scattered radiopacities.

Effects on surrounding structures. Seen from a lateral perspective, the nasopalatine cyst may expand the labial or palatal cortices of the maxilla (Fig. 23.20). If the cyst is large enough, the floor of the nasal fossa may be displaced in a superior direction. It should also be noted that the canal can expand asymmetrically, resulting in an asymmetric nasopalatine cyst (Fig. 23.21).

Effects on adjacent teeth. The nasopalatine cyst can displace the roots of the central incisors so they diverge, and occasionally root resorption occurs.

Differential Interpretation

The horizontal diameter of the incisive canal can be as large as 10 mm, so the most common differential interpretation is a large incisive foramen. However, a clinical examination should reveal the expansile features characteristic of a cyst and other changes that occur with a space-occupying lesion, such as tooth displacement. Two periapical images made at different horizontal angulations may show the cyst to be located palatal to the adjacent teeth. An occlusal image or a limited field-of-view CBCT examination centered in the maxillary midline may demonstrate the size change and expansion in the palatal direction. Rarefying osteitis

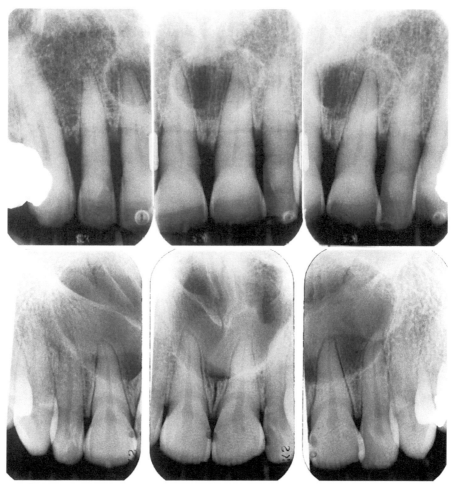

Fig. 23.19 Two examples of nasopalatine cysts. Note the uniform periodontal ligament space around all the apices of the adjacent tooth roots.

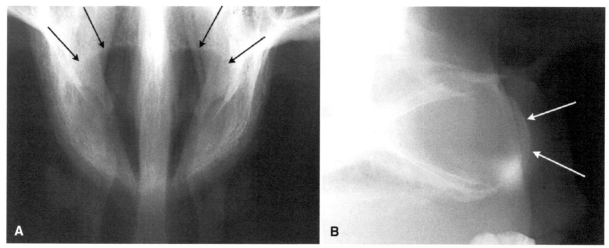

Fig. 23.20 An incisive canal cyst viewed from two perspectives *(arrows)*: a standard occlusal view (A) and a tangential occlusal view (B), created by placing the image receptor outside the mouth against the cheek and directing the x-ray beam at a tangent to the labial surfaces of the central incisors.

associated with a central incisor can appear similar to an asymmetric nasopalatine cyst; however, the absence of the lamina dura with enlargement of the periodontal ligament space around the apex of the central incisor indicates an inflammatory lesion. A vitality test of the central incisor tooth pulp may also be useful.

Management

The management of a nasopalatine cyst is enucleation, preferably from the palate to avoid the nasopalatine nerve. If the cyst is large and there is danger of devitalizing the tooth or creating a nasooral or antro-oral fistula, the surgeon may elect to perform marsupialization.

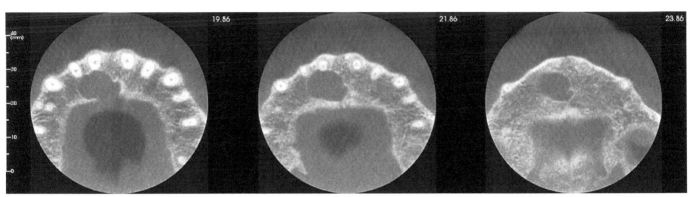

Fig. 23.21 Axial cone beam computed tomographic images of an asymmetric incisive canal cyst. Note the continuity of the cyst cavity with the midline incisive canal.

PSEUDOCYSTS

Simple Bone Cyst

Disease Mechanism

The SBC is not a true cyst because it lacks an epithelial lining. Rather, the SBC is lined with connective tissue, and it may be empty or contain a small amount of blood or serosanguinous fluid. The etiology of the SBC is not known; therefore it has been referred to by many different names, including hemorrhagic bone cyst, idiopathic bone cyst/cavity, traumatic bone cyst, solitary bone cyst/cavity, and unicameral bone cyst/cavity.

There are several hypotheses regarding the pathogenesis of SBCs; however, the one that makes the most biologic sense is that SBCs arise from a local disturbance in normal osteoblast differentiation during bone growth and development and osteoclastic coordination. The dysregulation of these processes is believed to give rise to the empty bone cavity. There is no evidence to support a traumatic etiology for the SBC.

Clinical Features

Solitary SBCs are very common, with most occurring in the first 2 decades of life; the mean age is approximately 18 years. One or more SBCs can develop in association with bone dysplasias; however, when this occurs with the cemento-osseous dysplasias, the mean age of occurrence is in the fifth decade of life with a striking female preponderance of 4:1.

SBCs are asymptomatic in most cases, but occasionally pain or tenderness may be present, especially if the cyst has become secondarily infected in association with a cemento-osseous dysplasia. Expansion of the mandible is also possible; however, tooth movement is unusual. If teeth are involved, the pulps of these teeth remain vital.

Most SBCs are found incidentally, during imaging examinations made for other purposes, particularly in adolescents. Although SBCs can become quite large, there is no evidence that they cause fractures of the jaws, unlike cysts in the appendicular skeleton.

Imaging Features

Location. Almost all SBCs are found in the mandible; they rarely develop in the maxilla. The lesion can occur anywhere in the mandible but is more commonly found in the posterior mandible and in older patients when it is associated with an osseous dysplasia.

Periphery. SBCs have well-defined, delicately corticated borders. In some instances the border may be so delicate that it is difficult to see, even on intraoral images. The boundary is usually better seen in the alveolar process around the teeth than in the inferior aspect of the body of the mandible. When the SBC encounters a tooth root, the periphery scallops around the roots of the teeth with a gentle, smooth curve (Fig. 23.22A).

Internal structure. The internal structure is totally radiolucent, although occasionally a larger SBC may appear to display delicate internal septation. These septa, often referred to as pseudosepta, are the result of pronounced scalloping of the SBC border into the endosteal surfaces of either the buccal or lingual cortices of the mandible (see Fig. 23.22B). The ridging of the internal surface of the bone cortex produced by the scalloping effect gives rise to the appearance of septa on panoramic or periapical images.

Effects on surrounding structures. Although some SBCs may expand the bone surface (see Fig. 23.22B), they have a general propensity to scallop the endosteal surface of a bone cortex. SBCs also have a tendency to grow along the long axis of the bone; however, larger lesions can cause expansion (Figs. 23.23 and 23.24).

Effects on adjacent teeth. In most cases, SBCs have no effect on adjacent teeth, although rare cases of tooth displacement and resorption have been documented. Most commonly SBCs leave the lamina dura intact or only partly disrupted (see Fig. 23.28A). Similarly, the lesion spares the cortical boundary of the follicle around a developing tooth; this is a highly characteristic feature.

Differential Interpretation

SBCs may have an appearance similar to that of a central giant cell lesion; however, the giant cell lesion has a greater propensity to displace teeth and develop areas of internal mineralization. Because smaller SBCs may grow through the bone and scallop bone borders, they may appear similar to OKCs. However, OKCs usually have a more definite cortical boundary, resorb and displace teeth, and disrupt the integrity and shape of tooth follicles. Because the SBC may displace bone from around teeth without affecting the teeth themselves, there may be a tendency to include a malignant lesion in the differential interpretation. However, the maintenance of some lamina dura and the lack of an invasive periphery and bone destruction should be enough to remove this category of disease from consideration.

The diagnosis of the SBC relies primarily on radiographic interpretation or the surgical finding of no epithelial lining. These lesions occasionally heal spontaneously; when they do, the formation of the new, immature bone may appear reminiscent of a bone dysplasia such as fibrous dysplasia or a benign tumor like an ossifying fibroma (Fig. 23.25). Therefore it is important for the oral and maxillofacial pathologist to make a radiologic correlation.

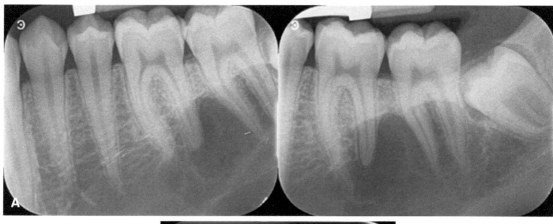

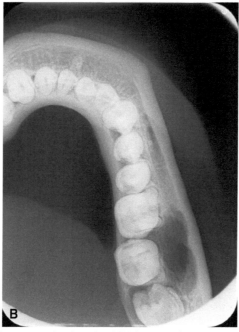

Fig. 23.22 Periapical (A) and cross-sectional occlusal (B) images of a simple bone cyst (SBC). The SBC has scalloped around the teeth, the buccal cortex of the mandible is thinned, but the lamina dura is present and intact.

Management

The management of SBCs may be observation with follow-up imaging or a conservative entry into the lesion to elicit bleeding and subsequent healing by secondary intention. Spontaneous healing has also been reported for SBCs. Solitary SBCs do not recur, although those associated with a cemento-osseous dysplasia may.

HEALING

When an intraosseous cyst is treated, the cavity fills in with bone and healing occurs by secondary intention. Some of the features of healing are discussed in Chapter 22. When a cyst that develops adjacent to the floor maxillary sinus heals, the osmotic pressure within the lesion cavity slowly decreases. Without the positive intraluminal pressure from within the cavity to support the displaced sinus floor, the borders of the lesion take on the appearance of a deflated balloon as the cavity fills with bone during healing (Fig. 23.26). This is referred to as a "collapsed cyst." Radiographically, new bone forms first at the periphery of the lesion; with time, the central radiolucent focus decreases in size as new bone

grows toward the center. Histopathologically, the new bone that is formed may appear similar to that seen in an ossifying fibroma or a dysplastic lesion of bone.

MANDIBULAR LINGUAL BONE DEPRESSION

Disease Mechanism

The mandibular lingual bone depression or Stafne defect is a pseudocyst because it is not a cavity in the bone and is not lined by epithelium. Rather, it is a depression within the lingual surface of the mandible, lined by the lingual cortex. It is classified as a pseudocyst because of its shape; the often round or oval appearance of the depression simulates the appearance of a cyst.

The Stafne defect is not a congenital anomaly. First described by Stafne in the posterior mandible in an adult cohort of patients, the depressions were once thought to arise from growth of the adjacent submandibular salivary gland. Although the pathogenesis of the depression is not known, surgical exploration and imaging studies of the depressions have revealed the presence of a number of different tissues within the defect, including salivary gland tissue.

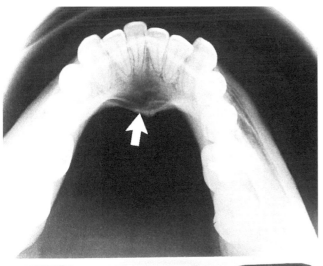

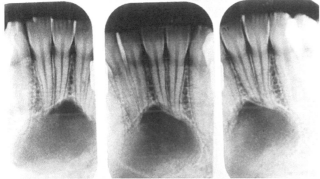

Fig. 23.23 Simple bone cyst *(arrow)* positioned in the anterior of the mandible. The superior aspect of the peripheral cortex is better defined than the inferior border, and there is evidence of some expansion of the lingual surface of the mandible, which may be due in part to muscle attachment at the genial tubercles.

Clinical Features

The depression is developmental in origin, with a peak incidence in the fourth and fifth decades of life; it is not a congenital anomaly. Over time the defect may increase in size. However, the ultimate size of the defect can vary. Although rare, the lingual cortical bone depression in the posterior mandible has an incidence of between 0.10% and 0.48%, although many likely go unseen. In the premolar area of the mandible, the incidence is much lower, at 0.009%.

Imaging Features
Location

All lingual cortical depressions are found in the mandible. The more posterior variant of the depression has an epicenter located inferior to the inferior alveolar canal and anterior to the antegonial notch. In the premolar area of the mandible, the depression is located in the periapical region of the mandibular premolars, superior to the mylohyoid ridge.

Periphery

The mandibular lingual cortical depression has a well-defined periphery and is corticated. The width of the cortex can, however, vary from one that mimics an odontogenic cyst to one that is very thick and reminiscent of the thickness of the lingual cortex of the mandible (Fig. 23.27). Often, continuity of the cortex of the depression with the inferior cortex of the mandible can be seen (Fig. 23.28).

Internal Structure

The internal structure is totally radiolucent.

Effects on Surrounding Structures

In addition to the change in the contour of the lingual surface of the mandible, there may be thinning of the lingual mandibular cortex within the depression, depending on the depth of the depression. When the depression is substantial, the lingual cortex may abut the endosteal surface of the buccal cortex.

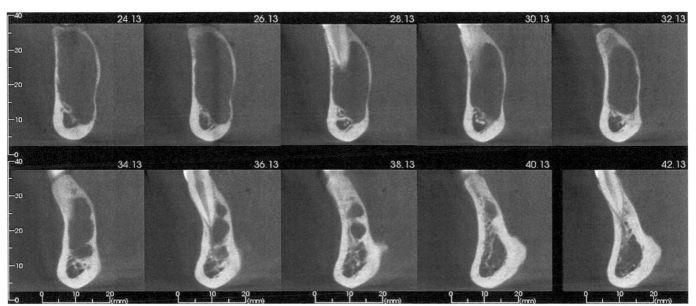

Fig. 23.24 Buccal-lingual cross-sectional cone beam computed tomographic images of a simple bone cyst. Note the thinning of the buccal and lingual cortices of the mandible and the subtle expansion of the lingual surface of the bone.

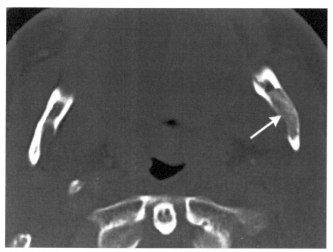

Fig. 23.25 Axial multidetector computed tomography image with a bone algorithm displaying a small simple bone cyst in the process of healing *(arrow)*. Note the fine internal granular bone and very slight expansion of the ramus.

Effects on Adjacent Teeth

There are no effects on the teeth.

Differential Interpretation

When the cortex of the depression is thick, it should not be confused with any other lesion occurring centrally within the bone. If the depression enlarges and overlaps the inferior alveolar canal or develops a thinner cortex, benign odontogenic and nonodontogenic entities should be considered. These may include OKCs or central giant cell lesions, depending on their location.

Management

Recognition of the depression should preclude the need for surgical intervention or advanced imaging.

CYSTS ORIGINATING IN SOFT TISSUES

Nasolabial Cyst

Disease Mechanism

The origin of the nasolabial or nasoalveolar cyst is not known. The epithelial component of these cysts may arise from remnant epithelial

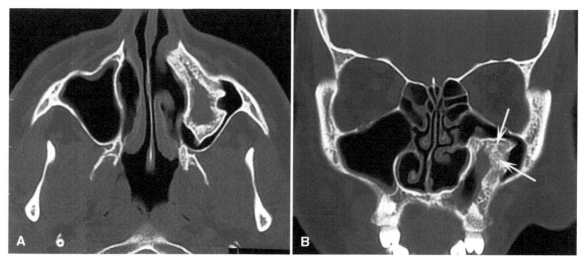

Fig. 23.26 Bone window axial (A) and coronal (B) multidetector computed tomography images of a collapsing cyst within the sinus. Note the unusual shape and contour of this entity and the new bone that is being formed from the periphery *(arrows* in B) toward the center. (Courtesy Drs. S. Ahing and T. Blight, University of Manitoba.)

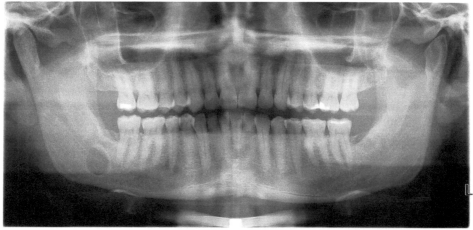

Fig. 23.27 Panoramic image of a mandibular lingual cortical depression (Stafne defect) in the right posterior mandible. Note the thickness of the cortex.

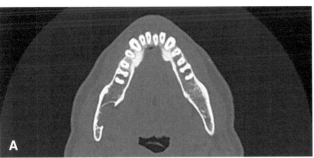
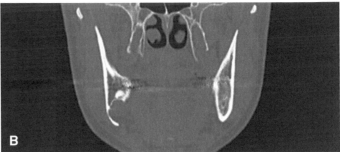

Fig. 23.28 Axial (A) and coronal (B) multidetector computed tomography images showing a large mandibular lingual cortical depression in the right posterior mandible. There has been substantial thinning of the mediolateral dimensions of the ramus.

rests during the merging or fusion of the embryonic nasal and maxillary processes. Alternatively, the source of the epithelium may be the embryonic nasolacrimal duct, which initially lies on the bone surface.

Clinical Features

The age of detection of the nasolabial cyst ranges from 12 to 75 years, with a mean age of 44 years, and approximately 75% of these lesions occur in females. When this rare lesion is small, it may produce a very subtle, unilateral swelling of the nasolabial fold and may elicit pain or discomfort. When large, it may distend the overlying soft tissues, flaring the nasal alae, distorting the nostrils, and creating fullness of the upper lip. In addition, the floor of the nasal cavity may become displaced, causing some obstruction. If infected, the cyst may drain into the nasal cavity. Although the nasolabial cyst is usually unilateral, some bilateral lesions have been reported.

Imaging Features

Location. Nasolabial cysts are primarily soft tissue lesions located adjacent to the alveolar process above the roots of the incisor teeth. Because this is a soft tissue lesion and plain radiographs may not show any detectable changes, the investigation could include either MDCT or MRI (Fig. 23.29).

Periphery. MDCT images with contrast enhancement viewed using the soft tissue algorithm will reveal a circular or oval lesion with slight soft tissue enhancement of the periphery.

Internal structure. In enhanced MDCT images, the cavity of the cyst will appear homogeneously low-attenuation/radiolucent with respect to the surrounding soft tissues.

Effects on surrounding structures. Occasionally a cyst may resorb the underlying bone (Fig. 23.30), producing an increased radiolucency of the alveolar process underlying the cyst and apical to the incisor teeth. Also, the outline of the floor of the nasal fossa may become distorted, resulting in a posterior bowing of this surface.

Differential interpretation. The swelling caused by an infected nasolabial cyst may simulate an acute dentoalveolar abscess. Therefore it is important to establish the vitality of the adjacent tooth pulps. This cyst may also resemble a nasal furuncle if it pushes upward into the floor of the nasal cavity. A large minor salivary gland mucocele or a cystic salivary adenoma should also be considered in the differential diagnosis of an uninfected nasolabial cyst.

Management. The nasolabial cyst should be excised through an intraoral approach. These cysts do not tend to recur.

Thyroglossal Duct Cyst
Disease Mechanism

The thyroglossal duct cyst develops from epithelial remnants of the embryonic thyroglossal duct, which extends from the foramen cecum

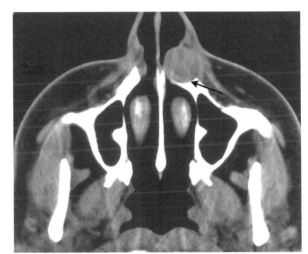

Fig. 23.29 Nasolabial cyst shown in an axial multidetector computed tomography image with a soft tissue algorithm. Note the well-defined periphery and the erosion of the labial aspect of the alveolar process *(arrow)*.

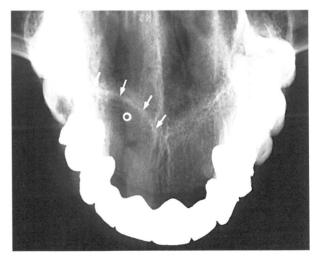

Fig. 23.30 Occlusal image of a nasolabial cyst. The image shows erosion of the alveolar bone *(o)* and elevation of the floor of the nasal fossa *(arrows)*. (From Chinellato LE, Damante JH. Contribution of radiographs to the diagnosis of naso-alveolar cyst. *Oral Surg Oral Med Oral Pathol.* 1984;58:729–735.)

in the midline of the dorsal surface of the tongue to the isthmus of the thyroid gland. This cyst is the most common congenital cyst and midline soft tissue mass in the head and neck.

Clinical Features

The cyst manifests as a slow-growing, painless mass, unless it is secondarily infected; it is found in the midline of the neck and most are detected in the first and second decades of life. Such cysts may occur along any portion of the former track of the duct and extend from below the hyoid bone to the tongue.

Imaging Features

Many of thyroglossal duct cysts have a close proximal relationship with the hyoid bone. The periphery of the cyst is usually well defined, and the curved outline is characteristic of a cyst. The shape of the cyst may

be influenced by the impingement of the surrounding structures. The internal structure on MDCT images is homogeneous and of low attenuation, equivalent to fluid (Fig. 23.31A).

Branchial Cleft Cyst
Disease Mechanism

The etiology for these cysts is controversial but seems to be related to remnants of epithelium from the embryonic first to fourth branchial arches. The cyst wall usually has a lining of stratified squamous cells with some lymphoid tissue elements.

Clinical Features

Branchial cleft cysts occur in the lateral aspect of the neck, anterior to the sternocleidomastoid muscle, in the second and third decades of life. If the cyst is related to the first branchial arch, it may be located

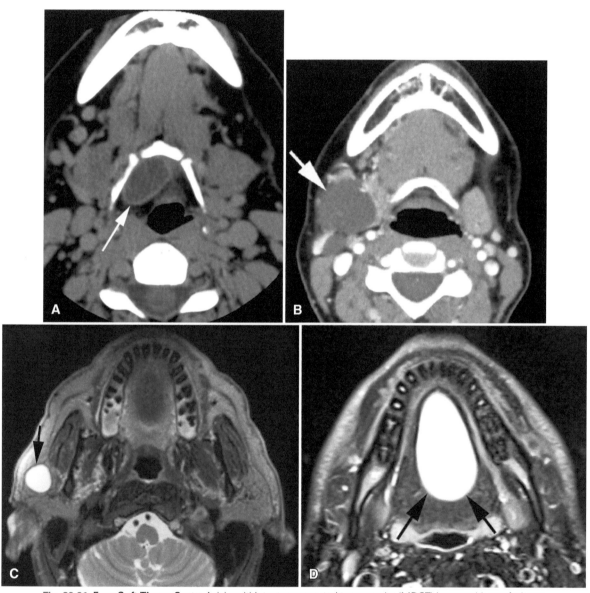

Fig. 23.31 Four Soft Tissue Cysts. Axial multidetector computed tomography (MDCT) image with a soft tissue algorithm of a thyroglossal duct cyst *(arrow)* positioned adjacent to the hyoid bone. Note the cystic shape and homogeneous low attenuation of the internal structure (A). Axial MDCT scan using soft tissue algorithm of a branchial cleft cyst *(arrow)* positioned just inferior the angle of the mandible and displacing the submandibular salivary gland medially (B). Axial T2-weighted magnetic resonance image of a lymphoepithelial cyst *(arrow)* positioned in the right parotid gland (C). Note the homogeneous high-signal *(white)* internal structure, indicating fluid. Axial T2-weighted magnetic resonance image of a dermoid cyst *(arrows)* in the floor of the mouth (D).

in an area extending from the angle of the mandible to the parotid and preauricular regions. This cyst usually manifests as a slow-growing, painless, fluctuant swelling unless it is secondarily infected.

Imaging Features

The imaging appearance of the branchial cleft cyst is very similar to that of the thyroglossal duct cyst in terms of both shape and internal image density (see Fig. 23.31B). The lateral position of the branchial cleft cyst in the neck differentiates it from a thyroglossal duct cyst. When it is associated with the parotid gland, it may be difficult to differentiate from a lymphoepithelial cyst.

Lymphoepithelial Cyst of the Parotid Gland
Disease Mechanism

Once also known as a branchial cyst, authors now believe this cyst to not be of branchial origin. It is commonly located within the parotid gland and its histopathologic appearance is very similar to that of a branchial cleft cyst.

Clinical Features

The mean age of the appearance of this cyst is the fifth decade with a slight female predominance. Usually manifesting as a slow-growing enlargement in the parotid gland, such a cyst may be associated with human immunodeficiency virus infections.

Imaging Features

Most commonly these cysts, located within the parenchyma of the parotid gland, have spherical or circular shapes with internal densities in advanced imaging examinations that are reminiscent of fluid (see Fig. 23.31C).

Dermoid Cyst
Disease Mechanism

Dermoid cysts are a cystic form of a teratoma thought to be derived from entrapped pluripotent embryonic cells. The resulting cysts are lined with epidermis and cutaneous appendages and are filled with keratin or sebaceous material. In rare cases they may contain bone, teeth, muscle, or hair, in which case they are properly called teratomas.

Clinical Features

Dermoid cysts usually become clinically apparent between ages 12 and 25 years, and manifest as slow, painless swellings. Although few (up to 10%) arise in the head and neck with the orbital region being the most common, only 1% to 2% develop in the oral cavity. Of these, approximately 25% occur in the floor of the mouth and on the tongue. When located in the neck or floor of the mouth, these cysts may interfere with breathing, speaking, and eating. On palpation, cysts may be fluctuant or doughy, according to their contents.

Imaging Features

Dermoid cysts have well-defined peripheries and a cystic shape. The internal aspect of the cyst may have a density equivalent to fluid, or it may have a soft tissue multilocular appearance (see Fig. 23.31D). If teeth or bone form in the cyst, these densities may become apparent on conventional imaging.

Differential Interpretation

Lesions that are clinically similar to dermoid cysts include ranulas in the floor of the mouth, thyroglossal duct cysts, cystic hygromas, and branchial cleft cysts.

REFERENCES

El-Naggar AK, Chan JKC, Grandis JR, et al. *WHO Classification of Tumors No 9*. 4th ed. Lyon: IARC Press; 2017.

Johnson NR, Gannon OM, Savage NW, et al. Frequency of odontogenic cysts and tumors: a systematic review. *J Investig Clin Dent*. 2014;5:9–14.

Ward JP, Magar V, Franks SJ, et al. A mathematical model of the dynamics of odontogenic cyst growth. *Anal Quant Cytol Histol*. 2004;26:39–46.

Odontogenic Cysts–*Buccal Bifurcation Cyst*

Bohay RN, Weinberg S. The paradental cyst of the mandibular permanent first molar: report of a bilateral case. *J Dent Child*. 1992;59:361–365.

David LA, Sandor GK, Stoneman DW. The buccal bifurcation cyst: is non-surgical treatment an option? *J Can Dent Assoc*. 1998;64:712–716.

Packota GV, Hall JM, Lanigan DT, et al. Paradental cysts on mandibular first molars in children: report of five cases. *Dentomaxillofac Radiol*. 1990;19:126–132.

Philipsen HP, Reichert PA, Ogawa I, et al. The inflammatory paradental cyst: a critical review of 342 from a literature survey, including 17 new cases from the author's files. *J Oral Pathol Med*. 2004;33:147–155.

Pompura JR, Sandor GK, Stoneman DW. The buccal bifurcation cyst: a prospective study of treatment outcomes in 44 sites. *Oral Surg Oral Med Oral Pathol Oral Radiol Endod*. 1997;83:215–221.

Odontogenic Cysts–*Calcifying Odontogenic Cyst*

Johnson A III, Fletcher M, Gold L, et al. Calcifying odontogenic cyst: a clinicopathologic study of 57 cases with immunohistochemical evaluation for cytokeratin. *J Oral Maxillofac Surg*. 1997;55:679–683.

Moleri AB, Moreira LC, Carvalho JJ. Comparative morphology of 7 new cases of calcifying odontogenic cysts. *J Oral Maxillofac Surg*. 2002;60:689–696.

Yoshiura K, Tabata O, Miwa K, et al. Computed tomographic features of calcifying odontogenic cysts. *Dentomaxillofac Radiol*. 1998;27:12–16.

Odontogenic Cysts–*Dentigerous Cyst*

Costa FW, Viana TS, Cavalcante GM, et al. A clinicoradiographic and pathological study of pericoronal follicles associated to mandibular third molars. *J Craniofac Surg*. 2014;25:e283–e287.

Xu GZ, Jiang Q, Yu CQ, et al. Clinicopathologic features of dentigerous cysts in the maxillary sinus. *J Craniofac Surg*. 2012;23:e226–e231.

Odontogenic Cysts–*Glandular Odontogenic Cyst*

MacDonald-Jankowski DS. Glandular odontogenic cyst: systematic review. *Dentomaxillofac Radiol*. 2010;39:127–139.

Noffke C, Raubenheimer EJ. The glandular odontogenic cyst: clinical and radiologic features: review of the literature and report of nine cases. *Dentomaxillofac Radiol*. 2002;31:333–338.

Odontogenic Cysts–*Lateral Periodontal Cyst*

Shear M, Pindborg JJ. Microscopic features of the lateral periodontal cyst. *Scand J Dent Res*. 1975;83:103–110.

Weathers DR, Waldron CA. Unusual multilocular cysts of the jaws (botryoid odontogenic cysts). *Oral Surg Oral Med Oral Pathol*. 1973;36:235–241.

Wysocki GP, Brannon RB, Gardner DG, et al. Histogenesis of the lateral periodontal cyst and the gingival cyst of the adult. *Oral Surg Oral Med Oral Pathol*. 1980;50:327–334.

Odontogenic Cysts–*Odontogenic Keratocyst*

Brannon RB. The odontogenic keratocyst: a clinicopathological study of 312 cases, I: clinical features. *Oral Surg Oral Med Oral Pathol*. 1976;42:54–72.

Guo YY, Zhang JY, Li XF, et al. PTCH1 gene mutations in Keratocystic odontogenic tumors: a study of 43 Chinese patients and a systematic review. *PLoS ONE*. 2013;8:e77305. doi:10.1371/journal.pone.0077305.

Odontogenic Cysts–*Nevoid Basal Cell Carcinoma Syndrome*

Kakarantza-Angelopoulou E, Nicolatou O. Odontogenic keratocysts: clinicopathologic study of 87 cases. *J Oral Maxillofac Surg*. 1990;48:593–599.

MacDonald D. Lesions of the jaws presenting as radiolucencies on cone beam CT. *Clin Radiol*. 2016;71:972–985.

Myoung H, Hong SP, Hong SD, et al. Odontogenic keratocyst: review of 256 cases for recurrence and clinicopathologic parameters. *Oral Surg Oral Med Oral Pathol Oral Radiol Endod.* 2001;91:328–333.

Donatsky O, Hjörting-Hansen E, Philipsen HP, et al. Clinical, radiographic, and histologic features of the basal cell nevus syndrome. *Int J Oral Surg.* 1976;5:19–28.

Evans DC, Farndon PA, Burnell LD, et al. The incidence of Gorlin syndrome in 173 consecutive cases of medulloblastoma. *Br J Cancer.* 1991;64:959–961.

Gorlin RJ. Nevoid basal cell carcinoma syndrome. *Medicine (Baltimore).* 1987;66:98–113.

Lam EWN, Lee L, Perschbacher SE, et al. The occurrence of keratocystic odontogenic tumours in nevoid basal cell carcinoma syndrome. *Dentomaxillofac Radiol.* 2009;38:475–479.

Odontogenic Cysts–*Residual Cyst*

High AS, Hirschmann PN. Age changes in residual cysts. *J Oral Pathol.* 1986;15:524–528.

Nonodontogenic Cysts–*Nasolabial Cyst*

Sheikh AB, Chin OY, Fang CH, et al. Nasolabial cysts: a systematic review of 311 cases. *Laryngoscope.* 2016;126:60–66.

Yuen H, Julian CY, Samuel CL. Nasolabial cysts: clinical features, diagnosis and treatment. *Br J Oral Maxillofac Surg.* 2007;45:293–297.

Nonodontogenic Cysts–*Nasopalatine Cyst*

Elliott KA, Franzese CB, Pitman KT. Diagnosis and surgical management of nasopalatine duct cysts. *Laryngoscope.* 2004;114:1336–1340.

Mraiwa RJ, Jacobs R, Van Cleynenbreugel J, et al. The nasopalatine duct cyst revisited using 2D and 3D CT imaging. *Dentomaxillofac Radiol.* 2004;33:396–402.

Swanson KS, Kaugars GE, Gunsolley JC. Nasopalatine duct cyst: an analysis of 334 cases. *J Oral Maxillofac Surg.* 1991;49:268–271.

Soft Tissue Cysts–*Branchial Cleft Cyst*

Glosser JW, Pires CA, Feinberg SE. Branchial cleft or cervical lymphoepithelial cysts: etiology and management. *J Am Dent Assoc.* 2003;134:81–86.

Prosser JD, Myer CM 3rd. Branchial cleft anomalies and thymic cysts. *Otolaryngol Clin North Am.* 2015;48:1–14.

Soft Tissue Cysts–*Dermoid Cyst*

Pryor SG, Lewis JE, Weaver AL, et al. Pediatric dermoid cysts of the head and neck. *Otolaryngol Head Neck Surg.* 2005;132:938–942.

Seward GR. Dermoid cysts of the floor of the mouth. *Br J Oral Surg.* 1965;3:36–47.

Soft Tissue Cysts–*Lymphoepithelial Cyst*

Shah GV. MR imaging of salivary glands. *Magn Reson Imaging Clin N Am.* 2002;10:631–662.

Sujatha D, Babitha K, Prasad RS, et al. Parotid lymphoepithelial cysts in human immunodeficiency virus: a review. *J Laryngol Otol.* 2013;127:1046–1049.

Wu L, Cheng J, Maruyama S, et al. Lymphoepithelial cyst of the parotid gland: its possible histopathogenesis based on clinicopathologic analysis of 64 cases. *Hum Pathol.* 2009;40:683–692.

Soft Tissue Cysts–*Thyroglossal Duct Cyst*

Ahuja AT, Wong KT, King AD, et al. Imaging for thyroglossal duct cyst: the bare essentials. *Clin Radiol.* 2005;60:141–148.

Ibrahim M, Hammoud K, Maheshwari M, et al. Congenital cystic lesions of the head and neck. *Neuroimaging Clin N Am.* 2011;21:621–639.

Pseudocysts–*Mandibular Lingual Bone Depression*

Stafne EC. Bone cavities situated near the angle of the mandible. *JADA.* 1942;29:1969–1972.

Pseudocysts–*Simple Bone Cyst*

Chadwick JW, Alsufyani NA, Lam EW. Clinical and radiographic features of solitary and cemento-osseous dysplasia-associated simple bone cysts. *Dentomaxillofac Radiol.* 2011;40:230–235.

Damante JH, Da S, Guerra EN, et al. Spontaneous resolution of simple bone cysts. *Dentomaxillofac Radiol.* 2002;31:182–186.

Perdigao AF, Silva EC, Sakurai E, et al. Idiopathic bone cavity: a clinical, radiographic and histological study. *Br J Oral Maxillofac Surg.* 2003;41:407–409.

Saito Y, Hoshina Y, Nagamine T, et al. Simple bone cyst: a clinical and histopathologic study of fifteen cases. *Oral Surg Oral Med Oral Pathol.* 1992;74:487–491.

Sapp PJ, Stark ML. Self-healing traumatic bone cysts. *Oral Surg Oral Med Oral Pathol.* 1990;69:597–602.

24

Benign Tumors and Neoplasms

Ernest W.N. Lam

DISEASE MECHANISM

A benign neoplasm is an abnormal mass of tissue that develops as a result of uncontrolled cell proliferation. Moreover, the potential for cell proliferation in a neoplasm is unlimited. Although the term tumor is often used synonymously for neoplasm, a tumor is a more generic term that refers to a tissue mass. So while all neoplasms are tumors, not all tumors are neoplasms. The loss of growth control in neoplasia is often the result of an identifiable gene mutation that regulates cell proliferation. The molecular abnormality is then propagated through cell division, which results in a population of cells, each of which contains the same genetic abnormality. This type of propagation, or clonal proliferation, is a hallmark of neoplasia. In contrast to malignant neoplasms, benign neoplasms lack the ability to metastasize; that is, benign neoplastic cells do not have the ability to form satellite masses at distant sites.

Benign neoplasms tend to resemble the tissue of origin histologically. For example, an ameloblastoma, a neoplasm that is derived from odontogenic epithelium, is composed of cells that resemble ameloblasts. A benign neoplasm should, however, be differentiated from a hyperplasia, metaplasia, and hamartoma. While these processes may produce a tissue mass, cell proliferation is limited. Hyperplasia is a proliferation of cells that develops in response to a stimulus. When the stimulus is removed, the mass regresses. In metaplasia, one mature cell type is transformed into another mature cell type. When the stimulus is removed, the metaplastic cell type reverts to its native cell type. A hamartoma is a mass of disorganized normal tissue that would normally be found at the site of growth.

CLINICAL FEATURES

Benign neoplasms may be found incidentally on radiologic examinations made for other purposes, or they may be detected clinically by an enlargement of the jaws or movement of teeth. Sometimes the radiologic examination is performed to try to discover the reason for the lack of eruption of a tooth. Benign neoplasms typically have an insidious onset, and grow slowly. These neoplasms are painless, but they can be locally aggressive should they extend into adjacent tissue spaces.

APPLIED DIAGNOSTIC IMAGING

If an abnormal enlargement of the jaw is suspected, a radiologic examination should be performed to document the extent and imaging characteristics of the lesion. This examination often begins with a panoramic image to identify the site and extent of the lesion, and intraoral periapical and/or occlusal images to evaluate the effects of the abnormality on the teeth and the surrounding structures. For lesions developing centrally within the bone, the addition of multidetector computed tomographic (MDCT) or cone beam CT (CBCT) imaging is essential

for further refining radiologic feature identification. If on panoramic or intraoral imaging, the lesion appears to extend into the surrounding tissues, or if clinically, it is determined that the lesion has developed in the soft tissue, MDCT or magnetic resonance imaging (MRI) may be required to characterize soft tissue involvement.

A systematic, thorough imaging examination provides important information regarding the extension of the lesion in or around the jaws. Furthermore, important radiologic features may be identified, allowing the clinician to differentiate the benign neoplasm from another disease process. On the one hand, some imaging features are so specific of a particular benign neoplasm that a preliminary diagnosis of the type of benign neoplasm can be made. On the other hand, should the imaging features overlap with other similar appearing entities and a preliminary diagnosis cannot be made, other diagnostic testing must be initiated. A thorough imaging examination may also direct the clinician to the most favorable biopsy site, should biopsy be necessary. In all cases, however, the imaging examination should be performed prior to biopsy, as the biopsy procedure could alter the radiologic appearances of the tissues in such a way as to mask characteristic features.

IMAGING FEATURES

Location

Some benign neoplasms have a specific anatomic predilection, so the location of a particular neoplasm may be important in establishing a preliminary differential interpretation. For example, lesions that develop from odontogenic cell sources occur in the alveolar processes superior to the inferior alveolar nerve canal, where odontogenic cells and teeth reside. Lesions of vascular and neural origin develop within the inferior alveolar canal, and cartilaginous neoplasms occur in locations where chondrocytes may reside, such as around the mandibular condyle.

Periphery

Benign neoplasms grow slowly as their cell population increases in number (Fig. 24.1). As a result, the borders of benign neoplasms are well defined. The amount of cortication at the lesion periphery can, however, vary. If the neoplasm exhibits a slower or more indolent growth pattern, the cortex is often more apparent. In contrast, if the neoplasm grows more quickly or aggressively, the cortex will be less clearly seen or there may be discontinuities or breaks.

The clonal nature of cell proliferation in a benign neoplasm often results in what appears to be a concentric pattern of enlargement of the neoplasm. This type of growth pattern is different than the hydraulic pattern that is seen with cysts. As the neoplastic cells proliferate, different subpopulations of cells may experience different microenvironments that support or retard the growth of the neoplasm. For example, in areas where the vascular supply is richer, the cells may proliferate at a faster rate and this region of the neoplasm may enlarge more quickly

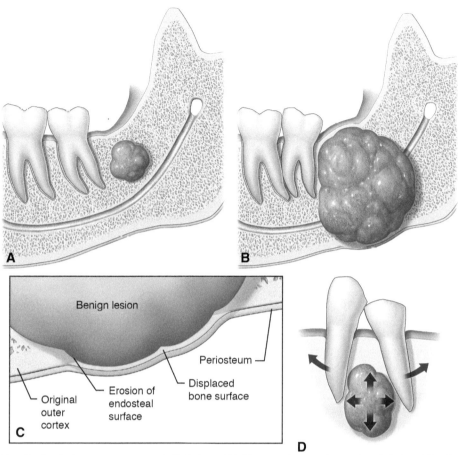

Fig. 24.1 Benign lesions grow concentrically in bone (A). They can be round to oval, or lobulated (B). As they grow, benign lesions can displace adjacent bone borders (C) and teeth (D), and externally resorb tooth roots.

than an adjacent area that may be less well vascularized. This type of differential growth may be appreciated radiologically as a lobulated periphery, where larger lobules reflect areas of faster growth and smaller lobules as areas of slower growth.

Internal Structure

The internal structure may be completely radiolucent or radiopaque, or it may be a mixture of both radiolucent and radiopaque areas. Normal bone that is trapped between growing adjacent lobules of a benign neoplasm are called septa (or a septum, if there is just one). These septa can be linear, curvilinear, or curved depending on the neoplasm, and can vary in thickness. Curved septa are a characteristic feature of ameloblastoma. While the cells in an ameloblastoma do not produce bone, the trapped residual bone between the lobules of the neoplasm is remodeled into curvilinear or curved structures by internal changes to the mass during growth. Should the sizes of adjacent lobules be larger and the entrapped bone becomes more significantly compressed, the septum will appear thinner. In contrast, smaller adjacent lobules will produce a thicker septum. Although residual bone in the form of septa may give rise to a mixed radiolucent and radiopaque internal structure, some clinicians differentiate septa (residual bone) from mineralized matrices produced de novo by the tumor cells themselves.

Some neoplasms have developed the capability to produce a mineralized matrix if the cells have reached an appropriate level of differentiation or maturation. These "true" mixed radiolucent and radiopaque lesions contain mineralized areas that can take the form of tooth material or

bone. Because the most mature part of the neoplasm is located more centrally, mineralization often occurs centrally first, before it spreads to more peripheral areas within the neoplasm. An ossifying fibroma often has an internal granular radiopaque pattern produced by the abnormal or immature bone that is actually being manufactured by the neoplastic cells. Often the internal pattern is characteristic for specific types of neoplasms, and this may aid in the interpretation. A neoplasm with a totally radiolucent internal structure is not as useful as an aid to the interpretation.

Effects on Surrounding Structures

The manner in which a neoplasm affects adjacent tissues may suggest a behavior that is benign, or behaviors that are more indolent or aggressive. As a benign neoplasm enlarges, it may displace its neighboring structures. If the growth pattern is indolent or slow, adjacent structures may respond by remodeling around the enlarging mass. For example, the surface of the bone may enlarge and the cortex may thin as the bone is remodeled to accommodate the growing mass. This appearance is caused by simultaneous resorption of bone along the inner surface (endosteal) of the cortex and deposition of bone along the outer cortical surface by the periosteum (see Fig. 24.1C). Because the remodeling process is slow, the cortex maintains its integrity and resists perforation, although faster, more aggressively growing neoplasms may exceed the capacity of the bone to remodel resulting in perforation of the cortex. Internal structures such as the inferior alveolar canal or the floor of the maxillary sinus may also be displaced to accommodate a developing adjacent benign neoplasm.

Effects on Adjacent Teeth

Benign neoplasms may also cause bodily displacement of adjacent teeth (see Fig. 24.1D). This very slow process is the result of stresses and strains on tooth roots by a growing adjacent benign neoplasm. The roots of teeth may also be resorbed in a directional manner as the edge of the neoplasm encounters the tooth root. Benign neoplasms tend to resorb the adjacent root surfaces in a smooth fashion.

ODONTOGENIC TUMORS AND NEOPLASMS

Disease Mechanism

Odontogenic neoplasms arise from odontogenic tissues in the jaws. According to the World Health Organization (WHO), these neoplasms can be classified on the basis of the cell of origin of each neoplasm: neoplasms composed of odontogenic epithelium, mixed neoplasms composed of both odontogenic epithelium and odontogenic ectomesenchyme (connective tissue), and neoplasms composed of primarily ectomesenchyme. Odontogenic neoplasms account for 1.3% to 15% of all oral neoplasms. Benign jaw neoplasms are presented in this chapter according to their tissues of origin. This format should assist the reader in learning to correlate the radiographic appearance of neoplasms with the underlying pathologic basis of the disease process.

ODONTOGENIC EPITHELIAL NEOPLASMS

Ameloblastoma

Disease Mechanism

Ameloblastomas are by far the most common odontogenic neoplasm. This neoplasm arises from odontogenic epithelium derived from remnants of the dental lamina and the enamel organ. Although a number of different subtypes have been described, all involve the localized or generalized proliferation of these cell remnants. The unicystic ameloblastoma may develop as a single entity or may form within the epithelial lining of a dentigerous cyst; this is also called a mural (within the wall) ameloblastoma (Fig. 24.2). More commonly, ameloblastomas are solid cell masses developing within the bone, or they may develop peripheral to the bone. For those ameloblastomas that develop within the bone, such neoplasms can develop cystic internal areas (cystic or multicystic) or induce the proliferation of fibrous connective tissue (desmoplastic).

Clinical Features

The age range for the diagnosis of ameloblastoma is very broad. While the unicystic ameloblastoma occurs in younger people, ameloblastomas may be found in children as young as 3 years, and adults over 80 years. Most patients are, however, between 20 and 50 years of age, with the average age at discovery about 40 years.

Ameloblastomas grow slowly, and few, if any, symptoms occur in the early stages. When small, the neoplasm may be an incidental finding, discovered during a routine dental examination. As the lesion increases in size, the patient eventually notices a gradually increasing facial asymmetry. Swelling of the cheek, gingiva, or hard palate has been reported as the chief complaint in 95% of untreated maxillary ameloblastomas. The mucosa over the mass is normal, and in most cases, patients do not report pain or paresthesia. The teeth in the involved region may be displaced and become mobile. As the neoplasm enlarges, palpation may elicit a bony hard sensation or crepitus as the bone surface thins. If the overlying bone becomes perforated, the swelling may feel firm or fluctuant, and there may be extension into the adjacent soft tissues.

An untreated neoplasm may grow to a great size, and is more of a concern in the maxilla where it can impinge on vital structures as it extends to the paranasal sinuses, orbit, nasopharynx, or vital structures at the skull base. Recurrence rates are higher in older patients and in patients with multilocular lesions. As seen with other jaw neoplasms, local recurrence, whether detected radiographically or histopathologically, may have a more aggressive character than the original neoplasm.

Imaging Features

Worth, in his 1963 text, describes four patterns of ameloblastoma: a unilocular radiolucent cavity (Fig. 24.3), a unilocular radiolucent cavity with partial division by coarse septa (Fig. 24.4), multilocular radiolucent cavities separated by curved septa of variable lengths (Fig. 24.5), and a honeycomb pattern consisting of many radiolucent compartments separated by small curved septa (Figs. 24.6 and 24.7). It should be noted that although a unicystic ameloblastoma is a unilocular entity, the unilocular appearance of ameloblastoma does not necessarily represent a unicystic ameloblastoma.

Location. Although remnants of odontogenic epithelium may be located anywhere within the jaws, most ameloblastomas (80%) develop in the molar/ramus region of the mandible. Most lesions that occur in

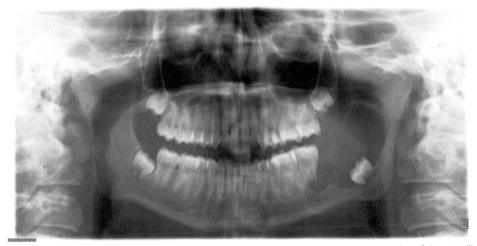

Fig. 24.2 Unicystic ameloblastoma developing in the left posterior mandible causing expansion of the mandibular body and ramus to the sigmoid notch and inferior displacement of the mandibular left third molar and root resorption of the mandibular left second molar.

the maxilla are in the third molar area, subjacent to the floor of the maxillary sinus or more anteriorly, the nasal floor (Fig. 24.8).

Periphery. The ameloblastoma has well-defined borders, although the thickness of the cortex as well as its continuity peripherally can vary depending on the relative aggressiveness of the neoplasm. For example, a faster, more aggressively growing neoplasm may exhibit a less visible cortex. The borders are often curved, and for smaller lesions, an ameloblastoma may be indistinguishable from a cyst (see Fig. 24.3). The periphery of lesions in the maxilla is usually less well defined, and this may be due to the native cancellous bone pattern in the maxilla and relative aggressiveness of maxillary lesions.

Internal structure. The internal structure of ameloblastomas can vary from one that is unilocular and radiolucent (see Fig. 24.3) to one that has many small locules separated by radiopaque septa (see Fig. 24.6). Indeed, the presence of a septum within a larger cyst-like cavity or when a septum produces partial loculation within a cavity add greatly to the possibility of ameloblastoma (see Figs. 24.4 and 24.5).

Most commonly, the septa in ameloblastomas are coarse and curved, partially dividing a unilocular cavity into multiple smaller, variably sized cavities (see Fig. 24.5C). Because this neoplasm frequently has internal cystic cavities, in some cases, the septa are remodeled into curves creating a soap bubble (larger compartments of variable size) or a honeycomb (numerous small compartments) pattern (see Fig.

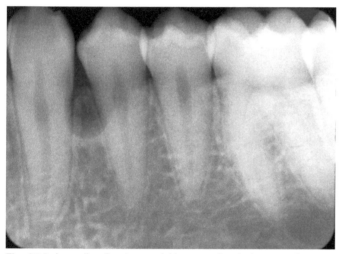

Fig. 24.3 A small unilocular ameloblastoma developing near the crest of the alveolar process of the mandible.

24.6). Generally, the loculations are larger in the posterior mandible and smaller in the anterior mandible. In the desmoplastic variety, the internal structure can be composed of very irregular sclerotic bone resembling a bone dysplasia or bone-forming neoplasm (Fig. 24.9).

Effects on surrounding structures. Occlusal imaging may demonstrate the often cyst-like expansion of the bone, and thinning of an adjacent cortical plate leaving a thin "eggshell" of remnant bone (see Fig. 24.5C). Where the crest of the alveolar process of the mandible in the retromolar area or the anterior border of the mandibular ramus has been perforated or lost, the probability of ameloblastoma is greatly increased. Unicystic ameloblastomas, for example, may cause extreme expansion of the mandibular ramus (Fig. 24.10). CT images often reveal regions of perforation of the displaced bone cortex owing to the inability of the production of periosteal new bone as the ameloblastoma expands (Fig. 24.11A). The value of MDCT in this instance is that soft tissue window images can demonstrate extension of the tumor mass into the adjacent soft tissues (see Fig. 24.11B).

Effects on adjacent teeth. There is a pronounced tendency for ameloblastomas to cause extensive root resorption (see Fig. 24.6). Tooth displacement is also common, and in some cases, this displacement can be apical.

Recurrent ameloblastoma. Ameloblastomas may recur when the initial surgical excision inadequately removes the entire neoplasm. Recurrent neoplasm has a characteristic appearance of multiple small cyst-like structures with very coarse, almost sclerotic borders (Fig. 24.12). Depending on how the neoplasm recurs, these small cyst-like areas may be separated by normal bone.

Additional imaging. If a preliminary interpretation of ameloblastoma is made on the basis of plain imaging, MDCT imaging is highly recommended. MDCT may help confirm the interpretation, but also more accurately demonstrates the anatomic extent and effects on the adjacent bone borders and soft tissues (see Fig. 24.12). In this regard, MDCT imaging has an advantage over CBCT imaging in that it can display the extension of the neoplasm's soft tissue out of the bone and into the adjacent and overlying structures. If soft tissue extension is extensive, an MRI can provide superior images of the nature and extent of the invasion. MDCT is also an essential tool in the postsurgical follow-up assessment of ameloblastoma.

Differential interpretation. Small unilocular ameloblastomas that are located around the crown of an unerupted tooth often cannot be differentiated from a dentigerous cyst. Because the appearance of internal septa is important for the interpretation of ameloblastoma, other types of lesions that also have internal septa, such as odontogenic keratocyst,

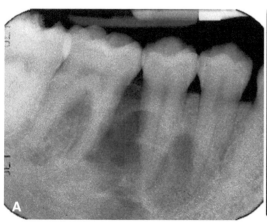
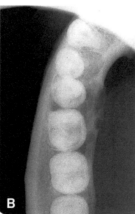
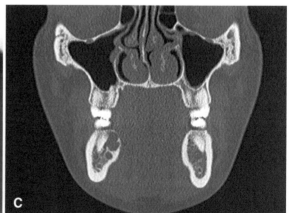

Fig. 24.4 Periapical (A) and cross-sectional occlusal images (B) showing short septa developing in an ameloblastoma. The partial loculations are seen in the coronal multidetector computed tomographic image (C).

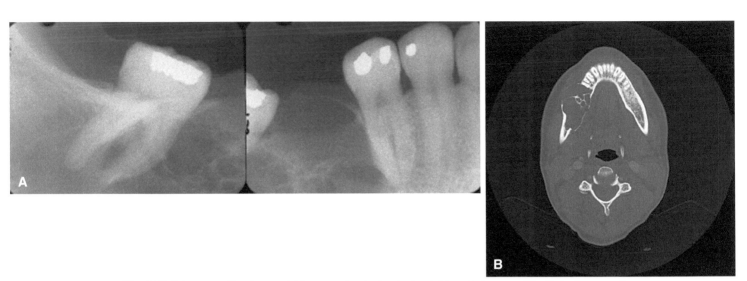

Fig. 24.5 A large multilocular ameloblastoma developing in the right posterior mandible. Note the curved septations dividing the larger cavity into smaller, more discrete regions on the periapical images (A). The multidetector computed tomographic image of the same patient (B) shows the variability in the sizes of these cavities.

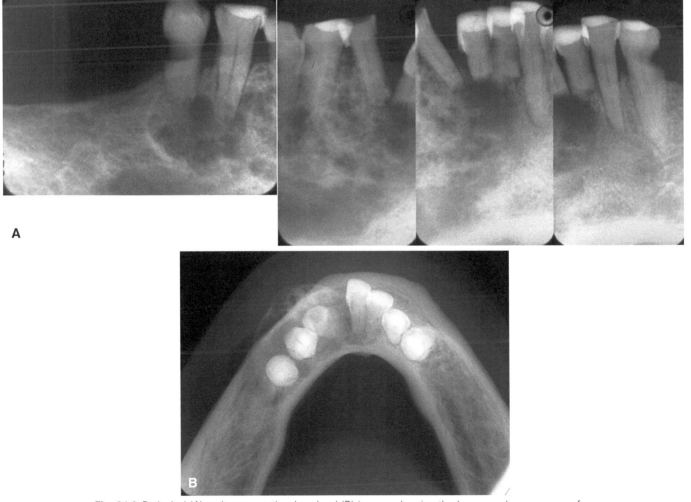

Fig. 24.6 Periapical (A) and cross-sectional occlusal (B) images showing the honeycomb appearance of an ameloblastoma. Note the short, curved septa and the small, closely spaced compartments of tumor reminiscent of honeycombs in a beehive.

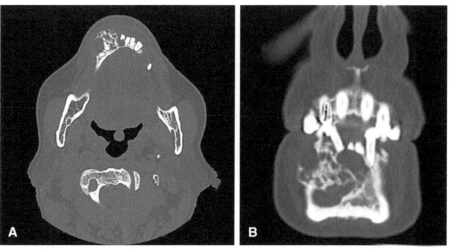

Fig. 24.7 Axial (A) and coronal (B) multidetector computed tomographic images of the same patient in Fig. 24.6 showing the short, curved septa and the small, closely spaced tumor compartments.

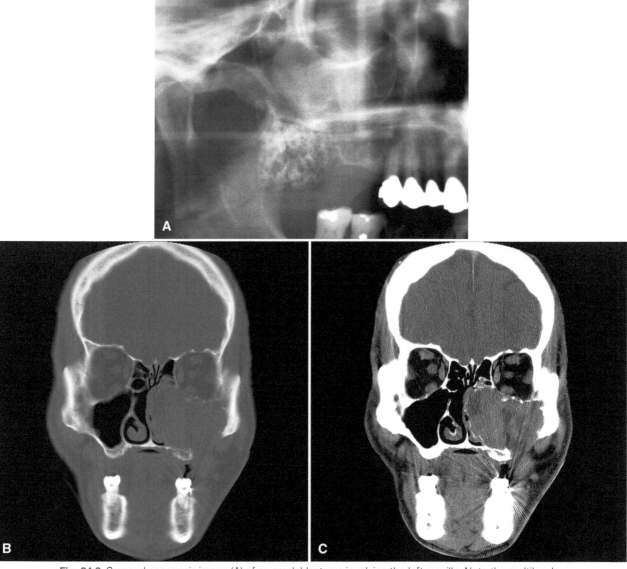

Fig. 24.8 Cropped panoramic image (A) of an ameloblastoma involving the left maxilla. Note the multilocular appearance in the tuberosity region. It is impossible to determine the extent of the lesion with the panoramic image. The same coronal computed tomographic image slices using both bone (B) and soft tissue (C) algorithms. Note the aggressive nature of the tumor as it has displaced both the sinus and nasal fossa floors, and perforated the lateral border of the maxilla.

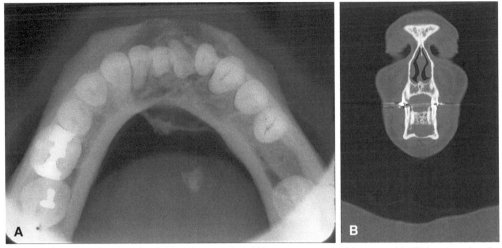

Fig. 24.9 Cross-sectional occlusal (A) and coronal multidetector computed tomographic (B) images showing the irregular sclerotic bone developing around the teeth in a desmoplastic ameloblastoma.

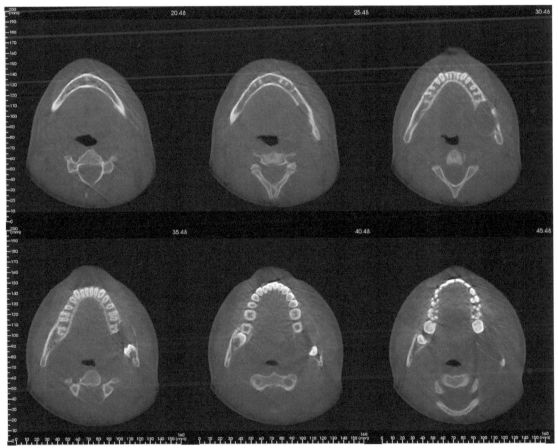

Fig. 24.10 Axial cone beam computed tomographic image shows significant medial and lateral expansion of the left posterior body and ramus of the mandible from a unicystic ameloblastoma.

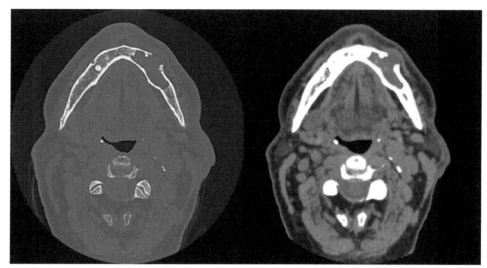

Fig. 24.11 Axial bone *(left)* and soft tissue *(right)* windowed multidetector computed tomographic images of an ameloblastoma in the mandible showing perforation of the buccal cortex of the bone, and outgrowth of the tumor into the adjacent soft tissues.

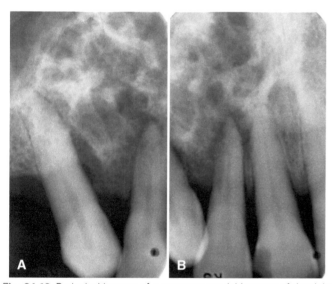

Fig. 24.12 Periapical images of a recurrent ameloblastoma of the right maxilla. Note the sclerotic margins of the small locules.

central giant cell (CGC) lesion, and odontogenic myxoma, may have a similar appearance. An odontogenic keratocyst may contain curved septa, but usually the odontogenic keratocyst tends to grow along the bone without marked buccal/lingual bone expansion, which is characteristic of ameloblastomas. Giant cell lesions, in addition to occurring in a younger age group, have more granular or wispy ill-defined septa that are produced de novo by the cells within the lesion. Odontogenic myxomas may have similar-appearing septa; however, there are usually one or two thin sharp, straight septa, which is characteristic of the myxoma. The presence of straight septa oriented perpendicularly to one another greatly adds to the probability of myxoma. Also, myxomas are not as expansile as ameloblastomas, and like odontogenic keratocysts, tend to grow along the bone.

Management. The size of the ameloblastoma often dictates the aggressiveness of its management. The most common treatment is en bloc surgical resection. The surgical procedure should take into account the tendency of the neoplasm to perforate an adjacent bone border, and extend into the adjacent soft tissues. The maxilla is usually treated more aggressively because of the tendency of ameloblastoma to encroach upon adjacent vital structures. Radiation therapy has been used for inoperable neoplasms, especially neoplasms in the posterior maxilla.

Calcifying Epithelial Odontogenic Tumor
Disease Mechanism
The calcifying epithelial odontogenic tumor (CEOT) or Pindborg tumor is a rare neoplasm, accounting for about 1% of odontogenic neoplasms. These neoplasms usually are located within bone, and its cells may produce a mineralized substance within an amyloid-like material.

Clinical Features
A CEOT is a less aggressive neoplasm than an ameloblastoma, and is found in about the same age group: 8 to 92 years, with an average age of about 42 years. Rarely does this neoplasm have an extraosseous location. Jaw expansion is a regular feature and usually the only symptom. Palpation of the swelling reveals a hard tumor.

Imaging Features
Location. Similar to ameloblastomas, CEOTs have a predilection for the mandible, with a ratio of at least 2:1. Most develop in the premolar and molar areas, and approximately 52% have an association with an unerupted or impacted tooth. In about half of cases, images made early in the development of these neoplasms reveal a radiolucent area associated with the crown of a mature, unerupted tooth.

Periphery. The periphery has a well-defined and corticated border resembling a cyst. In some neoplasms, however, the boundary may be irregular and poorly defined.

Internal structure. Internally, the CEOT may appear unilocular or multilocular with numerous scattered radiopaque internal foci of variable sizes and densities. Some of these foci may have a crescent or a doughnut shape, with a radiolucent center. The most characteristic finding is the appearance of the radiopacities close to the crown of the unerupted or impacted tooth (Fig. 24.13). In addition, small, thin, opaque trabeculae may cross the radiolucency in many directions.

Effects on surrounding structures. There may be expansion of the bone; however the cortical boundary is often maintained.

Effects on surrounding teeth. CEOTs may displace a developing tooth or prevent its eruption as a result of its pericoronal epicenter.

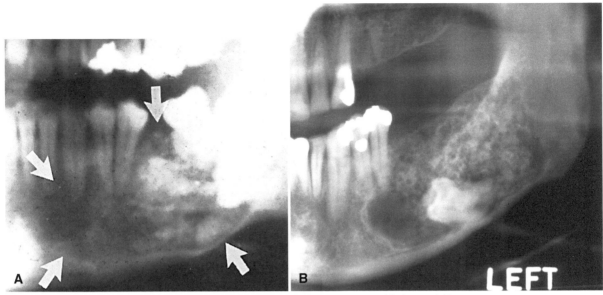

Fig. 24.13 Calcifying epithelial odontogenic tumor or Pindborg tumor (A) *(arrows)*. The tumor appears as a mixed radiolucent and radiopaque lesion (B) associated with an unerupted tooth. (A, Courtesy Dr. M. Gornitsky, Montreal, Canada. B, Courtesy Dr. D. Lanigan, University of Saskatchewan.)

Differential Interpretation

Lesions with a completely radiolucent internal structure may resemble a dentigerous cyst or odontogenic keratocyst. Lesions with radiopaque foci may resemble adenomatoid odontogenic tumor, ameloblastic fibro-odontoma, and calcifying odontogenic cyst. However, the prominent location of the CEOT and the age of the patient help in the differential interpretation.

Management

The management of a CEOT is local resection: a more conservative treatment than ameloblastoma.

MIXED EPITHELIAL AND MESENCHYMAL ODONTOGENIC TUMORS AND NEOPLASMS

Ameloblastic Fibroma

Disease Mechanism

Ameloblastic fibromas are benign mixed neoplastic proliferations of odontogenic epithelium and primitive mesenchymal components resembling the dental papilla. These cells do not deposit a mineralized matrix on the tumor cell bed.

Clinical Features

Ameloblastic fibromas occur in the first and second decades of life during the period of tooth formation, with an average age of about 15 years. They usually produce a painless, slow-growing soft tissue mass overlying the bone, and unerupted or impacted teeth (Fig. 24.14). Although the most common sign is swelling or a missing tooth, this neoplasm may also be discovered on imaging made for another purpose.

Imaging Features

Location. Ameloblastic fibromas usually develop in the posterior mandible, extending as far posteriorly as the mandibular ramus and as far mesially as the premolar/molar areas. A common location is

coronal to an unerupted tooth and near the crest of the alveolar process (Fig. 24.15), or it may arise in an area where a tooth has failed to develop.

Periphery. The borders of an ameloblastic fibroma are well defined and often corticated in a manner similar to that of a cyst.

Internal structure. An ameloblastic fibroma is more commonly totally radiolucent, and unilocular (see Figs. 24.14 and 24.15). Less commonly, these lesions may have a multilocular appearance with indistinct curved septa (Fig. 24.16).

Effects on surrounding structures. If the lesion is large, there may be expansion with an intact cortical plate.

Effects on adjacent teeth. The associated tooth or teeth may be inhibited from normal eruption or may be displaced in an apical direction.

Differential Interpretation

It may be difficult to differentiate a small tumor with a coronal relationship to an unerupted tooth from a hyperplastic follicle or a small dentigerous cyst. Unfortunately, the radiologic features may not allow differentiation between these three entities.

Although the ameloblastic fibroma may have similar features to an ameloblastoma, the ameloblastic fibroma occurs at an earlier age, and the septa in an ameloblastoma are more defined and coarse. In comparison, the septa in ameloblastic fibroma are infrequent and often very fine. CGC lesions may appear multilocular, but these neoplasms usually have an epicenter anterior to the mandibular first molar in young patients, and the internal radiopacities are characteristically more granular and poorly defined. Odontogenic myxomas can appear multilocular, but usually a few sharp straight septa can be identified, which are not characteristic of ameloblastic fibromas, and myxomas usually occur in an older age group.

Management

The management of ameloblastic fibromas is conservative surgical enucleation and mechanical curettage of the surrounding bone. This approach is reported to be successful, and there is no recurrence.

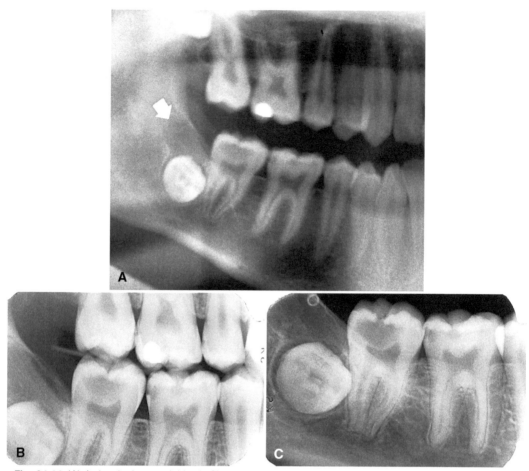

Fig. 24.14 (A) A developing ameloblastic fibroma is seen as a radiolucency coronal to the unerupted third molar *(arrow)*. Bite-wing (B) and periapical (C) images of the same lesion (B). (Courtesy Dr. G. Sanders, La Crosse, WI.)

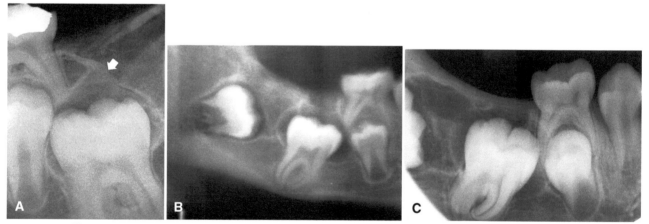

Fig. 24.15 Ameloblastic fibroma appearing as a unilocular outgrowth of the follicle of the unerupted first permanent molar (A). Periapical and cropped panoramic (B) images illustrating an ameloblastic fibroma associated with the crowns of the first and second molars.

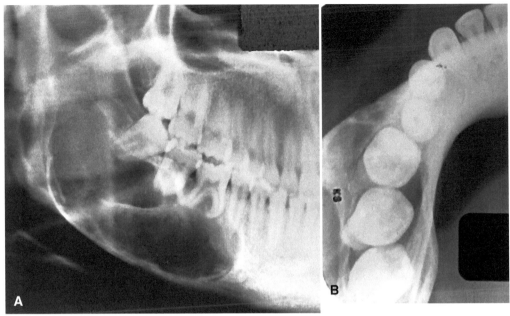

Fig. 24.16 Panoramic (A) and cross-sectional occlusal (B) images of an ameloblastic fibroma in the body and ramus of the right mandible. Note the expansion of the mandible on the occlusal image.

Ameloblastic Fibro-Odontoma

Disease Mechanism

An ameloblastic fibro-odontoma is a benign mixed neoplasm consisting of proliferations of odontogenic epithelium and primitive mesenchymal components with collections of enamel and dentin. Some authorities consider the ameloblastic fibro-odontoma to be a more mature stage of development of the ameloblastic fibroma.

Clinical Features

The clinical features are similar to ameloblastic fibromas, often located in an area of the jaws with a missing tooth or associated with a tooth that has failed to erupt. This neoplasm is found in the first and second decades of life, in an age range that is similar to ameloblastic fibromas and odontomas, and with no particular sex predilection.

Imaging Features

Location. Most cases occur in the posterior mandible, with the lesion epicenter located usually occlusal to a developing tooth or toward the alveolar crest (Fig. 24.17).

Periphery. The borders of an ameloblastic fibro-odontoma are well defined and often corticated.

Internal structure. The internal structure may have a radiolucent or a mixed radiolucent and radiopaque appearance. Small lesions may appear as enlarged follicles with only one or two small, discrete radiopaque foci while larger lesions may have a more extensive calcified internal structure (Fig. 24.18). In some cases, these small calcifications may have a round shape with a radiopaque enamel-like margin with a shape similar to that of a small doughnut or some may appear as small malformed teeth.

Effects on surrounding structures. If the lesion is large, there may be expansion with an intact cortical plate.

Effects on adjacent teeth. The coronal epicenter of the ameloblastic fibro-odontoma may inhibit the eruption of a permanent tooth, or the tooth may be displaced in an apical direction.

Differential Interpretation

If there are no internal calcifications, this neoplasm cannot be differentiated from an ameloblastic fibroma. Differentiation from a developing odontoma may be difficult, but generally these neoplasms have a larger soft tissue component than an odontoma, and this may be seen as a substantially sized radiolucent area. It may be argued that given time, the foci of internal mineralization will increase; however, the distribution of mineralized tissue between the ameloblastic fibro-odontoma and the odontoma is different. A complex odontoma, which shares a common location, usually has one single large mass of disorganized tissue in the center of the lesion with a thin radiolucent rim. In contrast, the ameloblastic fibro-odontoma usually has more randomly dispersed mature small pieces of dental hard tissue. Although the compound odontoma may contain multiple denticles, the posterior mandible is a rare location, and the organization of the tooth material in ameloblastic fibro-odontomas never appears organized enough to resemble a tooth.

Treatment

Usually conservative enucleation is used, although recurrence has been reported.

Odontoma

Disease Mechanism

The term *odontoma* is used to describe a hamartoma that is characterized by the production of mature enamel, dentin, cementum, and pulp tissue. Some authors consider the odontoma as being the final developmental stage of the ameloblastic fibroma and fibro-odontoma. However, unlike these other entities, the odontoma does not demonstrate uncontrolled and unlimited cell proliferation.

The structure of the component tissues may vary from being a nondescript, but heterogeneous mass of the dental hard tissues referred to as a complex odontoma, to more discrete, multiple well-formed teeth (denticles) referred to as a compound odontoma. A dilated odontoma has been described as another type of odontoma; however, this is a

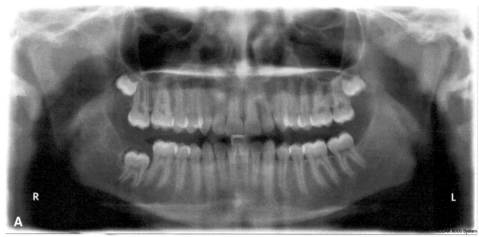

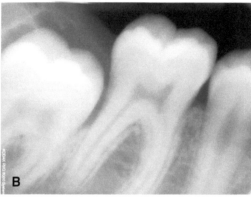

Fig. 24.17 A small developing ameloblastic fibro-odontoma developing coronal to the mandibular right second molar (A). The area of mineralization is faint, and can only be fully appreciated on the periapical image (B). (Courtesy Dr. H. Grubisa, Oakville, ON.)

single entity that actually may be a severe expression of a dens invaginatus or a dens in dente.

Clinical Features

Odontomas are very common, and often, they will interfere with the eruption of permanent teeth (Fig. 24.19). The odontoma shows no sex predilection, and most form while the dentition is developing in the second decade of life. As with ameloblastic fibroma and ameloblastic fibro-odontoma, odontomas may be found during investigations of retained primary teeth or delayed eruption of permanent teeth. In rare cases, odontomas are associated with primary teeth.

Left unidentified or untreated, odontomas will not increase in size, so they may remain undetected in the jaws until an image is made for other reasons. Compound odontomas are about twice as common as the complex type. Although the compound variety forms equally between men and women, 60% of complex odontomas occur in women. In very rare circumstances, a compound odontoma may erupt into the mouth.

Imaging Features

Location. The majority of compound odontomas (62%) occur in the anterior maxilla in association with the crown of an unerupted canine tooth. In contrast, 70% of complex odontomas are found in the mandibular first and second molar area.

Periphery. The borders of odontomas are well defined, with a smooth but irregular periphery. These lesions have a cortical border.

Internal structure. The contents of these lesions are heterogeneously radiopaque. Compound odontomas have a number of variably sized toothlike structures or denticles that have the appearance of deformed

teeth (Fig. 24.20). In some cases, enamel, dentin, and pulp spaces can be visualized (Fig. 24.21), thereby contributing to the heterogeneous appearance. Complex odontomas contain an irregular, but somewhat more homogeneous mass of calcified tissue (Figs. 24.22 and 24.23). The density of the mineralized matrix within these lesions may vary, reflecting differences in the amount and type of hard tissue that has been formed. A dilated odontoma has a single calcified structure with a more radiolucent central portion that has an overall form similar to a doughnut (see Fig. 24.23). The radiopaque component of odontomas is surrounded by a thin, radiolucent rim that has a similar appearance to the follicle surrounding a developing tooth crown.

Effects on surrounding structures. Large odontomas may cause expansion of bone, but with maintenance of the cortical boundary.

Effects on adjacent teeth. Odontomas can interfere with the normal eruption of teeth, and most (70%) are associated with impacted or malposed teeth, diastema, aplasia, malformation, or devitalization of adjacent teeth.

Differential Interpretation

The appearance of small, tooth-like radiopaque structures within a well-defined lesion leads to easy recognition of a compound odontoma. Complex odontomas differ from ossifying fibromas by their tendency to be associated with an unerupted tooth, and because they usually are more radiopaque than ossifying fibromas.

The fully mature stage of periapical cemento-osseous dysplasia may resemble complex odontomas but the cemento-osseous dysplasias may be associated with multiple teeth with epicenters at the root apices. Furthermore, odontomas are more radiopaque than the dysplastic bone

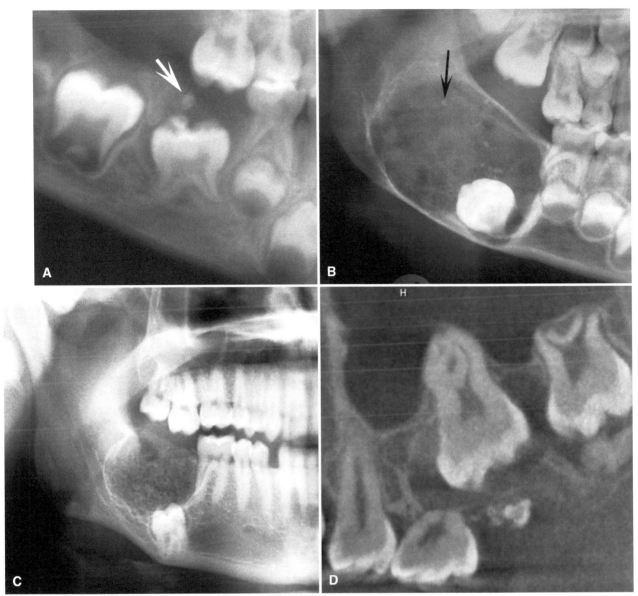

Fig. 24.18 Examples of Ameloblastic Fibro-Odontoma. (A) Cropped panoramic film with a lesion occlusal to a second deciduous molar. The lesion is ill-defined and radiolucent except for two small radiopacities *(arrow)*. (B) Cropped panoramic image of a well-defined radiolucent lesion with only a few scattered radiopacities. (C) Cropped panoramic image of a lesion with numerous radiopacities. (D) Sagittal cone beam computed tomographic image of an ameloblastic fibroma impeding the eruption of the first and second maxillary molars. Note the radiopacities with toothlike density occlusal to both teeth.

found in periapical cemento-osseous dysplasia. Dense bone islands, while radiopaque, lack the radiolucent rim surrounding the radiopaque focus that odontomas do.

Management
Odontomas are removed by simple excision. They do not recur and are not locally invasive.

Adenomatoid Odontogenic Tumor
Disease Mechanism
Adenomatoid odontogenic tumors (AOTs) are uncommon, nonaggressive neoplasms of odontogenic epithelium, and have a variety of patterns. Although the cells of origin of AOTs may be from enamel organ epithelium, it is classified as a mixed tumor because it also contains connective tissue

elements and sometimes calcifications that have been interpreted as dentin- or enamel-like material. Adenomatoid odontogenic tumors account for 3% of all oral tumors, and these can occur both centrally within the bone, and peripherally. Furthermore, the central tumors may be divided into a follicular type, associated with the crown of an unerupted or impacted tooth, and the extrafollicular type, not associated with a tooth. Approximately 73% of central lesions are the follicular type.

Clinical Features
Adenomatoid odontogenic tumors occur in a wide age range: 5 to 50 years. A majority develop in the second decade of life, with an average age of 16 years. In addition, the tumor has a 2:1 female predilection.

The follicular type is identified earlier than the extrafollicular type, probably because there is often an association with a missing tooth.

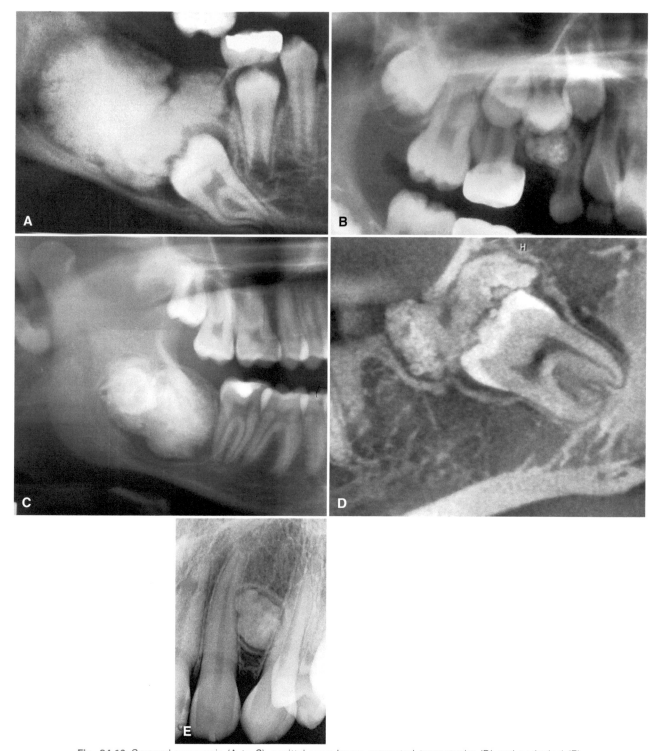

Fig. 24.19 Cropped panoramic (A to C), sagittal cone beam computed tomography (D) and periapical (E) images of complex odontomes. Note the toothlike density of the radiopaque mass, the thin radiolucent rim surrounding the mineralized tissue, and interference with the eruption of associated teeth.

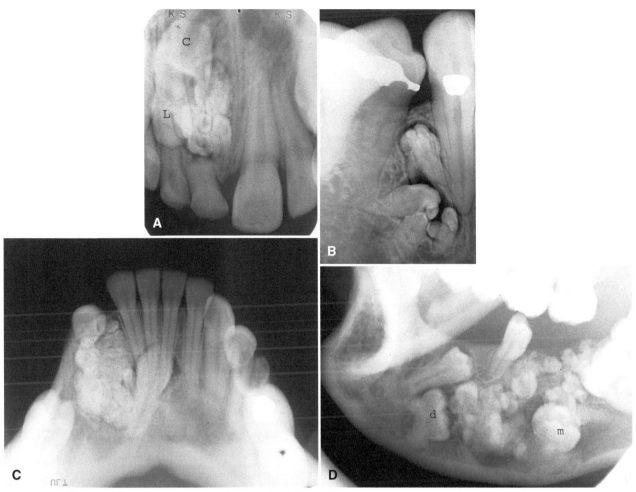

Fig. 24.20 Periapical (A and B), anterior occlusal (C), and lateral oblique (D) images of compound odontomas. Note the numerous internal, radiopaque denticles and the radiolucent periphery.

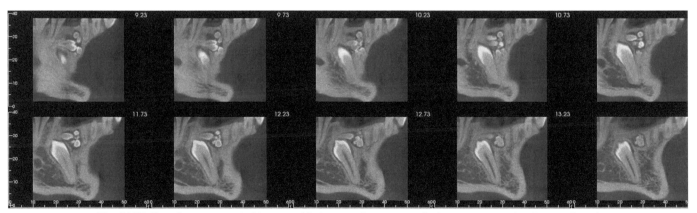

Fig. 24.21 Cone beam computed tomographic images of a compound odontoma preventing the eruption of a mandibular permanent canine. Note the small tooth-like morphologies within the lesion.

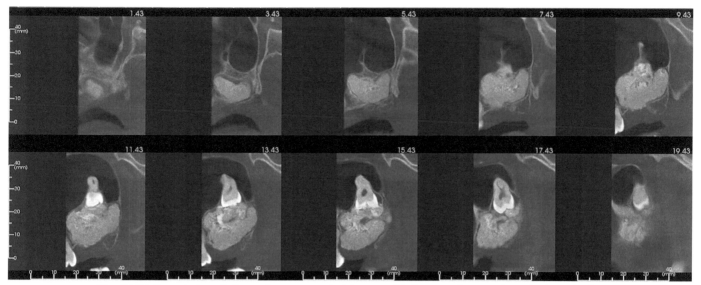

Fig. 24.22 Corrected sagittal cone beam computed tomographic images of a complex odontoma in the posterior maxilla. Note the thin radiolucent rim that surrounds the mass.

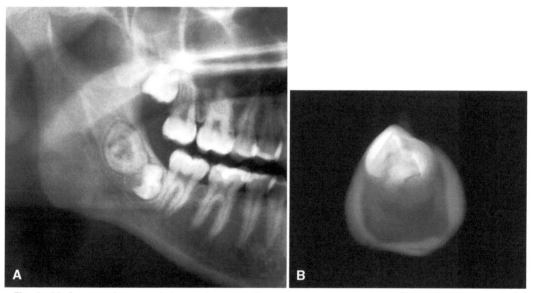

A   B

Fig. 24.23 A cropped panoramic image demonstrating a dilated odontoma located distal to the unerupted third molar (B). The image of the excised specimen shows the crown like morphology of the lesion.

The tumor is slow growing and manifests as a gradually enlarging, painless swelling or asymmetry.

Imaging Features

Location. At least 75% of AOTs occur in the anterior maxilla and mandible (Fig. 24.24). The incisor-canine-premolar region and especially the cuspid region is the usual area involved in both jaws. Although the follicular type may have a relationship with an impacted tooth, it may often not have an association with the cementoenamel junction but rather, surrounds a greater part of the tooth crown and root, most often a canine (Fig. 24.25).

Periphery. The periphery is well defined and corticated, although the cortex may show some variation in thickness.

Internal structure. The internal appearance may be radiolucent (see Fig. 24.25), or mixed radiolucent and radiopaque; the mixed type may

be up to two-thirds of cases. The appearance of the mixed type may vary from an appearance of faint, delicate radiopaque foci to more dense clusters of ill-defined radiopacities. Occasionally, the calcifications may have well-defined borders, similar to a cluster of small pebbles (see Fig. 24.25B). Intraoral imaging may be required to demonstrate these calcifications which may not be visible on panoramic or advanced imaging due to poorer image resolution. Microscopic studies have verified that the size, number, and density of small radiopacities may vary from tumor to tumor, and these seem to increase with age.

Effects on adjacent structures. As the tumor enlarges, some expansion of the jaw may occur; however the outer cortex is maintained.

Effects on surrounding structures. AOTs may cause the displacement of adjacent teeth; however, root resorption is rare. If the epicenter of the lesion is located coronal to a developing tooth, it may inhibit eruption of the tooth.

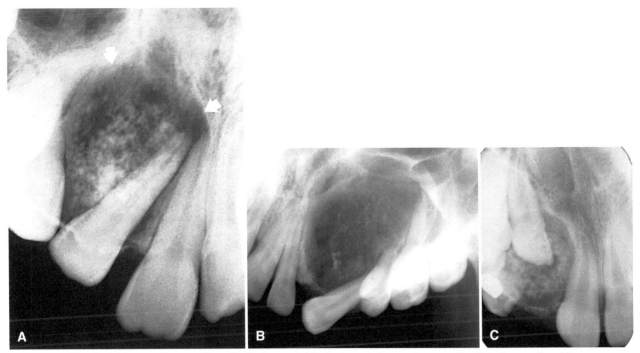

Fig. 24.24 Intraoral images (A to C) of adenomatoid odontogenic tumors (*arrows,* A) within the maxilla with varying amounts of calcification, some of which have a pebble-like shape. (A, Courtesy Dr. R. Howell, Morgantown, WV.)

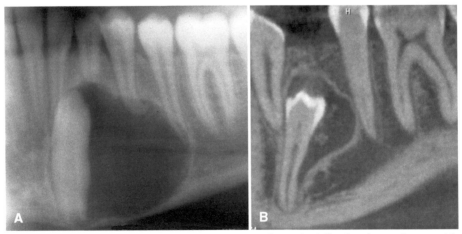

Fig. 24.25 Cropped panoramic image (A) shows no apparent internal calcifications in an adenomatoid odontogenic tumor. Cone beam computed tomographic image (B) of an adenomatoid odontogenic tumor related to the first premolar. Note the pebble-like calcifications distal to the premolar. (Courtesy Dr. M. Madhavji, Toronto, ON.)

Differential Interpretation

When this tumor is completely radiolucent and has a follicular relationship with an impacted tooth, differentiation from a dentigerous cyst or an odontogenic keratocyst may be difficult. If the relationship of the radiolucent entity is located more apical to the cementoenamel junction, a dentigerous cyst can be discounted; however, this would not exclude an odontogenic keratocyst. If there are radiopaque foci within the tumor, other lesions with calcifications might be entertained in the differential interpretation. The maxillary and mandibular anterior regions are also common sites for the calcifying odontogenic cyst, and it may be difficult to differentiate the extrafollicular type of AOT from a calcifying odontogenic cyst. Ameloblastic fibro-odontoma and CEOT may be considered; however, they may more commonly develop in the posterior mandible.

Management

Conservative surgical excision is adequate because the tumor is not locally invasive, is well encapsulated, and is easily separable from the bone. The recurrence rate is very low at approximately 0.2%.

MESENCHYMAL ODONTOGENIC TUMORS

Odontogenic Myxoma

Disease Mechanism

Myxomas resemble the mesenchymal portion of the dental papilla, which arises from odontogenic ectomesenchyme. They are so named for their loose, gelatinous, internal matrix of connective and mucoid tissues. Although nonodontogenic myxomas arise in the other areas of the skeleton, the presence of odontogenic epithelium that can be identified microscopically is the rationale behind its inclusion as an odontogenic tumor.

Clinical Features

Odontogenic myxomas are uncommon, accounting for only 3% to 6% of odontogenic tumors, and they have a slight female predilection. Although the lesion can occur at any age, more than half arise in individuals between 10 and 30 years; it rarely occurs before age 10 or after age 50. These tumors are slow growing, although they may be locally aggressive, particularly in the maxilla. Recurrence rates of 25% have been reported, and this high rate may be explained by the lack of encapsulation of the tumor, and the ability of the myxomatous matrix within the tumor to extend into marrow spaces, where it may be difficult to detect and remove surgically.

Imaging Features

Location. Myxomas are more commonly found in the mandible by a margin of 3:1. In the mandible, these tumors occur in the premolar and molar areas, and only rarely in the ramus and condyle. Myxomas in the maxilla usually involve the alveolar process in the premolar and molar regions, and the zygomatic process.

Periphery. The lesion usually is well defined, and it may have a corticated margin but most often is poorly defined, especially in the maxilla.

Internal structure. When it occurs in a pericoronal area, an odontogenic myxoma may appear cystlike and radiolucent internally. Residual bone trapped within the tumor may impart a multilocular appearance to the tumor, and characteristic features of these septa are straight, thin, and "etched" (Fig. 24.26). The sometimes linear appearance of septa in odontogenic myxomas have been described as having a tennis-racket-like or stepladder-like appearance, but this pattern is rarely seen. In reality, most septa are curved and coarse, but the finding of one or two straight septa often helps in the interpretation of this tumor (Fig. 24.27).

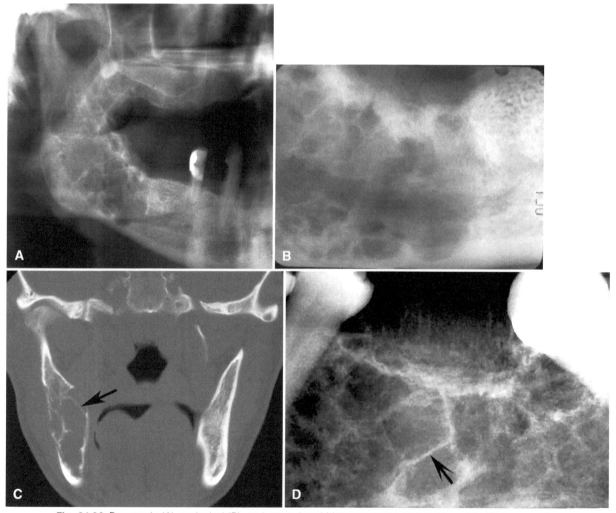

Fig. 24.26 Panoramic (A), periapical (B), and coronal multidetector computed tomographic (C) images of a large myxoma in the body and ramus of the right mandible. Notice the presence of a few straight septa, especially visible on the computed tomographic (CT) image *(arrow)*. The CT image also shows some, albeit modest expansion of the bone, considering the overall size of the tumor. A periapical image (D) of a different lesion shows one straight, sharp septum *(arrow)*.

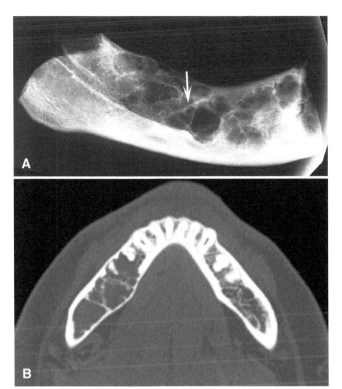

Fig. 24.27 Image of an excised surgical specimen (A) and the tumor, in situ (B), of an odontogenic myxoma. Note the sharp straight septum *(arrow)*.

Effects on adjacent structures. In the mandible, the odontogenic myxoma has a tendency to grow along the bone like an odontogenic keratocyst, without the same amount of expansion seen with other benign tumors; however, when they become very large, there may be considerable expansion.

Effects on adjacent teeth. When the odontogenic myxoma arises in a tooth-bearing area of the jaws, it displaces teeth and they may become mobile. Myxomas rarely cause resorption of tooth roots. The lesion also frequently scallops between the roots of adjacent teeth similar to a simple bone cyst.

Additional Imaging

MDCT imaging and, in particular, MRI can help in establishing the intraosseous involvement of the tumor, and guide the surgeon in planning the resection margins. The myxomatous matrix within the tumor produces a very characteristic high tissue signal on T2-weighted magnetic resonance (MR) images, and this is particularly useful in establishing both extension of the tumor in bone, and the presence of a recurrent tumor (Fig. 24.28).

Differential Interpretation

Because odontogenic myxomas most often have a multilocular internal pattern, the differential interpretation should include other multilocular lesions, such as ameloblastomas, odontogenic keratocysts, CGC lesions, and central hemangiomas. The finding of characteristic thin, straight septa with less than expected bone expansion is very useful in the differential interpretation. Occasionally, a small area of expansion with straight septa may be projected over an intact outer bony cortex and give a spiculated appearance. Careful inspection of this area of expansion, however, reveals a thin but intact outer cortex. An odontogenic fibroma occasionally has the same radiographic characteristics and cannot be reliably differentiated from a myxoma.

Management

Odontogenic myxomas are treated by resection with a generous amount of surrounding bone to ensure removal of the myxomatous material that may infiltrate the adjacent marrow spaces. With appropriate treatment, the prognosis is good.

Cementoblastoma

Disease Mechanism

Cementoblastomas are slow-growing, mesenchymal neoplasms of cementoblasts. The tumor manifests as a bulbous growth of cementum that develops around the root and root apex of a tooth.

Clinical Features

Cementoblastomas are uncommon, although likely, they occur more often than published accounts indicate. The lesion is more common in males than females, and in ages of reported patients range from 12 to 65 years, although most patients are younger.

The tumor most often develops in association with permanent teeth but in rare cases occurs with primary teeth. The tumor usually is a solitary lesion that is slow growing that may eventually displace teeth. The involved tooth pulp is vital, but pain is often reported that can be relieved by antiinflammatory drugs.

Imaging Features

Location. Cementoblastomas develop on the root surfaces of the mandibular dentition (78%), notably the premolar or first molar (90%).

Periphery. The lesion has a well-defined and corticated border.

Internal structure. Cementoblastomas are mixed radiolucent and radiopaque lesions in which most of the internal structure is radiopaque (Fig. 24.29). The resulting pattern may be amorphous, or a wheel-spoke pattern may be seen with the radiopaque structures emanating from the center of the mass. The density of the cemental mass usually obscures the outline of the enveloped root. This central radiopaque mass is surrounded by a radiolucent band indicating that the tumor is maturing from the center to the periphery.

Effects on adjacent structures. If large enough, this tumor can cause expansion of the bone, and in some cases there is a perforation through the outer cortical plate without periosteal reaction.

Effects on adjacent teeth. If the root outline is apparent, in most cases, varying amounts of external resorption of the root can be seen.

Differential Interpretation

The most common lesion to simulate a cementoblastoma is a solitary lesion of periapical cemento-osseous dysplasia. The differential interpretation may be difficult in some cases, and the presence or absence of symptoms or observation of the lesion over a period of time may be required. Generally, the radiolucent band around the cementoblastoma is usually better defined and uniform than with cemento-osseous dysplasia. Also, owing to the pattern of concentric growth of the cementoblastomas, the overall shape is more uniform and spherical than the more irregular undulating outline of the cemento-osseous dysplasia. Other lesions that may be included in the differential interpretation may include periapical sclerosing osteitis, dense bone island, and hypercementosis. However, sclerosing osteitis and dense bone islands do not have a radiolucent internal periphery. Although a periodontal ligament space may be seen surrounding a region of hypercementosis, the width of the ligament space is usually thinner than the internal radiolucent rim of the cementoblastoma, and there is no root resorption or jaw expansion with hypercementosis.

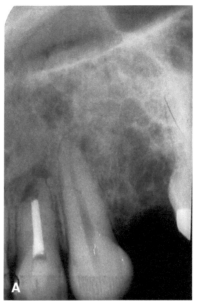

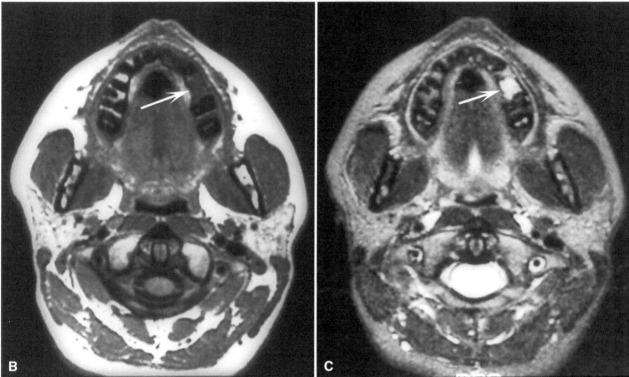

Fig. 24.28 Periapical image (A) obtained to investigate a possible recurrence of an odontogenic myxoma in the maxillary left premolar area after treatment by surgical curettage. (B) Axial T1-weighted magnetic resonance image shows a low *(black)* signal from the segment of the alveolar process (C) while the T2-weighted image shows a high *(white)* signal, which is characteristic of an odontogenic myxoma, confirming the presence of a recurrence.

Management

Cementoblastomas are managed with endodontic treatment and root amputation. In very large cases, excision and extraction of the associated tooth may be necessary.

Central Odontogenic Fibroma
Disease Mechanism

Central odontogenic fibromas are rare neoplasms that resemble the odontogenic myxoma. Indeed, some authors theorize that these entities represent two processes along a spectrum of connective tissue-type tumors. Two types of central odontogenic fibromas have been described

according to histopathologic appearances: the simple type, which contains mature fibrous connective tissue with sparsely scattered odontogenic epithelial rests, and the WHO type, which is more cellular, has more epithelial rests and may contain dysplastic mineralization.

Clinical Features

Most cases of central odontogenic fibromas occur between the ages of 11 and 39 years, and there is a definite female preponderance with a reported ratio of 2.2:1. An unusual, but rather distinctive feature of some maxillary cases is a cleft or depression in the palatal mucosa where expansion by the tumor would be expected (Fig. 24.30A).

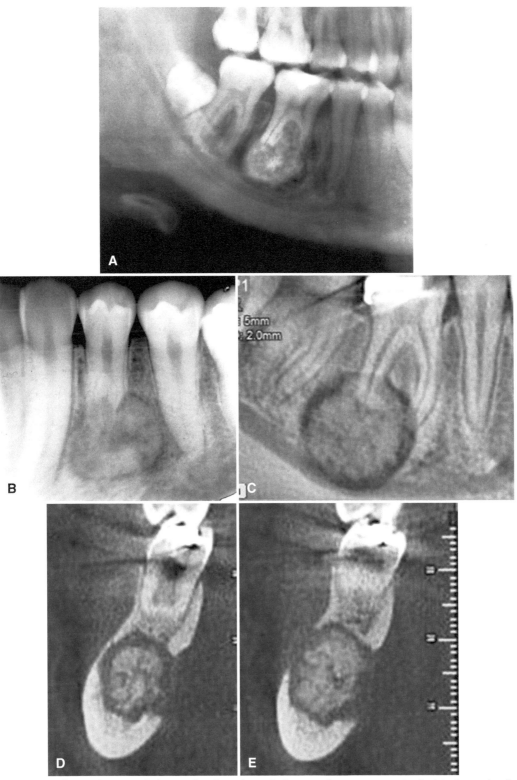

Fig. 24.29 Cropped panoramic image showing a large, bulbous, radiopaque mass attached to the roots of the mandibular right first molar (A). A radiolucent rim can be seen surrounding the mass, and root resorption of the molar roots has occurred. Periapical image of a lesion associated with a premolar (B). Cropped panoramic (C) and buccal lingual cross-sectional cone beam computed tomographic images of a cementoblastoma related to the roots of a mandibular first molar (D and E). There is perforation of the buccal and lingual cortical plates without evidence of periosteal bone formation. (A and B, Courtesy Dr. B. Pynn, Toronto, ON. C-E, Courtesy Dr. M. Amintavakoli, Tehran, Iran.)

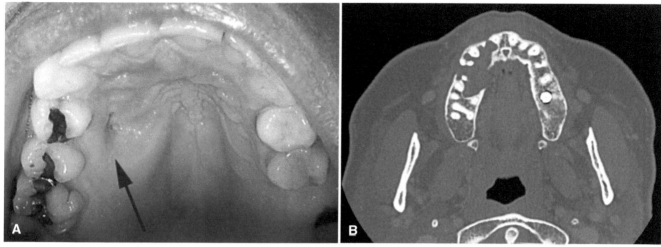

Fig. 24.30 Clinical photograph (A) of an odontogenic fibroma of the maxilla demonstrating a cleft *(arrow)* in the palatal mucosa. Axial computed tomographic image (B) of the same case showing loss of both the buccal and the palatal cortical plates without extension into the surrounding tissues and resorption of bone around the roots of the maxillary teeth with displacement or root resorption.

Imaging Features

Location.   Central odontogenic fibromas occur slightly more often in the mandible. The most common site is the molar-premolar region in the mandible and anterior to the first molar in the maxilla.

Periphery.   The periphery usually is well defined, and there may be a corticated border.

Internal structure.   Smaller lesions usually are unilocular, and larger lesions have a multilocular pattern. The internal septa may be fine and straight, as in odontogenic myxomas, or may be granular, resembling the internal structure seen in giant cell lesions. Some lesions are totally radiolucent, whereas unorganized internal calcification has been reported in others.

Effects on adjacent structures.   A central odontogenic fibroma may cause expansion with maintenance of a thin cortical boundary, or occasionally can grow along the bone with minimum expansion similar to an odontogenic keratocyst or myxoma.

Effects on adjacent teeth.   Tooth displacement is common, and root resorption has been reported. Some maxillary lesions have a distinctive behavior of resorbing the bone around teeth without tooth displacement or resorption (see Fig. 24.30B).

Differential Interpretation

The histopathologic features may resemble those of a central desmoplastic fibroma if no epithelial rests are apparent. Desmoplastic fibromas, however, are more aggressive and tend to break through the peripheral cortex and invade surrounding soft tissue. The septa in desmoplastic fibroma are very thick, straight, and angular. If thin, straight septa are present in the odontogenic fibroma, it may be impossible to differentiate this neoplasm from an odontogenic myxoma on radiographic criteria alone. If granular septa are present, the appearance may be identical to a giant cell lesion.

Management

Central odontogenic fibromas are treated with simple excision. These lesions have a very low recurrence rate.

NONODONTOGENIC TUMORS AND NEOPLASMS

Neuroma

Disease Mechanism

Despite its name, a neuroma is not a neoplasm. Rather, it is a reactive, but abnormal proliferation of scar tissue following trauma of a peripheral nerve. This trauma may be the result of mechanical or chemical injury caused by bone fracture, surgery, biopsy or excision of a cyst or tumor, extrusion of endodontic material, dental implant placement, or tooth extraction. Consequently, neuromas have also been referred to as traumatic or amputation neuromas. The proliferating nerve cells form a disorganized network of nerve fibers composed of varying proportions of axons, perineural connective tissue, Schwann cells, and scar tissue.

Clinical Features

Neuromas are slow-growing, reactive hyperplasias that seldom become large; they rarely exceed 1 cm in diameter. They may cause various symptoms, including severe pain resulting from pressure applied as the tangled mass enlarges within the bone, or as the result of external trauma. The patient may also develop a neuralgia, with pain referred to the eyes, face, and head.

Imaging Features

The imaging features of a neuroma relate to the extent and shape of the proliferating mass of neural tissue within the bone.

Location.   The most common location is the mental foramen, followed by the anterior maxilla and the posterior mandible.

Periphery.   Neuromas usually have well-defined, corticated borders. They may occur in various shapes, depending on the amount of resistance to expansion offered by the surrounding bone. In the mandible, the tumor usually forms in the mandibular canal, and therefore its periphery takes on the cortication of the canal's borders.

Internal structure.   The internal structure is totally radiolucent.

Effects on adjacent structures.   Fusiform expansion of the inferior alveolar nerve canal may occur.

Effects on adjacent teeth.   There are no effects on the teeth.

Differential Interpretation

It is impossible to differentiate this lesion from other benign neural tumors including schwannomas and neurofibromas.

Management

Treatment is recommended because neuromas tend to continue to enlarge, and they may also cause pain. Regardless of the type of injury that precipitates development of the neuroma, recurrence is uncommon after simple excision.

Neurofibroma

Disease Mechanism

Neurofibromas are caused by proliferations of Schwann cells in a disorderly pattern that includes portions of nerve fibers, such as peripheral nerves axon, and connective tissue of the sheath of Schwann. As neurofibromas grow, they may incorporate axons. In contrast, a Schwannoma is composed entirely of Schwann cells, and grows by displacing axons.

Clinical Features

The intraosseous neurofibroma may be the same lesion as those that develop in neurofibromatosis or von Recklinghausen disease. Although intraosseous lesions may also occur in von Recklinghausen disease, they are more rare. Neurofibromas can occur at any age but usually are found in young patients. Neurofibromas associated with the mandibular nerve may produce pain or paresthesia, and they may expand and perforate the bone cortex, causing swelling that is firm or hard to palpation.

Imaging Features

Location. Intraosseous neurofibromas may occur within the inferior alveolar canal, the cancellous bone, and underlying the periosteum.

Periphery. As with neurilemomas, the margins of the radiolucency in neurofibromas are usually very well defined and may be corticated. However, despite the slow growth rate of the neurofibroma, some lesions may have indistinct margins.

Internal structure. The tumors usually appear unilocular but occasionally may have a multilocular appearance.

Effects on adjacent structures. A neurofibroma of the inferior alveolar nerve shows a fusiform enlargement of the canal (Fig. 24.31).

Effects on adjacent teeth. There are no effects on the teeth.

Differential Interpretation

Differentiation from other types of neural lesions may be impossible. This tumor can be differentiated from vascular lesions because the expansion of the canal is both focal and fusiform shape, whereas vascular lesions enlarge the whole canal and alter its path.

Management

Solitary intraosseous neurofibromas that have been excised seldom recur. However, it is wise to reexamine the area periodically because these tumors are not encapsulated, and some undergo malignant change.

Schwannoma

Disease Mechanism

The schwannoma or neurilemoma is a tumor of neuroectodermal origin, arising from Schwann cells that produce the myelin sheath surrounding the axons of peripheral nerves. The exact cause is unknown.

Clinical Features

Schwannomas grow slowly, can occur at any age (but most commonly arise in the second and third decades), and occur with equal frequency in males and females. The mandible and sacrum are the most common sites. These lesions cause few symptoms other than those related to the location and size of the tumor. The usual chief complaint is an unexplained swelling. Although pain is uncommon unless the tumor encroaches on adjacent nerves, paresthesia may arise, especially with lesions originating in the inferior alveolar canal. Pain, when present, usually develops at the site of the tumor. If paresthesia occurs, it is felt distal (i.e., more peripheral) to the tumor.

Imaging Features

Location. Schwannomas most often involve the mandible, with less than 1 in 10 cases occurring in the maxilla. The tumor most often is located within an expanded inferior alveolar nerve canal between the mandibular foramen and the mental foramen (Fig. 24.32).

Periphery. In keeping with the slow growth rate, the borders of these tumors are well defined, and cortical walls of the inferior alveolar canal encompass the lesion. Small lesions may appear cystlike, but more commonly the shape of the tumor expands the canal in a more fusiform manner.

Internal structure. The internal structure is uniformly radiolucent. When lesions have a scalloping outline, this may give a false impression of a multilocular pattern.

Effects on surrounding structures. If the tumor reaches either the mandibular foramen or the mental foramen, it can cause enlargement of these foramina. Expansion of the inferior alveolar canal is slow, and the outer cortex of the canal is maintained and the expansion of the canal is usually localized with a definite epicenter unless the lesion is large.

Effects on surrounding structures. If the tumor becomes large, it may extend superiorly to involve the tooth-bearing areas of the jaws and cause root resorption of adjacent teeth (Fig. 24.33).

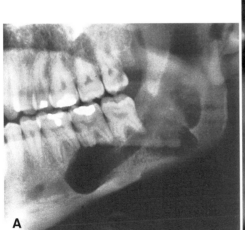
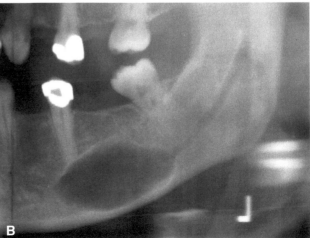

Fig. 24.31 Neurofibroma. (A) Portion of a panoramic radiograph shows a neurofibroma forming in the mandibular body along the path of the mandibular canal. (B) Cropped panoramic image of a neurofibroma within the body of the left mandible. Note the fusiform shape as the tumor expands the canal.

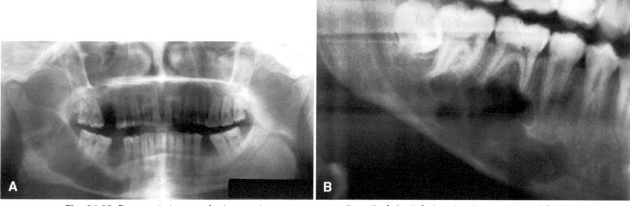

Fig. 24.32 Panoramic image of a large schwannoma expanding all of the inferior alveolar nerve canal from the mandibular to the mental foramen (A). Cropped panoramic image of a smaller tumor (B).

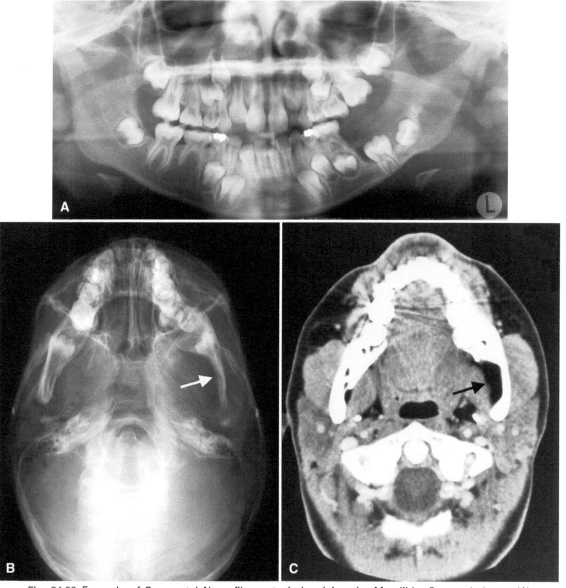

Fig. 24.33 Example of Segmental Neurofibromatosis Involving the Mandible. Panoramic image (A) demonstrates enlargement of the left coronoid notch, enlargement of the mandibular foramen, and interference of the eruption of the first and second molars. Basal skull view (B) of the same case reveals thinning and bowing of the ramus in a lateral direction *(arrow)*. The axial multidetector soft tissue window computed tomographic image (C) shows fat to be located adjacent to the abnormal mandibular ramus *(arrow)*.

Differential Interpretation

Because schwannomas most commonly originate within the inferior alveolar canal, vascular lesions, such as hemangioma or arteriovenous (A-V) malformations, should also be considered. Schwannomas have, however, a distinct epicenter within the canal, whereas vascular lesions usually cause a more uniform widening of the entire length of the canal without an obvious epicenter. Furthermore, vascular lesions may alter the course of the canal, and it may take on a serpiginous appearance. Only neural tumors and vascular lesions originate within the inferior alveolar canal, but malignant lesions may develop within the canal as a consequence of perineural spread. With a malignant lesion, the canal is often irregularly widened, and there is destruction of the canal cortex.

Management

Excision is usually the treatment of choice. These lesions generally do not recur if completely removed. A soft tissue capsule usually is present, facilitating surgical removal, although occasionally preservation of the nerve may not be possible. However, periodic examination is indicated to check for recurrence.

Neurofibromatosis
Disease Mechanism

Neurofibromatosis is one of the phakomatoses; a group of multisystem diseases that may involve the central nervous system, the eyes, and the skin. Three disease processes have been defined: neurofibromatosis type 1 (NF1), neurofibromatosis type 2 (NF2), and schwannomatosis. The *NF1* gene encodes a protein called neurofibromin which behaves as a tumor suppressor protein, and is produced by Schwann cells in the periphery and oligodendrocytes centrally. Mutations in *NF1* result in uncontrolled proliferation of Schwann cells and/or fibroblasts along peripheral nerves. In contrast, *NF2* encodes a protein called merlin or schwannomin, which also has tumor-suppressor qualities, and controls cell shape, growth, and adhesion. Mutations of *NF2* result in unmediated control of cell cycle progression, enhancing cell division and proliferation. Little is known currently of schwannomatosis; however, mutations of two genes have been identified, *SMARCB1* and *LZTR1*, both of which function as tumor growth suppressor genes.

Clinical Features

Neurofibromatosis type 1 or von Recklinghausen disease is the form of neurofibromatosis that can commonly involve the oral and maxillofacial region. Furthermore, it is one of the most common genetic diseases, affecting approximately 1 : 3000 births. The most common manifestations are the development of cutaneous and subcutaneous neurofibromas, and larger plexiform neurofibromas. Skin pigmentation called café au lait spots can also be identified, with the spots becoming larger and more numerous with age; most patients eventually have more than six spots larger than 1.5 cm in diameter. The expression of NF1 may also include dysplasias of the bones of the head and neck, including the ramus of the mandible and the greater and lesser wings of the sphenoid bone.

Imaging Features

The morphologic changes in the jaws with NF1 can be characteristic. These changes include the following alterations in the shape of the mandible: enlargement of the coronoid notch in the horizontal and/or the vertical dimensions, the development of an obtuse angle between the body and the ramus, lengthening and deformity of the condylar head, and lateral bowing and thinning of the mandibular ramus (see Fig. 24.33A). Changes in mandibular morphology can continue to increase in severity through the second decade. Other radiographic changes include enlargement of the mental and mandibular foramina, the inferior alveolar canal, and an increased incidence of branched canal branching. Erosive changes to the outer contour of the mandible and interference with normal eruption of the molars also may occur. Dysplasia of the sphenoid wing can result in an increase in the medial/lateral width of the superior orbital fissure and the appearance on occipto-mental (Water) view as an "empty orbit." Abnormal accumulations of fatty tissue within deformities of the mandible and sphenoid bone have been observed in images produced by MDCT imaging (see Fig. 24.33C).

Management

Most patients live a normal life with none or few symptoms. Small cutaneous and subcutaneous neurofibromas can be removed if they are painful, but large plexiform neurofibromas should be left alone. Malignant conversion of these lesions has occurred in rare cases.

MESENCHYMAL TUMORS AND NEOPLASMS

Dense Bone Island
Disease Mechanism

Dense bone islands, otherwise known as enostosis or idiopathic osteosclerosis, are the "internal counterparts" of exostoses; they represent localized hamartomatous growths of cortical bone into the cancellous bone space.

Clinical Features

DBIs are asymptomatic.

Imaging Features

Location. DBIs are more common in the mandible than in the maxilla. They occur most often in the premolar and molar areas (Fig. 24.34A), although their presence does not correlate with the presence or absence of teeth.

Periphery. DBIs directly abut adjacent normal bone. The periphery is usually well defined, and occasionally, the periphery blends with the trabeculae of the surrounding bone.

Internal structure. The internal pattern of DBIs can vary from a ground glass-like pattern to one that is uniformly radiopaque (see Fig. 24.34B). In some cases, heterogeneous radiolucent areas may be visualized, depending on the thickness of the DBI.

Effects on adjacent structures. There are no effects on adjacent structures.

Effects on adjacent teeth. A DBI located periapical to a tooth root can induce external root resorption (see Fig. 24.34C). The tooth most often involved is the mandibular first molar. In all circumstances, the tooth pulp is vital, and the root resorption appears to be self-limiting. A visible periodontal ligament space may be visible between the resorbed tooth root and the DBI. In very rare cases, DBIs can inhibit the eruption of a tooth and even displace a tooth.

Differential Interpretation

Several radiopaque entities must be considered in forming a differential interpretation. When a DBI is located at a root apex, it may resemble periapical sclerosing osteitis. However, in sclerosing osteitis, there is an associated widening of the periapical periodontal ligament space. As well, sclerosing osteitis should have an epicenter just apical to the root apex of the tooth. Finally, periapical inflammatory disease may have an apparent etiology, such as a large restoration or carious lesion.

Dense bone islands may also have similarities to periapical cemento-osseous dysplasia, or hypercementosis or cementoblastoma. In these cases, there should be a radiolucent periphery between the radiopaque center of these lesions and the adjacent normal bone.

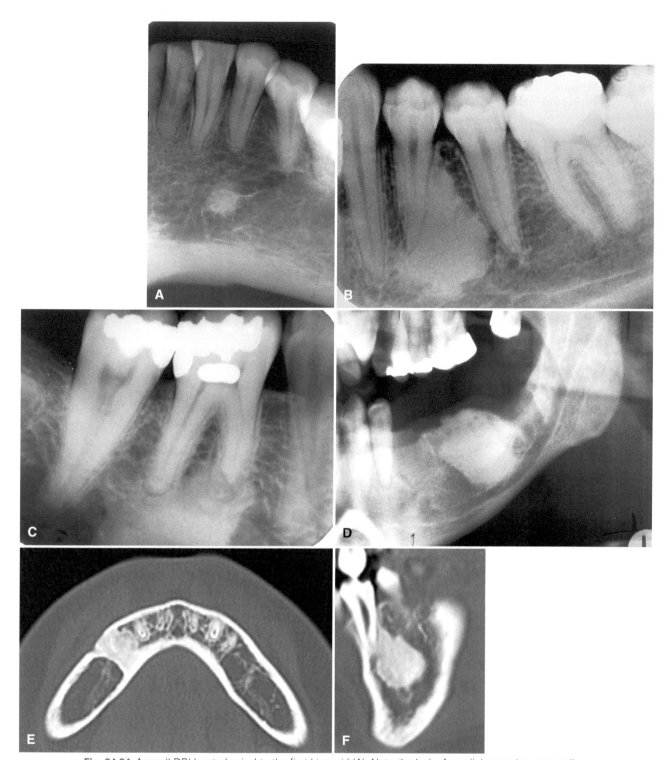

Fig. 24.34 A small DBI located apical to the first bicuspid (A). Note the lack of a radiolucent rim surrounding the DBI. Also, some of the surrounding trabeculae appear to merge into the radiopacity. A larger DBI between the premolar teeth (B). Note the normal-appearing periodontal ligament spaces and the continuity with the lamina dura. DBI located apical to a mandibular first molar (C) causing external root resorption. Large DBI occupying the body of the left mandible (D). Axial (E) and sagittal (F) cone beam computed tomographic images of DBI. Note the sharp margin that abuts and blends into the surrounding bone.

DBIs are often static in size, but they may increase in size, especially when there is active growth of the jaws. If five or more DBIs are present, adenomatous polyposis coli should be considered.

Management

DBI does not require treatment. If multiple DBIs are present, the patient's family history should be reviewed for the presence of colonic polyps.

Hyperostosis
Disease Mechanism

Hyperostoses and exostoses are exophytic, hamartomatous masses of mostly cortical bone, arising from the bone surface. Occasionally, hyperostoses may incorporate a small amount of internal cancellous bone. In the dental literature, the terms exostosis and hyperostosis are used to refer to the same entity, but in the medical literature the term exostosis is often used to refer to an osteochondroma, a benign neoplasm of cartilage and bone.

Clinical Features

Hyperostoses develop most commonly on the buccal surfaces of the maxillary alveolar processes, usually in the canine or molar area (Fig. 24.35). They may also occur on the palatal surface or crest, and less commonly on the mandibular alveolar process, where they may develop under the pontic of a fixed partial denture. They are less common than palatal or mandibular tori; however like tori, hyperostoses may attain a large size, and may be solitary or multiple. Hyperostoses may be flat prominences on the bone surface, or they may be nodular or pedunculated. In all cases, hyperostoses are covered with normal mucosa, and are bony hard on palpation. Published studies suggest a male predominance and an increase in frequency with age.

Imaging Features

Location. The maxillary alveolar process is the most common location, and the image of hyperostoses is superimposed over the roots of the adjacent teeth.

Periphery. The periphery of a hyperostosis is usually well defined and smoothly contoured with a curved border (see Fig. 24.35). However, some may have poorly defined borders that blend into the surrounding normal bone.

Internal structure. The internal structure of a hyperostosis usually is homogeneous and radiopaque. Although large hyperostoses can have an internal cancellous bone pattern, they most often consist only of cortical bone.

Effects on adjacent structures. Hyperostoses are continuous with the bone surface. This continuity may be difficult to visualize on plain imaging as hyperostoses may be small.

Effects on adjacent teeth. Hyperostoses have no effects on the teeth.

Management

Hyperostoses do not require treatment.

Torus
Disease Mechanism

A torus is an idiopathic protuberance of bone that may occur in the midline of the hard palate (torus palatinus) or the lingual surface of the mandible (torus mandibularis). It has been hypothesized that genetic and environmental factors may be involved in the development of torus mandibularis, with masticatory forces being reported as an essential factor underlying formation. The high prevalence among the Inuit and other subarctic peoples who make extraordinary chewing demands on their teeth and jawbones seems to support this suggestion.

Clinical Features

The torus palatinus (Fig. 24.36) is the most common hyperostosis, and occurs in about 20% of the population. Tori occur less often on the lingual surface of the mandible, in approximately 8% of the population. Interestingly, various studies have shown marked differences between the sexes, and ethnic groups. For example, tori develop commonly in the Asian population, and about twice as often in women as in men. Furthermore, in women, the occurrence of torus mandibularis correlates with occurrences of torus palatinus, but this apparently is not the case in men. Although tori may be discovered at any age, it is rare in children. They usually develop in young adults before 30 years of age, and they may continue to enlarge slowly during a lifetime.

The number, size, and shape of tori can vary broadly. In the hard palate, the base of the bony mass extends along the roof of the hard palate, and the bulk extends downward into the oral cavity. These lesions have been described as being flat, lobulated, nodular, or mushroom-like. In the mandible, single or multiple tori can develop, and they can be unilateral or bilateral, most often developing in the premolar region (see Fig. 24.37). Mandibular tori can also vary in size, ranging from an outgrowth that is barely palpable to one that contacts a torus on the opposite side. In contrast to palatal tori, mandibular tori develops later, in middle-aged adults. Normal mucosa covers the bony mass, and the mucosa may be thin and appear pale. Consequently, if traumatized, the mucosa may easily ulcerate. Patients often are unaware of having tori, and sometimes, patients who do discover them may insist that they have arisen suddenly and have grown rapidly.

Imaging Features

Location. On maxillary periapical or panoramic images, a torus palatinus appears as a dense radiopaque structure superimposed over the crowns and/or roots of the maxillary premolar and molar dentition (Fig. 24.38). The recognition of mandibular tori relies on their appearance and location. Their presence bilaterally reinforces this impression, although they can occur unilaterally. On mandibular periapical images, a torus mandibularis appears as a radiopaque entity, usually superimposed on the roots of premolars and molars and occasionally over a canine or incisor (Fig. 24.39).

Periphery. The periphery of tori are well defined, and they will appear convex or as a lobulated outline (Fig. 24.40). Mandibular tori in particular can appear very sharply demarcated on intraoral images.

Internal structure. The internal aspect is homogeneously radiopaque.

Effects on adjacent structures. Tori are continuous with the bone surface from which they are arising. This continuity may be difficult to visualize in the maxilla unless they appear on CBCT or MDCT images. In the mandible, this continuity may be visualized on cross-sectional occlusal images.

Effects on adjacent teeth. Tori have no effects on the teeth.

Management

Tori do not usually require treatment, although removal may be necessary to accommodate a removable denture.

Osteoma
Disease Mechanism

The etiology of the slow-growing osteoma is obscure, and it is unclear whether osteomas are hamartomas or neoplasms. Consequently, the behavior and radiologic appearances overlap considerably with dense bone islands, hyperostoses, and tori. Osteomas develop from the periosteum and may occur either externally on a bone surface or within the paranasal sinuses from cartilage or embryonal periosteum.

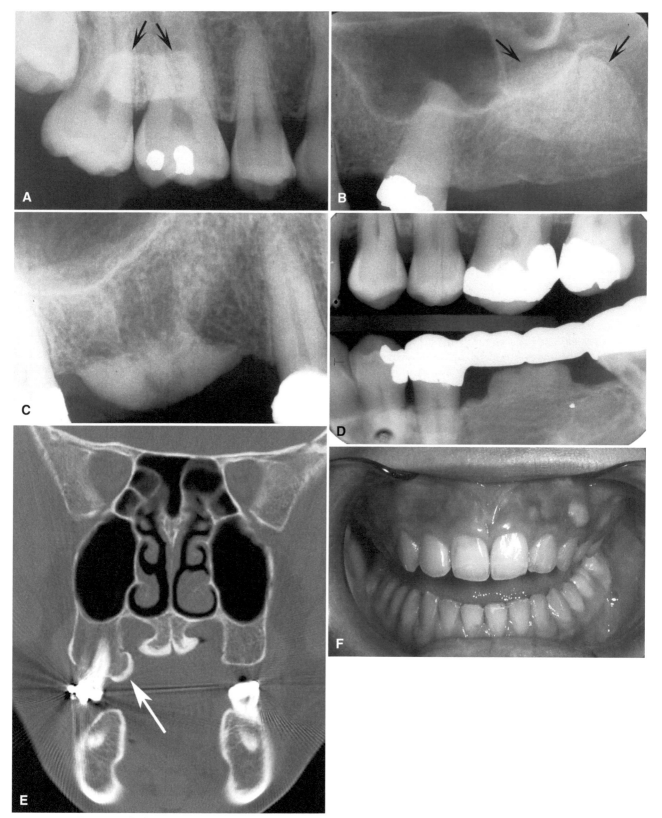

Fig. 24.35 Periapical image of a region of hyperostosis on the buccal surface of the maxillary alveolar process (A), seen as a region of radiopacity overlapping the roots of the molars *(arrows)*. Another example of hyperostosis superimposed over the edentulous posterior left maxilla (B). Periapical (C) and bite-wing (D) images of hyperostosis on the crest of the alveolar process and beneath a bridge pontic. Coronal cone beam computed tomographic image (E) of hyperostosis located on the palatal surface of the right maxillary alveolar process. Note the presence of a maxillary torus as well. Clinical photograph (F) of a small hyperostosis occurring on the labial surface of the maxillary alveolar ridge.

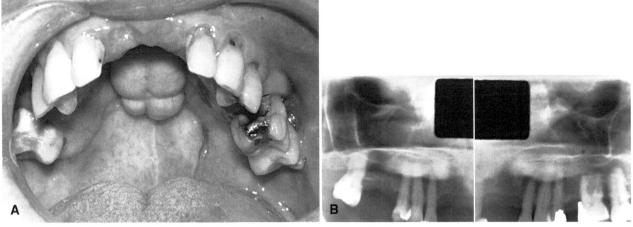

Fig. 24.36 Clinical photograph (A) of torus palatinus. Cropped panoramic image (B) shows the radiopaque image of torus palatinus superimposed over the root apices of the maxillary premolars and canine. (Courtesy Dr. R. Baker, Chapel Hill, NC.)

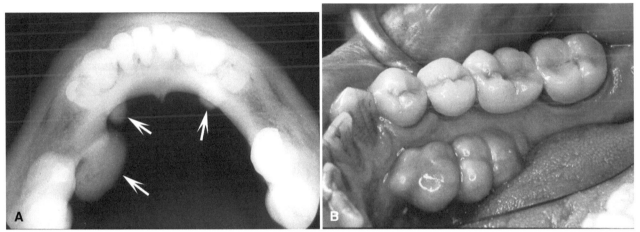

Fig. 24.37 Cross-sectional occlusal image (A) shows asymmetric mandibular tori *(arrows)*. Clinical photograph (B) of a different case. The tori extend from the region of the cuspid to the first molar. (B, Courtesy Dr. B. Friedland, Boston, MA.)

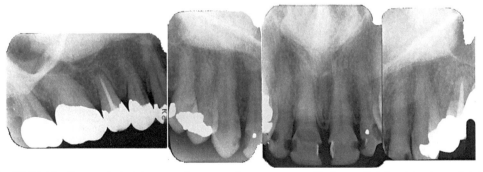

Fig. 24.38 Maxillary periapical images show a radiopaque area with the well-defined borders of torus palatinus.

Clinical Features

Osteomas can occur at any age but are most frequently found in individuals older than 40 years. Osteomas can develop as a solitary entity, or in multiples, occurring on a single bone or on numerous bones. Although most osteomas are small, some may become large enough to impact anatomy or function in the oral and maxillofacial region. Osteomas that arise within the frontal sinus and ethmoid air cells may do so without any clinical signs or symptoms. If they become large enough, they can block the outflow of mucous secretions from these air spaces creating the conditions for the formation of a mucocele.

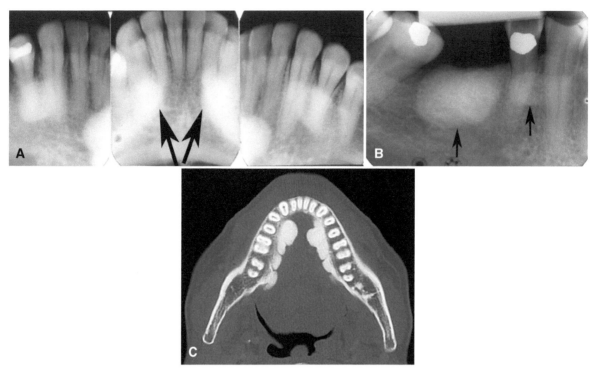

Fig. 24.39 Mandibular tori usually are seen as dense radiopacities on periapical images (A and B), superimposed over the tooth roots *(arrows)*. Axial computed tomographic image (C) with bilateral mandibular tori.

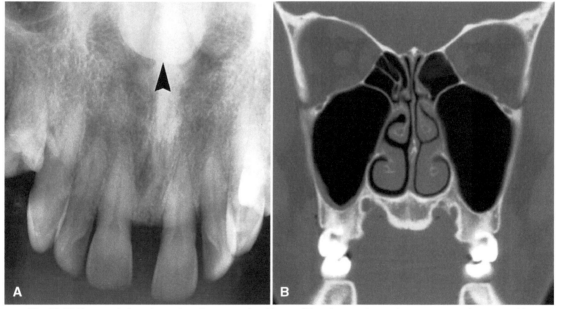

Fig. 22.40 Torus palatinus *(arrowhead)* on an occlusal image (A) and coronal cone beam computed tomographic image (B).

Osteomas originate from the periosteum and may occur either externally on a bone surface, or within the paranasal sinuses (Fig. 24.41). When osteomas develop on a bone surface, a patient may perceive a hard swelling. The swelling is painless until its size or position interferes with function. The osteomas are attached to the cortex of the jaw by a pedicle or along a wide base. Structurally, osteomas can be divided into three types: lesions composed of cortical bone (also called ivory osteomas); lesions composed of cancellous bone; and lesions composed of a combination of both.

Imaging Features

Location. The mandible is more commonly involved than the maxilla. This entity is found most frequently on the medial surface of the mandibular ramus or on the inferior border of the mandible in the molar area (Fig. 24.42). The mandibular lesions are exophytic, and may be either pedunculated or sessile, extending into adjacent soft tissues (Fig. 24.43). Osteomas also occur in the paranasal sinuses, especially the frontal sinus and ethmoid air cells.

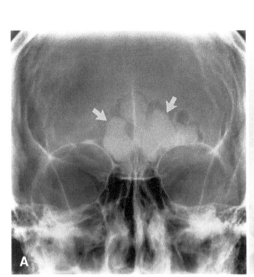
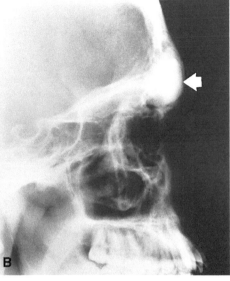

Fig. 24.41 A posterior-anterior skull (A) view shows an osteoma as a large, amorphous mass in the frontal sinus *(arrows)*. Lateral skull (B) view shows an osteoma occupying most of the space in the sinus *(arrow)*. (Courtesy Dr. G. Himadi, Chapel Hill, NC.)

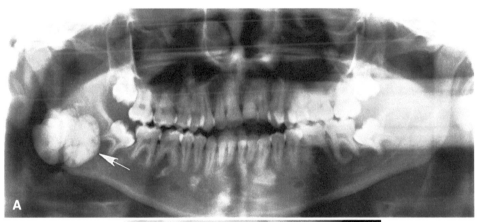
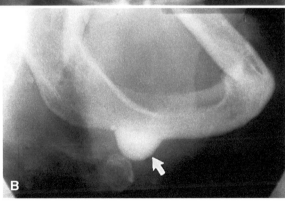

Fig. 24.42 Panoramic image shows an osteoma in the right mandibular angle region *(arrow)*. A lateral oblique image of the mandible (B) shows an osteoma as a sessile, exophytic, radiopaque mass attached to the inferior border of the mandible *(arrow)*. (A, From Matteson SR. *Dent Radiogr Photogr.* 1985;57(1–4):3–16, 53–59.)

Periphery. Osteomas have well-defined borders. Cortical osteomas lack a visible cortex while osteomas with a cancellous bone core may have a corticated periphery.

Internal structure. Osteomas composed solely of cortical bone are uniformly radiopaque, whereas osteomas containing cancellous bone show evidence of internal trabecular structure.

Effects on surrounding structures. Large lesions can displace adjacent soft tissues, such as the muscles of mastication, and cause jaw dysfunction. In some cases, there is a sclerotic bone reaction within the cancellous portion of the parent bone and adjacent to the base of the osteomas. The appearance of this sclerotic bone reaction is identical to a DBI.

Differential Interpretation

Usually the appearance of an osteoma is characteristic. A small osteoma may be similar in appearance to large hyperostosis or torus. Osteomas involving the condylar head can be difficult to differentiate from osteochondromas, osteophytes, or condylar hyperplasia. Furthermore, osteomas involving the coronoid process may be similar to osteochondromas.

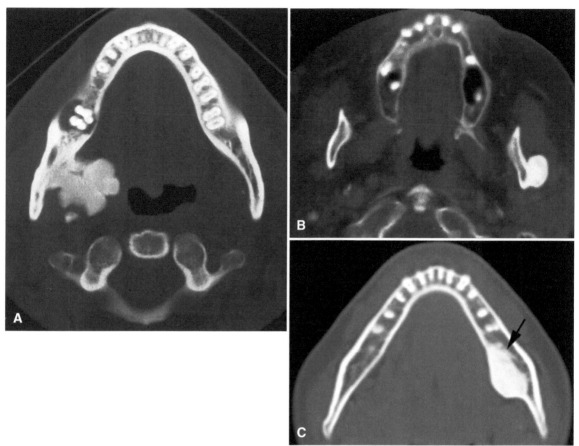

Fig. 24.43 Axial multidetector computed tomographic images of an osteoma on the medial surface of the mandibular ramus (A), the lateral side of the ramus (B), and on the lingual surface of the mandibular body (C) with the formation of adjacent dense bone within the mandible *(arrow)*.

Management

Unless the osteoma interferes with normal function or presents a cosmetic problem, this lesion may not require treatment. In such cases, the osteoma should be kept under observation. Resection of osteomas is possible, but may be difficult if the osteoma is of the cortical (ivory) type.

Familial Adenomatous Polyposis Syndrome
Disease Mechanism

Gardner syndrome is a subtype of familial adenomatous polyposis, a genetic disorder caused by a mutation of adenomatous polyposis coli *(APC)* gene. This mutation results in the development of multiple colonic polyps, and such patients are at a higher risk for developing colon cancers. These polyps can become malignant at an average age of 39 in the classic form, or at an average age of 59 years in the attenuated form.

Multiple osteomas are a feature of Gardner syndrome, as are multiple dense bone islands, epidermoid cysts, and subcutaneous desmoid tumors. The associated osteomas appear during the second decade, and are most common in the frontal and sphenoid bones, and the maxillae and mandible (Fig. 24.44). Because osteomas and DBIs often develop before intestinal polyps are identified, early recognition of the syndrome may be a lifesaving event. Occasionally, osteomas may not be present but the presence of five or more DBIs may indicate a familial multiple polyposis syndrome (Fig. 24.45). Also, dental abnormalities include an increased frequency of supernumerary and impacted teeth, and odontomas may also occur in Gardner syndrome.

Management

Generally, the removal of osteomas is unnecessary unless the tumors interfere with normal function or present a cosmetic concern. It is most important to recognize the relationship of multiple osteomas and multiple DBIs with familial adenomatous polyposis for early diagnosis. A family history of colorectal cancer may also help. These patients should be referred to their family physician for examination for intestinal polyposis and management.

Osteoblastoma
Disease Mechanism

An osteoblastoma is benign neoplasm of osteoblasts. These osteoblasts have the capacity to deposit osteoid and immature bone within the neoplasm.

Clinical Features

Osteoblastomas arise most commonly in the vertebrae of a young person with a male-to-female ratio of 2:1. The average age of occurrence is 17 years, with most lesions occurring in the second and third decades of life. Clinically, patients often report pain and swelling of the affected region.

Imaging Features

Location. Osteoblastomas are found in the tooth-bearing regions and the temporomandibular joint (within the condylar or the temporal bone components).

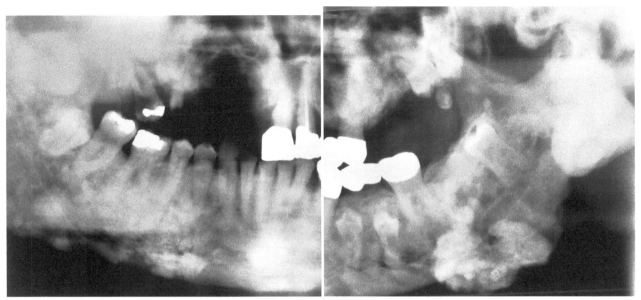

Fig. 24.44 Panoramic image shows several osteomas and DBIs throughout both jaws in a patient with Gardner syndrome. Note the impacted mandibular left second premolars.

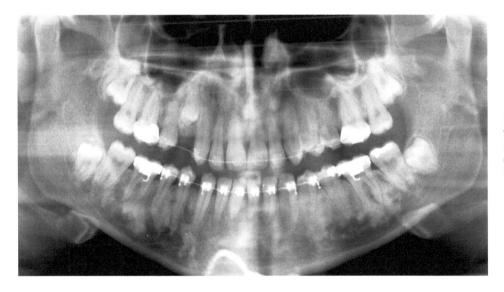

Fig. 24.45 Panoramic image of a patient with familial adenomatous polyposis syndrome. Note the multiple DBIs throughout the jaws; one has interfered with the eruption of the maxillary right first bicuspid.

Periphery. The periphery may be diffuse or may show evidence of a cortex. Lesions often have an internal radiolucent border surrounding the more central areas of abnormal bone deposition (Fig. 24.46).

Internal structure. The internal structure may be entirely radiolucent in early developing tumors, or there may be areas of varying central mineralization. The internal calcification may take the form of fine granular bone trabeculae.

Effects on adjacent structures. Osteoblastomas can expand bone, but usually a thin outer cortex is maintained. This lesion may invaginate the maxillary sinus or the middle cranial fossa.

Effects on adjacent teeth. If osteoblastomas develop in a tooth-bearing area within the jaws, there may be movement of teeth or external root resorption.

Differential Interpretation

Osteoblastomas and osteoid osteomas have very similar, if not identical appearances. Agreement is, however, increasing that osteoblastomas and osteoid osteomas are different lesions; they differ only in size, and in their morphologic histopathologic features. Osteoid osteomas are usually smaller and have an associated sclerotic bone reaction at the periphery.

An important differential interpretation may include osteosarcoma. This differentiation may rely on the benign features of the osteoblastoma as revealed in the diagnostic images. Osteoblastomas do not normally break through cortical boundaries or invade adjacent soft tissue. Sometimes the appearance of an osteoblastoma may be similar to a large area of cemento-osseous dysplasia. Both may have internal radiolucent peripheries that surround central radiopaque foci, but the osteoblastoma behaves more aggressively like a tumor.

Management

Osteoblastomas are treated with curettage or local excision and recurrences have been described.

Osteoid Osteoma
Disease Mechanism

The osteoid osteoma is a benign neoplasm of osteoblasts that bears a close resemblance to osteoblastoma. The core consists of osteoid and immature bone within highly vascularized, osteogenic connective tissue. The tumor usually develops within the outer bone cortex but may also form within the cancellous bone.

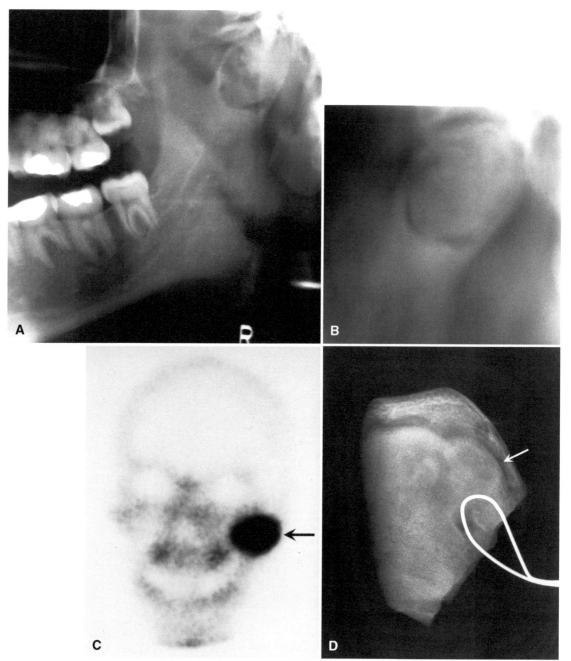

Fig. 24.46 Cropped panoramic image (A) of an osteoblastoma arising within the left mandibular condyle. Note the enlargement of the condyle and presence of the radiolucent rim that surrounds an internal structure of granular bone. Conventional tomograph (B) of the left condyle. ^{99m}Tc nuclear medicine image (C) demonstrates increased bone activity in the left condyle *(arrow)*. Image of the surgical specimen (D). Note the internal granular bone and the radiolucent rim *(arrow)*.

Clinical Features

Osteoid osteomas occur most often in young people, between the ages of 10 and 25 years with a 2:1 male-to-female predilection; they seldom occur before age 4 years or after age 40. Most of the lesions occur in the femur and tibia; the jaws are rarely involved. The osteoid osteoma has a small, oval or round, tumor-like core approximately 1 cm in diameter. Larger osteoid osteomas have been reported to reach approximately 5 or 6 cm. The osteoid trabeculae in an osteoid osteoma are generally smaller with more narrow trabecular spacing. In addition, the soft tissue over the involved bony area may be swollen and tender.

Osteoid osteomas produce severe bone pain that can be characteristically relieved with antiinflammatory drugs.

Imaging Features

Location. The lesion is most common in the cortex of the appendicular skeleton and spine. In the jaws osteoid osteomas are more common in the body of the mandible.

Periphery. The borders are well defined by a rim of sclerotic bone (Fig. 24.47).

Internal structure. The internal structure of young lesions is composed of a small round or ovoid radiolucent area. In more mature

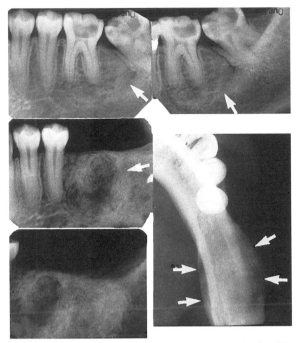

Fig. 24.47 Osteoid osteoma *(single arrow)* appears as a mixed radiolucent-radiopaque lesion in the molar region. The lesion has caused expansion of the buccal and lingual cortex of the mandible *(multiple arrows)*. (Courtesy Dr. A. Shawkat, Radcliff, KY.)

lesions, the appearance may have a mixed radiolucent and radiopaque appearance as abnormal bone is deposited.

Effects on adjacent structures. As previously mentioned, this tumor can stimulate a sclerotic bone reaction within the peripheral bone, and cause thickening of the cortex by stimulating periosteal new bone formation.

Differential Interpretation

The differential interpretation of osteoid osteoma, particularly because of the peripheral sclerotic bone reaction, should include sclerosing osteitis, ossifying fibroma, cementoblastoma, and cemento-osseous dysplasia. The presence of a central radiolucency usually eliminates dense bone island from the differential. Bone scintigraphy may assist in the interpretation by revealing considerable vascularity in the blood pool phase and a very high comparative bone metabolism.

Management

Spontaneous remission has been reported, although the data are insufficient for identifying such cases in advance. Complete excision currently is the recommended treatment because it often relieves the pain. A new, more conservative treatment involving radiofrequency thermoablation is obtaining success rates of 76% to 100%.

Cemento-Ossifying Fibroma
Disease Mechanism

This bone neoplasm consists of highly cellular, fibrous tissue that contains varying amounts of abnormal, immature bone and cementum-like tissue. Other internal regions of this tumor can have irregular trabeculae of woven or lamellar bone.

Clinical Features

The clinical behavior of ossifying fibroma can vary from indolent to aggressive. Cemento-ossifying fibroma can occur at any age but

usually is found in young adults. Females are more often affected than males. Juvenile ossifying fibroma is a very aggressive form of cemento-ossifying fibroma that occurs in the first two decades of life. Although the pathogenesis of this juvenile ossifying fibroma is controversial, the radiologic appearance has similarities to that of ossifying fibroma but may be much more expansile.

Cemento-ossifying fibroma is usually asymptomatic at the time of discovery. Occasionally, facial asymmetry develops. Displacement of the teeth may be an early clinical feature, although most lesions are discovered during routine dental examinations. In cases of juvenile ossifying fibroma, rapid growth may occur in a young patient, resulting in deformity of the involved jaw.

Imaging Features

Location. Cemento-ossifying fibroma appears almost exclusively in the facial bones and most commonly in the mandible where it arises apical to the premolars and molars, and superior to the inferior alveolar canal. In the maxilla, cemento-ossifying fibroma occurs most often in the canine fossa and in the region of the zygomatic process of the maxilla.

Periphery. The borders are usually well defined, and the cortex may appear thickened to the point of sclerosis.

Internal structure. The internal structure is mixed radiolucent and radiopaque with a pattern that depends on the amount and form of the manufactured bone. In some instances, the internal structure may appear almost totally radiolucent with just a hint of calcified material. In the type that contains mainly abnormal trabeculae of bone, the pattern may appear as being ground glass, similar fibrous dysplasia, or wispy (similar to stretched tufts of cotton), or flocculent (similar to large, heavy snowflakes) (Fig. 24.48). Lesions that produce more amorphous bone may contain solid, homogeneously radiopaque regions that do not have any intrinsic pattern (Fig. 24.49). A thin, radiolucent line, representing connective tissue, separates the more centrally occurring radiopaque area from the normal surrounding bone (see Fig. 24.49).

Effects on adjacent structures. Cemento-ossifying fibroma can be distinguished from bone dysplasias by its tumor-like behavior. Enlargement of the lesion is concentric within the medullary part of the bone, with outward growth approximately equal in all directions. This growth can result in displacement of the inferior alveolar canal and expansion of the adjacent bone cortices. A significant point is that the outer cortices, although displaced and thinned, remain intact. Cemento-ossifying fibroma that develops in the maxilla can cause significant displacement of the borders of the maxillary sinus and almost completely efface the sinus (Fig. 24.50). There is, however, a bony partition that separates the air-filled space with the tumor.

Effects on adjacent teeth. Cemento-ossifying fibroma can displace teeth. In addition, the lamina dura of involved teeth usually is missing, and resorption of teeth may occur.

Differential Interpretation

The differential interpretation of cemento-ossifying fibroma includes lesions with a mixed radiolucent and radiopaque internal structure. The differentiation from fibrous dysplasia can be very difficult. The boundaries of cemento-ossifying fibroma usually are better defined, and these lesions occasionally have a cortex with an adjacent internal radiolucent rim, whereas the periphery of fibrous dysplasia usually blends with surrounding bone. The internal structure of fibrous dysplasia lesions in the maxilla may be more homogeneous, and show less pattern variation. Both types of lesions can displace teeth, but cemento-ossifying fibroma displaces from a specific point or epicenter. Fibrous dysplasia rarely resorbs teeth.

The expansion of the jaws associated with cemento-ossifying fibroma is more concentric about a definite epicenter than fibrous

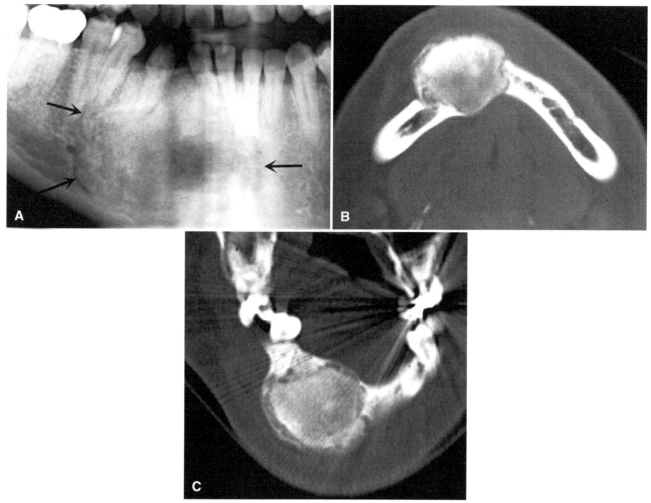

Fig. 24.48 Panoramic image *(arrows)* shows a cemento-ossifying fibroma (A). The expansile nature of the lesion is better depicted on axial (A) and (B) coronal multidetector computed tomographic images. Note the homogeneous, radiopaque internal structure of amorphous bone and the radiolucent band at the periphery.

dysplasia which enlarges the bone while distorting the overall shape to a smaller degree; in other words, the expanded bone still resembles normal morphology. In the maxilla, great difficulty may arise in differentiating cemento-ossifying fibroma from fibrous dysplasia when the lesion involves the maxillary antrum. Fibrous dysplasia usually displaces the lateral wall of the maxilla into the maxillary antrum; however, the pyramidal shape of the air cavity is maintained. The periphery of cemento-ossifying fibroma has a more convex shape, and therefore imparts a concavity to the floor of the air-filled antrum (see Fig. 24.50; also see Chapter 26). With respect to the teeth, fibrous dysplasia may alter the bone pattern around the teeth without displacing the teeth from an obvious epicenter of a concentrically growing benign tumor. The importance of this differentiation lies in the treatment, which is resection for an cemento-ossifying fibroma and observation for fibrous dysplasia.

The differential interpretation of the type of cemento-ossifying fibroma that produces a mainly homogeneous amorphous bone from periapical cemento-osseous dysplasia (PCOD) may be difficult, especially with large single lesions of PCOD. However, PCOD is often multifocal, whereas cemento-ossifying fibroma is not. Also, the presence of a simple bone cyst is a characteristic of either florid cemento-osseous dysplasia or PCOD but not cemento-ossifying fibroma. A wider sclerotic border is more characteristic of the slow-growing cemento-osseous dysplasia as well as a more undulating expansion.

Other lesions to be considered include those that have internal calcifications similar to the pattern seen in cemento-ossifying fibroma. These include giant cell lesions, calcifying odontogenic cysts, calcifying epithelial odontogenic (Pindborg) tumor, and adenomatoid odontogenic tumor.

Occasionally, the interpretation of osteogenic sarcoma is considered. However, characteristics suggesting a malignant lesion should be seen, such as cortical bone destruction and invasion into the surrounding soft tissues and along the periodontal ligament space.

Management

The prognosis of cemento-ossifying fibroma is favorable with surgical enucleation or resection. Large lesions require a detailed determination of the extent of the lesion, which can be obtained with MDCT or CBCT imaging. Even if the lesion has reached appreciable size, it usually can be separated from the surrounding tissue and completely removed. Recurrence after removal is unlikely.

Central Giant Cell Lesions
Disease Mechanism

There is debate as to whether CGC lesions are reactive or neoplastic lesions in origin. Despite the name, CGC lesions consist primarily of fibroblasts, with numerous vascular channels; giant cells are a minority of the cell population in these lesions. Because the behavior and imaging

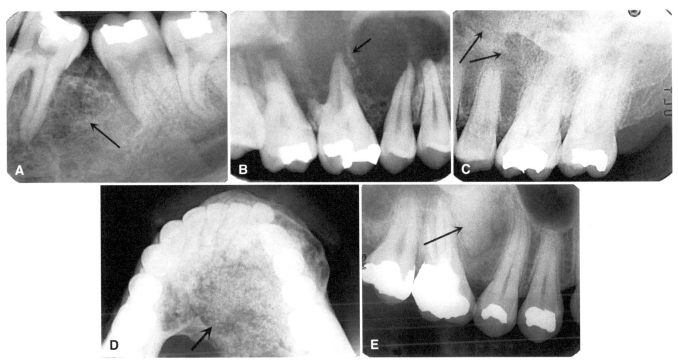

Fig. 24.49 Variations of the Bone Pattern Seen in Cemento-ossifying Fibroma. These may range from wispy trabecular patterns (A) *(arrow)* and (B), to a granular pattern *(arrows)* (C) reminiscent of fibrous dysplasia. Also, there may be a flocculent pattern with larger tufts of bone formation *(arrow)* (D) and a more solid, radiopaque pattern *(arrow)* (E).

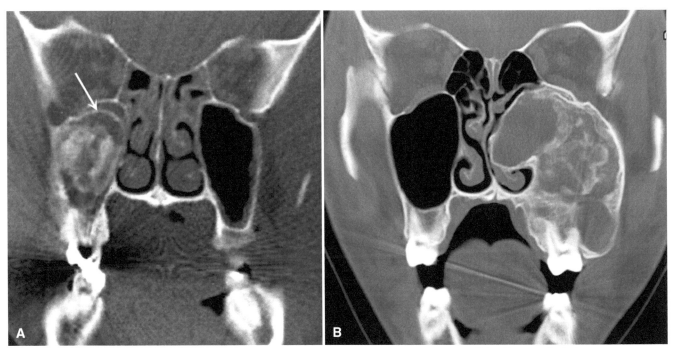

Fig. 24.50 Coronal multidetector computed tomographic images of large cemento-ossifying fibromas displacing the floor of the maxillary sinus. In contrast to fibrous dysplasia, the altered contour of the sinus cavity *(arrow)* does not parallel the original shape of the antrum (A). A larger lesion (B) expanding the maxilla, occupying all of the maxillary antrum, and extending into the nasal fossa.

characteristics of CGC lesions are similar in many respects to benign tumors, they are included in this chapter.

Clinical Features

CGC lesions affect mostly adolescents and young adults; at least 60% of cases occur in individuals younger than 20 years old. Many CGC lesions are asymptomatic; however when on the surface of the bone, the most common presenting sign is a swelling. Palpation of the area may elicit tenderness, and in some cases, the patient may complain of pain. Because of the highly vascular nature of these lesions, the overlying mucosa may have a purple color. The rate of lesion growth is variable with faster growing lesions creating the suspicion of a malignancy.

Imaging Features

Location. CGC lesions develop in the mandible twice as frequently as in the maxilla. Within the first two decades of life, there is a tendency for the epicenter of the lesion to be located mesial to the first molar in the mandible, and mesial to the canine in the maxilla. In older individuals, CGC lesions can occur with greater frequency in the posterior regions of the jaws.

Periphery. Slower growing lesions have a well-defined periphery, but in most cases, the periphery shows no evidence of a cortex. They may have more poorly defined borders, an appearance that may appear more aggressive, even malignant.

Internal structure. Some CGC lesions show no evidence of internal structure, and may be radiolucent (Fig. 24.51). This is especially true of small lesions. Other lesions have a subtle granular pattern of calcification that may require a change in image brightness to perceive, and occasionally, this granular bone pattern is organized into wispy striations or septa (Fig. 24.52). Unlike conventional septa, those seen in CGC lesions are manufactured by the cells within the lesion; they do not represent remnant normal bone. When present, these newly formed septa are characteristic of CGC lesions, especially if they emanate at right angles from the periphery of the lesion. This characteristic appearance is further brought to prominence if a small indentation of the expanded cortex is seen at the point where this right-angled septum

originates (Fig. 24.53). In some instances, the septa are better defined and divide the internal aspect into compartments, creating a multilocular appearance.

Effects on adjacent structures. CGC lesions have a strong propensity to expand bone borders and displace anatomic structures. The expansion usually is uneven or undulating in nature, which may give the appearance of a double boundary when the expansion is assessed using an occlusal image. The bone forming the border of the expanded mandible often has a more granular quality compared with cortical bone. In some instances, the bone cortex is destroyed and not expanded; this occurs more often in the maxilla, where the cortical bone destruction may give the lesion a malignant appearance. The inferior alveolar canal may be displaced in an inferior direction.

Effects on adjacent teeth. CGC lesions often displace and resorb tooth roots (see Fig. 24.53). Resorption of tooth roots is not, however, a consistent feature, but when it occurs, it may be profound and irregular in outline. The lamina dura of teeth within the lesion are usually lost.

Differential Interpretation

A small CGC lesion that is totally radiolucent may appear similar to a cyst, especially a simple bone cyst. Evidence of tooth displacement or root resorption of an adjacent tooth or expansion is more characteristic of neoplastic behavior.

If the internal structure of the CGC lesion contains radiopaque striations or septa, the differential interpretation may include odontogenic myxoma, aneurysmal bone cyst (ABC), and ameloblastoma. If the internal structure appears less striated, cemento-ossifying fibroma may be considered. Useful characteristics for differentiating an ameloblastoma may include the thickness and curvature of the septa compared to what is seen with CGC lesions; they tend to be more coarse, curved, and well defined, whereas CGC lesions are more delicate, wispy, straight, and poorly defined septa, some of which are oriented at a right angle to the periphery. Odontogenic myxomas occur in an older age group, may have sharper and straighter (true) septa, and do not have the same propensity to expand bone as CGC lesions. ABCs can appear identical to CGC lesions, radiologically, especially the appearance of the internal striations or septa. ABCs are, however, comparatively rare lesions that occur more often in the posterior aspect of the jaws, and usually cause profound expansion.

The radiologic appearance of a brown tumor of hyperparathyroidism are identical to a CGC lesion. Also, the appearance may also be identical to the bilateral lesions seen in cherubism. However, the lesions in cherubism are multiple and have epicenters that are located in the posterior maxilla, and mandibular body and ramus.

Management

MDCT may be useful to identify the presence of internal structures, particularly, the radiopaque striations or septa within the lesion. In addition, advanced imaging may show the quality of these septa more clearly than plain imaging. MDCT imaging is required for large lesions to determine whether the lesion has extended through the cortex to involve the overlying soft tissue. Occasionally, CGC lesions can behave very aggressively. If a CGC lesion occurs after the second decade of life, hyperparathyroidism should be considered, and serum testing for elevated parathyroid hormone should be ordered.

Treatment may include intralesional delivery of corticosteroids and/ or calcitonin if the lesion is large, followed by enucleation and curettage. Some lesions are also resected. The patient should be followed carefully to rule out recurrence, especially if a more conservative management strategy is used. Although recurrences are rare, they tend to be more common in the maxilla.

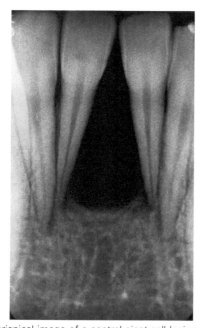

Fig. 24.51 Periapical image of a central giant cell lesion in the anterior mandible with no evidence of internal structure.

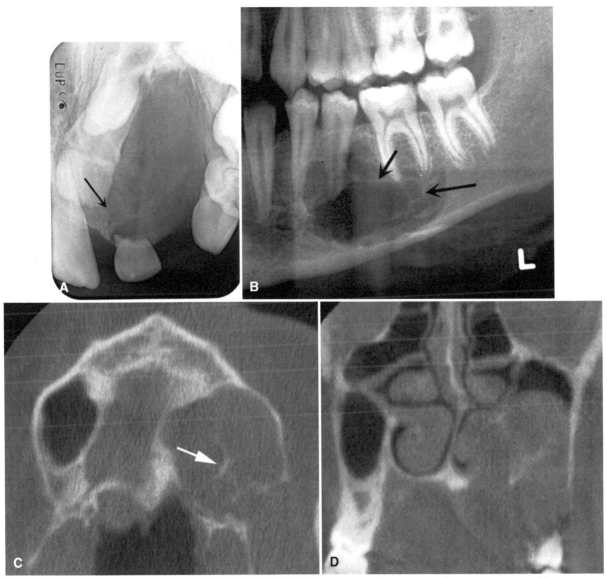

Fig. 24.52 Central giant cell lesions in the anterior maxilla may demonstrate a very fine, internal pattern (A). In the posterior mandible, the internal pattern may show wispy, ill-defined granular septa (B). Axial (C) and coronal (D) cone beam computed tomographic images of a central giant cell lesion of the maxilla. Note the poorly calcified, barely visible internal radiopacities *(arrow)*.

Cherubism

Disease Mechanism

Cherubism is a rare, inherited disease caused by a mutation of the *SH3BP2* gene located on the short arm of chromosome 4 in the 16.3 position. It is, however, likely that other mutations are also involved. The lesions that develop are identical histopathologically and radiologically to CGC lesions.

Clinical Features

Cherubism develops in early childhood, between the ages of 2 and 6 years. The most common presenting sign is a firm, painless, bilateral enlargement of the lower face. Enlargement of the submandibular lymph nodes may occur, but no systemic abnormalities are involved. In addition, the lesions may produce bilateral swelling of the cheeks due to the expansile nature of these lesions in the maxilla. Because children's faces are often chubby, mild cases may go undetected for some time. Profound

swelling of the maxilla may result in stretching of the skin of the cheeks, which depresses the lower eyelids, exposing a thin line of sclera and causing the appearance of upturned eyes, "raised to heaven." Cherubism is, however, a time-limited disease, and the lesions involute and heal without treatment around the time of skeletal maturity.

Imaging Features

Location. The lesions of cherubism are bilateral, and both jaws can be affected. When present in only one jaw, the mandible is the most common location. The epicenters of these lesions are always in the posterior body and ramus of the mandible, or in the tuberosity of the maxilla (Fig. 24.54). The lesions grow concentrically, and in severe cases can extend to the midline.

Periphery. The periphery is well defined, and corticated.

Internal structure. The internal appearance is very similar to the appearance within CGC lesions. That is, there may be fine, granular

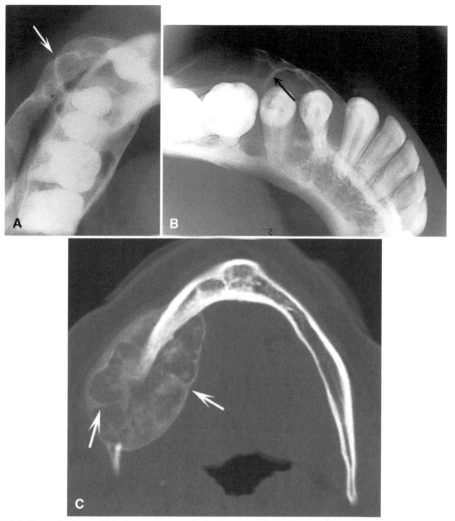

Fig. 24.53 Central giant cell lesions characteristically expand the bone, although the expansion may be uneven (A). Surface indentations with right-angled septa (B) may be useful features to identify. Axial multidetector computed tomographic image (C) shows a central giant cell lesion causing undulating expansion and containing two right-angled septa.

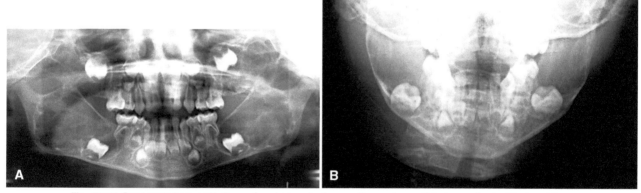

Fig. 24.54 Panoramic image (A) shows four lesions in the maxillae and mandible in a patient with cherubism. The epicenters of the lesions are in the maxillary tuberosity and mandibular ramus. Note the mesial displacement of the unerupted maxillary first molars. Internally, the mandibular lesions contain ill-defined septa. A posterior-anterior view of the mandible (B) shows the expanded mandible.

bone oriented in wispy striations, imparting a multilocular pattern to the lesions.

Effects on adjacent structures. Expansion of the surfaces of the maxilla and mandible by cherubism can result in severe enlargement of the jaws. Maxillary lesions can displace the maxillary sinus floors, and in the mandible, there may be substantial displacement of the medial and lateral surfaces of the ramus. Of particular concern is that extensive medial displacement of the soft tissues can compromise the airway.

Effects on adjacent teeth. Because the epicenters of these lesions are in the posterior mandible and maxilla, the teeth are displaced toward the midline. The degree of displacement can be severe, and developing tooth buds may be aggressively disrupted with some lesions.

Differential Interpretation

Although the radiologic appearance of cherubism are similar to CGC lesions, the fact that cherubism is bilateral with an epicenter in the posterior mandible and maxilla should provide a clear differentiation. The differentiation of cherubism from fibrous dysplasia should not present any difficulties because fibrous dysplasia is more commonly a unilateral disease. Also, the sometimes multilocular appearance of cherubism, and the aggressive displacement of teeth and disruption of tooth follicles are more characteristic of cherubism. Cherubism may also have some similarities to odontogenic keratocysts in nevoid basal cell carcinoma syndrome. The bilateral symmetry of cherubism, anterior displacement of teeth, and multilocular appearance are characteristics that help with the differential interpretation.

Management

The distinctive radiologic features of cherubism may be more diagnostic than the histopathologic findings; therefore the diagnosis can rely on the radiologic findings alone. Treatment can be delayed because the lesions may cease their growth, and infill with granular bone during adolescence and at skeletal maturity. After skeletal growth has stopped, conservative surgical procedures, if required, may be done for cosmetic problems. Surgery also may be required to uncover displaced teeth, and orthodontic treatment may be needed.

Aneurysmal Bone Cyst
Disease Mechanism

The ABC has been considered to be a reactive lesion of bone, although recently, a number of chromosomal translocations have been described that all lead to activation of the *USP6* gene on chromosome short arm of chromosome 17 at the 13 position, which gives some credence to a neoplastic etiology. As this lesion has both clinical and radiologic features that mimic an aggressive, benign neoplasm, we have included the ABC in this chapter. The ABC represents a proliferation of fibroblasts and small vessels; osteoclast-like cells; and reactive, poorly calcified woven bone.

Clinical Features

More than 90% of ABCs that arise within the jaws occur in individuals younger than 30 years old, and the condition appears to have a predilection for females. An ABC in the jaw usually manifests as a fairly rapid bony swelling. Pain is an occasional complaint, and the involved area may be tender on palpation. ABCs occasionally develop in association with other primary lesions, such as fibrous dysplasia, central hemangioma, CGC lesions, and osteosarcoma.

Imaging Features

Location. The mandible is involved more often than the maxilla by a ratio of 3:2. Furthermore, the molar and ramus regions are more often involved than the anterior regions of the jaws (Fig. 24.55).

Periphery. The periphery of ABCs is well defined, and it may be partially corticated, depending on the aggressiveness of its growth. The shape is usually circular or "hydraulic," resembling the classical shape of a cyst.

Internal structure. Small initial lesions may show no evidence of an internal structure. Larger lesions, however, develop internal areas of mineralization that bear a striking resemblance to CGC lesions. These wispy, sometimes granular-appearing striations or septa represent new bone formed by the lesion rather than residual bone, and may give the ABC a multilocular type of appearance (Figs. 24.55 and 24.56). Septa positioned at right angles to the outer expanded border are another similar finding. In MDCT soft tissue algorithm images, the low-attenuation or radiolucent areas may have a somewhat circular shape, and represent large vascular spaces within the lesion.

Effects on adjacent structures. When an ABC becomes large, there can be extreme expansion of the bone surface with displacement and thinning of the bone cortices (see Figs. 24.55 and 24.56). This characteristic is more dramatic in ABCs than in almost any other lesion.

Effects on adjacent teeth. ABCs can displace and resorb tooth roots.

Differential Interpretation

The radiologic appearance of the ABC and the CGC lesions may be identical. ABCs may expand the bone to a far greater degree, and they are more common in the posterior regions of the mandible than the anterior. ABCs may also show a similarity to the lesions in cherubism; however, cherubism is a multifocal, bilateral disease. Ameloblastoma may be considered, but generally, ameloblastomas occur in an older age group. The diagnosis is based on biopsy results. A hemorrhagic aspirate favors the diagnosis of ABC.

Management

MDCT or MRI are recommended to determine the extent of the lesion better, and to characterize the very vascular nature of these lesions. Surgical curettage and partial resection are the primary means of treatment. The recurrence rate ranges from 19% to about 50% after curettage, and approximately 11% after resection. Careful follow-up is needed.

Desmoplastic Fibroma
Disease Mechanism

A desmoplastic fibroma arising in bone is an aggressive, infiltrative neoplasm that produces abundant collagen fibers. The lack of pleomorphism of the fibroblast-like cells that may display ovoid or elongated nuclei is an important histopathologic feature.

Clinical Features

Patients usually complain of facial swelling, pain (in rare cases), and sometimes dysfunction, especially when the neoplasm is located close to the temporomandibular joint. The lesion occurs most often in the first two decades of life, with a mean reported age of 14 years. Although it originates in bone, the tumor may invade the surrounding soft tissue extensively. Desmoplastic fibroma may occur as part of Gardner syndrome.

Imaging Features

Location. Desmoplastic fibromas of bone may occur in the mandible or maxilla, but the most common site is the posterior mandible and ramus.

Periphery. The periphery most often is poorly defined, and has an invasive characteristic commonly seen in malignant tumors.

Internal structure. Internally, the desmoplastic fibroma may be totally radiolucent, especially when the lesion is small. Larger lesions appear

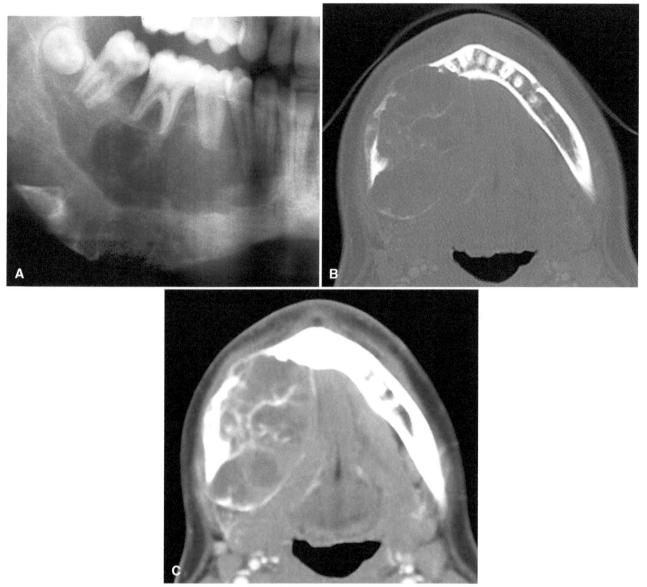

Fig. 24.55 Cropped panoramic image (A) of an aneurysmal bone cyst occupying the right mandibular body. Axial bone (B) and soft tissue (C) window multidetector computed tomographic images show the exuberant expansion of the bone, and faint, wispy septa within the lesion. Also note the low-attenuation *(dark)* areas on the soft tissue window image that demonstrate a fluid-like density.

to be multilocular with very coarse, thick septa. These wide septa may be straight or may have an irregular shape (Fig. 24.57).

Effects on surrounding structures. Desmoplastic fibromas of bone can expand bone and often break through the outer cortex, extending into the adjacent soft tissue. Usually CT scan or MRI is required to determine the exact soft tissue extent of the lesion.

Differential Interpretation

Distinguishing desmoplastic fibroma from a fibrosarcoma may be difficult both radiologically and histopathologically. However, the presence of coarse, irregular, and sometimes straight septa may help support the correct diagnosis. The appearance of these septa also helps differentiate the lesion from other multilocular tumors. Very small lesions may resemble simple bone cysts.

Management

Resection of this neoplasm with adequate margins is recommended because of its high recurrence rate. Patients who have been treated for the condition should be followed closely with frequent radiologic examinations.

Central Hemangioma
Disease Mechanism

The etiology of hemangiomas is not known, although they may be developmental or traumatic in origin. A hemangioma is a proliferation of blood vessels creating a mass that resembles a neoplasm, although in many cases it is actually a hamartoma. Hemangiomas can occur anywhere in the body but are most frequently noticed on the skin and

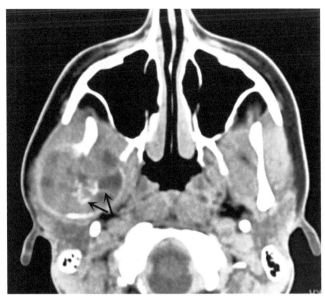

Fig. 24.56 Axial soft tissue window multidetector computed tomographic image of an aneurysmal bone cyst in the left mandibular condylar head. Note the very significant expansion of the bone, and the wispy septa *(arrows)*.

subcutaneous tissues. The central (intraosseous) type most often is found in the vertebrae and skull, and rarely in the jaws.

Clinical Features

Hemangiomas occur most commonly in the first decade of life, although they may also occur later in life, and with a strong 2:1 female prevalence. Enlargement of the bone is slow, producing a nontender expansion of the jaw that occurs over several months or years. Pain, if present, is of the throbbing type. Some tumors may be compressible or pulsate should they involve adjacent soft tissues, and a bruit may be detected on auscultation. Anesthesia of the skin can also occur should the lesion compress an adjacent peripheral nerve. Bleeding may occur from the gingiva around affected teeth, and teeth may be loosened or displaced. Some teeth may demonstrate rebound mobility; that is, when depressed into their sockets, they return to their original position within several minutes because of pressure from the vascular network around the tooth roots. Aspiration with a syringe produces arterial blood that may be under considerable pressure.

Imaging Features

Location. Hemangiomas affect the mandible about twice as often as the maxilla. In the mandible, the most common site is the posterior body and ramus, and within the inferior alveolar canal.

Periphery. The range of appearances of intraosseous hemangiomas may be quite variable. In some instances, the periphery is well defined and corticated; however, some lesions may exhibit a poorly defined periphery, even simulate the appearance of a malignant neoplasm.

Internal structure. Intraosseous hemangiomas may be totally radiolucent; however, when there is residual bone trapped around the proliferating blood vessels, hemangiomas can take on a multilocular appearance. Small radiolucent locules may resemble enlarged marrow spaces surrounded by coarse, dense, and well-defined trabeculae (Fig. 24.58). These internal trabeculae may produce a honeycomb pattern composed of small circular radiolucent spaces that represent blood vessels that are oriented along the path of the incident x-ray beam.

Effects on adjacent structures. When the inferior alveolar canal is involved, the entire canal may appear enlarged, and often the normal path of the canal may develop a serpiginous course (Fig. 24.59). The mandibular and mental foramen may also be enlarged. In addition, the involved bone may be enlarged and have coarse, internal trabeculae. When an intraosseous hemangioma extends beyond the bone surface and displaces the periosteum, linear spicules of bone can be seen emanating from bone in a sunray-like pattern (Fig. 24.60).

When a hemangioma involves soft tissue, focal areas of mineralization can be seen on imaging. These entities, known as phleboliths, represent calcifications that are formed in regions where there are disruptions to the normal flow velocity within a vessel (Fig. 24.61). Phleboliths develop from thrombi that become organized and mineralized, and consist of calcium phosphate and calcium carbonate. With time, phleboliths can take on a "target-like" appearance, with alternating, concentric layers of radiolucency and radiopacity.

Effects on adjacent teeth. The roots of teeth are often resorbed or displaced by an adjacent vascular lesion. Also, developing teeth may be larger and erupt earlier when in an intimate relationship with a hemangioma (Fig. 24.62).

Differential Interpretation

Contrast-enhanced MDCT, or conventional and MR angiography are useful modalities for aiding the differential interpretation of any vascular lesion and other neoplasms of the jaws. Conventional angiography is a radiologic procedure performed by injecting a radiopaque contrast agent into an artery. The distribution of the contrast agent in the vascular neoplasm can by seen in real time, and provide important information about both size and extent, and vessels involved in feeding the lesion. MR angiography is now being used routinely for the same purposes without the necessity of an intra-arterial injection of contrast. When a hemangioma produces a sunray, spiculated bone pattern at its periphery, the appearance may be difficult to differentiate from a bone-forming malignancy.

Management

Central hemangiomas should be treated without delay because trauma that disrupts the integrity of the affected jaw may result in lethal exsanguination. Specifically, embolization (introduction of inert materials into the lesion through the vasculature), surgery (en bloc resection with ligation the feeder vessel), and sclerosing techniques have been used singly or together.

Arteriovenous Malformation
Disease Mechanism

The arteriovenous malformation or fistula is not a neoplasm or tumor, but a direct communication between an artery and a vein that bypasses the intervening capillary system. It usually results from trauma but in rare instances may be a developmental anomaly. An A-V malformation can occur anywhere in the body. The head and neck are the most common sites, and A-V malformations can arise centrally in the jaw and the adjacent soft tissues.

Clinical Features

The clinical appearance of a central A-V malformation can vary considerably, depending on the extent of bone or soft tissue involvement. The lesion may expand bone, and a mass may be present in the overlying soft tissue. The soft tissue swelling may have a purple discoloration, and palpation or auscultation of the swelling may reveal a pulse. Furthermore, aspiration produces blood. Recognition of the hemorrhagic nature of these lesions is of utmost importance because extraction of an associated tooth may be immediately followed by life-threatening bleeding.

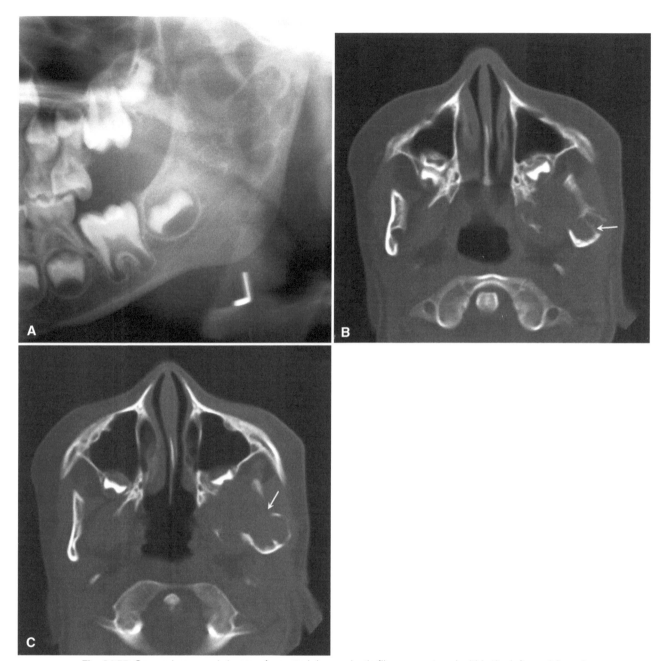

Fig. 24.57 Cropped panoramic image of a central desmoplastic fibroma centered within the left condyle and ramus (A). Axial bone window multidetector computed tomographic image (B) reveals thick straight septa *(arrows)*. More superiorly, (C) computed tomographic images reveal that the tumor has perforated the anterior cortex of the condylar head.

Imaging Features

Location. These lesions most commonly develop in the retromolar area of the mandible and ramus, and involve the mandibular canal.

Periphery. The borders are usually well defined and corticated.

Internal structure. The A-V malformation is radiolucent, although the tortuous path of an enlarged vessel in bone may give it a multilocular appearance (Fig. 24.63).

Effects on surrounding structures. Both central lesions and lesions in adjacent soft tissue can resorb bone. The inferior alveolar canal may take on a serpiginous appearance in a manner similar to a hemangioma.

Effects on adjacent teeth. The roots of teeth may be resorbed or displaced by an adjacent vascular lesion.

Differential Interpretation

As with hemangiomas, contrast-enhanced MDCT, or conventional and MR angiography are useful modalities for aiding the differential interpretation of A-V malformations as well as the identification of a feeder vessel (Fig. 24.64). The differential interpretation is similar to hemangiomas and includes multilocular lesions.

Management

An A-V malformation is treated surgically.

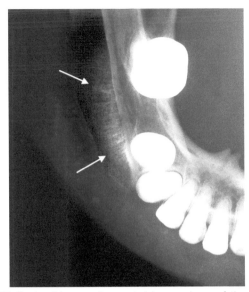

Fig. 24.58 Occlusal image of a central hemangioma of the mandible with adjacent spiculation *(arrows)*. This pattern has a very similar appearance to the spiculation seen in osteosarcoma.

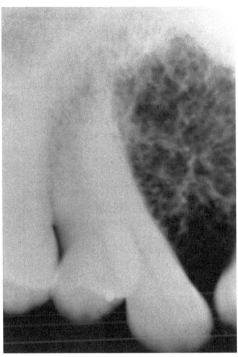

Fig. 24.59 Hemangioma in the anterior maxilla shows a coarse trabecular pattern. (Courtesy Dr. E. J. Burkes, Chapel Hill, NC.)

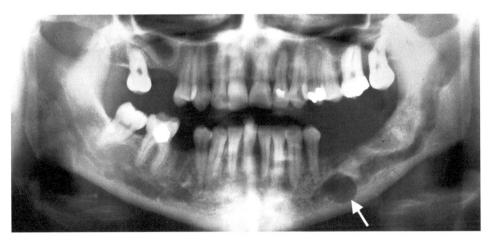

Fig. 24.60 Panoramic image of a vascular lesion within the left inferior alveolar canal. The canal is enlarged, and has an irregular, serpiginous path and the mental foramen is enlarged *(arrow)*.

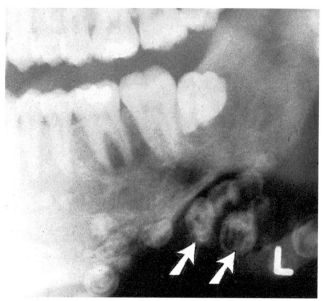

Fig. 24.61 A soft tissue hemangioma with phleboliths *(arrows).*

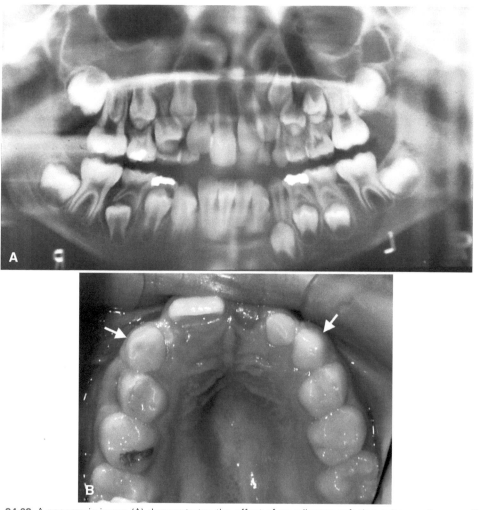

Fig. 24.62 A panoramic image (A) demonstrates the effect of an adjacent soft tissue hemangioma on the developing dentition. The root development and eruption of the canine and premolar teeth on the right side are significantly advanced compared with the left side. A clinical photograph (B) from the same case shows the size asymmetry of the maxillary deciduous canine teeth.

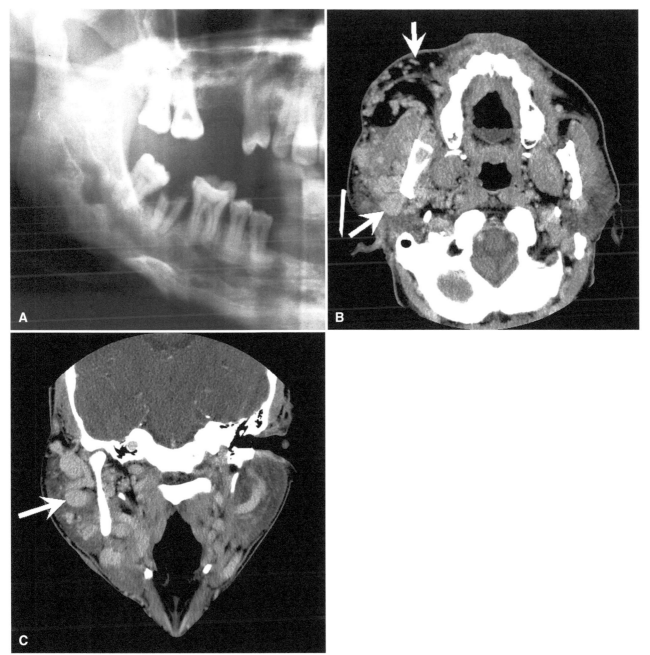

Fig. 24.63 Panoramic image of a patient with an A-V malformation. Note the enlarged, serpiginous inferior alveolar canal (A). Axial (B) and coronal (C) soft tissue multidetector computed tomographic images obtained after administration of intravascular contrast medium fills the feeder vessels of the malformation, and causes the blood vessels to be more radiopaque *(arrows)*.

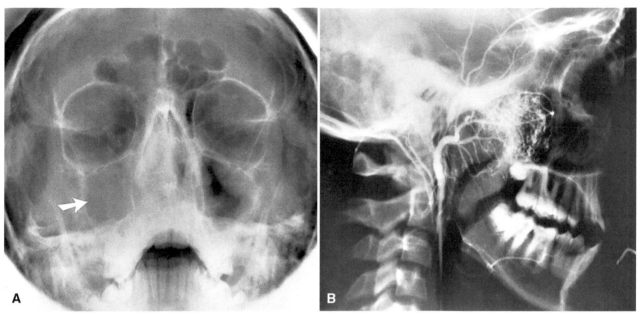

Fig. 24.64 Waters image radiograph shows a radiopacified right maxillary antrum *(arrow)* due to the presence of an A-V malformation (A). The lateral skull view (B) was made following the injection of radiopaque contrast medium as part of an angiographic examination. The contrast agent serves to enhance visualization. (Courtesy Dr. G. Himadi, Chapel Hill, NC.)

REFERENCES

Bilodeau EA, Prasad JL, Alawi F, et al. Molecular and genetic aspects of odontogenic lesions. *Head Neck Pathol.* 2014;8:400–410.

Bilodeau EA, Collins BM. Odontogenic cysts and neoplasms. *Surg Pathol Clin.* 2017;10:177–222.

El-Naggar AK, Chan JKC, Grandis JR, et al. *WHO Classification of Tumors No 9.* 4th ed. Lyon: IARC Press; 2017.

Daley TD, Wysocki GP, Pringle GA. Relative incidence of odontogenic tumors and oral and jaw cysts in a Canadian population. *Oral Surg Oral Med Oral Pathol.* 1994;77:276–280.

Harmon M, Arrigan M, Toner M, et al. A radiological approach to benign and malignant lesions of the mandible. *Clin Radiol.* 2015;7: 335–350.

Hoffman S, Jacoway JR, Krolls SO. Intraosseous and parosteal tumors of the jaws. In: *Atlas of Tumor Pathology, Series 2, Fascicle 24.* Washington, DC: Armed Forces Institute of Pathology; 1987;36:771–778, 1978.

Unni KK. *Dahlin's Bone Tumors: General Aspects and Data on 11,087 Cases.* 5th ed. Philadelphia: Lippincott-Raven; 1996.

Adenomatoid Odontogenic Tumor

Dare A, Yamaguchi A, Yoshiki S, et al. Limitation of panoramic radiography in diagnosing adenomatoid odontogenic tumors. *Oral Surg Oral Med Oral Pathol.* 1994;77:662–668.

Philipsen HP, Reichart PA. Adenomatoid odontogenic tumor: facts and figures. *Oral Oncol.* 1998;35:125–131.

Reichart PA, Philipsen HP, Kongkhuntian P, et al. Immune profile of the adenomatoid odontogenic tumor. *Oral Dis.* 2016;doi:10.1111/odi.12572.

Ameloblastic Fibroma

Buchner A, Vered M. Ameloblastic fibroma: a stage in the development of a hamartomatous odontoma or a true neoplasm? Critical analysis of 162 previously reported cases plus 10 new cases. *Oral Surg Oral Med Oral Pathol Oral Radiol.* 2013;116:598–606.

Dallera P, Bertoni F, Marchetti C, et al. Ameloblastic fibroma: a follow-up of six cases. *Int J Oral Maxillofac Surg.* 1996;25:199–202.

Ameloblastoma

Effiom OA, Odukoya O. Desmoplastic ameloblastoma: analysis of 17 Nigerian cases. *Oral Surg Oral Med Oral Pathol Oral Radiol Endod.* 2011;111:e27–e31.

Kim S, Jang HS. Ameloblastoma: a clinical, radiographic, and histopathologic analysis of 71 cases. *Oral Surg Oral Med Oral Pathol Oral Radiol Endod.* 2001;91:649–653.

Nagi R, Sahu S, Rakesh N. Molecular and genetic aspects in the etiopathogenesis of ameloblastoma: an update. *J Oral Maxillofac Pathol.* 2016;20:497–504.

Sun ZJ, Wu YR, Cheng N, et al. Desmoplastic ameloblastoma - a review. *Oral Oncol.* 2009;45:752–759.

Ueta E, Yoneda K, Ohno A, et al. Intraosseous carcinoma arising from mandibular ameloblastoma with progressive invasion and pulmonary metastasis. *Int J Oral Maxillofac Surg.* 1996;25:370–372.

Weissman JL, Snyderman CH, Yousem SA, et al. Ameloblastoma of the maxilla: CT and MR appearance. *AJNR Am J Neuroradiol.* 1993;14:223–226.

Worth HM. *Principles and Practice of Oral Radiologic.* Chicago: Year Book Medical Publishers Inc; 1963:476–487.

Aneurysmal Bone Cyst

Buraczewski J, Dabska P. Pathogenesis of aneurysmal bone cyst: relationship between the aneurysmal bone cyst and fibrous dysplasia of bone. *Cancer.* 1971;28:597–604.

Struthers P, Shear M. Aneurysmal bone cyst of the jaws. I. Clinicopathological features. *Int J Oral Surg.* 1984;13:85–91.

Struthers P, Shear M. Aneurysmal bone cyst of the jaws. II. Pathogenesis. *Int J Oral Surg.* 1984;13:92–100.

Triantafillidou K, Venetis G, Karakinaris G, et al. Variable histopathological featrues of 6 cases of aneurysmal bone cysts developed in the jaws: review of the literature. *J Craniomaxillofac Surg.* 2012;40:33–38.

Calcifying Epithelial Odontogenic Tumor

Franklin CD, Pindborg JJ. The calcifying epithelial odontogenic tumor: a review and analysis of 113 cases. *Oral Surg Oral Med Oral Pathol.* 1976;42:753–765.

Kaplan I, Buckner A, Caleron S, et al. Radiological and clinical features of calcifying epithelial odontogenic tumor. *Dentomaxillofac Radiol.* 2001;30:22–28.

Pñtino B, Fernández-Alba J, Garcia-Rozado A, et al. Calcifying epithelial odontogenic (Pindborg) tumor: a series of 4 distinctive cases and review of the literature. *J Oral Maxillofac Surg.* 2005;63:1361–1368.

Cementoblastoma

Brannon RB, Fowler CB, Carpenter WM, et al. Cementoblastoma: an innocuous neoplasm? A clinicopathological study of 44 cases and review of the literature with special emphasis on recurrence. *Oral Surg Oral Med Oral Pathol Oral Radiol Endod.* 2002;93:311–320.

Jelic JS, Loftus MJ, Miller AS, et al. Benign cementoblastoma: report of an unusual case and analysis of 14 additional cases. *J Oral Maxillofac Surg.* 1993;51:1033–1037.

Ruprecht A, Ross AS. Benign cementoblastoma (true cementoblastoma). *Dentomaxillofac Radiol.* 1983;12:31–33.

Central Central Giant Cell Lesions

Carlos R, Sedano HO. Intralesional corticosteroids as an alternative treatment for central giant cell granuloma. *Oral Surg Oral Med Oral Pathol Oral Radiol Endod.* 2002;93:161–166.

de Lange J, van den Akker HP. Clinical and radiological features of central giant-cell lesions of the jaw. *Oral Surg Oral Med Oral Pathol Oral Radiol Endod.* 2005;99:464–470.

de Lang J, van den Akker HP, Veldhujzen van Zanten GO, et al. Calcitonin therapy in central giant cell granuloma of the jaw: a randomized double-blind placebo-controled study. *Int J Oral Maxillofac Surg.* 2006;35:791–795.

Kaffe I, Ardekian L, Taicher S, et al. Radiologic features of central giant cell granuloma of the jaws. *Oral Surg Oral Med Oral Pathol Oral Radiol Endod.* 1996;81:720–726.

Kruse-Lösler B, Diallo R, Gaertner C, et al. Central giant cell granuloma of the jaws: a clinical, radiologic and histopathologic study of 26 cases. *Oral Surg Oral Med Oral Pathol Oral Radiol Endod.* 2006;101:346–354.

Central Odontogenic Fibroma

Brannon RB. Central odontogenic fibroma, myxoma (odontogenic myxoma, fibromyxoma) and central odontogenic granular cell tumor. *Oral Maxillofac Surg Clin North Am.* 2004;16:359.

Handlers JP, Abrams AM, Melrose RJ, et al. Central odontogenic fibroma: clinicopathologic features of 19 cases and review of the literature. *J Oral Maxillofac Surg.* 1991;49:46–54.

Kaffe I, Buchner A. Radiologic features of central odontogenic fibroma. *Oral Surg Oral Med Oral Pathol.* 1994;78:811–818.

Cherubism

Bianchi SD, Boccardi A, Mela F, et al. The computed tomographic appearances of cherubism. *Skeletal Radiol.* 1987;16:6–10.

Hyckel P, Berndt A, Schleier P, et al. Cherubism-new hypotheses on pathogenesis and therapeutic consequences. *J Craniomaxillofac Surg.* 2005;33:61–68.

Tsodoulos S, Ilia A, Antoniades K, et al. Cherubism: a case report of a three generation inheritance and literature review. *J Oral Maxillofac Surg.* 2014;72:405.e1–405.e9.

Dense Bone Island

McDonnel D. Dense bone island: a review of 107 patients. *Oral Surg Oral Med Oral Pathol.* 1993;76:124–128.

Petrikowski GC, Peters E. Longitudinal radiographic assessment of dense bone islands of the jaws. *Oral Surg Oral Med Oral Pathol Oral Radiol Endod.* 1997;83:627–634.

Desmoplastic Fibroma

Hopkins KM, Huttula CS, Kahn MA, et al. Desmoplastic fibroma of the mandible: review and report of two cases. *J Oral Maxillofac Surg.* 1996;54:1249–1254.

Said-Al-Naief N, Fernandes R, Louis P, et al. Desmoplastic fibroma of the jaw: a case report and review of literature. *Oral Surg Oral Med Oral Pathol Oral Radiol Endod.* 2006;101:82–94.

Hemangioma

Lund BA, Dahlin DC. Hemangiomas of the mandible and maxilla. *J Oral Surg.* 1964;22:234–242.

Fan X, Qiu W, Zhang Z, et al. Comparative study of clinical manifestation, plain-film radiography and computed tomographic scan in arteriovenous malformations of the jaws. *Oral Surg Oral Med Oral Pathol Oral Radiol Endod.* 2002;94:503–509.

Zlotogorski A, Buchner A, Kaffe I, et al. Radiological features of central haemangioma of the jaws. *Dentomaxillofac Radiol.* 2005;34:292–296.

Hyperostosis

Jainkittivong A, Langlais RP. Buccal and palatal exostosis: prevalence and concurrence with tori. *Oral Surg Oral Med Oral Pathol Oral Radiol Endod.* 2000;90:48–53.

Odontogenic Myxoma

Cohen MA, Mendelsohn DB. CT and MR imaging of myxofibroma of the jaws. *J Comput Assist Tomogr.* 1990;14:281–285.

Peltola J, Magnusson B, Happonen RP, et al. Odontogenic myxoma: a radiographic study of 21 tumours. *Br J Oral Maxillofac Surg.* 1994;32:298–302.

Simon EN, Merkx MA, Vuhahula E, et al. Odontogenic myxoma: a clinicopathological study of 33 cases. *Int J Oral Maxillofac Surg.* 2004;33:333–337.

Sumi Y, Miyaishi O, Ito K, et al. Magnetic resonance imaging of myxoma in the mandible: a case report. *Oral Surg Oral Med Oral Pathol Oral Radiol Endod.* 2000;90:671–676.

Neurofibromatosis

D'Ambrosio JA, Langlais RP, Young RS. Jaw and skull changes in neurofibromatosis. *Oral Surg Oral Med Oral Pathol.* 1988;66:391–396.

Lee L, Yan YH, Pharoah MJ. Radiographic features of the mandible in neurofibromatosis: a report of 10 cases and review of the literature. *Oral Surg Oral Med Oral Pathol Oral Radiol Endod.* 1996;81:361–367.

Odontoma

Kaugars GE, Miller ME, Abbey LM. Odontomas. *Oral Surg Oral Med Oral Pathol.* 1989;67:172–176.

Pippi R. Odontomas and supernumerary teeth: is there a common origin? *Int J Med Sci.* 2014;11:1282–1297.

Soluk Tekkesin M, Pehlivan S, Olgac V, et al. Clinical and histopathological investigation of odontomas: review of the literature and presentation of 160 cases. *J Oral Maxillofac Surg.* 2012;70:1358–1361.

Osteoblastoma

Alvares Capelozza AL, Gião Dezotti MS, Casati Alvares L, et al. Osteoblastoma of the mandible: systematic review of the literature and report of a case. *Dentomaxillofac Radiol.* 2005;34:1–8.

Jones AC, Prihoda TJ, Kacher JE, et al. Osteoblastoma of the maxilla and mandible: a report of 24 cases, review of the literature, and discussion of its relationship to osteoid osteoma of the jaws. *Oral Surg Oral Med Oral Pathol Oral Radiol Endod.* 2006;102:639–650.

Lucas DR, Unni KK, McLeod RA, et al. Osteoblastoma: clinicopathologic study of 306 cases. *Hum Pathol.* 1994;25:117–134.

Osteoma

Bilkay U, Erdem O, Ozek C, et al. Benign osteoma with Gardner syndrome: review of the literature and report of a case. *J Craniofac Surg.* 2004;15:506–509.

Earwaker J. Paranasal osteomas: a review of 46 cases. *Skeletal Radiol.* 1993;22:417–423.

Matteson S, Deahl ST, Alder ME, et al. Advanced imaging methods. *Crit Rev Oral Biol Med.* 1996;7:346–395.

Thakker NS, Evans DG, Horner K, et al. Florid oral manifestations in an atypical familial adenomatous polyposis family with late presentation of colorectal polyps. *J Oral Pathol Med.* 1996;25:459–462.

Schwannoma

Chi AC, Carey J, Muller S, et al. Intraosseous schwannoma of the mandible: case report and review of the literature. *Oral Surg Oral Med Oral Pathol Oral Radiol Endod.* 2003;96:54–65.

Minowa K, Sakakibara N, Yoshikawa K, et al. CT and MRI findings of intraosseous schwannoma of the mandible: a case report. *Dentomaxillofac Radiol.* 2007;36:113–116.

Torus

Eggen S, Natvig B. Concurrence of torus mandibularis and torus palatinus. *Scand J Dent Res.* 1994;102:60–63.

Eggan S, Natvig B, Gåsemyr J. Variation in torus palatinus prevalence in Norway. *Scand J Dent Res.* 1994;102:54–59.

Gorsky M, Raviv M, Kfir E, et al. Prevalence of torus palatinus in a population of young and old Israelis. *Arch Oral Biol.* 1996;41:623–625.

25

Diseases Affecting the Structure of Bone

Ernest W.N. Lam

DISEASE MECHANISM

Coordination of the activities of bone-forming (i.e., osteoblasts), bone-maintaining (i.e., osteocytes), and bone-removing (e.g., osteoclasts) cells regulates the normal structure of bone in the skeleton. Indeed, it has been estimated that approximately 5% to 10% of total bone volume in the adult skeleton is replaced per year. Disease processes may produce abnormalities in the bone through disturbances in the balance of serum concentrations of calcium and phosphate while others may dysregulate osteoblasts, osteocytes, and osteoclasts (Fig. 25.1). A disease that alters the balance of calcium and phosphate levels can result in the abnormal formation of bone and teeth. For example, a low serum calcium concentration can mobilize calcium from bone, thus depleting bone. The resultant reduced calcium level in bone can alter the pattern of trabeculation within the bone, producing bone of low density in the radiologic image.

Bone dysplasias are also characterized by a dysregulation of the normally coordinated activities of osteoblasts and osteocytes; however, here the normal bone is replaced with an exuberant proliferation of fibrous connective tissue and immature and abnormal bone. These lesions, sometimes referred to by the descriptive histopathologic term "fibro-osseous lesions", encompass a broad group of disease processes ranging from conditions of bone cell dysregulation to neoplasms. In oral and maxillofacial radiology, the term "fibro-osseous" is therefore discouraged, and the more specific terminology reflecting the nature of this disease process (bone dysplasia) is preferred.

APPLIED DIAGNOSTIC IMAGING

Diagnostic imaging has many important roles in the assessment and follow-up of diseases that affect bone and bone turnover. Imaging may be useful to describing the extent of disease and to determine if one or more bones are involved. Furthermore, imaging, particularly intraoral imaging, may be useful in characterizing change in the bone pattern of the jaws.

Various diagnostic imaging modalities may be used to aid in these diagnoses. Intraoral images are often the first line of imaging. They provide the best image resolution and may reveal subtle changes to the intraosseous architecture of the jaws as well as involvement of the periodontal ligament (PDL) space and lamina dura. Panoramic imaging and skull imaging can determine if adjacent bones are involved and may reveal changes to the paranasal sinuses. Cone beam computed tomography (CBCT) and multidetector computed tomography (MDCT) can demonstrate the three-dimensional involvement of the bone, and nuclear medicine may provide useful information as to the current metabolic state of the bone.

Because these diseases may affect the entire body, the changes manifested in the appearance of the jaws in diagnostic images are usually generalized and often nonspecific, making it difficult to identify the diseases based on imaging characteristics alone (Table 25.1). The general changes that can be seen in the jaws may include the following:
1. Change in size and shape of the bone
2. Change in the number, size, and orientation of trabeculae
3. Altered thickness and density of cortical structures
4. Increase or decrease in overall bone density

Changes to the bone cortex or trabeculae can result in a decrease or increase in bone density. Because many of the parameters used to produce diagnostic images influence the density of the image, it may be difficult to detect genuine changes in the density of bone caused by systemic disease. Systemic conditions that result in a decrease in bone density do not affect mature teeth; the image of the teeth may stand out with normal density against a generally radiolucent jaw. In severe cases, the teeth may appear to lack any bony support. Also, cortical structures appear thin, are less defined, and occasionally cannot be visualized. A true increase in bone density may be detected by a loss of contrast of the inferior cortex of the mandible as the radiopacity of the cancellous bone approaches that of cortical bone. Often the radiolucent outline of the inferior alveolar nerve canal appears more distinct in contrast to the surrounding radiopaque dense bone.

Some systemic diseases that occur during tooth formation may result in dental alterations. Lamina dura is part of the bone structure of the alveolar process, but because it is usually examined in conjunction with the periodontal membrane space and roots of teeth, it is included with the description of the dental structures (Table 25.2). Changes to teeth and associated structures include the following:
1. Accelerated or delayed eruption
2. Hypoplasia
3. Hypocalcification
4. Loss of a distinct lamina dura

The teeth and their supporting structures often exhibit no detectable changes associated with systemic diseases. However, the first symptoms of a disease may occasionally manifest as a dental problem.

METABOLIC BONE ABNORMALITIES

Osteopenia

Disease Mechanism

Osteopenia is an imbalance of bone deposition and resorption that results in a net decrease in bone formation. Although the histopathologic appearance of the bone may seem normal, there are changes in the trabecular architecture and the size and thickness of individual trabeculae.

Osteopenia occurs as part of the aging process of bone and can be considered a variation of normal. Bone mass normally increases from infancy to about 30 years of age; however, after this age, there is a gradual and progressive decline in bone mass, occurring at a rate of about 8% per decade in females and 3% per decade in males. The loss of bone mass with age is so gradual that it is virtually imperceptible until it reaches significant proportions.

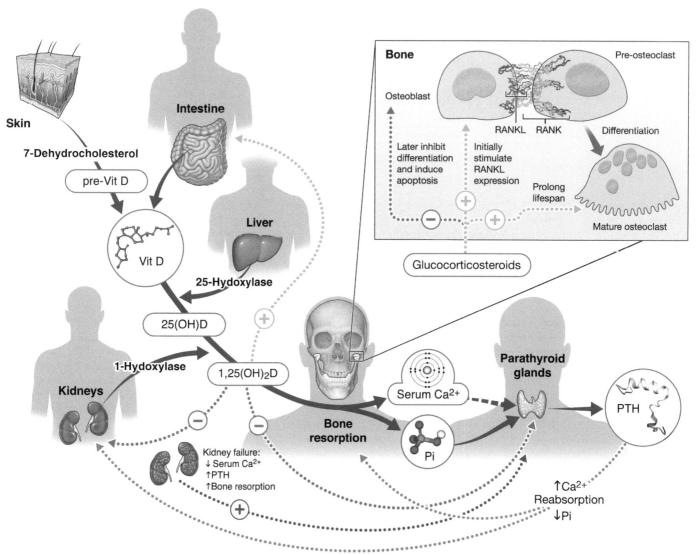

Fig. 25.1 This figure shows the activity of vitamin D, parathyroid hormone *(PTH)*, and glucocorticosteroids in bone and other tissues and outlines their roles in maintaining normal serum levels of calcium *(Ca²⁺)* and inorganic phosphate *(Pi)* in bone metabolism. Bone metabolism is a balance of osteoblastic bone formation and osteoclastic bone resorption. A plus *(+)* sign indicates a promotion effect, and a minus *(–)* sign indicates an inhibitory effect. Vitamin D, either ingested or produced in the skin, undergoes a series of hydroxylation reactions, first in the liver and then in the kidneys, to the active form of 1,25-dihydroxy vitamin D *(1,25(OH)₂D)* *(solid dark gray arrows)*. 1,25(OH)₂D promotes Ca²⁺ and Pi absorption in the intestine *(dotted green line)* and tips the balance of bone metabolism in favor of resorption, releasing Ca²⁺ and Pi from the bone to the serum. Bone resorption is accomplished through the expression of receptor activator of nuclear factor kappa B ligand *(RANKL)* by osteoblasts, which interacts with a receptor activator of nuclear factor-kappa B *(RANK)* receptor on preosteoclasts. This induces differentiation of these cells into active osteoclasts that can resorb the bone *(upper right inset box)*. 1,25(OH)₂D can also inhibit the last hydroxylation of its precursor (25(OH)D) within the kidneys *(dashed red arrow)* and inhibit the parathyroid glands from producing PTH *(dashed red arrow)*. PTH can increase serum Ca²⁺ by directly increasing bone resorption through promoting the expression of RANKL and the differentiation of osteoclasts *(dashed blue arrow)*. PTH also increases serum Ca²⁺ by increasing reabsorption of Ca²⁺ in the kidneys and promoting the hydroxylation of vitamin D to its active form in the kidneys *(dashed blue arrow)*. However, elevated serum Ca²⁺ can reduce production of PTH by the parathyroid glands *(dashed dark gray arrow)*. In the event of kidney failure, PTH may be upregulated to increase serum calcium *(dashed purple arrow)*. Glucocorticosteroids initially increase bone resorption through increased osteoblastic expression of RANKL, thus increasing osteoclast differentiation; thus they can prolong the life span of the osteoclast. Later, glucocorticosteroids reduce bone formation by limiting differentiation and inducing apoptosis of osteoblasts.

TABLE 25.1   Changes in Bone Observed in Systemic Disease[a]

Systemic Disease	BONES Density	Size of Jaws	TRABECULAE Increase	Decrease	Granular
Hyperparathyroidism	Decrease	No	Yes	Yes	Yes
Hypoparathyroidism	Rare increase	No	No	No	No
Hyperpituitarism	No	Large	No	No	No
Hypopituitarism	No	Small	No	No	No
Hyperthyroidism	Decrease	No	No	No	No
Hypothyroidism	No	Small	No	No	No
Cushing syndrome	Decrease	No	No	Yes	Yes
Osteoporosis	Decrease	No	No	Yes	No
Rickets	Decrease	No	No	Yes	No
Osteomalacia	Rare decrease	No	No	Rare decrease	No
Hypophosphatasia	Decrease	No	No	Yes	No
Renal osteodystrophy	Decrease; rare increase	Large	Rare	Yes	Yes
Hypophosphatemia	Decrease	No	No	Yes	Yes
Osteopetrosis	Increase	Large			
Sickle cell anemia	Decrease	Large maxilla			
Thalassemia	Decrease	Large maxilla			

[a]This table summarizes the major imaging changes to bone with endocrine and metabolic bone diseases. It does not include all the possible variable appearances.

TABLE 25.2   Effects on Teeth and Associated Structures[a]

Systemic Disease	Hypocalcification	Hypoplasia	Large Pulp Chamber	Loss of Lamina Dura	Loss of Teeth	Eruption
Hyperparathyroidism	No	No	No	Yes	Rare	No
Hypoparathyroidism	No	Yes	No	No	No	Delayed
Hyperpituitarism	No	No	No	No	No	Supereruption
Hypopituitarism	No	No	No	No	No	Delayed
Hypothyroidism	No	No	No	No	Yes	Early
Hyperthyroidism	No	No	No	Thin	Yes	Delayed
Cushing syndrome	No	No	No	Partial	No	Premature
Osteoporosis	No	No	No	Thin	No	No
Rickets	Yes, enamel	Yes, enamel	No	Thin	No	Delayed
Osteomalacia	No	No	No	Thin	No	No
Hypophosphatasia	Yes	Yes	Yes	Yes	Yes	Delayed
Renal osteodystrophy	Yes	Yes	No	Yes	No	No
Hypophosphatemia	Yes	Yes	Yes	Yes	Yes	No
Osteopetrosis	Yes	Rare	No	Thick	Yes	Delayed

[a]This table summarizes the major imaging changes that can occur to teeth and associated structures with endocrine and metabolic bone diseases. It does not include all the possible variable appearances.

Clinical Features

When loss of bone mass becomes significant, patients may undergo a diagnostic test known as dual x-ray photon absorptiometry (DEXA), and they may be clinically diagnosed with osteoporosis. The most important clinical manifestation of osteoporosis is fracture, which may involve the distal radius, proximal femur, ribs, and vertebrae. Patients may have bone pain. Postmenopausal women are most at risk.

Imaging Features

Effects on the teeth and jaws. Osteopenia results in an overall reduction of bone density, and this change can be observed by comparing the bone to the adjacent teeth. There may also be evidence of reduced density and thinning of bone cortices, such as the inferior cortex of the mandible (Fig. 25.2). The reduction in the number of trabeculae is the least evident in the alveolar processes, possibly because of the forces applied to bone in this area by the teeth. Occasionally the lamina dura may appear thinner than normal. In other regions of the mandible, a reduction in the number of trabeculae may be evident.

Attempts have been made to use commonly acquired periapical and panoramic images to determine the risk of osteoporosis; however, this has proven unreliable. Novel techniques to analyze the trabecular pattern in intraoral images are, however, being developed.

Management

The administration of estrogens and calcium and vitamin D supplements after menopause helps to reduce the rate of bone mineral loss. Weight-bearing exercise programs are an effective adjunct to the development of osteopenia, and more recently oral antiresorptive medications have been used to slow down bone loss in osteoporotic patients.

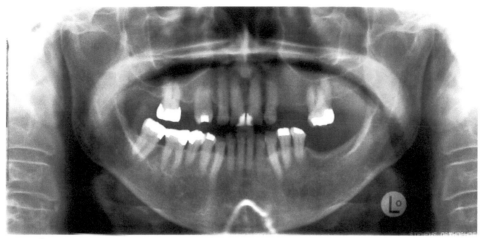

Fig. 25.2 Generalized osteopenia is evident as a loss of the normal trabecular bone pattern. Also, there is heterogeneity and thinning of the normal inferior cortex of the mandible. Note the prominence of the dentition on the background of the demineralized bone.

Rickets and Osteomalacia
Disease Mechanism
Both rickets and osteomalacia result from a defect in the normal activity of the metabolites of vitamin D, especially 1,25-dihydroxy vitamin D (1,25(OH)$_2$D), which is required for the absorption of calcium in the gastrointestinal tract. The term *rickets* is applied when the disease affects the growing skeleton in infants and children, whereas the term osteomalacia is used when this disease affects the mature skeleton in adults.

Rickets and osteomalacia may develop as a result of a lack of vitamin D or calcium in the diet, malabsorption of vitamin D in the gastrointestinal tract, or an inability to synthesize the active metabolite 1,25(OH)$_2$D, which is required for the gastrointestinal absorption of calcium. In more northerly climates, lack of exposure to ultraviolet light may reduce the body's ability to form 1,25(OH)$_2$D from 7-dehydrocholesterol and provitamin D. Liver and kidney disease may impair the synthesis of 25-hydroxy vitamin D (25(OH)D) and 1,25(OH)$_2$D, respectively. Finally, a defect of the gastrointestinal cell response to 1,25(OH)$_2$D may also impair calcium absorption.

Clinical Features
Rickets. In the first 6 months of life, tetany or convulsions are the most common clinical signs of rickets. Later in infancy, the skeletal effects of the disease may be more clinically prominent. Craniotabes, a softening of the posterior portions of the parietal bones, may be the initial sign of the disease. Children with rickets usually have short stature and deformity of the extremities, and there may be swelling of the wrists and ankles. Eruption and development of the dentition is delayed, and the enamel and dentin may be hypocalcified.

Osteomalacia. Most patients with osteomalacia have some degree of bone pain as well as muscle weakness of varying severity. Other clinical features include a peculiar waddling or "penguin" gait, tetany, and greenstick fractures of the bone.

Imaging Features
Effects on the teeth and jaws. Rickets in infancy or early childhood may result in the hypoplasia of developing dental teeth, including the enamel (Fig. 25.3). If the disease occurs before the age of 3 years, enamel hypoplasia is fairly common. This early manifestation of rickets can be demonstrated in diagnostic images to involve both unerupted and erupted teeth. Diagnostic images may also document retarded tooth

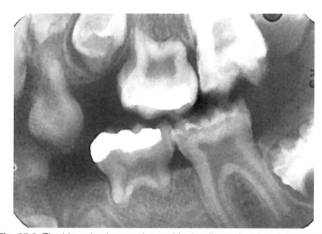

Fig. 25.3 The bite-wing image shows thinning (hypoplasia) and decreased mineralization (hypocalcification) of the enamel in a child with rickets. (Courtesy H. G. Poyton, DDS, Toronto, ON, Canada.)

eruption in early rickets. The lamina dura and the cortical borders of tooth follicles may be thin or missing.

Changes in the jaws generally occur after changes in the ribs and long bones. Jaw cortices such as the inferior cortex or the borders of the inferior alveolar canals may be thin. Within the cancellous portion of the jaws, the trabeculae are reduced in density, number, and thickness; this imparts a generalized radiolucency to the jaws. In severe cases, the jaws appear so radiolucent that the teeth appear to lack bony support.

Osteomalacia does not alter the teeth or the jaws because they are already fully developed before the onset of the disease. However, when manifestations are present in diagnostic images, there may be an overall radiolucent appearance to the bone, and the trabeculae may be sparse. In patients with long-standing or severe osteomalacia, the lamina dura may be thin.

Effects on the skeleton. The earliest and most prominent feature of rickets is widening of the epiphyses of the long bones. This is a manifestation of the wide uncalcified osteoid seams that are seen histologically. The resultant abnormal biomechanics leads to cupping and fraying of the metaphases of the long bones, and the soft weight-bearing bones such as the femur and tibia undergo a characteristic bowing. Greenstick fractures, which are incomplete fractures through the bone, occur in many patients with rickets.

In osteomalacia, the cortex of bone may be thin. Pseudofractures, which are poorly calcified, ribbon-like zones extending into bone at approximate right angles to the margin of the bone, may also be present. Pseudofractures occur most commonly in the ribs, pelvis, and weight-bearing bones and rarely in the mandible.

Management

Because the cause of rickets and osteomalacia is vitamin D deficiency, the treatment of choice is vitamin D supplementation. Cholecalciferol is a vitamin D supplement that is stored in the body and released over several weeks. Signs of healing are seen in as few as 6 to 7 days after treatment.

Hypophosphatemic Rickets
Disease Mechanism

Hypophosphatemic or vitamin D–resistant rickets is a group of inherited conditions that produce renal tubular disorders causing an inability to resorb phosphorus in the distal renal tubules and resulting in a decrease in serum phosphorus (hypophosphatemia). Multiple myeloma may also induce hypophosphatemia as a result of secondary damage to the kidneys.

Normal calcification of the osseous structures requires the correct amount and ratio of serum calcium and phosphorus. Hypophosphatemia

can result in low-density bone development because of low calcium content. This results in the abnormal formation of trabeculae, which are sometimes short and irregular, and the appearance of a granular bone pattern. Hypophosphatemia also interferes with the normal calcification of dentin, resulting in larger than normal pulp chambers and root canals.

Clinical Features

Children with hypophosphatemic rickets show reduced growth and bony changes similar to rickets, including bowing of the legs, enlarged epiphyses, and skull changes. Adults have bone pain, muscle weakness, and vertebral fractures.

Imaging Features

Effects on the teeth and jaws. The teeth may be poorly formed, with thin enamel and large pulp chambers and root canals (Fig. 25.4B and C). In addition, periapical and periodontal abscesses may occur frequently. The occurrence of rarefying osteitis without an apparent etiology may be a result of defects in the dentin and large pulp chambers allowing for the ingress of oral microorganisms and subsequent pulp necrosis. If the disease is severe, the patient will have premature loss of the teeth. The lamina dura may be sparse, and the cortices around tooth crypts may be thin or entirely absent.

The jaws are usually osteopenic and in extreme cases may be remarkably radiolucent. Cortical boundaries may be unusually thin or not

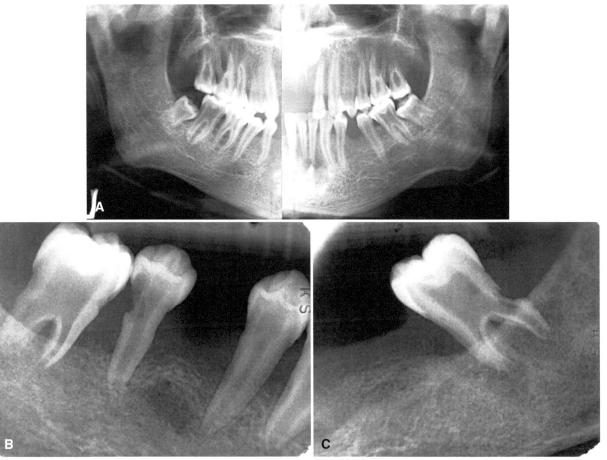

Fig. 25.4 Panoramic image of a patient with hypophosphatemic rickets (A). Note the generalized osteopenic appearance of the jaws, the lack of bone density, and the large pulp chambers. Periapical images (B and C) of a different patient demonstrate apparent bone loss around the teeth, a granular bone pattern, large pulp chambers, and external root resorption.

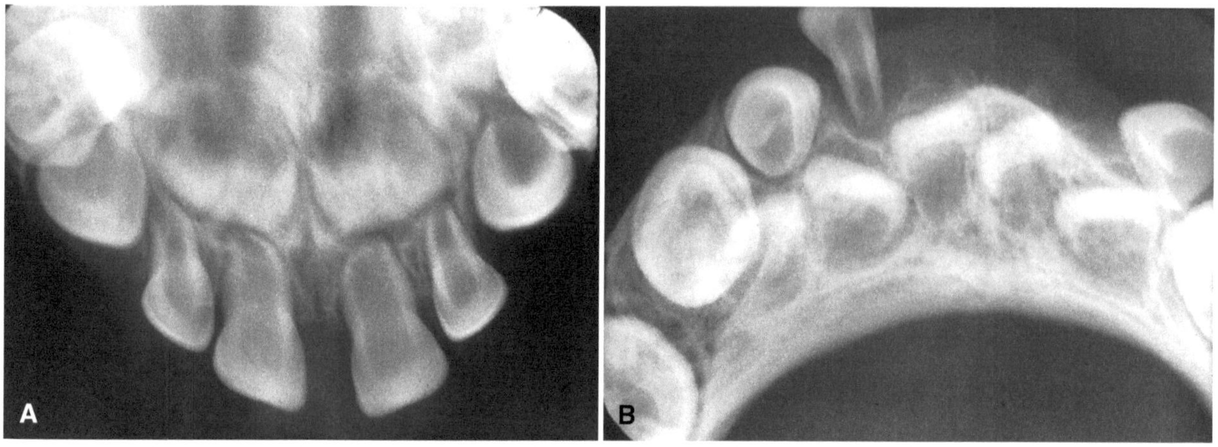

Fig. 25.5 Note the very large pulp chambers in the deciduous dentition in a patient with hypophosphatasia (A) and premature loss of the mandibular incisors (B) on these anterior occlusal images. (Courtesy Dr. H. G. Poyton, Toronto, ON, Canada.)

apparent at all (see Fig. 25.4). Other manifestations include fewer visible trabeculae and a granular bone pattern.

Effects on the skeleton. In children with hypophosphatemic rickets, the radiologic findings are indistinguishable from rickets. In adults, the long bones may show persistent deformity, fractures, or pseudofractures.

Management

Treatment consists of administering vitamin D supplements, phosphates, and anticalciurics. Serum calcium concentrations must be closely monitored to prevent hypercalcemia and its complications. Nephrocalcinosis is a long-term complication that may arise from treatment.

Hypophosphatasia
Disease Mechanism

Hypophosphatasia is a rare inherited disorder caused by a reduction in the activity of the tissue nonspecific alkaline phosphatases, one of a family of enzymes produced by osteoblasts and odontoblasts that is required for the normal mineralization of osteoid and teeth. When deficient, the enzyme fails to cleave phosphate-containing substances, such as inorganic pyrophosphate, and results in the extracellular accumulation of inorganic pyrophosphate, a known inhibitor of hydroxyapatite formation.

Six clinical forms of the disease are recognized, depending on the age at diagnosis: a perinatal form which is lethal; a perinatal form that is nonlethal (benign); infantile, childhood, and adult forms; and odontohypophosphatasia. The disease in individuals with homozygous involvement is usually severe, has an early onset (in utero), and leads to death within the first year. The severe forms of the condition have an autosomal recessive mode of disease transmission, whereas the milder forms have a variable pattern of inheritance.

Clinical Features

Infants demonstrate bowed limb bones and a marked deficiency of skull ossification. Individuals with the milder forms of the disease show poor growth and deformities similar to rickets. There may be a history of fractures, delayed walking, or bone pain. Approximately 85% of these children show premature loss of the primary teeth, particularly the incisors, and delayed eruption of the permanent dentition. Dental findings are often the first clinical sign of hypophosphatasia and the only sign of odontohypophosphatasia.

Imaging Features

Effects on the teeth and jaws. Both primary and permanent teeth have a thin enamel layer and large pulp chambers and root canals (Fig. 25.5). The teeth may also be hypoplastic and may be lost prematurely. In the jaws, there is a generalized osteopenic appearance to the bones. The cortical bone and lamina dura are thin, and the alveolar processes are poorly calcified and may appear deficient.

Effects on the skeleton. In young children with hypophosphatasia, the long bones show irregular defects in the epiphyses, and the skull is poorly calcified. In older children, premature closure of the skull sutures results in gyral impressions on the inner table of the skull that resemble hammered metal. The skull may assume a brachycephalic shape. In adults, a generalized reduction in bone density may be seen.

Management

There is no curative treatment for hypophosphatasia. However, enzyme replacement therapy is currently being investigated and has demonstrated improvement in children with life-threatening hypophosphatasia.

Osteopetrosis
Disease Mechanism

Osteopetrosis, otherwise known as marble bone disease or Albers-Schönberg disease, is an inherited disorder of bone that results from a defect in the differentiation and function of osteoclasts. The disorder is inherited in an autosomal recessive (osteopetrosis congenita) or autosomal dominant (osteopetrosis tarda) manner. The lack of normally functioning osteoclasts results in abnormal formation of the primary skeleton and abnormal bone turnover thereafter. The failure of bone to remodel causes the bones to become densely mineralized, fragile, and susceptible to fracture and infection.

Clinical Features

The more severe, recessive form of osteopetrosis is seen in infants and young children; it is invariably fatal early in life. The patient has progressive deposition of bone, resulting in narrowing of bony canals and foramina. These changes create morphologic defects as well as sensorineural and sensorimotor deficits, including hydrocephalus, blindness, deafness, vestibular nerve dysfunction, and facial nerve paralysis. The benign, dominant form appears in adults and may be entirely asymptomatic or accompanied by mild signs and symptoms. It may be discovered at any time from childhood into adulthood as an incidental finding, or it may manifest as a bone fracture. The loss of marrow spaces secondary to the deposition of bone in patients with osteopetrosis may also affect the hematopoietic development of red and white blood cells and platelets, resulting in anemia, leukopenia, and thrombocytopenia. Consequently patients may develop lethargy, be prone to infection, and have longer than normal bleeding times.

In some more chronic cases, bone pain and cranial nerve palsies caused by neural compression may be clinical problems. The increased bone density and relatively poor vascularity result in an increased susceptibility to osteomyelitis, usually from odontogenic inflammatory lesions. This problem is more common in the mandible, where periapical and periodontal inflammatory conditions are common.

Imaging Features

Effects on the teeth and jaws. Effects on teeth may include early tooth loss, missing teeth, malformed roots and crowns, and teeth that are poorly calcified and prone to caries. The normal eruption pattern of the primary and secondary dentitions may be delayed as a result of the increased bone density or ankylosis. The lamina dura and cortical borders may appear thicker than normal.

The increased radiopacity of the jaws may be so great that the diagnostic image may fail to reveal any internal structure, and even the roots of the teeth may not be apparent. The normal interface between cortical and cancellous bone may be lost, and in the mandible, the inferior alveolar canal may appear very prominent. On plain imaging, the image of the bone may appear underexposed due to failure of the incident x-ray beam to penetrate the bone.

Effects on the skeleton. All bones may become mildly enlarged and show greatly increased radiopacity. Because this condition is systemic, the changes affect all bones bilaterally (Fig. 25.6). The bones can become so radiopaque that the trabecular pattern may not be visible. The homogeneous radiopacity of the cancellous bone also reduces the contrast between the bone cortex and the cancellous portion of the bone.

Management

Treatment of osteopetrosis consists of bone marrow transplantation to attempt to stimulate the formation of functional osteoclasts. The hematologic complications are managed with systemic steroids. When

osteomyelitis develops (Fig. 25.7), it is difficult to treat, and a combination of antibiotics and hyperbaric oxygen therapy is used. It is therefore imperative that odontogenic inflammatory disease not develop in these individuals.

Endocrine Disturbances
Diagnostic Imaging Features

Endocrine disturbances affect the entire body, and the changes manifested in the appearances of the teeth and jaws in diagnostic images are usually generalized and often nonspecific. Therefore it may be difficult to identify the diseases based on imaging characteristics alone (see Table 25.1).

When systemic diseases manifest during tooth formation, teeth may appear hypoplastic or hypocalcified, and their eruption may be accelerated or delayed. Because the lamina dura is often examined in conjunction with the PDL space and the roots of teeth, the lamina dura may become less distinct or lost. If the teeth have developed, no detectable changes to the teeth or lamina dura may be visible. However, the first symptoms of a disease may occasionally manifest as a dental problem.

The general changes that can be seen in the jaws can include alterations in bone density; the number, size, and orientation of trabeculae; the thickness of bone cortices; and the size and shape of the bone. Because both technical and patient factors can determine the appearance of bone on a diagnostic image, it may be difficult not only to detect but also to quantify genuine changes in the density of bone when they arise. For example, systemic conditions that may decrease bone density generally do not affect mature teeth, and the images of the teeth may develop greater prominence and stand out against a generally more radiolucent bone pattern in the jaws. In severe cases, the normal supporting structures around the teeth may not be visible. Also, cortical structures may appear thin and less well defined; occasionally they may disappear. In contrast, a true increase in bone density may be detected by a loss of contrast of the cortical/cancellous bone interface as the radiopacity of the cancellous bone approaches that of cortical bone. Moreover, the radiolucent outline of the inferior alveolar nerve canal may appear more distinct in contrast to the surrounding radiopaque dense bone.

Hyperparathyroidism
Disease Mechanism

Hyperparathyroidism is an endocrine abnormality in which there is an excess of circulating parathyroid hormone (PTH). This excess favors

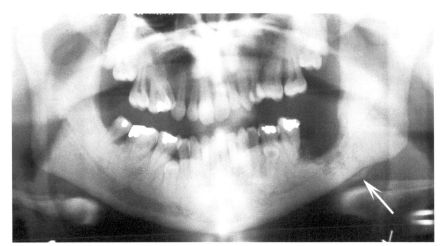

Fig. 25.6 A significant and generalized increase in the radiopacity of the bones is seen on this panoramic image of a patient with osteopetrosis. The inferior alveolar canals are prominently seen and narrowed. Also, there is osteomyelitis in the body of the left mandible with periosteal new bone formation *(arrow)*.

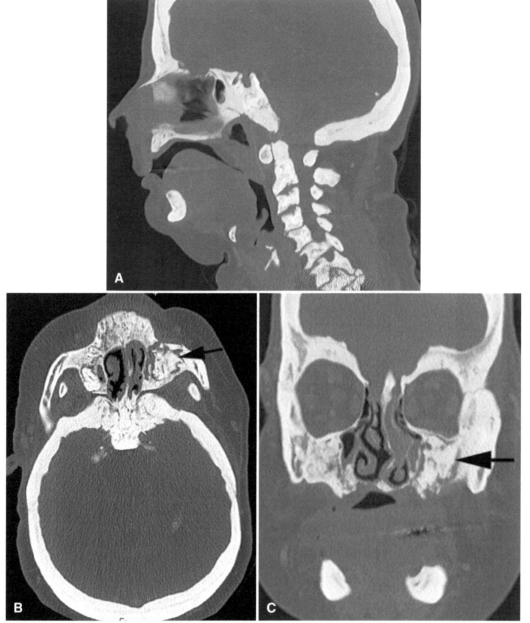

Fig. 25.7 Sagittal (A), axial (B), and coronal (C) multidetector computed tomography images show dense calcification of the bones in a patient with osteopetrosis. Note the loss of definition of the cortical and cancellous bone interfaces and the uniformly increased density of all the bones. The case is complicated by osteomyelitis of the left maxilla with development of sequestra (*arrows* in B and C).

osteoclastic resorption of bone, which mobilizes calcium from the skeleton. This change can alter the normal morphology of bone trabeculae and increase renal tubular reabsorption of calcium and the production of 1,25$(OH)_2$D. The net result of these changes is an increase in serum calcium levels (Fig. 25.8).

In 80% to 85% of cases, primary hyperparathyroidism is usually the result of PTH overproduction from a benign secretory tumor (adenoma) of one of the four parathyroid glands. The incidence of primary hyperparathyroidism is about 0.1%, and the condition can be sporadic or part of a hereditary syndrome, such as hyperparathyroidism-jaw tumor syndrome, which involves tumors of parathyroid glands, jaws, and kidneys. Less frequently, in 10% to 15% of cases, patients may have hyperplastic parathyroid glands that secrete excess PTH.

Secondary hyperparathyroidism results from a compensatory increase in the output of PTH in response to hypocalcemia. The underlying hypocalcemia may result from inadequate dietary intake, poor intestinal absorption of vitamin D, or deficient metabolism of vitamin D in the liver or kidneys (renal osteodystrophy). Chronic renal failure produces bone changes by interfering with the hydroxylation of 25-hydroxy vitamin D to 1,25$(OH)_2$D, a process that occurs in the kidneys. The various biologic functions of 1,25$(OH)_2$D outlined in Fig. 25.1 are hindered, especially the absorption of calcium from the intestines. The result is a state of hypocalcemia and hyperphosphatemia. This imbalance of serum concentrations of calcium and phosphate prevents the normal calcification of bone and teeth and stimulate the parathyroid gland to secrete PTH so that more calcium can be liberated into the blood.

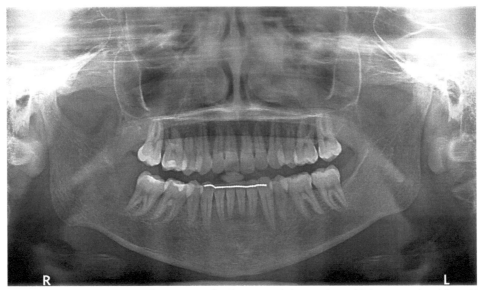

Fig. 25.8 This panoramic image shows generalized osteopenia in a patient with hyperparathyroidism. Note how the teeth stand out in contrast to the osteopenic bone.

Clinical Features

Primary hyperparathyroidism affects females two to three times more commonly than males. The condition occurs mainly in adults 30 to 60 years of age. The clinical manifestations of the disease are related to hypercalcemia. They cover a broad range of signs and symptoms often summarized as the triad of "stones, bones, and groans": renal calculi; bone complications including osteoporosis, arthritis, and fracture; and gastrointestinal symptoms including peptic ulcers. In the jaws, gradual loosening, drifting, and loss of teeth may occur. The combination of hypercalcemia and an elevated serum level of PTH is diagnostic of primary hyperparathyroidism. Serum alkaline phosphatase level, a reliable indicator of bone turnover, may also be elevated in hyperparathyroidism.

The clinical features of secondary hyperparathyroidism are the same as those seen in chronic renal failure. In children, growth retardation and frequent bone fractures may occur. Adults may have a gradual softening and bowing of the bones.

Imaging Features

Effects on the teeth and jaws. The imaging features of primary (see Fig. 25.7) and secondary hyperparathyroidism (see Fig. 25.8) are similar. In children, there may be hypoplasia and hypocalcification of the teeth, sometimes resulting in loss of any evidence of enamel in diagnostic images. One of the earliest manifestations of hyperparathyroidism is the loss of lamina dura in approximately 10% of patients. Depending on the duration and severity of the disease, the loss of lamina dura may be partial or involve an entire tooth, and one or more teeth can be affected. The result of lamina dura loss may give the root a tapered appearance because of loss of image contrast. Although PTH mobilizes minerals from the skeleton, mature teeth are immune to this systemic demineralizing process.

Only about one in five patients with hyperparathyroidism has observable bone changes. In the jaws, there may be demineralization and thinning of bone cortices including the inferior border of the mandible, the cortical borders of the inferior alveolar canal, and the cortical borders of the maxillary sinuses. The density of the jawbones is decreased, resulting in a radiolucent appearance that contrasts with the normal density of the teeth (see Fig. 25.8). The elevated rate of bone remodeling can result in an abnormal bone pattern wherein normal trabeculae are replaced by numerous small, more randomly oriented trabeculae, resulting in a ground-glass appearance in the diagnostic image (Fig. 25.9). In the skull, the calvarium may take on a granular appearance that is classically known as the "salt and pepper" skull. This appearance is caused by loss of the central (diploic) trabeculae and thinning of the cortical tables (Fig. 25.10).

Brown tumors of hyperparathyroidism, which are giant cell lesions, may also appear in bone, and these are frequently found in the facial bones and jaws, particularly in cases of long-standing disease (Figs. 25.11 and 25.12). The lesions are called brown tumors because of their brown or reddish-brown appearances on gross examination. Brown tumors may be solitary or multiple within a single bone. If a giant cell lesion occurs later than the second decade of life, the patient should be screened for increases in serum calcium, PTH, and alkaline phosphatase.

Effects on the skeleton. One of the earliest and most reliable changes with hyperparathyroidism is subtle erosions of bone from the subperiosteal surfaces of the phalanges of the hands. Demineralization of the skeleton may result in an unusual generalized radiolucent appearance (generalized osteopenia); the bone may appear "gray." Osteitis fibrosa cystica is seen in advanced cases as localized regions of bone loss produced by osteoclastic activity, as are brown tumors. And finally, the increased levels of serum calcium may precipitate in the soft tissues, forming punctate or nodular calcifications in the joints and kidneys.

The features of secondary hyperparathyroidism are quite variable. Some changes of the skeleton resemble changes seen in rickets, and other changes are consistent with primary hyperparathyroidism, including generalized loss of bone density and thinning of bony cortices. Interestingly, one may occasionally see an increase in bone density in some patients. There may also be brown tumors, but these are less frequently seen compared with primary hyperparathyroidism.

Management

After successful surgical removal of the causative parathyroid adenoma, almost all changes revert to normal. The only exception may be the site of a brown tumor, which often heals with bone that is more sclerotic than normal. Many people with this disease are being diagnosed earlier,

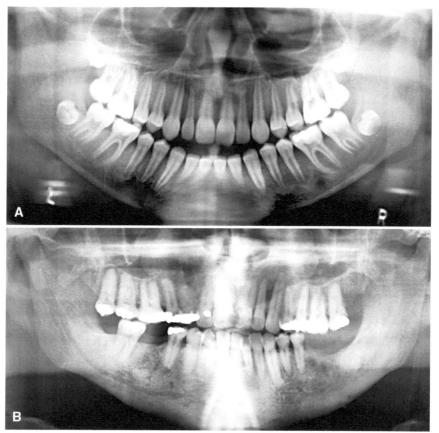

Fig. 25.9 Two Cases of Renal Osteodystrophy. (A) Panoramic image reveals radiolucent areas of bone loss, loss of distinct lamina dura and a sclerotic pattern around the roots of teeth. (B) Panoramic image reveals a generalized sclerotic bone pattern. Note the loss of a clear interface between the cancellous bone and cortical bone.

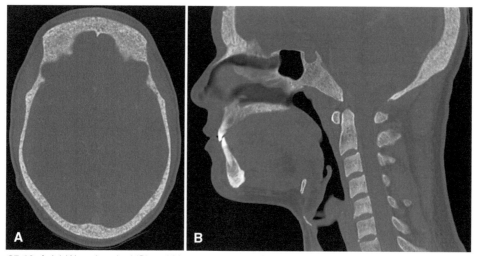

Fig. 25.10 Axial (A) and sagittal (B) multidetector computed tomography images in a patient with secondary hyperparathyroidism. Note the generalized thinning and loss of definition of the cortical bone and the internal granular pattern of the bone.

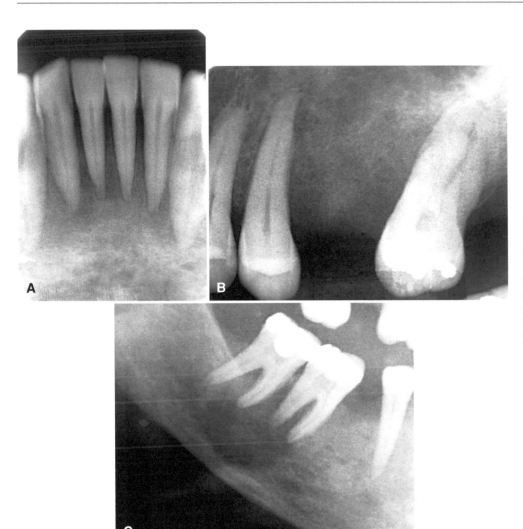

Fig. 25.11 Periapical images (A and B) show loss of lamina dura around the teeth in a patient with hyperparathyroidism. Also, note the loss of definition of the floor of the maxillary antrum. The cropped panoramic image (C) of the same patient reveals a central giant cell lesion (brown tumor) developing apical to the mandibular right second and third molars.

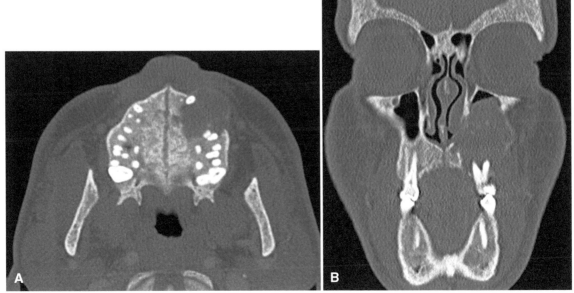

Fig. 25.12 Axial (A) and coronal (B) multidetector computed tomography images in a patient with secondary hyperparathyroidism and a central giant cell lesion (brown tumor) involving the left maxilla.

resulting in fewer severe cases. In secondary hyperparathyroidism, patients with renal osteodystrophy are given vitamin D supplements and phosphate binders. The imaging features of secondary hyperparathyroidism may persist even after a successful renal transplant because of hyperplasia of the parathyroid glands secondary to the previous chronic low serum levels of calcium.

Hypoparathyroidism and Pseudohypoparathyroidism
Disease Mechanism
Hypoparathyroidism is an uncommon condition in which insufficient secretion of PTH occurs. Several causes exist, but the most common is unintended damage or removal of the parathyroid glands during thyroid surgery. In pseudohypoparathyroidism, there is a defect in the response of the target tissue cells to normal levels of PTH. In both cases, the result is low serum levels of calcium.

Clinical Features
There are a variety of clinical manifestations. Although some patients may show no changes, those that do may report sharp flexion (tetany) of the wrist and ankle joints (carpopedal spasm). Some patients experience sensorineural abnormalities consisting of paresthesia of the hands or feet or the area around the mouth. Neurologic changes may include anxiety and depression, epilepsy, parkinsonism, and chorea. Chronic forms may produce a reduction in intellectual capacity. Patients with pseudohypoparathyroidism often have early closure of certain bony epiphyses and manifest short stature or disproportionate extremities.

Imaging Features
Effects on the teeth and jaws. Imaging of the jaws may reveal dental enamel hypoplasia, external root resorption, delayed eruption, or root dilaceration (Fig. 25.13).

Effects on the skeleton. On skull images, the calcifications may appear flocculent and bilateral within the cerebral hemispheres on posteroanterior skull images. Centrally there is calcification of the basal ganglia.

Management
These conditions are managed with orally administered supplemental calcium and vitamin D.

Hyperpituitarism
Disease Mechanism
Hyperpituitarism in the form of gigantism and acromegaly results from hyperfunction of the anterior lobe of the pituitary gland. These conditions develop in response to an increased production of growth hormone.

In skeletally immature children, the condition is known as gigantism; in skeletally mature adults, the condition is known as acromegaly. An excess of growth hormone causes overgrowth of all tissues in the body, including bone, still capable of growth. The usual cause of this problem is a benign functional, secretory tumor of the somatotrophs (growth hormone-secreting cells) in the anterior lobe of the pituitary gland.

Clinical Features
In children, there is generalized overgrowth of most hard and soft tissues. Active growth occurs in bones in which the epiphyses have not fused with the bone shaft. During adolescence, generalized skeletal growth is excessive and may be prolonged, and affected individuals may ultimately attain heights of 7 to 8 feet or more, but with remarkably normal proportions. The eyes and other parts of the central nervous system do not enlarge except in rare cases in which the condition manifests in infancy.

In adults, acromegaly has an insidious clinical course, quite different from what is seen in children. In adults, the clinical effects of a pituitary adenoma develop quite slowly because many types of tissues have lost the capacity for growth. This is also true of much of the skeleton. Interestingly, an excess of growth hormone can stimulate the mandible and the phalanges of the hand. Also, the supraorbital ridges and the underlying frontal sinus may enlarge. Excess growth hormone in adults also results in hypertrophy of some soft tissues including the lips, tongue, nose, and soft tissues of the hands and feet, sometimes to a striking degree.

Imaging Features
Effects on the teeth and jaws. The tooth crowns are usually normal in size, although the roots of premolar and molar teeth often enlarge as a result of hypercementosis. This condition may be the result of functional and structural demands on teeth instead of a secondary hormonal effect. Supraeruption of the posterior teeth may occur in an attempt to compensate for the growth of the mandible.

Hyperpituitarism causes enlargement of the jaws, most notably the mandible (Fig. 25.14). Mandibular condylar growth may be very prominent, and patients can develop a prominent skeletal class III appearance with a strongly prognathic mandible. The increase in the length of the dental arch results in spacing of the teeth. The mandibular angle may also increase. This change, in combination with the flaring of the anterior teeth caused by enlargement of the tongue (macroglossia), may result in the development of an anterior open bite. The sign of incisor flaring is a helpful point of differentiation between acromegalic prognathism and inherited prognathism. The thickness and height of the alveolar processes may also increase.

Effects on the skeleton. Functional adenomas of the pituitary gland may not enlarge the sella turcica at all. However, in some cases there

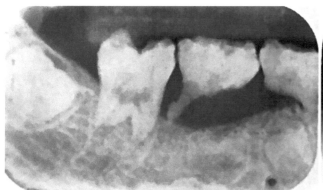
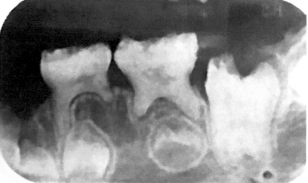

Fig. 25.13 Anomalies of Tooth Development in a Patient With Pseudohypoparathyroidism. (Courtesy Dr. S. Bricker, San Antonio, TX.)

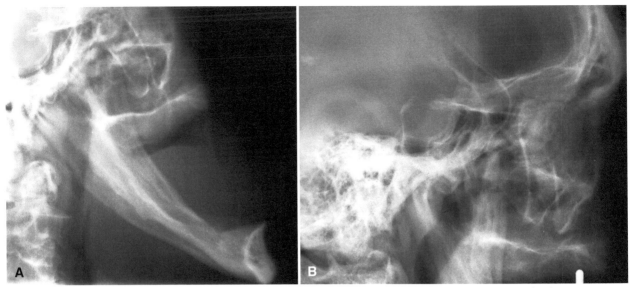

Fig. 25.14 A patient with acromegaly manifesting in growth of the mandible and the development of a class III skeletal relationship of the jaws (A). A portion of a lateral skull image of the same patient demonstrates enlargement of the sella turcica (B).

is an enlargement or "ballooning" of the sella (see Fig. 25.7B). Skull images characteristically reveal enlargement of the paranasal sinuses (especially the frontal sinus). These air sinuses are more prominent in acromegaly than in pituitary gigantism because sinus growth in gigantism tends to be more in step with the generalized enlargement of the facial bones. Acromegaly also produces diffuse thickening of the outer cortex of the skull.

Management

Surgical removal of the pituitary gland is the first line of treatment. If surgery fails or is not possible, medications may be used to reduce growth hormone levels. Radiation therapy may also be considered, but this usually takes several years to show an effect.

Hypopituitarism
Disease Mechanism

Hypopituitarism is the result of decreased secretion of pituitary hormones, the most common of which is growth hormone.

Clinical Features

Individuals with this condition exhibit dwarfism but have relatively well-proportioned bodies. One study reported a marked failure of development of the maxilla and mandible, and the dimensions of these bones in adults with this disorder were approximately the same as those in normal children 5 to 7 years of age.

Imaging Features

Effects on the teeth and jaws. Eruption of the primary dentition occurs at the normal time, but exfoliation is delayed by several years. The crowns of the permanent teeth also develop normally, but their eruption is delayed several years. The third molar buds may be completely absent.

Effects on the skeleton. In hypopituitarism, the jaws, especially the mandible, are small, which results in crowding and malocclusion.

Management

Treatment is usually directed toward removal of the cause or replacement of the pituitary hormones or hormones of its target gland. The response

of the dentition to treatment with growth hormone is variable but seems to parallel the skeletal response.

Hyperthyroidism
Disease Mechanism

Hyperthyroidism is a disease process that involves excessive production of thyroxine in the thyroid gland. The most common forms of hyperthyroidism are diffuse toxic goiter (Graves disease), toxic nodular goiter (Plummer disease), and toxic adenoma, a benign tumor of the thyroid gland. Each of these conditions results in increased levels of circulating thyroxine.

Clinical Features

Excessive thyroxine causes a generalized increase in the metabolic rate of all body tissues, resulting in tachycardia, increased blood pressure, sensitivity to heat, and irritability. Hyperthyroidism is more common in females.

Imaging Features

Effects on the teeth and jaws. Hyperthyroidism results in an advanced rate of dental development and early eruption, with premature loss of the primary teeth.

Effects on the skeleton. Hyperthyroidism results in an increased rate of bone turnover that is imbalanced in favor of excessive bone resorption. This resorption is manifest in adults as a generalized loss of bone density or bone volume in edentulous areas.

Management. Radioactive ^{131}I is the most common treatment for hyperthyroidism followed by antithyroid medications and surgical removal of the thyroid gland.

Hypothyroidism
Disease Mechanism

Hypothyroidism or cretinism usually results from insufficient secretion of thyroxine by the thyroid glands despite the levels of circulating thyroid-stimulating hormone.

Clinical Features

In children, hypothyroidism may result in retarded mental and physical development. The base of the skull shows delayed ossification, and the paranasal sinuses show only partial development. Dental development is delayed, and the primary teeth are slow to exfoliate.

Hypothyroidism in an adult results in myxedematous swelling but not the dental or skeletal changes seen in children. Adult symptoms may range from lethargy, poor memory, inability to concentrate, constipation, and cold intolerance to the more florid clinical picture of a dull and expressionless face, periorbital edema, large tongue, sparse hair, and skin that feels "doughy" to the touch.

Imaging Features

Effects on the teeth and jaws. There may be delayed eruption of teeth, teeth with short roots, and thinning of the lamina dura. The maxilla and mandible may be relatively small. Patients with adult hypothyroidism may develop periodontal disease and diastemas of the teeth as a result of enlargement of the tongue. There may also be external root resorption and premature tooth loss. In the calvarium, skull sutures may exhibit wormian bone formation—that is, the formation of one or more islands of bone within a suture.

Effects on the skeleton. Features in children include delayed closure of the epiphyses.

Management

Patients with hypothyroidism are managed with hormone replacement and careful monitoring to prevent the development of iatrogenic hyperthyroidism.

Hypercortisolism
Disease Mechanism

Hypercortisolism arises from prolonged exposure to elevated levels of either exogenous or endogenous glucocorticoids. Hypersecretion of endogenous glucocorticoids may be the result of an adrenal hyperplasia, adenoma, or adenocarcinoma or it may be due to a pituitary adenoma secreting adrenocorticotrophic hormone (Cushing disease). The increased concentration of glucocorticoid results in a loss of bone mass from reduced osteoblastic function and either directly or indirectly increased osteoclastic function.

Clinical Features

This condition affects females 3 to 5 times as frequently as males, and onset may occur at any age but is usually seen in the third or fourth decades of life. Patients with hypercortisolism often exhibit obesity that spares the extremities and is more pronounced in the face ("moon facies") and upper back ("buffalo hump"). These patients also demonstrate violaceous striae and muscle weakness and may have hypertension and concurrent diabetes.

Imaging Features

Effects on the teeth and jaws. The teeth may erupt prematurely, and partial loss of the lamina dura may occur (Fig. 25.15).

Effects on the skeleton. The altered osteoblastic and osteoclastic activity can result in thinning of the skull, which may be accompanied by a mottled appearance. There may be generalized osteopenia secondary to reduced osteoblastic and increased osteoclastic activity, and the bone may also exhibit a granular pattern as a result of the abnormal formation of numerous short and randomly oriented bone trabeculae. Skeletal osteopenia may also result in fractures.

Progressive Systemic Sclerosis
Disease Mechanism

Progressive systemic sclerosis (PSS) or scleroderma is a generalized connective tissue disease that causes excessive collagen deposition resulting in hardening (sclerosis) of the skin and other tissues. Involvement of the

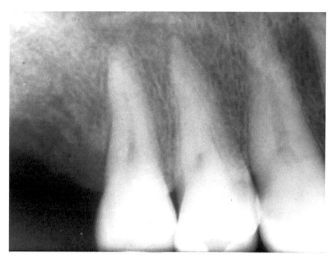

Fig. 25.15 Cushing disease manifested in the jaws as thinning or loss of the lamina dura around the teeth and generalized osteopenia. (Courtesy Dr. H.G. Poyton, Toronto, ON, Canada.)

gastrointestinal tract, heart, lungs, and kidneys usually results in more serious complications. The cause of the disease is unknown.

Clinical Features

PSS is a disease of middle age, with the greatest incidence between 30 and 50 years of age; it is rarely seen in adolescents and elderly adults. Females are affected about three times as often as males.

In most patients with moderate to severe PSS, the involved skin has a thickened, leathery quality that drapes the underlying tissues tightly. Involvement of the facial region may restrict normal mandibular opening. Patients with diffuse disease are also likely to have xerostomia and increased numbers of decayed, missing, or filled teeth. Also, patients are more likely to have deeper periodontal pockets and higher gingivitis scores. Patients with cardiac and pulmonary involvement may have varying degrees of heart failure and respiratory insufficiency. Renal involvement usually leads to some degree of uremia with or without hypertension.

Imaging Features

Effects on the teeth and jaws. The most common manifestation of PSS in images of the jaws is a generalized increase in the width of the PDL spaces around the teeth, with approximately two-thirds of patients exhibiting this feature (Fig. 25.16). The PDL spaces are usually at least twice as wide, although this is more pronounced around the posterior teeth. The lamina dura remains normal. Despite the widening of the PDL spaces, the clinician finds that the involved teeth are often not mobile, and their gingival attachments are usually intact. Almost half of patients with PDL space thickening also have some mandibular erosive bone changes.

A characteristic feature in some cases of PSS is an unusual pattern of mandibular erosion at the sites of masticatory muscle attachment, such as the angles of the mandible, the coronoid processes, the digastric region, and the condylar heads (Fig. 25.17). This type of resorption is typically bilateral and fairly symmetric. Most of these erosive borders are smooth and sharply defined, and the resorption may progress with the disease.

Differential Interpretation

Other causes of PDL space widening include "traumatic occlusion," orthodontic tooth movement, intermaxillary fixation with arch bars,

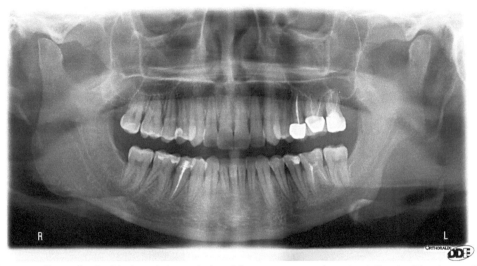

Fig. 25.16 Generalized widening of the periodontal ligament spaces throughout the dentition in a patient with progressive systemic sclerosis. (Courtesy Dr. B. Friedland, Boston, MA.)

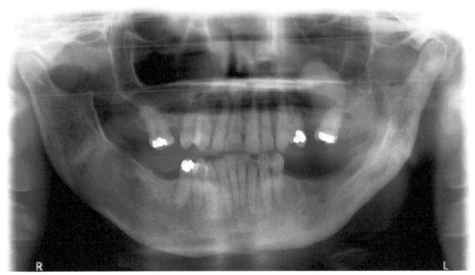

Fig. 25.17 Resorption of the mandibular angles, the insertion sites of the masseter, and medial pterygoid muscles in a patient with progressive systemic sclerosis. (Courtesy Dr. H. Grubisa, Oakville, ON.)

and invasion of the PDL by malignant neoplasms. Widening of the PDL space with malignant neoplasia differs in that it is localized, asymmetric, and accompanied by destruction of the lamina dura.

Management
The progressive loss of bone in the region of the mandibular angle is more serious because of potential fracture. It is reasonable to obtain initial and periodic panoramic images in all patients with PSS to assess mandibular integrity.

Bone Dysplasias
Disease Mechanism
Bone dysplasias include a group of conditions in which normal bone is replaced with fibrous connective tissue and abnormal, immature bone (Fig. 25.18). Although the mechanism is not well understood, it has been hypothesized that osteoblast and osteoclast function becomes dysregulated, favoring one cell type's activity over the other. It is important to understand

that in the context of bone, the term "dysplasia" does not imply that the process is premalignant. This is in stark contrast to the use of the term in the context of epithelium. Furthermore, bone dysplasias are not neoplasms and therefore should not be managed like a neoplasm.

Cemento-Osseous Dysplasia
Disease Mechanism
The cemento-osseous dysplasias are disease processes whereby one or more focal areas of normal bone metabolism are altered and cancellous bone is replaced by a mixture of fibrous connective tissue containing varying amounts of immature, abnormal bone. Periapical cemento-osseous dysplasia (PCOD) is the more localized form, affecting one sextant of the jaws, while florid cemento-osseous dysplasia (FCOD) is the more generalized form. No clear definition exists as to when multiple foci of PCOD should be termed FCOD. However, if multiple sextants of the jaws are involved, it is usually considered FCOD. In some cases a familial trend can be seen in FCOD. As the lesions mature and more abnormal

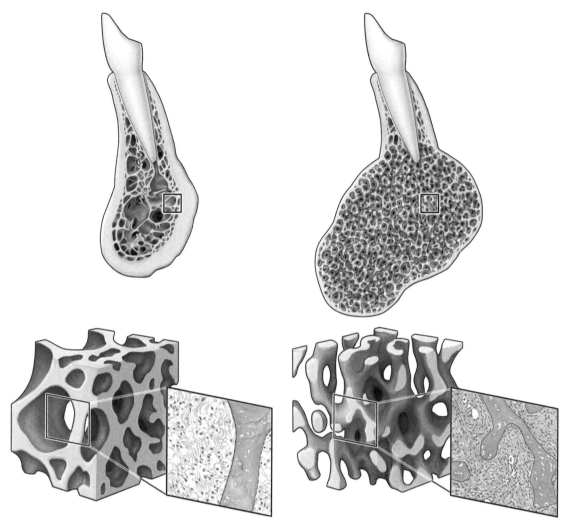

Fig. 25.18 Dysplastic Lesions of Bone Alter the Normal Bone Architecture. Normal bone is replaced by fibrous connective tissue and numerous short, irregularly shaped trabeculae.

bone is deposited, the vascular supply can be compromised—a condition that likely contributes to its increased susceptibility to infection.

Lesions of cemento-osseous dysplasia occur in the periapical areas of the teeth. The replacement process undergoes three stages: in the first, the normal bone is resorbed and in the second and third the new bone is deposited in increasing amounts, first centrally and then more peripherally within the resorptive area.

Clinical Features

PCOD is a common bone dysplasia that typically occurs during the fourth and fifth decades of life. It occurs more often in women than men and commonly affects non-Caucasian populations. Lesions of PCOD are often identified as incidental findings on images made for other purposes. The pulps of the involved teeth are vital, and the patient usually has no history of pain or sensitivity. In some patients, the lesions can become quite large, causing a notable expansion of the alveolar process and thinning of adjacent cortices. The lesions may continue to enlarge slowly. Occasionally patients may note the development of a swelling or an area of low-grade, intermittent, poorly localized pain, especially when a simple bone cyst has developed within the lesion. Extensive lesions often have an associated bony swelling.

Should lesions of FCOD become secondarily infected, some of the features of osteomyelitis may develop; these may include mucosal ulceration and fistulous tracts with suppuration and pain. Histopathologically FCOD that has been secondarily infected has been diagnosed as osteomyelitis, particularly when the lesions are in their most mature, radiopaque states. If osteomyelitis is suspected, a cone beam computed tomography (CBCT) or multidetector computed tomography (MDCT) examination should be ordered to determine the extent of involvement.

Imaging Features

Location. The epicenter of an cemento-osseous dysplasia lesion is located in the periapical areas of the teeth, within the alveolar processes of the jaws (Fig. 25.19). In rare cases, the epicenter is located slightly more coronally and may be nearer to the apical third of the root. In the mandible, the epicenters of the lesions are located superior to the inferior alveolar canal.

PCOD may be multiple and bilateral, but occasionally a solitary lesion arises. FCOD lesions are usually bilateral and present in both jaws (Fig. 25.20). However, when they are present in only one jaw, the mandible is the more common location. If the involved tooth is extracted, this lesion can still develop, but the periapical location is less clear (Fig. 25.21).

Periphery. In most cases, the periphery of a PCOD lesion is well defined, and the cortex can vary in width to the point of appearing sclerotic. Internally there may be a variably wide radiolucent rim surrounding the radiopaque center, which sometimes may be difficult to

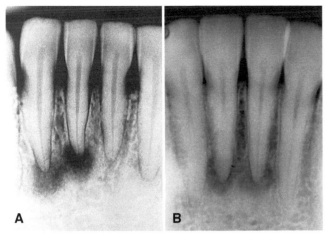

Fig. 25.19 Periapical images of early lesions of periapical cemento-osseous dysplasia showing loss of the periodontal ligament spaces around the root apices of some anterior teeth (A) and retention of the periodontal ligament space in another patient (B).

visualize in mature lesions (Fig. 25.22). As the lesions mature, a band of variably thick, almost sclerotic bone can appear. The lesion may be irregularly shaped or may have an overall round or oval shape centered at the apex of the tooth.

Internal structure. The internal appearance of PCOD can vary, depending on the degree of maturity of the lesion. In the early stage, normal bone is resorbed and replaced with fibrous connective tissue that is usually continuous with the PDL space (causing loss of the lamina dura). This appears as a radiolucency at the apex of the involved tooth (see Fig. 25.19).

In the second, more mature stage, radiopaque foci appear within the center of the radiolucent zone, and these can vary in their appearance from small oval and circular regions (cotton-wool appearance) to large, irregular, amorphous areas of calcification. Sometimes the bone forms a swirling pattern (see Fig. 25.22), whereas in other cases the radiopaque pattern resembles the abnormal trabecular patterns seen in fibrous dysplasia (Fig. 25.23). The internal density of larger FCOD lesions can vary from an equal mixture of radiolucent and radiopaque regions to almost complete radiopacity. Some prominent radiolucent regions may

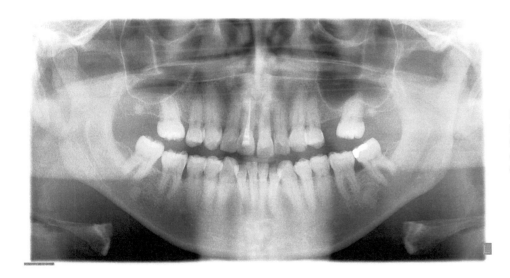

Fig. 25.20 Panoramic Image Showing Four Small Foci of Mature Florid Cemento-Osseous Dysplasia. Note the appearance of the peripheral radiolucent border encircling the dysplastic bone.

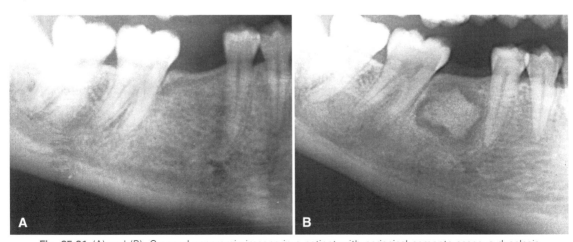

Fig. 25.21 (A) and (B), Cropped panoramic images in a patient with periapical cemento-osseous dysplasia (PCOD) made 3 years apart. Note the interval development of a solitary lesion of PCOD in the edentulous first molar area.

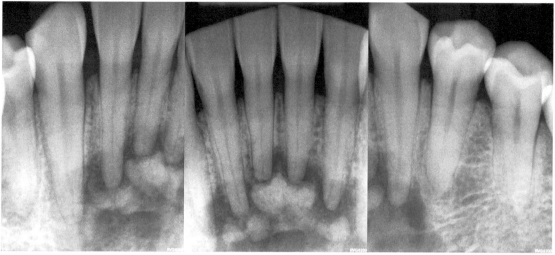

Fig. 25.22 The mixed radiolucent and radiopaque appearance of a more mature stage of periapical cemento-osseous dysplasia. Note the radiolucent rim encircling the radiopaque foci of dysplastic bone.

be present, which usually represent the development of a simple bone cyst (Fig. 25.24). These cysts may enlarge with time even beyond the boundary of the lesion into the surrounding normal bone or may fill in with abnormal dysplastic bone.

In the third and most mature stage, the internal pattern may be completely radiopaque without any obvious pattern. A variably wide radiolucent border can usually be seen at the periphery of the radiopacity because the lesion mineralizes from the center to the periphery (Fig. 25.25). Occasionally this radiolucent margin is not apparent, which makes the differential interpretation more difficult. The internal structure may appear dramatically radiolucent if a simple bone cyst (Fig. 25.26) develops in association with cemento-osseous dysplasia; in some cases the simple bone cyst may extend beyond the original border of the cemento-osseous dysplasia.

Effects on adjacent structures. Some lesions stimulate a sclerotic bone reaction from the surrounding bone. Small lesions do not expand the jawbone; however, larger lesions can cause expansion of the jaw (Fig. 25.27). In such cases, a thin intact outer cortex can be visualized similar to that seen in fibrous dysplasia. The surface of the expanded bone is not usually fusiform as in fibrous dysplasia but rather undulating. Lesions of cemento-osseous dysplasia can displace the floor of the maxillary sinus superiorly. When large enough, they can displace the inferior alveolar canal inferiorly and cause enlargement of the alveolar bone by displacement of the buccal and lingual cortical plates.

Effects on adjacent teeth. The lamina dura around the involved area of the tooth roots of teeth involved with the lesion is lost, making the PDL space either less apparent or apparently wider (see Fig. 25.19). The tooth structure is usually not affected, although roots may develop hypercementosis, particularly in FCOD, making extraction difficult.

Differential Interpretation

Early lesions of PCOD are radiolucent, and the most important differential interpretation is rarefying osteitis. Occasionally PCOD cannot be distinguished from this inflammatory lesion by radiologic characteristics alone. In these cases, the final diagnosis must rely on clinical information, such as testing of the vitality of the involved tooth pulp.

In the case of a solitary, mature lesion of PCOD, the differential interpretation may include a cementoblastoma, especially when periapical to a mandibular first molar tooth. This tumor is usually attached to the surface of the root, which may be partially resorbed. Also, the peripheral radiolucency may be better defined in cementoblastoma, and there may

be a unique pattern to the internal structure, such as a radiating pattern. Expansion of the bone caused by the tumor is more concentric, without the surface undulation seen in PCOD. The presence or absence of clinical symptoms may help to distinguish PCOD from cementoblastoma. Another lesion to consider is an odontoma. Although odontomas often arise occlusal to a tooth and prevent its eruption, some odontomas may have a periapical position. The appearance of tooth-like structures and the identification of enamel (which is very radiopaque) can help in the differential interpretation. Also, the peripheral cortex of an odontoma is often better defined, and the internal radiolucent periphery is more uniform in width. Mature PCOD lesions may resemble a dense bone island. The appearance of a radiolucent periphery in PCOD, even if very slight, points to PCOD. Solitary lesions, particularly those that expand the bone, may be difficult to differentiate from cemento-ossifying fibroma.

The fact that FCOD is bilateral and centered in the alveolar processes helps in differentiating it from other lesions. Paget disease of bone may also display cotton-wool radiopaque regions with associated hypercementosis. However, Paget disease affects the bone of the entire mandible, is more focal, and located superior to the inferior alveolar canal. Furthermore, Paget disease of bone is often polyostotic, involving other bones as well as the jaws. The well-defined nature of FCOD, with its radiolucent periphery and surrounding sclerotic border, is also useful in making the differential diagnosis. Another disease that may resemble FCOD is osteomyelitis, particularly if large areas of sclerosis develop. The radiopaque foci in FCOD may appear similar to the sequestra seen in osteomyelitis. This should not, however, be confused with a situation where FCOD has become secondarily infected, resulting in osteomyelitis. The foci of an amorphous bone that has become secondarily infected have a wider and more profound radiolucent border (Fig. 25.28). CBCT or MDCT imaging is essential for the diagnosis and to determine the extent of the osteomyelitis within the FCOD.

Management

The interpretation of cemento-osseous dysplasia can be made on the basis of the appropriate radiologic features and clinical findings. The cemento-osseous dysplasias do not require treatment, although there is value in obtaining a panoramic image to establish the extent of the disease. Because of the propensity for the most mature lesions to become secondarily infected, the patient should be encouraged to maintain an effective oral hygiene program to avoid odontogenic infections and bone loss due to periodontal disease. However, if the teeth have been

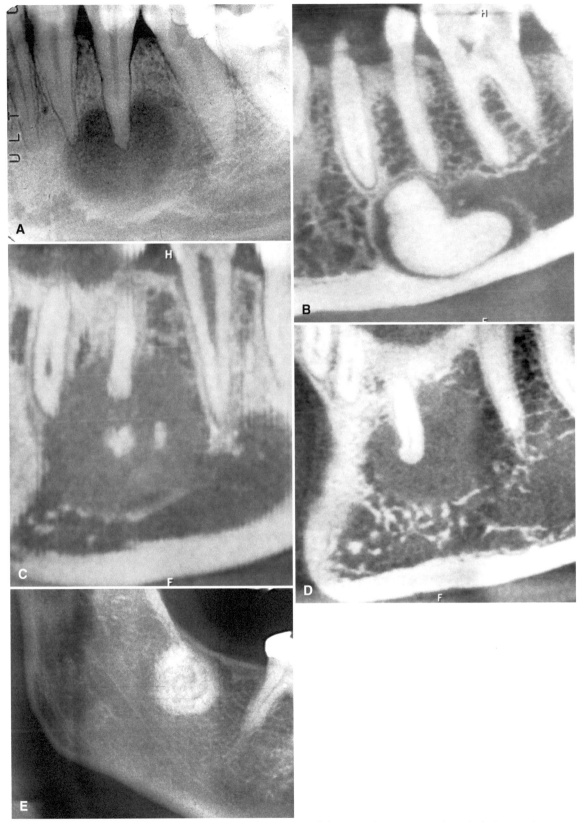

Fig. 25.23 The ground-glass internal pattern is a variant of the normal pattern seen in periapical cemento-osseous dysplasia (A). Sagittal cone beam computed tomography images of variations of internal patterns of periapical cemento-osseous dysplasia. These may range from a homogeneous amorphous bone pattern (B), to a mix of fine granular bone with two foci of amorphous bone (C), to a totally granular pattern (D). A cropped panoramic image shows a swirling internal pattern of periapical cemento-osseous dysplasia (E).

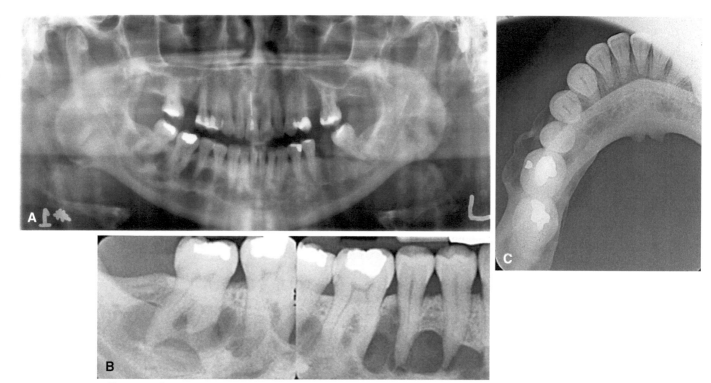

Fig. 25.24 Panoramic image (A) shows simple bone cysts developing with florid cemento-osseous dysplasia. The scalloping feature around the roots of the molar teeth in the right mandible is very characteristic of simple bone cyst (B). The cross-sectional occlusal image (C) shows the change in the buccal surface of the mandible induced by the simple bone cyst.

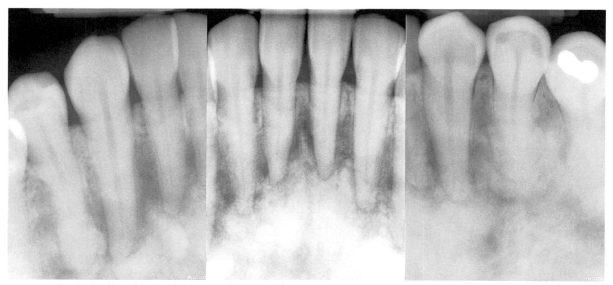

Fig. 25.25 Very Mature Lesions of Periapical Cemento-osseous Dysplasia. The radiopaque component dominates the images and the radiolucent periphery is very thin.

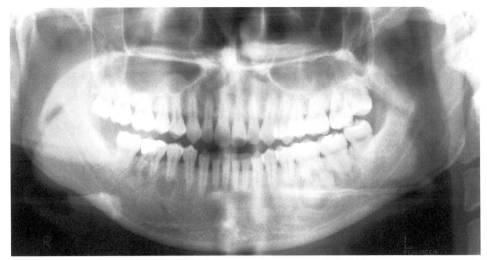

Fig. 25.26 Panoramic Image Showing Multiple Stages of Maturation of Florid Cemento-osseous Dysplasia. A simple bone cyst is developing at the apex of the mandibular right second premolar. (Courtesy Dr. C. Poon-Woo, Toronto, ON, Canada.)

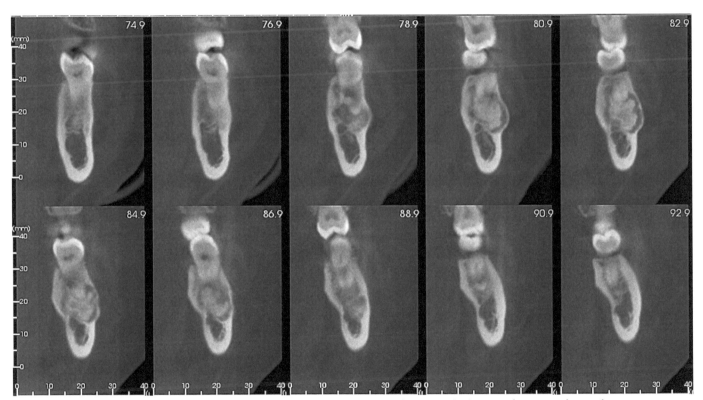

Fig. 25.27 Buccal lingual cross-sectional cone beam computed tomography images of a mature focus of periapical cemento-osseous dysplasia causing expansion of the buccal cortex of the mandible.

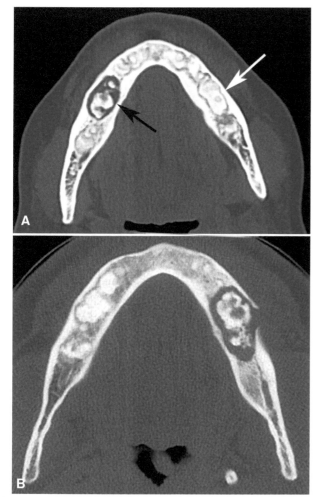

Fig. 25.28 Axial Multidetector Computed Tomography Images of Florid Cemento-osseous Dysplasia. Note the radiolucent rim *(white arrow)* on the patient's left side around a mature focus of dysplastic bone and the focus on the right side with a more pronounced radiolucent border (A). The latter appearance suggests that the focus is secondarily infected *(black arrow)*. A different case (B) of osteomyelitis caused by a secondarily infected focus of cemento-osseous dysplasia. Note the discontinuity of buccal cortex where the lesion is draining into the adjacent soft tissues.

removed and if considerable atrophy of the alveolar ridge has occurred, these foci of dysplastic bone may reach the mucosal surface, much in the same way stones become exposed in old worn concrete. These foci of abnormal bone can perforate the mucosa, particularly when located under a denture, and can become secondarily infected. If osteomyelitis occurs, the avascular foci of amorphous bone become large sequestra. The osteomyelitis may spread slowly throughout the jaw from one region of FCOD to another, and the infection may spread to adjacent areas. Biopsy of lesions of cemento-osseous dysplasia is not required, although a possible complication is secondary infection following biopsy.

Fibrous Dysplasia
Disease Mechanism
Fibrous dysplasia is a disease process wherein normal bone metabolism is altered, and cancellous bone is replaced by a mixture of fibrous connective tissue containing varying amounts of immature, abnormal bone. Recently mutations of the *GNAS1* gene, located on the long arm of chromosome 20 at position 13.32, have been detected in 93% of cases of fibrous dysplasia tested. At the histopathologic level, the result is the appearance of numerous short, irregularly shaped trabeculae of woven bone. Unlike normal bone,

where trabeculae are oriented in response to stresses and strains placed on the bone, trabeculae in fibrous dysplasia are oriented randomly. Compared with normal bone, there are more trabeculae per unit volume within the cancellous component of the involved bone.

Clinical Features
Fibrous dysplasia commonly affects the skeleton unilaterally, and can affect multiple bones in the body. The most common sites include the ribs, femur, tibia, maxilla, and mandible. The solitary or monostotic form of fibrous dysplasia accounts for approximately 70% of all cases and is the most commonly identified type in the jaws. *Polyostotic fibrous dysplasia* is the term given to the disease process when multiple bones are affected. When polyostotic fibrous dysplasia is accompanied by cutaneous pigmentation (café au lait spots), the disease entity is referred to as *the Jaffe type*. And when polyostotic involvement is accompanied by café au lait spots and endocrine hyperfunction abnormalities, this is termed *McCune-Albright syndrome*.

Polyostotic fibrous dysplasia is usually found in children younger than 10 years of age, whereas monostotic disease is typically discovered in a slightly older age group. The lesions usually become static when skeletal growth ceases, but bone changes may continue, particularly in the polyostotic form. Furthermore, lesions may become active during pregnancy or with the use of oral contraceptives. Studies of the sex distribution of fibrous dysplasia show no sexual predilection except for McCune-Albright syndrome, which affects females almost exclusively.

Symptoms of fibrous dysplasia may be absent or mild, depending on the degree of involvement. Monostotic fibrous dysplasia is often discovered as an incidental finding in dental diagnostic images made for other purposes. Patients with jaw involvement may first complain of unilateral facial swelling or an enlarging deformity of the alveolar process. Pain and pathologic fractures are rare. If craniofacial lesions involve the skull base, the bone changes may impinge on neural foramina, and peripheral sensorineural deficits may arise.

Imaging Features
Location. Fibrous dysplasia affects the maxilla almost twice as often as the mandible and is more frequently seen in the more posterior regions of the jaw. Lesions in the axial skeleton are more commonly unilateral (Fig. 25.29), but when fibrous dysplasia affects a single midline bone such as the mandible or the frontal or sphenoid bones, the changes can cross the midline. This pattern has led some to characterize lesions in the head and neck as craniofacial fibrous dysplasia.

Periphery. The periphery of fibrous dysplasia lesions is most commonly poorly defined, with a gradual and broad transition between the dysplastic and normal bone. Some refer to this broad zone of transition as "blending" of the fibrous dysplastic bone into the normal trabecular pattern. Occasionally the boundary between the dysplastic and normal bone can appear better defined and even corticated, especially in young lesions (Fig. 25.30).

Internal structure. The density and internal pattern of fibrous dysplasia lesions vary considerably, with the variation being more pronounced in the mandible and more homogeneous in the maxilla. The internal density of the dysplastic bone may be radiolucent, radiopaque, or a mixture of both compared with normal bone. Early lesions may be more radiolucent (Fig. 25.31) than mature lesions. In the maxilla and skull base, where the bone changes tend to be more homogeneous, the bone may appear more radiopaque. In the mandible, where the lesions may be more heterogeneous, one may appreciate granular internal septa, giving a multilocular appearance to the abnormal bone.

The abnormal trabeculae are usually shorter, thinner, and more irregularly shaped. In addition, these may be more numerous in number than the normal trabeculae they are replacing. These changes create a

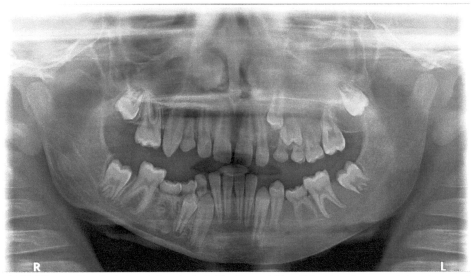

Fig. 25.29 Fibrous Dysplasia Involving the Left Maxilla and Mandible. Note the ground-glass bone pattern in both bones as well as the expansion of the left maxillary tuberosity and the inferior surface of the mandible. (Courtesy Dr. H. Grubisa, Oakville, ON, Canada.)

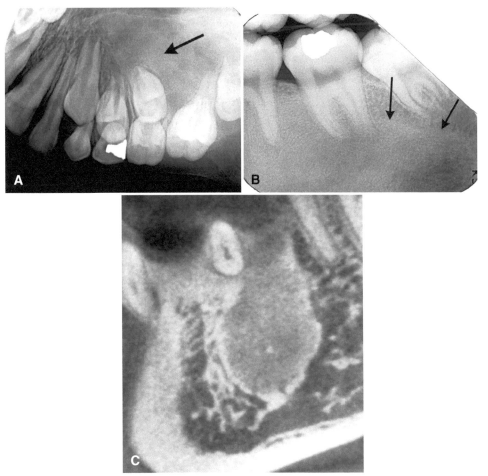

Fig. 25.30 This dysplastic granular bone pattern blends into the adjacent normal bone pattern in the region of the unerupted maxillary canine (A). In contrast (B), the border in this case of fibrous dysplasia of the mandible has a better-defined, almost corticated border *(arrows)*. This sagittal cone beam computed tomography image of a small focus of fibrous dysplasia (C) has a border that appears more definitively corticated.

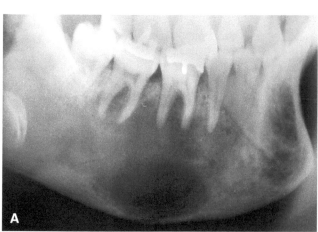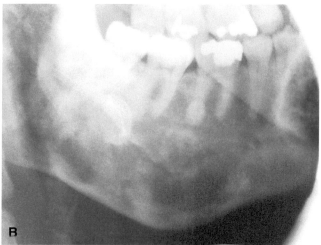

Fig. 25.31 Cropped panoramic images showing an earlier, more radiolucent stage of fibrous dysplasia (A) and, after 18 years, a more radiopaque appearance (B).

series of classical radiologic patterns that can be seen in fibrous dysplasia (Fig. 25.32). The patterns can include an appearance referred to as granular or ground-glass, resembling the appearance of sand-blasted or etched glass. Another common pattern is one that resembles the surface texture of a citrus fruit, particularly an orange—*peau d'orange*. And still a third pattern has a wispy arrangement that resembles loose to dense cotton. A distinctive characteristic is the organization of the abnormal trabeculae into a swirling pattern similar to a fingerprint. Occasionally radiolucent regions may occur in mature lesions of fibrous dysplasia; these are simple bone cysts (Fig. 25.33).

Effects on adjacent structures. When a lesion of fibrous dysplasia is small, it may have no effect on surrounding structures, and this is referred to as subclinical fibrous dysplasia. As the lesion increases in size, bone expansion results, with maintenance of a thinned cortex (Fig. 25.34). In the mandible, this pattern of enlargement affects the bone more evenly along its length; this is referred to as fusiform enlargement. This pattern of enlargement should be contrasted with the more concentric type of expansion seen with benign tumors.

Fibrous dysplasia arising in the maxilla can displace the cortical borders of the maxillary sinus, reducing the size of the air cavity. The lateral wall of the maxillary sinus is often the first to be impacted; the last region of the sinus to be involved is usually the most posterosuperior border. A characteristic of involvement of the maxilla and maxillary sinus, in particular, is a miniaturized airspace that approximates the normal anatomic shape of the antrum (Fig. 25.35).

Cortical boundaries, such as the floor of the antrum, may also become less distinct when the dysplastic bone involves the bone cortex. And when the growth epicenter of fibrous dysplasia occurs inferior to the inferior alveolar canal, it may displace the canal in a superior direction (see Fig. 25.35).

Effects on adjacent teeth. Often the bone surrounding the teeth is altered without affecting the dentition, and a distinct lamina dura disappears as the dysplastic bone engages this structure (see Fig. 25.32). If the fibrous dysplasia increases the bone density, the PDL space may appear to be narrow. Fibrous dysplasia can displace teeth or interfere with normal eruption, complicating orthodontic therapy. In rare cases, some root resorption or hypercementosis may occur.

Differential Interpretation

Other disease processes can alter bone patterns in a manner that is similar to fibrous dysplasia. The ground-glass appearance is often seen where there has been healing by secondary intention, when immature new bone grows into the connective tissue matrix of granulation tissue. Commonly this may be seen following tooth extraction or orthograde endodontic treatment of a lesion of rarefying osteitis. Occasionally PCOD may show a similar bone pattern, but these lesions are often multifocal and bilateral, with an epicenter in the periapical area of the tooth. PCOD also occurs in an older age group. Healing of a simple bone cyst may also create a similar pattern; indeed, both the histopathologic and radiologic appearances of the bone may mimic that which is seen in fibrous dysplasia.

Metabolic bone diseases such as hyperparathyroidism may produce a ground-glass type of pattern in the bone, however these lesions are often bilateral and polyostotic and, unlike fibrous dysplasia, do not cause bone expansion. Paget disease of bone may produce a cotton-wool type of pattern, and there may be expansion with bilateral bone involvement.

Of paramount importance is the differentiation of osteomyelitis, cemento-ossifying fibroma, and osteosarcoma from fibrous dysplasia. Although these four entities can have very similar histopathologic and radiologic appearances, their management is dramatically different. Whereas osteomyelitis may cause a bone to enlarge, the additional bone is generated at the bone surface by the periosteum. The new bone that is laid down on the surface of the outer cortex in osteomyelitis may reveal evidence of the original cortex and lamellar periosteal new bone formation. In contrast, fibrous dysplasia enlarges the bone from the inside, displacing and thinning the outer cortex as the bone grows so that the remaining cortex maintains its position at the outer surface of the bone. The identification of sequestra aids in the differentiation of osteomyelitis from fibrous dysplasia. Osteosarcoma may produce a similar internal pattern depending on the degree of differentiation of the malignant osteoblasts, but it should show other malignant and more aggressive radiologic features (see Chapter 26). Some difficulty may arise in differentiating ossifying fibroma of the maxilla, especially the juvenile type of ossifying fibroma. Cemento-ossifying fibroma grows in a more concentric manner. If the bone pattern is altered around the teeth, and the teeth are displaced from a specific epicenter, the lesion is likely ossifying fibroma rather than fibrous dysplasia. In the maxilla, the shape of the enlarged bone of fibrous dysplasia adjacent to the antrum maintains the contour of the antral wall, which is different from the more convex pattern of expansion of a neoplasm.

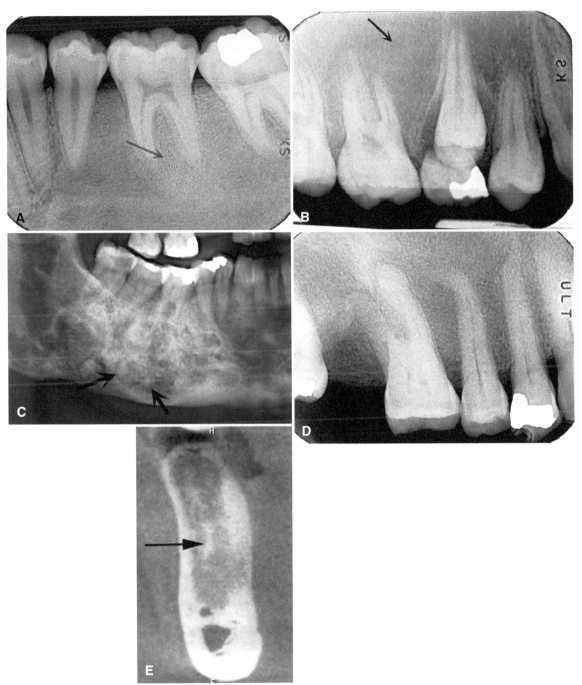

Fig. 25.32 A Series of Images Showing the Range of Internal Patterns of Fibrous Dysplasia. A periapical image (A) shows the fingerprint-like pattern around the roots of the first molar *(arrow)*. Note the change in the lamina dura around the molars into the abnormal bone pattern. A periapical image (B) shows a granular or ground-glass pattern *(arrow)*. The cropped panoramic image (C) shows a more heterogeneous cotton-wool pattern. Note the almost circular radiopaque regions *(arrows)*. The periapical image (D) shows the more stippled orange-peel pattern. A buccolingual cone beam computed tomography image (E) shows a granular internal bone pattern with strands of more amorphous bone *(arrow)*.

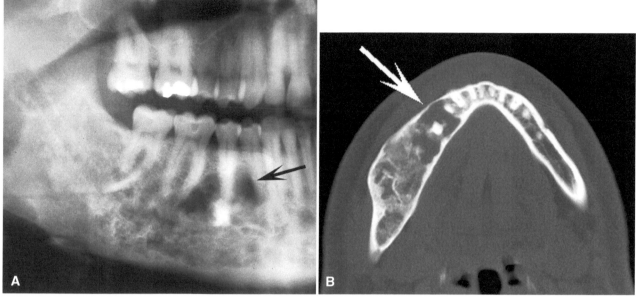

Fig. 25.33 Cropped panoramic (A) and axial mutlidetector computed tomography (B) images showing a simple bone cyst developing within a focus of fibrous dysplasia *(arrow).*

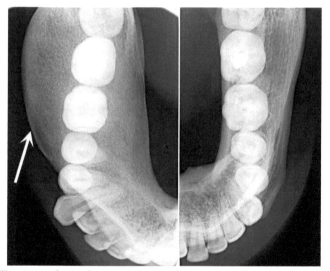

Fig. 25.34 Cross-Sectional Occlusal Images of Both Sides of the Mandible of the Same Patient. Note the expansion of the right side of the mandible, which is caused by fibrous dysplasia. The buccal surface of the mandible has been displaced, and the cortex has been thinned but is still intact *(arrow).*

Management

In most cases, the clinical and radiologic features of fibrous dysplasia are sufficient to allow the practitioner to make a diagnosis without a biopsy. However, consultation with an oral and maxillofacial radiologist is advisable. The radiologist may supplement a conventional imaging examination with CBCT or MDCT, so that features not seen on plain imaging may become more apparent. Such an examination may also serve as a precise baseline for future comparisons.

It is reasonable to continue occasional monitoring of the lesion or ask the patient to report any changes. With many lesions, bone enlargement slows at skeletal maturation; orthodontic treatment and cosmetic surgery may be delayed until this time. Sarcomatous changes are unusual but have been reported, especially if radiation therapy has been administered.

Paget Disease of Bone
Disease Mechanism

Paget disease of bone, or osteitis deformans, is a polyostotic skeletal disorder that may involve a paramyxovirus infection and subsequent changes to the host cell genome. Mutations have been identified in three genes involved in bone remodeling: *SQSTM1*, *TNFRSF11A*, and *TNFRSF11B*. Of these, the most commonly identified mutation involves the *SQSTM1* gene. Abnormal osteoclasts produce an intense wave of bone resorption; after a period of time, this is followed by vigorous osteoblastic activity, forming poor-quality woven bone. The disease may involve many bones simultaneously, but it is not a generalized skeletal disease.

Clinical Features

Paget disease of bone is seen most frequently in Great Britain and Australia and less often in North America; it has an incidence of approximately 3.5% of individuals above 40 years of age. At age 65, the incidence of involvement in men is approximately twice that in women.

The affected bone is enlarged and commonly deformed because of the poor quality of bone formation. This can result in bowing of the legs, curvature of the spine, and enlargement of the skull. Also, there is enlargement of the jaws, which can cause tooth movement, diastema, and malocclusion. Dentures may become tight or may fit poorly in edentulous patients.

Bone pain is an inconsistent symptom and is most often directed toward the weight-bearing bones; facial or jaw pain is uncommon. Patients with Paget disease of bone may also have ill-defined sensorineural pain due to the impingement neural foramina and canals. They also often have severely elevated levels of serum alkaline phosphatase (greater than with any other disorder) during osteoblastic phases of the disease. These patients also often have high levels of hydroxyproline in the urine; a marker of collagen degradation.

Imaging Features

Location. Paget disease of bone occurs most often in the pelvis, femur, skull (Figs. 25.36 and 25.37), and vertebrae and infrequently in the jaws. Whenever the jaws are involved, the maxilla is affected approximately twice as often as the mandible. Although disease involvement is generally

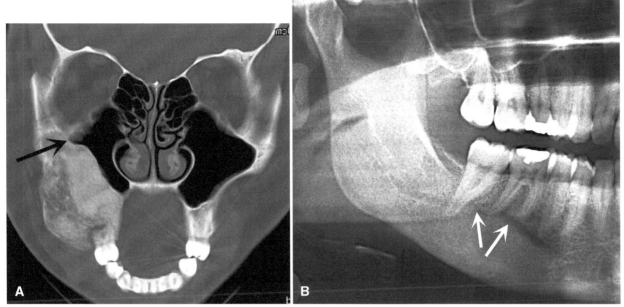

Fig. 25.35 Coronal multidetector computed tomography image of a region of fibrous dysplasia in the right maxilla (A) shows nonconcentric expansion of the lateral surface of the maxilla and the residual airspace within the maxillary sinus. Note that the right maxillary sinus appears as a smaller version of the unaffected left maxillary sinus and the retained right zygomatic recess *(arrow)*. The cropped panoramic image (B) shows superior displacement of the inferior alveolar nerve canal by a focus of fibrous dysplasia *(arrows)*.

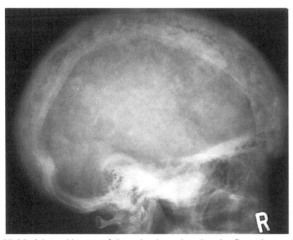

Fig. 25.36 A lateral image of the calvarium showing the flocculent cotton-wool appearance of the bone and substantial thickening of the skull bones. (Courtesy Dr. K. Dolan, Iowa City, IA.)

bilateral, occasionally only one maxilla is involved or the involvement may be significantly greater on one side. In the mandible, the entire bone is usually involved.

Internal structure. The internal appearance of the bone is variable and depends on the developmental stage of the disease. The overall density of the jaws may decrease or increase, depending on the number of trabeculae. Classically, Paget disease of bone has three radiographic stages, although these may often overlap. In the early stage of primarily osteoclastic activity, the bone appears radiolucent. In the intermediate stage of the disease, granular or ground-glass–patterned bone appears within the radiolucent areas. Finally, in the most mature stage, the bone becomes dense and radiopaque. These stages are less apparent in the jaws.

The trabeculae are altered in number and shape. In the early stage, they are decreased. During the intermediate and late stages, the trabeculae may become elongated and align themselves in a linear pattern—an appearance that is more common in the mandible. Trabeculae may be short, with random orientations, and may have a granular pattern similar to that which is seen in fibrous dysplasia. A third pattern occurs when the trabeculae are organized into rounded, radiopaque patches of abnormal bone, creating a cotton-wool appearance (Fig. 25.38).

Effects on adjacent structures. Paget disease of bone always enlarges an affected bone to some extent, even in the early stage. Often the bone enlargement is impressive. Prominent pagetic skull bones may increase to three or four times their normal thickness. In enlarged jaws, the cortex may be thinned but remains intact; it may have a laminated appearance in occlusal images (see Fig. 25.38). When the maxilla is involved, the disease invariably involves the sinus floor. However, the airspace is usually not diminished to a great extent. The sinus floor may appear more granular and less apparent as sharp boundaries.

Effects on adjacent teeth. The lamina dura may become less evident and may be altered into the abnormal bone pattern. Hypercementosis often develops on a few or most of the teeth in the involved jaw. This hypercementosis may be exuberant and irregular, which is characteristic of Paget disease (Fig. 25.39).

Differential Interpretation

Paget disease of bone may appear similar to fibrous dysplasia; however, the disease occurs in an older age group and is almost always bilateral. In the maxilla, fibrous dysplasia has a tendency to encroach on the sinus airspace, whereas Paget disease does not. The linear trabeculae and cotton-wool appearance of Paget disease are distinctive. Lesions of osseous dysplasia are more focal and less generalized than Paget disease of bone, and there are areas of normal intervening bone between the foci of osseous dysplasia. The cemento-osseous dysplasias may also have an internal cotton-wool pattern, but these lesions are centered

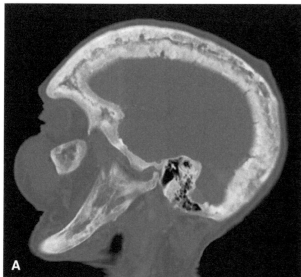

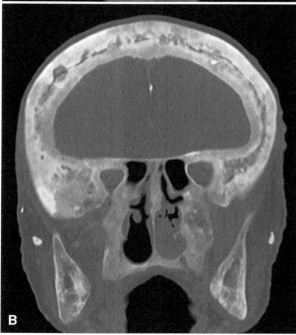

Fig. 25.37 Sagittal (A) and coronal (B) multidetector computed tomography images in a patient with Paget disease of bone. Note increase in thickness of the bones and the bone density.

There are complications of this disease that are of concern. Extraction sites heal slowly, and the incidence of osteomyelitis is higher. Approximately 10% of cases with polyostotic disease develop osteosarcoma.

Sickle Cell Anemia
Disease Mechanism
Sickle cell anemia is an autosomal recessive chronic hemolytic blood disorder. Patients have abnormal hemoglobin that, under low oxygen tension, results in a change to the morphology of the red blood cells, causing them to acquire the shape of a sickle. In addition, red blood cells have a reduced capacity to carry oxygen to tissues; they adhere to vascular endothelial cells and obstruct capillaries because of damage to their membrane lipids and proteins. The spleen traps and readily destroys these abnormal red blood cells, resulting in anemia. The hematopoietic system responds to the resultant anemia by increasing the production of red blood cells by inducing a compensatory hyperplasia of the bone marrow in regions of the skeleton that no longer have the capacity for this to occur.

Clinical Features
The homozygous recessive genotype of sickle cell anemia occurs in approximately 1 in every 400 African-Americans. Although the heterozygous genotype is present in about 6% to 8% of African-Americans, these individuals do not show related clinical findings.

The signs and symptoms of sickle cell anemia vary considerably, and most patients with the disease normally manifest mild, chronic features. Prolonged, quiet episodes of hemolytic quiescence occur, occasionally punctuated by exacerbations known as sickle cell crises. During the crisis state, patients often have severe abdominal, muscle and joint pain and a high temperature; they may also experience circulatory collapse. During milder periods, a patient may complain of fatigue, weakness, shortness of breath, and muscle and joint pain. As in other chronic anemias, the heart is usually enlarged, and a murmur may be present. The disease occurs mostly in children and adolescents, and although it is compatible with a normal life span, many patients die of complications of the disease before the age of 40 years.

Imaging Features
The hyperplasia of the bone marrow at the expense of cancellous bone is the primary reason for the abnormal manifestations of sickle cell anemia seen in diagnostic images. The extent of bone changes in sickle cell anemia relates to the degree of this hyperplasia.

Effects on the teeth and jaws. The manifestations of sickle cell anemia in the jaws include generalized osteopenia. Osteopenia occurs because of a decrease in the volume of trabecular bone and, to a lesser extent, thinning of the cortical plates as the jawbones are recruited to produce new red blood cells. In most cases, the change is mild or moderate; extreme manifestations are unusual.

Images of the jaws of children with sickle cell anemia have been reported to show a high frequency of severe osteopenia. The bone pattern may be altered to one with fewer but coarser trabeculae. Rarely, bone marrow hyperplasia may cause enlargement and protrusion of the maxillary alveolar ridge.

Effects on the skeleton. The thinning of individual cancellous trabeculae and cortices is most common in the vertebral bodies, long bones, skull, and jaws. The skull may show widening of the diploic space and thinning of the inner and outer cortices (Fig. 25.40). In extreme cases (5%), the surface cortex of the skull is not apparent, and a "hair-on-end" appearance may occur as a compensatory change to increase the volume of bone available to produce new red blood cells. Small areas of infarction may be present within bones after blockage of the microvasculature; these are seen as areas of localized bone sclerosis.

above the inferior alveolar nerve canal, and a radiolucent internal periphery may be appreciated. The bone pattern in Paget disease of bone may show some similarities to the bone pattern in metabolic bone diseases, and both conditions may be bilateral. However, Paget disease enlarges bone, and metabolic diseases do not. The specific bone pattern changes, the late age of onset, the enlargement of the involved bone, and the extreme elevation of serum alkaline phosphatase aid in the differential diagnosis.

Management
Paget disease of bone is usually managed medically, using calcitonin or, more recently, bisphosphonates. The medication relieves pain and reduces the serum alkaline phosphatase levels and osteoclastic activity. Surgery may be required to correct deformities of the long bones and treat fractures.

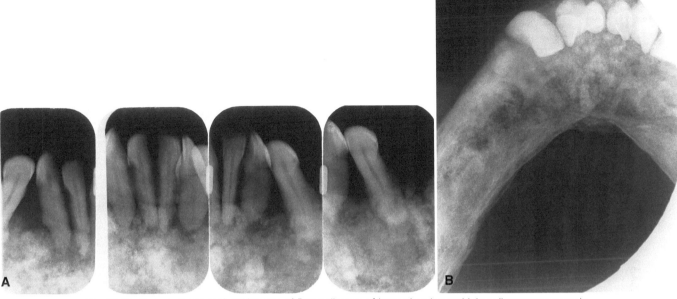

Fig. 25.38 Periapical and occlusal images of Paget disease of bone showing multiple radiopaque masses in the mandible with a cotton-wool appearance (A) and mandibular expansion (B). Note maintenance of the thin cortices on the occlusal image.

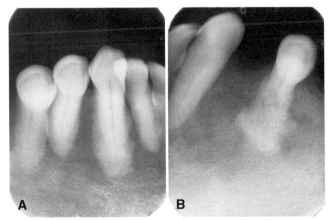

Fig. 25.39 Two periapical images Paget disease of bone showing exuberant hypercementosis of the roots.

Osteomyelitis may complicate sickle cell anemia if infection begins in an area of pronounced hypovascularity. There also may be retardation of generalized bone growth.

Management

Management of patients with sickle cell anemia is supportive and aims to control the symptoms and prevent the complications of this multisystem disease. Bone marrow transplantation is a curative option, but its applicability is limited because of the associated risks.

Thalassemia
Disease Mechanism

Thalassemia or Mediterranean anemia is a hereditary disorder that results in a defect in either the α-globulin or β-globulin genes. The resultant red blood cells have reduced hemoglobin content, are thin, and have a shortened life span. The heterozygous form of the disease (thalassemia minor) is mild, whereas the homozygous form (thalassemia

major) may be severe. A less severe form, thalassemia intermedia, also occurs. As in sickle cell anemia, the result is hyperplasia of the bone marrow component of bone, which results in fewer trabeculae per unit area and can change the overall shape of the bone.

Clinical Features

In the severe form of the disease, the onset is in infancy and the survival time may be short. The face develops prominent cheekbones and a protrusive premaxilla, resulting in a "rodent-like" face. The milder form of the disease occurs in adults.

Imaging Features

Effects on the teeth and jaws. The roots of the teeth may be short, and the lamina dura is thin. Severe bone marrow hyperplasia prevents development of the paranasal sinuses, especially the maxillary sinus, and causes an expansion of the maxilla resulting in malocclusion. The jaws appear radiolucent, with thinning of the cortical borders and enlargement of the marrow spaces as bone marrow is recruited to produce more red blood cells. The trabeculae are large and coarse. In the skull, the diploic space exhibits marked thickening, especially in the frontal region. The skull also shows a generalized granular appearance (Fig. 25.41) and occasionally a "hair on end" effect may develop.

Effects on the skeleton. As with sickle cell anemia, the features of thalassemia generally result from hyperplasia of the ineffective bone marrow and its subsequent failure to produce normal red blood cells. However, these changes are usually more severe than with other anemias (Fig. 25.42). There is a generalized radiolucency of the long bones with cortical thinning.

Management

Patients with thalassemia minor require no treatment except for iron supplementation when iron deficiency is confirmed. Patients with thalassemia major require regular hypertransfusion to maintain their hemoglobin levels and iron chelation to prevent iron overload complications such as cardiomyopathy and liver cirrhosis.

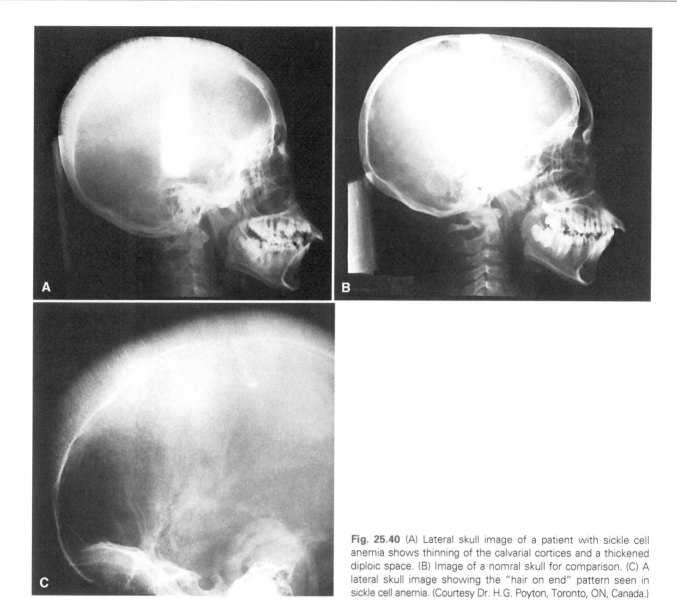

Fig. 25.40 (A) Lateral skull image of a patient with sickle cell anemia shows thinning of the calvarial cortices and a thickened diploic space. (B) Image of a nomral skull for comparison. (C) A lateral skull image showing the "hair on end" pattern seen in sickle cell anemia. (Courtesy Dr. H.G. Poyton, Toronto, ON, Canada.)

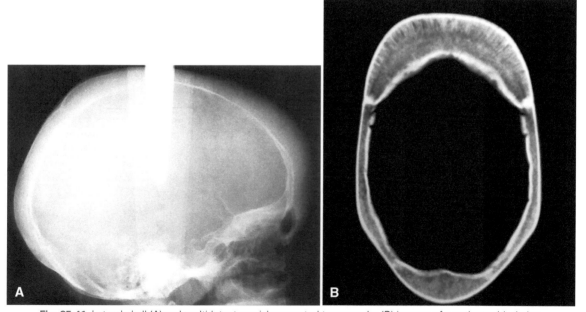

Fig. 25.41 Lateral skull (A) and multidetector axial computed tomography (B) images of a patient with thalassemia. Note the granular appearance of the skull and thickening of the diploic space. The computed tomography image shows a linear pattern in the frontal bone. (A, Courtesy Dr. H.G. Poyton, Toronto, ON, Canada.)

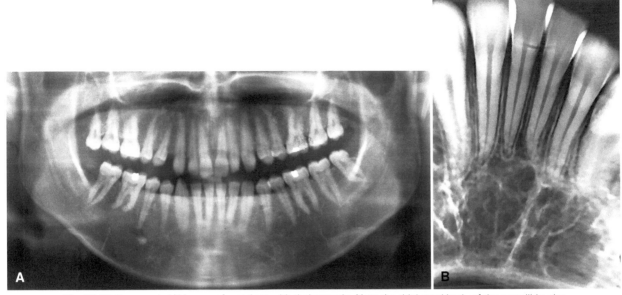

Fig. 25.42 Panoramic (A) image of a patient with thalassemia. Note the thickened body of the mandible, the sparse trabeculae, and absent maxillary sinuses. In the periapical image (B) of a different patient, note the thick trabeculae and large bone marrow spaces. (Courtesy Dr. H.G. Poyton, Toronto, ON, Canada.)

BIBLIOGRAPHY

Fibrous Dysplasia

Cohen MM, Howell RE. Etiology of fibrous dysplasia and McCune-Albright syndrome. *Int J Oral Maxillofac Surg.* 1999;28:366–371.

Couturier A, Aumaître O, Gilain L, et al. Craniofacial fibrous dysplasia: a 10-case series. *Eur Ann Otorhinolaryngol Head Neck Dis.* 2017;doi:10.1016/j.anorl.2017.02.004.

MacDonald-Jankowski DS, Yeung R, Li TK, et al. Computed tomography of fibrous dysplasia. *Dentomaxillofac Radiol.* 2004;33:114–118.

Michou L, Brown JP. Genetics of bone diseases: Paget disease, fibrous dysplasia, osteopetrosis, and osteogenesis imperfecta. *Joint Bone Spine.* 2011;78:252–258.

Petrikowski CG, Pharoah MJ, Lee L, et al. Radiographic differentiation of osteogenic sarcoma, osteomyelitis and fibrous dysplasia of the jaws. *Oral Surg Oral Med Oral Pathol Oral Radiol Endod.* 1977;50:1–7.

Tokano H, Sugimoto T, Noguchi Y, et al. Sequential computed tomography images demonstrating characteristic changes in fibrous dysplasia. *J Laryngol Otol.* 2001;115:757–759.

Hypercortisolism

Kaltsas G, Makras P. Skeletal diseases in Cushing's syndrome: osteoporosis versus arthropathy. *Neuroendocrinology.* 2010;92(suppl 1):60–64.

Lodish M, Stratakis CA. A genetic and molecular update on adrenocortical causes of Cushing's syndrome. *Nat Rev Endocrinol.* 2016;12:255–265.

Hyperthyroidism

Little JW. Thyroid disorders. Part I: hyperthyroidism. *Oral Surg Oral Med Oral Pathol Oral Radiol Endod.* 2006;101:276–284.

Hyperparathyroidism

Aldred MJ, Talacko AA, Savarirayan R, et al. Dental findings in a family with hyperparathyroidism-jaw tumor syndrome and a novel HRPT2 gene mutation. *Oral Surg Oral Med Oral Pathol Oral Radiol Endod.* 2006;101:212–218.

Daniels JM. Primary hyperparathyroidism presenting as a palatal brown tumor. *Oral Surg Oral Med Oral Pathol Oral Radiol Endod.* 2004;98:409–413.

Hata T, Irei I, Tanaka K, et al. Macrognathia secondary to dialysis-related renal osteodystrophy treated successfully by parathyroidectomy. *Int J Oral Maxillofac Surg.* 2006;35:378–382.

Pappu R, Jabbour SA, Regianto AM, et al. Musculoskeletal manifestations of primary hyperparathyroidism. *Clin Rheumatol.* 2017;35:3081–3087.

Proctor R, Kumar N, Stein A, et al. Oral and dental aspects of chronic renal failure. *J Dent Res.* 2005;84:199–208.

Rosenberg EH, Guralnick W. Hyperparathyroidism: a review of 220 proved cases with special emphasis on findings in the jaws. *Oral Surg Oral Med Oral Pathol.* 1962;15(suppl 2):84–94.

Raubenheimer EJ, Noffke CE, Hendrik HD. Recent developments in metabolic bone diseases: a gnathic perspective. *Head Neck Pathol.* 2014;8:475–481.

Scutellari PN, Orzincolo C, Bedani PL, et al. Radiographic manifestations in teeth and jaws in chronic kidney insufficiency. *Radiol Med (Torino).* 1996;92:415–420.

Zanocco KA, Yeh MW. Primary hyperparathyroidism: effects on bone health. *Endocrinol Metab Clin North Am.* 2017;46:87–104.

Hypoparathyroidism

Abate EG, Clarke BL. Review of hypoparathyroidism. *Front Endocrinol (Lausanne).* 2017;7:doi:10.3389/fendo.2016.00172.

Frensilli J, Stoner R, Hinrichs E. Dental changes of idiopathic-hypoparathyroidism: report of three cases. *J Oral Surg.* 1971;29:727–731.

Hypophosphatasia

Jedrychowski JR, Duperon D. Childhood hypophosphatasia with oral manifestations. *J Oral Med.* 1979;34:18–22.

Macfarlane JD, Swart JGN. Dental aspects of hypophosphatasia: a case report, family study, and literature review. *Oral Surg Oral Med Oral Pathol.* 1989;67:521–526.

Whyte MP. Hypophosphatasia - aetiology, nosology, pathogenesis, diagnosis and treatment. *Nat Rev Endocrinol.* 2016;12:233–246.

Hypopituitarism

Conley H, Steflik DE, Singh B, et al. Clinical and histologic findings of the dentition in a hypopituitary patient: report of case. *ASDC J Dent Child.* 1990;57:376–379.

Edler RJ. Dental and skeletal ages in hypopituitary patients. *J Dent Res.* 1977;56:1145–1153.

Kosowicz J, Rzymski K. Abnormalities of tooth development in pituitary dwarfism. *Oral Surg Oral Med Oral Pathol.* 1977;44:853–863.

Myllarniemi S, Lenko HL, Perheentupa J. Dental maturity in hypopituitarism, and dental response to substitution treatment. *Scand J Dent Res.* 1978;86:307–312.

Cemento-osseous Dysplasias

Alsufyani NA, Lam EW. Osseous (cemento-osseous) dysplasia of the jaws: clinical and radiographic analysis. *J Can Dent Assoc.* 2011;77:b70.

Alsufyani NA, Lam EW. Cemento-osseous dysplasia of the jaw bones: key radiographic features. *Dentomaxillofac Radiol.* 2011;40:141–146.

Chadwick JW, Alsufyani NA, Lam EW. Clinical and radiographic features of solitary and cemento-osseous dysplasia-associated simple bone cysts. *Dentomaxillofac Radiol.* 2011;40:230–235.

MacDonald-Jankowski DS. Florid cemento-osseous dysplasia: a systematic review. *Dentomaxillofac Radiol.* 2003;32:141–149.

Mahomed F, Altini M, Meer S, et al. Cemento-osseous dysplasia with associated simple bone cysts. *J Oral Maxillofac Surg.* 2005;63:1549–1554.

Noffke CE, Raubenheimer EJ, MacDonald D, et al. Fibro-osseous disease: harmonizing terminology with biology. *Oral Surg Oral Med Oral Pathol Oral Radiol Endod.* 2012;114:388–392.

Osteoporosis

Lee BD, White SC. Age and trabecular features of alveolar bone associated with osteoporosis. *Oral Surg Oral Med Oral Pathol Oral Radiol Endod.* 2005;100:92–98.

Taguchi A, Suei Y, Ohtsuka M, et al. Usefulness of panoramic radiography in the diagnosis of postmenopausal osteoporosis in women: width and morphology of inferior cortex of the mandible. *Dentomaxillofac Radiol.* 1996;25:263–267.

White SC. Oral radiographic predictors of osteoporosis. *Dentomaxillofac Radiol.* 2002;31:84–92.

Osteopetrosis

Barry CP, Ryan CD, Stassen LF. Osteomyelitis of the maxilla secondary to osteopetrosis: a report of two cases in sisters. *J Oral Maxillofac Surg.* 2007;65:144–147.

Ruprecht A, Wagner H, Engel H. Osteopetrosis: report of a case and discussion of the differential diagnosis. *Oral Surg Oral Med Oral Pathol.* 1988;66:674–679.

Waguespack SG, Hui SL, Dimeglio LA, et al. Autosomal dominant osteopetrosis: clinical severity and natural history of 94 subjects with a chloride channel 7 gene mutation. *J Clin Endocrinol Metab.* 2007;92:771–778.

Younai F, Eisenbud L, Sciubba JJ. Osteopetrosis: a case report including gross and microscopic findings in the mandible at autopsy. *Oral Surg Oral Med Oral Pathol.* 1988;65:214–221.

Paget Disease of Bone

Alsonso N, Calero-Paniagua I, Del Pino-Montes J. Clinical and genetic advances in paget disease of bone: a review. *Clin Rev Bone Miner Metab.* 2017;15:37–48.

Rao V, Karasick D. Hypercementosis: an important clue to Paget disease of the maxilla. *Skeletal Radiol.* 1982;9:126–128.

Sofaer J. Dental extractions in Paget disease of bone. *Int J Oral Surg.* 1984;13:79–84.

Van Staa TP, Selby P, Leufkens HGM, et al. Incidence and natural history of Paget disease in bone in England and Wales. *J Bone Miner Res.* 2002;17:465–471.

Progressive Systemic Sclerosis

Alexandridis C, White SC. Periodontal ligament changes in patients with progressive systemic sclerosis. *Oral Surg Oral Med Oral Pathol.* 1984;58:113–118.

Auluck A, Pai KM, Shetty C, et al. Mandibular resorption in progressive systemic sclerosis: a report of three cases. *Dentomaxillofac Radiol.* 2005;34:384–386.

Rout PG, Hamburger J, Potts AJ. Orofacial radiological manifestations of systemic sclerosis. *Dentomaxillofac Radiol.* 1996;25:193–196.

Wood RE, Lee P. Analysis of the oral manifestations of systemic sclerosis (scleroderma). *Oral Surg Oral Med Oral Pathol.* 1988;65:172–178.

Rickets

Harris R, Sullivan HR. Dental sequelae in deciduous dentition in vitamin-D resistant rickets: case report. *Aust Dent J.* 1960;5:200–203.

Marks SC, Lindahl RL, Bawden JW. Dental and cephalometric findings in vitamin D resistant rickets. *J Dent Child.* 1965;32:259.

Opsahl VS, Gaucher C, Bardet C, et al. Tooth dentin defects reflect genetic disorders affecting bone mineralization. *Bone.* 2012;50:989–997.

Sickle Cell Anemia

Javed F, Correa FO, Nooh N, et al. Orofacial manifestations in patients with sickle cell disease. *Am J Med Sci.* 2013;345:234–237.

Sears RS, Nazif MM, Zullo T. The effects of sickle-cell disease on dental and skeletal maturation. *ASDC J Dent Child.* 1981;48:275–277.

White SC, Cohen JM, Mourshed FA. Digital analysis of trabecular pattern in jaws of patients with sickle cell anemia. *Dentomaxillofac Radiol.* 2000;29:119–124.

Thalassemia

Hazza'a AM, Al-Jamal G. Radiographic features of the jaws and teeth in thalassaemia major. *Dentomaxillofac Radiol.* 2006;35:283–288.

Poyton HG, Davey KW. Thalassemia: changes visible in radiographs used in dentistry. *Oral Surg Oral Med Oral Pathol.* 1968;25:564–576.

26

Malignant Neoplasms

Ernest W.N. Lam

DISEASE MECHANISM

Malignant neoplasms or cancers are abnormal growths of tissue that develop as a result of uncontrolled and unlimited cell proliferation. In contrast to benign neoplasms, malignant neoplasms show generally more aggressive growth patterns, invade adjacent normal tissues, and have the ability to metastasize to regional lymph nodes or distant sites via the lymphatic or vascular systems, or through perineural spread. Malignant neoplasms that arise de novo are referred to as primary neoplasms, and a lesion that originates from a distant primary malignant neoplasm is termed a metastasis.

The loss of control of cell proliferation and cell adhesion in malignant neoplasia are the result of now often identifiable gene mutations. Such mutations can be caused by viruses, high-dose radiation exposure, or exposure to carcinogenic agents. For example, tobacco is strongly associated with oral squamous cell carcinoma. As with benign neoplasia, the molecular abnormality in a malignant cell is propagated through cell division, resulting in a clonal population of abnormal cells.

The most practical method of classification of malignant neoplasms is based on the cell of origin. In this chapter, malignancies that commonly affect the jaws have been divided into four categories: (1) lesions of epithelial origin or carcinomas, (2) lesions of mesenchymal origin or sarcomas, (3) lesions of hematopoietic origin, and (4) metastatic lesions. Of these, carcinomas are by far the most common in the head and neck. The prognosis for the patient is related to early detection. Often, malignant lesions are not recognized early enough, are misdiagnosed as other disease processes such as inflammation, and are mismanaged. Discussions of unusual malignant neoplasms have been omitted from this chapter to concentrate on more common lesions that a general practitioner may encounter.

CLINICAL FEATURES

Clinical signs and symptoms that suggest a lesion may be malignant may include a rapidly developing mass, ulceration and hemorrhage, and the presence of a firm (indurated) or rolled border. The mass may develop without any overt dental cause, and teeth may become mobile. The lesion may develop a foul smell if it is colonized by bacterial microorganisms and the patient may have difficulty swallowing (dysphagia), speaking (dysphonia), and tasting (dysguesia). There may also be weight loss, sensorineural or sensorimotor deficits, and lymphadenopathy.

Dentists should vigilantly watch for signs of malignant disease in their patients, particularly those who may engage in high-risk behaviors or have a genetic predisposition. Because the incidence of oral malignancies (primarily carcinomas) can vary widely around the world, some general dentists may rarely or never see a patient with a malignant neoplasm. This scarcity may make a dentist less likely to recognize a malignant condition when it is present. The failure to identify a malignancy in its early stages may result in delayed diagnosis and treatment, and an increased need for aggressive treatment with added morbidity, and, in the worst case, premature death. Indeed, it has been said that *it is better to suspect a malignancy and to be wrong, than to not suspect one and be wrong.*

APPLIED DIAGNOSTIC IMAGING

Diagnostic imaging has many important roles in the assessment and management of a patient with a malignant neoplasm. First, imaging may aid in the establishment of an initial diagnosis of a neoplasm. Second, imaging also aids in describing the extent of disease; specifically, local and lymph node involvement, and more distant sites of spread. Appropriate radiologic investigations assist the oncologist and surgeon to determine the anatomic spread of the neoplasm so a plan can be developed for treatment or follow-up. Radiologic investigations may also help to determine the presence of osseous involvement from a soft tissue neoplasm, assist in determining the best site for biopsy, and stage the neoplasm for prognosis. Finally, a thorough diagnostic imaging examination is part of the management of a patient who has survived cancer, who often is rendered xerostomic, neutropenic, and susceptible to dental caries, periodontal disease, and systemic infection.

Various diagnostic imaging modalities may be used to aid in the diagnosis. Intraoral images provide the best image resolution, and may reveal subtle changes, such as periodontal ligament space widening that computed tomography (CT) or magnetic resonance imaging (MRI) may be incapable of demonstrating. Panoramic imaging can provide an overall assessment of the osseous structures of the jaws, and can reveal relevant changes such as the destruction of the borders of the maxillary sinus. Either cone beam computed tomography (CBCT) or multidetector computed tomography (MDCT) images can demonstrate the three-dimensional involvement of osseous structures, while MDCT and MRI may show the extent of the soft tissue component of a neoplasm and the involvement of adjacent tissues. MRI has been found to be particularly useful for demonstrating perineural spread of disease and lymph node involvement. Positron emission tomographic (PET) imaging, a technique capable of detecting abnormal cellular metabolic activity associated with malignant neoplasms, has been used with MDCT and MRI for localizing a neoplasm for surgery and radiation therapy.

IMAGING FEATURES

Malignant neoplasms grow quickly and aggressively, leaving little if any time for the normal tissues around it to respond. Consequently, the imaging features of malignancy are, by and large, destructive in nature.

Location

Primary and metastatic malignant neoplasms may occur anywhere in the oral and maxillofacial region. Primary malignant neoplasms of epithelium (i.e., squamous cell carcinomas) are the most common malignancy of the head and neck, and these may arise from any mucosal surface (e.g., the floor of the mouth, the tongue, the retromolar area in the mandible, the oropharyngeal tonsillar area, the soft palate, the lip, and the gingiva). Consequently, malignant neoplasms arising from any of these sites may involve the jaws by direct extension. Sarcomas, arising from cells with a mesenchymal lineage are more common in the mandible and in the posterior regions of both jaws, while metastatic malignant disease is most common in the posterior mandible and maxilla. Rarely, metastases may develop at the apices of teeth or in the follicles of developing teeth (Fig. 26.1D).

Periphery

The shape of a malignant neoplasm of the jaw is commonly irregular, and their peripheries can vary from those that are more well defined to those that are very poorly defined. This variation often reflects the aggressiveness of the neoplasm's growth characteristics. Moreover, malignant neoplasms lack the border cortication associated with slower growing, benign masses that allow bone the opportunity to remodel as the mass enlarges. For example, some oral squamous cell carcinomas invading the mandible may have more well-defined borders, particularly if the invading neoplasm has a very broad surface. Other malignancies may create more irregular, poorly defined borders, as smaller populations of malignant cells invade the bone in a more piecemeal-like manner; this is referred to as an infiltrative pattern (see Fig. 26.1A). Evidence of destruction of a cortical boundary with an adjacent soft tissue mass is highly suggestive of malignancy (see Fig. 26.1B). Such a mass may exhibit a smooth or ulcerated peripheral border if cast against a radiolucent background, such as the air within the maxillary sinus.

Internal Structure

Most malignancies that develop in or around the jaws do not produce bone and do not stimulate the formation of reactive bone. Consequently, such neoplasms are internally radiolucent. Occasionally, residual islands of bone may be visualized, resulting in a pattern of patchy destruction. Sarcomas and metastases, particularly from the breast or the prostate, can produce abnormal bone giving the appearance of a somewhat irregular or disorganized, patchy, radiopaque pattern internally. Also, should these lesions extend to the bone surface, there may be effects associated with displacement of the periosteum.

Effects on Adjacent Structures

Malignant neoplasia is a destructive process—often rapidly so. And the effects on surrounding structures mirrors this behavior. The normal trabecular bone pattern is destroyed, as are cortical boundaries such as the sinus floor (see Fig. 26.1B), the inferior border of the mandible, the cortex of the inferior alveolar canal, and the follicular cortices of developing teeth. Malignant neoplasms invade structures through the path of least resistance, and these may include the maxillary antrum, the inferior alveolar canal or the periodontal ligament space resulting in irregular widening with destruction of the lamina dura (see Fig. 26.1C). Usually no periosteal reaction occurs where the neoplasm has destroyed the outer cortex of bone; however, some neoplasms may lift the periosteum from the bone surface giving rise to a pattern of alternating linear radiolucent and radiopaque lines emanating from the bone surface (see Fig. 26.1E). These patterns have been referred to as "hair-on-end" or "sunburst" patterns. If there is a secondary inflammatory lesion coexisting with the malignancy, an "onion skin" type of periosteal reaction normally associated with an inflammatory lesion may be seen.

Effects on Adjacent Teeth

Slower growing benign growths may resorb tooth roots or displace teeth in a bodily manner without causing the teeth to loosen. In contrast, rapidly growing malignant lesions generally destroy the supporting bone and associated structures around the teeth so that the teeth may appear to be floating in space (see Fig. 26.1F).

Occasionally, root resorption can occur, although this is more common with hematogenous malignancies like multiple myeloma and sarcomas such as osteosarcoma. Malignant neoplasms can also invade the periodontal ligament space around teeth resulting in irregular, nonconcentric widening of the space with destruction of the lamina dura, sometimes referred to as "Garrington sign" (see Fig. 26.1C).

CARCINOMAS

Squamous Cell Carcinoma Arising in Soft Tissue

Disease Mechanism

Squamous cell carcinoma is the most common primary malignancy in the head and neck, accounting for over 95% of malignancies. These malignant neoplasms arise from the surface epithelium lining the upper aerodigestive tract, and their etiology appears to be multifactorial, with chronic tobacco and alcohol use implicated as risk factors. Although a number of different gene mutations have been identified in both human and animal cell models of oral cancer, none have been definitively linked to disease pathogenesis. The human papillomavirus and Epstein-Barr virus (EBV) have also been implicated in playing a role in the development of some tonsillar, tongue, and laryngeal carcinomas.

Histopathologically, squamous cell carcinoma is characterized initially by invasion of malignant epithelial cells through the basement membrane into the underlying connective tissue with subsequent spread into deeper soft tissues and occasionally into adjacent bone, regional lymph nodes, and to even more distant sites in the lung, liver, and skeleton.

Clinical Features

Squamous cell carcinoma appears initially as white and/or red surface lesion in mucosa. With time, these lesions may exhibit central ulceration and necrosis, a rolled or indurated border (which represents invasion of malignant cells), and palpable infiltration into adjacent muscle or bone. Pain may be variable, and regional lymphadenopathy with hard, nonpainful lymph nodes that may or may not be fixed to underlying structures may be present. Other clinical features may include the presence of a soft tissue mass, altered sensation, foul smell, trismus, grossly loosened teeth, or hemorrhage. Large lesions can obstruct the airway, the opening of the Eustachian tube orifice (leading to diminished hearing) or the nasopharynx. Patients often report significant weight loss and feel unwell, and the condition is often fatal if untreated.

Imaging Features

Location. Squamous cell carcinoma commonly involves the floor of the mouth, the retromolar trigone area of the mandible, and the dorsum of the tongue. A common site of bone invasion is the posterior lingual surface of the mandible. Lesions involving the attached gingiva may mimic inflammatory disease such as periodontal disease. This malignancy is also seen on the tonsils, soft palate, and buccal vestibule.

Periphery. Squamous cell carcinoma may invade into the underlying bone from any direction, producing a radiolucency that may appear more broadly based at the bone surface, and this has been described as a "cookie bite" type of pattern of bone destruction. Invasion is characterized most commonly by a noncorticated border that is usually poorly defined (Fig. 26.2). Lesions that have a broader surface may have a more well-defined border, with a narrow transition zone between abnormal and normal bone (Fig. 26.3). Other lesions have an irregular and poorly defined border with a wider transition zone with finger-like extensions into the surrounding bone. Should the bone become structurally compromised by the invading mass, fracture can occur, and the borders will show sharpened thinned bone ends with displacement of segments. Sclerosis in underlying osseous structures (likely

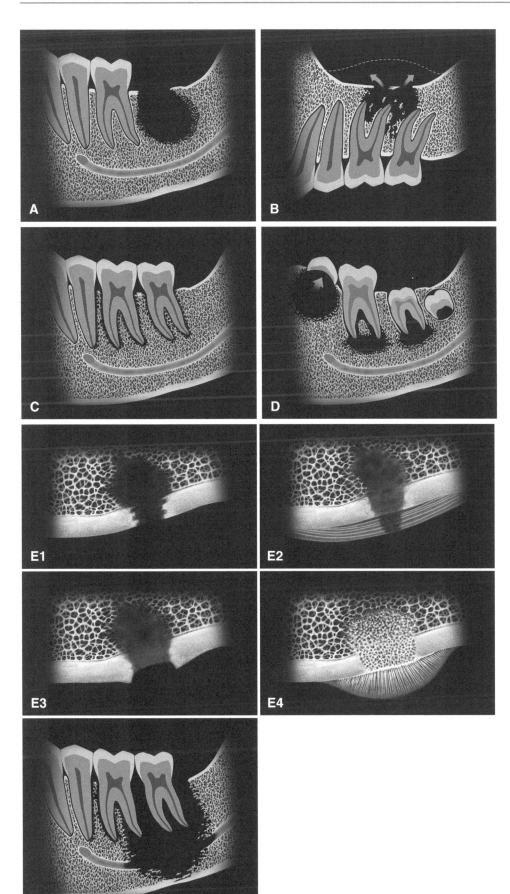

Fig. 26.1 Diagrammatic Representations of Some of the Important Radiologic Features of Malignant Neoplasia. (A) The poorly defined borders of a malignancy are the result of piecemeal bone destruction at the lesion's periphery. (B) Destruction of cortical boundaries (e.g., the floor of maxillary sinus) with an adjacent soft tissue mass *(arrows)*. (C) Invasion into the periodontal ligament space causing nonconcentric widening of this space. (D) Multifocal lesions located at root apices and in the papilla of a developing tooth destroying the crypt cortex, and displacing the developing tooth in an occlusal direction *(arrow)*. (E) Four types of effects on cortical bone and periosteal reaction: *(1)* cortical bone destruction, *(2)* destruction of the cortical bone and new periosteal bone formation, *(3)* destruction of cortical bone with Codman triangles, and *(4)* a spiculated or sunray type of periosteal reaction. (F) Bone destruction around teeth producing the appearance of teeth floating in space.

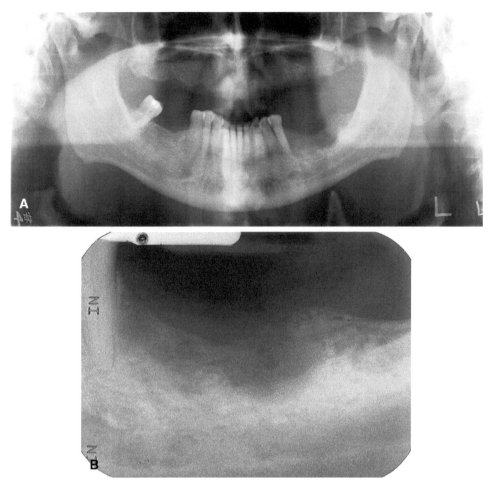

Fig. 26.2 Panoramic (A) and periapical (B) images of a squamous cell carcinoma invading the alveolar process of the left posterior mandible.

Fig. 26.3 Panoramic image of a squamous cell carcinoma destroying the floor of the left maxillary sinus and the adjacent alveolar process of the maxilla. The teeth have been left "floating in space" by the bone destruction. (Courtesy Dr. I. Hernandez, Edmonton, AB, Canada.)

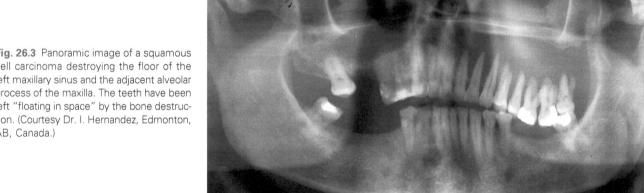

from secondary inflammatory disease) may be seen in association with erosions from surface carcinomas.

Internal structure. The internal structure of the invaded bone is radiolucent; the original osseous structure can be completely lost. Occasionally, small islands of residual normal trabecular bone are visible within this central radiolucency.

Effects on adjacent structures. Neoplasms may grow through neural foramina and along the inferior alveolar canal, resulting in an increase

in canal width and loss of the cortical boundary (Fig. 26.4). Destruction of adjacent internal cortical boundaries, such as the floor of the nose and maxillary sinus can occur, and bone cortices may be thinned or lost resulting in fracture of the bone.

Effects on adjacent teeth. Evidence of the invasion of bone around teeth may first appear as widening of the periodontal ligament space with loss of adjacent lamina dura. Teeth may appear to float in space, bereft of any bony support (Fig. 26.5). In extensive neoplasms, a rapidly

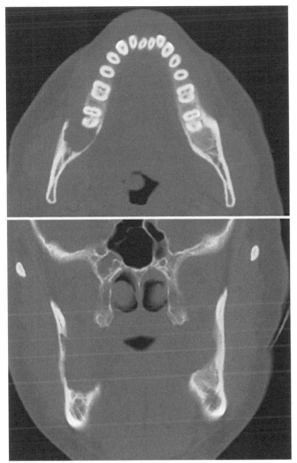

Fig. 26.4 Axial and coronal multidetector computed tomography images of bone destruction in the mandibular retromolar area by a squamous cell carcinoma.

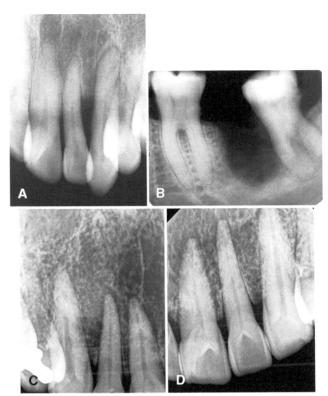

Fig. 26.5 Periapical image reveals bone destruction similar to periodontal disease around the lateral incisor from a squamous cell carcinoma originating in the soft tissues of the alveolar process (A). Note the lack of a sclerotic bone reaction at the periphery. The tooth socket from an extracted second molar has enlarged in size, and has not healed because of the presence of a squamous cell carcinoma (B). Periapical images (C and D) of a squamous cell carcinoma invading the alveolar process from the nasal cavity. In (C), note the wide transition zone from the bone destruction near the midline to the more normal bone pattern distal to the canine tooth.

growing soft tissue mass may carry the teeth from their normal positions resulting gross displacement.

Differential Interpretation

Squamous cell carcinoma is discernible from other malignancies by its clinical and histopathologic features. The bone loss from squamous cell carcinoma originating in the soft tissues of the alveolar process may appear very similar to periodontal disease (see Fig. 26.5A). Enlargement of a recent extraction socket instead of evidence of healing new bone formation can indicate the presence of an alveolar squamous cell carcinoma (see Fig. 26.5B)

Occasionally, it may be difficult to differentiate an inflammatory lesion, such as osteomyelitis, from squamous cell carcinoma, especially when oral bacterial microorganisms have gained entry to the bone through the neoplasm. Both osteomyelitis and squamous cell carcinoma can be destructive, leaving remnant islands of bone. Evidence of profound bone destruction or virulent invasion can help to differentiate malignancy from inflammation, but even this may sometimes be problematic. Osteomyelitis usually produces a periosteal reaction, whereas squamous cell carcinoma does not. In cases of radiation-induced necrosis in which the patient has had a prior malignancy, a periosteal reaction is absent. If bone destruction is present, the differentiation of this condition from squamous cell carcinoma requires advanced imaging and biopsy.

Management

Head and neck squamous cell carcinoma is usually managed by radiation therapy and surgery. The choice of which modality is used, and in what sequence, depends on the protocol of the treatment facility, and the location and severity of the neoplasm. Generally, chemotherapy is not a common treatment modality.

Squamous Cell Carcinoma Originating in the Maxillary Sinus
Disease Mechanism

Risk factors for developing squamous cell carcinoma originating in the mucosal lining of the maxillary sinus include chronic sinusitis, organic chemicals used in manufacturing, wood dust, and metals such as nickel and chromium.

Clinical Features

These malignancies occur most commonly in patients of African and Asian heritage, with men affected more commonly than women. The initial signs may be very similar to inflammatory disease and may include recurrent sinusitis, nasal obstruction, epistaxis, sinus pain, and facial paresthesia.

Imaging Features

Squamous cell carcinoma arising in the mucosal lining of the maxillary sinus may manifest as opacification of the maxillary sinus with soft tissue, and destruction of sinus cortical border and the adjacent maxillary alveolar process (Fig. 26.6). An associated soft tissue mass may also project into the oral cavity.

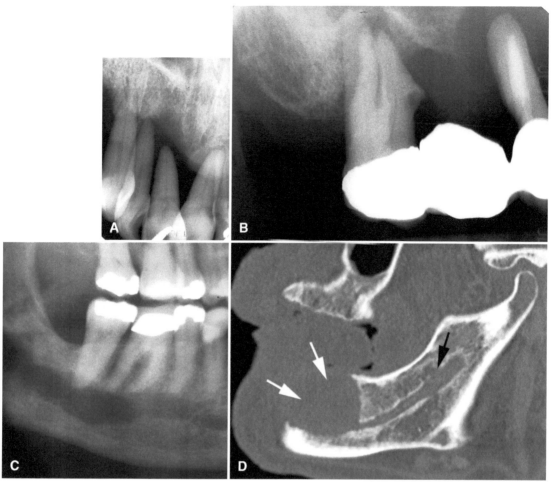

Fig. 26.6 Periapical images (A and B) of two cases of squamous cell carcinoma involving the maxillary alveolar processes. Bone destruction around the tooth roots leaves the teeth bereft of any bone support. Cropped panoramic image of a squamous cell carcinoma involving the inferior alveolar canal (C). Note the irregular width of the canal and destruction of its cortical borders. Sagittal multidetector computed tomography image of another case of a squamous cell carcinoma destroying the mandible in the region of the mental foramen *(white arrows)* and growing down the canal. Again, note the destruction of the peripheral cortex of the canal *(black arrow)* (D).

Squamous Cell Carcinoma Originating in Bone
Disease Mechanism
Primary squamous cell carcinoma arising within the jaw has no connection with the surface epithelium of the oral mucosa. Consequently, the surface epithelium is invariably normal in appearance. Such primary intraosseous carcinomas are presumed to arise from intraosseous remnants of odontogenic epithelium, such as the dental lamina, and carcinomas from surface epithelium, the lining of an odontogenic cyst, or metastases, must be excluded.

Clinical Features
These neoplasms are very rare, and may remain clinically silent until they have reached a fairly large size. Pain or other sensorineural changes such as lip paresthesia, jaw fracture, and lymphadenopathy may accompany the neoplasm. It is more common in men and in patients in their fourth to eighth decade of life.

Imaging Features
Location. The mandible is far more commonly involved than the maxilla, with most cases being present in the molar region (Fig. 26.7A). The lesions are less frequently seen in the anterior aspect of the jaws.

Because the lesion is, by definition, associated with remnants of the dental lamina, it originates only in tooth-bearing parts of the jaw.

Periphery. The periphery of most lesions is poorly defined. They are most often rounded or irregular in shape and have a border that demonstrates osseous destruction with varying degrees of extension into the bone. The degree of raggedness of the border may reflect the aggressiveness of the lesion. If sufficient in size, the bone cortices may be thinned, and jaw fracture can occur with an associated step defect in the bone surface.

Internal structure. The internal structure within the bone is radiolucent with no evidence of bone production and very little residual bone left within the center of the lesion. If the lesion is small, the adjacent buccal or lingual cortices may superimpose over the lost bone and mimic the appearance of an internal bone pattern.

Effects on adjacent structures. These lesions are capable of causing extensive destruction of the nasal and antral borders, the cortical outline of the inferior alveolar canal, and loss of the lamina dura.

Effects on adjacent teeth. Teeth that lose bone support and lamina dura appear to be floating in space. Root resorption is unusual.

Differential Interpretation
If the lesions are not aggressive and have a smooth border and radiolucent area, they may be mistaken for periapical inflammatory disease.

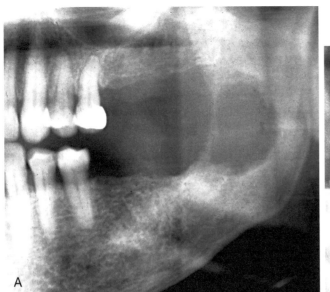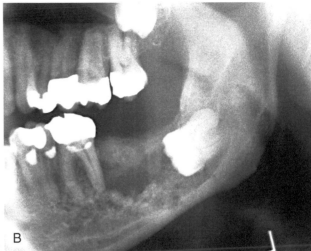

Fig. 26.7 Rare cases of primary intraosseous carcinoma developing in the left mandibular ramus (A) and within a dentigerous cyst (B) associated with the mandibular left third molar. In (B), note the absence of the cyst cortex, the invasion into adjacent bone, and the poorly defined borders.

Alternatively, if lesions are not centered about the apex of a tooth, occasionally it may be difficult to differentiate this condition from an odontogenic cyst or neoplasm. If the border is infiltrative with extensive bone destruction, a hematogenous malignancy, such as multiple myeloma or a metastatic lesion, must be excluded. Examination of the oral cavity and especially the surface epithelium assists in differentiating this condition from surface squamous cell carcinoma.

Management

Such lesions are managed in much the same way as squamous cell carcinoma arising from the oral soft tissues.

Squamous Cell Carcinoma Originating in a Cyst
Disease Mechanism

Squamous cell carcinoma may develop from the lining of an odontogenic cyst (periapical inflammatory lesion, residual cyst, dentigerous cyst, and odontogenic keratocyst).

Clinical Features

The development of squamous cell carcinoma from the lining of an odontogenic cyst is exceptionally rare. Such a malignancy must be differentiated from invasion from a surface epithelial carcinoma, metastatic disease, and primary intraosseous carcinoma. The most common presenting sign or symptom associated with this condition is pain. The pain may be characterized as dull and of several months' duration. Swelling is occasionally reported. Jaw fracture, fistula formation, and regional lymphadenopathy may occur. If the maxilla is involved, sinus pain, epistaxis or, swelling may be present.

Imaging Features

Location. This neoplasm may occur anywhere that odontogenic epithelium may be present and where an odontogenic cyst may be found; that is, the tooth-bearing areas of the jaws. Most cases occur in the mandible (see Fig. 26.7B), with a few cases reported in the anterior maxilla.

Periphery. The appearance of squamous cell carcinoma arising within a cyst wall may not be visible until the abnormality attains a size that is large enough to impact adjacent bone. As the malignant cells progressively replace the cyst lining, the smooth, well-defined, and corticated cyst border is lost or becomes poorly defined. In the more advanced lesion, the shape of the cyst becomes less "hydraulic" and the border takes on a poorly defined, infiltrative quality that lacks any cortication.

Internal structure. This lesion is radiolucent, perhaps more so than invasive surface carcinoma, owing to prior osteolysis from the cyst.

Effects on adjacent structures. There is destruction of adjacent bone surfaces including the inferior border of the mandible or floor of the nose or maxillary sinus. It can also produce complete destruction of the alveolar process.

Effects on adjacent structures. Carcinoma arising in a dental cyst can thin and destroy the lamina dura of adjacent teeth.

Differential Interpretation

If a dental cyst is infected, it may lose its normal cortical boundary and appear ragged and identical to a malignant lesion arising in a preexisting cyst. However, with inflammation, there will be a peripheral sclerotic response in the bone. This sclerosis is not normally present in a cyst that has undergone malignant transformation. Nevertheless, the two may be difficult to differentiate radiologically, and the epithelium from an excised cyst should always be submitted for histopathologic examination. Multiple myeloma may appear as a solitary lesion and may be difficult to distinguish, especially if it has a well-defined periphery and a cyst-like shape. Metastatic disease may be similar, although it is commonly multifocal.

Management

The treatment of squamous cell carcinoma originating in a cyst is identical to the treatment described for primary intraosseous carcinoma.

Central Mucoepidermoid Carcinoma
Disease Mechanism

Central mucoepidermoid carcinoma is an epithelially derived malignant salivary gland neoplasm arising in bone. It is histologically indistinguishable from its soft tissue counterpart. The malignant cells are believed to arise from metaplasia of odontogenic epithelium. The clinician must exclude the possibility of an invasive overlying mucoepidermoid carcinoma or odontogenic neoplasm.

Clinical Features

In contrast to other malignant neoplasms of the jaws, the central mucoepidermoid carcinoma is more likely to mimic a benign neoplasm or cyst. The most common patient complaint is a painless or tender swelling that may have been present for months or years, which has caused a facial asymmetry. Occasionally, patients may feel as if teeth have been displaced, or a denture no longer fits. Paresthesia involving the distribution of the inferior alveolar nerve and spreading of the lesion to regional lymph nodes have been reported. In contrast to other oral malignancies, central mucoepidermoid neoplasm is more common in females than males.

Imaging Features

Location. The lesion is three to four times more common in the mandible than the maxilla, and usually develops in the premolar and molar regions. The lesion most commonly occurs above the inferior alveolar canal in the tooth-bearing areas of the jaws, similar to odontogenic cysts and neoplasms.

Periphery. Mucoepidermoid carcinoma manifests as a unilocular or multilocular expansile mass (Fig. 26.8). The border is most often well defined and corticated with a crenated or undulating periphery, which is similar to the appearance of a benign odontogenic neoplasm.

The peripheral cortication may be impressively thick, which belies its malignant nature.

Internal structure. The internal structure has features similar to a benign odontogenic neoplasm such as a recurrent ameloblastoma. Lesions are often described as being multilocular, or having either soap bubble- or a honeycomb-like internal structure. This is often seen as round radiolucent areas without or with thick or sclerotic bony peripheries. Also, there may be regions of adjacent sclerotic bone, although this bone is not produced by the neoplasm; it is merely remodeled residual bone.

Effects on adjacent structures. Central mucoepidermoid carcinoma is capable of causing bone expansion and displacement of adjacent cortices, often with perforation and sometimes extension into the surrounding soft tissues. Similar to benign odontogenic neoplasms, the inferior alveolar canal may be displaced.

Effects on adjacent structures. Teeth remain largely unaffected by this disease, although adjacent lamina dura may be lost.

Differential Interpretation

Some imaging characteristics of this neoplasm may appear similar to a benign odontogenic neoplasm. Its malignant nature is revealed if there is expansion with perforation of the outer cortex with extension of the neoplasm into the surrounding soft tissues. The primary differential interpretation is a recurrent ameloblastoma, with which it shares similarities in its peripheral and internal features; it may be impossible to differentiate the two. The features of odontogenic myxoma and central

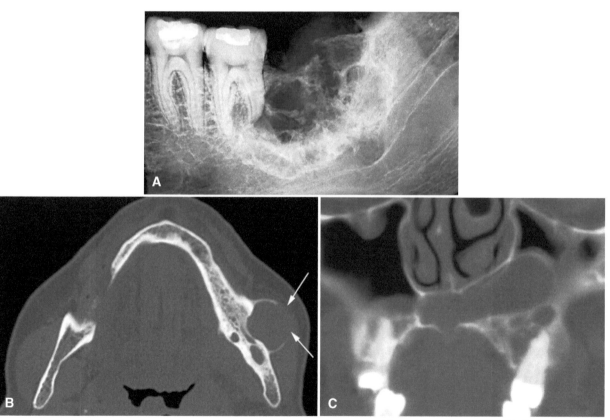

Fig. 26.8 Multilocular radiolucency is characteristic of central mucoepidermoid carcinoma (A). This lesion has destroyed the crest of the alveolar process and the bone distal to the second molar, and has displaced the mandibular canal inferiorly. Axial multidetector computed tomography (MDCT) image reveals multiple cyst-like epicenters, some surrounded by sclerotic bone and expansion of the mandible with extension into the surrounding soft tissue *(arrows)* (B). Coronal MDCT image (C) of a central mucoepidermoid carcinoma in the maxilla with a multilocular internal structure.

giant cell lesion may also overlap with mucoepidermoid carcinoma, as may other odontogenic cysts or neoplasms.

Management

Central mucoepidermoid carcinoma is treated surgically with *en bloc* resection encompassing a margin of adjacent normal bone. Neck dissection and postoperative radiation therapy may be required to control the spread to the lymph nodes.

"Malignant Ameloblastoma" and Ameloblastic Carcinoma

Disease Mechanism

"Malignant ameloblastoma" is defined as a classic ameloblastoma with typical benign histologic features, which is deemed malignant because of its biologic behavior; that is, metastasis. Indeed, the histopathologic features may not correlate with the clinical behavior. Ameloblastic carcinoma is a classic ameloblastoma exhibiting the histopathologic criteria of a malignant neoplasm, such as increased and abnormal mitosis and hyperchromatic, large, pleomorphic nuclei.

Clinical Features

Malignant ameloblastoma and ameloblastic carcinoma are exceptionally rare neoplasms. Clinically and radiologically, these lesions may be impossible to differentiate from the classic ameloblastoma. They present as a hard expansile mass with displaced and perhaps loosened teeth, and normal overlying mucosa. Tenderness of the overlying soft tissue has been reported. Metastatic spread may be to the cervical lymph nodes, lung, or other viscera, and the skeleton—especially the spine. Local extension may occur into adjacent bones, connective tissue, or salivary glands. These neoplasms occur most commonly between the first and sixth decades of life and are more common in males than in females.

Imaging Features

Location. These lesions are more common in the mandible than in the maxilla. Most occur in the premolar and molar region, where classic ameloblastoma is typically found.

Periphery. These lesions may appear similar to classic ameloblastoma with a well-defined and corticated border, and crenations or scalloping of the border. Malignant ameloblastoma may show more evidence of the aggressive behavior commonly seen in malignant neoplasm, that is, loss of, and subsequent breaching of, the cortical boundary invading into the surrounding soft tissue.

Internal structure. The lesions are either unilocular or more commonly multilocular, giving the appearance of a honeycomb- or soap bubble-like pattern that is seen in classic ameloblastomas. Most of the septa are robust and thick.

Effects on adjacent structures. The bone borders may be breached or lost, and as with classic ameloblastoma, the lesions may displace anatomic boundaries such as the floor of the nasal fossa and maxillary sinus. The inferior alveolar canal may be displaced or the cortices lost.

Effects on adjacent teeth. Teeth may be moved bodily by the neoplasm and may exhibit root resorption similar to a benign neoplasm.

Differential Interpretation

The differential interpretation of this lesion should include classic ameloblastoma, odontogenic keratocyst, odontogenic myxoma, and central mucoepidermoid carcinoma, from which it may not be distinguishable radiologically. If the lesion is locally invasive and this is apparent radiologically, the interpretation of carcinoma arising from an odontogenic cyst should be considered. If the patient is young and the location of the lesion is anterior to the second permanent molar, central giant cell lesions may mimic some of its radiologic features. The final diagnosis often is the result of histopathologic evaluation or the detection of metastatic lesions.

Management

These lesions are most often treated with *en bloc* surgical resection. However, many may not be identified as being malignant until the time of biopsy. Because the histopathologic appearance of these lesions may indicate classic ameloblastoma the initial treatment often is inadequate. In addition, the metastatic lesions may not appear for many months or years after treatment of the primary neoplasm, adding another reason for treatment failure.

METASTATIC DISEASE

Disease Mechanism

Metastasis is the establishment of new foci of malignant disease from a distant primary malignant neoplasm. For patients, metastasis is often the terminal event in the clinical course of cancer. Metastatic disease that involves the jaws usually occurs when the distant primary lesion, usually located anatomically inferior to the clavicles, is already known, although occasionally the presence of a metastasis may reveal the presence of a silent primary malignancy.

Less than 0.1% of cells within a primary malignant neoplasm develop the phenotypic ability to undergo metastasis, and most often, this process involves the vascular system. Although the process is complex, two broad sets of events occur. The first of these occurs within the primary tissue or organ (the proximal metastatic event) and the second, which occurs within the distant tissue or organ (the distal metastatic event). During the proximal event, the neoplastic cell loses its adhesion to adjacent cells within the neoplasm and migrates through the basement membrane (if present) into the underlying connective tissue where it may encounter a blood vessel. The neoplastic cell passes through the basement membrane and endothelial cell layer of the vessel wall, and enters the circulation. Once in the circulation, the neoplastic cell must evade the body's immune system, and travel through the vasculature until it adheres to a distant endothelial cell, where the distal metastatic event occurs. The series of events that occurs in the distant tissue or organ is the reverse of what has already occurred during the proximal event. That is, the cell moves across the basement membrane and the vascular endothelial cell junction into the adjacent tissue. Should the microenvironment in this location be favorable, the malignant cell is able to proliferate, and a metastatic focus develops. It should also be noted that spread of malignant disease through the lymphatic system and along nerve axons are other important means of disease dissemination.

Metastatic disease in the jaws accounts for less than 1% of metastatic malignancies found in bone, with most affecting the bones of the vertebrae, pelvis, skull, ribs, and humerus. Most metastases arise from carcinomas—the most common being from breast, lung, prostate, colorectal, kidney, thyroid, gastrointestinal, melanoma, testicle, bladder, ovarian, and cervical cancers. In children, metastatic disease may arise from neuroblastoma, retinoblastoma, and Wilms' neoplasm.

Clinical Features

Metastatic disease is the most common malignancy that develops in bone. Women have almost twice the number of metastatic neoplasms as men. Metastatic disease is more common in patients in their fifth to seventh decade of life, and breast metastases outnumber all other types. Patients may complain of dental pain, develop unexplained paresthesia or anesthesia involving the third branch of the trigeminal nerve, or hemorrhage from the tumor site. Patients may also experience

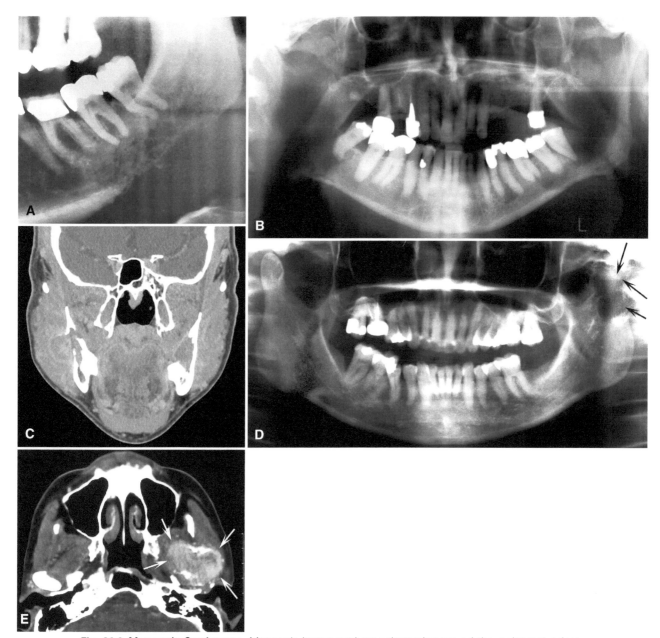

Fig. 26.9 Metastatic Carcinomas. Metastatic breast carcinoma destroying around the molar root apices, and extending to the inferior border of the mandible (A). Bilateral metastatic lung lesions destroying the mandibular rami (B), and (C) a coronal soft tissue multidetector computed tomography image of the case shown in (B). Destruction of the left mandibular condyle *(arrows)* from a thyroid metastatic lesion (D). (E) Axial soft tissue multidetector computed tomography image of the case shown in (D) demonstrates invasion into surrounding soft tissue *(arrows)*.

a change to their occlusion should the neoplasm grow large enough for teeth to lose their bone support or from jaw fracture.

Imaging Features
Location
The posterior mandible is most commonly affected (Fig. 26.9) given the rich vascular supply to this area of the bone. The maxilla and maxillary sinus may be the next most common sites, followed by the anterior hard palate and mandibular condyle. Frequently, metastatic lesions of the mandible are seen bilaterally (see Fig. 26.9B and C). Also, occasionally, lesions may develop in the periodontal ligament space (sometimes at the root apex), mimicking periapical or periodontal inflammatory disease, or in the papilla of a developing tooth.

Periphery
Metastatic lesions may have moderately well-defined to poorly defined peripheries, without any cortex (see Fig. 26.9A). The lesions typically exhibit a lobular or polymorphous shape owing to the microenvironment of the bone. In general, areas with a richer microenvironment may see a greater proliferation of neoplastic cells, while areas with a less rich microenvironment may see less proliferation—thus, the contours of adjacent regions within the same neoplasm may appear heterogeneous.

Internal Structure
Metastatic lesions are generally radiolucent relative to bone, although some residual normal trabecular bone may be appreciated in association

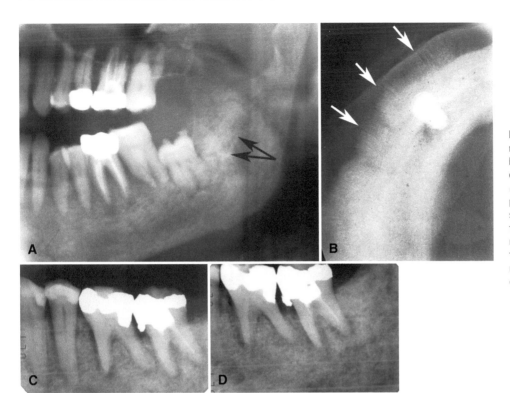

Fig. 26.10 Cropped panoramic image of metastatic prostate lesions involving the body and ramus of the body (A). Note the osteoblastic (sclerotic) bone reaction *(arrows)*. Occlusal image (B) of a metastatic prostate lesion producing sclerosis and a spiculated surface sunray periosteal reaction *(arrows)*. Two periapical images of a metastatic breast lesion (C and D) showing the sclerotic bone reaction around the molar roots as well as the nonconcentric widening of the periodontal ligament spaces.

with the more osteolytic areas. Some metastatic lesions from prostate and breast lesions may also stimulate osteoblasts within the bone to produce an osteoblastic response that produces sclerosis.

The metastatic focus may begin as a few smaller areas of bone destruction separated by normal bone. As the metastatic cell populations begin to proliferate and coalesce, smaller regions may develop into a larger, poorly defined region over time, and the jaw may become enlarged. If osteoblastic metastases are present, the normally poorly defined radiolucent focus may develop areas of patchy sclerosis as the result of new bone formation (Fig. 26.10). If the neoplasm is seeded into multiple regions of the bone, the result may be multiple variably sized radiolucent lesions with normal bone between the metastatic foci. Significant dissemination of metastatic neoplasm may give the jaws a general radiolucent appearance, or one that appears osteopenic.

Effects on Adjacent Structures

The cortical borders of adjacent structures, including neurovascular canal and airspaces, may be destroyed. Occasionally, the metastatic lesion may breach the outer cortex of the jaws and extend into surrounding soft tissues, and manifest as an intraoral mass.

Some metastatic carcinomas, namely from the prostate and breast, may stimulate a periosteal reaction on the bone surface that usually takes the form of a spiculated pattern (see Fig. 26.10). When a metastatic focus increases in size to reach the bone surface and cortex, the neoplasm may lift the periosteum from the bone surface, stimulating progenitor osteoblasts to deposit a mineralized matrix along Sharpey fibers and vascular channels, which are perpendicularly oriented relative to the bone surface.

Effects on Adjacent Teeth

Typical of malignancy, a metastasis can efface the lamina dura and can cause an irregular increase in the width of the periodontal ligament space. If the neoplasm has seeded the papilla of a developing tooth, the

cortices of the crypt may be totally or partially destroyed. Teeth may seem to be floating in a soft tissue mass, and their position may be altered because of a loss of bony support. Extraction sockets may fail to heal and may increase in size. Resorption of teeth is generally rare, although this is sometimes seen with multiple myeloma, chondrosarcoma, and osteosarcoma—a feature more common in benign lesions.

Differential Interpretation

In most cases, if a known primary malignancy has been identified, the diagnosis of metastasis is straightforward. Hematogenous malignancies including multiple myeloma may be confused with metastatic disease; however, the border of multiple myeloma is usually better defined than a metastatic focus. When a lesion originates within the periodontal ligament space of a tooth, the appearance may be identical to that of periapical inflammatory disease. A point of differentiation is that the periodontal ligament space widening from inflammation occurs in a more concentric manner at the apex of a tooth root. In contrast, the metastatic disease usually causes irregular ligament space widening, which may extend up the side of the root. Odontogenic cysts, if secondarily infected, may have a poorly defined border giving a similar appearance to a metastatic lesion; however, if multiple lesions are seen, the possibility of a metastasis is more likely. Invasion of the jaws by head and neck squamous cell carcinoma may be difficult to distinguish from metastatic disease. In general, the epicenter of squamous cell carcinoma will be nearer the surface of the bone, and a "cookie bite" defect of the bone surface may be appreciated. In contrast, a metastasis should have an epicenter within the bone, and the shape of the lesion would be more circular or oval.

Management

The identification of a metastasis in the jaws indicates a poor prognosis. If the appearance in the images is suspicious, an opinion from an oral and maxillofacial radiologist should be sought, and the tissue biopsied and submitted for histopathology. A radiologic examination of the body with plain imaging or nuclear medicine may be employed to detect other metastatic lesions.

Isolated malignant deposits, if symptomatic, may be treated with localized radiation therapy. On the rare occasion that the jaw is the first diagnosed site of metastasis, it is imperative that the patient be referred quickly to the appropriate physician specialist so that treatment can be promptly rendered.

SARCOMAS

Osteosarcoma
Disease Mechanism
Osteosarcoma is a malignant neoplasm of osteoblasts in which osteoid is produced directly by the malignant cells. As with all malignancies, the cause of osteosarcoma is due to the loss of control of cell proliferation, which is the result of gene mutations. In osteosarcoma, it is interesting to note that these neoplasms can arise within Paget disease of bone and fibrous dysplasia after radiation therapy.

Clinical Features
Osteosarcoma of the jaws is quite rare, and accounts for approximately 7% of all osteosarcomas. The lesion occurs in in males twice as frequently as females, and jaw lesions typically occur with a peak in the fourth decade, about 10 years later, on average, than long bone osteosarcomas.

The dentist may be the first health professional to identify an osteosarcoma developing in the jaws, with the most commonly reported sign or symptom being a rapidly enlarging swelling that may be present 6 months before diagnosis. Other signs and symptoms may include pain, tenderness, erythema of the overlying mucosa, ulceration, loose teeth, epistaxis, hemorrhage, nasal obstruction, exophthalmos, trismus, and blindness. Hypoesthesia has also been reported in cases where peripheral nerves have become involved.

Imaging Features
Location. The mandible is more commonly affected than the maxilla. Although the lesion can occur in any part of either jaw, the posterior mandibular alveolar process, angle, and ramus is most commonly affected. The molar areas are also more commonly affected in the maxilla, with the most frequent sites being the alveolar ridge, antrum, and palate. In the anterior parts of the jaws, the lesion may cross the midline.

Periphery. In most instances, osteosarcoma has a poorly defined border with no cortex.

Internal structure. Osteosarcoma may be entirely radiolucent, mixed radiolucent-radiopaque, or radiopaque, depending on the ability of the malignant cells to produce bone. The internal structure may have the appearance of granular- or sclerotic-appearing bone, cotton, wisps of bone, or honeycombs with adjacent destruction of the normal osseous architecture. Whatever the resultant internal structure, the normal trabecular structure of the jaws is lost.

Effects on adjacent structures. Mandibular lesions may destroy the cortex of the inferior alveolar canal, and the antral or nasal wall cortices may be lost with maxillary lesions. Alternatively, the neurovascular canal may be symmetrically widened and enlarged if the malignant cells invade this space. If the lesion extends to the bone surface, a soft tissue mass may be seen emanating from the bone. Should the overlying periosteum be lifted and displaced, a mineralized triangle called a Codman triangle may be seen at the periphery of the elevated periosteum. Also, the typical "sunray" or "hair-on-end" appearance, caused by mineralization of Sharpey fibers and/or small vessels, may also be seen within the adjacent soft tissues (Fig. 26.11).

Effects on adjacent teeth. Nonconcentric widening of the periodontal ligament space is associated with osteosarcoma, but is also seen in other malignancies (Fig. 26.12). This appearance, sometimes referred to as Garrington sign, arises when malignant cells invade the periodontal ligament space and produce osteolysis of the adjacent bone and external resorption of the tooth root.

Differential Interpretation
It is impossible to differentiate osteosarcoma from chondrosarcoma. If no osseous structure is visible, the practitioner should also consider fibrosarcoma. If the sunray or speculated bone pattern is seen at the bone surface, prostate and breast metastases should be considered. A comprehensive physical examination and laboratory tests may be useful in the differentiation of a primary bone-forming malignancy from metastatic disease.

Benign neoplasms, such as ossifying fibroma and fibrous dysplasia, are better demarcated than osteosarcoma. In general, they are more uniform in their internal structure, and both lack invasive, destructive characteristics. The histopathology of a biopsy specimen of osteosarcoma may be interpreted as a bone dysplasia, and the correct diagnosis in these cases may rely on the imaging characteristics. Ewing sarcoma, solitary plasmacytoma, and osteomyelitis share some of the radiographic characteristics of osteosarcoma, although osteosarcoma is generally not associated with signs of infection.

Management
The management of osteosarcoma is resection with a large border of adjacent normal bone. Such resection may be possible in orthopedic cases but may be complicated by the myriad of important adjacent anatomic structures in the head and neck. Generally, radiation therapy and chemotherapy are used only for controlling metastatic spread or for palliation.

Chondrosarcoma
Disease Mechanism
Chondrosarcoma is a malignant neoplasm of mesenchymal origin where the malignant cells produce cartilage. These neoplasms may occur centrally within bone, on the bone surface, or, less commonly, in soft tissue. Some form directly from malignant mesenchymal cells, and some form from preexisting cartilaginous lesions. In the case of the latter, they are termed secondary chondrosarcomas.

Clinical Features
Chondrosarcomas are quite rare in the facial bones, accounting for about 10% of all cases. Generally, these neoplasms occur at any age, although they are more common in adults with a mean age of 47 years. Males and females are affected equally. A patient with chondrosarcoma may have a firm or hard mass of relatively long duration. Enlargement of these lesions may cause pain, headache, and deformity. Less frequent signs and symptoms include hemorrhage from the neoplasm, or from the supporting structures around teeth. As with osteosarcoma, there may also be sensory nerve deficits, proptosis, and visual disturbances. The neoplasms invariably are covered with normal overlying skin or mucosa unless secondarily ulcerated. If chondrosarcoma occurs in or near the temporomandibular joint region, trismus or abnormal joint function may result.

Imaging Features
Location. Chondrosarcomas occur in the mandible and maxilla with equal frequency. Maxillary lesions typically occur in the anterior region in areas where cartilage may be present, while mandibular lesions involve the coronoid process, condylar head and neck (Fig. 26.13B and C), and occasionally the symphysis.

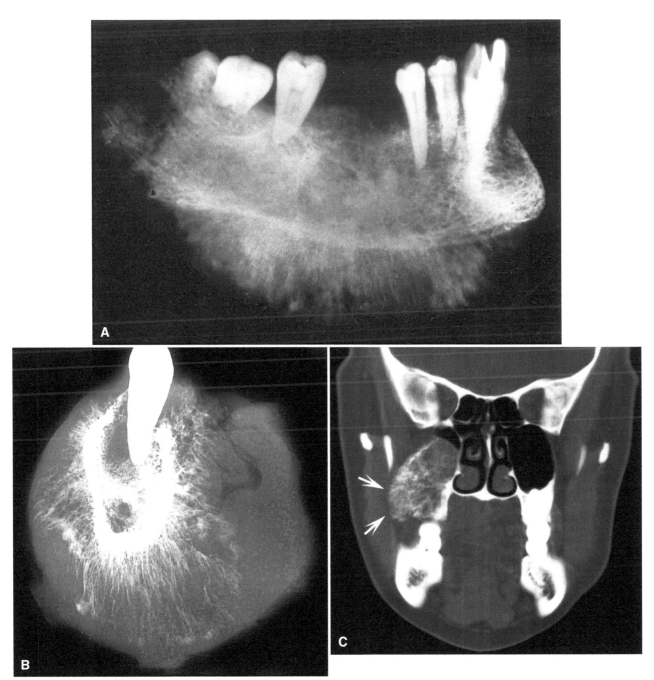

Fig. 26.11 Images of a resected mandible (A and B) of an osteosarcoma from a 25-year-old male, showing the characteristic sunray spicules at the bone surface. Coronal multidetector computed tomography image of an osteosarcoma of the maxilla (C). Again, note the spiculated new bone extending laterally from the maxilla *(arrows)*.

Periphery. Chondrosarcomas are slow-growing neoplasms, and their radiologic signs may be misleading and benign in nature. The lesions are generally round, ovoid, or lobulated. Their borders are generally well defined and at times corticated; at other times blend with adjacent normal bone. Occasionally, a sunray or hair-on-end appearance may be seen. Uncommonly, these lesions have more aggressive appearances, and their peripheries may appear poorly defined and infiltrative with noncorticated borders.

Internal structure. Chondrosarcomas are rarely radiolucent, but usually exhibit some form of internal calcification, giving them a mixed radiolucent and radiopaque appearance. The internal pattern may be quite variable. The appearance can take the form of moth-eaten bone alternating with islands of residual bone unaffected by neoplasm. Alternatively, when the malignant cells produce mineralization, the central radiopaque pattern has been described as "flocculent," implying snow-like features. This type of diffuse calcification may be superimposed on a background that resembles granular or ground-glass-appearing abnormal bone (see Fig. 26.13A). Careful examination of these areas of flocculence may reveal a central radiolucent nidus, which is probably cartilage surrounded by calcification.

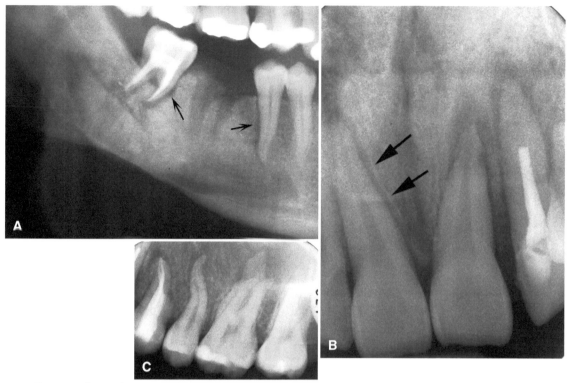

Fig. 26.12 Cropped panoramic image shows the widened periodontal ligament spaces around teeth *(arrows)*, and that the increased radiopacity of the mandible in the first molar region due to an osteosarcoma (A). Periapical images (B and C) of another case of osteosarcoma show nonconcentric widening of the periodontal ligament space of the teeth of the right and left maxilla in osteosarcoma *(arrows)*.

Effects on adjacent structures. Chondrosarcoma, being relatively slow growing, often expands normal cortical boundaries rather than rapidly destroying them. In mandibular cases, the inferior border or alveolar process may be grossly expanded, while still maintaining its cortical covering. Maxillary lesions may displace the walls of the maxillary sinus or nasal fossa, and impinge on the infratemporal fossa. Lesions of the condyle may cause expansion, and remodel the adjacent glenoid fossa and articular eminence. If lesions arise in the articular disk region, a widened joint space may be present with corresponding remodeling of the condylar neck. Erosion of the articular fossa may also occur.

Effects on adjacent teeth. When chondrosarcoma develops near teeth, external root resorption and tooth displacement may occur, as may widening of the periodontal ligament space.

Differential Interpretation

Chondrosarcoma is indistinguishable from osteosarcoma on diagnostic images. Although the calcifications may be absent from osteosarcoma, the neoplasms share many other radiologic features. Fibrous dysplasia may have a similar internal pattern to chondrosarcoma, although generally, the periphery of fibrous dysplasia is more well defined without signs of bone destruction, and its borders with adjacent teeth differs from chondrosarcoma. For instance, fibrous dysplasia alters the bone pattern up to and including the lamina dura, leaving a normal or thin periodontal ligament space. Because chondrosarcomas may be slow growing and displace teeth and other surrounding structures, these characteristics may be misinterpreted as benign features.

Management

The management of chondrosarcoma is surgical. Radiation therapy and chemotherapy generally have no role to play. Patients with

chondrosarcomas have a relatively good 5-year survival rate, but 10-year survival is poor.

Ewing Sarcoma
Disease Mechanism

Ewing sarcoma is a small round cell neoplasm that appears to have a common origin with primitive neuroectodermal neoplasms. It is a neoplasm of long bones and is relatively rare in the jaws. Lesions arise in the medullary portion of the bone and spread to the endosteal, and later periosteal, surfaces.

Clinical Features

Ewing sarcoma is most common in the second decade of life with most patients between 5 and 30 years of age. Males are twice as likely to develop the disease as females. However, Ewing sarcoma rarely occurs in the jaws. The patient's signs and symptoms may include, in descending frequency, swelling, pain, loose teeth, paresthesia, exophthalmos, ptosis, epistaxis, ulceration, displaced teeth, trismus, and sinusitis. Multicentric lesions have been reported, as has cervical lymphadenopathy.

Imaging Features

Location. Mandibular cases outnumber maxillary cases by about 2:1, with the highest frequency found in the posterior areas of both jaws. Generally, the lesions develop centrally within the marrow spaces, and expand to the adjacent bone cortices.

Periphery. Ewing sarcoma may be round or ovoid but generally has no typical shape. They have a poorly defined periphery, and are never corticated. Its advancing edge destroys bone in an uneven fashion, resulting in a ragged border. The neoplasm can cause jaw fracture with an adjacent radiographically visible soft tissue mass (Fig. 26.14).

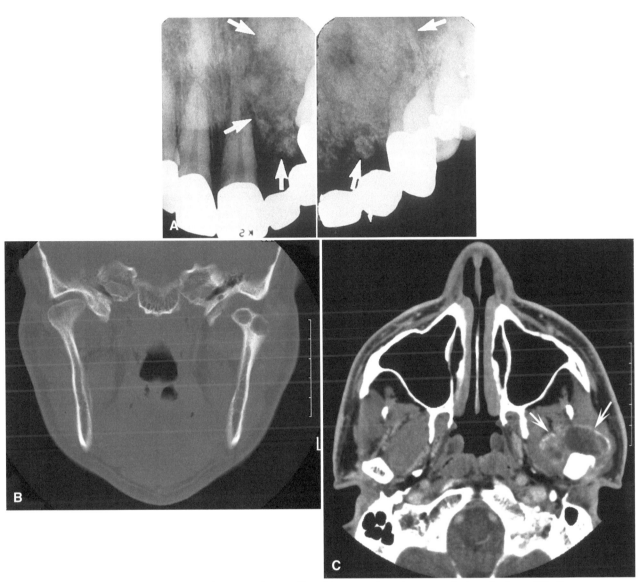

Fig. 26.13 Chondrosarcoma of the anterior maxilla, with sparse, irregular areas of mineralization within the neoplasm *(arrows)* (A). Coronal multidetector computed tomography (MDCT) image of a chondrosarcoma involving the mandibular condyle (note the two areas of bone destruction) (B). Axial soft tissue MDCT image demonstrating the soft tissue component *(arrows)* of a chondrosarcoma, which cannot be appreciated on the bone window MDCT image (C). (A, Courtesy Dr. L. Hollender, Seattle, WA.)

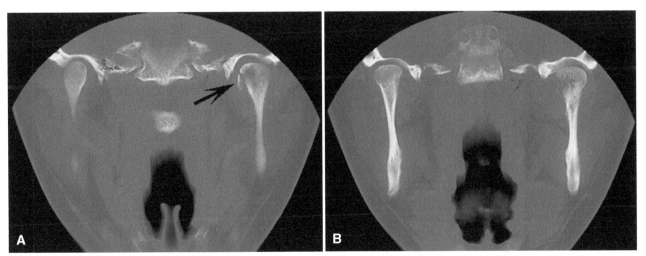

Fig. 26.14 Coronal multidetector computed tomography images (A and B) demonstrate a Ewing sarcoma involving the left mandibular condyle. Note the irregular borders of the lesion, destruction of the medial cortex of the condyle, and a small fracture fragment *(arrow)*.

Internal structure. Ewing sarcoma is primarily osteolytic, with little internal bone formation. Because it grows from within the bone, and only involves the endosteal and periosteal surfaces later in its course, it is usually entirely radiolucent.

Effects on adjacent structures. Ewing sarcoma grows rapidly, and can engage the bone surface and periosteum quickly. This may stimulate progenitor osteoblasts in the periosteum, and Codman triangle and "sunray" or "hair-on-end" spiculation may be seen. Laminar periosteal new bone formation, similar to that seen in osteomyelitis, has been reported to occur, but is not a common feature of Ewing sarcoma lesions in the jaws. Adjacent normal structures, including the inferior alveolar canal, inferior border of the mandible, and alveolar cortices, may be lost. If the lesion abuts teeth or tooth follicles, the lamina dura and follicular cortices are destroyed. This neoplasm does not characteristically cause root resorption, although it does destroy the supporting bone of adjacent teeth.

Effects on adjacent teeth. If the lesion abuts teeth or tooth follicles, the lamina dura and follicular cortices are destroyed. This neoplasm does not characteristically cause root resorption, although it does destroy the supporting bone of adjacent teeth.

Differential Interpretation

Osteomyelitis may share some of the radiographic features of Ewing sarcoma. Although both lesions are radiolucent, osteomyelitis is likely to have demonstrable sequestra present within the confines of the lesion, whereas Ewing sarcoma does not. Inflammatory lesions contain some sign of reactive bone formation, resulting in a sclerosis occurring internally or at the periphery.

Chronic localized Langerhans cell histiocytosis (LCH) of the jaw is also a destructive process, which can occur in the same part of the bone. This disease process can be associated with laminar periosteal new bone formation, whereas Ewing sarcoma in the jaws may not be. Other central primary malignancies of bone, such as osteosarcoma, chondrosarcoma, and fibrosarcoma, may be difficult to differentiate from this condition.

Management

Too few cases of maxillofacial Ewing sarcoma are available at any single treatment center for any specific treatment policy to have been adopted. Surgery, radiation therapy, and chemotherapy may be used alone or in combination.

Fibrosarcoma
Disease Mechanism

Fibrosarcoma is a neoplasm composed of malignant fibroblasts that produce collagen and elastin. The etiology is unknown; mutations may develop secondarily in cells that have received therapeutic levels of radiation.

Clinical Features

These lesions occur equally in males and females with a mean age in the fourth decade. The usual presenting symptom is an enlarging mass within bone, in which case it is usually accompanied by pain. Peripheral lesions or lesions exiting from bone may invade local soft tissues, causing a bulky, clinically obvious lesion. If such lesions reach a large size, jaw fracture may occur. If fibrosarcomas involve the course of peripheral nerves, sensorineural abnormalities may arise. Overlying mucosa, although initially normal, may become erythematous or ulcerated. Involvement of the temporomandibular joint or the muscles of mastication is often accompanied by trismus.

Imaging Features

Location. Most cases of fibrosarcoma of the jaws occur in the mandible, with the greatest number of these occurring in the premolar and molar region.

Periphery. Fibrosarcomas have noncorticated, poorly defined borders that are best described as being ragged (Fig. 26.15). These neoplasms are generally shaped in a fashion that suggests that they have grown along a bone, and so they tend to be somewhat elongated through the marrow space. The radiographic border may underestimate the extent of the neoplasm because these lesions typically are infiltrative. If soft tissue lesions occur adjacent to bone, they may cause a saucer-like depression in the underlying bone or invade it as would a squamous cell carcinoma. Finally, sclerosis may occur in the adjacent normal bone whether the fibrosarcoma is peripheral to bone or central.

Internal structure. Fibrosarcomas are radiolucent. If the lesions have been present for some time and are not overly aggressive, either residual jawbone or reactive osseous bone formation occurs.

Effects on adjacent structures. The most common effect on adjacent structures is destruction. In the mandible, the alveolar process, the inferior border of the jaw, and the cortices of neurovascular canal are lost. In the maxilla, the floor of the maxillary sinus, posterior wall of

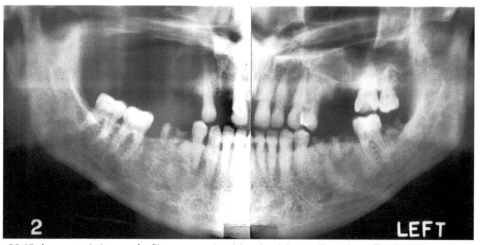

Fig. 26.15 A panoramic image of a fibrosarcoma involving the right maxillary sinus. The lesion has destroyed the floor of the maxillary sinus, the zygomatic process of the maxilla, the hard palate, and the alveolar process.

the maxilla and floor of the nasal fossa can be destroyed. Periosteal new bone formation is uncommon; however, if the lesion disrupts the periosteum, a Codman triangle or "sunray" or "hair-on-end" type of spiculation may be evident.

Effects on adjacent teeth. In either jaw, lamina dura and follicular cortices are obliterated. Teeth are more likely to be grossly displaced and lose their support bone so that they appear to be floating in space. Root resorption is rare. In addition, widening of the periodontal ligament space occurs with this neoplasm, as in other malignancies.

Differential Interpretation

Fibrosarcoma is difficult to differentiate from other central malignancies. If the lesion does not cause enlargement of the jaw, the practitioner must rule out metastatic carcinoma, multiple myeloma, and primary or secondary intraosseous carcinoma. If there is substantial enlargement of the jaw with an associated soft tissue mass, other sarcomas such as chondrosarcoma and osteosarcoma should be considered, although both usually have some internal structure. Ewing sarcoma and squamous cell carcinoma share many imaging characteristics with fibrosarcoma, and therefore may not be distinguishable.

Management

The management of fibrosarcoma is primarily surgical. A wide margin of adjacent normal bone is taken if anatomically possible. Radiation therapy and chemotherapy are usually palliative treatments.

MALIGNANCIES OF THE HEMATOPOIETIC SYSTEM

Multiple Myeloma

Disease Mechanism

Multiple myeloma is a malignant neoplasm of cells derived from plasma cells. A solitary lesion is referred to as a plasmacytoma while multiple lesions are called multiple myeloma. One common finding is the partial deletion of chromosome 13, although chromosomal translocations have also been reported.

Clinical Features

Multiple myeloma is the most common malignancy in bone. Most patients are male, and present between 35 and 70 years of age, with a mean age of 60 years. The patient may complain of fatigue, weight loss, fever, and bone pain, although the typical presenting feature is lower back pain. Orally, patients may complain of dental pain, swelling, hemorrhage, dysesthesia, or paresthesia. Secondary signs may include anemia, amyloidosis, and hypercalcemia. In half of all patients, the characteristic Bence-Jones protein can be detected in the patient's urine, which causes it to be foamy. When this clonal proliferation of plasma cells occurs, the cells first occupy cancellous bone spaces, and later cortical bone as the population of cells increases. These abnormal cells accumulate in the bone marrow and interfere with normal hematopoiesis.

Imaging Features

Location. The number of patients with demonstrable radiologic findings of multiple myeloma of the jaws at the time of diagnosis is relatively small. When multiple myeloma involves the jaws, it is more frequently seen in the mandible than the maxilla. In the mandible, lesions may be commonly seen in the posterior body, ramus, and condyle. Maxillary lesions usually appear in posterior sites. Soft tissue lesions have also been reported in the jaws and the nasopharynx

Periphery. The periphery of multiple myeloma lesions is well defined, but the lesions are not corticated (Fig. 26.16). The lack of cortication or any response of the adjacent bone to the lesion results in a nonexistent zone of transition between the lesion and the normal adjacent bone. Consequently, these appearances have led to the adaptation of the descriptor, "punched out" to these lesions (Fig. 26.17). However, many lesions have ragged borders, and may even appear infiltrative. Solitary lesions have an oval or cystic shape; however, untreated or aggressive areas of bone destruction may develop confluence, giving the appearance of multilocularity. In osteopenic patients, lesions may be difficult to detect.

Internal structure. Lesions of multiple myeloma are radiolucent. Occasionally islands of residual bone, yet unaffected by neoplasm, may give the appearance of mineralization with the radiolucency.

Effects on adjacent structures. The borders of the inferior alveolar canal may become less clear as it loses its cortical boundary, in whole or in part. These changes are profound when there is associated renal disease. Mandibular lesions can produce a localized area of osteolysis involving the endosteal surface of the inferior cortex of the mandible, which has been referred to as a "cookie bite" or scallop of the cortex. Any cortical boundary may be effaced if lesions involve them. Periosteal reaction is uncommon, but if present, it takes the form of a single radiopaque line parallel to the bone surface.

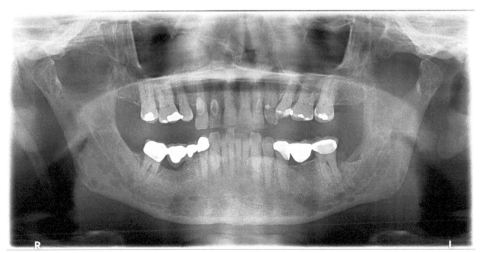

Fig. 26.16 Multiple myeloma lesions in the mandible showing the "punched-out" nature of the lesions. Note the absence of any bone reaction at the peripheries of the lesions. (Courtesy Dr. L. Lee, Toronto, ON, Canada.)

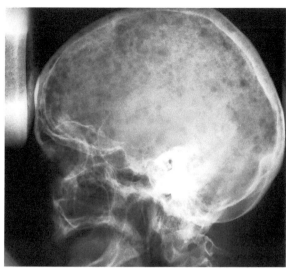

Fig. 26.17 There are multiple circular radiolucent lesions of multiple myeloma in the skull.

Effects on adjacent teeth. If a good deal of bone is lost, teeth may appear relatively radiopaque, and may stand out conspicuously against the osteopenic background of the bone. Lamina dura and the follicles of impacted teeth may lose their corticated peripheries in a manner analogous to that seen in hyperparathyroidism. In rare cases, there may be irregular root resorption.

Differential Interpretation

The most likely disease to be mistaken for multiple myeloma is metastasis, particularly when the metastases are osteolytic. Knowledge of a prior malignancy in a patient may help differentiate multiple myeloma from metastatic disease. Severe osteomyelitis may appear similar to multiple myeloma; however, a visible cause for the inflammatory response usually exists. Furthermore, inflammatory disease is generally accompanied by sclerosis, which is not the case with multiple myeloma. Simple bone cysts may be bilateral in the mandible and may be mistaken for multiple myeloma. They are usually corticated in part and characteristically interdigitate or scallop between the roots of the teeth in a much younger population. Also, the periodontal ligament spaces and lamina dura are preserved adjacent to a simple bone cyst.

Generalized osteopenia of the jaws may be caused by hyperparathyroidism, but it can be differentiated based on abnormal blood chemistry. However, brown tumors of hyperparathyroidism, if present with generalized osteopenia and similar symptoms, can readily be confused with multiple myeloma. Other metabolic diseases, such as Gaucher disease or oxalosis, may also cause many changes similar to multiple myeloma observed on images made for dental purposes.

Management

Multiple myeloma is treated with chemotherapy, without or with autologous or allogeneic bone marrow transplantation. Radiation therapy may be used for the treatment of symptomatic osseous lesions when palliation is required.

Lymphoma
Disease Mechanism

Lymphomas are malignant neoplasms of lymphocytes, at various levels of maturation. In general, lymphomas arise within lymph nodes; however,

extranodal sites, such as bone, skin, gastrointestinal mucosa, tonsils, and Waldeyer ring can be involved. The term non-Hodgkin lymphoma describes a family of heterogeneous neoplasms of varying type and severity based on their histopathologic appearances into low-, intermediate-, and high-grade neoplasms, with the last being the most aggressive. Hodgkin lymphoma is defined by the identification of the Reid-Sternberg cell in histopathology.

Clinical Features

Non-Hodgkin lymphoma occurs in all age groups, but is rare in patients in the first decade of life. The maxillary sinus, palate, tonsillar area, and bone may be sites of lymphoma spread. Lesions occurring outside lymph nodes in the head and neck may be present in one of five cases. Patients may feel unwell, experience night sweats, pruritus, and weight loss. A palpable, nonpainful swelling, lymphadenopathy, and sensorineural deficits may accompany isolated lesions of the jaws. Lesions present for some time may cause pain and ulceration.

Imaging Features

Location. Most cases of non-Hodgkin lymphomas of the head and neck occur in the lymph nodes. Extranodal non-Hodgkin lymphoma is more likely to affect the maxilla, including the maxillary sinus and the posterior mandible. A few cases have originated within the inferior alveolar nerve canal.

Periphery. When bone is involved, non-Hodgkin lymphomas initially take the shape and form of the host bone. If these lesions are untreated, they are capable of causing destruction of the overlying cortex (Fig. 26.18). Lymphoma lesions may appear round or multiloculated, and lack a cortex. The borders generally are poorly defined, with an invasive quality. Occasionally, lymphoma may show multifocal areas of bone destruction, which likely appear as finger-like extensions of malignant neoplasm cells in a buccal or lingual direction. When the lesions involve the soft tissues, their borders are smooth.

Internal structure. The internal structure of lymphoma is almost always entirely radiolucent. It is rare to see internal radiopacities or reactive bone formation at the periphery of lesions.

Effects on adjacent structures. In the maxillary sinus, a soft tissue mass may be visible on imaging, either internally or externally, and the antral walls may be lost. Lesions developing within the mandible will destroy the cortex of the inferior alveolar canal and the cortices of the bone. Periosteal reaction is uncommon, but when seen, it may take the form of a laminated or spiculated bone formation. With the advent of MRI, it has become apparent that lymphoma has a tendency of growing along fat planes, and along the surface of bone.

Effects on adjacent teeth. Lymphoma has a propensity to grow into the periodontal ligament space of erupted teeth (Fig. 26.19). In developing teeth, the cortex of the crypts may be lost when the malignant cells infiltrate the developing papilla, and the developing teeth may be displaced in an occlusal direction and exfoliated from their crypts.

Differential Interpretation

Multiple myeloma and metastatic disease can be easily confused with lymphoma when it arises in the jawbones. However, Ewing sarcoma and LCH, although also capable of producing the same effects, occur in a slightly younger age group. Osteolytic osteosarcoma and any of the central carcinomas may not be distinguishable from lymphoma on imaging examinations. Squamous cell carcinoma arising in the maxillary sinus may be difficult to differentiate from lymphoma of the maxillary sinus. Other lesions that can displace developing teeth in an occlusal direction include leukemia and LCH. Differentiation from periapical rarefying osteitis may be difficult; however, careful inspection of the

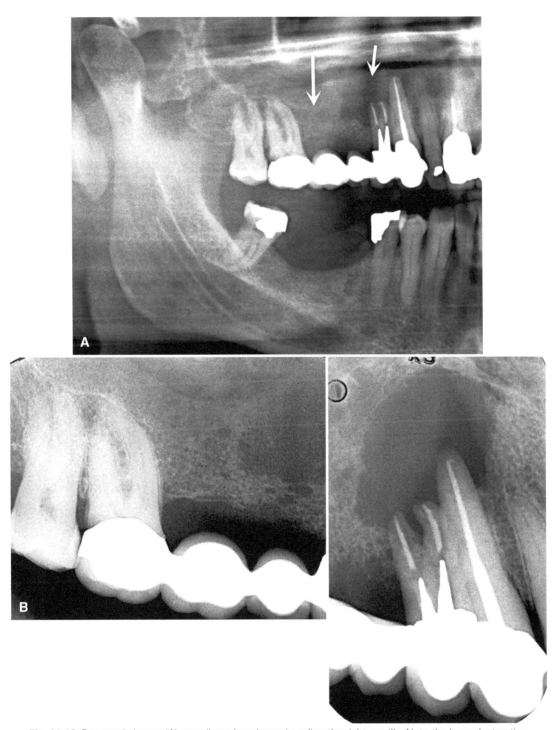

Fig. 26.18 Panoramic image (A) revealing a lymphoma invading the right maxilla. Note the bone destruction, and the poorly defined periphery of the lesion. Also, there has been destruction of the floor of the maxillary sinus *(arrows)*. Intraoral images also show bone destruction, and the lack of any bone reaction surrounding the lesion (B).

image may reveal the presence of an infiltrative border with adjacent bone destruction not seen in inflammation.

Management

The management of extranodal or isolated nodal disease is radiation therapy and/or chemotherapy. Treatment depends on the histopathologic variant, and the location and extent of disease.

Burkitt Lymphoma
Disease Mechanism

Burkitt lymphoma is a high-grade B-cell lymphoma that differs from other B-cell lymphomas with respect to its histologic appearance and clinical behavior. First described in East Africa as African jaw lymphoma, two types of the disease have now been described: the endemic African

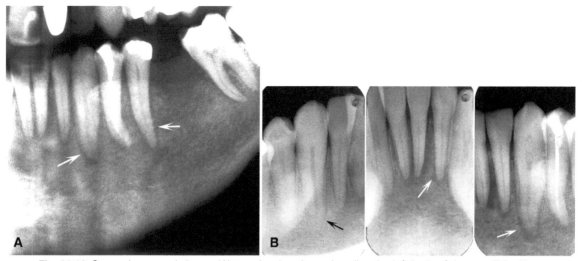

Fig. 26.19 Cropped panoramic image (A) reveals a lymphoma invading the left body of the mandible. Note the poorly defined periphery of the lesion as well as the nonconcentric widening of the periodontal ligament spaces *(arrows)*. Intraoral images (B) of the same case demonstrate widened periodontal ligament spaces *(white arrows)* compared with the normal periodontal ligament space of the right mandibular canine *(black arrow)*.

Burkitt lymphoma and the non-African form. The African form is linked to previous infections of malaria parasites and EBV; however, the role of EBV in the non-African form is uncertain. The infections are believed to facilitate a well-described translocation of chromosome 8 that involves the *Myc* oncogene, which controls cell function and proliferation. The latter is not characterized by jaw involvement (although it occurs), but there is involvement of abdominal viscera. African Burkitt lymphoma affects young children, whereas American Burkitt lymphoma affects adolescents and young adults. Cases of both have been described throughout the world.

Clinical Features

Burkitt lymphoma affects more males than females, and clinically, the hallmark of this neoplasm is its rapidity of growth with a neoplasm doubling time of less than 24 hours. The disease may involve children as young as 2 years, and adults in their seventh decade, although it is primarily a disease of youth.

Jaw neoplasms are rapidly growing; however, this feature is more characteristic of the African form. The neoplasms can cause facial deformity very early in their course, and they may block nasal passages, displace orbital contents, and ulcerate through skin. The African type can also cause pain and paresthesia, with paresthesia of the inferior alveolar nerve or other sensory facial nerves being more common.

Imaging Features

Location. Extranodal disease is the norm in Burkitt lymphoma. African cases may involve one jaw or both, primarily affecting the posterior parts of the jaws. In contrast, American cases may not involve the facial bones, but they are more likely to affect the abdominal viscera and testes.

Periphery. The lesions may begin as multiple, poorly defined, non-corticated radiolucencies, which later coalesce into larger areas. The lesions may be of no specific shape; however, they can expand the bone rapidly and have been likened to a balloon. This type of expansion can thin and breach bone cortices, and a soft tissue neoplasm may develop adjacent to the bone lesion. Lesions that abut the orbital contents or the maxillary sinus may radiologically show a smooth surface soft tissue mass.

Internal structure. Burkitt lymphoma developing in the bone is particularly radiolucent in children. In adults, there is rarely production of reactive bone.

Effects on adjacent structures. Cortical boundaries, such as the maxillary sinus, nasal floor, orbital walls, and inferior border of the mandible, are thinned and later destroyed. The cortex of the inferior alveolar canal is lost, although the canal cortex may be difficult to evaluate in children. If the periosteum is involved, the border may show "sunray" type of spiculation, although this is rare. Cases that impinge on the orbit can displace the orbital contents, and this may be seen both clinically and radiologically.

Effects on adjacent teeth. Erupted teeth adjacent to a Burkitt neoplasm are grossly displaced, as are developing tooth crypts. Neoplastic cells invading the crypts of developing tooth crowns may displace the developing tooth bud to one side of the crypt or superiorly. A neoplasm that is located apical to a developing tooth may cause the tooth to be displaced so it appears to erupt with little if any root formation. After neoplasm involvement of the developing dental structures occurs, root development ceases. Lamina dura of teeth in the area are destroyed.

Differential Interpretation

Burkitt lymphoma may be indistinguishable from Ewing sarcoma and osteolytic osteosarcoma both clinically and radiologically. Cherubism is bilateral, has more internal structure, does not breach bony borders and grows much more slowly. Finally, non-Hodgkin lymphoma must be considered, although it occurs in a much older age group in most cases.

Management

Burkitt lymphoma is treated with chemotherapy.

Leukemia
Disease Mechanism

Leukemia is a malignant neoplasm of hematopoietic stem cells, and associated with a number of nonrandom chromosomal abnormalities. A number of histopathologic subtypes have been defined based on their cell of origin. These malignant cells displace normal bone marrow constituents and spill out into the peripheral blood. Acute leukemias

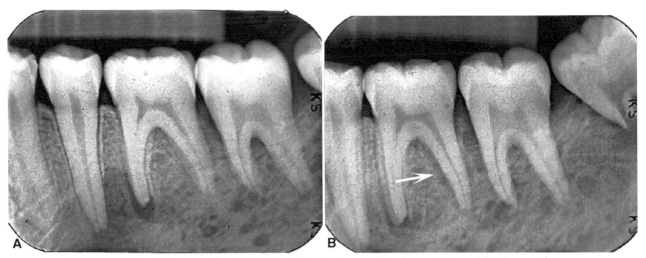

Fig. 26.20 Periapical images (A and B) of the left posterior mandible demonstrate multifocal areas of bone destruction and widening of portions of the periodontal ligament spaces *(arrow)* in leukemia. Note the infiltrative appearance of the bone destruction.

occur with a bimodal age distribution, in very young patients and very old patients. Most cases of leukemia are associated with nonrandom chromosomal abnormalities, although the exact etiology is not known.

Clinical Features

Leukemia is broadly classified as being either acute or chronic. Patients with acute leukemia generally feel unwell with weakness and bone pain. They may exhibit pallor, spontaneous hemorrhage, hepatomegaly, splenomegaly, lymphadenopathy, and fever. Oral symptoms are generally absent, but if present they include loose teeth, petechiae, ulceration, and boggy enlarged gingiva. A patient with chronic leukemia may have no presenting signs or complaints.

Imaging Features

Radiologic signs associated with chronic leukemia are comparatively rare.

Location. Leukemia affects the entire body, as the malignant cells are disseminated throughout the bone marrow via the circulating blood. Manifestations in the jaws may be seen more often in areas of developing teeth with rare involvement of the jaws of adults.

Periphery. As leukemia is a systemic malignancy, its radiologic features may be present bilaterally as poorly defined, radiolucent areas. With time and lack of treatment, these smaller, patchy areas of disease may coalesce to form larger areas radiolucent regions within bone (see Fig. 26.19).

Internal structure. The internal structure of leukemia is radiolucent, and there is generalized radiolucency of the bone. Rarely, granular bone may be seen within these lesions. Occasionally, foci of leukemic cells may be present outside of the jaws as a mass called chloromas, which may behave like a solitary, localized, malignant neoplasm.

Effects on surrounding structures. Leukemia does not cause expansion of bone, although occasionally a single layer of periosteal new bone may be seen in association with this disease; however, this is uncommon in chronic leukemia. If lesions affect the periodontal structures, the crestal bone may be lost.

Effects on adjacent teeth. The teeth may appear to stand out conspicuously from the surrounding osteopenic bone. Should the lesions involve the periodontal ligament space, there may be nonconcentric widening (Fig. 26.20). Developing teeth in their crypts and teeth undergoing eruption may be displaced in an occlusal direction (Fig. 26.21) or into the oral

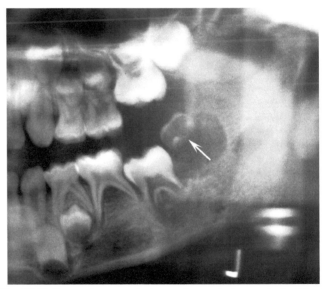

Fig. 26.21 Cropped panoramic image demonstrates unusual occlusal displacement of the developing mandibular second molar from its follicle *(arrow)*.

cavity before root development is completed. Less commonly, developing teeth may be displaced from their normal position. The result of this is premature loss of teeth. The lamina dura and cortical outlines of follicles may be effaced.

Differential Interpretation

Generally, a medical diagnosis has been reached by the time radiologic signs of leukemia are present in the jaws. However, the development of radiologic changes may be the first indication of the relapse of disease. Occasionally, lymphoma may mimic some of the features of destruction seen in leukemia. A metabolic disorder may be considered in cases in which generalized rarefaction of bone is seen; however, these conditions can be excluded on the basis of blood testing. With periapical lesions, careful clinical and radiologic examination of the involved tooth typically shows no apparent cause for rarefying osteitis.

Management

The management of leukemia is primarily through a combination of chemotherapy with or without allogeneic or autologous bone marrow transplantation. Some chronic leukemias are managed with low-dose chemotherapy.

Langerhans Cell Histiocytosis

Disease Mechanism

Langerhans cells are specialized cells of the histiocytic cell line that normally are found in the skin. The disorders included in LCH are abnormalities that result from the abnormal proliferation of Langerhans-like cells or their precursors due to mutations affecting the proto-oncogene $BRAF^{V600E}$. This proto-oncogene encodes a protein, B-Raf, which plays a role in the control of cell proliferation.

The abnormal proliferation of Langerhans cells and eosinophils results in a spectrum of clinical diseases; chronic localized histiocytosis (eosinophilic granuloma), chronic disseminated histiocytosis (Hand-Schüller-Christian disease) and acute disseminated histiocytosis (Letterer-Siwe disease). More recently, a newly proposed classification scheme designates two types: (1) nonmalignant unifocal or multifocal eosinophilic granuloma and (2) malignant Letterer-Siwe disease and variants of histiocytic lymphoma. Although lesions of LCH often have a prominent inflammatory component, more recently, all forms of LCH have been shown to be clonal and of a neoplastic nature.

Clinical Features

Head and neck, and oral lesions, are common on initial presentation, with approximately 10% of all patients with LCH having oral lesions. LCH usually involves the skeleton (ribs, pelvis, long bones, skull, and jaws), and—rarely—soft tissue. This condition occurs most commonly in older children and young adults.

The lesions often form quickly and may cause a dull, steady pain. In the jaws, LCH may cause bony swelling, a soft tissue mass, gingivitis, bleeding gingiva, and ulceration. LCH may have a single focus or may develop into a multifocal, more aggressive disease. The disseminated form, previously known as Hand-Schüller-Christian disease, may involve multiple bone lesions, diabetes insipidus, and exophthalmos.

Letterer-Siwe disease is the most aggressive form of LCH that most often occurs in children younger than 3 years of age. Soft tissue and bony granulomatous reactions disseminate throughout the body, and the condition is marked by intermittent fever, hepatosplenomegaly, anemia, lymphadenopathy, hemorrhage, and failure to thrive. Lesions in bone are rare. Death usually occurs within several weeks of the onset of the disease.

Imaging Features

Location. LCH lesions within the alveolar processes are commonly multiple, whereas intraosseous lesions usually are solitary. The mandible is a more commonly affected site than the maxilla, and the posterior regions are more involved than the anterior regions (Fig. 26.22). The mandibular ramus is a common site of intraosseous lesions. Solitary lesions of the jaws may be accompanied by lesions in other bones.

Periphery. The periphery of LCH lesions varies from moderately well defined to well defined, but without cortication. In some cases, the periphery can appear punched out (Fig. 26.23). The borders may be smooth or irregular. Lesions within the alveolar processes have an epicenter in the midroot regions of the teeth. The bone destruction progresses in a somewhat oval or round shape until the alveolar process appears scooped out (Figs. 26.24 and 26.25).

Internal structure. The internal structure usually is radiolucent.

Effects on adjacent structures. LCH destroys bone. These lesions are able to stimulate periosteal new bone formation; this occurs more commonly with the intraosseous type of lesion (Fig. 26.26). The periosteal new bone formation is indistinguishable from the lamellar appearance seen with inflammatory lesions of the jaws. This lesion can destroy the outer cortical plate and in rare cases extends into the surrounding soft tissues in the CT examination.

Effects on adjacent teeth. With lesions centered in the alveolar processes, the bone around teeth, including the lamina dura, is destroyed, and the teeth appear to be floating in space. The lesion does not displace teeth, although teeth may move because they are bereft of bone support (see Fig. 26.25). Only minor root resorption has been reported.

Differential Interpretation

The major differential interpretation of alveolar lesions of LCH is advanced stage periodontitis and squamous cell carcinoma. An important characteristic to differentiate LCH from advanced stage periodontitis is that the epicenter of the bone destruction in LCH is approximately in the midroot region, which produces the scooped-out appearance. In contrast, the bone destruction in periodontal disease begins at the alveolar crest, and extends apically down the root surface. Differentiation of a squamous cell carcinoma may be impossible by imaging characteristics

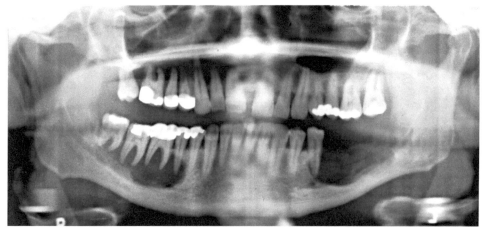

Fig. 26.22 Panoramic image of multiple lesions of Langerhans cell histiocytosis. Note the "scooped-out" shape of the bone destruction, as well as the destruction of the floor of the right maxillary sinus.

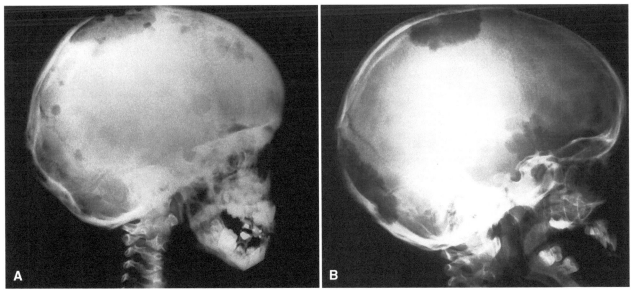

Fig. 26.23 Skull lesions of Langerhans cell histiocytosis showing the variably sized radiolucent lesions (A and B).

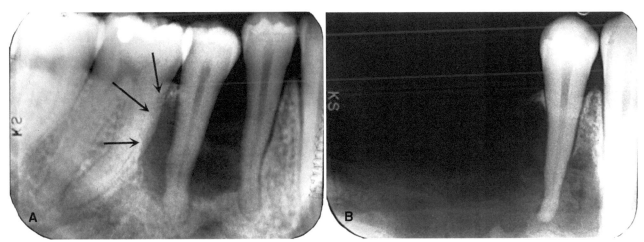

Fig. 26.24 Periapical Images of the Same Region of the Mandible Approximately 1 Year Apart. The earlier image (A) shows the scooped-out appearance of the lesion with an epicenter near the mid-root level of the involved teeth (in contrast to periodontal disease). The later image (B) shows much more extensive bone destruction, and the loss of teeth. (Courtesy Dr. D. Stoneman, Toronto, ON, Canada.)

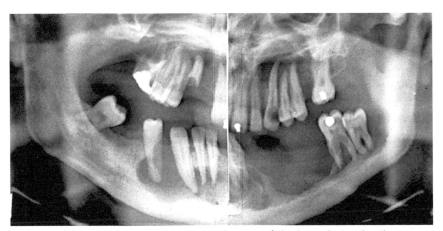

Fig. 26.25 Panoramic image shows the bone extensiveness of the bone destruction that can occur with Langerhans cell histiocytosis, and the appearance of the remaining teeth to be "floating in space." (Courtesy Dr. D. Stoneman, Toronto, ON, Canada.)

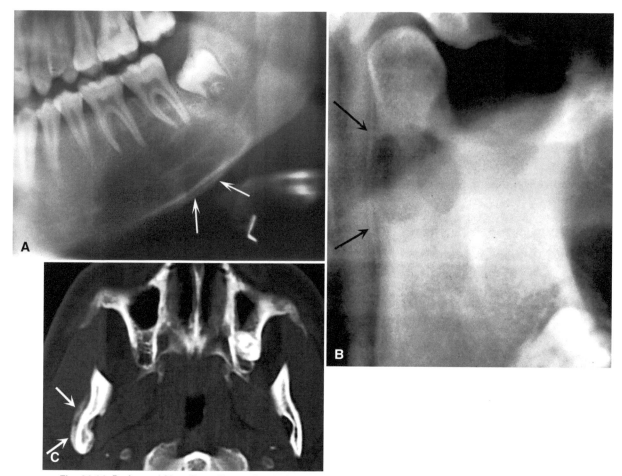

Fig. 26.26 Periosteal New Bone Formation in Langerhans Cell Histiocytosis. Note the early destruction of bone around the molar teeth on the cropped panoramic image (A) and the lamellar periosteal new bone formation adjacent to the inferior cortex of the mandible. A similar appearance can be seen along the posterior border of the right ramus (B). Axial multidetector computed tomography image (C) shows the lamellar periosteal new bone formation along the lateral surface of the right mandibular ramus.

alone, although the borders of an LCH lesion typically are better defined. Multiple lesions in a younger age group (usually the first three decades) are more likely to be LCH than squamous cell carcinoma, which typically appears as a single lesion in middle-aged or elderly patients.

The differential interpretation of solitary intraosseous lesions includes metastatic disease and malignant neoplasms extending into bone from adjacent soft tissues. However, the well-defined borders and the periosteal reaction seen in LCH help in the differential interpretation.

Management

Patients suspected to have LCH should be referred to an oral and maxillofacial radiologist for a complete work-up, which may include nuclear medicine to detect other possible bone lesions. If confirmed, the lesion should undergo biopsy. Because the histopathologic appearance of histiocytosis may be hidden by changes caused by secondary infection from the oral cavity in alveolar lesions, it is important to correlate the radiologic and histopathologic findings from the biopsy.

Management of localized lesions usually consists of surgical curettage or limited radiation therapy. Surgical management of jaw lesions usually is preferable because these lesions have a low recurrence rate. The earlier LCH lesions of the mandible are diagnosed and controlled, and fewer teeth are lost to bone destruction. Disseminated disease is treated with chemotherapy.

ORAL AND MAXILLOFACIAL IMAGING FOR CANCER SURVIVORS

Patients who have survived cancer treatment require dental treatment just like any other patient. For a cancer survivor, an oral and maxillofacial radiologic examination may be more important than for a healthy patient to receive a recall examination. Some patients who have received a full course of radiation therapy are concerned about the additional radiation dose from an oral and maxillofacial radiologic examination. However, this is not a valid concern because the relatively minuscule dose associated with oral and maxillofacial radiologic imaging examinations is negligible compared with the dose received from radiation therapy for a malignancy.

A patient treated for head and neck malignancy with radiation therapy—even with today's advanced radiotherapeutic methods—is prone to develop postradiation dental caries and radiation-induced bone necrosis. Careful clinical examination and a thorough oral and maxillofacial radiologic examination may be periodically required to ensure that the remaining dentition and periodontal apparatus is in good shape. Radiation caries occurs in many patients and appears clinically different from typical dental caries. If untreated, these carious teeth can develop nonvital pulps, and there may be extension of the inflammatory response to the jaw more widely. If such a patient requires tooth extraction, healing can be expected to be slow, and occasionally osteoradionecrosis may result. Also, bisphosphonates and other related therapies are now used extensively with some chemotherapy regimens, as in multiple myeloma. Changes seen with either radiation therapy or medication may mimic odontogenic inflammatory disease and should be differentiated to avoid unnecessary treatment and secondary osteonecrosis (see Chapter 22).

The role of oral and maxillofacial radiology in these patients should not be restricted to examination only of the teeth and supporting structures. Equally important is monitoring of the outcome of treatment and specifically the examination of oral and maxillofacial images for evidence of neoplasm recurrence, and the development of metastases and osteonecrosis.

BIBLIOGRAPHY

Burkitt Lymphoma

Adatia AK. Significance of jaw lesions in Burkitt lymphoma. *Br Dent J.* 1978;145:263–266.

Burkitt DA. Sarcoma involving the jaws in African children. *Br J Surg.* 1958;46:218–223.

England CG, Rui L, Cai W. Lymphoma: current status of clinical and preclinical imaging with radiolabeled antibodies. *Eur J Nucl Med Mol Imaging.* 2017;44:517–532.

Sariban E, Donahue A, Magrath IT. Jaw involvement in American Burkitt lymphoma. *Cancer.* 1984;53:1777–1782.

Central Squamous Cell Carcinoma

Ariji E, Ozeki S, Yonetsu K, et al. Central squamous cell carcinoma of the mandible: computed tomographic findings. *Oral Surg Oral Med Oral Pathol.* 1994;77:541–548.

Lin YJ, Chen CH, Wang WC, et al. Primary intraosseous carcinoma of the mandible. *Dentomaxillofac Radiol.* 2005;34:112–116.

Suei Y, Tanimoto K, Taguchi A, et al. Primary intra-osseous carcinoma: review of the literature and diagnostic criteria. *J Oral Maxillofac Surg.* 1994;52:580–583.

Chondrosarcoma

Garrington GE, Collett WK. Chondrosarcoma. I. A selected literature review. *J Oral Pathol.* 1988;17:1–11.

Garrington GE, Collett WK. Chondrosarcoma. II. Chondrosarcoma of the jaws: analysis of 37 cases. *J Oral Pathol.* 1988;17:12–20.

Gorsky M, Epstein JB. Craniofacial osseous and chondromatous sarcomas in British Columbia—a review of 34 cases. *Oral Oncol.* 2000;36:27–31.

Hayt MW, Becker L, Katz DS. Chondrosarcoma of the maxilla: panoramic radiographic and computed tomographic with multiplanar reconstruction findings. *Dentomaxillofac Radiol.* 1998;27:113–116.

Hertzanu Y, Mendelsohn DB, Davidge-Pitts K, et al. Chondrosarcoma of the head and neck—the value of computed tomography. *J Surg Oncol.* 1985;28:97–102.

Vener J, Rice D, Newman AN. Osteosarcoma and chondrosarcoma of the head and neck. *Laryngoscope.* 1984;94:240–242.

Ewing Sarcoma

Becker M, Stefanelli S, Rougemont AL, et al. Non-odontogenic neoplasms of the facial bones in children and adolescents: role of multiparametric imaging. *Neuroradiology.* 2017;doi:10.1007/s00234-017-1798-y.

Guimarāres JB, Rigo L, Lewin F, et al. The importance of PET/CT in the evaluation of patients with Ewing neoplasms. *Radiol Bras.* 2015;48:175–180.

Fibrosarcoma

Pereira CM, Jorge J Jr, Di Hipólito O Jr, et al. Primary intraosseous fibrosarcoma of jwa. *Int J Oral Maxillofac Surg.* 2005;34:579–581.

Langerhans Cell Histiocytosis

Dagenais M, Pharoah MJ, Sikorski PA, et al. The radiographic characteristics of histiocytosis X. *Oral Surg Oral Med Oral Pathol Oral Radiol Endod.* 1992;74:230–236.

Haroche J, Cohen-Aubart F, Rollins BJ, et al. Histiocytoses: emerging neoplasia behind inflammation. *Lancet Oncol.* 2017;18:e113–e125.

Wong GB, Pharoah MJ, Weinberg S, et al. Eosinophilic granuloma of the mandibular condyle: report of three cases and review of the literature. *J Oral Maxillofac Surg.* 1997;55:870–878.

Leukemia

Curtis AB. Childhood leukemias: initial oral manifestations. *J Am Dent Assoc.* 1971;83:159–164.

Miyagi T, Nagasaki A, Taira T, et al. Extranodel adult T-cell leukemia/lymphoma of the head and neck: a clinicopathological study of nine cases and a review of the literature. *Leuk Lymphoma.* 2009;50:187–195.

Morgan L. Infiltrate of chronic lymphocytic leukemia appearing as a periapical radiolucent lesion. *J Endod.* 1995;21:475–478.

Sugihara Y, Wakasa T, Kameyama T, et al. Pediatric acute lymphocytic leukemia with osseous changes in jaws: literature review and report of a case. *Oral Radiol.* 1989;5:25–31.

"Malignant Ameloblastoma" and Ameloblastic Carcinoma

Dissanayake RK, Jayasooriya PR, Siriwardena DJ, et al. Review of metastasizing (malignant) ameloblastoma (METAM): pattern of metastasis and treatment. *Oral Surg Oral Med Oral Pathol Oral Radiol Endod.* 2011;111:734–741.

Yunaev M, Abdul-Razak M, Coleman H, et al. A rare case of ameloblastic carcinoma. *Ear Nose Throat J.* 2014;93:E34–E36.

Metastatic Neoplasms

D'Silva NJ, Summerlin DJ, Cordell KG, et al. Metastatic neoplasms in the jaws: a retrospective study of 114 cases. *J Am Dent Assoc.* 2006;137:1667–1672.

Fidler IJ. The pathogenesis of cancer metastasis: the 'seed and soil' hypothesis revisted. *Nat Rev Cancer.* 2003;3:453–458.

Hirshberg A, Berger R, Allon I, et al. Metastatic neoplasms to the jaws and mouth. *Head Neck Pathol.* 2014;8:463–474.

Van der Waal RI, Buter J, Van der Waal I, et al. Oral metastases: report of 24 cases. *Br J Oral Maxillofac Surg.* 2003;41:3–6.

Mucoepidermoid Carcinoma

Chan KC, Pharoah M, Lee L, et al. Intraosseous mucoepidermoid carcinoma: a review of diagnostic imaging features of four jaw cases. *Dentomaxillofac Radiol.* 2013;42:20110162.

Inagaki M, Yuasa K, Nakayama E, et al. Mucoepidermoid carcinoma in the mandible. *Oral Surg Oral Med Oral Pathol Oral Radiol Endod.* 1998;85:613–618.

Raut D, Khedkar S. Primary intraosseous mucoepidermoid carcinoma of the maxilla: a case report and review of the literature. *Dentomaxillofac Radiol.* 2009;38:163–168.

Strick MJ, Kelly C, Soames JV, et al. Malignant neoplasms of the minor salivary glands—a 20 year review. *Br J Plast Surg.* 2004;57:624–631.

Multiple Myeloma

Furutani M, Ohnishi M, Tanaka Y. Mandibular involvement in patients with multiple myeloma. *J Oral Maxillofac Surg.* 1994;52:23–25.

Kaffe I, Ramon Y, Hertz M. Radiographic manifestations of multiple myeloma in the mandible. *Dentomaxillofac Radiol.* 1986;15:31–35.

Raza S, Leng S, Lentzsch S. The critical role of imaging in the management of multiple myeloma. *Curr Hematol Malig Rep.* 2017;doi:10.1007/s11899-017-0379-9.

Witt C. Radiographic manifestations of multiple myeloma in the mandible: a retrospective study of 77 patients. *J Oral Maxillofac Surg.* 1997;55:450–453.

Non-Hodgkin Lymphoma

Maxymiw WG, Goldstein M, Wood RE. Extranodal non-Hodgkin's lymphoma of the maxillofacial region: analysis of 88 consecutive cases. *SADJ.* 2001;56:524–527.

Pazoki A, Jansisyanont P, Ord RA. Primary non-Hodgkin's lymphoma of the jaws: report of four cases and review of the literature. *J Oral Maxillofac Surg.* 2003;61:112–117.

Yamada T, Kitagawa Y, Ogasawara T, et al. Enlargement of the mandibular canal without hypesthesia caused by extranodal non-Hodgkin's lymphoma. *Oral Surg Oral Med Oral Pathol Oral Radiol Endod.* 2000;89:388–392.

Osteosarcoma

Bainchi SD, Boccardi A. Radiological aspects of osteosarcoma of the jaws. *Dentomaxillofac Radiol.* 1999;28:42–47.

Chindia ML. Osteosarcoma of the jaw bones. *Oral Oncol.* 2001;37: 545–547.

Clark JL, Unni KK, Dahlin DC, et al. Osteosarcoma of the jaw. *Cancer.* 1983;51:2311–2316.

Gardner DG, Mills DM. The widened periodontal ligament of osteosarcoma of the jaws. *Oral Surg Oral Med Oral Pathol.* 1976;41: 652–656.

Givol N, Buchner A, Taicher S, et al. Radiological features of osteogenic sarcoma of the jaws: a comparative study of different radiographic modalities. *Dentomaxillofac Radiol.* 1998;27:313–320.

Stewart BD, Reith JD, Knapik JA, et al. Bone- and cartilage-forming neoplasms and ewing sarcoma: an update with gnathic emphasis. *Head Neck Pathol.* 2014;8:454–462.

Wang S, Shi H, Yu Q. Osteosarcoma of the jaws: demographic and CT imaging features. *Dentomaxillofac Radiol.* 2012;41:37–42.

Squamous Cell Carcinoma

Brown JS, Lowe D, Kalavrezos N, et al. Patterns of invasion and routes of neoplasm entry into the mandible by oral squamous cell carcinoma. *Head Neck.* 2002;24:370–383.

O'Brien CJ, Carter RL, Soo KC, et al. Invasions of the mandible by squamous carcinomas of the oral cavity and oropharynx. *Head Neck Surg.* 1986;8:247–256.

Rao LP, Das SR, Mathews A, et al. Mandibular invasion in oral squamous cell carcinoma: investigation by clinical examination and orthopantomogram. *Int J Oral Maxillofac Surg.* 2004;33:454–457.

Squamous Cell Carcinoma Originating in a Cyst

Cavalcanti MGP, Veltrini VC, Ruprecht A, et al. Squamous-cell carcinoma arising from an odontogenic cyst—the importance of computed tomography in the diagnosis of malignancy. *Oral Surg Oral Med Oral Pathol Oral Radiol Endod.* 2005;100:365–368.

Eversole LR, Sabre WR, Lovin S. Aggressive growth and neoplastic potential of odontogenic cysts. *Cancer.* 1975;35:270–282.

Kaffe I, Ardekian L, Peled M, et al. Radiological features of primary intra-osseous carcinoma of the jaws: analysis of the literature and report of a new case. *Dentomaxillofac Radiol.* 1998;27:209–214.

van der Wal KGH, de Visscher JGAM, Eggink HF. Squamous cell carcinoma arising in a residual cyst. *Int J Oral Maxillofac Surg.* 1993;23:350–352.

27

Trauma

Sanjay M. Mallya

Radiologic examination is an integral component of the diagnostic evaluation of the patient with trauma to the teeth and jaws. It provides essential information about the presence, location, and orientation of fracture planes and fragments; the involvement of adjacent vital anatomic structures; and the presence of foreign objects that have may have become embedded within the soft tissues. Posttherapeutic images allow for the monitoring of healing and detection of long-term changes resulting from the trauma.

APPLIED RADIOLOGY

The initial assessment of a patient with craniofacial trauma is directed toward developing a prioritized treatment plan based on the severity of the trauma and to determine the presence of any life-threatening injuries. Diagnostic imaging is an important component guiding this management. Depending on the extent of the injuries and the clinical context, the imaging examination may encompass the brain, facial bones, dentoalveolar arches, and cervical spine. In acute trauma settings, this is typically accomplished with multidetector computed tomography (MDCT) and magnetic resonance imaging (MRI), depending on the clinical presentation, and may be supplemented with conventional oral and maxillofacial images. However, the choice of the imaging examination may be limited by the extent of the patient's injuries and the availability of imaging modalities.

Dentoalveolar Fractures

Patients with trauma to the teeth and supporting alveolar processes of the jaws must be evaluated with imaging. Such examinations are necessary prior to definitive management, especially in pediatric patients where manipulation of a traumatized deciduous tooth root could potentially damage the underlying permanent tooth bud. Intraoral images are the first choice and provide the best image resolution with regard to the detection of coronal and root fractures and the potential displacement of the tooth within its socket. To effectively identify root fractures, at least two periapical images should be made at different horizontal angulations of the x-ray beam. Furthermore, the examination must include intraoral images of teeth in the opposing arch. When mouth opening is limited because of trauma, cross-sectional occlusal images (see Chapter 7) may be used instead of periapical images. In pediatric patients, an American National Standards Institute (ANSI) size 2 receptor may be used to obtain such occlusal images.

Panoramic imaging is a convenient approach to examine a broad anatomic region in order to localize dentoalveolar injuries and detect mandibular fractures. However, the image resolution is often inadequate to critically evaluate traumatic injuries to the teeth and supporting bone, especially in the anterior regions of the jaws. Small or limited field-of-view (FOV) cone beam computed tomography (CBCT) provides high-resolution multiplanar imaging and may facilitate the identification of fractures involving the teeth and alveolar processes.

If a tooth or a large fragment of a tooth is missing, a chest or abdominal image can provide information on accidental aspiration or ingestion. If there are lacerations in the lips or cheek, the soft tissues must be evaluated for potential embedded foreign bodies or tooth fragments. This can be accomplished relatively simply by exposing an intraoral receptor placed adjacent to the traumatized soft tissue. If the laceration is in the tongue, an imaging examination can be accomplished with a mandibular occlusal projection image. Alternatively, the tongue can be protruded and then imaged with a receptor placed adjacent to the laceration site.

Mandibular Fractures

Panoramic imaging is often the initial examination performed to evaluate suspected or clinically evident mandibular fractures in a conscious patient. Where involvement of the mandibular body or alveolar process is suspected, cross-sectional mandibular occlusal images can provide additional information about the orientation of the fracture plane and potential displacement of the fractured segments. Likewise, panoramic imaging is often supplemented by an open-mouth Towne view to evaluate the mandibular condylar head and neck, especially in cases of nondisplaced greenstick fractures of the condylar neck. Patients with suspected multiple or complex fractures of the mandible are best imaged with CBCT or preferably MDCT. Where soft tissue injuries to the temporomandibular joint capsule and disk are present or suspected, MRI is the modality of choice.

Maxillofacial Fractures

Computed tomography (CT) is the method of choice for imaging fractures of the maxillofacial skeleton, particularly when they involve multiple bones. Because of its superior soft tissue detail, MDCT is preferred to CBCT.

Radiologic Signs of Fracture

Fractures are often erroneously referred to as "lines," despite their three-dimensional nature. Fractures represent planes of cleavage through a tooth or bone, and these planes can extend deep into the tissues. A fracture may be missed if the plane of the fracture is not aligned with the direction of the incident x-ray beam on a single planar image.

The following are general signs that may indicate the presence of a fracture of a tooth or bone:
1. **The presence of one or two usually sharply defined radiolucent lines within the anatomic boundaries of a structure.** Radiolucent line(s) that extend beyond the boundaries of the mandible most likely represent an superimposed structure. If a line extends beyond the boundaries of a tooth root, it may represent a superimposed neurovascular canal.

2. **A change in the normal anatomic outline or shape of the structure.** Noticeable asymmetry or a change in the contour of the occlusal plane may indicate the presence and location of a fracture.
3. **A loss of continuity of an outer border.** This may appear as a gap in the continuity of the otherwise smooth tooth or cortical border. Such a gap may also produce a "step-type" defect, where the two fragments have become displaced relative to one another.
4. **An increase in the radiopacity of a structure.** When two fragments of tooth or bone overlap, that region may appear "doubly" radiopaque. The region adjacent to this radiopaque zone must be scrutinized for discontinuity of borders or step deformities as described earlier.

DENTOALVEOLAR TRAUMA

Dentoalveolar injuries can affect all age groups and are caused by falls, contact sports and playground activities, and child abuse. Injuries may also occur as part of more extensive facial trauma caused by motor vehicle accidents. Trauma to the teeth may be iatrogenic; indeed, dental trauma is the most frequent general anesthesia–related claim in litigation. Andreasen's classification system of dentoalveolar injuries is widely used to facilitate communication and treatment planning of injuries to the primary and permanent dentition. The system categorizes the hard tissue injuries into three groups: tooth fractures, periodontal tissue injury, and injuries to the supporting bone (Box 27.1).

DENTAL FRACTURES

Dental Crown Fractures
Definition
Fractures of the dental crown account for approximately 25% of traumatic injuries to the permanent teeth and 40% of injuries to the deciduous teeth. The most common event responsible for the fracture of permanent teeth is a fall, followed by accidents involving vehicles (e.g., bicycles, motorcycles, and automobiles), and impacts from foreign objects striking the teeth. Fractures involving only the crown are divided into three categories:
1. **Crown infraction:** Fractures and cracks confined to enamel without the loss of enamel substance (Fig. 27.1A).

2. **Uncomplicated crown fractures:** Fractures confined to enamel or enamel and dentin with no pulp exposure (see Fig. 27.1B).
3. **Complicated crown fractures:** Fractures that involve enamel, dentin, and pulp (see Fig. 27.1C).

Clinical Features
Fractures of the dental crowns most frequently involve anterior teeth. Infractions and cracks in the enamel are best detected by indirect light or transillumination. Histologic studies have shown that such cracks extend through the enamel but do not involve dentin.

Uncomplicated crown fractures that involve dentin can be recognized by the contrast in color between dentin and the peripheral layer of enamel. The exposed dentin is usually sensitive to chemical, thermal, or mechanical stimulation. In the permanent dentition, uncomplicated crown fractures are more common than complicated ones. In contrast, complicated and uncomplicated fractures occur with nearly equal frequencies in the deciduous teeth. When the fracture extends deeper into the tooth, the pink blush of the pulp may be evident through the thin remaining dentin wall. Complicated crown fractures are distinguishable by bleeding from the exposed pulp or by droplets of blood forming from pinpoint exposures. The pulp is visible and may extrude from the open pulp chamber if the fracture is not recent. The exposed pulp is sensitive to most forms of stimulation.

Imaging Features
The objectives of imaging are to identify the location and extent of the fracture, and its relationship to the pulp chamber (Fig. 27.2). Imaging also provides a baseline record for comparison with future images made to monitor the development of the pathologic consequences of dental trauma, such as periapical inflammation, disruption of root development, and root resorption. The initial assessment of tooth trauma is usually made with intraoral imaging. Imaging of the adjacent soft tissues may be needed to locate embedded tooth fragments or foreign objects (Fig. 27.3).

Management
Crown infractions typically do not require management beyond smoothing of rough edges or restoration of form and function to the traumatized tooth. The vitality of the tooth should be determined at the initial visit and after approximately 6 to 8 weeks following pulpal recovery and secondary dentin formation. The prognosis for teeth with fractures limited to the enamel is good, and pulpal necrosis develops in less than 2% of such cases. If a fracture involves both dentin and enamel, the frequency of pulpal necrosis is approximately 3%. Oblique fractures have a worse prognosis than horizontal fractures because potentially a greater amount of dentin is exposed. Concomitant concussion and luxation disturb the blood supply and increase the frequency of subsequent pulpal necrosis.

When complicated crown fractures occur in immature, developing permanent teeth, attempts should be made to maintain pulp vitality to allow for subsequent root development. If development of the root apex is completed, endodontic therapy is typically the treatment of choice, although pulp capping and partial pulpectomy may be acceptable depending on the size of the pulp exposure and the amount of elapsed time since the trauma. In the primary dentition, complicated crown fractures are managed by pulp capping and pulpectomy to attempt to retain pulp vitality. Depending on the child's maturity and cooperation, extraction may, however, be an acceptable option.

Dental Crown and Root Fractures
Definition
Fractures involving both the crown and roots (i.e., crown-root fractures) are most often complicated by pulp exposure. The permanent teeth are

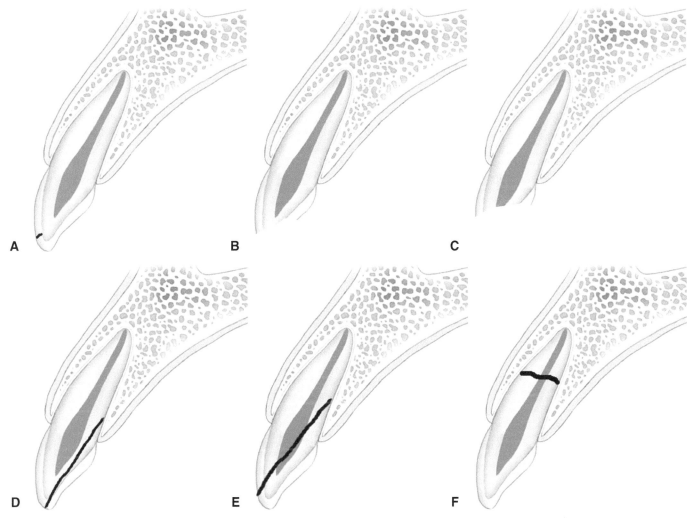

Fig. 27.1 Classification of dental fractures. (A) Crown infraction. (B) Uncomplicated crown fracture. (C) Complicated crown fracture. (D) Uncomplicated crown-root fracture. (E) Complicated crown-root fracture. (F) Horizontal root fracture.

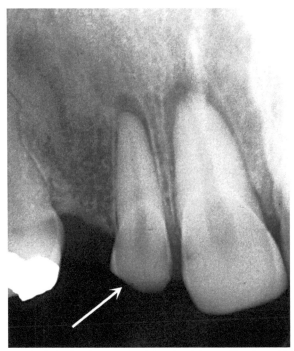

Fig. 27.2 Incisal-edge fracture involving the right maxillary lateral incisor *(arrow)* and subluxation of both the central and the lateral incisors. Note the increases to the widths of the apical periodontal ligament spaces.

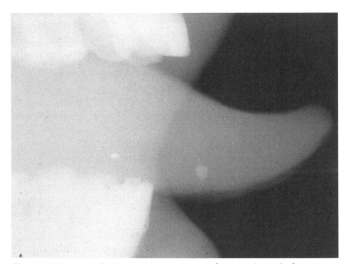

Fig. 27.3 Image of the tongue to locate fractured tooth fragments embedded in the soft tissue. The image is underexposed to highlight contrast between the small radiopaque fragments and the soft tissue of the tongue. (Courtesy Dr. A. Tadinada, University of Connecticut School of Dental Medicine, Farmington, CT.)

affected about twice as frequently as the deciduous teeth. Most crown and root fractures of the anterior teeth are the result of direct trauma. Many posterior teeth are predisposed to such fractures by large restorations or extensive caries.

Clinical Features

The fracture plane of a typical crown-root fracture of an anterior tooth extends obliquely from the labial surface near the gingival third of the crown to a position apical to the gingival attachment on the palatal or lingual surface. The involved teeth are tender to percussion, and the patient may experience pain with separation of the fractured tooth fragments when the tooth is loaded (e.g., during mastication). Displacement of the fragments is usually minimal, and the coronal fragment may be mobile. Crown-root fractures occasionally manifest with bleeding from the pulp.

Imaging Features

Manifestation of a fracture on conventional two-dimensional imaging depends on the relative angulation of the incident x-ray beam to the fracture plane and the degree of separation of the fragments. If the x-ray beam is aligned along the fracture plane, the root fracture is depicted as a single well-defined radiolucent line confined to the anatomic limits of the root. However, if the x-ray beam traverses the fracture plane in a more oblique manner, the root fracture appears as a poorly defined single line or as two discrete lines that converge at the mesial and distal surfaces of the root.

The identification of crown-root fractures can be challenging. Periapical and cross-sectional occlusal images are used for the initial assessment, with multiple images made at different horizontal and vertical angulations to maximize detection of the fracture plane.

Management

Emergency management involves temporary stabilization of the involved teeth. Management options include fragment removal and restoration, often after endodontic therapy. If the pulp is not exposed and the fracture does not extend more than 3 to 4 mm below the epithelial attachment, restorative treatment is likely to be successful. Orthodontic extrusion and crown lengthening may be necessary. In partially developed teeth, pulp capping should be considered to retain pulp vitality until the completion of root development. If only a small amount of root is lost with the coronal fragment but the pulp has been compromised, it is likely that the tooth can be restored after endodontic treatment. Fractures that extend deeper into the root, especially in the vertical direction, have a poor prognosis and are managed by extraction, with subsequent implant-supported or conventional prosthetic rehabilitation.

Dental Root Fractures
Definition

Root fractures are categorized as horizontal or vertical, depending on the orientation of the fracture plane, and they all involve the pulp. For horizontal fractures, the plane of cleavage can vary in angulation from one that is more oblique to one that is more horizontal through the thickness of the root. In contrast, the fracture planes in vertical root fractures run lengthwise from the crown toward the apex of the tooth, usually through the facial and lingual root surfaces.

Clinical Features

Horizontal root fractures occur more commonly in maxillary central incisors and are usually the result of a direct application of traumatic force to the face, alveolar processes, or teeth. In contrast, vertical fractures most commonly occur in endodontically treated premolar and molar

teeth. They may also be iatrogenic, following the insertion of retention screws or pins into teeth, or result from high occlusal forces, particularly in teeth with large restorations.

The mobility of the fractured tooth crown relates to the level of the fracture. When the fracture plane is located toward the apex, the tooth is relatively more stable. The mobility of a traumatized tooth is tested by placing a finger firmly over the alveolar process; if movement of only the crown is detected, a root fracture is likely. Fractures of the root may occur with fractures of the alveolar process and are often not detected. This situation is most commonly observed in the anterior region of the mandible, where root fractures are infrequent. Although root fracture is usually associated with temporary loss of sensitivity (by all usual criteria), the sensitivity of most teeth returns to normal within about 6 months.

Imaging Features

As described earlier, manifestation of a root fracture on conventional two-dimensional imaging depends on the relative angulation of the incident x-ray beam to the fracture plane and on the degree of separation of the fragments. A root fracture may manifest as a single well-defined radiolucent line, a poorly defined single line, or as two discrete lines that converge at the mesial and distal surfaces of the root. Horizontal root fractures may occur at any level and involve one (Fig. 27.4) or more roots of multiroot teeth. Most of the fractures occur in the apical and middle thirds of the root. The fracture plane is often diagonal through the root. Comminuted root fractures may also be less well defined.

The imaging appearance of nondisplaced root fractures is usually subtle and may necessitate multiple image exposures made at different angulations. These fractures may, however, not be evident on periapical images, particularly immediately following the traumatic episode. Subsequent inflammation of the adjacent periodontal ligament and resorption may increase the visible separation between the fragments and facilitate image detection. In some instances when the fracture plane is not visible, the only evidence of a fracture may be a localized increase in the width of the periodontal ligament space adjacent to the fracture site (Fig. 27.5A). With longer-standing fractures, the width of the fracture plane tends to increase with resorption of the fractured surfaces (see Fig. 27.5B). Over time, calcification and obliteration of the pulp chamber and canal may be seen.

In vertical root fractures, the fracture plane is along the vertical axis of the root (Fig. 27.6). Nondisplaced fractures, and fractures in the mesiodistal plane are often undetectable on periapical images and pose a diagnostic challenge. More recently, high-resolution, small FOV CBCT imaging has been used to evaluate teeth with root fractures (Fig. 27.7). CBCT imaging offers multiplanar views of the tooth and thus overcomes the limitation of x-ray beam orientation (Fig. 27.8). Additionally, CBCT also provides better depictions of the adjacent periradicular bone and the supporting alveolar process (see Figs. 27.7 and 27.8). Guidelines from the American Academy of Oral and Maxillofacial Radiology and the American Association of Endodontics recommend that small-FOV CBCT be considered the imaging modality of choice when clinical examination and two-dimensional intraoral images are inconclusive in the detection of a vertical root fracture. However, vertical root fractures are more frequent in teeth that have been endodontically treated and potentially in those with metal post-core restorations. Artifacts from highly attenuating materials (e.g., gutta percha and metal) can degrade image quality, making fracture identification difficult and often impossible (Fig. 27.9). The presence of a vertical root fracture may, however, be identified indirectly by the presence of focal widening of the periodontal ligament space adjacent to the fracture site (Fig. 27.10).

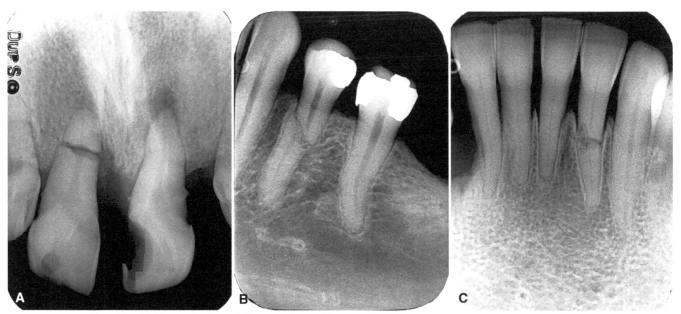

Fig. 27.4 (A) Recent horizontal fracture of the right maxillary central incisor and apical rarefying osteitis involving the adjacent left central incisor. (B) Healed fracture with slight displacement of the fragments. (C) Healed fracture with root resorption and separation of the fractured segments.

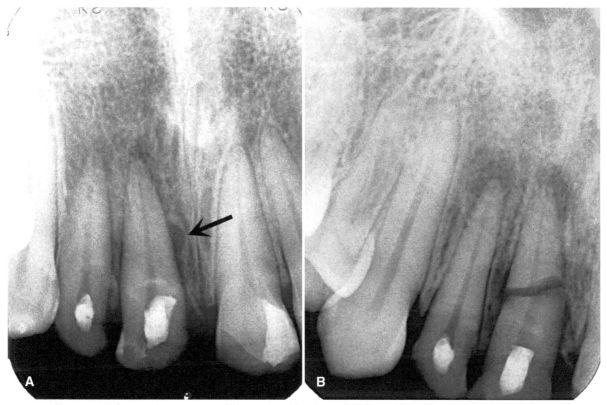

Fig. 27.5 (A) Subtle evidence of a root fracture involving the root of the maxillary right central incisor. Although a fracture plane is not apparent on the mesial aspect of the root because of malalignment of the x-ray beam, there is widening of the periodontal membrane space on the mesial surface *(arrow)* at the site of the fracture. (B) Later dislocation of the root fragments.

Differential Interpretation

Superimposition of the image of a fracture of the alveolar process, or small neurovascular canals, or soft tissue structures such as the lip, ala of the nose, or nasolabial fold over the image of a root may mimic a root fracture.

Management

Horizontal fractures in the coronal third of the root have a poor prognosis and are typically managed by extraction unless the residual root fragment can be orthodontically extruded and restored. Horizontal fractures in the middle or apical thirds of the roots of permanent teeth are manually

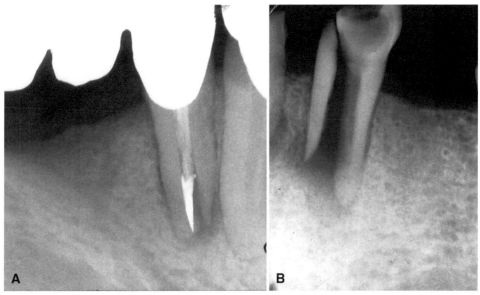

Fig. 27.6 (A) Vertical fracture through the root of a mandibular first premolar that has been endodontically treated. The fracture plane extends through the root canal, and there is more displacement between the root fragments at the apex of the root. (B) Vertical root fracture through the root of a mandibular canine with significant displacement of the fragments.

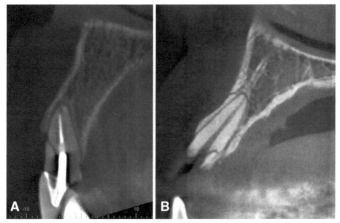

Fig. 27.7 (A) Cone beam computed tomography (CBCT) section shows a vertical fracture through the root of a maxillary incisor that has been endodontically treated and restored with a postcore restoration. The fracture plane begins at the base of the metal post. (B) CBCT section shows a fractured root of a maxillary incisor with exposure of the pulp.

repositioned and immobilized with a splint. The prognosis is generally favorable because of the relatively low incidence of pulpal necrosis. Fractures located closer to the apex have a better prognosis. Fractured deciduous tooth roots may be retained with the expectation that they will be normally resorbed, as attempts at removal may result in damage to the developing succedaneous tooth.

It is important to determine pulp vitality on follow-up visits. Notably, false-negative responses may persist for as long as 3 months. Endodontic therapy is performed when there is evidence of pulpal necrosis. It is also common for bone resorption to occur at the site of the fracture rather than at the apex.

The prognosis of teeth with vertical root fractures is poor. Single-rooted teeth with vertical root fractures must be extracted. Multirooted teeth may be hemisected and the intact fragment of the tooth may be restored with endodontic therapy and a crown.

PERIODONTAL TISSUE INJURY

Patients with dentoalveolar trauma must be examined clinically and radiologically to assess the nature and extent of injury to the periodontal tissues.

Concussion
Definition

The term concussion refers to a crush injury to the vascular structures at the tooth root apex and the periodontal ligament, resulting in inflammatory edema. The affected tooth is minimally loosened with no displacement. The injury may result in mild extrusion of the tooth from its socket, causing its occlusal surface to make premature contact with an opposing tooth during mandibular closing.

Clinical Features

The patient usually complains that the traumatized tooth is tender to touch, and this can be confirmed by gentle horizontal or vertical percussion of the tooth. The tooth may also be sensitive to biting forces, although patients usually try to modify their occlusion to avoid contacting the traumatized tooth.

Imaging Features

The imaging appearance of a dental concussion may be subtle. No changes may be visible, or there may be localized widening of the apical periodontal ligament space (Fig. 27.11). Changes to the size of the pulp chamber and root canals may develop in the months and years after traumatic injury to the teeth, and this may be particularly evident in teeth that are still developing. Should pulpal necrosis occur after trauma, there may be no further deposition of (secondary) dentin as the odontoblasts and the pulpal and pulpal stem cell populations die.

Teeth that have undergone trauma before apical closure may develop a morphologically abnormal apex called an osteodentin cap. As the

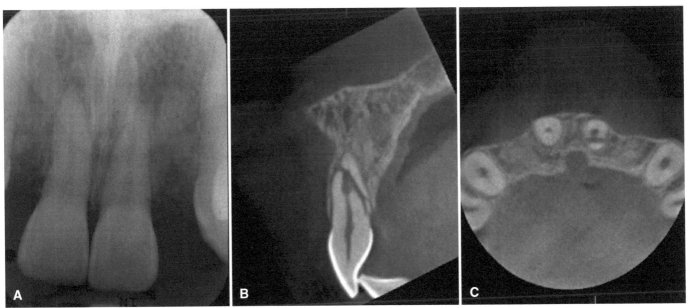

Fig. 27.8 (A) Periapical image of the maxillary central incisors with no evidence of a root fracture. (B) In the same patient, cone beam computed tomography (CBCT) section through the maxillary left central incisor shows an angular fracture through the root. Resorption of the fractured edges has caused separation of the fragments. Resorption of the pulp canal in the distal fragment is evident. (C) Axial CBCT section through the apical third of the roots shows a fracture of the maxillary left central incisor root.

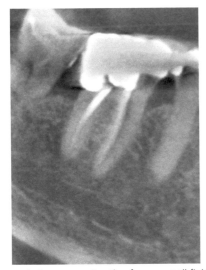

Fig. 27.9 Panoramic-type reconstruction from a small field-of-view cone beam computed tomography volume shows a dark line running parallel to the root canal filling material in the mesial root of the mandibular molar. This "cupping" or "beam hardening" artifact could be misinterpreted as a vertical root fracture.

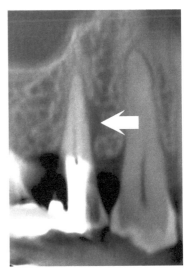

Fig. 27.10 Vertical fracture through the root of a maxillary second premolar that has been endodontically treated. The fracture is barely perceptible and extends to the middle third of the root. Localized widening of the periodontal ligament space *(arrow)* is present as a consequence of the inflammation caused by the root fracture.

process of pulpal necrosis begins coronally and progresses apically, vital odontoblasts may remain at the developing root apex and tertiary dentin (osteodentin) may be deposited ahead of the advancing front of pulpal necrosis. This disorganized and irregularly mineralized matrix may resemble bone in structure and morphologically "caps" the end of the root. The osteodentin cap in some instances may appear on an image to be continuous with the developing root apex or appear separate from it. In contrast to the pattern of internal resorption, where the root canal is focally widened (Fig. 27.12), the root canal seen in association with a tooth that has developed an osteodentin cap appears uniformly widened from the pulp chamber to the apex (Fig. 27.13).

The development of the canal and deposition of dentin in a tooth that has developed an osteodentin cap appears "frozen in time" at the developmental stage at which pulpal necrosis occurred. When the image of the cap is covered or "hidden" from view, the apex of the root resembles that of a developing tooth (see Fig. 27.13C).

Management

Because significant displacement of the tooth or teeth does not occur, the appropriate treatment is conservative and may include occlusal adjustment of the opposing tooth or teeth (if necessary) or the application of a flexible splint. Periodic monitoring in the first year with repeated vitality testing and images are indicated. Should rarefying osteitis develop, endodontic treatment is appropriate.

Subluxation
Definition
The term subluxation refers to periodontal tissue injury that causes abnormal loosening more than with concussion but with no displacement.

Clinical Features
The traumatized tooth is tender to horizontal or vertical percussion and is sensitive to biting forces. Bleeding at the gingival crevice is indicative of the damage to the periodontal tissues.

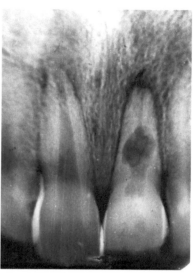

Fig. 27.12 Consequences of dental trauma. An incisal fracture of the maxillary left central incisor is present. Note obliteration of the pulp chamber but not the root canal and internal root resorption. Also note the periapical radiolucency involving the maxillary right central incisor and the widened pulp chamber and canal.

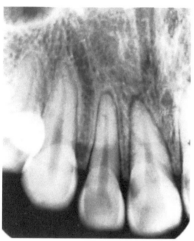

Fig. 27.11 Widening of the periodontal ligament spaces of the incisors after dental concussion.

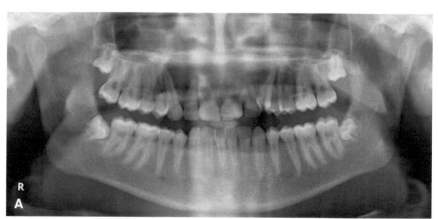

Fig. 27.13 Panoramic (A) and periapical (B) images showing an osteodentin cap associated with the maxillary right central incisor. There is a large area of rarefying osteitis extending from the maxillary midline to the mesial surface of the maxillary right canine. Note the uniformly wide root canal of the incisor. When the osteodentin cap is "obscured," the apex of the root is reminiscent of a developing root apex (C).

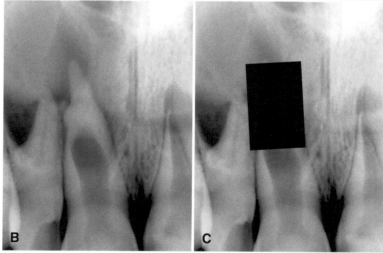

Imaging Features

As with dental concussion, the imaging manifestations are subtle, with no visible changes or with localized widening of the apical periodontal ligament space.

Management

Treatment is conservative, with occlusal adjustments of the opposing dentition and a splint as needed. Periodic monitoring in the first year—with repeated vitality testing and images—is indicated. Approximately 26% of teeth with subluxations will require endodontic treatment due to the development of pulpal necrosis.

Luxation

Definition

Luxation is a dislocation of the tooth from its socket after severing of the periodontal attachment. Such teeth are abnormally mobile and displaced.

Depending on their magnitude and direction, traumatic forces can cause intrusive luxation (displacement of a tooth into the alveolar process), extrusive luxation (partial displacement of a tooth out of its socket), or lateral luxation (movement of a tooth in a direction other than intrusive or extrusive displacement). In intrusive and lateral luxation, comminution or crushing of the alveolar process may accompany tooth dislocation.

The movement of the apex and disruption of the circulation to the traumatized tooth that accompanies luxation can produce either temporary or permanent changes to the dental pulp, and these changes may result in pulpal necrosis. If the pulp survives the traumatic incident, the rate of dentin formation may accelerate and continue until it obliterates the pulp chamber and root canal. This process may occur in both permanent and deciduous teeth.

Clinical Features

Clinical history is helpful in identifying luxation and ordering the appropriate images. The clinical crowns of intruded teeth may appear reduced in height. Maxillary incisors may be intruded so deeply into the alveolar process that they appear to be completely avulsed or lost. The displaced tooth may cause some damage to adjacent teeth, and particularly to underlying developing permanent teeth.

Depending on the orientation and magnitude of the force and the shape of the root, the tooth may be displaced through the buccal or, less commonly, the lingual cortex of the alveolar process, where it may be seen and palpated. On repeated vitality testing, the sensitivity of a luxated tooth may be temporarily decreased or undetectable, especially shortly after the injury. Vitality may return weeks or several months later.

Usually two or more teeth are involved in luxation injuries, and the teeth most frequently affected are the deciduous and permanent maxillary incisors. The mandibular teeth are seldom affected. The type of luxation appears to vary with age; this may reflect changes to the nature of maturing bone. Both intrusions and extrusions occur in the deciduous dentition. In the permanent dentition, the intrusive type of luxation is less frequent.

Imaging Features

Imaging examinations of luxated teeth demonstrate the extent of injury to the root, periodontal ligament, and alveolar process. An image made at the time of injury can serve as a valuable reference point for comparison with subsequent images. Luxation injuries are often accompanied by damage to the bony socket and alveolus.

The depressed position of the crown of an intruded tooth is often apparent on an image (Fig. 27.14), although a minimally intruded tooth may be difficult to demonstrate. Intrusion may result in partial or total obliteration of the apical periodontal ligament space. Multiple radiologic projections, including occlusal views, may be necessary to show the direction of tooth displacement and the relationship of the displaced tooth to adjacent teeth and the outer cortex of bone.

A tooth that has been extruded may demonstrate varying degrees of apical widening of the periodontal ligament space, depending on the magnitude of the extrusive force (Fig. 27.15). A laterally luxated tooth with some degree of extrusion may show a widened periodontal ligament space with greater width on the side of impact.

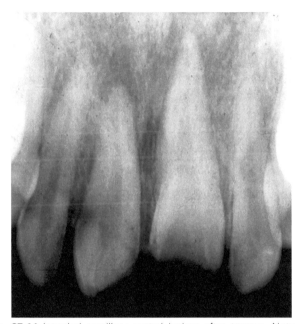

Fig. 27.14 Intruded maxillary central incisor after trauma. Note the fractured incisal edges of both central incisors.

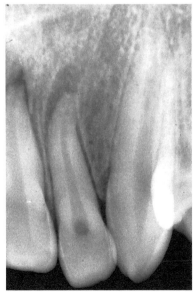

Fig. 27.15 Extruded maxillary lateral incisor after trauma. Note the localized increase to the width of the apical periodontal ligament space.

Management

Management of intrusive luxation is dictated by root development. Teeth with partially developed roots can be allowed to reerupt, with orthodontic extrusion as needed. Teeth with completely developed roots may be repositioned and stabilized, followed by initiation of endodontic treatment.

Teeth with extrusive luxation may be gently repositioned and splinted. Pulp necrosis is a common sequela, occurring in approximately 65% of teeth with such injuries. Thus periodic vitality testing and follow-up imaging are essential.

Lateral luxation is managed by digital manipulation to reposition the displaced teeth to reestablish occlusion, with splinting as needed. Follow-up imaging and vitality testing of the traumatized tooth and adjacent teeth are continued for several months.

Avulsion

Definition

The term avulsion refers to complete displacement of a tooth from the alveolar process. Teeth may be avulsed when a force is applied directly to the tooth or by indirect trauma, such as a force applied as a result of sudden jaw closure. Avulsion occurs in approximately 15% of traumatic injuries to the teeth, with fights being responsible for the avulsion of most permanent teeth and accidental falls accounting for the traumatic loss of most deciduous teeth.

Clinical Features

Maxillary central incisors are the most commonly avulsed teeth from both dentitions. Most often only a single tooth is lost. This injury typically occurs in a relatively young age group when the permanent central incisors are just erupting. Fractures of the alveolar process and lip lacerations may also be seen with an avulsed tooth.

Imaging Features

In a recent avulsion, the lamina dura of the empty socket is apparent and usually persists for several months. The missing tooth may be displaced into the adjacent soft tissue and its image may project over the image of the alveolar process, giving the false impression that it lies within the bone. To differentiate between an intruded tooth and an avulsed tooth lying within the adjacent soft tissues, a soft tissue image of the lacerated lip or tongue should be made. In some instances, new bone within the healing socket may be very dense and resemble a retained root tip (Fig. 27.16).

Management

If the avulsed tooth cannot be found by clinical or radiologic examination, a chest or abdominal image may be considered to localize it within the airway or gastrointestinal tract. Avulsed teeth can be reimplanted into the dentoalveolar socket. The success of reimplantation is determined by the viability of the periodontal tissues that remain attached to the tooth surface, the condition of the tooth, and the length of time it is out of its socket. Optimally, teeth must be reimplanted within 2 hours of avulsion. Commercially available solutions, such as Hanks solution, provide a compatible osmolarity and pH to store teeth for as long as 24 hours. Milk has often been used as a medium to store avulsed teeth but is effective for only approximately 6 hours.

Endodontic therapy may be necessary after reimplantation, and external root resorption is a common complication. Avulsed deciduous teeth are not reimplanted, as the procedure can damage the underlying developing permanent tooth.

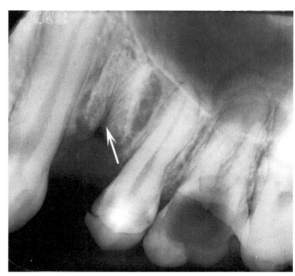

Fig. 27.16 Bone formation during healing of a first premolar tooth socket. Note how the bone is developing from the lateral walls of the socket. The central radiolucent line *(arrow)* may have a similar appearance to that of a root canal, falsely giving the impression of a retained tooth fragment.

ALVEOLAR PROCESS INJURY

Definition

Simple fractures of the alveolar process may involve the buccal or lingual cortical plates of the maxillae or mandible. These fractures are commonly associated with luxation injuries with or without dislocation. Several teeth are usually affected, and the fracture plane is most often horizontal in orientation. The fracture may involve a single cortical plate or extend through the entire alveolar process; the fracture plane may also be located apical to the teeth or involve the tooth socket. Alveolar process injuries are commonly associated with luxation injuries, often with tooth fractures.

Clinical Features

Alveolar fractures are more common in the anterior and premolar regions and are relatively rare in the posterior segments of the arches. In the posterior region, fracture of the buccal plate usually occurs during removal of a maxillary posterior tooth.

A characteristic feature of an alveolar process fracture is marked malocclusion with displacement and mobility of the fragment, with several teeth moving as a block. The teeth in the fragment have a recognizable dull sound when percussed, and the attached gingiva may have lacerations. The detached bone may include the floor of the maxillary sinus, in which case bleeding from the nose on the involved side may occur as well as ecchymosis of the buccal vestibule. Misalignment or displacement of the fractured segments may result in altered occlusion.

Imaging Features

Patients with limited dentoalveolar trauma are often imaged with periapical and occlusal images. These images may show radiolucent fracture lines located at any level between the crest of the alveolar process and the periapical region. Fractures of a single cortical plate are difficult to detect, especially when the fractured segments are nondisplaced. However, a fracture of the anterior labial cortical plate may be apparent on an occlusal image if bone displacement has occurred and the x-ray beam is oriented at nearly right angles to the direction of bone displacement. Fractures of both cortical plates of the alveolar process are usually apparent (Fig. 27.17).

Small-FOV CBCT imaging provides better depiction of the location, extent, and displacement of the fractured bone plates (Fig. 27.18). The AAOMR-AAE imaging guidelines recommend that in the absence of other maxillofacial or soft tissue injuries that may require other advanced imaging modalities, small-FOV CBCT should be considered the imaging modality of choice for the diagnosis of limited dentoalveolar trauma.

The closer the proximity of the fracture is to the alveolar crest, the greater the possibility that a root fracture is also present. On conventional imaging, it may be difficult to differentiate a root fracture from an overlapping fracture line of the alveolar process. Multiple images made at different projection angles may help with this differentiation; if the fracture plane is truly associated with the tooth, the radiolucent line should not shift relative to the tooth. Fractures of the posterior alveolar process may involve the floor of the maxillary sinus and result in abnormal thickening of the sinus mucosa or the accumulation of blood and sinus secretions, in which case an air-fluid level may be apparent.

The location of the fracture line relative to the apices is an indicator of risk of subsequent complication. When the fracture plane is in contact with the root apices, the risk for internal or external resorption is high.

Management

Treatment of limited injury to the alveolar process is directed toward fracture reduction and stabilization. Closed reduction by digital manipulation and rigid splints are often adequate. Fracture segments that are markedly displaced may need open reduction.

TRAUMATIC INJURIES TO THE FACIAL BONES

Facial fractures most frequently affect the mandible and midface and, to a lesser extent, the maxillae. Radiologic examinations play a crucial role in the diagnosis and management of traumatic injuries to these and the other facial bones. Superficial signs of injury, such as soft tissue swelling, hemorrhage, or hematoma formation from a laceration or abrasion, may focus the radiologic examination. Localized injuries may be investigated with plain imaging. Imaging of a maxillofacial fracture is conducted primarily using MDCT.

Mandibular Fractures

The mandible is the most commonly fractured facial bone. Eighty percent of mandibular fractures occur in males. Assaults, motor vehicle accidents, and falls are the three most frequent causes of injury. Most mandibular fractures occur in the 18- to 54-year age group. Fractures of the symphysis, body, and angle are most frequent, followed by the condyle, condylar neck, and ramus. Fractures of the alveolar and coronoid processes are less frequent. Fractures are more likely to occur on weekend days than on other days of the week. Trauma to the mandible is often associated with other injuries, most commonly concussion (loss of consciousness) and other fractures, usually of the maxillae, zygomatic bones, and cranial vault.

The locations and patterns of the fractures vary with the mechanism of injury and the direction the force of impact. Depending on its anatomic location, fractures of the mandible can be classified as dentoalveolar, symphyseal, parasymphyseal, body, angle, ramal, coronoid, or condylar (Fig. 27.19). A second clinically relevant categorization is based on the pattern of the fracture. *Simple fractures* consist of single fracture planes that do not communicate with the external environment. In contrast,

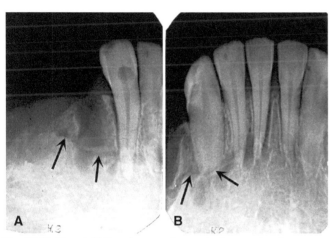

Fig. 27.17 (A and B) Two images demonstrating an alveolar process fracture extending from the distal aspect of the mandibular right cuspid in an anterior direction *(arrows)* and through the tooth socket of the right central incisor.

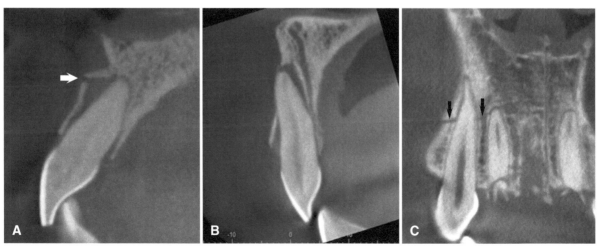

Fig. 27.18 (A and B) Cone beam computed tomography (CBCT) sections through the long axes of the maxillary central incisors showing fractures of the buccal cortical plate *(white arrow)* and asymmetric widening of the periodontal ligament spaces, indicating luxation injuries and alveolar fractures. (C) Coronal CBCT section through the maxillary anterior region shows an alveolar fracture, manifested as a horizontal radiolucent line *(black arrows)*.

compound fractures communicate with the exterior, either via the periodontal ligament space or lacerations of the oral mucosa or facial skin. *Comminuted fractures* involve multiple bone fragments at one fracture site and are often the consequence of a higher-impact force. *Greenstick fractures* are incomplete fractures that involve only one cortical plate, leading to distortion of the bone shape without separation of

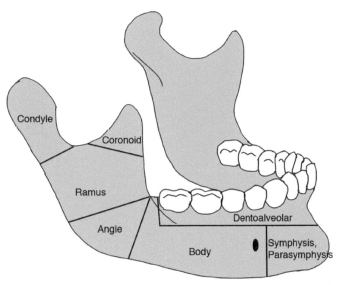

Fig. 27.19 Classification of mandibular fractures based on anatomic location.

bone fragments. The term *complex fracture* or *complicated fracture* is used to describe fractures with damage to adjacent major vessels and nerves (e.g., the inferior alveolar neurovascular bundle). Fractures that arise distant to the site of direct traumatic impact are called *indirect fractures.* Indirect fractures may occur in the mandible because of its unique morphology: the bone is curved and there are regional differences in cortical thickness and buccolingual width. Consequently tensile forces from an impact can be transmitted through the bone to sites distant from the site of primary impact. For example, a fracture of the mandibular body on one side can be accompanied by a fracture of the condylar neck on the opposite side. Likewise, trauma to the anterior mandible often results in unilateral or bilateral fractures of the condylar necks. When a localized heavy force is directed posteriorly to the mandible, there may be fractures of the angle, ramus, or coronoid process. In children, fractures of the mandibular body usually occur in the anterior region. A "pathologic fracture" is one that has developed in normal bone from minimal trauma or with normal functional forces in a bone that has been compromised by a pathologic process. For example, cysts and tumors in the jaw can become large and compromise the structural integrity of the mandible.

Fractures of the Mandibular Symphysis, Body, Angle, and Ramus

Definition. Most mandibular fractures involve the symphysis, body, and ramus. Mandibular fractures are classified as being either favorable or unfavorable, depending on the orientation of the fracture plane and the displacement of the bone fragments (Fig. 27.20). Unfavorable fractures are fractures in which the contractile action of the adjacent muscles

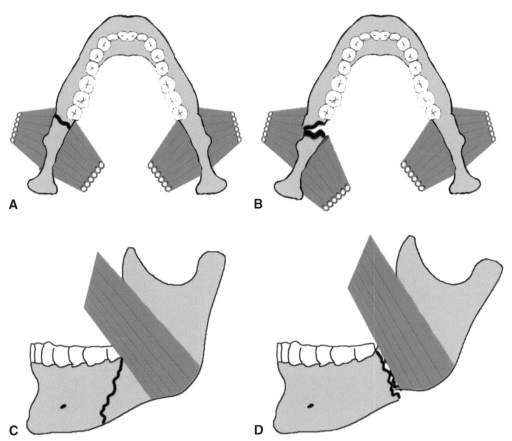

Fig. 27.20 (A) Vertically favorable fracture. (B) Vertically unfavorable fracture, with the medial pterygoid muscle pull causing separation of the fragments. (C) Horizontally favorable fracture of the mandibular body. (D) Horizontally unfavorable fracture, with the masseter muscle pull causing separation of the fragments.

displaces the fragments away from one another and the width of the fracture plane increases. In favorable fractures, the muscle action tends to reduce the fracture, drawing the fragments together. Fractures may be further categorized as being vertically or horizontally favorable or unfavorable. In a vertically favorable fracture, the orientation of the fracture plane resists the medial displacement of the more posterior fragment by the medial pterygoid muscle. In contrast, a horizontally favorable fracture resists displacement of the more posterior fragment by the contractile action of the masseter muscle (see Fig. 27.20).

Clinical features. A history of injury is typically substantiated by some evidence of the trauma that caused the fracture, such as injury to the overlying skin. The patient frequently has swelling and a deformity that is accentuated when the patient opens his or her mouth. A discrepancy is often present in the occlusal plane, and manipulation may produce crepitus or abnormal mobility. Intraoral examination may reveal ecchymosis in the floor of the mouth. In the case of bilateral fractures to the mandible, a risk exists that the digastric, mylohyoid, and omohyoid muscles will displace the anterior mandibular fragment posteriorly and inferiorly, causing impingement on the airway.

Imaging features. The examination of a suspected mandibular fracture may include panoramic or CT imaging. If the patient is cooperative and conscious, intraoral periapical, and occlusal images may be beneficial, given their higher resolution, especially when dentoalveolar fractures are suspected.

The margins of fracture planes usually appear as sharply defined radiolucent lines of separation that are confined to the structure of the mandible (Fig. 27.21). Displacement of the fragments results in a cortical discontinuity or "step-type defect," or an irregularity in the occlusal plane. Occasionally the margins of the adjacent fracture fragments overlap, resulting in an area of increased radiopacity at the fracture site.

Nondisplaced mandibular fractures may involve one or both buccal and lingual cortical plates (Fig. 27.22). When the x-ray beam is not directed through the fracture plane, the fracture lines in the buccal and lingual plates are not superimposed and may appear as two lines that converge at the periphery (Fig. 27.23).

Differential interpretation. The superimposition of soft tissue images on a panoramic image of the mandible may simulate a fracture. A narrow airspace between the dorsal surface of the tongue and the soft palate superimposed across the angle of the mandible on a panoramic image may simulate a fracture. The airspace between the dorsal surface of the tongue and the posterior pharyngeal wall can mimic a fracture on lateral views of the mandible. Similar appearances can occur in the region of the soft palate where it is superimposed on the ramus.

Management. The management goals of a mandibular symphysis or body fracture are to restore a stable occlusion and the range of mandibular opening and excursive movements.

Most mandibular fractures can be managed by closed reduction and intermaxillary fixation. Fractures with more severely displaced fragments may require open reduction. Treatment for mandibular body fractures often includes antibiotic therapy, because a tooth root may be in the line of the fracture. When the fracture line involves third molars, severely mobile teeth, or teeth with at least half their roots exposed in the fracture line, the involved teeth are often extracted to reduce the risk of infection and problems with fixation.

Mandibular Condyle Fractures

Definition. Fractures of the mandibular condylar process may occur at the condylar neck or the condylar head. Condylar neck fractures are more common and typically result in displacement of the condylar head in a medial, inferior, and anterior direction as a result of the contractile action of the lateral pterygoid muscle (Fig. 27.24). Fractures of the condylar head may result in a vertical cleft dividing the condylar head fragments or produce multiple fragments in a compression-like injury (Fig. 27.25). Almost half of patients with condylar fractures also have fractures in the mandibular body (Fig. 27.26).

Clinical features. The clinical symptoms of a fractured mandibular condylar head are not always apparent, so the preauricular area must be carefully examined and palpated. The patient may have pain on opening or closing the mouth or trismus from local swelling. An anterior open bite may be present with only distal molar contacts, and there may be deviation of the mandible on opening. A significant feature may be the patient's inability to protrude the mandible because the lateral pterygoid muscle is attached to the condyle.

Imaging features. Nondisplaced fractures of the mandibular condylar head may be difficult or often impossible to detect on a panoramic image (Fig. 27.27). CT imaging is the modality of choice because it enables the clinician to visualize the three-dimensional relationship of the displaced condylar head to the glenoid fossa and to adjacent anatomic structures in the skull base and infratemporal fossa (see Figs. 27.24–27.26).

Children and adolescents have much greater remodeling potential than adults. In children younger than 12 years, most fractured condyles regain normal morphology after healing, whereas the remodeling is less complete in teenagers. In adults, only minor remodeling is observed. The extent of remodeling is also greater with fractures of the condylar head than with condylar neck fractures with displacement of the condylar head. The most common deformities are medial inclination of the condyle, abnormal shape of the condyle, shortening of the neck, erosion, and flattening. Early condylar fractures commonly result in hypoplasia of the ipsilateral side of the mandible.

Management. Condylar fractures can be successfully managed by closed reduction in both adults and children. This is accomplished with a period of intermaxillary fixation to allow for the reestablishment of

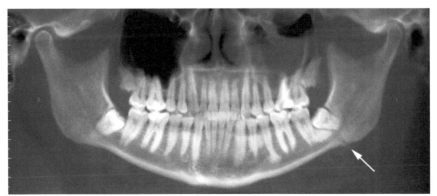

Fig. 27.21 Reconstructed panoramic image from a large field-of-view cone beam computed tomography volume shows an oblique fracture through the left posterior mandible *(arrow).*

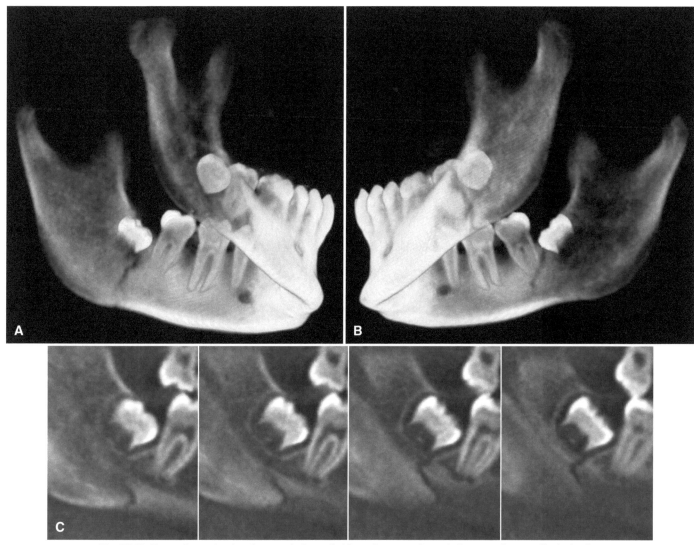

Fig. 27.22 Three-dimensional surface renderings of oblique fractures through the posterior mandibular bodies and rami (A and B) and sagittal cone beam computed tomography images through the fracture on the right side (C).

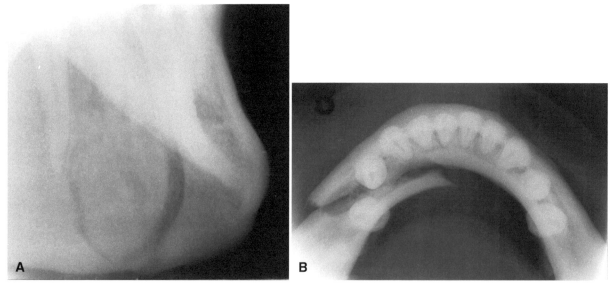

Fig. 27.23 (A) Lateral oblique image of the right mandible in the premolar region shows what appear to be two fracture lines that converge at the inferior cortex. (B) True occlusal image of the mandible of the same case demonstrates only a single fracture plane. The two lines seen in (A) reflect the obliquity of the fracture plane relative to the x-ray beam.

Sagittal   Frontal

Left

Right

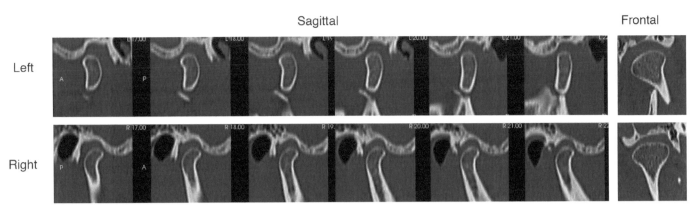

Fig. 27.24 Corrected sagittal and coronal computed tomography images through the right and left temporomandibular joints show a condylar neck fracture. The corrected sagittal images of the left temporomandibular joint *(top panel)* show anterior and slight inferior displacement of the condylar head. The coronal images show medial rotation of the condylar head. Sections through the contralateral side *(bottom panel)* show normal condylar morphology.

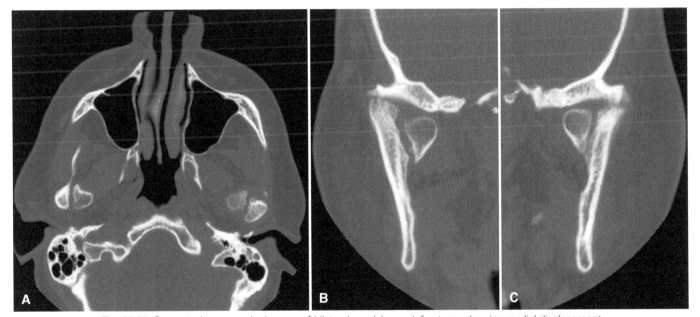

Fig. 27.25 Computed tomography images of bilateral condylar neck fractures showing medial displacement of the condylar heads in line with the lateral pterygoid muscles in the axial image (A) and medial displacement in the coronal images (B and C); also, in (C) there is osseous ankylosis between the residual condylar neck and the temporal bone.

the occlusion. Factors that dictate treatment decisions include whether one or both condyles are involved, the extent of displacement, and the occurrence and severity of concomitant fractures. The treatment is directed to relieve acute symptoms, restore proper anatomic relationships, and prevent bony ankylosis. If a malocclusion develops, intermaxillary fixation may be provided to restore proper occlusion. Open reduction of condylar neck fractures is limited by the risk of procedure-related morbidity and the size and position of the fracture fragments.

Midfacial Fractures Including Maxillary Fractures

Midface fractures are caused by falls, motor vehicle accidents, and assaults; they can involve one or multiple bones in the midface skeleton.

Orbital Wall Blowout Fractures

Definition. Blowout fractures of the orbital walls result from a direct blow to the orbit by an object that is too large to enter the orbital cavity,

such as a fist or a baseball. The force of the impact travels through the bone and is transferred to one or more of the very thin walls of the orbit. By definition, the orbital rim remains intact in a blowout fracture. The most common fractures involve the medial wall of the orbit, which is formed by the lamina papyracea of the ethmoid bone and the floor of the orbit, which separates this space from the maxillary sinus.

Clinical features. Periorbital edema is a common feature of the orbital blowout fracture, as is enophthalmos. Eye movements may be restricted if one or more of the periorbital muscles becomes entrapped in the bony defect created by the fracture. If the ethmoid air cells are involved, there may be epistaxis.

Imaging features. The imaging modality of choice to evaluate orbital blowout fractures is thin-section MDCT with multiplanar reformats in bone and soft tissue kernels. Coronal reconstructions best demonstrate discontinuities of the lamina papyracea in a medial wall or the orbital floor. In orbital floor blowout fractures, herniation of the orbital cavity soft tissues can be seen through the roof of the maxillary sinus. Coronal MDCT imaging may show the classic "trapdoor" appearance of the displaced orbital floor (Fig. 27.28A). MDCT imaging may also show soft tissue densities or air-fluid levels in the adjacent ethmoid air cells or maxillary sinus (see Fig. 27.28B) or herniation of periorbital fat and entrapment of periorbital muscle through the bony defect in the orbital floor (see Fig. 27.28C).

Management. Surgical repair may be attempted for patients who have severely affected eye movements because of muscle entrapment or unacceptable enophthalmos.

Zygomatic Fractures

Definition. Fractures involving the zygomatic bone may include tripod fractures, in which the zygomatic bone and adjacent areas of the maxillary, frontal, sphenoid, and temporal bones may be involved; zygomatic arch fractures, in which the zygomatic process of the temporal bone is fractured; and Le Fort type II and III fractures (described in the following section).

Injuries to the zygomatic bone or arch usually result from a forceful blow to the cheek or side of the face. Although a zygomatic bone fracture may rotate or displace the fragments medially, support by the adjacent temporalis and masseter muscles may limit displacement.

Clinical features. Flattening of the upper cheek with tenderness and dimpling of the skin over the side of the face may occur, although some of the clinical characteristics of zygomatic fractures may not be apparent much longer than an hour after trauma because they may be masked by edema. In most cases, periorbital ecchymosis and hemorrhage into the sclera (near the outer canthus) occur. Additional symptoms may include unilateral epistaxis (for a short time after the accident), anesthesia or paresthesia of the cheek, and compromised eye movements. The presence of diplopia suggests a significant injury to the floor of the orbit. Mandibular movement may be limited if the displaced zygomatic bone impinges on the coronoid process.

Imaging features. Because of edema obscuring the clinical features, the imaging examination may provide the only means of determining the presence and extent of the injury (Fig. 27.29). MDCT is the modality of choice for imaging these fractures (Fig. 27.30).

The zygomatic arch may fracture at its weakest point, about 1 cm posterior to the zygomaticotemporal suture. Separation or fracture through the frontozygomatic suture may also occur. Fractures do not usually occur through the zygomaticomaxillary suture; however, in some cases, a fracture plane may extend obliquely, involving the inferior rim of the orbit and the lateral wall of the maxilla. If the fracture plane involves the maxillary sinus, the sinus may exhibit increased radiopacity subsequent to accumulation of blood and mucous secretions or an air-fluid level.

It is important to consider that on panoramic images, the zygomaticotemporal suture appears as a radiolucent line that may have the appearance of a discontinuity in the inferior border. This is a variation of normal anatomy and should not be misinterpreted as a fracture.

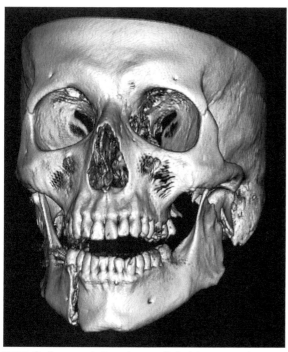

Fig. 27.26 Surface rendering of a maxillofacial computed tomography examination showing fractures of the left condylar neck and the right mandibular body.

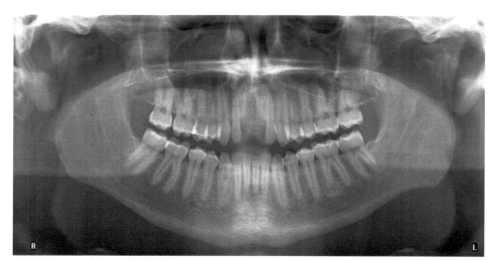

Fig. 27.27 Panoramic image showing bilateral condylar fractures with anterior displacement of the fractured condylar fragments.

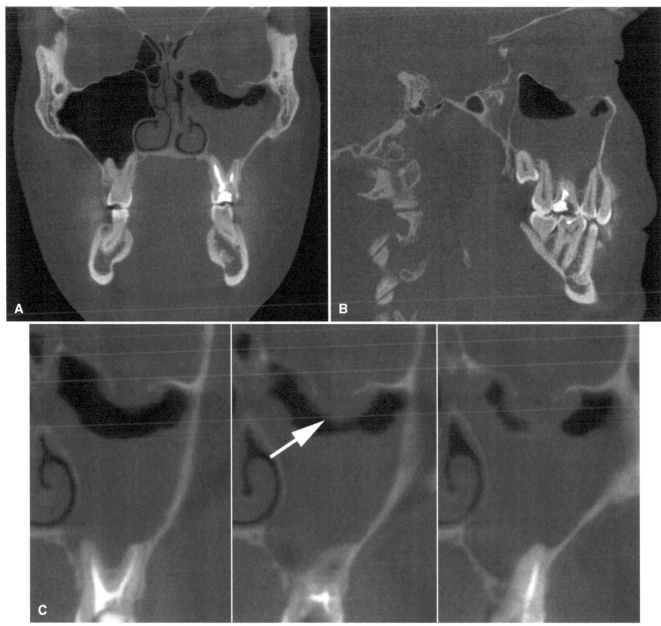

Fig. 27.28 Cone beam computed tomography images show orbital blowout fractures involving the lamina papyracea of the left ethmoid bone and the orbital floor in the coronal (A) and sagittal (B) planes. Note the fluid/soft tissue densities in the adjacent ethmoid air cells and the air-fluid level in the left maxillary sinus. (C) Computed tomography reconstructions made perpendicular to the track of the optic nerve show the "trapdoor" appearance of the orbital floor blowout fracture with herniation of soft tissue into the maxillary sinus *(arrow)*.

Management. When symptoms include minimal displacement of the zygomatic arch and there are no cosmetic deformities or any impairment of eye movement, no treatment may be required. Otherwise reduction is usually indicated. Fractures of the zygomatic bone and arch may be reduced through an intraoral or extraoral approach.

Le Fort Fractures

Complex fractures involving multiple facial bones may be quite variable but often follow general patterns classified by the French surgeon René Le Fort. By definition, all Le Fort fractures include fractures of one or more of the pterygoid plates of the sphenoid bone. Although Le Fort fractures may be bilateral, they are most often unilateral.

The detection of fractures of the midface in images is difficult because of the complex anatomy and the multiple superimpositions of structures. MDCT is the diagnostic imaging modality of choice for complex facial fractures because it provides multiple image slices in orthogonal planes through the face, allowing for the display of osseous structures without the complication of overlapping anatomy, which is problematic with plain imaging. MDCT also provides suitable image detail to detect secondary changes associated with trauma, including herniation of orbital fat and extraocular muscle, soft tissue swelling or emphysema, and blood or fluid accumulation. As an aid in determining the spatial orientation of fractures or bone fragments, MDCT images may be rendered to produce three-dimensional surface renderings.

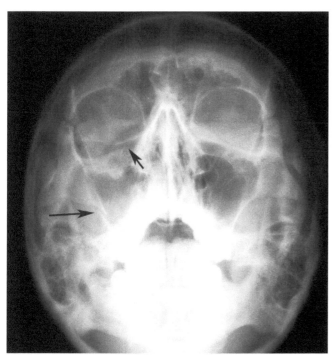

Fig. 27.29 Waters view shows a tripod fracture involving the right zygomatic bone. Note the fracture through the right orbital rim *(short arrow)* and lateral wall of the maxillary sinus *(long arrow)*. Also, there is radiopacification of the right maxillary sinus.

Le Fort I (Horizontal Fracture)

Definition. The Le Fort I fracture plane extends through the maxillary body in a relatively horizontal orientation that results in detachment of the alveolar process and adjacent bone of the maxilla from the midface. This fracture is the result of a horizontally directed traumatic force directed posteriorly at the base of the nose. The fracture plane passes superior to the roots of the teeth and nasal floor and posteriorly through the base of the maxillary sinus and the tuberosity to the pterygoid processes (Fig. 27.31). In the unilateral fracture, there is an auxiliary fracture in the midline of the palate. The unilateral fracture must be distinguished from a fracture within the alveolar process (discussed previously) that does not extend to the midline or involve the pterygoid plates posteriorly. Concomitant fractures of the mandible (54%) and zygomatic bone (23%) are frequent in these patients.

Clinical features. If the fragment is not distally impacted, it can be manipulated by holding on to the teeth. If the fracture line is at a high level, the fragment may include the pterygoid muscle attachments, which pull the fragment posteriorly and inferiorly. As a result, the posterior maxillary teeth contact the mandibular teeth first, resulting in an anterior open bite, retruded chin, and long face. If the fracture is at a low level, no displacement may occur. Other symptoms may include associated swelling and bruising about the eyes, pain over the nose and face, deformity of the nose, and flattening of the middle of the face. Epistaxis is inevitable, and occasionally double vision and varying degrees of paresthesia over the distribution of the infraorbital nerve may occur. Manipulation may reveal a mobile maxilla and crepitation.

Imaging features. MDCT imaging reveals an air-fluid level or radiopacification in the maxillary sinus (Fig. 27.32A). Coronal images may reveal the plane of the fracture extending posteriorly through the maxilla, whereas coronal or axial images together may reveal involvement of the pterygoid plates posteriorly. Three-dimensional reconstructions of the MDCT data set may show the plane of the fracture to greatest advantage (see Fig. 27.32B).

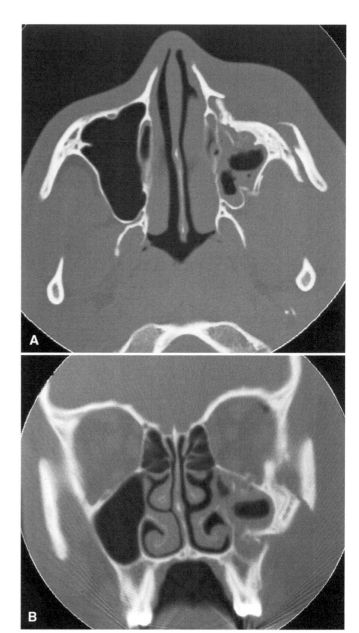

Fig. 27.30 Axial (A) and coronal (B) computed tomography images show depression and rotation of a left tripod fracture. An air-fluid level is also visible in the left maxillary sinus.

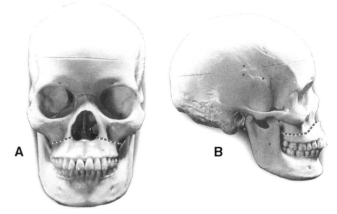

Fig. 27.31 Usual position of a Le Fort I fracture on frontal (A) and lateral (B) views.

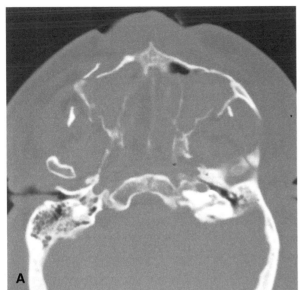

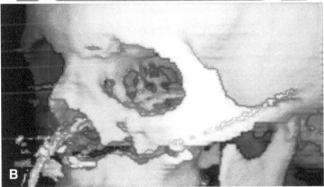

Fig. 27.32 (A) Axial image of Le Fort I fractures involving the anterior and posterolateral walls of the right and left maxilla and the pterygoid plates. Opacification of the maxillary sinuses is also seen, with a small retained collection of air in the left maxillary sinus. (B) Three-dimensional reconstruction of the image data shows extension of the fracture plane from above the base of the nose posteriorly through the maxillary tuberosity.

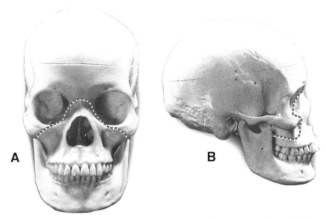

Fig. 27.33 Usual position of the Le Fort II fracture on frontal (A) and lateral (B) views.

Management. If the fracture is not displaced and is at a relatively low level in the maxilla, it can be treated by intermaxillary fixation. Fractures that are high, with the fragment displaced posteriorly or with pronounced separation, require craniomaxillary fixation in addition to intermaxillary fixation.

Le Fort II (Pyramidal Fracture)

Definition. A Le Fort II fracture has a pyramidal shape on postero-anterior skull images, and hence the name. It results from a violent force applied posteriorly and superiorly through the base of the nose. This force separates the maxilla from the base of the skull. The fracture plane extends from the bridge of the nose inferiorly, laterally, and posteriorly through the nasal and lacrimal bones, the orbital floor and inferior rim obliquely, inferiorly across the maxilla, and posteriorly to the pterygoid processes (Figs. 27.33 and 27.34). The frontal and ethmoid sinuses are involved in about 10% of cases, especially in severe com-minuted fractures.

Clinical features. In contrast to the Le Fort I fracture, which may be characterized by only slight swelling about the upper lips, a Le Fort II fracture results in massive edema and marked swelling of the middle third of the face. Typically ecchymosis develops around the eyes within

minutes of the injury. The edema is likely to be so severe that it is impossible to see the globes. The conjunctivae over the inner quadrants of the eyes are bloodshot; if the zygomatic bones are involved, this ecchymosis will extend to the outer quadrant.

The broken nose is displaced because the face has fallen, and the nose and face are lengthened. An anterior open bite occurs. Epistaxis is inevitable, and cerebrospinal fluid rhinorrhea may occur. Palpation reveals the discontinuity of the lower borders of the orbits. By applying pressure between the bridge of the nose and the palate, the "pyramid" of bone can be moved. Other common symptoms include double vision and variable degrees of paresthesia over the distribution of the infraorbital nerve.

Imaging features. The radiologic examination reveals fractures of the nasal bone, frontal process of the maxilla, infraorbital rim, and orbital floor. More inferiorly and posteriorly, there would be involvement of the zygomatic bone or zygomatic process of the maxilla, separation of the zygomaticomaxillary suture, and fracture of the lateral wall of the maxillary sinus and the pterygoid plates. Involvement of the ethmoid air cells and frontal and maxillary sinuses would result in thickening of the sinus mucosa or the accumulation of blood-fluid levels in the airspaces. CT imaging is the modality of choice for imaging such complex fractures.

Management. Le Fort II fractures are managed by reduction of the displaced maxilla via intermaxillary fixation, open reduction, and interosseous wiring of the infraorbital rims as well as plating of the accompanying fractures of the nose, nasal septum, and orbital floor. Repair of the detached medial canthal ligaments may also be required. Leakage of cerebrospinal fluid requires neurosurgical intervention if the posterior or superior walls of the frontal sinuses are involved.

Le Fort III (Craniofacial Disjunction)

Definition. A Le Fort III midface fracture results when the traumatic force is of sufficient magnitude to separate the middle third of the facial skeleton completely from the cranium. The fracture plane usually extends from the nasal bone and frontal process of the maxilla or nasofrontal and maxillofrontal sutures across the orbital floor, through the ethmoid air cells and sphenoid sinus, to the zygomaticofrontal sutures (Fig. 27.35). More posteriorly and inferiorly, the fracture plane passes across the pterygomaxillary fissure and separates the bases of the pterygoid plates from the sphenoid bone. If the maxilla is displaced and freely movable, a fracture must also have occurred at the zygomaticotemporal suture. Because the zygomatic bone or zygomatic arch is involved, these injuries are associated with multiple other maxillary fractures. Mandibular fractures are also observed in half the cases.

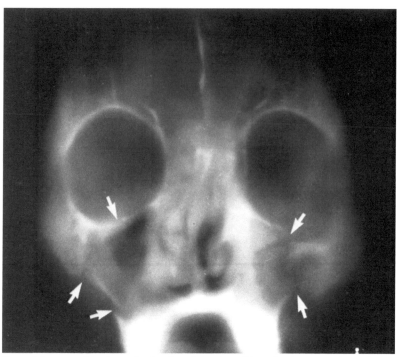

Fig. 27.34 Coronal tomographic view of a Le Fort II fracture. Note the fractures through the orbital rims bilaterally. Also, there are fractures through the ethmoid bones and the lateral walls of the maxillae *(arrows)*. (Courtesy Dr. C. Schow, Galveston, TX.)

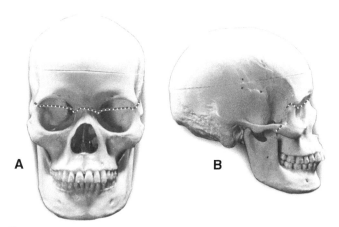

Fig. 27.35 Usual position of a Le Fort III fracture on frontal (A) and lateral (B) views.

Clinical features. Craniofacial disjunction produces a clinical appearance similar to that of a pyramidal fracture; however, this injury is considerably more extensive. The soft tissue injuries are severe, with massive edema. The nose may be blocked with blood or blood clot, or cerebrospinal fluid rhinorrhea may be present. Bleeding may occur into the periorbital tissues and the conjunctiva, and numerous eye signs of neurologic importance are likely to be present. A "dished-in" or concave deformity of the face is characteristic of this fracture pattern, as is an anterior open bite because of the retroclined positions of the maxillary incisors with only the posterior teeth in occlusion. Even on mandibular opening, the patient is unable to separate the molars. Intraoral and extraoral palpation reveals irregular contours and step deformities, and crepitation is apparent when the fragments are moved.

Imaging features. It is virtually impossible to document these multiple fractures with plain films, and CT imaging in concert with the clinical information is required. The main radiologic findings are distractions of the frontonasal, frontomaxillary, zygomaticofrontal, and zygomaticotemporal sutures and fractures through the nasal bone, frontal process of the maxilla, orbital floor, and pterygoid plates (Fig. 27.36). Associated fractures involving the walls of all the paranasal sinuses result in radiopaque air-fluid levels with mucosal thickening. Three-dimensional reconstructions show the fracture planes and large bone fragments (see Fig. 27.36D and E).

Management. The associated severe soft tissue injury necessitates airway management, initial hemorrhage control, and repair of lacerations. Surgery may be delayed until the edema has sufficiently resolved. Fixation of the loose middle third of the facial skeleton is difficult due to concurrent fractures of the zygomatic arch. The only possibilities are external immobilization or immobilization within the tissues. In the former, the loose maxilla is suspended by wires through the cheeks from a metal head frame (halo) or fixed by external pins anchored in bone. The other possibility is immobilization within the tissues by using internal wiring to the closest solid bone superior to the fracture. Many complications may develop during or after this treatment.

MONITORING THE HEALING OF FRACTURES

The goals of imaging following management of facial trauma are to confirm adequate reduction of the fracture and monitor the continued immobilization of the fracture site during repair. Typically monitoring of this type is accomplished by the use of conventional imaging and is directed to evaluation of the alignment of the cortical plates of the involved bone and remodeling and remineralization of the fracture site. During normal healing, the fracture plane increases in width about 2 weeks after reduction of the fracture. This increase in width results from the resorption of the fractured ends and small sequestered fragments of bone. Evidence of remineralization usually occurs 5 to 6 weeks after treatment. In contrast to the long bones of the skeleton, callus formation

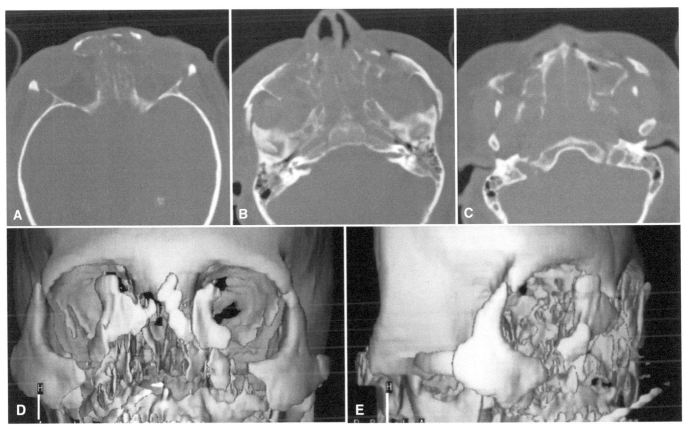

Fig. 27.36 Axial computed tomography (CT) images show a bilateral Le Fort III fracture with distractions of the frontonasal (A), frontomaxillary, zygomaticofrontal, and zygomaticotemporal sutures (B) and fractures of the nasal bone, frontal process of the maxilla, orbital floor, and pterygoid plates (C). Note the near-total radiopacification of the maxillary sinuses. Three-dimensional reconstructions, frontal view (D) and lateral view (E), of the axial CT images reveal substantial fragmentation of the periorbital bones, zygomatic bone, and arch posteriorly.

during healing of jaw fractures is rare. The complete remodeling of the fracture site with obliteration of the fracture line may take several months. Fracture lines may persist for years on rare occasions, even when the patient has made a clinically complete recovery. Possible complications of healing include malalignment of the fracture segments and inflammatory lesions related to teeth with nonvital pulps near or in the line of the fracture. Other complications include nonunion of the fractured segments, which is seen as increased width of fracture line, cortication of the fractured surfaces, and rounding of the sharp edges of the segments. The development of osteomyelitis of the fracture site appears as an increase in sclerosis of the surrounding bone, inflammatory periosteal new bone, and the development of sequestra.

BIBLIOGRAPHY

Boffano P, Kommers SC, Karagozoglu KH, et al. Aetiology of maxillofacial fractures: a review of published studies during the last 30 years. *Br J Oral Maxillofac Surg.* 2014;52(10):901–906.

Brook IW, Wood N. Aetiology and incidence of facial fractures in adults. *Int J Oral Surg.* 1983;12:293–298.

Curtis W, Horswell BB. Panfacial Fractures: An Approach to Management. *Oral and Maxillofacial Surgery Clinics of North America.* 2013;25(4):649–660.

Gelesko S, Markiewicz MR, Bell RB. Responsible and Prudent Imaging in the Diagnosis and Management of Facial Fractures. *Oral and Maxillofacial Surgery Clinics of North America.* 2013;25(4):545–560.

Haug RH, Foss J. Maxillofacial injuries in the pediatric patient. *Oral Surg Oral Med Oral Pathol Oral Radiol Endod.* 2000;90(2):126–134.

Krishnan DG. Systematic Assessment of the Patient with Facial Trauma. *Oral and Maxillofacial Surgery Clinics of North America.* 2013;25(4):537–544.

Dental Fractures

Andreasen JO. *Traumatic Injuries of the Teeth.* Philadelphia: Saunders; 1981.

Andreasen JO, Andreasen FM, Skeie A, et al. Effect of treatment delay upon pulp and periodontal healing of traumatic dental injuries—a review article. *Dent Traumatol.* 2002;18:116–128.

Malmgren B, Andreasen JO, Flores MT, et al. International Association of Dental Traumatology guidelines for the management of traumatic dental injuries: 3. Injuries in the primary dentition. *Dent Traumatol.* 2012;28(3):174–182.

Ravn JJ. Follow-up study of permanent incisors with enamel fractures as a result of acute trauma. *Scand J Dent Res.* 1981;89:213–217.

Ravn JJ. Follow-up study of permanent incisors with enamel-dentin fracture after acute trauma. *Scand J Dent Res.* 1981;89:355–365.

Tooth Root Fracture

Chavda R, Mannocci F, Andiappan M, et al. Comparing the in vivo diagnostic accuracy of digital periapical radiography with cone-beam computed tomography for the detection of vertical root fracture. *J Endod.* 2014;40(10):1524–1529.

Cvek M, Mejare I, Andreason JO. Healing and prognosis of teeth with intra-alveolar fractures involving the cervical part of the root. *Dent Traumatol.* 2002;18:57–65.

Edlund M, Nair MK, Nair UP. Detection of vertical root fractures by using cone-beam computed tomography: a clinical study. *J Endod.* 2011;37(6):768–772.

Hovland EJ. Horizontal root fractures: treatment and repair. *Dent Clin North Am.* 1992;36:509–525.

Majorana A, Pasini S, Bardellini E, et al. Clinical and epidemiological study of traumatic root fractures. *Dent Traumatol.* 2002;18:77–80.

Neves FS, Freitas DQ, Campos PS, et al. Evaluation of cone-beam computed tomography in the diagnosis of vertical root fractures: the influence of imaging modes and root canal materials. *J Endod.* 2014;40(10):1530–1536.

Schetritt A, Steffensen B. Diagnosis and management of vertical root fractures. *J Can Dent Assoc.* 1995;61:607–613.

Sim IG, Lim TS, Krishnaswamy G, et al. Decision Making for Retention of Endodontically Treated Posterior Cracked Teeth: A 5-year Follow-up Study. *J Endod.* 2016;42(2):225–229.

Walton RE, Michelich RJ, Smith GN. The histopathogenesis of vertical root fractures. *J Endodont.* 1984;10:48–56.

Fractures of the Alveolar Process

Andreasen JO. Fractures of the alveolar process of the jaw: a clinical and radiographic follow-up study. *Scand J Dent Res.* 1970;78:263–272.

Giovannini UM, Goudot P. Radiologic evaluation of mandibular and dentoalveolar fractures. *Plast Reconstr Surg.* 2002;109:2165–2166.

Luxation

Andreasen JO. Luxation of permanent teeth due to trauma: a clinical and radiographic follow-up study of 189 injured teeth. *Scand J Dent Res.* 1970;78:273–286.

Diangelis AJ, Andreasen JO, Ebeleseder KA, et al. International Association of Dental Traumatology guidelines for the management of traumatic dental injuries: 1. Fractures and luxations of permanent teeth. *Dent Traumatol.* 2012;28(1):2–12.

Avulsion

Andersson L, Andreasen JO, Day P, et al. International Association of Dental Traumatology guidelines for the management of traumatic dental injuries: 2. Avulsion of permanent teeth. *Dent Traumatol.* 2012;28(2):88–96.

Donaldson M, Kinirons MJ. Factors affecting the time of onset of resorption in avulsed and replanted incisor teeth in children. *Dent Traumatol.* 2001;17:205–209.

Trauma to the Mandible

Afrooz PN, Bykowski MR, James IB, et al. The Epidemiology of Mandibular Fractures in the United States, Part 1: A Review of 13,142 Cases from the US National Trauma Data Bank. *J Oral Maxillofac Surg.* 2015;73(12):2361–2366.

Braasch DC, Abubaker AO. Management of Mandibular Angle Fracture. *Oral and Maxillofacial Surgery Clinics of North America.* 2013;25(4):591–600.

Escott EJ, Branstetter BF. Incidence and characterization of unifocal mandible fractures on CT. *AJNR Am J Neuroradiol.* 2008;29:890–894.

Goodday RHB. Management of Fractures of the Mandibular Body and Symphysis. *Oral and Maxillofacial Surgery Clinics of North America.* 2013;25(4):601–616.

Kaeppler G, Cornelius CP, Ehrenfeld M, et al. Diagnostic efficacy of cone-beam computed tomography for mandibular fractures. *Oral Surg Oral Med Oral Pathol Oral Radiol.* 2013;116(1):98–104.

Condylar Fractures

Consensus Conference on Open or Closed Management of Condylar Fractures, 12th ICOMS, Budapest, 1995. *Int J Oral Maxillofac Surg.* 1998;27:243–267.

Dahlström L, Kahnberg KE, Lindahl L. 15 years follow-up on condylar fractures. *Int J Oral Maxillofac Surg.* 1989;18:18–23.

Davis B. Late Reconstruction of Condylar Neck and Head Fractures. *Oral and Maxillofacial Surgery Clinics of North America.* 2013;25(4):661–681.

Dimitroulis G. Condylar injuries in growing patients. *Aust Dent J.* 1997;42:367–371.

Kisnisci R. Management of Fractures of the Condyle, Condylar Neck, and Coronoid Process. *Oral and Maxillofacial Surgery Clinics of North America.* 2013;25(4):573–590.

Trauma to the Maxilla

Ceallaigh PO, Ekanaykaee K, Beirne CJ, et al. Diagnosis and management of common maxillofacial injuries in the emergency department. Part 4: orbital floor and midface fractures. *Emerg Med J.* 2007;24(4):292–293.

Hopper RA, Salemy S, Sze RW. Diagnosis of midface fractures with CT: what the surgeon needs to know. *Radiographics.* 2006;26(3):783–793.

Winegar BA, Murillo H. Tantiwongkosi B. Spectrum of critical imaging findings in complex facial skeletal trauma. *Radiographics.* 2013;33(1):3–19.

Zygomatic Complex Fractures

Kochhar A, Byrne PJ. Surgical management of complex midfacial fractures. *Otolaryngol Clin North Am.* 2013;46(5):759–778.

Moreira Marinho RO, Freire-Maia B. Management of Fractures of the Zygomaticomaxillary Complex. *Oral and Maxillofacial Surgery Clinics of North America.* 2013;25(4):617–636.

28

Paranasal Sinus Diseases

Sotirios Tetradis

The paranasal sinuses are the four paired sets of air-filled cavities of the maxillofacial complex, and they consist of the maxillary, frontal, and sphenoid sinuses and the ethmoid air cells. The maxillary sinuses are of particular importance to the dentist because of their proximity to the teeth and their associated structures. Abnormalities arising from within the maxillary sinuses can cause symptoms that may mimic diseases of odontogenic origin, and conversely, abnormalities that arise in and around the teeth may affect the sinuses or mimic the symptoms of sinus disease. Because the paranasal sinuses may appear on many diagnostic images used in the practice of dentistry, the dentist should be familiar with variations in the normal appearance of the sinuses and the more common diseases that may affect them.

NORMAL DEVELOPMENT AND VARIATIONS

The paranasal sinuses develop as invaginations from the nasal fossae into their respective bones (maxillary, frontal, sphenoid, and ethmoid) and continue to enlarge until skeletal maturity. Like the nasal cavities, the paranasal sinuses are lined with respiratory mucosa composed of pseudostratified ciliated columnar epithelium. The cilia move sinus secretions through the ostia and into the nasal fossae. The maxillary sinuses or antra are the first to develop in the second month of intrauterine life. An invagination develops in the lateral wall of the nasal fossa in the middle meatus, and the sinus cavity enlarges laterally into the body of the maxilla. At birth, each sinus is a thin, small slit, no more than 8 mm in length in its anteroposterior dimension. With time, the maxilla becomes progressively more pneumatized as the air cavity expands further into the bone both laterally under the orbits toward the zygomatic process and inferiorly into the alveolar process. Pneumatization into the alveolar process drapes the maxillary sinus floor over the roots of the premolar or molar teeth to varying degrees. The imaging appearance of the floor of the maxillary sinus is a thin, well-defined radiopaque line. If the alveolar process of the maxilla is not well pneumatized, the floor of the sinus may not be visible on periapical images (Fig. 28.1A), or it may be seen superior to the roots of the maxillary premolar or molar teeth (see Fig. 28.1B). With greater pneumatization, the floor of the sinus may appear to undulate around or drape over the roots of the teeth or be superimposed over the tooth roots, giving the false impression that the roots have penetrated the sinus floor (see Fig. 28.1C and D). Closer examination of the periapical areas reveals intact laminae durae and periodontal ligament spaces.

In patients with considerable pneumatization of the alveolar process of the maxilla, the lamina dura of a premolar or molar tooth may form a portion of the sinus floor. Maxillary pneumatization may also extend into the palatal, zygomatic, and frontal processes of the maxilla; this can be appreciated on plain images and advanced imaging examinations such as cone beam computed tomography (CBCT), multidetector

computed tomography (MDCT), or magnetic resonance imaging (MRI) (Fig. 28.2A). In some instances the appearance of the normally pneumatized maxilla may be mistakenly confused with a benign space-occupying lesion, particularly on plain images (Fig. 28.3).

Hypoplasia of the maxillary sinuses occurs unilaterally in approximately 1.7% of patients (see Fig. 28.2B and C), and bilaterally in 7.2%. In plain images of these patients, the affected sinus may appear more radiopaque than normal because of the relatively large amount of surrounding maxillary bone. The configuration of the maxillary sinus walls frequently helps to distinguish between a hypoplastic sinus and a sinus that is pathologically radiopaque. Asymmetry in the size of the right and left maxillary sinuses is seen not only in the presence of a unilateral hypoplastic sinus but can also appear in silent sinus syndrome (SSS) (see Fig. 28.2D).

SSS is a rare pathologic entity believed to be caused by sinus hypoventilation due to obstruction of the ostium of the involved maxillary sinus, eventually leading to a decrease in the size of the sinus. SSS is associated with clinical symptoms such as enopthalmos and hypoglobus. Radiographically, SSS is characterized by reduced sinus size with bowing of the sinus walls and an inferiorly displaced orbital floor with increased orbital content.

Development of the frontal sinus usually begins around the fifth or sixth year of life. This sinus either develops directly in extension from the nasal fossae or from the anterior ethmoid air cells (Fig. 28.4B). In approximately 4% of the population, the frontal sinuses fail to develop. As with the other paranasal sinuses, the right and left frontal sinus cavities develop separately; as they expand, they approach each other in the midline. In such instances, a thin bony septum may partially or completely separate the two asymmetric cavities. In adults, frontal sinus pneumatization may also extend posteriorly into the orbital roofs.

The sphenoid sinus begins growing in the fourth fetal month as invaginations from the sphenoethmoidal recesses of the nasal fossae. Located in the body of the sphenoid bone, the sinuses are usually separated by a partial or complete bony septum and are asymmetric in size and shape. As with the other sinuses, the sphenoid sinuses may extend beyond the body of the bone into the dorsum sella, the clinoid processes, the greater or lesser wings, and the pterygoid processes. The ostium of the sphenoid sinus is a relatively large-diameter opening; this may explain why blockages of the sphenoid sinus ostium are uncommon (see the section on mucoceles later in this chapter).

The ethmoid air cells extend into the developing ethmoid bones during the fifth fetal month. They consist of multiple separate or interconnected air-filled chambers that border the medial and sometimes inferior aspects of the orbital cavities (see Fig. 28.4A and B). The number of air cells varies considerably, with each ethmoid bone containing 8 to 15 cells. In some cases, the ethmoid air cells may encroach into the neighboring maxillary, lacrimal, frontal, sphenoid, and palatine bones.

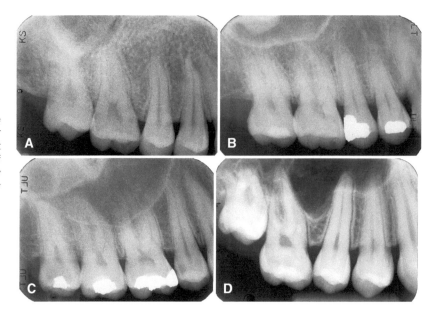

Fig. 28.1 (A–D) The range of the normal positions of the maxillary sinus floor relative to the premolar and molar teeth is shown in periapical images. There is no apparent floor in (A), with progressively more pneumatization of the alveolar process in (B) and (C); draping of the maxillary sinus border over the apices of the teeth is particularly evident in (D).

The function of the paranasal sinuses has been controversial. However, many authorities now believe the role of the paranasal sinuses is to insulate or protect deeper vital structures from external trauma.

DISEASES ASSOCIATED WITH THE PARANASAL SINUSES

The maxillary sinuses are of greatest concern to the dentist because of their proximities to the teeth and supporting structures. Therefore the emphasis in this chapter is be on diseases related to the maxillary sinus.

Definition

Diseases associated with the maxillary sinuses include those originating primarily from tissues within the sinus (intrinsic diseases) and those originating outside the sinus (commonly of odontogenic origin) that either impinge on or infiltrate the sinus (extrinsic diseases).

Clinical Features

The clinical signs and symptoms of maxillary sinus disease include pain and a sensation of pressure, altered voice characteristics, pain on head movement, percussion sensitivity of the teeth, regional dysesthesia, paresthesia or anesthesia, and swelling and tenderness of the facial structures adjacent to the maxilla.

Applied Diagnostic Imaging

When maxillary sinus disease is suspected, it may be reasonable for the dentist to proceed with the initial radiologic investigation. A periapical image provides a detailed view of the periapical structures of the teeth and their relationships to the alveolar recess and floor of the maxillary antrum. If an abnormality is suspected, a panoramic image can provide a view of a greater region of the sinus as well as parts of the inferior, posterior, and anteromedial walls. In some cases it may be difficult to compare the floors of the right and left sinuses on a panoramic image because of the overlapping of adjacent anatomic structures or ghost images. If there are positive findings on these images, the patient should be referred to an oral and maxillofacial radiologist for a more comprehensive imaging examination.

Advanced imaging has become increasingly important for the evaluation of sinus disease. CBCT and MDCT examinations contribute significantly to delineating the extent of disease, particularly in patients who have chronic or recurrent sinusitis. Coronal MDCT and CBCT images provide superior visualization of the ostiomeatal complex (the region of the ostia of the maxillary sinus and ethmoid air cells) and nasal cavities and for demonstrating any reaction in the surrounding bone to sinus disease. MRI provides superior visualization of the soft tissues, especially the extension of neoplasms developing or infiltrating the sinuses or surrounding soft tissues, or the differentiation of retained fluid secretions from soft tissue masses in the sinuses.

INTRINSIC DISEASES OF THE PARANASAL SINUSES

This section describes abnormalities that originate from tissues within the sinuses.

Inflammatory Disease

Inflammation may result from various causes, such as infection, chemical irritation, allergy, introduction of a foreign body, or facial trauma. These conditions can produce thickening of the sinus mucosa, which can be captured on imaging. Viral infections may, however, not produce any imaging change in a sinus.

Mucositis

Disease mechanism. The mucosal lining of the paranasal sinuses is normally less than 1 mm thick and cannot be visualized on imaging. However, when the mucosa becomes thickened due to inflammation, it may increase in thickness 10 to 15 times, and this may be seen with imaging. Localized inflammatory change is referred to as mucositis.

Clinical features. Many patients may be unaware of a change to their sinus mucosa, and these changes are often discovered as incidental findings on images made for other purposes. Consequently the discovery of thickened mucosa in an individual who is otherwise asymptomatic does not imply that further investigations are warranted or that treatment is required.

Imaging features. Thickened mucosa is readily detectable on imaging as a well-defined, noncorticated radiopaque band of soft tissue density that follows the contour of the bony wall of the sinus (Fig. 28.5).

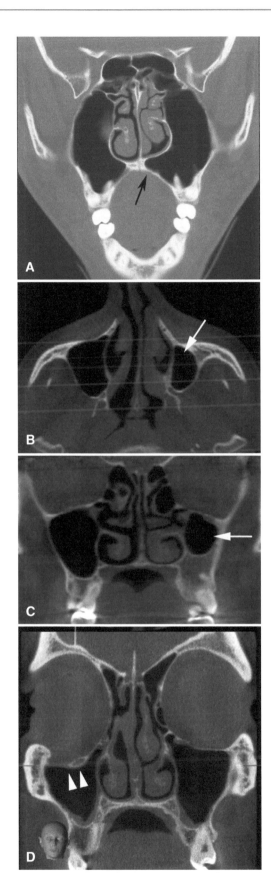

Fig. 28.2 (A) Pneumatization of the palatal process of the maxilla *(arrow)* by the maxillary sinus in a coronal multidetector computed tomography image. (B) Axial and (C) coronal cone beam computed tomography (CBCT) images demonstrating a hypoplastic left maxillary sinus *(arrows)*. (D) Coronal CBCT image of a patient with silent sinus syndrome. Note the inferiorly positioned floor of the right orbit *(arrowheads)* and enlarged size of the orbit.

Sinusitis

Disease mechanism. Sinusitis is a generalized inflammatory condition of the sinus mucosa caused by an allergen, bacterium, or virus. Inflammatory changes may lead to ciliary dysfunction and the retention of sinus secretions as well as, on occasion, blockage of the ostiomeatal complex. The term pansinusitis describes sinusitis affecting all the paranasal sinuses. In children with pansinusitis, the possibility of cystic fibrosis should be considered. Sinusitis is often categorized as acute or chronic based on the length of time the disease has been present. If the disease has been present for 4 weeks or less, it is termed *acute sinusitis*. If sinus disease has been present for more than 12 consecutive weeks, it is considered *chronic*. For sinusitis lasting from more than 4 weeks up to 12 weeks, the term *subacute* may be used.

Clinical features. Acute sinusitis is the most common of the sinus conditions that cause pain and is often a complication of the common cold. After a few days, nasal congestion accompanied by a clear discharge can increase, and the patient may complain of pain and tenderness to pressure or swelling over the involved sinus. The pain may also be referred to the premolar and molar teeth on the affected side, and these teeth may develop sensitivity to percussion. In the case of a bacterial sinusitis, a green or greenish-yellow discharge may accompany the other aforementioned signs and symptoms. In such circumstances, it is important that the teeth be ruled out as a possible source of the pain or infection.

Chronic maxillary sinusitis is a sequela of an acute infection that fails to resolve by 12 weeks. Generally no external signs occur except during periods of acute exacerbation, when increased pain and discomfort become apparent. Chronic sinusitis may develop with anatomic derangements, including deviation of the nasal septum and the presence of concha bullosa (pneumatization of the middle concha), which inhibits the outflow of mucus, or with allergic rhinitis, asthma, cystic fibrosis, and dental infections.

Imaging features. Thickening of the sinus mucosa and the accumulation of secretions, both of which accompany sinusitis, reduce the airspace of the sinus and cause it to become increasingly radiopaque. The most common radiopaque patterns are generalized thickening of the mucosal lining around the entire sinus cavity wall, and nearly complete or complete radiopacification of the sinus (Figs. 28.6 and 28.7). Mucosal thickening, when present, may also cause blockage of the sinus ostium. Mucosal thickening in just the base of the sinus may not represent sinusitis. Rather, it may represent the more localized thickening or mucositis that can occur in association with rarefying osteitis from a tooth with a nonvital pulp. If untreated, this condition may progress to involve the entire sinus.

The image of thickened sinus mucosa may be uniform or polypoid. In the case of an allergic reaction, the mucosa tends to be more lobulated. In contrast, in cases of infection, the thickened mucosal outline tends to be smoother, with its contour following that of the sinus wall. The inability to perceive the delicate walls of the ethmoid air cells is a particularly sensitive sign of ethmoid sinusitis.

An air-fluid level resulting from the accumulation of secretions may also be present. Because the radiopacities of transudates, exudates, blood, and pathologically altered mucosa are similar, differentiation among them relies on their shape and distribution. When present, fluid appears radiopaque and occupies the inferior or so-called dependent region of the sinus. The border between the radiopaque fluid and the relatively radiolucent air in the antrum is horizontal and straight, and a meniscus may be seen at the periphery where the fluid meets the sinus wall (see Fig. 28.6). Chronic sinusitis may result in persistent radiopacification of the sinus with sclerosis and thickening of the bony walls as osteoblasts in the bone respond to inflammatory mediators and the sinus periosteum is stimulated (Fig. 28.8).

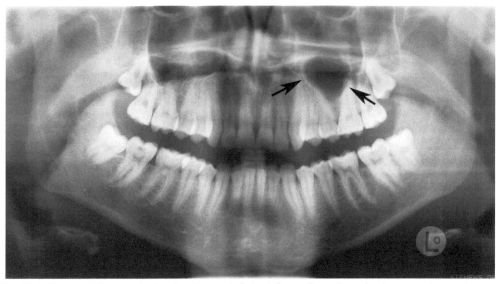

Fig. 28.3 Panoramic image of a loculus *(arrows)* of the left maxillary sinus draping over the tooth roots, mimicking a benign space-occupying lesion.

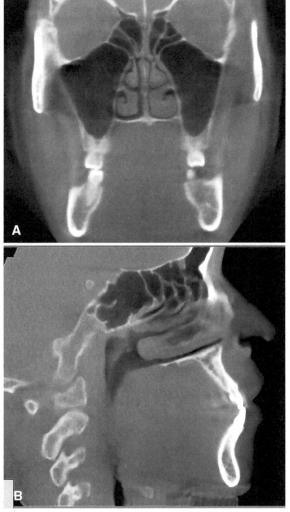

Fig. 28.4 (A) Coronal cone beam computed tomography (CBCT) image of normal maxillary sinuses and ethmoid air cells. (B) Sagittal CBCT image of normal frontal and sphenoid sinuses and ethmoid air cells.

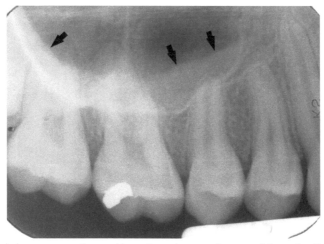

Fig. 28.5 Thickened sinus mucosa *(arrows)* is portrayed as a radiopaque ribbon of soft tissue that parallels the contour of the maxillary sinus floor.

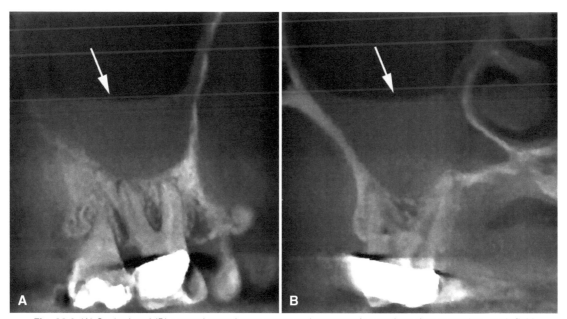

Fig. 28.6 (A) Sagittal and (B) coronal cone beam computed tomography sections demonstrating an air-fluid level in the right maxillary sinus *(arrows)*.

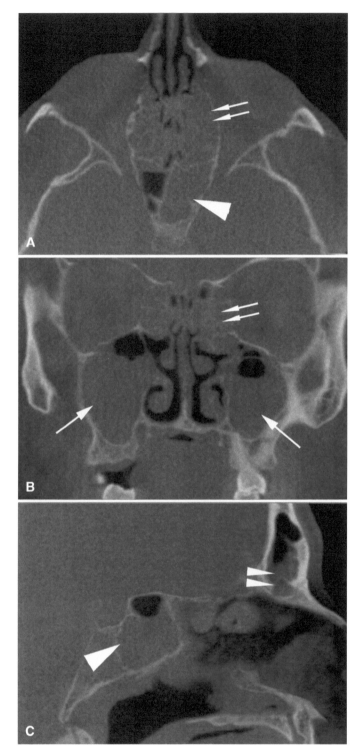

Fig. 28.7 (A) Axial, (B) coronal, and (C) sagittal cone beam computed tomography images showing opacification of the maxillary *(arrows)*, ethmoid *(double arrows)*, sphenoid *(arrowheads)*, and frontal *(double arrowheads)* paranasal sinuses.

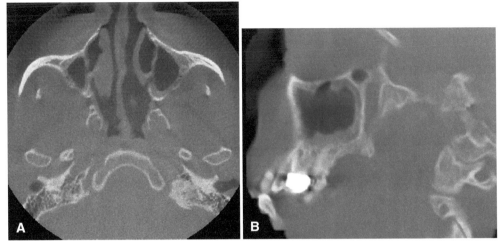

Fig. 28.8 Axial (A) and sagittal (B) cone beam computed tomography images show bony thickening of the left maxillary sinus walls due to chronic sinusitis.

Resolution of acute sinusitis becomes apparent on the image as a gradual increase in the radiolucency of the sinus. This can first be recognized when a small clear area appears in the interior of the sinus; the thickened mucosa gradually shrinks so that it begins to follow the outline of the bony wall. In time, the image of the mucosa becomes invisible and the sinus returns to a normal appearance. In chronic sinusitis, the changes to the sinus wall may persist.

Management. The treatment goals of sinusitis are to control the infection, promote drainage, and relieve pain. Acute sinusitis is usually treated pharmacologically with decongestants to reduce mucosal swelling and with antibiotics in the case of a bacterial sinusitis. Chronic sinusitis is primarily a disease of obstruction of the ostia; the goal is ventilation and drainage. Endoscopic surgery is often performed to enlarge obstructed ostia, or an alternative path of drainage may be established.

Retention Pseudocyst

Disease mechanism. The term retention pseudocyst is used to describe several related conditions that result in the development of cyst-like lesions that are not lined by epithelium. The pathogenesis of these lesions is controversial, but because their clinical and imaging features are similar, no attempt is made to distinguish among them. As such, many synonyms have been used for this entity: antral pseudocyst, benign mucous cyst, mucous retention cyst, mucous retention pseudocyst, mesothelial cyst, pseudocyst, interstitial cyst, lymphangiectatic cyst, false cyst, retention cyst of the maxillary sinus, benign cyst of the antrum, benign mucosal cyst of the sinus, serous nonsecretory retention pseudocyst, and mucosal antral cyst.

One etiology suggests that blockage of the secretory ducts of seromucous glands in the sinus mucosa may result in a pathologic submucosal accumulation of secretions, resulting in swelling of the tissue. A second theory suggests that the serous nonsecretory retention pseudocyst arises as a result of cystic degeneration within an inflamed, thickened sinus lining.

Clinical features. Retention pseudocysts can be found in any of the sinuses at any time of the year, although they may occur more often in the early spring or fall. This occurrence suggests that the development of retention pseudocysts may be related to changes in seasonal allergies, colds, humidity, or temperature. Most studies have found that retention pseudocysts are more common in males.

A retention pseudocyst rarely causes any signs or symptoms, and the patient is usually unaware of the lesion. It often is noticed as an incidental finding on images obtained for other purposes. Retention pseudocysts may range widely in size—from the size of a fingertip to a size large enough to fill the sinus completely and make it radiopaque. However, when a pseudocyst completely fills the maxillary sinus cavity, it may prolapse (extrude) through the ostium and cause nasal obstruction. The retention pseudocyst may also rupture as a result of abrupt pressure changes caused by sneezing or blowing of the nose, producing postnasal discharge. These symptoms may be the only clinical evidence of the presence of the pseudocyst. The pseudocyst may be present on an imaging examination of the maxillary sinus and be absent only a few days later, only to reappear on subsequent examinations.

The maxillary sinus is the most common site of retention pseudocysts. Pseudocysts are occasionally found in the sphenoid sinus and less often in the frontal sinuses and ethmoid air cells. Antral retention pseudocysts are not related to dental extractions or associated with periapical inflammatory disease.

Imaging features

Location. Partial images of retention pseudocysts of the maxillary antrum may appear on maxillary posterior periapical images (Fig. 28.9A), but they are best demonstrated on views acquired extraorally (see Fig. 28.9B). One or more pseudocysts may occur within the same or different sinus cavities. These pseudocysts usually form on the floor of the sinus (see Fig. 28.9A and B), although they may form on any wall or the roof, or they may fill most of the sinus cavity (see Fig. 28.9C–E).

Periphery. Retention pseudocysts usually appear as well-defined mostly sessile radiopaque masses that are noncorticated, smooth, and dome-shaped. Because the lesion originates from within the sinus, it does not have a radiopaque corticated border.

Internal structure. The internal structure is homogeneous and more radiopaque than the surrounding air of the sinus cavity (see Fig. 28.9). The radiopacity of the lesion is caused by the accumulation of fluid in the soft tissue lining of the sinus together with the thickened mucosa, both of which are relatively more radiopaque than air.

Effects on adjacent structures. There are no effects on the surrounding structures. The adjacent sinus floor is always intact.

Effects on adjacent teeth. When a retention pseudocyst occurs adjacent to the root of a tooth, the lamina dura surrounding the root is intact and the width of the periodontal ligament space is unaffected.

Differential interpretation. It is important to distinguish retention pseudocysts from antral polyps, odontogenic cysts, or neoplasms arising in the maxilla adjacent to the sinus. In contrast, the floor of the maxillary

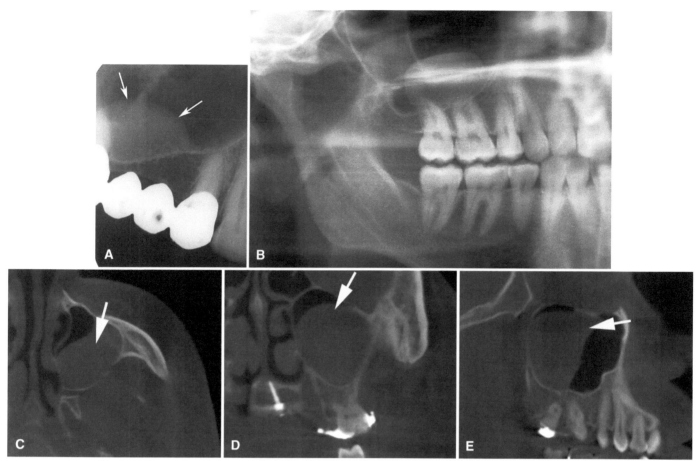

Fig. 28.9 Noncorticated dome-shaped retention pseudocysts *(arrows)* seen in periapical (A) and panoramic (B) images and axial (C), coronal (D), and sagittal (E) cone beam computed tomography images. Retention pseudocysts have noncorticated borders, indicating that they arise from within the sinus. They can reach various sizes and can occupy most of the sinus cavity.

sinus may be displaced by a developing odontogenic cyst or neoplasm as the border of the lesion becomes coincident with the bony sinus floor. In some instances, periodic fenestrations can be seen through the bony sinus floor, depending on the growth rate or aggressiveness of the cyst or neoplasm. The retention pseudocyst is dome-shaped but lacks the thin marginal radiopaque line representing the corticated border characteristic of the odontogenic cyst or neoplasm.

Antral polyps of infectious or allergic origin may be difficult to distinguish from retention pseudocysts, but when there is concurrent mucositis and multiple soft tissue masses, the possibility of polyps should be considered. Benign neoplasms may also mimic retention pseudocysts. If benign neoplasms originate from outside the sinus, they are separated from the cavity of the sinus by a radiopaque border, similar to odontogenic cysts. Malignant neoplasms may destroy the osseous border of the sinus, whether they arise from within the sinus or from the alveolar process. However, a malignant neoplasm is less likely to appear as dome-shaped as a retention pseudocyst.

Management. Retention pseudocysts in the maxillary sinus require no treatment because they customarily resolve spontaneously without any residual effect on the antral mucosa.

Polyps

Disease mechanism. The thickened mucosa of a chronically inflamed sinus frequently forms into irregular folds called *polyps*. Polyposis of

the sinus mucosa may develop in an isolated area or in many areas throughout the sinus.

Clinical features. Polyps may cause displacement or destruction of bone. In the ethmoid air cells, polyps may cause destruction of the medial wall of the orbit (lamina papyracea of the ethmoid bone) and an ipsilateral proptosis.

Imaging features. A polyp may be differentiated from a retention pseudocyst on an image by noting that a polyp usually occurs with a thickened mucosal lining because the polypoid mass is no more than an accentuation of mucosal thickening. In the case of a retention pseudocyst, the adjacent mucosa is usually not apparent. If multiple retention pseudocysts are seen within a sinus, the possibility of sinus polyposis should be considered.

The image of the bone displacement or destruction associated with polyps may mimic a benign or malignant neoplasm. Because many sinus neoplasms are asymptomatic, examination of a paranasal sinus that reveals bone destruction associated with increased radiopacity is an indication for additional imaging and biopsy; management should not be delayed by initial conservative treatment.

Antrolith

Disease mechanism. Antroliths occur within the maxillary sinuses and are the result of the deposition of mineral salts—such as calcium phosphate, calcium carbonate, and magnesium—around a nidus. Such

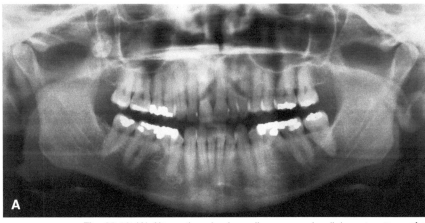
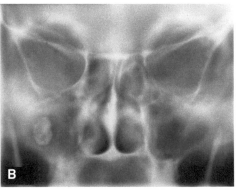

Fig. 28.10 (A) Alternating circular radiopaque and radiolucent pattern of an antrolith is seen on a panoramic image superimposed over the posterior wall of the right maxillary sinus. (B) Coronal multidirectional conventional tomographic image confirms the location of the antrolith within the sinus and shows the antrolith embedded in the soft tissue lining of the sinus.

an antrolith may be intrinsic, as when masses of stagnant or inspissated mucus or cellular debris collect at sites of previous inflammation, or it may be extrinsic, when materials are introduced into the sinus from the outside.

Clinical features. Small antroliths are usually asymptomatic and discovered incidentally on an imaging examination done for another purpose. If they continue to grow, the patient may have associated sinusitis, a blood-stained nasal discharge, nasal obstruction, or facial pain.

Imaging features

Location. Antroliths occur within the maxillary sinus above the floor of the maxillary antrum in either periapical or panoramic images (Fig. 28.10).

Periphery. Antroliths have a well-defined periphery and may have a smooth or irregular shape.

Internal structure. The internal pattern may vary from a barely perceptible radiopacity to an extremely radiopaque structure. The internal radiopacity may be homogeneous or heterogeneous. In some instances, alternating layers of concentric radiolucency and radiopacity in the form of laminations may be seen.

Differential interpretation. Antroliths may be distinguished from root fragments in the sinus by inspection of the mass for the usual root anatomy, such as the presence of a root canal. Unless it is lodged between the bone and the sinus lining, a displaced root fragment in the sinus may move when imaging is performed with the head in different positions. Rhinoliths are similar calcifications found within the nasal fossae.

Management. An otolaryngologist may have to remove symptomatic antroliths.

Mucocele

Disease mechanism. A mucocele is an expanding, destructive lesion that results from a blocked sinus ostium. The blockage may result from intra-antral or intranasal inflammation, polyp, or neoplasm, and the entire sinus becomes the pathologic cavity. As mucous secretions accumulate and the sinus cavity fills, the increase in pressure within the cavity results in thinning and displacement of the sinus walls and, in some cases, sinus wall destruction. When the cavity is filled with pus, it is termed an empyema, pyocele, or mucopyocele.

Clinical features. A mucocele in the maxillary sinus may exert pressure on the superior alveolar nerves and cause radiating pain. The patient may first complain of a sensation of fullness in the cheek, and the area

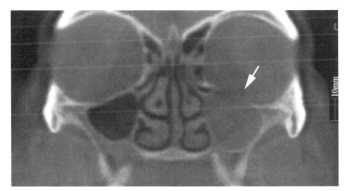

Fig. 28.11 Coronal cone beam computed tomography image demonstrating a mucocele that has caused complete radiopacification of the left maxillary sinus. Note the lack of a distinct border and displacement of the orbital floor *(arrow)* and the medial wall of the sinus.

may swell. This swelling may first become apparent over the anteroinferior aspect of the antrum—the area where the wall is thin or destroyed. If the lesion expands inferiorly, it may cause loosening of the adjacent posterior teeth. If the medial wall of the sinus is expanded, the lateral wall of the nasal cavity deforms and the nasal airway may become obstructed. If the lesion expands into the orbit, it may cause diplopia (double vision) or proptosis (protrusion of the globe of the eye).

Imaging features

Location. About 90% of mucoceles occur in the ethmoid air cells and frontal sinuses; they are rarely found in the maxillary and sphenoid sinuses.

Periphery. The normal shape of the sinus is changed into a more circular, "hydraulic" shape as the mucocele enlarges.

Internal structure. Internally, the sinus cavity is uniformly radiopaque (Fig. 28.11).

Effects on adjacent structures. The shape of the sinus changes as its borders are displaced outward and the bone expands. Septa and the bony walls may be severely thinned. When the mucocele is associated with the maxillary antrum, teeth may be displaced or roots resorbed. In the frontal sinus, the usually scalloped border is smoothed by the expanding mucocele, and any septa may be displaced. The superomedial border of the orbit may be displaced or destroyed. In the ethmoid air cells, displacement of the lamina papyracea may occur, displacing the contents of the orbit. In the sphenoid sinus, the expansion may be in a superior direction, suggesting a pituitary neoplasm.

Differential interpretation. Although it may be impossible to distinguish between a mucocele in the maxillary antrum and a cyst or neoplasm, any suggestion that the lesion is associated with an occluded ostium should strengthen the likelihood of a mucocele. Blockage of the ostium is usually the result of a previous surgical procedure, although a deviated nasal septum or polyps may be a factor. A large odontogenic cyst displacing the maxillary antral floor may mimic a mucocele. One should look for any remnants of an airspace between the wall of the cyst and the wall of the antrum. MDCT or CBCT is the imaging method of choice for making these distinctions.

Management. Treatment of the mucocele is usually surgical, through a transnasal endoscopic or a Caldwell-Luc approach to allow excision of the lesion. The prognosis is excellent.

Fungus Balls

Disease mechanism. Fungus balls, also referred to as fungal sinusitis, aspergillosis, and mycetoma, develop from the entrapment and growth of fungal hyphae and spores within the affected sinus and are associated with abnormal function of the cilia in the sinus mucosa. *Aspergillus fumigatus, Aspergillus flavus, Alternaria* spp. and *Pseudallescheria boydii* are the most common associated fungi. Interestingly, the presence of fungus balls in the maxillary sinus has been associated with endodontic treatment of maxillary teeth and the use of zinc containing endodontic sealers.

Clinical features. Usually fungus balls are seen in older individuals (60 to 70 years of age) although the age range is wide (28 to 86 years). They usually affect only one sinus and are more commonly found in the maxillary and less frequently in the sphenoid sinuses. The symptoms are similar to those of chronic sinusitis and include nasal discharge, pain, and nasal obstruction. Sometimes the patient may be asymptomatic and the diagnosis may be an incidental finding.

Imaging features

Location. Fungus balls usually affect the maxillary sinuses and less commonly, the sphenoid sinus. The ethmoid air cells may be affected by extension of the maxillary sinus disease.

Periphery. Fungus balls may cause partial or complete radiopacification of the maxillary sinus (Fig. 28.12). Thickening of the walls of the affected sinus might be present. However, minimal or no sinus expansion is observed.

Internal structure. Most of the sinus demonstrates a uniform radiopacification with soft tissue density. Central, focal areas of increased attenuation within the fungus ball represent calcified fungal debris and hyphae (see Fig. 28.12, *arrows*).

Effects on adjacent structures. Usually adjacent structures are not affected. The disease may extend to the sinus ostium. Thickening of the sinus walls may be present.

Differential interpretation. The differential interpretation of fungus balls includes other forms of rhinosinusitis, or a mucocele. The presence of internal calcifications on imaging aids in the diagnosis. The presence of fungi is confirmed by biopsy.

Management. Treatment usually involves the surgical removal of the fungus ball and reestablishment of sinus drainage by middle meatus antrostomy.

Neoplasms

Benign neoplasms of the paranasal sinuses are rare. The imaging features of such benign neoplasms are nonspecific. The involved portion of the sinus cavity appears radiopaque because of the presence of a mass, and there may be displacement of adjacent sinus borders.

The most common malignant neoplasms of the paranasal sinuses are squamous cell carcinoma and, to a lesser extent, malignant salivary

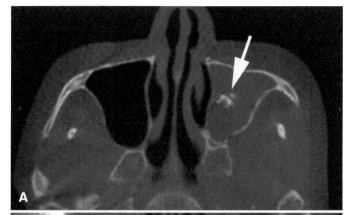

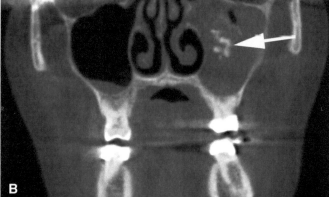

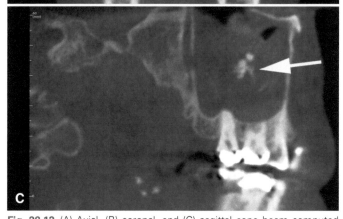

Fig. 28.12 (A) Axial, (B) coronal, and (C) sagittal cone beam computed tomography images demonstrating complete radiopacification of the left maxillary sinus and the presence of discrete radiopacities *(arrows)* representing calcified fungal debris and hyphae in a patient with a fungus ball.

gland neoplasms. Of carcinomas of the paranasal sinuses, 74% originate in the maxillary sinus. Although radiopacification is a feature of both inflammatory conditions and neoplasms, bone destruction is more common with malignant neoplasms.

Benign Neoplasms of the Paranasal Sinuses
Papilloma

Disease mechanism. Epithelial papilloma is a rare neoplasm of respiratory epithelium that occurs in the nasal cavity and paranasal sinuses. It occurs predominantly in men.

Clinical features. Unilateral nasal obstruction, nasal discharge, pain, and epistaxis may occur. The patient may have complained of recurring sinusitis for years, and a subsequent nasal obstruction on the same side as the sinusitis may develop. The epithelial papilloma, although benign, has a 10% incidence of associated carcinoma.

Imaging features. Imaging features are nonspecific; the diagnosis can be made only by histopathologic examination of the tissue.

Location. The epithelial papilloma usually occurs in the maxillary sinus or ethmoid air cells. It may also appear as an isolated polyp in the nose or sinus.

Internal structure. This neoplasm appears as a homogeneous radiopaque mass of soft tissue density.

Effects on adjacent structures. If bone destruction is apparent, it is the result of pressure erosion.

Osteoma

Disease mechanism. The osteoma is the most common mesenchymal neoplasm in the paranasal sinuses. For a detailed description, see Chapter 24.

Clinical features. Osteomas are almost twice as common in males as in females and are most common in the second, third, and fourth decades. Most are usually slow-growing and asymptomatic; they are usually detected incidentally in an examination performed for another purpose. When symptoms do occur, they are the result of obstruction of the sinus ostium or infundibulum or of erosion or deformity, orbital involvement, or intracranial extension. Osteomas growing in the maxillary sinus may extend into the nose and cause nasal obstruction or swelling of the side of the nose. They may also expand the sinus and produce swelling of the cheek or hard palate. In cases extending to the orbit, the patient may have proptosis.

Imaging features

Location. Although osteomas occasionally develop in the maxillary sinus, they more often occur in the frontal sinus and ethmoid air cells. The incidence in the maxillary antrum ranges from 3.9% to 28.5% of the incidence in all paranasal sinuses.

Periphery. An osteoma is usually round or lobulated and has a well-defined border (Fig. 28.13).

Internal structure. The internal pattern is homogeneous, and extremely radiopaque.

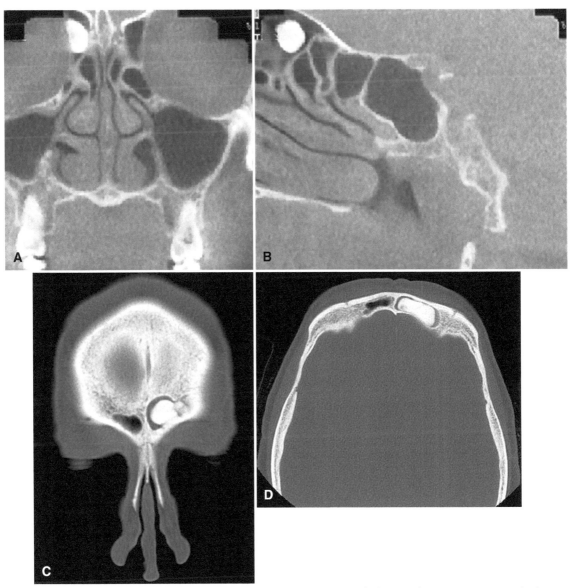

Fig. 28.13 Coronal (A) and sagittal (B) cone beam computed tomography images show an osteoma attached to the lateral wall of an anterior ethmoid air cell. Coronal (C) and axial (D) computed tomography images of an osteoma in the frontal sinus. (Courtesy Dr. E. Yu, Toronto, ON.)

Differential interpretation. The differential interpretation includes antrolith, mycolith, teeth, odontomas, or odontogenic neoplasms, although these lesions are usually not as homogeneous in appearance as osteomas.

Malignant Neoplasms of the Paranasal Sinuses

Malignant neoplasms of the paranasal sinuses are exceptionally rare, accounting for less than 1% of all malignancies in the body. Squamous cell carcinoma accounts for 80% to 90% of the cancers in this site and is the most common primary malignant neoplasm of the paranasal sinuses. Other primary neoplasms include adenocarcinoma, carcinomas of salivary gland origin, soft and hard tissue sarcomas, melanoma, and lymphoma. Factors that contribute to a poor prognosis for cancers of the paranasal sinuses include the advanced stage of the disease when it is finally diagnosed and the close proximity of vital anatomic structures.

The clinical signs and symptoms of a sinus malignancy may masquerade as an inflammatory sinusitis. The early primary lesions may appear only as a soft tissue mass in the sinus before they cause bone destruction. The lesion may become extensive, involving the entire sinus, with evidence of bone destruction before symptoms become apparent. Therefore any unexplained radiopacity in the maxillary sinus in an individual older than 40 years should be investigated thoroughly.

Squamous Cell Carcinoma

Disease mechanism. Squamous cell carcinoma likely originates from metaplastic epithelium of the sinus mucosal lining.

Clinical features. The most common symptoms of cancer in the maxillary sinus are facial swelling, epistaxis, dysesthesia, paresthesia, nasal obstruction, and the presence of a lesion in the oral cavity. The mean patient age is 60 years (range, 25 to 89 years). Twice as many men as women are affected. Lymph nodes are involved in about 10% of cases, and symptoms are present for approximately 5 months before diagnosis.

The symptoms produced by malignant neoplasms in the maxillary sinus depend on which wall of the sinus is involved. The medial wall is usually the first to become eroded, leading to nasal signs and symptoms such as obstruction, discharge, bleeding, and pain. These symptoms may appear trivial and their significance may be unappreciated. Lesions that arise on the floor of the sinus may first produce dental signs and symptoms, including enlargement of the alveolar process, unexplained pain, and altered sensation of the teeth, loose teeth, swelling of the palate or alveolar process, and ill-fitting dentures. The neoplasm may erode the sinus floor and penetrate the oral cavity. Such oral manifestations appear in 25% to 35% of patients with malignancies developing in the maxillary sinus. When the lesion penetrates the lateral wall, facial and vestibular swelling becomes apparent, and the patient may complain of pain and hyperesthesia of the maxillary teeth. Involvement of the sinus roof and the floor of the orbit causes signs and symptoms related to the eye, including diplopia, proptosis, pain, and hyperesthesia or anesthesia and pain over the cheek and maxillary teeth. Invasion and penetration of the posterior wall of the antrum can lead to invasion of the muscles of mastication, causing painful trismus and obstruction of the eustachian tube, causing a "stuffy ear," It may also cause referred pain and hyperesthesia over the distribution of the second and third divisions of the fifth cranial nerve.

Imaging features. Sometimes the imaging findings, especially in the early stages of malignant disease of the paranasal sinuses, are nonspecific. It may be impossible to differentiate the early manifestations in images of the maxillary sinus from the radiopacity of the sinus that develops in sinusitis and polyp formation. Evidence relies on changes seen in the surrounding bone, the sinus walls, and the alveolar process.

Location. Most carcinomas occur in the maxillary sinuses, but involvement of the frontal and sphenoid sinuses is also comparatively common.

Internal structure. The internal structure of the maxillary sinus has a soft tissue radiopaque appearance.

Effects on adjacent structures. As the lesion enlarges, it may destroy sinus walls and in general cause irregular radiolucent areas in the surrounding bone. A detailed examination of the adjacent alveolar process may reveal bone destruction around the teeth. Frequently the medial wall of the maxillary sinus is thinned or destroyed, although there may also be destruction of the floor, or the medial or posterior walls, which may be detected in the panoramic image. Destruction of the nasal cavity outline may be present.

Effects on adjacent teeth. A detailed examination of the adjacent alveolar process may reveal irregular widening of the periodontal ligament space and loss of lamina dura.

Additional imaging. If plain imaging of any radiopacified sinus reveals the slightest suggestion of bone destruction, advanced imaging, MDCT or MRI, is imperative (Fig. 28.14). On MDCT, the most characteristic sign of malignancy is invasion into the adjacent soft tissue spaces beyond the sinus walls (see Fig. 28.14). Consequently MDCT is useful in revealing the extent of paranasal sinus neoplasms, especially when extension into the orbit, infratemporal fossa, or cranial cavity has occurred. MRI is excellent for revealing the extent of soft tissue penetration into adjacent structures and in differentiating an accumulation of mucus from the soft tissue mass of the neoplasm.

Differential interpretation. The differential interpretation includes all the conditions that may cause radiopacity of the antrum, such as sinusitis, a large retention pseudocyst, and odontogenic cysts or tumors. Bone destruction may also occur in infectious conditions and some benign conditions. A neoplasm should be suspected in any older patient in whom chronic sinusitis develops for the first time without an obvious cause.

Management. Treatment of squamous cell carcinoma in the paranasal sinuses may include radiation therapy, surgery, or a combination of these. Malignant neoplasms in the paranasal sinuses usually have a poor prognosis because they tend to be well advanced by the time of diagnosis. Other factors contributing to the poor prognosis include frequently inaccurate preoperative staging and the complex anatomy of the region.

Pseudotumor

Disease mechanism. *Pseudotumor* is a descriptive name for any nonspecific inflammatory expansile lesion; this may include inflammatory pseudotumor, plasmocytic cell granuloma, fibroinflammatory pseudotumor, inflammatory myofibroblastic tumor, fibroblastoma, xanthogranuloma, and plasma cell granuloma. The exact etiopathogenesis is unknown, but as reflected in the multitude of synonyms, the lesion is considered an exaggerated inflammatory reaction.

Clinical features. Pseudotumor often occurs after a series of recurrent infections. The symptoms may not be very specific. There may be recurring pain and a mass simulating a neoplasm. The latter may cause erosion of the walls of the involved sinus and proptosis if the orbit is involved. Altered nerve function resulting from involvement of the nerve or occlusion of blood vessels by the mass has also been reported. Although cases have been reported in otherwise healthy individuals, many appear in patients who are immunocompromised or have systemic diseases, such as diabetes mellitus, von Willebrand disease, or myelodysplasia.

Imaging features. The imaging findings in pseudotumor include masses simulating malignant neoplasms that cause erosion of bony walls of the involved sinuses.

Differential interpretation. The differential interpretation includes benign and malignant neoplasms.

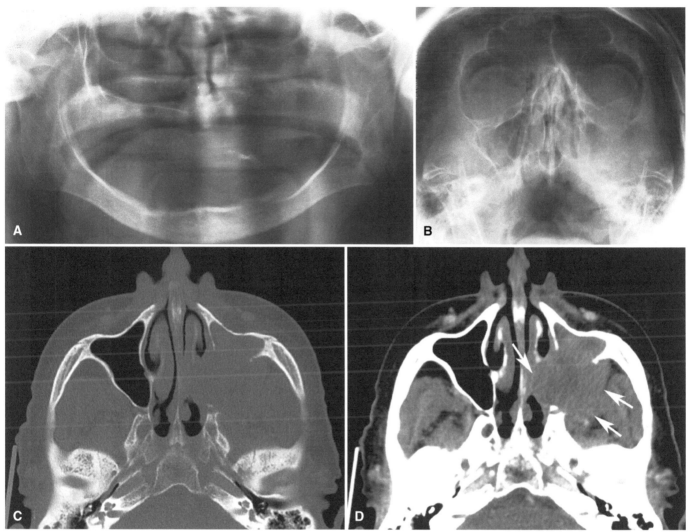

Fig. 28.14 (A) Panoramic image of a squamous cell carcinoma shows loss of definition of the cortex of the left maxillary sinus, nasal floor, and alveolar crest. (B) Waters view of the same patient shows a similar loss of cortical integrity to the lateral wall of the left maxilla and radiopacification of the left maxillary sinus. (C) Axial bone algorithm computed tomography image of a squamous cell carcinoma of the left maxillary sinus shows destruction of the posterolateral and medial walls of the sinus. (D) Same axial image slice with soft tissue algorithm demonstrates extension of the malignant neoplasm into the surrounding soft tissues *(arrows)*. ([B], Courtesy Dr. K. Dolan, Iowa City, IA.)

Management. The treatment of pseudotumor, which can include debridement of the sinuses by a Caldwell-Luc surgical approach or the administration of antifungal medication or other medicines, reflects the differences in the specific lesions included under the term *pseudotumor of the sinuses*, the exact location of the disease, the organism involved, and the medical status of the patient.

EXTRINSIC DISEASES INVOLVING THE PARANASAL SINUSES

Inflammatory Diseases

Perhaps 10% of inflammatory episodes of the maxillary sinuses are extensions of dental infections. Dental inflammatory lesions, such as periodontal or periapical inflammatory disease, may cause a localized mucositis in the adjacent floor of the maxillary antrum. This mucositis is a result of the inflammatory mediators diffusing beyond the floor of the antrum and into the periosteum and the mucosal lining of the sinus; it manifests as a homogeneous radiopaque, ribbon-like thickening

of the soft tissue that follows the contour of the maxillary sinus (see Fig. 28.5) and usually resolves in days or weeks after successful treatment of the underlying cause. The thickened mucosa is usually centered directly above the inflammatory lesion.

Periostitis and Periosteal New Bone Formation

Disease mechanism. As previously described, the exudate from a dental inflammatory lesion can diffuse through the cortical boundary of the antral floor. These products can strip and elevate the periosteal lining of the cortical bone of the floor of the maxillary antrum, stimulating the differentiation of pluripotential stem cells found within the cambium or osteogenic layer of the periosteum to produce an elevated thin layer of new bone adjacent to the root apex of the involved tooth (Fig. 28.15). The presence of one or more halo-like layers of new bone is a characteristic feature of inflammation of the periosteum.

Imaging features. Although the periosteal tissue is not visible on the image per se, this process is referred to as periosteal new bone formation. Such new bone may take the form of one or more thin radiopaque

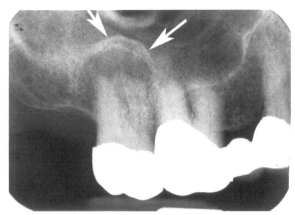

Fig. 28.15 The halo-like appearance of bone surrounding the roots of a maxillary second molar is the result of periosteal new bone formation and displacement of the adjacent maxillary sinus floor *(arrows)*.

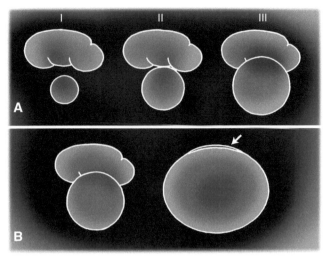

Fig. 28.16 (A) An odontogenic cyst or neoplasm develops adjacent to the floor of a sinus *(I)*. As the lesion enlarges, it abuts the maxillary sinus floor *(II)*; ultimately, as it continues to enlarge, it displaces the floor superiorly *(III)*. The border of the cyst and the border of the sinus are now the same line of bone. (B) As it continues to enlarge, the lesion may encroach on almost all the space of the sinus, leaving a small saddle-like sinus over it *(arrow)*. The appearance may mimic sinusitis.

lines, or the line may be thick. The new bone should be centered directly above the inflammatory lesion.

Benign Odontogenic Cysts and Neoplasms

The appearances of benign odontogenic cysts and neoplasms on the maxillary sinuses may be similar. Odontogenic cysts, and particularly radicular and dentigerous cysts, are the most common extrinsic lesions that encroach on the maxillary sinuses. For detailed descriptions of specific odontogenic cysts and benign neoplasms, see Chapters 23 and 24, respectively. Some odontogenic neoplasms, particularly ameloblastoma and odontogenic myxoma, show a more aggressive pattern of growth in the maxilla because of the richer blood supply in the maxilla compared with the mandible and their closer proximity to vital structures. As the cyst or neoplasm grows, its border becomes indistinguishable from the sinus border. With continued growth, the lesion encroaches on the space of the sinus, displacing its borders, and the air-filled space decreases in volume (Fig. 28.16). A thin radiopaque line divides the contents of the cyst from the sinus cavity. This appearance is in contrast to a retention pseudocyst, which, being inside the sinus, does not have a cortex around its periphery.

Imaging Features

Periphery. The enlarging cyst or benign neoplasm can have a round or oval shape with a curved or "hydraulic" contour. Both groups of lesions may have well-defined thin cortical borders, although more aggressively growing lesions may lack areas of cortication.

Internal structure. The internal structure of the cyst is homogeneous and radiopaque relative to the air-filled sinus cavity. Some neoplasms may also develop fine or coarse internal septation and appear multilocular or have regions of dystrophic calcification, depending on the histopathologic nature of the neoplasm. MDCT may be particularly useful in such situations to differentiate the area of increased radiopacity from bone.

Effects on adjacent structures. Both odontogenic cysts and neoplasms may displace the floor of the maxillary antrum and cause thinning of the peripheral cortex. These lesions may enlarge to the point where they almost completely encroach on the sinus airspace. This residual airspace may appear as a thin saddle over the cyst or neoplasm (see Fig. 28.16).

Effects on adjacent teeth. A cyst or benign neoplasm can cause displacement of adjacent teeth as well as external resorption of roots, often producing a sharp, curved edge that mirrors the growth front of

the cyst or neoplasm. Also, the lamina dura and periodontal ligament space may be lost.

Differential interpretation. An antral loculation may occasionally have a round shape and sometimes appear to have a cortex. However, because it contains air, the loculation appears as radiolucent as the surrounding sinus or more so.

Odontogenic cysts, in particular, must be differentiated from the common retention pseudocyst. Although odontogenic cysts may have a shape that is similar to that of a retention pseudocyst, only an odontogenic cyst demonstrates a peripheral cortex (Fig. 28.17). If the odontogenic cyst were to become infected, the cortex may become thickened, developing a sclerotic periphery; or it may be lost. Should the cortex become lost, it may be difficult to determine whether the lesion has arisen from outside or from within the sinus. However, in most cases, careful scrutiny of the lesion reveals some remaining cyst cortex, and the relationship to neighboring teeth may help to make this decision (Fig. 28.18). It may be difficult to differentiate a dentigerous cyst from an odontogenic keratocyst if the latter develops in a pericoronal relationship to a tooth. The differentiation may be aided by locating the association of the lesion with a tooth's cementoenamel junction on CBCT or MDCT.

Large cysts or neoplasms can completely efface the sinus cavity. When this occurs, little or no imaging evidence of residual airspace may exist, and it may appear as if the cyst had developed within the sinus. In this case, because of the radiopacity of the cyst, the appearance may resemble sinusitis with radiopacification of the sinus. Evaluation of such a situation is aided by locating a region where both the displaced sinus floor and the unaffected sinus wall meet—the "double cortex" appearance (see Fig. 28.17C). Additionally, the wall of the cyst often has a more "hydraulic" contour than the wall of the sinus. A cyst that occupies the entire sinus usually causes expansion of the medial wall (middle meatus) of the sinus and alters the sigmoid contour of the posterolateral wall of the sinus as viewed in axial CBCT or MDCT images.

With or sometimes without treatment, an odontogenic cyst involving the sinus may "collapse" and heal. The end result is the appearance of

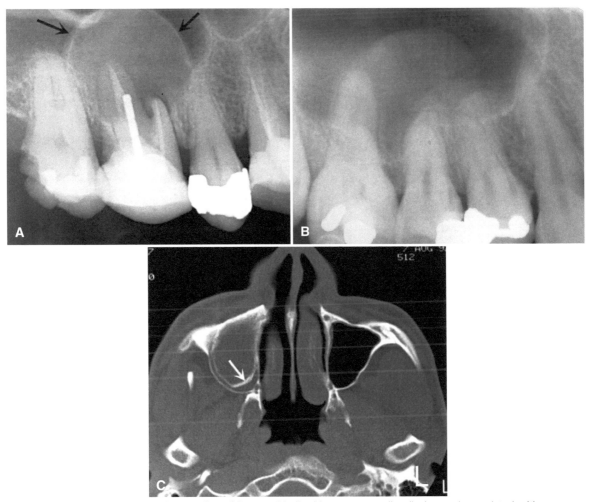

Fig. 28.17 (A) Periapical image of rarefying osteitis (in this case, a small radicular cyst) associated with a maxillary molar tooth. Note the peripheral cortex *(arrows)*. (B) Periapical image of a pseudocyst; note the lack of a peripheral cortex. (C) Axial computed tomography image of a large radicular cyst; note the peripheral cortex *(arrow)* inside the outer cortex of the sinus.

an irregularly shaped bone formation with a radiolucent center projecting from the floor of the sinus (see Chapter 23). This bone formation should be differentiated from a bone-forming neoplasm, such as an osteoma or ossifying fibroma.

Bone Dysplasias

Periapical and florid osseous dysplasias, when they develop near the root apices of the maxillary premolar and molar teeth, behave in much the same way radiographically as cysts or benign neoplasms (Fig. 28.19). Fibrous dysplasia may arise adjacent to any of the paranasal sinuses, causing expansion of the bone as well as displacement of sinus borders, which can result in a smaller sinus on the affected side. For a detailed description of bone dysplasias, see Chapter 25.

Clinical Features

Involvement of the facial skeleton with fibrous dysplasia can result in facial asymmetry, nasal obstruction, proptosis, pituitary gland compression, impingement on cranial nerves, or sinus obliteration. Obliteration of the airspace results when the expanding dysplastic bone encroaches on it. The lesion may displace the roots of teeth and cause teeth to separate or migrate, but it usually does not cause root resorption. Fibrous

dysplasia is more common in children and young adults, and growth of the dysplastic bone usually ceases at the age of skeletal maturity.

Imaging Features

Location. The posterior maxilla is the most common location for fibrous dysplasia.

Periphery. The lesion itself is usually not well defined, tending to blend into the surrounding bone. The external cortex of the bone and the sinus border are intact but displaced.

Internal structure. The normal radiolucent maxillary sinus may be partially or totally replaced by the increased radiopacity of this lesion. The degree of radiopacity depends on its stage of development and the relative amounts of bone and fibrous tissue present. Usually the radiopaque areas have a uniform characteristic ground-glass appearance on extraoral images or an orange-peel appearance on intraoral views (Fig. 28.20).

Effects on adjacent structures. Fibrous dysplasia may expand the alveolar process superiorly, elevating the orbital floor inferiorly and causing asymmetry of the alveolar process medially, facially, or posterolaterally. The new bone may also encroach on the dimensions of the air cavity, causing it to appear smaller in size but maintaining a resemblance to a normal shape.

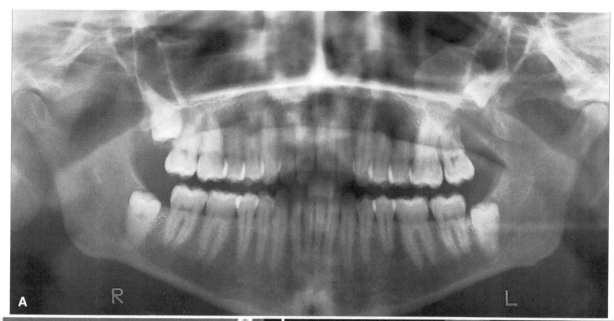

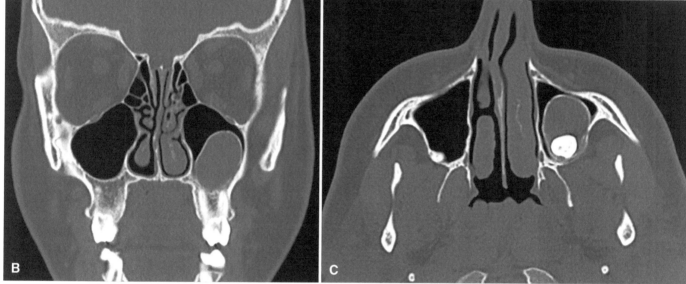

Fig. 28.18 Series of images showing displacement of the left maxillary sinus floor as a result of a developing dentigerous cyst associated with the maxillary left third molar. (A–C) The corticated periphery of the cyst is well seen in the panoramic image (A). (B) Coronal multidetector computed tomography (MDCT) image shows the displaced floor of the left maxillary sinus. (C) Axial MDCT image shows the bowing of the posterior sinus wall and the adjacent impacted tooth.

Effects on adjacent teeth. There may be no effects on the dentition. In some cases, when the radiopacity of the dysplastic bone increases, the periodontal ligament space may appear narrowed, with the lamina dura being lost as continuity develops between it and the dysplastic bone.

Differential Interpretation

The diagnosis of fibrous dysplasia in a relatively young person is usually not difficult. In contrast, Paget disease of bone does not usually obliterate the sinus. Ossifying fibroma, which may have an appearance similar to that of fibrous dysplasia, may have an internal radiolucent periphery and be more expansile. In some cases, however, the differential interpretation of ossifying fibroma involving the antrum and fibrous dysplasia can be difficult. In fibrous dysplasia, the shape of the dysplastic bone

encroaching on the sinus can result in a smaller airspace. In such instances, however, the shape of the airspace is maintained.

Iatrogenic Effects of Dental Procedures on the Maxillary Sinus
Mechanism

Dental procedures involving the posterior maxilla may have adverse effects on the appearance and function of the maxillary sinuses (Fig. 28.21). The continuity of the maxillary sinus floor may be lost during tooth extraction, resulting in an oroantral communication. Tooth roots may be fractured as a result of various forms of trauma, including tooth extraction, and may be displaced into the airspace of the sinus. Exuberant extrusion of restorative material during endodontic treatment

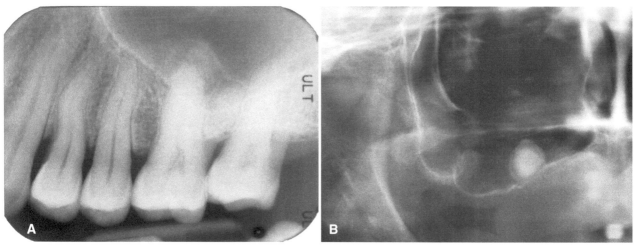

Fig. 28.19 (A) Periapical image demonstrates elevation of the maxillary sinus floor by a focus of periapical cemento-osseous dysplasia located at the apices of the maxillary left first molar. (B) Cropped panoramic image reveals a small region of cemento-osseous dysplasia invaginating the inferior aspect of the sinus. Note the thin radiolucent soft tissue capsule and cortex at the periphery.

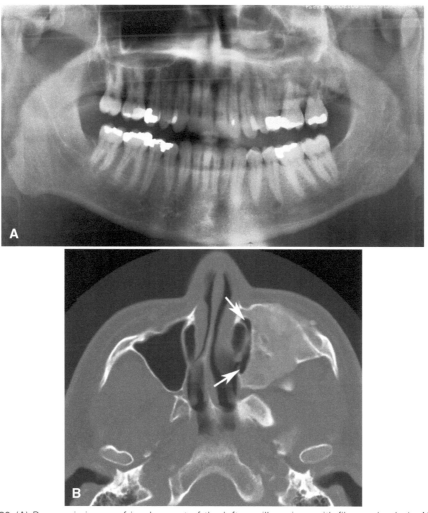

Fig. 28.20 (A) Panoramic image of involvement of the left maxillary sinus with fibrous dysplasia. Note the radiopacification of the left maxillary sinus compared with the right sinus. (B) Axial multidetector computed tomography image of the same case reveals almost complete encroachment on the sinus; a small portion of the medial airspace remains *(arrows)*. Note the very fine homogeneous bone pattern of fibrous dysplasia.

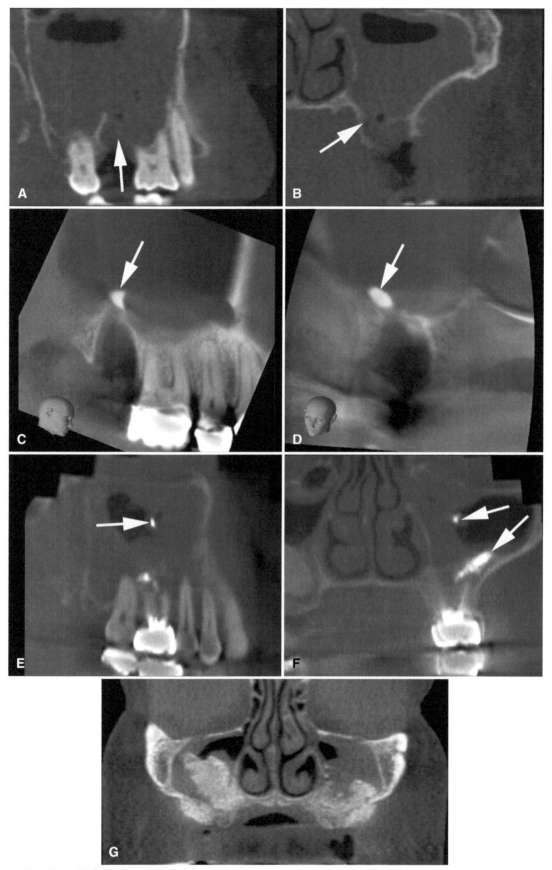

Fig. 28.21 (A) Sagittal and (B) coronal cone beam computed tomography (CBCT) images demonstrating loss of the continuity of the sinus floor *(arrow)* after extraction of the maxillary left second molar. Note the presence of air bubbles and an air-fluid level. (C) Sagittal and (D) coronal CBCT images showing a root fragment *(arrows)* intruding through the base of the extraction socket of the maxillary right second molar and displacement through the floor of the maxillary sinus. (E) Sagittal and (F) coronal CBCT images demonstrating endodontic material *(arrows)* displaced into the maxillary sinus after endodontic treatment of the maxillary left second molar. Note the associated mucosal thickening. (G) Coronal CBCT image demonstrating bone graft material within the right and left maxillary sinuses after an alveolar ridge augmentation procedure. Note the nearly complete radiopacification of both sinuses and the punctate spicules of the graft in the left sinus.

of posterior maxillary teeth may lead to its deposition in the maxillary sinus. Finally, ridge augmentation procedures during implant placement may disrupt the integrity of the sinus mucosal lining and result in the intrusion of bone graft material into the sinus cavity.

Clinical Features

No specific features may be present if the integrity of the sinus wall has been acutely violated. In case of tooth extraction, the dentist may note the absence of the root fragment on examining the extracted tooth and may be unable to locate it anywhere else. Sometimes asking the patient to hold his or her nose while attempting to breathe out, similar to a Valsalva maneuver, causes bubbles to appear within the blood contained within the fresh extraction socket. If the insult has occurred in the more distant past, the presenting symptom may be that of sinusitis (see the previous discussion of sinusitis).

Imaging Features

Location. Teeth, root fragments, endodontic material, or osseous grafts may be displaced into the sinus. These may be found anywhere within the sinus but are more often located near the floor of the sinus because of gravity (Fig. 28.22A). Sometimes they may be located submucosally, between the osseous wall of the sinus and the mucoperiosteum.

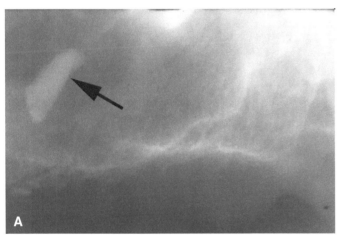

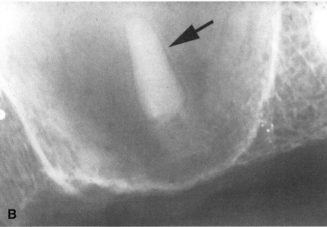

Fig. 28.22 (A) Periapical image revealing a portion of tooth root *(arrow)* within the maxillary sinus. (B) Another periapical image of a retained root tip outside the sinus, but its image is superimposed over the sinus *(arrow)*. The presence of a periodontal ligament space indicates that it is in the alveolar process and not in the sinus.

Periphery. Disruption of the sinus wall may be difficult or impossible to see on conventional images. CBCT avoids superimposition of anatomic structures and is recommended for assessment of the integrity of the sinus walls.

Internal structure. Most displaced objects are radiopaque and, if large enough, can be seen on an imaging examination. However, owing to the limitations of two-dimensional images, their exact location can be difficult to identify.

Effects on adjacent structures. Usually no effect on surrounding structures is noted other than the altered anatomy during the dental procedure or the violation of the sinus floor's integrity during the intrusion of a tooth fragment. At later stages and if sinusitis ensues, partial or complete opacification of the involved sinus might be present.

Differential Interpretation

In most cases the history of a surgical procedure and the relevant clinical symptoms and signs lead to the correct diagnosis. However, the diagnostic challenge focuses on identifying the exact location of the displaced objects, their relation to anatomic landmarks such as the sinus ostium, and the possible concomitant sinus inflammation.

Bony masses that represent hyperostosis of the sinus wall, floor, or septa within the sinus may mimic dental root fragments or even whole teeth. Antroliths may also have a similar appearance. The shape of the radiopacity, the presence of a pulp chamber or root canal, a layer of enamel, or the high radiopacity of endodontic material may help in the differential interpretation. If the root tip remains in its socket, it may be superimposed over the maxillary sinus, but the presence of a lamina dura and periodontal ligament space indicates a position within the alveolar process (see Fig. 28.22B).

Management

Management ranges from follow-up with the patient to see whether the object will be removed from the sinus through the ostium by ciliary action to entering the sinus surgically by a Caldwell-Luc procedure. Sinusitis may develop and should be managed with the appropriate treatment.

For other trauma involving the paranasal sinuses, see Chapter 27.

BIBLIOGRAPHY

Normal Development and Variations

Dodd GD, Jing BS. *Radiology of the Nose, Paranasal Sinus and Nasopharynx.* Baltimore: Williams & Wilkins; 1977.

DuBrul EL. *Sicher's Oral Anatomy.* 7th ed. St Louis: Mosby; 1980.

Grant JCB. *A Method of Anatomy.* Baltimore: Williams & Wilkins; 1958.

Guillen DE, Pinargote PM, Guarderas JC. The silent sinus syndrome: protean manifestations of a rare upper respiratory disorder revisited. *Clin Mol Allergy.* 2013;11:5.

Hengerer AS. Embryonic development of the sinuses. *Ear Nose Throat J.* 1984;63:134–136.

Karmody CS, Carter B, Vincent ME. Developmental anomalies of the maxillary sinus. *Trans Sect Otolaryngol Am Acad Ophthalmol Otolaryngol.* 1977;84:723–728.

Lusted LB, Keats TE. *Atlas of Roentgenographic Measurement.* 3rd ed. Chicago: Year Book Medical Publishers; 1972.

Ritter FN. *The Paranasal Sinuses: Anatomy and Surgical Technique.* St Louis: Mosby; 1973.

Scuderi AJ, Harnsberger HR, Boyer RS. Pneumatization of the paranasal sinuses: normal features of importance to the accurate interpretation of CT scans and MR images. *AJR Am J Roentgenol.* 1993;160:1101–1104.

Shapiro R. *Radiology of the Normal Skull.* Chicago: Year Book Medical Publishers; 1981.

Som PM. The paranasal sinuses. In: Bergeron RT, Osborn AG, Som PM, eds. *Head and Neck Imaging: Excluding the Brain.* St Louis: Mosby; 1984.

Takahashi R. The formation of the human paranasal sinuses. *Acta Otolaryngol Suppl.* 1984;408:1–28.

Lloyd GA. Diagnostic imaging of the nose and paranasal sinuses. *J Laryngol Otol.* 1989;103:453–460.

Zinreich SJ. Imaging of chronic sinusitis in adults: x-ray, computed tomography, and magnetic resonance imaging. *J Allergy Clin Immunol.* 1992;90:445–451.

Inflammatory Changes

Nurbakhsh B, Friedman S, Kulkarni GV, et al. Resolution of maxillary sinus mucositis after endodontic treatment of maxillary teeth with apical periodontitis: a cone beam computerized tomography pilot study. *J Endod.* 2011;37:1504–1511.

Robinson K. Roentgenographic manifestations of benign paranasal disease. *Ear Nose Throat J.* 1984;63:144.

Thickened Mucous Membrane—*Mucositis*

Dolan K, Smoker W. Paranasal sinus radiology. Part 4A; maxillary sinuses. *Head Neck Surg.* 1983;5:345–362.

Killey HC, Kay LA. *The Maxillary Sinus and Its Dental Implications.* Bristol: John Wright; 1975.

Periostitis—*Sinusitis*

Druce HM. Diagnosis and medical management of recurrent and chronic sinusitis in adults. In: Gershwin ME, Incaudo GA, eds. *Diseases of the Sinuses.* Ottawa, Canada: Humana Press; 1996.

Fireman P. Diagnosis of sinusitis in children: emphasis on the history and physical examination. *J Allergy Clin Immunol.* 1992;90:433–436.

Incaudo G, Gershwin ME, Nagy SM. The pathophysiology and treatment of sinusitis. *Allergol Immunopathol (Madr).* 1986;14:423–434.

Kennedy DW. First-line management of sinusitis: a national problem? Surgical update. *Otolaryngol Head Neck Surg.* 1990;103:884–886.

Killey HC, Kay LA. *The Maxillary Sinus and Its Dental Implications.* Bristol: John Wright; 1975.

Palacios E, Valvassori G. Computed axial tomography in otorhinolaryngology. *Adv Otorhinolaryngol.* 1978;24:1–8.

Paparella MM. Mucosal cyst of the maxillary sinus. *Arch Otolaryngol.* 1963;77:650–670.

Poyton HG. Maxillary sinuses and the oral radiologist. *Dent Radiogr Photogr.* 1972;45:43–50.

Reilly JS. The sinusitis cycle. *Otolaryngol Head Neck Surg.* 1990;103:856–861.

Shapiro GG, Rachelefsky GS. Introduction and definition of sinusitis. *J Allergy Clin Immunol.* 1992;90:417–418.

Zinreich SJ. Imaging of chronic sinusitis in adults: x-ray, computed tomography, and magnetic resonance imaging. *J Allergy Clin Immunol.* 1992;90:445–451.

Empyema

Ash JE, Raum M. *An Atlas of Otolaryngic Pathology.* New York: American Registry of Pathology; 1956.

Groves J, Gray RF. *A Synopsis of Otolaryngology.* Bristol: John Wright; 1985.

Polyps

Potter GD. Inflammatory disease of the paranasal sinuses. In: Valvassori GE, Potter GD, Hanefee WN, eds. *Radiology of the Ear, Nose and Throat.* Philadelphia: Saunders; 1982.

Retention Pseudocysts

Allard RH, van der Kwast WA, van der Waal JI. Mucosal antral cysts: review of the literature and report of a radiographic survey. *Oral Surg Oral Med Oral Pathol.* 1981;51:2–9.

Dolan K, Smoker W. Paranasal sinus radiology. Part 4A: maxillary sinuses. *Head Neck Surg.* 1983;5:345–362.

Gothberg K, Little JW, King DR, et al. A clinical study of cysts arising from mucosa of the maxillary sinus. *Oral Surg.* 1976;41:52–58.

Kadymova MI. Lymphangiectatic (false) cysts of the maxillary sinuses and their relation with allergy. *Vestib Otorhinolaringol.* 1966;28:58.

Kaffe I, Littner MM, Moskona D. Mucosal-antral cysts: radiographic appearance and differential diagnosis. *Clin Prev Dent.* 1988;10:3–6.

Mills CP. Secretory cysts of the maxillary antrum and their relationship to the development of antrochoanal polypi. *J Laryngol Otol.* 1959;73:324–334.

Poyton HG. *Oral Radiology.* Baltimore: Williams & Wilkins; 1982.

Ruprecht A, Batniji S, el-Neweihi E. Mucous retention cyst of the maxillary sinus. *Oral Surg Oral Med Oral Pathol.* 1986;62:728–731.

Shafer WG, Hine MK, Levy BM. *A Textbook of Oral Pathology.* 4th ed. Philadelphia: Saunders; 1983.

van Norstrand AWP, Goodman WS. Pathologic aspects of mucosal lesions of the maxillary sinus. *Otolaryngol Clin North Am.* 1976;9:21–34.

Mucocele—*Fungus Balls*

Abdel-Aziz M, El-Hoshy H, Azooz K, et al. Maxillary sinus mucocele: predisposing factors, clinical presentations, and treatment. *Oral Maxillofac Surgery.* 2017;21:55–58.

Atherino C, Atherino T. Maxillary sinus mucopyoceles. *Arch Otolaryngol.* 1984;110:200.

Jones JL, Kaufman PW. Mucopyocele of the maxillary sinus. *J Oral Surg.* 1981;39:948.

Zizmor JK, Noyek AM. The radiologic diagnosis of maxillary sinus disease. *Otolaryngol Clin North Am.* 1976;9:93.

Hathiram BT, Khattar VS. Fungus balls of the paranasal sinuses. *Otolaryngol Clinics.* 2009;1:33–35.

Nicolai P, Mensi M, Marsili F, et al. Maxillary fungus ball: zinc-oxide endodontic materials as a risk factor. *ACTA otorhinolaryngologica italica.* 2015;35:93–96.

Odontogenic Cysts

Killey HC, Kay LA. *The Maxillary Sinus and Its Dental Implications.* Bristol: John Wright; 1975.

Poyton H. Maxillary sinuses and the oral radiologist. *Dent Radiogr Photogr.* 1972;45:43–50.

Van Alyea OE. *Nasal Sinuses.* Baltimore: Williams & Wilkins; 1951.

Odontogenic Keratocysts

MacDonald-Jankowski DS. The involvement of the maxillary antrum by odontogenic keratocysts. *Clin Radiol.* 1992;45:31–33.

Neoplasms

Goepfert H, Luna MA, Lindberg RD, et al. Malignant salivary gland tumors of the paranasal sinuses and nasal cavity. *Arch Otolaryngol.* 1983;109:662–668.

St-Pierre S, Baker SR. Squamous cell carcinoma of the maxillary sinus: analysis of 66 cases. *Head Neck Surg.* 1983;5:508–513.

Epithelial Papilloma

Rogers JH, Fredrickson JM, Noyek AM. Management of cysts, benign tumors, and bony dysplasia of the maxillary sinus. *Otolaryngol Clin North Am.* 1976;9:233–247.

Osteoma

Dolan K, Smoker W. Paranasal sinus radiology. Part 4B: maxillary sinuses. *Head Neck Surg.* 1983;5:428–446.

Goodnight J, Dulguerov P, Abemayor E. Calcified mucor fungus ball of the maxillary sinus. *Am J Otolaryngol.* 1993;14:209–210.

Reuben BM. Odontoma of the maxillary sinus: a case report. *Quintessence Int Dent Dig.* 1983;14:287–290.

Samy LL, Mostofa H. Osteoma of the nose and paranasal sinuses with a report of twenty-one cases. *J Laryngol Otol.* 1971;85:449–469.

Ameloblastoma

Hames RS, Rakoff SJ. Diseases of the maxillary sinus. *J Oral Med.* 1972;27:90–95.

Reaume C, Wesley RK, Jung B, et al. Ameloblastoma of the maxillary sinus. *J Oral Surg.* 1980;38:520–521.

Malignant Neoplasms of the Paranasal Sinuses

Batsakis JG. *Tumors of the Head and Neck.* 2nd ed. Baltimore: Williams & Wilkins; 1979.

St-Pierre S, Baker S. Squamous cell carcinoma of the maxillary sinus: analysis of 66 cases. *Head Neck Surg.* 1983;5:508–513.

Zizmor J, Noyek AM. Cysts, benign tumors and malignant tumors of the paranasal sinuses. *Otolaryngol Clin North Am.* 1973;6:487–508.

Squamous Cell Carcinoma

Batsakis JG, Rice DH, Solomon AR. The pathology of head and neck tumors: squamous and mucous-gland carcinomas of the nasal cavity, paranasal sinuses and larynx. Part 6. *Head Neck Surg.* 1980;2:497–508.

Bridger M, Beale F, Bryce D. Carcinoma of the paranasal sinuses: a review of 158 cases. *J Otolaryngol.* 1978;7:379–388.

Eddleston B, Johnson R. A comparison of conventional radiographic imaging and computed tomography in malignant disease of the paranasal sinuses and the post-nasal space. *Clin Radiol.* 1983;34:161–172.

Hasso AN. CT of tumors and tumor-like conditions of the paranasal sinuses. *Radiol Clin North Am.* 1984;22:119–130.

Larheim TA, Kolbenstvedt A, Lien H. Carcinoma of maxillary sinus, palate and maxillary gingiva, occurrence of jaw destruction. *Scand J Dent Res.* 1984;92:235–240.

Lund VJ, Howard DJ, Lloyd GA. CT evaluation of paranasal sinus tumors for cranio-facial resection. *Br J Radiol.* 1983;56:439–446.

Mancuso A, Hanafee WN, Winter J, et al. Extensions of paranasal sinus tumors and inflammatory disease: an evaluation by CT and pluridirectional tomography. *Neuroradiology.* 1978;16:449–453.

St-Pierre S, Baker SR. Squamous cell carcinoma of the maxillary sinus: analysis of 66 cases. *Head Neck Surg.* 1983;5:508–513.

Thomas GK, Kasper KA. Ossifying fibroma of the frontal bone. *Arch Otolaryngol.* 1966;83:43–46.

Tsaknis PJ, Nelson JF. The maxillary ameloblastoma: an analysis of 24 cases. *J Oral Surg.* 1980;38:336–342.

Weber A, Tadmore R, Davis R, et al. Malignant tumors of the sinuses: radiologic evaluation, including CT scanning, with clinical and pathologic correlation. *Neuroradiology.* 1978;16:443–448.

Pseudotumor

Muzaffar M, Hussain SI, Chughtai A. Plasma cell granuloma: maxillary sinuses. *J Laryngol Otol.* 1994;108:357–358.

Naveen J, Sonalika W, Prabhu S, et al. Inflammatory pseudotumor of maxillary sinus: Mimicking as an aggressive malignancy. *J Oral Maxillofac Pathol.* 2011;15:344–345.

Newlin HE, Werning JW, Mendenhall WM. Plasma cell granuloma of the maxillary sinus: a case report and literature review. *Head Neck.* 2005;27:722–728.

Ozhan S, Araç M, Isik S, et al. Pseudotumor of the maxillary sinus in a patient with von Willebrand's disease. *AJR Am J Roentgenol.* 1996;166:950–951.

Som PM, Brandwein MS, Maldjian C, et al. Inflammatory pseudotumor of the maxillary sinus: CT and MR findings in six cases. *AJR Am J Roentgenol.* 1994;163:689–692.

Fibrous Dysplasia

Malcolmson KG. Ossifying fibroma of the sphenoid. *J Laryngol Otol.* 1967;81:87–92.

Thomas GK, Kasper KA. Ossifying fibroma of the frontal bone. *Arch Otolaryngol.* 1966;83:43–46.

Wong A, Vaughan CW, Strong MS. Fibrous dysplasia of temporal bone. *Arch Otolaryngol.* 1965;81:131–133.

29

Craniofacial Anomalies

Carol Anne Murdoch-Kinch

Developmental disturbances can affect the normal growth and differentiation of craniofacial structures, resulting in observable craniofacial anomalies. These developmental craniofacial anomalies are usually first discovered in infancy or childhood. Some are caused by known and recently discovered genetic mutations, others result from environmental factors, and a third group are multifactorial. These conditions are manifested by a variety of abnormalities of the face and jaws, including abnormalities of structure, shape, organization, and function of hard and soft tissues. A multitude of conditions affect the morphogenesis of the face and jaws, many of which are rare syndromes. This chapter briefly reviews more common or significant craniofacial developmental anomalies that may be encountered in dental practice.

CLEFT LIP AND PALATE

Disease Mechanism

Facial clefts of various types are caused by a failure of fusion of the developmental processes of the face during fetal development. Cleft lip and cleft palate (CL/P), cleft lip (CL), and cleft palate (CP) together are the most common developmental craniofacial anomalies worldwide. Their incidence varies with geographic location, ethnic background, and socioeconomic status. Worldwide, the average birth prevalence of all orofacial clefts is 9.92 per 10,000. In Caucasian populations, the incidence of CL is 1 : 800 to 1 : 1000 live births, and the incidence of CP is approximately 1 : 1000. CL with or without CL/P and CP are two different conditions with different etiologies.

CL/P results from a failure of fusion of the medial nasal process with the maxillary process, and can range in severity from a unilateral CL to bilateral complete clefting through the lip, maxillary alveolar processes, and hard and soft palate in the most severe cases. CP develops from a failure of fusion of the lateral palatal shelves. The minimal manifestation of CP is a submucous cleft in which the palate appears to be intact except for notching of the uvula (bifid uvula) or notching in the posterior border of the hard palate, detectable by palpation. The most severe presentation of CP is complete clefting of the hard and soft palate. The precise etiology of orofacial clefting is not yet completely understood. However, most cases of non-syndromic CL/P and CP are considered to follow a multifactorial threshold model, with environmental risk factors and a strong genetic component.

Several genes are associated with orofacial clefting. CL/P and CP each can be associated with other abnormalities, as part of a genetic malformation syndrome, such as 22q.11 deletion syndrome (velocardiofacial syndrome—CP and facial and cardiac abnormalities) or van der Woude syndrome (CL or CP or both and lip pits). Other factors that are implicated in the development of orofacial clefts include nutritional disturbances (prenatal folate deficiency), environmental teratogenic agents (maternal smoking, *in utero* exposure to anticonvulsants), stress (which results in increased secretion of hydrocortisone), defects of vascular supply to the involved region, and mechanical interference with the fusion of the embryonic processes (CP in Pierre Robin sequence). Clefts involving the lower lip and mandible are extremely rare.

Clinical Features

The frequency of CL/P and CP vary with sex and ethnic background, but in general CL/P is more common in males, whereas CP is more common in females. Both conditions are much more common in east Asian and Indigenous American populations than those with European, south Asian and African ancestry, which have lower birth prevalence rates. The severity of CL/P varies from a notch in the upper lip, to a cleft involving only the lip, to extension into the nostril resulting in deformity of the ala of the nose. As CL/P increases in severity, the cleft includes the alveolar process and palate. Bilateral CL is more frequently associated with CP. CP also varies in severity, ranging from involvement of only the uvula or soft palate to complete extension through the palate to include the alveolar process in the region of the lateral incisor on one or both sides. With involvement of the alveolar process, there is an increase in frequency of dental anomalies in the region of the cleft, including missing, hypoplastic, and supernumerary teeth and enamel hypoplasia. Dental anomalies are also more prevalent in the mandible in these patients. In both CL/P and CP, the palatal defects interfere with speech and swallowing. Affected individuals with palatal clefts are also at increased risk for recurrent middle ear infections because of the abnormal anatomy and function of the eustachian tube.

Imaging Features

The typical imaging appearance is a well-defined vertical radiolucent defect in the alveolar process and numerous associated dental anomalies (Figs. 29.1 and 29.2). These anomalies may include the absence of the maxillary lateral incisor and the presence of supernumerary teeth in this region. The involved teeth often are malformed and poorly positioned. In patients with CL/P, there may be a mild delay in the development of maxillary and mandibular teeth and an increased incidence of hypodontia in both arches. The osseous defect may extend to include the floor of the nasal cavity. In patients with a repaired cleft, instead of a well-defined osseous defect, a vertically short alveolar process may be apparent at the cleft site.

Management

Management of CL/P and CP is complex, requiring the coordinated efforts of a multidisciplinary team known as a CP/craniofacial anomalies team. This team usually includes a plastic and reconstructive surgeon, an oral and maxillofacial surgeon, an ear, nose, and throat surgeon, an orthodontist, a dentist, a speech therapist, an audiologist, psychologist/ behaviorist, a nutritionist, and a social worker. Clefts of the palate are

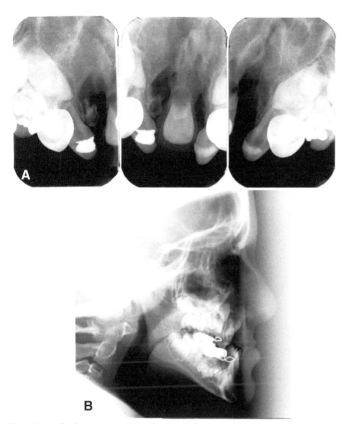

Fig. 29.1 Cleft lip/palate results in defects in the alveolar ridge and abnormalities of the dentition. (A) Bilateral clefts of the maxilla in the lateral incisor regions and defects of the dentition. (B) Lateral cephalometric skull image shows underdevelopment of the maxilla.

usually surgically repaired within the first year of life, whereas clefts of the lip are usually repaired within the first 3 months to aid in feeding and maternal-infant bonding. The bone in the cleft site is often augmented with bone graft material before replacement of missing teeth with either fixed or removable prosthodontics or dental implants. Orthodontic treatment, without or with orthognathic surgery, is usually necessary to re-create a normal arch form and functional occlusion.

CRANIOFACIAL DYSOSTOSIS (CROUZON SYNDROME)

Disease Mechanism

Craniofacial dysostosis (syndromic craniostenosis, premature craniostenosis) or Crouzon syndrome is an autosomal dominant skeletal dysplasia characterized by variable expressivity and almost complete penetrance. It is one of many diseases characterized by premature craniosynostosis (closure of cranial sutures), and has an incidence estimated at 1: 25,000 births. Of these cases, 33% to 56% may arise as a consequence of spontaneous mutations, with the remaining being familial.

Craniofacial dysostosis is caused by a mutation in fibroblast growth factor receptor II on chromosome 10. Mutations at this site are also responsible for other craniosynostosis syndromes with similar facial features but clinically visible limb abnormalities. In patients with this syndrome, the coronal suture usually closes first, and eventually all cranial sutures close early. There is also premature fusion of the synchondroses of the cranial base. The subsequent lack of bone growth perpendicular to the synchondroses and cranial coronal sutures produces the characteristic cranial shape and facial features.

Clinical Features

Patients characteristically have brachycephaly (short skull anterior to posterior), hypertelorism (increased distance between eyes), and orbital proptosis (protruding eyes) (Fig. 29.3A and B). In familial cases, the minimal criteria for diagnosis are hypertelorism and orbital proptosis. Patients may become blind as a result of early suture closure and increased intracranial pressure. The nose often appears prominent and pointed because the maxilla is narrow and short in a vertical and anteroposterior dimension. The anterior nasal spine is hypoplastic and retruded, failing to provide adequate support to the soft tissue of the nose. The palatal vault is high, and the maxillary arch is narrow and retruded, resulting in crowding of the dentition.

Imaging Features

The earliest radiologic signs of cranial suture synostosis are sclerosis and overlapping edges. Sutures that should normally appear radiolucent on a skull image are not detectable or show sclerotic changes. Rarely, the facial features may manifest before evidence of sutural synostosis. Premature fusion of the cranial base leads to diminished downward and forward facial growth. In some cases, prominent cranial markings are noted, which are also seen in normal growing patients, but are more prominent because of an increase in intracranial pressure from the growing brain. These markings may be seen as multiple radiolucencies appearing as depressions (so-called digital impressions) of the inner surface of the cranial vault, which results in a beaten metal or copper appearance (see Fig. 29.3C–E).

In the jaws, the lack of growth in an anteroposterior direction at the cranial base results in maxillary hypoplasia, creating a class III malocclusion in some patients. The maxillary hypoplasia contributes to the characteristic orbital proptosis because the maxilla forms part of the inferior orbital rim and, if severely hypoplastic, fails to support the orbital contents adequately. The mandible is typically smaller than normal but appears prognathic in relation to the severely hypoplastic maxilla.

Differential Diagnosis

Premature craniosynostosis, either isolated or as part of a genetic syndrome, is a common disorder. The incidence of craniofacial dysostosis is reported to range from 1:2100 to 1:2500 births. Other causes of craniosynostosis must be differentiated from Crouzon syndrome, including other syndromic forms of craniosynostosis and nonsyndromic coronal craniosynostosis. The characteristic facial features must be present to suggest Crouzon syndrome.

Management

The craniofacial features of craniofacial dysostosis worsen over time because of the abnormal craniofacial growth. Early diagnosis permits surgical and orthodontic treatment from infancy through adolescence, coordinated by a multidisciplinary CP/craniofacial anomalies team. The objectives of these treatments are to allow normal brain growth and development by preventing increased intracranial pressure, protect the eyes by providing adequate bony support, and improve facial esthetics and occlusal function. Because of early diagnosis and improvements in medical and dental care, most patients have normal intelligence and good functional outcomes and can expect a normal life span.

HEMIFACIAL MICROSOMIA

Hemifacial microsomia is known by a number of different terms, including hemifacial hypoplasia, craniofacial microsomia, lateral facial dysplasia, Goldenhar syndrome, and oculoauriculovertebral (OAV) dysplasia spectrum.

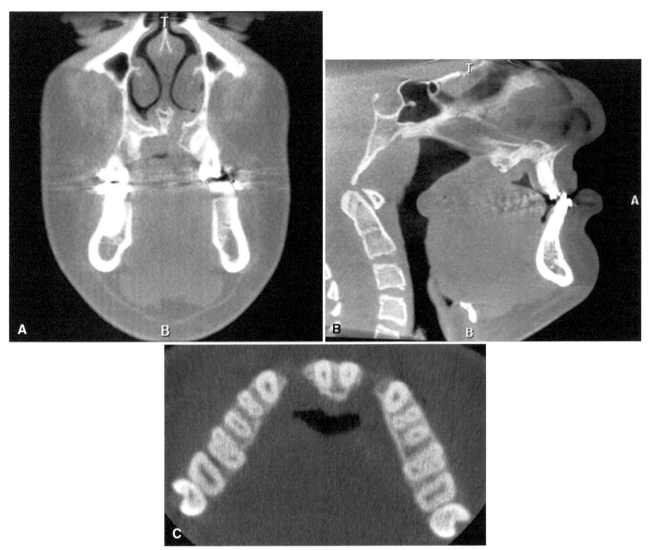

Fig. 29.2 Cone beam computed tomography (CBCT) images of a patient with left unilateral cleft lip/palate. (A) Coronal view. Note the discontinuity in the nasal floor visible on the patient's left side. (B) Sagittal view of the same patient shows maxillary hypoplasia and deficient palatal anatomy. (C) Axial CBCT image of a different patient with bilateral clefts shows bilateral defects in the maxillary alveolar processes. ([A and B], Courtesy Dr. S. Edwards, Ann Arbor, MI.)

Disease Mechanism

Hemifacial microsomia is a common birth defect involving the first and second branchial arches. It is the second most common developmental craniofacial anomaly after CL/P, and affects approximately 1:5600 live births. Hemifacial microsomia is a feature of Goldenhar syndrome. This syndrome can also include a broader array of anomalies within the OAV dysplasia complex. Patients with hemifacial microsomia typically display reduced growth and development of half of the face owing to abnormal development of the first and second branchial arches. This malformation sequence is usually unilateral but may occasionally be bilateral (craniofacial microsomia). When the whole side of the face is involved, the mandible, maxilla, zygomatic bone, external and middle ear, hyoid bone, parotid gland, vertebrae, fifth and seventh cranial nerves, musculature, and other soft tissues are reduced in size and sometimes fail to develop. Delayed eruption of teeth and hypodontia on the affected side also have been reported. Most cases occur spontaneously, but familial cases demonstrating autosomal dominant inheritance, and occasionally, autosomal recessive inheritance have been reported. There is a male predominance of 3:2 and a right-side predominance of 3:2.

Cases have been reported with epibulbar dermoids, preauricular skin appendages, preauricular fistulas, additional vertebral anomalies, as well as cardiac, cerebral, and renal malformations (Goldenhar syndrome and OAV complex). Genetic mutations involving chromosome 14q32 and microdeletions at 22q11 have been associated with some cases of Goldenhar syndrome. In most cases, however, a clear genetic cause cannot be found. The pathogenesis is not known; however, hemifacial microsomia (HFM) is thought to be caused by a disruption of vascular supply during embryonic development. There is some limited evidence that assisted reproductive technologies are associated with an increased risk of OAV dysplasias, including patients with hemifacial macrosomia. A recent large study demonstrated that systemic malformations including vertebral, genitourinary, cardiovascular, and cerebral anomalies were common, and seen in a total of 73/86 patients in one institution; therefore multidisciplinary team-based care is essential.

Clinical Features

Hemifacial microsomia is usually apparent at birth. Patients with this condition have facial asymmetry and ear malformations. Aplasia or hypoplasia of the external ear (microtia) is common, and the ear canal

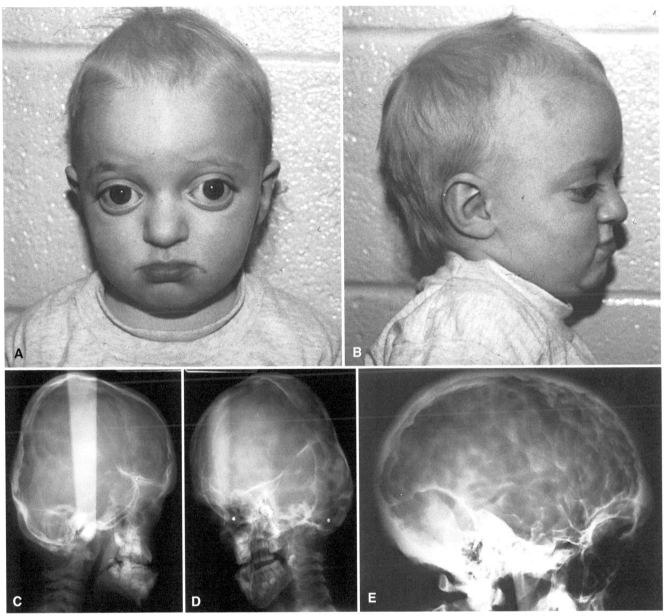

Fig. 29.3 (A and B) Characteristic facial features of craniofacial dysostosis (Crouzon syndrome) in this 2-year-old boy include orbital proptosis, hypertelorism, and midfacial hypoplasia. Rarely, these facial features may precede the radiographic features of sutural synostosis. (C) Mandibulofacial dysostosis results in early closure of the cranial sutures and depressions (digital impressions) on the inner surface of the calvaria from growth of the brain. (D and E) Closure of the cranial sutures in another patient. Note also the prominent digital markings. ([D and E], Courtesy Department of Radiology, Baylor University Hospital, Dallas, TX.)

is often missing. In some patients, the skull is diminished in size. In about 90% of cases, there is malocclusion on the affected side. The midsagittal plane of the patient's face is curved toward the affected side. The occlusal plane often is canted up to the affected side.

Imaging Features

The primary radiologic finding is a reduction in the sizes of the bones on the affected side. This change is clearest in the mandible, which may show a reduction in the size or, in severe cases, lack of any development of the condyle, coronoid process or ramus. The body is reduced in size, and a portion of the distal aspect may be missing (Fig. 29.4). The dentition on the affected side may show a reduction in the number or size of the teeth. Multidetector computed tomography (MDCT) shows

a reduction in the sizes of the muscles of mastication and muscles of facial expression, and hypoplasia or atresia of the auditory canal and ossicles of the middle ear. The course of the facial nerve is often shown to be abnormal on MDCT examination of the temporal bone. Magnetic resonance imaging (MRI) can also be useful in demonstrating the extent of inner ear abnormalities and involvement of the facial nerve and other soft tissues of the mouth and eyes. Thin section MDCT imaging of the temporal bone is often performed to assess the degrees of stenosis of the external auditory meatus and middle and inner ear malformations to plan treatment, including the use of cochlear implants, bone-anchored hearing aids, or implant-retained ear prostheses. This imaging is particularly important for patients with Goldenhar syndrome and the broader OAV complex. A multimodality approach to imaging can be

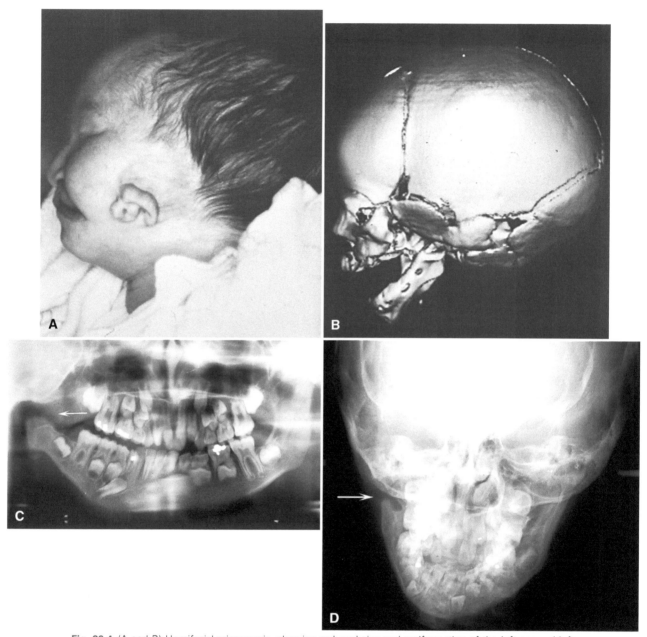

Fig. 29.4 (A and B) Hemifacial microsomia, showing reduced size and malformation of the left ear and left side of the mandible. (A) Clinical photograph of an infant with hemifacial microsomia. (B) Three-dimensional multidetector computed tomography (MDCT) reconstruction of the affected side shows the extent of the bony malformation. Note the complete absence of the temporomandibular joint and coronoid process as well as auditory canal atresia. (C and D) Panoramic image (C) and posteroanterior skull image (D) of other cases show lack of development of the ramus, coronoid process, and condyle *(arrows)*. ([A and B], Courtesy Dr. A. Rozzelle, Detroit, MI.)

optimal, including panoramic images to demonstrate dental development, cephalometric images and cone beam computed tomography (CBCT) to assess the facial asymmetry and plan orthognathic and orthodontic treatment, MDCT imaging of the temporal bones to assess the external and internal ear anatomy, and 3D reconstructions of MDCT images for surgical treatment planning.

Differential Interpretation

The features of hemifacial microsomia are characteristic. Condylar hypoplasia, especially caused by a fracture at birth or progressive condylar

resorption may be similar, but it does not produce the ear changes. Exposure of the face of a child to radiation therapy during growth also may result in underdevelopment of the irradiated tissues. In progressive hemifacial atrophy (Parry-Romberg syndrome), the changes become more severe over time but are generally not present at birth, and the ears are normal.

Management

The mandibular abnormalities may be corrected by conventional orthognathic surgery or distraction osteogenesis to lengthen the ramus on the affected side. Orthodontic intervention may correct or prevent malocclusion. The ear abnormalities may be repaired by plastic surgery or corrected with prosthetic ears, and the hearing loss may be partly corrected by hearing aids, such as bone-anchored hearing aids. In bilateral cases with profound hearing loss (Goldenhar syndrome and OAV complex), cochlear implants may be used to correct severe hearing loss. Because of the range of craniofacial anomalies as well as systemic anomalies associated with this condition, management by a multidisciplinary team is recommended.

MANDIBULOFACIAL DYSOSTOSIS (TREACHER COLLINS SYNDROME)

Disease Mechanism

Mandibulofacial dysostosis or Treacher Collins syndrome is an autosomal dominant disorder of craniofacial development. It is the most common type of mandibulofacial dysostosis, with an incidence of 1:50,000.

Mandibulofacial dysostosis has variable expressivity and complete penetrance. Approximately half of cases arise as the result of sporadic mutation, and the rest are familial. Mandibulofacial dysostosis is caused by a mutation in the *TCOF1* gene on chromosome 5.

Clinical Features

Individuals with mandibulofacial dysostosis have a wide range of anomalies, depending on the severity of the condition. The most common clinical findings are relative underdevelopment or absence of the zygomatic bones resulting in a small, narrow face, a downward inclination of the palpebral fissures, underdevelopment of the mandible resulting in a downturned, wide mouth, malformation of the external ears, absence of the external auditory canal, and occasional facial clefts (Fig. 29.5A and B). The palate develops with a high arch or cleft in 30% of cases. Hypoplasia of the mandible and a steep mandibular angle results in an Angle class II malocclusion with anterior open bite. Hypoplasia or atresia of the external ear, auditory canal, and ossicles of the middle ear may result in partial or complete deafness.

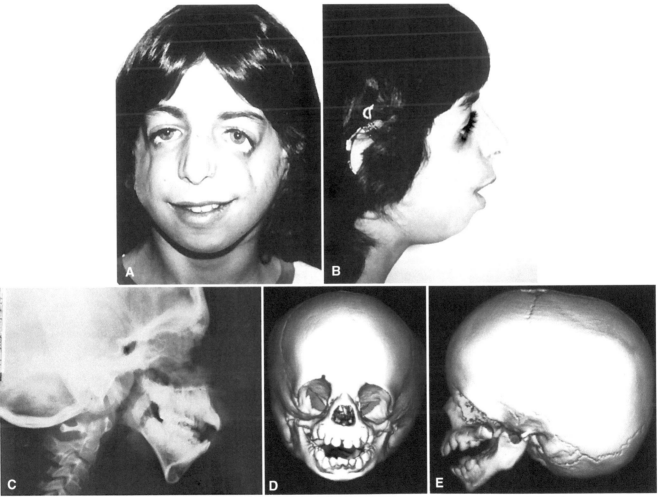

Fig. 29.5 Mandibulofacial dysostosis (Treacher Collins syndrome). (A and B) Note the characteristic facies: downward-sloping palpebral fissures, colobomas of the outer third of the lower lids, depressed cheekbones, receding chin, little if any nasofrontal angle, and a nose that appears relatively large. (C) Correlation of radiographic features with clinical features: short mandibular rami, steep mandibular angle, and anterior open bite. The zygomas are poorly formed. (D and E) Three-dimensional multidetector computed tomography reconstruction of young child with mandibulofacial dysostosis show the extent of the bony abnormalities, including bilateral auditory canal atresia, aplasia of the zygomatic arch, and hypoplasia of the mandibular ramus with characteristic "curved" shape of the mandibular body and pronounced antegonial notching.

Imaging Features

A striking finding is the hypoplastic or absent zygomatic bones, and hypoplasia of the lateral aspects of the orbits. The auditory canal, mastoid air cells, and articular eminence often are smaller than normal or absent. The maxilla and especially the mandible are hypoplastic, showing accentuation of the antegonial notch and a steep mandibular angle, which gives the impression that the body of the mandible is bending in an inferior and posterior direction (see Fig. 29.5C–F). The ramus is especially short. The condyles are positioned posteriorly and inferiorly. The maxillary sinuses may be underdeveloped or absent.

Cervical spine anomalies have also been reported in 18% of patients with mandibulofacial dysostosis, including spina bifida occulta, dysmorphic C1, and reduced C2-C3 space. In one case series, five of seven patients with cervical spine anomalies also had CP. This finding suggests that patients with mandibulofacial dysostosis and CP may be at higher risk for cervical spine anomalies and should be targeted for assessment. A more recent study has also reported dysplasia or aplasia of major salivary glands, as detected by ultrasound imaging, in half of patients with mandibulofacial dysostosis followed at a major craniofacial anomalies center. This finding is important because these salivary gland anomalies could significantly increase risk for dental caries in patients with this syndrome.

Differential Interpretation

Other disorders that may result in severe hypoplasia of the entire mandible include condylar agenesis, Hallermann-Streiff syndrome, Nager syndrome, and Pierre Robin sequence, which can be a part of several other genetic syndromes or an isolated anomaly.

Management

Comprehensive treatment of patients with mandibulofacial dysostosis is optimally provided by a multidisciplinary CP/craniofacial anomalies team. Growth of the facial bones during adolescence may result in some cosmetic improvement. Surgical intervention, including bilateral distraction osteogenesis of the mandible, may improve the osseous defects. Treatment of the external ear defects may involve plastic and reconstructive surgery or prostheses or both. Hearing aids or cochlear implants may be used to treat the hearing loss, depending on the severity. Coordinated orthodontics and orthognathic surgery are often used to treat malocclusion and improve function and esthetics.

CLEIDOCRANIAL DYSPLASIA

Disease Mechanism

Cleidocranial dysplasia is an autosomal dominant malformation syndrome affecting bones and teeth. The prevalence is estimated at 1:1 million, and it affects both sexes equally. Cleidocranial dysplasia is caused by a mutation in the *RUNX2* gene on chromosome 6; a gene that codes for an osteoblast-specific transcription factor. The mutation has variable expressivity and almost complete penetrance, and can be inherited or arise as a result of sporadic mutation.

Clinical Features

Although the disease affects the entire skeleton, cleidocranial dysplasia primarily affects the dentition, skull, and clavicles. Affected individuals have been shown to be of shorter stature than unaffected relatives but not short enough for this to be considered a form of dwarfism. The face appears small in contrast to the cranium because of hypoplasia of the maxilla and a brachycephalic skull (reduced anteroposterior dimension with increased skull width) and the presence of frontal and parietal bossing. The paranasal sinuses may be underdeveloped and there is an increased risk of sinusitis. Hearing loss and recurrent otitis media have also been reported. There is delayed closure of the cranial sutures, and the fontanels may remain patent years beyond the normal time of closure. The bridge of the nose may be broad and depressed, with hypertelorism (excessive distance between the eyes). The complete absence (aplasia) or reduced size (hypoplasia) of the clavicles allows excessive mobility of the shoulder girdle (Fig. 29.6A and B).

The dental abnormalities produce most of the morbidity associated with cleidocranial dysplasia and are often the reason for diagnosis in mildly affected individuals. Characteristically, patients show prolonged retention of the primary dentition and delayed eruption of the permanent dentition. Extraction of primary teeth does not adequately stimulate eruption of underlying permanent teeth. A study of teeth from patients with cleidocranial dysplasia revealed a paucity or complete absence of cellular cementum on both erupted and unerupted teeth. Often unerupted supernumerary teeth are present, and considerable crowding and disorganization of the developing permanent dentition may occur. The number of supernumerary teeth has been correlated with a reduction in skeletal height in these patients.

Imaging Features

The characteristic skull findings are brachycephaly, delayed or failed closure of the fontanels, open skull sutures including a persistent open metopic suture, and multiple wormian bones (small, irregular bones in the sutures of the skull that are formed by secondary centers of ossification in the suture lines) (see Figs. 29.6C–G and 29.7). In the most severe cases, very little formation of the parietal and frontal bones may occur. Typically, the clavicles are underdeveloped to varying degrees, and they are completely absent in approximately 10% of cases. Other bones also may be affected, including the long bones, vertebral column, pelvis, and bones of the hands and feet.

In the jaws, the maxilla and paranasal sinuses are characteristically underdeveloped, resulting in maxillary micrognathia. The mandible is usually normal in size. A patent (open) mandibular symphysis has been reported in 3% of adults and 64% of children. Several investigators have described the alveolar processes overlying unerupted teeth as being denser than usual with a coarse trabecular pattern in the mandible. This finding correlates to the histologic findings of decreased resorption and multiple reversal lines, and it may account for the delayed eruption in teeth not mechanically obstructed by supernumerary and other unerupted teeth.

Characteristically, there is prolonged retention of the primary dentition and multiple unerupted permanent and supernumerary teeth (Fig. 29.8A and B). The number of supernumerary teeth varies—as many as 63 have been reported in one individual patient with the disorder. The unerupted teeth develop most commonly in the anterior maxilla and premolar regions of the jaws. Many resemble premolars, and these unerupted teeth may develop dentigerous cysts. The supernumerary teeth develop, on average, 4 years later than the corresponding normal teeth. Because of this delayed development, it has been proposed that the supernumerary teeth represent a third dentition.

Differential Interpretation

Cleidocranial dysplasia may be identified by the family history, excessive mobility of the shoulders, clinical examination of the skull, and pathognomonic radiographic findings of prolonged retention of the primary teeth with multiple unerupted supernumerary teeth. Other conditions associated with multiple unerupted and supernumerary

Text continued on p. 573

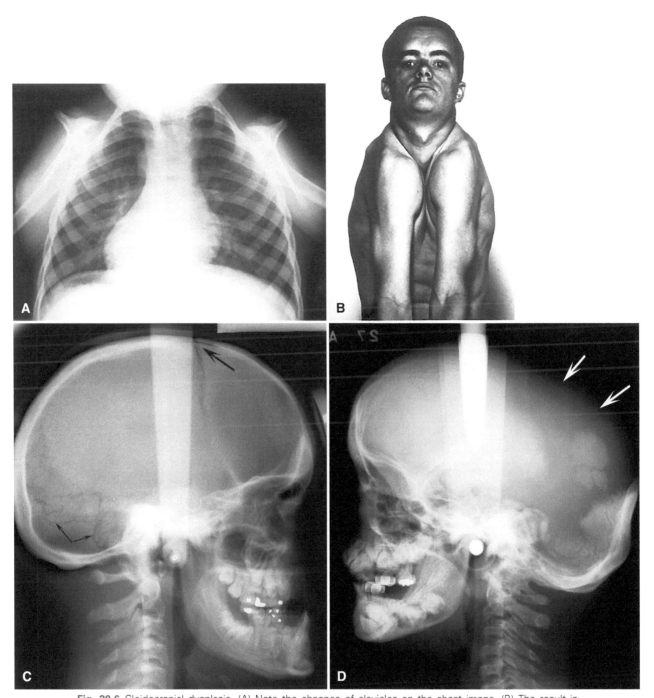

Fig. 29.6 Cleidocranial dysplasia. (A) Note the absence of clavicles on the chest image. (B) The result is excessive mobility of the shoulders. Note also the frontal bossing and underdeveloped maxilla. (C) Lateral skull image shows the wormian (sutural) bones in the occipital region *(small arrows)* and the open fontanel *(large arrow)*. (D) Lateral skull image shows a lack of development of the parietal bones *(arrows)*.

Continued

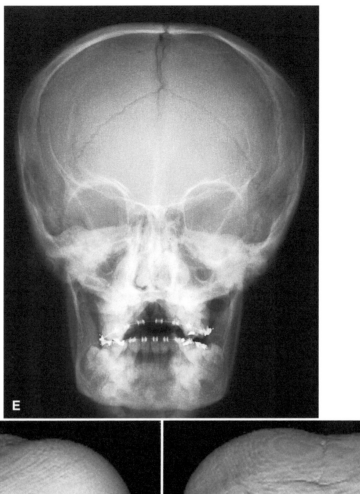

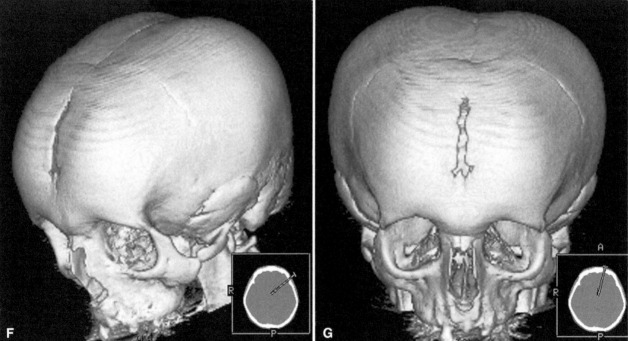

Fig. 29.6, cont'd (E) Posteroanterior skull image. Brachycephaly results in a light bulb–like shape to the silhouette of the skull and mandible. (F) Three-dimensional reconstruction of a multidetector computed tomography (MDCT) study with oblique orientation shows the typical skull shape seen in this condition. Note the parietal and frontal bossing and open metopic suture in this 18-year-old man. (G) Direct frontal view of the same 3D MDCT reconstruction shows the light-bulb shape of the skull and the open metopic suture. ([A], Courtesy Department of Radiology, Baylor University Hospital, Dallas, TX.)

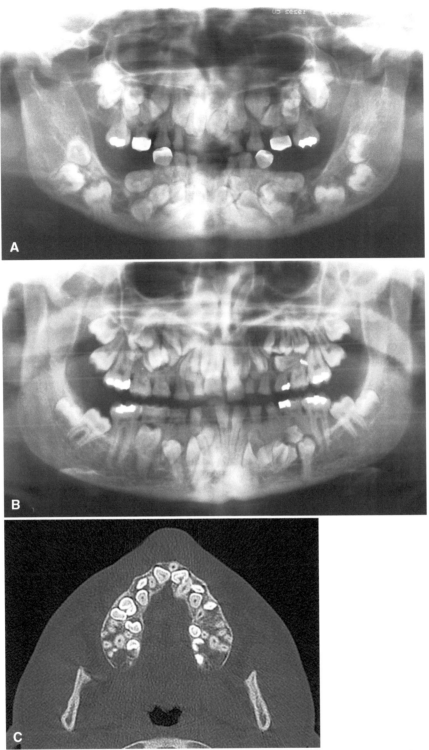

Fig. 29.7 (A and B) Panoramic images of cleidocranial dysplasia. Note the prolonged retention of the primary dentition and multiple unerupted supernumerary teeth and lack of normal coronoid notches. (C) Axial computed tomography image of the mandible demonstrates multiple unerupted teeth. This type of imaging can be used to localize the unerupted teeth to assist in treatment planning of extractions and orthodontic tooth movement. (Courtesy Dr. S. Edwards, Ann Arbor, MI.)

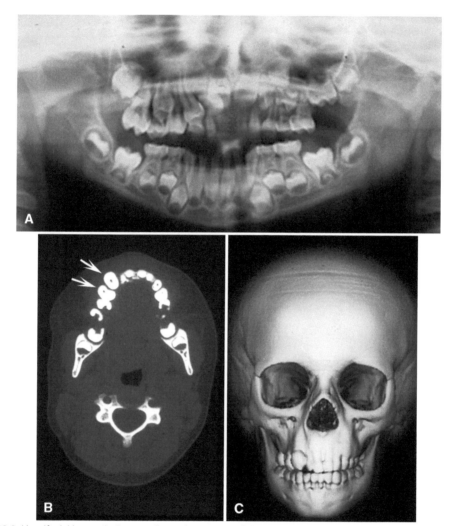

Fig. 29.8 Hemifacial hyperplasia, revealing enlargement of the right maxilla only. (A) Panoramic image shows accelerated dental development limited to the right maxilla in a 5-year-old boy. (B) Computed tomography axial image using bone algorithm of the same patient demonstrates enlargement of the maxillary canine and first premolar *(arrows)* compared with the contralateral side. (C) Three-dimensional multidetector computed tomography reconstruction shows subtle bony enlargement of the right maxilla and the right canine.

teeth, such as familial adenomatous polyposis (Gardner syndrome) and pyknodysostosis, must be considered in the differential interpretation.

Management

In cleidocranial dysplasia, dental care should include the removal of primary and supernumerary teeth to improve the possibility of spontaneous eruption of the permanent teeth. The bone overlying the normal permanent teeth should be removed to expose the crown when half of the root is formed to aid their eruption. Autotransplantation of teeth has been shown to be a successful strategy to treat older patients. Ideally, patients should be identified early, before age 5 years, to take advantage of combined orthodontic and surgical treatment, as well as address other problems including hearing loss. Prosthodontic rehabilitation with dental implants has been used in some cases. Patients should be monitored for development of distal molars and cysts until late adolescence. Surgical treatment of the bony defects of the skull is often performed to address esthetic concerns. In those cases, CT imaging is used to visualize the size and thickness of such defects and plan for harvesting of bone graft material from other parts of the skull (see Fig. 29.7A–C). As with other complex craniofacial anomalies, management is best provided by an experienced multidisciplinary craniofacial anomalies team.

HEMIFACIAL HYPERPLASIA

Disease Mechanism

Hemifacial hyperplasia (hemifacial hypertrophy, hemihyperplasia) is a condition in which there is unilateral enlargement of the region of the face from the frontal bone to the inferior border of the mandible, and from the midline to the pinna of the ear. There is enlargement of teeth, bone, and soft tissues within the affected region. This condition can be associated with enlargement of other parts of the body as well. The cause of this condition is unknown. Some cases are associated with genetic diseases such as Beckwith-Wiedemann syndrome.

Clinical Features

Hemifacial hyperplasia begins at birth and usually continues throughout the growing years. In some cases, it may not be recognized at birth but becomes more apparent with growth. It often occurs with other abnormalities, including mental deficiency, skin abnormalities, compensatory scoliosis, genitourinary tract anomalies, and various neoplasms, including Wilms' tumor of the kidney, adrenocortical tumor, and hepatoblastoma (Beckwith-Wiedemann syndrome). Females and males are affected with approximately equal frequency. The dentition of affected individuals may show unilateral enlargement, accelerated development, and premature loss of primary teeth. The tongue and alveolar bone enlarge on the involved side.

Imaging Features

Radiologic examination of the skulls of patients reveals enlargement of the bones on the affected side, including the mandible (see Fig. 29.8), maxilla, zygomatic, frontal and temporal bones. A few cases have been reported involving only one side of the maxilla or one side of the mandible.

Differential Diagnosis

The differential diagnosis should consider hemifacial hypoplasia of the opposite side, arteriovenous malformation, hemangioma, and congenital lymphedema. Also, severe condylar hyperplasia that may involve half of the mandible should be considered. The presence of enlarged teeth together with rapid eruption of the dentition suggests hemifacial hyperplasia. Cases limited to one side of the maxilla must be differentiated from monostotic fibrous dysplasia and segmental odontomaxillary dysplasia, both of which have characteristic changes in the radiographic appearance of the alveolar bone, not present in hemifacial hyperplasia.

Management

An insufficient number of cases of hemifacial hyperplasia with long-term follow-up have been reported to make definitive recommendations for treatment. Although most cases are isolated, a child with suspected hemifacial hyperplasia should be referred to a medical geneticist for diagnosis and early detection of one of several genetic syndromes that can be associated with this condition.

SEGMENTAL ODONTOMAXILLARY DYSPLASIA

Disease Mechanism

Segmental odontomaxillary dysplasia or hemimaxillofacial dysplasia is a developmental abnormality of unknown etiology that affects the posterior alveolar process of one side of the maxilla, including the teeth and attached gingiva.

Clinical Features

The abnormality is always unilateral and results in enlargement of the alveolar process, without or with enlargement of the gingiva, and dental anomalies. Teeth are frequently missing (most commonly the premolars) or hypoplastic, and some of the teeth that remain are unerupted. Ipsilateral hypertrichosis and other skin anomalies, including closely packed sebaceous glands in the upper lip, hyperpigmentation, hypopigmentation, Becker nevus, and clefting have also been reported in 23% of cases. Mild facial enlargement has also been reported in a few cases. Most cases are detected in childhood because a parent notices the lack of tooth eruption or mild facial asymmetry, or the dentist notices missing premolars on diagnostic images.

Imaging Features

The density of the maxillary alveolar process is increased, with a greater number of thick trabeculae that appear to be aligned in a vertical orientation (Fig. 29.9). There have been some reports of missing buccal cortical plate, but this is not a consistent feature. The roots of the deciduous teeth are larger than on the unaffected side and usually are splayed in shape. The crowns of the deciduous teeth and sometimes the permanent teeth are enlarged. Enlargement of pulp chambers and irregular resorption of the roots of deciduous teeth also may be seen. The alveolar process is not pneumatized by the maxillary sinus and appears smaller than on the contralateral side. There is often delayed eruption of the first and second permanent molars.

Differential Interpretation

Other conditions that must be differentiated from segmental odontomaxillary dysplasia include segmental hemifacial hyperplasia, monostotic fibrous dysplasia and regional odontodysplasia. Hemifacial hyperplasia is not associated with coarse vertically oriented trabeculae in the bone; monostotic fibrous dysplasia is not typically associated with missing teeth and, in contrast to segmental odontomaxillary dysplasia, will continue to show disproportionate growth of the affected side; and regional odontodysplasia typically is associated with ghost teeth and is not associated with expansion and alteration in trabecular pattern in the alveolar bone.

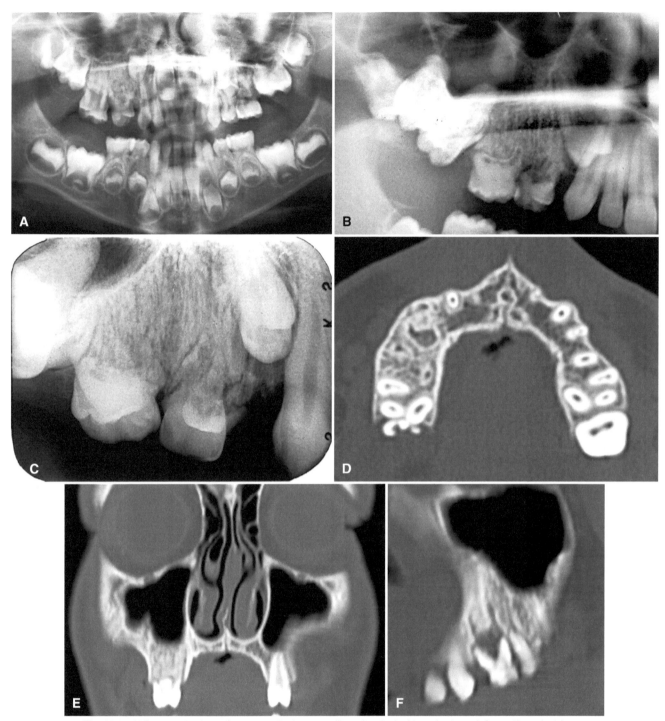

Fig. 29.9 (A) Panoramic view of segmental odontomaxillary dysplasia. Note the large left maxillary deciduous molars compared with the right side and the lack of formation of the premolars, delayed eruption of the first molar, and the dense bone pattern of the left maxillary alveolar process. (B and C) A second case demonstrating the coarse trabecular pattern of the right maxillary alveolar process and delayed eruption of the maxillary right first premolar and molars. (D–F) Cone beam computed tomography images of another case involving the right maxilla. (D) Axial image shows an increase in internal bone density within the right maxilla. (E) Coronal image shows increase in width of the alveolar process. (F) Multiple vertical radiolucent linear structures, which likely represent nutrient canals.

BIBLIOGRAPHY

Cohen MM Jr, McLean RE. *Craniosynostosis: Diagnosis, Evaluation, and Management*. 2nd ed. New York: Oxford University Press; 2000.

Gorlin RJ, Cohen MM Jr, Hennekam RCM. *Syndromes of the Head and Neck*. 4th ed. New York: Oxford University Press; 2001.

Neville BW, Damm DD, Allen CM, et al. *Oral and Maxillofacial Pathology*. 4th ed. Philadelphia: Saunders; 2015.

Worth HM. *Principles and Practice of Oral Radiologic Interpretation*. Chicago: Year Book Medical; 1963.

Cleft Lip and Cleft Palate

Beaty TH, Marazita ML, Leslie EJ. Genetic factors influencing risk to orofacial clefts: today's challenges and tomorrow's opportunities. *F1000Res*. 2016;5:2800. doi:10.12688/f1000research.9503.1.g.

Habel A, Sell D, Mars M, et al. Management of cleft lip and palate. *Arch Dis Child*. 1996;74:360.

Harris EF, Hullings JG. Delayed dental development in children with isolated cleft lip and palate. *Arch Oral Biol*. 1990;35:469.

Honein MA, Rasmussen SA, Reefhuis J, et al. Maternal and environmental tobacco smoke exposure and the risk of orofacial clefts. *Epidemiology*. 2007;18:226–233.

Shapira Y, Lubit E, Kuftinec MM. Hypodontia in children with various types of clefts. *Angle Orthod*. 2000;70:16–21.

Craniofacial Dysostosis (Crouzon Syndrome)

Murdoch-Kinch CA, Bixler D, Ward RE. Cephalometric analysis of families with dominantly inherited Crouzon syndrome: an aid to diagnosis in family studies. *Am J Med Genet*. 1998;77:405–411.

Tuite GF, Evanson J, Chong WK, et al. The beaten copper cranium: a correlation between intracranial pressure, cranial radiographs, and computed tomographic scans in children with craniosynostosis. *Neurosurgery*. 1996;39:691–699.

Hemifacial Microsomia

AlHadidi A, Cevidanes LHS, Mol A, et al. Comparison of two methods for quantitative assessment of mandibular asymmetry using cone beam computed tomography image volumes. *Dentomaxillofac Radiol*. 2011;40:351–357.

Cohen N, Cohen E, Gaiero A, et al. Maxillofacial features and systemic malformations in expanded spectrum hemifacial microsomia. *Am J Med Genet*. 2017;173:1208–1218.

Johnson JM, Moonis G, Green GE, et al. Syndromes of the first and second branchial arches, part 2: syndromes. *AJNR Am J Neuroradiol*. 2011;32:230–237.

Maruko E, Hayes C, Evans CA, et al. Hypodontia in hemifacial microsomia. *Cleft Palate Craniofac J*. 2001;38:15–19.

Monahan R, Seder K, Patel P, et al. Hemifacial microsomia: etiology, diagnosis and treatment. *J Am Dent Assoc*. 2001;132:1402–1408.

Senggen E, Laswed T, Meuwly J-Y, et al. First and second branchial arch syndromes: multimodality approach. *Pediatr Radiol*. 2011;41:549–561.

Mandibulofacial Dysostosis (Treacher Collins Syndrome)

Osterhus IN, Skogedal N, Akre H, et al. Salivary gland pathology as a new finding in Treacher Collins syndrome. *Am J Med Genet A*. 2012;158A:1320–1325.

Posnick JC. Treacher Collins syndrome: perspectives in evaluation and treatment. *J Oral Maxillofac Surg*. 1997;55:1120.

Pun AH-Y, Clark BE, David DJ, et al. Cervical spine in Treacher Collins syndrome. *J Craniofac Surg*. 2012;23:218–220.

Cleidocranial Dysplasia

Dalessandri D, Laffranchi L, Tonni I, et al. Advantages of cone beam computed tomography (CBCT) in the orthodontic treatment planning of cleidocranial dysplasia patients: a case report. *Head Face Med*. 2011;7:6.

Golan I, Baumert U, Hrala BP, et al. Dentomaxillofacial variability of cleidocranial dysplasia: clinicoradiological presentation and systematic review. *Dentomaxillofac Radiol*. 2003;32:347–354.

McGuire TP, Gomes PP, Lam DK, et al. Cranioplasty for midline metopic suture defects in adults with cleidocranial dysplasia. *Oral Surg Oral Med Oral Pathol Oral Radiol Endod*. 2007;103:175–179.

Seow WK, Hertzberg J. Dental development and molar root length in children with cleidocranial dysplasia. *Pediatr Dent*. 1995;17:101–105.

Yoshida T, Kanegane H, Osata M, et al. Functional analysis of RUNX2 mutations in Japanese patients with cleidocranial dysplasia demonstrates novel genotype-phenotype correlations. *Am J Hum Genet*. 2002;71:724–738.

Hemifacial Hyperplasia

Fraumeni JF, Geiser CF, Manning MD, et al. Wilms' tumor and congenital hemihypertrophy: report of five new cases and review of the literature. *Pediatrics*. 1967;40:886.

Hoyme HE, Seaver LH, Procopio F, et al. Isolated hemihyperplasia (hemihypertrophy): report of a prospective multicenter study of the incidence of neoplasia and review. *Am J Med Genet*. 1998;79:274–278.

Kogon SL, Jarvis AM, Daley TD, et al. Hemifacial hypertrophy affecting the maxillary dentition: report of a case. *Oral Surg Oral Med Oral Pathol*. 1984;58:549–553.

Segmental Odontomaxillary Dysplasia

Danforth RA, Melrose RJ, Abrams AM, et al. Segmental odontomaxillary dysplasia: report of eight cases and comparison with hemimaxillofacial dysplasia. *Oral Surg Oral Med Oral Pathol*. 1990;70:81.

Miles DA, Lovas JL, Clhen MM, et al. Hemimaxillofacial dysplasia: a newly recognized disorder of facial asymmetry, hypertrichosis of the facial skin, unilateral enlargement of the maxilla, and hypoplastic teeth in two patients. *Oral Surg Oral Med Oral Pathol*. 1987;64:445.

Minett CP, Daley TD. Hemimaxillofacial dysplasia (segmental odontomaxillary dysplasia): case study with 11 years of follow-up from primary to adult dentition. *J Oral Maxillofac Surg*. 2012;70:1183–1191.

Packota GV, Pharoah MJ, Petrikowski CG, et al. Radiographic features of segmental odontomaxillary dysplasia: a study of 12 cases. *Oral Surg Oral Med Oral Pathol Oral Radiol Endod*. 1996;82:577.

Whitt JC, Rokos JW, Dunlap CL, et al. Segmental odontomaxillary dysplasia: report of a series of 5 cases with long-term follow-up. *Oral Surg Oral Med Oral Pathol Oral Radiol Endod*. 2011;112:e29–e47.

30

Temporomandibular Joint Abnormalities

Susanne E. Perschbacher

DISEASE MECHANISM

Disorders of the temporomandibular joint (TMJ) include all abnormalities that interfere with the normal form or function of the TMJ. These disorders include developmental abnormalities that can result in an abnormal form of the osseous or soft tissue structures of the joint. Other disorders are acquired, such as dysfunction of the articular disc and associated ligaments, the muscles of mastication, joint arthritides, inflammatory lesions, trauma, and neoplasia.

CLINICAL FEATURES

A wide range of conditions can elicit disorders of the TMJ, and these may manifest with an extensive assortment of clinical features. Dysfunction of the joint is the most common disorder, and is most likely to manifest with pain in the TMJ or ear, or both; headache; muscle tenderness; joint stiffness; clicking or other joint noises; reduced range of motion; and locking and subluxation. Careful clinical examination can help identify which structures are likely contributing to the joint dysfunction. For example, pain to palpation of the muscles of mastication and headache suggest a myofascial pain disorder, while clicking or popping sounds in the joint, locking, or reduced range of motion are often associated with disc abnormalities. Crepitus and pain over the joint itself can commonly indicate arthritic involvement.

A higher incidence of TMJ dysfunction has been reported in females, especially in their reproductive years, although the reason for this preponderance is unclear. In most cases, the clinical signs and symptoms are transient, and often treatment is not indicated beyond patient reassurance and education. However, a small percentage (5%) of patients have severe dysfunction (e.g., severe pain, marked functional impairment, or both), which requires a thorough diagnostic workup, including diagnostic imaging, before treatment.

Other disorders of the TMJs are less common. A neoplasm may manifest with swelling of the area surrounding the joint, whereas redness and heat over the joint may indicate an inflammatory condition. Developmental abnormalities are most likely to be unilateral and manifest with facial asymmetry. Changes in occlusion also may be a sign of an abnormality in one or both of the TMJs.

IMAGING ANATOMY OF THE TEMPOROMANDIBULAR JOINT

A thorough understanding of the anatomy and morphology of the TMJ is essential so that a normal variant is not mistaken for an abnormality. Each joint is formed by the articulating components of the mandible and the temporal bone. The mandible is unique because the two TMJs must function together in a coordinated fashion as part of a single unit in order to facilitate mandibular movements. An articular disc composed of fibrocartilage is interposed between the articulating surface of the mandibular condylar head and the glenoid fossa of the temporal bone of each joint, and retrodiscal tissues and ligamentous attachments help maintain the normal position of the disc. A fibrous joint capsule lined with a synovial membrane surrounds and encloses the joint. The synovial tissue is present on non-load-bearing surfaces, and secretes synovial fluid which lubricates the joint. The muscles of mastication allow movement of the condyle, but the ligaments limit the extent of this movement.

Mandibular Component

The mandibular condyle is the mandibular component of the TMJ. The condyle is a bony ellipsoid process of the mandible that extends superiorly from the mandibular ramus by way of a narrow neck (Fig. 30.1). The condyle is approximately 20 mm in width mediolaterally and 8 to 10 mm in dimension, anteroposteriorly. The shape of the condyle varies considerably; the superior surface may be flat, round, or markedly convex, whereas the mediolateral contour is usually only mildly convex. These variations in shape may cause difficulty with radiographic interpretation, and it is this that underlines the importance of understanding the range of normal appearances (Fig. 30.2).

The extreme medial and lateral surfaces of the condyle are called the medial and lateral poles. The long axis of the condyle is formed by an imaginary line connecting these poles, and is slightly rotated on the condylar neck so that the medial pole is angled posteriorly, forming an angle of between 15 and 33 degrees with respect to the sagittal plane. The two condylar axes typically intersect near the anterior border of the foramen magnum in the axial or horizontal plane of the skull.

Most condyles have a pronounced ridge oriented mediolaterally on the anterior surface, marking the anteroinferior limit of the articulating area. This ridge is the upper limit of the pterygoid fovea, a small depression on the anterior surface at the junction of the condyle and condylar neck, which is the insertion site of the superior head of the lateral pterygoid muscle. The ridge should not be mistaken for an osteophyte (spur), which is a sign of degenerative joint disease (DJD).

Although the mandibular and temporal components of the TMJ are calcified by 6 months of age, complete calcification of the cortical borders may not be completed until 20 years of age. As a result, images of the mandibular condyles in children may show little or no evidence of a cortical border. In the absence of disease, the cortical borders in adults are visible in the diagnostic image. The layer of fibrocartilage overlying the condyle is not visible in conventional imaging or computed tomography (CT).

Temporal Component

The articular component of the temporal bone is formed by the inferior surface of the squamous process, and is composed of the glenoid or mandibular fossa posteriorly and the articular eminence and tubercle anteriorly (Fig. 30.3). As with the condyle, the mandibular fossa is covered with a thin layer of fibrocartilage. The posterior surface of the articular eminence is convex in shape, and its most inferior point is called the summit, apex, or crest. In the normal TMJ, the roof of the glenoid fossa, the posterior slope of the articular eminence and the summit form a gentle "S-shape" curve when viewed in the sagittal plane (Fig. 30.4A). The squamotympanic fissure and its medial extension, the petrotympanic fissure, form the posterior limit of the glenoid fossa. The roof of the glenoid fossa forms a small portion of the floor of the middle cranial fossa, and here, only a thin layer of cortical bone separates the joint cavity from the intracranial space. The spine of the sphenoid forms the medial limit of the fossa. Glenoid fossa depths vary, and the development of the articular eminence relies on a functional stimulus from the condyle. For example, the mandibular fossa is very shallow and underdeveloped in patients with micrognathia or condylar agenesis. Young infants also lack a definitive fossa and articular eminence. In this age group, the fossa and articular eminence develop during the first 3 years of life and reach a mature shape by age 4 years, although

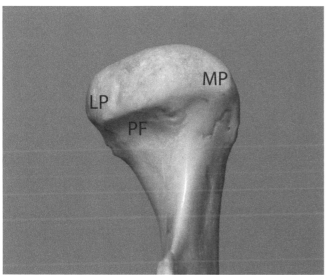

Fig. 30.1 Anterior view of the mandibular condyle. *LP,* Lateral pole; *MP,* medial pole; *PF,* pterygoid fovea.

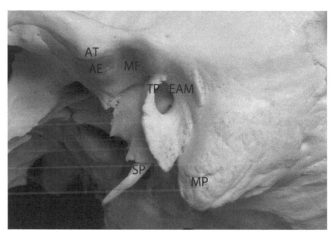

Fig. 30.3 Lateral and inferior view of the skull showing the temporal component of the temporomandibular joint. *AE,* Articular eminence; *AT,* articular tubercle; *EAM,* external auditory meatus; *MF,* mandibular fossa; *MP,* mastoid process; *SP,* styloid process; *TP,* tympanic plate.

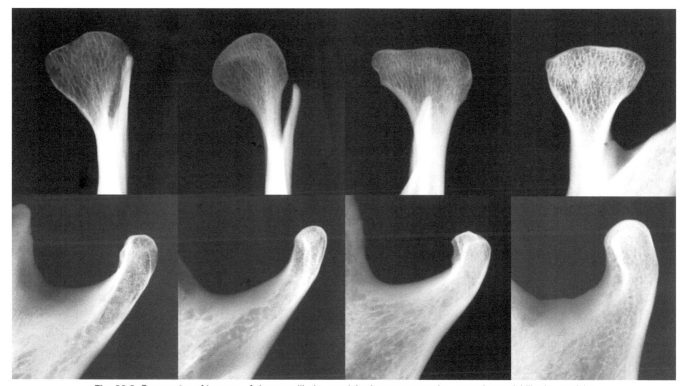

Fig. 30.2 Composite of images of the mandibular condyle demonstrates the extensive variability in condylar shape: heart-shaped, round, flat, and with large medial and lateral poles. The upper row are coronal views with the corresponding lateral views immediately below.

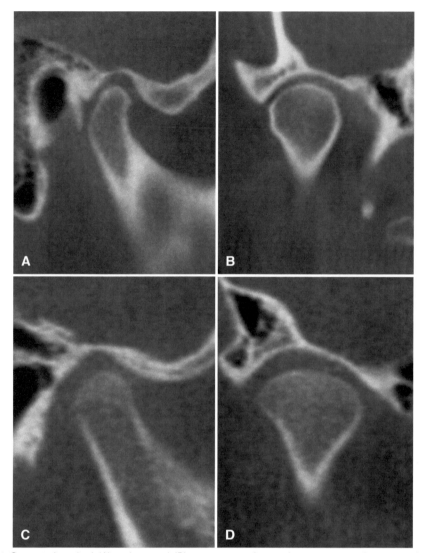

Fig. 30.4 Corrected sagittal (A) and coronal (B) reconstructed cone beam computed tomography (CBCT) images of the right temporomandibular joint (TMJ) in an adult. Note the thick regular cortication of all articulating surfaces and development of the glenoid fossa and articular eminence. Corrected sagittal (C) and coronal (D) reconstructed CBCT images of the right TMJ in a 7-year-old child. Note the thin cortication of the articulating surfaces, shallow glenoid fossa, and short articular eminence.

the cortices may remain indistinct until adulthood (see Fig. 30.4C and D, compared to A and B).

All aspects of the temporal bone, including the temporal component of the TMJ, may be pneumatized by small air cells derived from the mastoid air cell complex (Fig. 30.5A and B). Pneumatization of the articular eminence is seen radiographically in approximately 2% of patients.

Interarticular Disc

The interarticular disc (sometimes referred to as a meniscus) is composed of avascular fibrous connective tissue, and is positioned between the condylar and temporal components of the joint. The disc divides the joint cavity into two compartments; the inferior (lower) and superior (upper) joint spaces, which are located below and above the disc, respectively (Fig. 30.6). The normal disc has a biconcave shape with a thick anterior band, a thicker posterior band, and a thin middle or intermediate zone. The disc is also thicker medially than laterally. In the normal joint, the thin, biconcave central portion of the disc is in contact with the bony surfaces of the condyle and articular eminence. In the closed mouth position, the posterior band is located adjacent to the superior surface of the condyle, or slightly anterior to it, in the 11 o'clock position. The periphery of the disc blends with fibers of the inner surface of the joint capsule. Medial and lateral collateral ligaments also anchor the disc under the medial and lateral poles of the condyle. The anterior band is also thought to be attached to some fibers of the superior head of the lateral pterygoid muscle, while the posterior band attaches to the retrodiscal tissues.

During mandibular opening, as the condyle rotates and translates anteriorly and inferiorly, the disc is also carried forward so that its thin biconcave intermediate zone remains interposed between the articulating convexities of the condylar head and articular eminence. The disc attachments to the condylar neck laterally and medially by the collateral ligaments help to ensure passive movement of the disc with the condyle. On mandibular closing, this process reverses, with the disc moving posteriorly and superiorly with the condyle into the mandibular fossa.

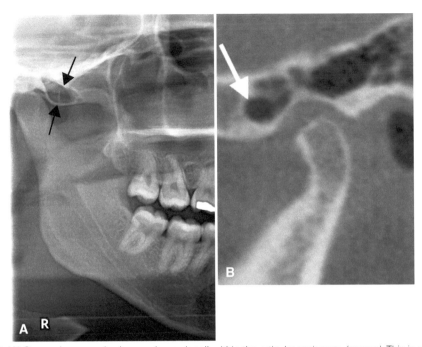

Fig. 30.5 (A) Cropped panoramic shows a large air cell within the articular eminence *(arrows)*. This is a variation of normal. (B) Note the pneumatization of the articular eminence on this reconstructed corrected sagittal CBCT image *(arrow)*.

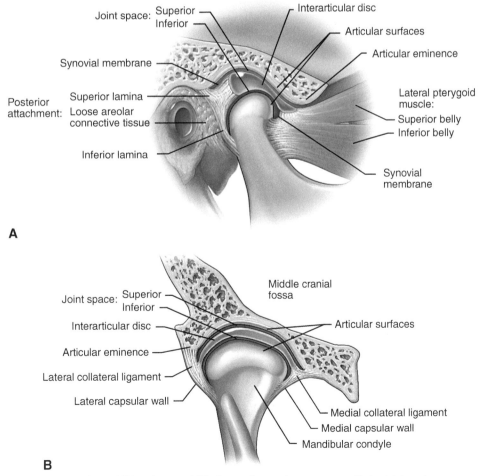

Fig. 30.6 Lateral (A) and coronal (B) views of normal temporomandibular joint anatomy.

Retrodiscal Tissues (Posterior Disc Attachment)

The retrodiscal tissues consist of superior and inferior lamellae enclosing a region of loose vascular tissue, and this is often referred to as the bilaminar zone. The superior lamina, which is rich in elastin, inserts into the posterior wall of the mandibular fossa. During opening movements of the jaw, the superior lamina distends, and allows the disc to move anteriorly with condylar translation. On closing, the superior lamina allows for the smooth recoil of the disc posteriorly. The inferior lamina attaches more tightly to the posterior surface of the condyle. As the condyle moves anteriorly and inferiorly, the retrodiscal tissues expand in volume, primarily as a result of venous distention, to fill the void created by the translated condyle. The retrodiscal tissues are well innervated and may be the source of pain when the posterior attachment becomes trapped between the condyle and articular eminence in cases of anterior disc displacement.

Temporomandibular Joint Bony Relationships

Joint space is a general term used to describe the radiolucent space located between the condyle and temporal component of the joint seen in conventional diagnostic images and CT. The radiographic joint space contains the articular disc and its attachments. This term should not be confused with the terms superior joint space and inferior joint

space described earlier, which refer to soft tissue spaces located superior and inferior to the disc. The anteroposterior position of the condyle within the glenoid fossa can be determined by examining the dimensions of the radiographic joint space viewed on lateral imaging projections of the joint that have been corrected for the angulation of the condylar head. Under normal conditions, the condyle is positioned centrally when the anterior and posterior recesses of the radiolucent joint space are uniform in width. The condyle is considered to be retruded when the anterior joint space width is greater than the posterior, and it is considered to be protruded when the anterior joint space is more narrow than the posterior. However, because the shapes of the glenoid fossa and the condyle do not necessarily match as a perfect "ball-and-socket," the dimensions of the joint spaces often vary from the medial to the lateral aspects of the normal joint (Fig. 30.7).

The diagnostic significance of mild or moderate condylar eccentricity is unclear. Condylar eccentricity is seen in one-third to one-half of asymptomatic individuals, and is not a reliable indicator of the soft tissue status of the joint, particularly because the shape of the condylar head does not always mirror the concavity of the fossa. Markedly eccentric condylar positioning usually represents an abnormality. For example, inferior positioning of the condyle where the joint space is widened superoinferiorly, may be seen in cases involving fluid or blood accumulation within the joint. In contrast, superior positioning of the condyle

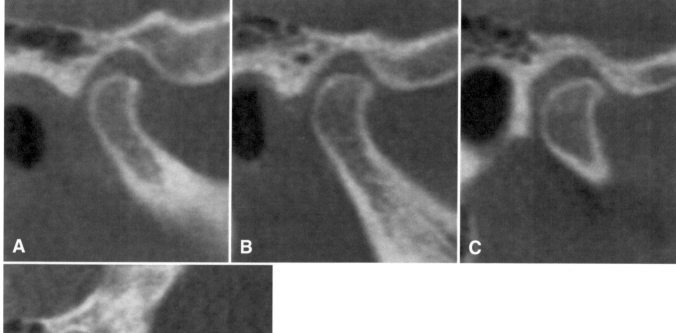

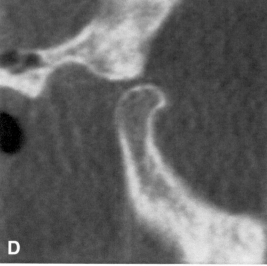

Fig. 30.7 Reconstructed corrected sagittal cone beam computed tomography image. (A–C) Closed position. Lateral image slice (A), central image slice (B), and medial image slice (C) of the same joint. The condyle appears retruded in the lateral slice, centered in the central slice, and anteriorly positioned in the medial slice. (D) Open view shows the condyle positioned at the summit of the articular eminence, which is a normal degree of translation.

where this space is narrowed or not visible, with apparent contact of osseous components, may indicate loss, displacement, or perforation of the disc or its attachments. Marked posterior condylar positioning is seen in some cases of anterior disc displacement, and pronounced anterior condylar positioning may be seen when there has been destruction of the articular eminence, such as in juvenile idiopathic arthritis (JIA).

Condylar Movement

The condyle undergoes complex rotational and translational movements during mandibular opening. A hinge-like, rotatory movement of the condylar head occurs between the superior surface of the condyle and the inferior surface of the disc, and this is followed by inferior (downward) and anterior (forward) translation (sliding) of the condyle, which occurs between the superior surface of the disc and the articular eminence. The extent of normal condylar translation varies considerably. In most individuals, at maximal opening, the condyle translates to the summit of the articular eminence or slightly anterior to it (see Fig. 30.7D). The condyle typically is found within a range of 2 to 5 mm posterior and 5 to 8 mm anterior to the crest of the eminence. Reduced condylar translation, in which the condyle has little or no downward and forward movement and does not leave the mandibular fossa, is seen in patients who clinically have a reduced degree of mouth opening. Hypermobility of the joint may be suspected if the condyle translates more than 5 mm anterior to the eminence. If a superior movement also occurs anterior to the articular eminence, anterior locking or dislocation of the condyle may occur.

APPLICATION OF DIAGNOSTIC IMAGING

Imaging of the TMJ may be necessary to supplement information obtained from the clinical examination. Diagnostic imaging should be considered when an osseous abnormality or infection is suspected, in patients with a history of trauma, significant dysfunction, alteration in range of motion, sensory or motor abnormalities, or significant changes in occlusion. TMJ imaging is not indicated for joint sounds if other signs or symptoms are absent, or for asymptomatic children and adolescents before orthodontic treatment. The purposes of TMJ imaging are to evaluate the integrity and relationships of the hard and soft tissues, confirm the extent or stage of progression of disease, and evaluate the effects of treatment. There is often poor correlation between the severity of findings on TMJ imaging and the severity of the patient's signs and symptoms. For example, severe degenerative changes may be noted on an imaging study, but the patient has only mild discomfort, or vice versa. The clinician must correlate the imaging information with the patient's history and clinical findings to arrive at a final diagnosis and to plan the management of the underlying disease process.

TEMPOROMANDIBULAR JOINT IMAGING MODALITIES

Several variables must be considered when selecting the type of imaging technique to use, including the specific clinical problem to be addressed; whether the imaging of hard or soft tissues is desired; the strengths and limitations of the modalities being considered; the cost of the examination; and the radiation dose. Both joints should be imaged during the examination for comparison. Images of the osseous structures of the joints may be obtained using panoramic imaging, cone beam computed tomography (CBCT) or multidetector computed tomography (MDCT). The soft tissues of the joints are best imaged with magnetic resonance imaging (MRI). The application of these techniques to the diagnosis of TMJ dysfunction is discussed further in the following sections.

Osseous Structures
Panoramic Imaging

The panoramic image is a useful tool for providing a broad overview of the anatomic structures of and around the TMJ. This form of imaging allows the clinician to rule out gross disease, and for some patients, it is the only imaging required before conservative therapy is initiated. Gross osseous changes involving the condyles may be identified, such as asymmetries, extensive erosions, large osteophytes, neoplasms, or fractures; however, panoramic imaging is less reliable for more subtle changes (Fig. 30.8). The panoramic image also provides a means of comparing left and right sides of the mandible, and can reveal odontogenic diseases and other disorders that may be the source of TMJ symptoms. However, no information about condylar position or function is provided because the mandible is partly opened and protruded when this image is made. Also, mild osseous changes may be obscured, and only marked changes in articular eminence morphology can be seen as a result of superimposition by the skull base and zygomatic arch. For these reasons, when a detailed assessment of the joint structures is desired, the panoramic image should be supplemented. The TMJ algorithms available on some panoramic machines do not provide the views required because of thick image layers and oblique, distorted views, and more advanced modalities are indicated.

Cone Beam Computed Tomography

CBCT creates image volumes that allow the user to reconstruct thin section views of anatomy in multiple, customizable planes. Thin sections allow the structures of the joints to be assessed without superimposition of surrounding anatomy. Classically, the joints are viewed in coronal and sagittal planes, corrected along the long axes of the condylar heads (Fig. 30.9). These "corrected" views provide the least distorted representations of the condylar and temporal components, and their relationship to one other. Panoramic and three-dimensional renderings of the jaws also can be created from a CBCT volume, and these may be useful for assessing skeletal asymmetries or other osseous deformities. A CBCT examination is usually acquired with the patient in the closed mouth position with the teeth in maximal intercuspation. Some CBCT systems allow low-resolution image acquisitions to be done in the open mouth or other positions (see Chapter 12) to evaluate range of motion. CBCT has the advantage of reduced radiation dose to the patient compared with MDCT. This reduced dose makes CBCT imaging ideal for imaging of osseous changes associated with DJD. CBCT imaging is also useful for determining the presence and extent of ankylosis and neoplasms, characterizing fractures, evaluating complications from the use of polytetrafluoroethylene or silicon sheet implants, and identifying heterotopic bone growth. Soft tissue structures including the discs cannot be visualized with CBCT imaging. Metallic implants in or around the joints may create streak artifacts, which can obscure the joint structures.

Multidetector Computed Tomography

MDCT (see Chapter 13) is capable of providing the same information as CBCT imaging, but additionally, it allows some—albeit limited—visualization of the soft tissues. This additional visualization is required only in a few situations, such as when a neoplasm is suspected to extend beyond bone borders. The articular disc cannot be visualized with this modality, and patients are exposed to higher radiation doses than CBCT imaging.

Soft Tissue Structures

The most common indication for soft tissue imaging is when clinical findings suggest disc displacement with symptoms such as TMJ pain and dysfunction, and when symptoms do not respond to conservative

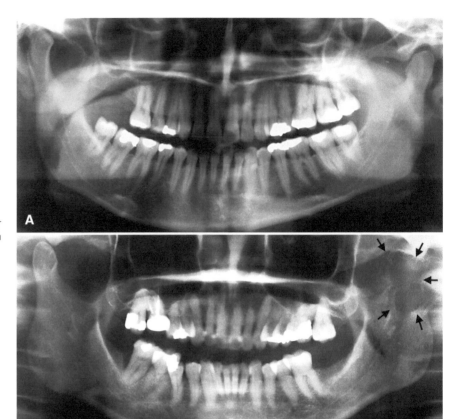

Fig. 30.8 Panoramic images reveal right condylar hyperplasia (A) and destruction of the condyle by a malignant tumor (B) (arrows).

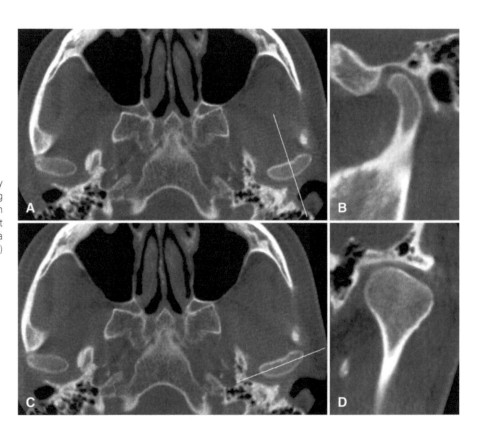

Fig. 30.9 Cone beam computed tomography images show reconstruction planes for evaluating the temporomandibular joints. (A) Axial image with line indicating corrected sagittal plane. (B) Resultant corrected sagittal image. (C) Axial image with a line indicating the corrected coronal plane. (D) Resultant corrected coronal image.

therapy. Soft tissue imaging also may be required to supplement osseous imaging in rare cases where infection or a neoplasm is suspected. As with any other modality, imaging should be prescribed only when the anticipated results are expected to influence patient management. MRI is the modality of choice for visualizing the disc and other soft tissues of the TMJ.

Magnetic Resonance Imaging

MRI uses static and gradient magnetic fields, and nonionizing electromagnetic radiation in the form of radiofrequency pulses to produce tomographic images (see Chapter 13). Specialized surface coils placed on the skin surface over the patient's TMJs improve image signal-to-noise, and therefore image quality. The examinations may be performed with the use of T_1-weighted, proton density or T_2-weighted pulse sequences, depending on the type of information required. Proton density images are slightly superior to T_1-weighted images in demonstrating osseous and discal tissues, whereas T_2-weighted images demonstrate inflammation and joint effusion. Furthermore, MRI allows the acquisition of images in the corrected sagittal and coronal planes without repositioning the patient (Fig. 30.10). These images usually are acquired in closed and opened mouth positions, with the aid of a bite block. Cinematic or cine MRI studies during opening and closing can be obtained by having the patient open the jaw incrementally, and using rapid image acquisition ("fast scan") techniques.

Depending on the radiofrequency pulse sequence selected, MRI creates contrast between different soft tissues, and this feature can be used to differentiate the articular disc from the other soft tissue components of the joint. Joint effusions can also be detected with MRI. MRI imaging displays the osseous structures of the TMJ but not with the detail comparable to CBCT or MDCT.

MRI is contraindicated in patients who have pacemakers or some other implanted devices, intracranial vascular clips, or metal particles in vital structures. Dental materials that contain stainless steel or its component metals, such as orthodontic hardware, may create image artifacts over the jaws, and may, in some cases, obscure the joints. Some patients may be unable to tolerate the procedure because of claustrophobia or an inability to remain motionless.

ABNORMALITIES OF THE TEMPOROMANDIBULAR JOINT

Developmental Abnormalities
Disease Mechanism

Developmental abnormalities are the result of disturbances in the normal growth and development of the TMJ. These abnormalities may affect the form or size of the joint components, most commonly the mandibular condyle. Because the condylar articular cartilage is considered a growth center for the mandible, disturbances involving this cartilage can result in altered growth of the mandibular condyle, ramus, body, and alveolar process on the affected side.

Condylar Hyperplasia

Disease mechanism. Condylar hyperplasia is a developmental abnormality that results in enlargement and occasionally deformity of the condylar head; this may have a secondary effect on the mandibular fossa as it remodels to accommodate the abnormal condyle. Proposed etiologic factors include hormonal influences, trauma, infection, heredity, intrauterine factors, and hypervascularity. The mechanism may involve overactive cartilage or persistent cartilaginous rests; the thickness of the entire cartilaginous and precartilaginous layers is increased. This condition usually is unilateral and may be accompanied by varying degrees of hyperplasia of the ipsilateral mandible.

Clinical features. Condylar hyperplasia is more common in females and is most frequently discovered before age 20 years. The condition is self-limiting and tends to arrest with the termination of skeletal growth; however, a few cases continue to grow, and adult onset has been reported. The condition may progress slowly or rapidly. Patients have a mandibular asymmetry that varies in severity, depending on the degree of condylar enlargement. The chin may be deviated to the unaffected side, or it may remain unchanged but with an increase in the vertical dimension of the ramus, mandibular body, or alveolar process of the affected side. As a result of this growth pattern, patients may have a posterior open bite on the affected side or a crossbite on the contralateral side with resultant problems with mastication or speech. Patients may also have

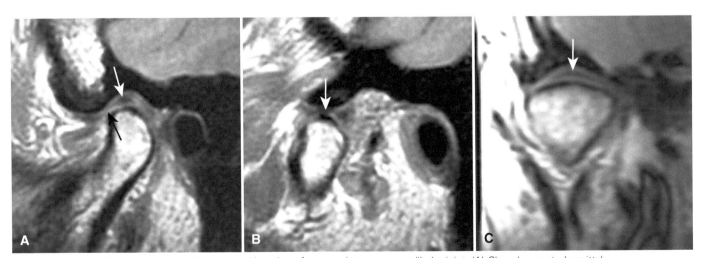

Fig. 30.10 Magnetic resonance imaging of a normal temporomandibular joint. (A) Closed corrected sagittal image shows the condyle and temporal component. The biconcave disc is located with its posterior band *(white arrow)* directly superior to the condyle and the thin intermediate part interposed between the articulating surfaces *(black arrow)*. (B) Open corrected sagittal image shows the condyle positioned at the summit of the articular eminence with the articular disc normally positioned between the osseous components *(white arrow)*. (C) Closed corrected coronal image shows the osseous components and disc *(white arrow)* superior to the condyle.

symptoms related to TMJ dysfunction and may complain of a limited or deviated mandibular opening caused by restricted mobility of the enlarged condyle.

Imaging features. The hyperplastic condyle may have a relatively normal shape but be enlarged, or its form could be altered (e.g., conical, spherical, elongated, lobulated) or irregular. It may appear to be more radiopaque in plain images because of the additional bone volume present. However, the cortical thickness and trabecular pattern of the enlarged condyle are usually normal, which helps to distinguish hyperplasia from a neoplasm. The glenoid fossa may be enlarged to compensate for the larger condylar head, usually as a result of remodeling of the posterior slope of the articular eminence. Secondary degenerative changes may be present because of the altered forces on the joint. The condylar neck also may be longer and thickened. Forward bending of the elongated condylar head and neck, to compensate for the increased bone volume, may result in an inverted "L shape" to these structures. The condylar neck also may bend laterally when viewed in the coronal (anteroposterior) plane (Fig. 30.11). Secondary enlargement of the ramus and mandibular body also may result in a characteristic downward bowing of the inferior mandibular border on the affected side. The ramus may have increased vertical and anteroposterior dimensions.

Differential interpretation. A condylar neoplasm, most notably an osteochondroma, is included in the differential interpretation. An osteochondroma usually results in a condyle with a more lobular and irregular shape compared with a hyperplastic condyle because this neoplasm creates a more localized, protruding growth. Surface irregularities and continued growth after cessation of skeletal growth should increase suspicion of neoplasia. Occasionally, a condylar osteoma or a large osteophyte occurring in chronic DJD may simulate condylar hyperplasia. Associated ipsilateral hyperplasia of the mandible would not be seen in these other conditions.

Management. The management of condyler hyperplasia consists of a combination of condylectomy, orthognathic surgery, and orthodontics. Condylectomy removes the source of abnormal growth, whereas orthognathic surgery and orthodontics aim to correct any resultant functional and esthetic deficits. The initiation of treatment before

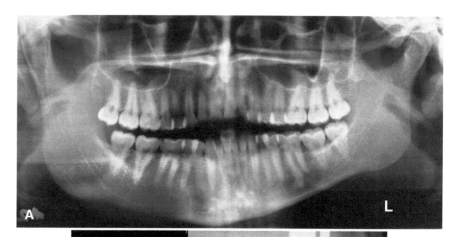

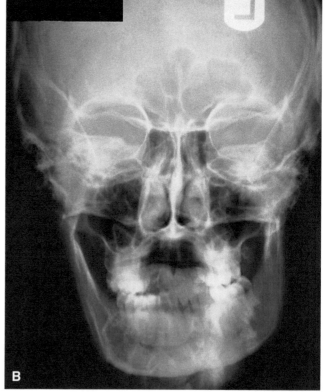

Fig. 30.11 (A) Panoramic image of condylar hyperplasia causing enlargement of the right condyle, ramus, and body of the mandible. (B) The resulting asymmetry of the mandible is apparent in the posteroanterior skull view.

condylar growth is complete helps limit the severity of mandibular deformation and compensatory changes in the maxilla and dentoalveolar structures. Management also may be delayed until growth is completed to avoid relapse and the need for additional interventions. A nuclear medicine examination with the radionuclide, technetium (^{99m}Tc) may be helpful in determining if condylar growth is still active or if it has ceased. However, nuclear medicine may be misleading because of its poor specificity, and particularly if there is increased activity secondary to concurrent remodeling or degenerative changes.

Condylar Hypoplasia

Disease mechanism. Condylar hypoplasia is an undersized mandibular condyle, which may be the result of congenital, developmental, or acquired diseases that affect condylar growth. Severe congenital malformations may result in complete lack of formation of the condyle (aplasia). Rare congenital conditions causing hypoplasia of the condyle often also present with abnormalities of other structures of the face, such as the ear, eye, and zygomatic arch (see Chapter 29). Trauma, infection, and therapeutic radiation exposure to the condyle during growth are potential acquired causes of hypoplasia.

Clinical features. Condylar hypoplasia is more commonly unilateral, unless it is a feature of a syndrome (e.g., mandibulofacial dysostosis or Treacher Collins syndrome, Pierre Robin sequence). The condyle is a mandibular growth center; therefore, condylar hypoplasia is usually associated with some degree of unilateral mandibular hypoplasia and facial asymmetry. Deviation of the mandibular midline to the affected side and accentuation of this deviation on mandibular opening and malocclusion may develop. The amount of growth disturbance of the mandible is related to how early the onset of the disturbance to condylar growth occurs; earlier onset results in more severe underdevelopment of the ramus and mandibular body. Patients with condylar hypoplasia may develop symptoms of TMJ dysfunction.

Imaging features. The condyle may be normal in shape and structure but is diminished in size, and the mandibular fossa is proportionally small. The condylar neck is thinner and may appear short or elongated. The coronoid process is usually slender. The posterior border of the ramus and condylar neck may have a posterior (dorsal) inclination, creating a concavity in the outline of the posterior surface of the mandibular ramus in the panoramic image. If there is an associated mandibular hypoplasia, it manifests with a deepened antegonial notch and decreased vertical height of the mandibular body (Fig. 30.12). Occasional dental crowding may also result. Degenerative changes in the affected joint may be detected (Fig. 30.13).

Differential interpretation. Juvenile idiopathic arthritis (JIA) may cause damage to the condyle, resulting in hypoplasia. However, other signs of joint destruction would also be seen. An examination of other joints or testing for rheumatoid factor may be helpful if there is uncertainty. Changes in condylar morphology in severe DJD or other arthritic conditions also may mimic a hypoplastic condyle, but other signs of arthritis are usually visible in the affected joint. Additionally, arthritis does not cause mandibular hypoplasia of the affected side unless it occurs during growth. Occasionally, it is difficult to determine if there is condylar hypoplasia or if the contralateral side is enlarged. Careful examination of the inferior border for a pronounced antegonial notch (hypoplasia) versus downward bowing (hyperplasia) is helpful.

Treatment. Orthognathic surgery, bone grafts, and orthodontic therapy may be required.

Coronoid Hyperplasia

Disease mechanism. Coronoid hyperplasia results from an elongation of the coronoid process of the mandible. The etiology may be acquired or developmental. The coronoid processes may impinge on the posterior surface of the maxilla or zygomatic bone during opening, restricting condylar translation. Sometimes a pseudojoint develops between the hyperplastic coronoid and the posterior surface of the zygoma, a condition called Jacob disease.

Clinical features. The developmental variant of coronoid hyperplasia is more commonly bilateral. This form is most often diagnosed in young men who have a long history of progressive limitation of mouth opening. The resulting restricted opening may simulate the features of an apparent closed lock owing to disc displacement. Acquired coronoid hyperplasia usually develops secondary to restricted movement of the condyle, such as in ankylosis. The condition is painless.

Imaging features. Coronoid hyperplasia is best seen in panoramic images and CT examinations. The coronoid processes are elongated, and the tips extend at least 1 cm above the inferior rim of the zygomatic arch (Fig. 30.14). The coronoid processes may have a large but normal shape, or may curve anteriorly and appear very radiopaque. Impingement of the coronoid against the zygomatic bone can be confirmed by performing CT imaging with the patient's mouth opened maximally. Remodeling of the posterior surface of the zygomatic process of the maxilla, to accommodate the enlarged coronoid process during function, also may be seen. Because this condition is often bilateral, both sides should be examined for abnormality. The radiographic appearances of the TMJs are usually normal.

Differential interpretation. Unilateral elongation of the coronoid process should be differentiated from a neoplasm such as an osteochondroma or osteoma. In contrast to coronoid hyperplasia, neoplasms usually have an irregular shape. Clinical presentation of limited opening most often prompts examination of the TMJs for abnormalities that

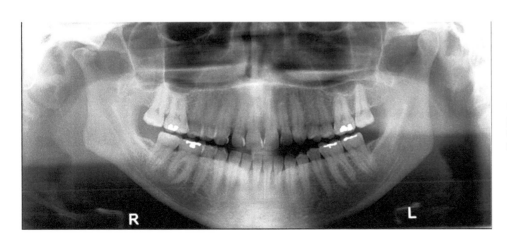

Fig. 30.12 Panoramic image reveals hypoplasia of the right condyle with the associated short vertical height of the right mandibular ramus and body.

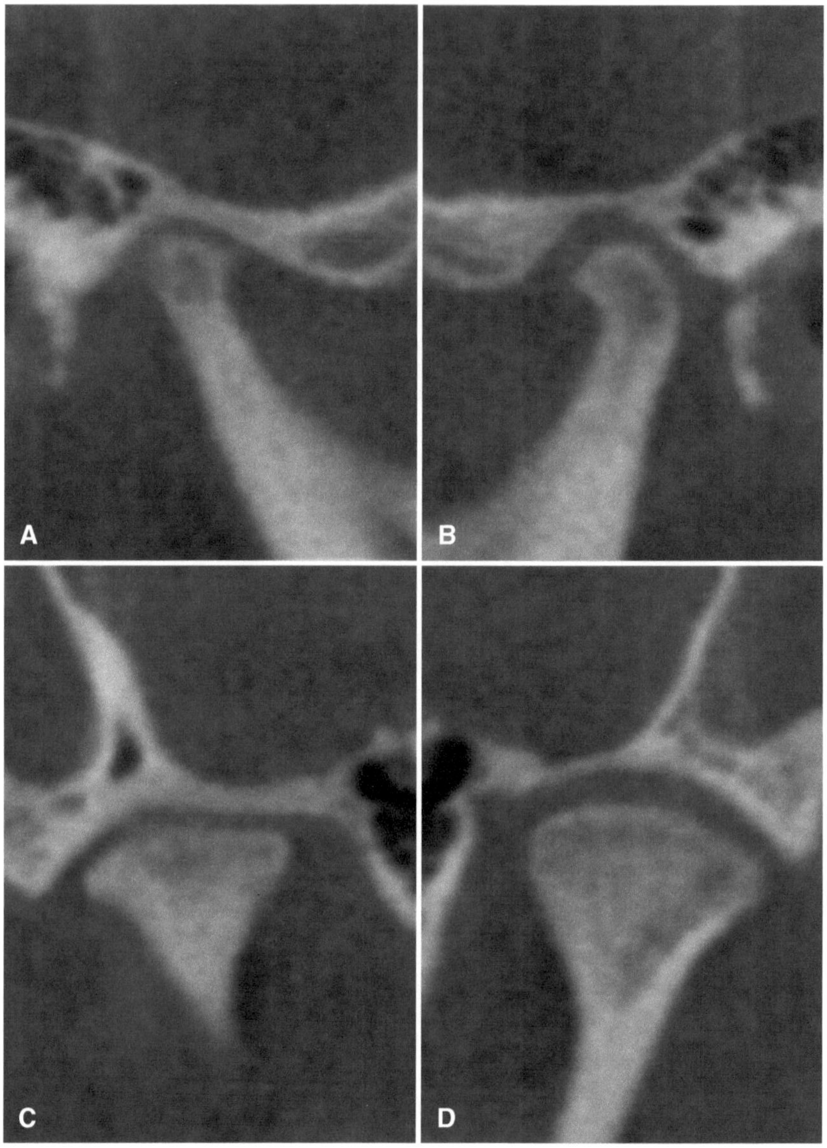

Fig. 30.13 Cone beam computed tomography images of unilateral condylar hypoplasia. Reconstructed sagittal (A and B) and coronal (C and D) images. (A and C) The right condyle is hypoplastic, and there is secondary remodeling. The articular surfaces of the condyle and anterior aspect of the glenoid fossa are flattened, and the superior joint space is thinner compared with the left. (B and D) Left side of the same patient showing normal condyle.

may restrict joint movement, such as internal derangement, neoplasm, or ankylosis. However, inclusion of the coronoid processes during TMJ imaging helps ensure that coronoid hyperplasia is not overlooked.

Management. Treatment consists of surgical removal of the coronoid process and postoperative physiotherapy. Regrowth of the coronoid process after surgery has been reported.

Bifid Condyle

Disease mechanism. A condyle that is bifid has a vertical depression, notch, or cleft in the surface of the condylar head. This feature is best seen in the corrected sagittal or coronal plane, and results in the appearance of a "double-headed" condyle. There may be actual duplication of the condyle. This condition is rare and is more often unilateral, although it may be bilateral. It may result from an obstructed blood supply during development or other embryopathy, although a traumatic cause has been postulated with the divided condyle resulting from a longitudinal fracture.

Clinical features. Bifid condyle is usually an incidental finding in panoramic images or anteroposterior plain imaging. Some patients have signs and symptoms of TMJ dysfunction, including joint noises and pain.

Imaging features. Although the orientation of the bifid condyle may be anteroposterior or mediolateral, commonly, a depression or notch is present on the superior condylar surface, giving a heart-shaped outline when viewed in corrected coronal plane (Fig. 30.15). The depth of the depression is variable. A more remarkable presentation is complete duplication of the condylar head in the sagittal plane. The mandibular fossa may remodel to accommodate the altered condylar morphology.

Differential interpretation. A slight medial depression on the superior condylar surface may be considered a normal variation; the point at which the depth of the depression signifies a bifid condyle is unclear. The differential interpretation also includes a vertical fracture through the condylar head.

Management. Treatment is not indicated unless pain or functional impairment is present.

Soft Tissue Abnormalities
Disc Displacement

Disease mechanism. The articular disc may become abnormally positioned or displaced relative to the condylar and temporal components of the TMJ. The disc most often is displaced in an anterior direction, but it may be displaced anteromedially, medially, or anterolaterally.

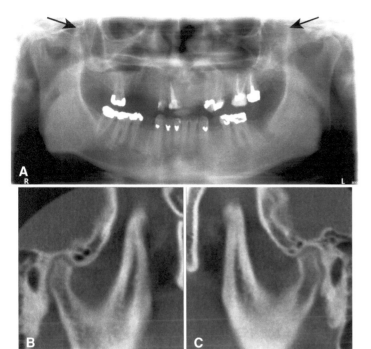

Fig. 30.14 (A) Panoramic image reveals bilateral coronoid hyperplasia *(arrows)* in a patient complaining of limited opening. (B and C) Reconstructed corrected sagittal cone beam computed tomography images of a different patient with bilateral coronoid hyperplasia. Note the pronounced elongation of the coronoid processes but with maintenance of a normal shape. ([B and C], Courtesy Dr. S. Fireman, Toronto, ON, Canada.)

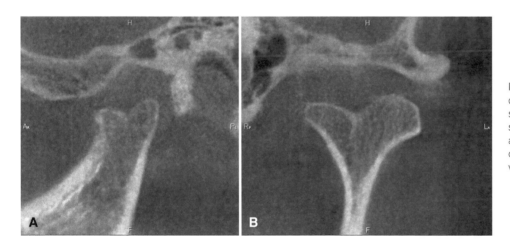

Fig. 30.15 Bifid condyle. Reconstructed corrected sagittal (A) and coronal (B) images show a central depression in the superior surface of the mandibular condyle creating a bilobed or heart-shaped outline. The osseous structures in this joint are otherwise normal.

Lateral and posterior displacements are extremely rare. A displaced disc may interfere with normal function of the joint or cause pain, although it is a common finding in asymptomatic patients, leading to the hypothesis that disc displacements may be considered a normal variation. A disc that is displaced in the closed position may resume a normal relationship with the condyle when the mouth is open, or it may remain displaced; the terms *reducing* and *nonreducing* are used to describe these situations, respectively (Fig. 30.16). A displaced disc may become deformed or be associated with other signs of TMJ dysfunction, including DJD, adhesion, effusion, and perforation. The cause of disc displacement is unknown, although parafunction, jaw injuries (e.g., direct trauma), whiplash injury, and forced opening beyond the normal range have been implicated. The term *internal derangement* is a nonspecific designation for an abnormality in the soft tissue components of the joint resulting in altered function, which may include disc displacement.

Clinical features. Disc displacement has been found both in symptomatic and asymptomatic patients, and it is unknown why some individuals progress to more severe dysfunction, whereas others do not. Joint noises, such as popping or clicking, are a common sign of disc

displacement but usually are not painful. Crepitus, a crunching or grinding sound, is suggestive of osseous degeneration associated with a long-term, nonreducing disc. Symptoms associated with a displaced disc include pain in the preauricular region, headaches, and closed or open locking of the joint. A decreased range of motion may be present, and when the displacement is unilateral, this may manifest as deviation of the mandible to the affected side on opening.

Imaging features

Normal disc position. The articular disc cannot be visualized with conventional imaging, CBCT, or MDCT; MRI is the technique of choice. On MRI, the normal disc has a low signal intensity relative to the signal from the joint space immediately surrounding it. In other words, the disc signal is lower (i.e., darker). In contrast, the signal intensity of the posterior attachment is usually higher (i.e., brighter).

In a corrected sagittal image, the normal biconcave disc has a "bow tie" shape. In the closed mouth position, the normal disc is positioned with the thick posterior band located either directly superior to or slightly anterior to the condylar head (around the 11 o'clock position). The thin intermediate zone of the disc is located between the

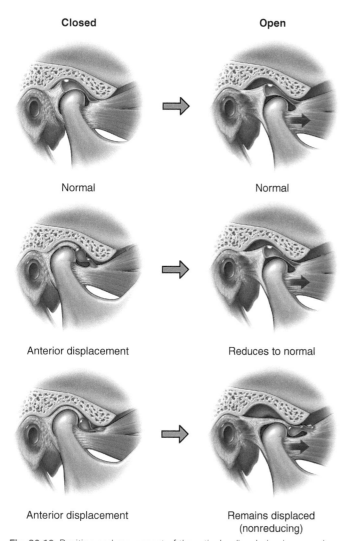

Closed

Open

Normal

Normal

Anterior displacement

Reduces to normal

Anterior displacement

Remains displaced (nonreducing)

Fig. 30.16 Position and movement of the articular disc during jaw opening. *Top,* Normal position. *Middle,* Partially displaced anteriorly (with reduction). *Bottom,* Severely displaced anteriorly (without reduction).

anterosuperior surface of the condyle and the posterior surface of the articular eminence (see Fig. 30.10). In all positions of mouth opening, the thin intermediate zone should remain the articulating surface of the disc between the condyle and the articular eminence.

Disc displacement. MRI is required for identification of a displaced disc. Although a retruded condylar position, seen in CBCT or MDCT, has been associated with an anteriorly displaced disc, condylar position in maximal intercuspation is an unreliable indicator of disc displacement. Anterior displacement is the most common disc displacement. A disc is considered anteriorly displaced when its posterior band is located anterior to the normal position and the thin intermediate zone is no longer positioned between the condyle and articular eminence (Fig. 30.17A). This displacement may range from partial to full displacement with the posterior band located between the condyle and articular eminence in a mild partial displacement to being located well anterior to the condylar head in a severe, full dislocation. When the disc is severely anteriorly displaced, partial folding of the disc within the anterior joint space may be seen. Sometimes identification of the posterior band is difficult because of deformation of this part of the disc.

When the disc is chronically anteriorly positioned, the posterior attachment is stretched between the articulating surfaces of the condyle and temporal bone, and owing to resulting fibrosis its MRI signal may become lower and approximate that of the posterior band. It is helpful to identify the position of the thin intermediate part of the disc to determine if it is anteriorly displaced from its normal position between the articulating surfaces of the condyle and articular eminence.

Medial, lateral, and anteromedial displacements also can be identified on MRI (see Fig. 30.17C). Anteromedial displacement is indicated in corrected sagittal images when the disc is in a normal position in the medial images of the joint, but is anteriorly positioned in the lateral images of the same joint. Medial or lateral displacement is indicated on corrected coronal MRI when the body of the disc is positioned at the medial or lateral aspect of the condyle, respectively. Posterior disc displacement is rare.

Disc reduction and nonreduction. During mouth opening, an anteriorly displaced disc may return to a normal relationship with the condylar head during any part of the opening movement. In motion studies, this is usually seen as a rapid posterior movement of the disc, and it is often accompanied by an audible click. This condition is referred to as disc reduction and can be diagnosed on MRI if the disc is anteriorly displaced in closed mouth views but is in a normal position in open mouth images (see Fig. 30.17). If the disc remains anteriorly displaced on opening, it is interpreted as being nonreducing. It may appear bent or deformed as the condyle pushes forward against it (Fig. 30.18). Fibrotic changes of the posterior attachment of a displaced disc may alter its tissue signal to approximate the signal of the disc. In such cases, the disc may be erroneously interpreted as occupying a normal position at maximal opening. Identification of excessive tissue with low signal intensity anterior to the condylar head, representing the true disc tissue, should help confirm the nonreducing state of the disc.

Deformities and perforation. If the disc remains chronically displaced, it undergoes permanent deformation, losing its biconcave shape. MRI can depict the alteration to the normal biconcave outline of the disc, which may vary from enlargement of the posterior band to a bilinear or biconvex disc outline. In cases of gross deformation or atrophy, identification of the disc may be difficult or impossible. Disc deformities may be accompanied by changes in its signal intensity, including an increase in signal. Changes to the condyle and temporal component of the joint consistent with DJD often accompany cases with long-standing displaced discs (Fig. 30.19). Perforations between the superior and inferior joint spaces most commonly occur in the retrodiscal tissue, just behind the posterior band of the disc (Fig. 30.20D), and can be detected in arthrographic investigations but are not reliably detected with MRI. Loss of the joint space, resulting in bone-to-bone contact between the osseous components, is suggestive of perforation of the disc or its attachment.

Fibrous adhesions and effusion. Fibrous adhesions are masses of fibrous tissue or scar tissue that form in the joint space, particularly after TMJ surgery. Adhesions may restrict normal movement of the disc during mandibular opening, resulting in a "stuck disc" and possible closed lock. Adhesions are best identified with arthrography by resistance to injection of contrast agent, or they may be detected on MRI studies as tissue with low signal intensity. Adhesions also may be suspected when there is no movement of the disc relative to the articular eminence in mandibular open position in MRI. Joint effusion (fluid in the joint) is considered to be an early change that may precede DJD. MRI can detect joint effusion, which appears as an area of high signal intensity in the joint spaces on T_2-weighted images (see Fig. 30.18B and D).

Management. Management of an asymptomatic displaced disc is not indicated. In symptomatic patients, conservative, noninvasive therapy should be initiated first. Most patients' symptoms resolve with time.

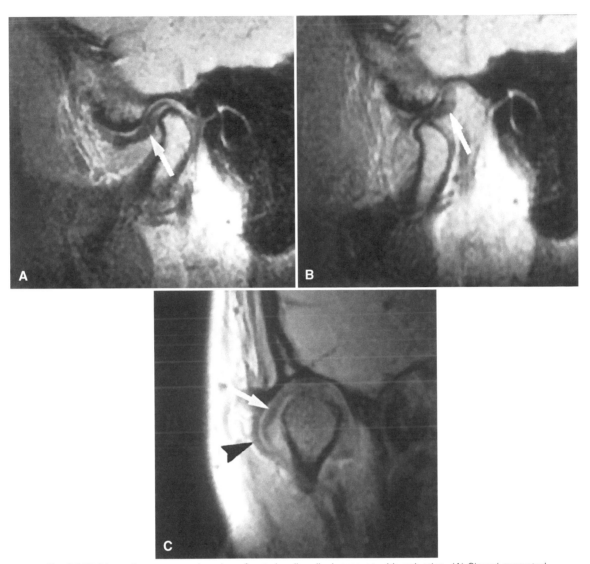

Fig. 30.17 Magnetic resonance imaging of anterior disc displacement with reduction. (A) Closed corrected sagittal view shows the disc with its posterior band *(arrow)* anterior to the condyle; note the anterior position of the thin intermediate section of the disc. (B) Open view shows the normal relationship of the disc and condyle and the posterior band of the disc *(arrow)*. (C) Corrected coronal view shows the disc *(arrow)* laterally displaced. The joint capsule *(arrowhead)* bulges laterally. ([B], Courtesy Dr. P.-L. Westesson, Rochester, NY.)

Arthroscopy or arthrocentesis may be helpful in releasing adhesions and improving joint mobility. Open joint surgery is reserved for refractory cases.

Remodeling and Arthritic Conditions
Remodeling

Disease mechanism. Remodeling is an adaptive response of cartilage and bone to loading forces applied to the joint that may exceed the normal tolerances of the tissues. This adaptive response results in alterations of the shape of the condyle and articular eminence, and may result in the flattening of curved joint surfaces. Such changes effectively redistribute the loading forces over a greater surface area. The number of trabeculae also increase, thereby increasing the density of subchondral cancellous bone (subchondral sclerosis) to resist applied forces better. No destruction or degeneration of fibrous articular tissue covering the bony components occurs. TMJ remodeling occurs throughout adult life and is considered abnormal only if it is accompanied by clinical signs and symptoms of pain or dysfunction, or if the degree of

remodeling seen on imaging is judged to be severe. Remodeling may be unilateral and does not invariably serve as a precursor to DJD.

Clinical features. Remodeling may be asymptomatic, or patients may have signs and symptoms of TMJ dysfunction that may be related to the soft tissue components, associated muscles, or ligaments. Accompanying disc displacement may be a factor.

Imaging features. Changes noted in the diagnostic images may affect the condyle, temporal bone, or both. Such changes first occur on the anterosuperior surface of the condyle and the posterior slope of the articular eminence. The lateral aspect of the joint also may be affected in the early stages, and the central and medial aspects become involved as the remodeling progresses. These changes may include one or a combination of the following: flattening, thickening of the cortex of the articulating surfaces, and subchondral sclerosis (see Fig. 30.20).

Differential interpretation. Severe joint flattening and subchondral sclerosis may be difficult to differentiate from early-onset DJD. The microscopic changes of degeneration occur before they can be detected in the diagnostic image. The appearance of bone erosions, osteophytes,

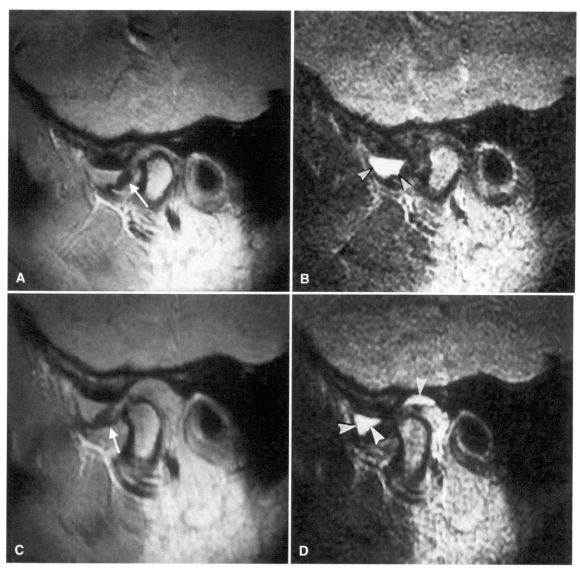

Fig. 30.18 Magnetic resonance imaging of disc displacement without reduction in the presence of joint effusion. (A) The disc *(arrow)* is anteriorly displaced in closed T_1-weighted image. (B) T_2-weighted image of the same section shows the collection of joint effusion *(arrowheads)* in the anterior recess of the upper joint space. (C) Open T_1-weighted image shows the disc remains anterior to the condyle. The posterior band of the disc is indicated with an *arrow*. (D) T_2-weighted image is at the same level as image in C. Note the joint effusion *(arrowheads)* in the anterior and posterior recesses of the upper joint space. (Courtesy Dr. P.-L. Westesson, Rochester, NY.)

and loss of joint space in the diagnostic image are signs of DJD. Joints affected by degenerative changes may also remodel to have flattened surfaces during nondestructive phases; significant loss of bone volume of the condyle or eminence suggests previous erosion as opposed to adaptive remodeling.

Management. When no clinical signs or symptoms are present, management is not indicated. Otherwise, management directed to reduce joint loading, such as splint therapy, may be considered. However, this should be preceded by an attempt to discover the cause of the joint overloading.

Degenerative Joint Disease

Disease mechanism. DJD or osteoarthritis is the breakdown of the articulating fibrocartilage covering the bony components of the joint leading to eventual deterioration of the osseous structures. DJD is

thought to occur when the ability of the joint to adapt to excessive joint loading forces, through remodeling, is exceeded. Numerous etiologic factors may be important, including acute trauma, hypermobility, and abnormal loading of the joint that may occur in parafunction. Disc displacement also may be a contributing element, and loss of normal lubrication within the joint has been suggested to play a part at the molecular level. It has been reported that joints with long-term nonreducing disc displacement have a higher incidence of progressive radiographic changes of DJD than joints with no disc displacement or reducing discs.

It should be noted that DJD is a noninflammatory disorder characterized by joint deterioration and bony proliferation. Joint deterioration is characterized by bone erosion, whereas new bone formation at the periphery of articular surfaces (osteophyte) and in the subchondral region (sclerosis) represents the proliferative component. Usually a variable combination of deterioration and proliferation occurs, but

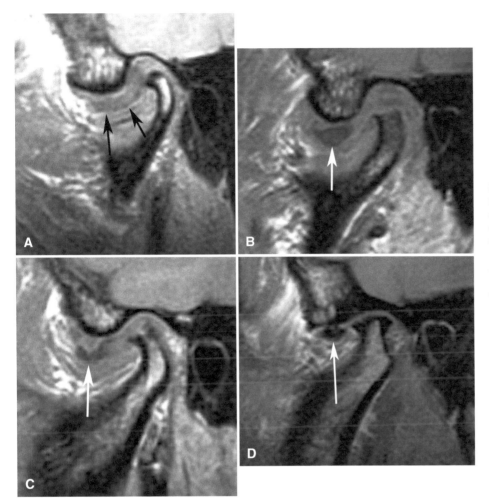

Fig. 30.19 Corrected sagittal magnetic resonance imaging of several cases of anteriorly displaced discs *(arrows)* with various stages of degenerative joint disease. (A) Example of severe deformation of the disc and an increase in the tissue signal. (B) Severe erosions of the superior aspect of the condyle. (C) Erosions involving the condyle and a small osteophyte on the anterior aspect. (D) Example of osteophytes forming on both the anterior and the posterior surfaces of the condyle.

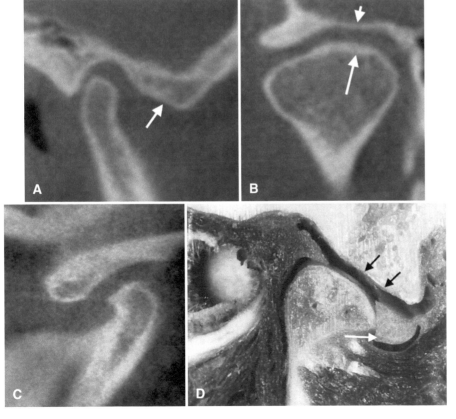

Fig. 30.20 Reconstructed corrected sagittal (A) and coronal (B) cone beam computed tomography (CBCT) images of the right temporomandibular joint show remodeling. (A) The right temporal component shows subchondral sclerosis and flattening of the articular eminence *(arrow)*. (B) The right condyle shows mild flattening of the lateral aspect and subchondral sclerosis of the medial aspect *(arrow)*. The right temporal component is also flattened *(arrowhead)*. (C) Reconstructed corrected sagittal CBCT image shows significant flattening of the condylar head. (D) Cadaver specimen. Note the flattening of the temporal component *(black arrows)* and large perforation posterior to a residual deformed disc *(white arrow)*.

occasionally one aspect predominates. Generally, deterioration is more common in acute disease, and proliferation predominates in chronic disease.

Clinical features. DJD can occur at any age, although the incidence increases with age. DJD has a female preponderance. The disease may be asymptomatic, or patients may complain of signs and symptoms of TMJ dysfunction, including pain on palpation and movement, joint noises (crepitus), limited range of motion, and muscle hyperactivity. The onset of symptoms may be sudden or gradual, and symptoms may disappear spontaneously, only to return in recurring cycles. Some studies report that the disease eventually "burns out," and symptoms disappear or decrease markedly in severity in long-standing cases.

Imaging features. Osseous changes in DJD are more accurately depicted on CT images, although osseous changes also may be seen on MRI, particularly T_1-weighted or proton density images. Erosions of the bone are a sign of the deteriorating component of DJD. These manifest as small to large "bites" or "scoops" out of the articulating surfaces of the joint, resulting in loss of the continuity of the cortices and eventual loss of bone volume (Fig. 30.21). In severe DJD, the glenoid fossa may appear grossly enlarged because of erosion of the posterior slope of the articular eminence. This erosion may allow the condylar

head to move forward and superiorly into an abnormal anterior position that may result in an anterior open bite. The condyle also may be markedly diminished in size and altered in shape because of severe erosions. In some cases, small, round, radiolucent areas with irregular margins surrounded by a varying area of sclerosis are visible, deep to the articulating surfaces. These lesions, referred to as subchondral or Ely cysts, are not true cysts but rather are areas of degeneration that contain fibrous connective tissue, granulation tissue, and osteoid (see Fig. 30.21A and B). When the patient is in maximal intercuspation, the joint space may be narrow or absent. This finding often correlates with a displaced disc and frequently with a perforation of the disc or posterior attachment, resulting in bone-to-bone contact of the joint components.

In the proliferative phase of the disease, bone formation occurs at the periphery of the articulating surfaces. These projections of new bone are called osteophytes, and although they may form on any part of the joint, they usually emanate from the anterosuperior surface of the condyle, the lateral aspect of the temporal bone or both (Fig. 30.22). Osteophytes create broader, flatter bony articulating surfaces, and serve to better distribute the biomechanical load on the joint over a greater area. In severe cases, osteophyte formation may extend from the articular eminence almost to encase the condylar head. Osteophytes may also

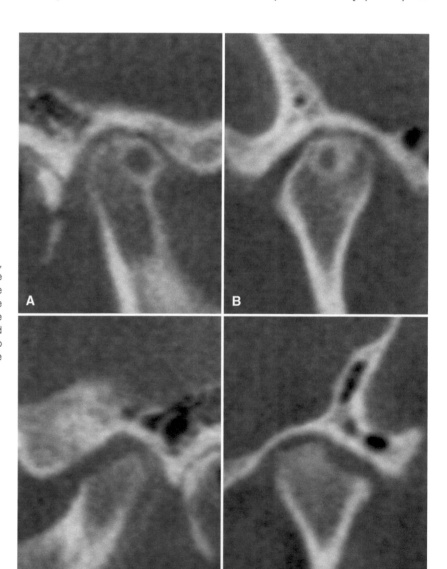

Fig. 30.21 Cone beam computed tomography image, closed position, depicting various erosions in degenerative joint disease. (A and B) Same patient, right side. Large subchondral cyst-like erosion (Ely cyst) of the condyle surrounded by a broad zone of sclerosis. Note also the thin joint space. (C and D) Same patient, left side. Broad erosion of the anterolateral condylar surface. Note also the lack of cortication of the remaining condylar surface and flattening of the temporal component.

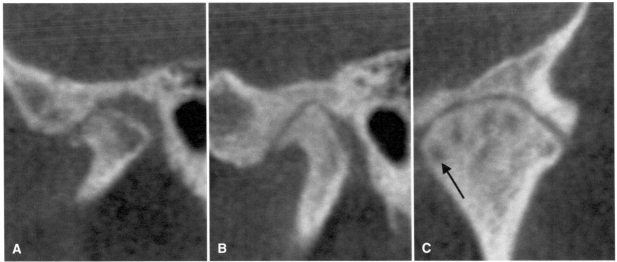

Fig. 30.22 Cone beam computed tomography image, closed position displaying two cases of degenerative joint disease (different patients). (A) Corrected sagittal reconstruction. Surface erosions and subchondral sclerosis of the condyle and articular eminence. There is also osteophyte formation at the anterior aspect of the condyle. The condyle is anteriorly positioned in the glenoid fossa. (B) Corrected sagittal reconstruction. Prominent osteophyte formation at the anterior aspect of the condyle, flattening, and subchondral sclerosis of all joint components, with decreased width of the joint space. (C) Corrected coronal reconstruction, same patient as B. Multiple subchondral erosions are seen, which are not visible in the sagittal reformat (one example indicated by *arrow*).

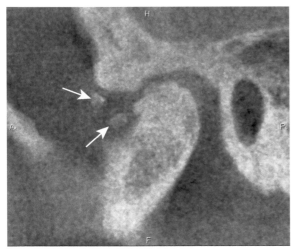

Fig. 30.23 Corrected sagittal reconstructed cone beam computed tomography image shows joint mice located anterior to the condyle *(arrows)*. Erosions, profound subchondral sclerosis, and osteophyte formation affecting the articulating surfaces are also noted, consistent with degenerative joint disease.

break off and lie free within the joint space. These fragments are known as "joint mice," and they must be differentiated from other conditions that cause joint space radiopacities (Fig. 30.23). Variable degrees of sclerosis of the subchondral bone may accompany any of the changes described.

Differential interpretation. DJD can have a spectrum of appearances ranging from extensive erosions (degenerative component) to substantial subchondral sclerosis and osteophyte formation (proliferative component). A more erosive appearance may simulate inflammatory arthritides, such as rheumatoid arthritis (RA), whereas a more proliferative appearance with extensive osteophyte formation may simulate a benign neoplasm, such as an osteoma or osteochondroma.

Management. The changes to the joint produced by DJD cannot be reversed by any known treatment. Treatment is directed toward unloading the forces on the abnormally loaded joint, relieving secondary inflammation with antiinflammatory drugs, and increasing joint mobility and function (e.g., physiotherapy).

Rheumatoid Arthritis

Disease mechanism. RA is a heterogeneous group of systemic disorders that manifests mainly as synovial membrane inflammation in several joints. The TMJ becomes involved in approximately half of affected patients. The characteristic imaging findings are a result of villous synovitis, which leads to formation of synovial granulomatous tissue (pannus) that grows into fibrocartilage and bone, releasing enzymes that destroy the articular surfaces and underlying bone.

Clinical features. RA is more common in females and can occur at any age but increases in incidence with increasing age. A juvenile variant is discussed separately. Usually the small joints of the hands, wrists, knees, and feet are affected in a bilateral, symmetric fashion. TMJ involvement is variable; when the TMJ is affected, involvement is often bilateral and often occurs later than in other joints. Patients with TMJ involvement complain of swelling, pain, tenderness, stiffness on opening, limited range of motion, and crepitus. The chin appears receded, and an anterior open bite is a common finding because the condyles settle in an anterosuperior position as the articulating components are progressively destroyed.

Imaging features. CT imaging allows detailed assessment of the osseous changes associated with RA. MRI may demonstrate the pannus, joint effusions, marrow edema, and disc abnormalities. The use of gadolinium as an MRI contrast agent has been shown to permit early detection of the inflammatory changes in joints with RA. The initial changes of RA may be generalized osteopenia (decreased density) of the condyle, and temporal component and synovial inflammation. The pannus that develops may destroy the disc resulting in diminished width of the joint space. Bone erosions by the pannus most often involve the articular eminence and the anterior aspect of the condylar head. Erosion

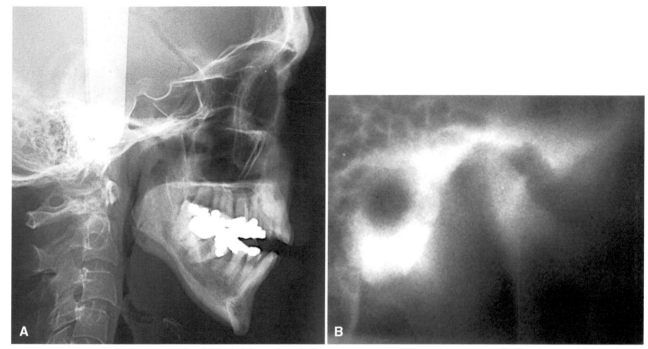

Fig. 30.24 Rheumatoid arthritis. (A) Lateral cephalometric image illustrates a steep mandibular plane and anterior open bite. (B) Lateral tomogram *(closed position)* illustrates a large erosion of the anterosuperior condylar head accompanied by severe erosions of the temporal component, including the articular eminence.

of the anterior and posterior condylar surfaces at the attachment of the synovial lining may result in a "sharpened pencil" appearance of the condyle. Erosive changes may be so severe that the entire condylar head is destroyed, with only the neck remaining as the articulating surface. Similarly, the articular eminence may be destroyed to the extent that a concavity replaces the normally convex eminence. Such erosions permit anterosuperior positioning of the condyle when the teeth are in maximal intercuspation, resulting in an anterior open bite (Fig. 30.24). Joint destruction eventually leads to secondary DJD. Subchondral sclerosis and flattening of articulating surfaces as well as subchondral cyst and osteophyte formation may occur. Fibrous ankylosis or, in rare cases, osseous ankylosis may occur (Fig. 30.25) with reduced mobility related to the duration and severity of the disease.

Differential interpretation. The differential interpretation includes severe DJD and psoriatic arthritis. Osteopenia and severe erosions, particularly of the articular eminence, are more characteristic of RA. Involvement of other joints is also suggestive; a medical workup is required when RA is suspected. Psoriatic arthritis may be considered when the patient has a history of skin lesions.

Management. Treatment is directed toward pain relief (analgesics), reduction or suppression of inflammation (e.g., nonsteroidal antiinflammatory drugs [NSAIDs], antirheumatic drugs, corticosteroids), and preservation of muscle and joint function (physiotherapy). Joint replacement surgery may be necessary in patients with severe joint destruction.

Juvenile Idiopathic Arthritis

Disease mechanism. JIA, formerly known as juvenile RA, juvenile chronic arthritis and Still disease, is a chronic rheumatologic inflammatory disease that manifests before age 16 years (mean age, 5 years). JIA is characterized by chronic, intermittent synovial inflammation that results in synovial hypertrophy, joint effusion, and swollen, painful joints. As the disease progresses, cartilage and bone are destroyed. The rheumatoid factor may be absent; hence the preferred terminology of

JIA rather than juvenile RA. JIA differs from adult RA in that it has an earlier onset, and systemic involvement usually is more severe. TMJ involvement occurs in approximately 40% of patients and may be unilateral or bilateral.

Clinical features. JIA more commonly affects females. Children with JIA may have systemic symptoms, including lethargy and pain. The TMJs in these patients are often asymptomatic, even when active disease affects the joints. When symptoms are present, they include pain in the muscles of mastication, pain and swelling over the joints, and limitations in mandibular movement. Unilateral onset is common, but contralateral involvement may occur as the disease progresses. Severe TMJ involvement results in the inhibition of mandibular growth. Affected patients may have micrognathia and posteroinferior chin rotation, resulting in a facial appearance known as "bird face," which also may be accompanied by an anterior open bite. The degree of micrognathia is proportional to the severity of joint involvement and is worse with earlier onset of the disease. Additionally, when only one TMJ is involved, or if one side is more severely affected, the patient may have a mandibular asymmetry with the chin deviated to the affected side.

Imaging features. MRI with gadolinium contrast agent is the modality of choice for assessing patients with JIA because it can demonstrate early synovial inflammation, even in asymptomatic patients, before bone destruction occurs. CT imaging can be performed for detailed assessment of osseous changes, whereas panoramic and cephalometric images are useful for evaluation of growth disturbances. Osteopenia (decreased density) of the affected TMJ components may be the only initial radiographic finding. Erosion of the articular eminence may result in the appearance of a large glenoid fossa. The condyle may be pointed (pencil-shaped) or concave, or completely destroyed. As a result of bone destruction, the condylar head typically is positioned anterosuperiorly in the mandibular fossa (Fig. 30.26).

Because the inflammatory response is intermittent, the cortex of the joint surfaces may reappear during quiescent periods, and the surfaces appear flattened. Secondary degenerative changes manifesting as sclerosis

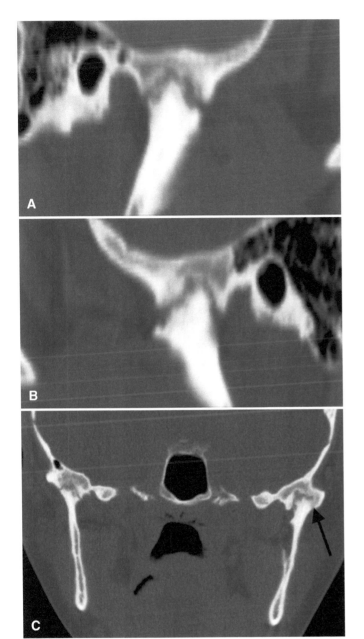

Management. Early, aggressive management of JIA has resulted in improved outcomes. Medical treatments include NSAIDs, methotrexate, and biologic agents. Orthodontics and orthognathic surgery are often required to improve dentofacial form and function.

Psoriatic Arthritis and Ankylosing Spondylitis

Psoriatic arthritis and ankylosing spondylitis are seronegative, systemic arthritides that may affect the TMJs. Psoriatic arthritis occurs in patients with psoriasis of the skin, with inflammatory joint disease occurring in 7% of patients. Ankylosing spondylitis occurs predominantly in males and progresses to spinal fusion. TMJ imaging changes seen in these disorders may be indistinguishable from changes caused by RA, although occasionally a profound sclerotic change is seen in psoriatic arthritis.

Progressive Condylar Resorption

Disease mechanism. Progressive condylar resorption (PCR), otherwise known as idiopathic condylar resorption or condylosis is a condition leading to loss of bone mass of the mandibular condyle, not attributable to other destructive conditions (i.e., RA, DJD, or septic arthritis). PCR also may be related to the condition first described in the 1960s by Boering as "Boering's arthrosis."

During the first decade of growth, the mandibular condyle appears normal, but there is significant resorption of the condylar head, typically during adolescence. The etiology of PCR is unknown, although it is theorized to be the result of decreased biologic adaptation to increased mechanical loading in a susceptible population of young females. Also, a hormonal influence has also been postulated. An association with specific skeletal relationships, namely steep mandibular plane angle and class II jaw relationship, have been noted. Displacement of the articular disc away from its normal position also may be a risk factor. Many cases have been reported to occur after orthognathic surgery.

Clinical features. PCR affects mainly females during the second decade of life. It usually is an incidental finding on a panoramic image, or the patient may develop a mandibular asymmetry, signs and symptoms of TMJ dysfunction, or both. PCR may be unilateral or bilateral. As the condylar changes progress, the patient often develops an anterior open bite.

Imaging features. On a panoramic image, the mandibular condyle often demonstrates flattening and apparent elongation of the anterior surface with a posterior inclination of the condylar head and neck (Fig. 30.27). In addition, there also may be bowing of the posterior surface of the ramus. Together these features have been described as having a "toadstool" appearance. Secondary hypoplasia of the ipsilateral mandible is seen due to loss of the normal growth center within the affected condyle. This is evident by shortening of the ramus and deepening of the antegonial notch. More detailed imaging with CBCT or MDCT may demonstrate erosion of the articulating surface of the condyle. Progressive erosion of bone mass leads to loss of the vertical height of the condyle, and eventual complete resorption of the condyle can occur in some cases. Involvement of the temporal component also may be seen. An anterior open bite can develop as condylar height is lost and the mandible counter-rotates.

Differential interpretation. None of the radiologic features of PCR are unique to this condition; rather, they overlap with other arthritic conditions affecting the TMJs. Diagnosis requires consideration of the clinical presentation with the imaging features, and elimination of other possible diagnoses, including resorption secondary to JIA and severe DJD.

Management. The management of PCR is difficult because orthognathic surgery and orthodontic therapy done to correct occlusal discrepancies or asymmetry may exacerbate the condition. Relapse after orthographic surgery is common. Disc repositioning, costochondral grafts, and alloplastic TMJ replacement also have been advocated.

Fig. 30.25 (A and B) Corrected sagittal reconstructed multidetector computed tomography (MDCT) images with bone algorithm of the right and left joints of a case of rheumatoid arthritis. Note the irregular surface of the condyle and articular eminence and that the shapes are similar to opposing pieces of a puzzle, suggesting the possibility of fibrous ankylosis. Because of erosion of the articular eminence, the condyles have an abnormal anterior position near the residual articular eminence. (C) Coronal MDCT image of the same case. Note osseous ankylosis on the lateral aspect of the left joint *(arrow).*

and osteophyte formation may be superimposed on the rheumatoid changes. Hypomobility at maximal opening is common, and fibrous ankylosis may occur in some cases. An abnormal disc shape is often observed in patients with long-term TMJ involvement. Manifestations of inhibited mandibular growth, such as deepening of the antegonial notch, diminished height of the ramus, and dorsal bending of the ramus and condylar neck, also may occur unilaterally or bilaterally, resulting in an obtuse angle between the mandibular body and the ascending ramus.

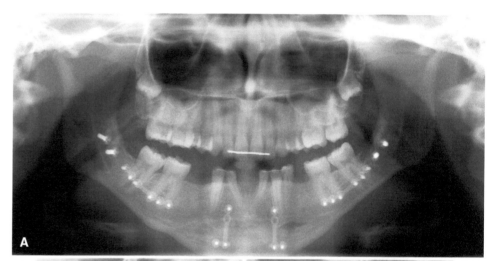

Fig. 30.26 (A and B) Corrected sagittal reconstructed multidetector computed tomography images of juvenile idiopathic arthritis. Note the severe erosion of the articular eminences and the condyles, and the abnormal anterior positioning of both condyles. (C) Coronal computed tomography image of the same case shows small remnants of the condylar heads after severe erosion.

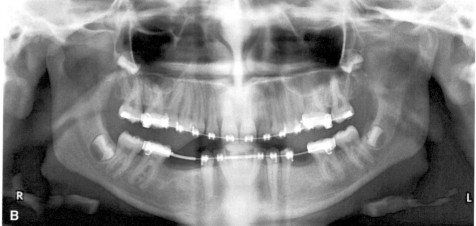

Fig. 30.27 (A) Panoramic image of progressive condylar resorption in a young female patient. There is loss of bone structure of the mandibular condyles due to severe resorption. The anterior surfaces of the condyles appear flattened and elongated. (B) Panoramic image of the same patient before orthognathic surgery shows normal condylar morphology.

Septic Arthritis

Disease mechanism. Septic or infectious arthritis is an inflammatory condition involving the TMJ that can result in joint destruction. Compared with the incidence of DJD and RA in the TMJ, septic arthritis is rare. Septic arthritis of the TMJ may be caused by direct spread of organisms from an adjacent cellulitis, or from parotid, otic, or mastoid infections. It also may occur by direct extension of osteomyelitis involving the mandibular body and ramus. Hematogenous spread from a distant, often occult, nidus also has been reported. Trauma and immunosuppression are also potential etiologic factors.

Clinical features. Individuals can be affected at any age, and the condition shows no sex predilection. It usually occurs unilaterally. The patient may have redness and swelling over the joint, trismus, severe pain on opening, inability to occlude the teeth, large, tender cervical lymph nodes, and fever and malaise. The mandible may be deviated to the unaffected side as a result of joint effusion.

Imaging features. CBCT, MDCT, and MRI are most useful for examining cases of suspected septic arthritis. No imaging signs may be present in the acute stages of the disease, although the space between the condyle and the roof of the mandibular fossa may be widened because of inflammatory exudate in the joint spaces. Osteopenic (radiolucent) changes involving the osseous components of the joint as well as the mandibular ramus may be evident. More obvious bony changes may be seen approximately 7 to 10 days after the onset of clinical symptoms. As a result of the osteolytic effects of inflammation, the condylar articular cortex may become slightly radiolucent, erosions of the surface of the condyle and articular eminence may be seen, sequestra may be identified, and there may be periosteal new bone formation (Fig. 30.28).

Inflammatory changes that may accompany septic arthritis can be seen in CT images, such as opacification of mastoid air cells, osteomyelitis of the mandible, and cellulitis of the surrounding soft tissue. MRI, with T_2-weighted images, may show muscle enlargement and edema, joint effusion, or abscess. Nuclear medicine may have a role in the diagnosis because ^{99m}Tc bone imaging shows increased bone metabolism within the involved osseous components, especially the condyle. Furthermore, a positive nuclear medicine examination with gallium (^{67}Ga) can confirm the presence of infection. As the disease progresses, the condyle and articular eminence, including the disc, may be destroyed. DJD is a common long-term sequela, and fibrous or osseous ankylosis may occur after the infection subsides. If the disease occurs during the period of mandibular growth, manifestations of inhibited mandibular growth may be evident in the diagnostic images.

Differential interpretation. The diagnosis of septic arthritis is ideally made by identification of organisms in joint aspirate, although cultures occasionally remain negative. The imaging changes caused by septic arthritis may mimic the changes of severe DJD or RA, although septic arthritis usually occurs unilaterally. Also, the patient often has clinical signs and symptoms of infection.

Management. Management can include antimicrobial therapy, drainage of effusion, arthrocentesis, and joint rest. Physiotherapy to reestablish joint mobility is initiated after the acute phase of infection has passed.

Articular Loose Bodies
Disease Mechanism

Articular loose bodies are calcifications of varying origin that may be located in the synovium, inside the capsule in the joint spaces, or outside the capsule in soft tissue. They appear on images as radiopaque entities

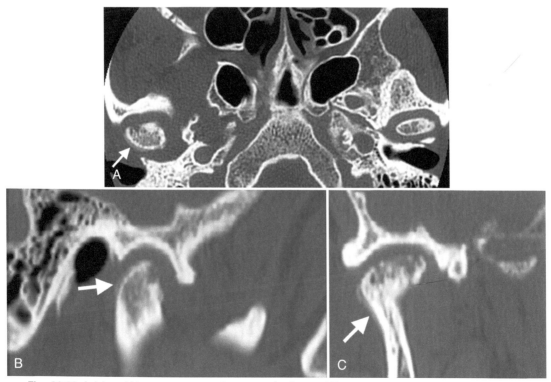

Fig. 30.28 Axial multidetector computed tomography image (A), corrected sagittal (B), and coronal (C) reconstructed computed tomography image of a case of septic arthritis involving the right joint. Note the erosions, sclerosis, and periosteal reaction that extends along the back of the condyle and lateral condylar neck *(arrows)*.

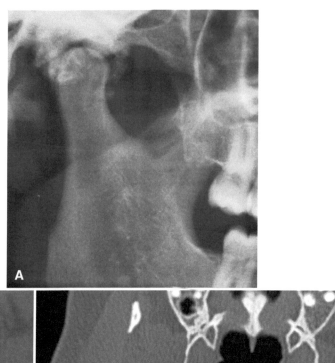

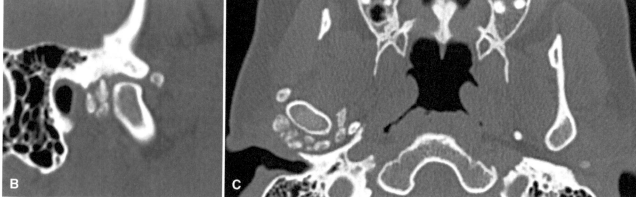

Fig. 30.29 (A) Cropped panoramic image of a right joint involved with synovial chondromatosis. (B) Sagittal computed tomography reformat image. (C) Axial multidetector computed tomography image revealing multiple ossified bodies surrounding the condyle and within the joint capsule.

seen around or superimposed over the condylar head. The loose bodies may represent bone that has separated from joint components in DJD (joint mice), hyaline cartilage metaplasia (calcification) that occurs in synovial chondromatosis, crystals deposited in the joint space in crystal-associated arthropathy (chondrocalcinosis), or tumoral calcinosis associated with renal disease. In rare cases, chondrosarcoma also may mimic the appearance of articular loose bodies.

Synovial Chondromatosis

Disease mechanism. Synovial chondromatosis, also known as osteochondromatosis or chondrometaplasia, is an uncommon benign disorder characterized by metaplastic formation of multiple cartilaginous and osteocartilaginous nodules within the synovial membrane of the joints. Some of these nodules may detach from the synovial tissues, and form loose bodies in the joint space where they persist and increase in size, being nourished by synovial fluid. This condition is more common in the axial skeleton than in the TMJ. When the cartilaginous nodules ossify, the term *synovial osteochondromatosis* is appropriate.

Clinical features. Females are more commonly affected in the TMJ ̖ males. Patients may be asymptomatic or may complain of preau- ̖ swelling, pain, a change in occlusion, and a decreased range of ̖ ̖Some patients have crepitus or other joint noises. The condition ̖ ̖urs unilaterally.

Imaging features. The osseous components may appear normal or may exhibit osseous changes similar to changes in DJD. The joint space may be widened, and if ossification of the cartilaginous nodules has occurred, a radiopaque body or several radiopaque loose bodies may be seen surrounding the condylar head (Fig. 30.29). There is considerable variation in the size of these ossified loose bodies. CT imaging can indicate the location of these calcifications and confirm that they represent ossifications. Morphological changes to the joint that are reminiscent of DJD may be seen, as well as reactive sclerosis of the glenoid fossa and condyle. Occasionally, erosion through the glenoid fossa roof into the middle cranial fossa may occur, which is best detected with CT imaging. MRI can detect joint space effusion and enlargement, and may be useful in defining the tissue planes between the synovial chondromatosis mass and the surrounding soft tissue.

Differential interpretation. The appearance of synovial osteochondromatosis cannot always be differentiated from chondrocalcinosis; however, the ossified bodies in osteochondromatosis are often larger and may have a peripheral cortex that identifies their bony nature. Conditions that appear similar include DJD with joint mice (detached osteophytes), or chondrosarcoma or osteosarcoma. Sarcomas may be accompanied by severe bone destruction, which would help in differentiating the condition from synovial chondromatosis.

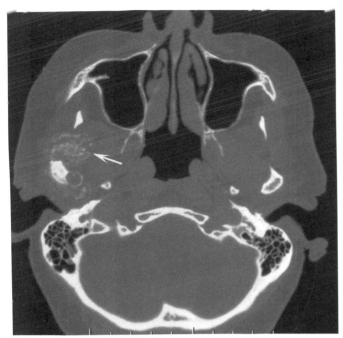

Fig. 30.30 Axial bone algorithm multidetector computed tomography image of chondrocalcinosis. Note the calcifications anterior to the right condyle *(arrow)* and the large erosion involving the medial pole of the condyle. There is also profound sclerosis of the lateral pole.

Treatment. Treatment consists of removal of the loose bodies and resection of the abnormal synovial tissue in the joint by arthroscopic or open joint surgery.

Chondrocalcinosis

Disease mechanism. Chondrocalcinosis or pseudogout is a condition that is characterized by acute or chronic synovitis and precipitation of calcium pyrophosphate dihydrate crystals in the joint space. It differs from classical gout, in which monosodium urate monohydrate crystals are precipitated; hence the term "pseudogout."

Clinical features. The more commonly affected joints are the knee, wrist, hip, shoulder, and elbow; TMJ involvement is uncommon and the condition occurs unilaterally. Patients most often complain of pain and swelling over the joint; however, some patients are asymptomatic.

Imaging features. The appearance of chondrocalcinosis may simulate synovial chondromatosis, described previously. Often the radiopacities within the joint space are finer and have a more even distribution than in osteochondromatosis (Fig. 30.30). Crystal deposition may also extend to tissues surrounding the joint. Bone erosions and profound sclerosis of the osseous components have been described. Erosions of the glenoid fossa may be present, which require CT imaging for detection. Soft tissue swelling and edema of the surrounding muscles may be seen with MRI.

Differential interpretation. The differential interpretation is the same as for synovial chondromatosis.

Management. Management consists of surgical removal of the large crystalline masses. Steroids, aspirin, and NSAIDs may provide relief. Colchicine may be used to alleviate acute symptoms and for prophylaxis.

Trauma
Effusion

Disease mechanism. Effusion is an influx of fluid into the joint and may be associated with trauma, soft tissue abnormalities, such as disc displacement, or arthritic conditions. Effusions within the joint after trauma most often represent hemorrhage into the joint spaces (hemarthrosis).

Clinical features. The patient may have swelling over the affected joint, pain in the TMJ preauricular region or ear, and limited range of motion. Patients may also complain of the sensation of fluid in the ear, tinnitus, hearing difficulties, and difficulty occluding the posterior teeth.

Imaging features. Joint effusions are best seen on T_2-weighted MRI as high signal (white) areas around the condyle. The involved joint spaces would be increased in width (see Fig. 30.18).

Differential interpretation. Effusion secondary to trauma must be differentiated from other conditions manifesting with effusion, including disc displacement and arthritis. Evidence of condylar fracture may be detected in cases of trauma. Patient history and clinical examination should be helpful.

Management. Treatment may include antiinflammatory drugs, although surgical drainage of the effusion occasionally is necessary.

Condylar Dislocation

Disease mechanism. Condylar dislocation is abnormal positioning of the mandibular condyle out of the mandibular fossa but within the joint capsule. It usually occurs bilaterally and most commonly, the dislocation is in an anterior direction. Dislocation may be caused by trauma and is often associated with a condylar fracture. Forced mouth opening, such as during an intubation procedure, also may lead to dislocation. Loose ligaments and joint capsule may predispose to chronic TMJ dislocation. Dislocation also may rarely occur superiorly through the roof of the glenoid fossa into the middle cranial fossa as a result of trauma.

Clinical features. In anterior dislocation, patients are unable to close the mandible to maximal intercuspation. Some patients cannot reduce the dislocation, whereas others may be able to reduce the mandible by manipulation. Associated pain and muscle spasm often are present.

Imaging features. CBCT and MDCT are most useful for evaluating the relationships of the osseous structures. Imaging shows the condyle positioned outside the glenoid fossa, most commonly anterior and superior to the summit of the articular eminence. Signs of an associated condylar fracture also may be present.

Differential interpretation. In patients with mandibular hypermobility, the condyles may translate anterior and superior to the articular eminence on opening. Clinical correlation to confirm that the patient cannot close the jaw normally is important to make the diagnosis of dislocation.

Management. Treatment consists of manual manipulation of the mandible to reduce the dislocation. Surgery occasionally is necessary to achieve reduction, especially in protracted cases.

Fracture

Disease mechanism. Fractures of the TMJ may occur within the condylar head (intracapsular) or in the condylar neck (extracapsular). Condylar neck fractures are most common and are often accompanied by dislocation of the condylar head. Condylar head fractures may be horizontal, vertical, or compression fractures. Rarely, the fracture may involve the temporal component. Unilateral fractures, which are more common than bilateral fractures, may be accompanied by a parasymphyseal or mandibular body fracture on the contralateral side.

Clinical features. The patient may have swelling over the TMJ, pain, limited range of motion, deviation to the affected side, and malocclusion or an anterior open bite. Some TMJ fractures may be asymptomatic and may not be discovered at the time of trauma. Instead, such traumatic injuries may come to light as incidental findings at a later time when images are obtained for other reasons. Condylar fractures should

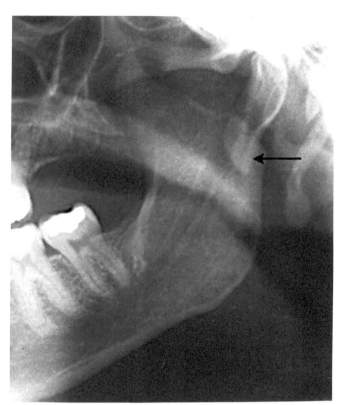

Fig. 30.31 Panoramic image of condylar neck fracture. *Arrow* points to overlapped fragments, as evidenced by increased radiopacity. There is also a step defect evident along the posterior border of the ramus.

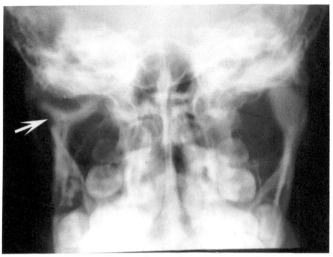

Fig. 30.32 Open mouth Towne image demonstrates a flattened appearance of the right mandibular condyle due to a compression fracture *(arrow)*.

ruled out if the patient has a history of an impact to the mandible, especially to the mental region.

If a condylar fracture occurs during the period of mandibular growth, growth may be disrupted because of damage to the condylar growth center. The degree of subsequent hypoplasia is related to the severity of the injury and the stage of mandibular development at the time of injury (younger patients have more profound hypoplasia). Patients younger than 10 years old have a higher remodeling potential and may have less deformity compared with older patients, although injuries in patients younger than 3 years old tend to produce severe asymmetries. Injury to the joint may result in hemorrhage or effusion into the joint spaces that may eventually form bone during the healing process, and this may result in ankylosis and limited joint function.

Imaging features. In relatively recent condylar neck fractures, a radiolucent line limited to the outline of the neck may be visible. This line may vary in width, depending on the amount of distraction between the fragments. When the bone fragments are well aligned, the line is narrow. However, when there is greater displacement between the fragments, the line may become wider line. If the bone fragments overlap, an area of apparent increased radiopacity may be seen (the "overlapping fragment sign") instead of the radiolucent line (Fig. 30.31). Careful examination of the cortical outline of the condyle and neck may reveal an irregularity to the normally smooth outline of the bone surface (i.e., a "step defect"). Approximately 60% of condylar fractures show evidence f fragment angulation and a variable degree of displacement of the ure fragments. Displacement of the condylar head most commonly ʼn an anterior and medial direction because of the muscle fiber s of the lateral pterygoid muscle. Fractures of the condylar ʼmmon and may be horizontal, vertical (responsible for ɔ of bifid condyle), or compressive (Fig. 30.32). CBCT

is the preferred imaging modality to evaluate condylar fractures because there is no superimposition of adjacent structures, and customizable renderings of the TMJs may demonstrate the fracture plane to better advantage. Two-dimensional and three-dimensional reformatted images are useful to localize a fractured fragment accurately.

The amount of remodeling seen in the TMJ after a condylar fracture with medial displacement varies considerably. In some cases, the bony fragments may remodel to a form that is essentially normal. Alternatively, the mandibular fossa may remodel, becoming more shallow, to compensate for the new condylar position. The condylar fragment may fuse to the condylar neck or ramus in a new, abnormal position. The condyle eventually may show degenerative changes, including flattening, erosion, osteophyte formation, and ankylosis. These changes are more severe if the condyle is displaced. Condylar fractures also can be associated with damage of the intracapsular soft tissues including the disc, the joint capsule, and the retrodiscal tissues, and with hemarthrosis and joint effusion.

Differential interpretation. The most common difficulty is determining whether a fracture is present or not. Panoramic images made as an initial examination may not disclose a fracture, especially greenstick fractures of the condylar neck because changes in the coronal plane of the bone cannot be appreciated. Supplementation of the panoramic image with a plain image at right angles such as an open-mouth Towne view or CBCT is often necessary to visualize displacements. Occasionally, old fractures that have remodeled may be difficult to differentiate from developmental abnormalities of the condyle.

Management. Management may not be indicated if mandibular function is adequate; otherwise, the fracture is reduced surgically. Physiotherapy may be important to maintain mobility and prevent the development of ankylosis.

Neonatal Fractures

Disease mechanism. The use of forceps during delivery of neonates may result in fracture and displacement of the rudimentary condyle, which later manifests as severe mandibular hypoplasia and lack of development of the glenoid fossa and articular eminence. Such cases have a characteristic radiographic appearance in the panoramic image, having the appearance of a partly opened pair of scissors in place of a normal condyle (Fig. 30.33). This presentation results from the overlapping images of the medially displaced carrot-shaped rudimentary condyle and remnants of the condylar neck.

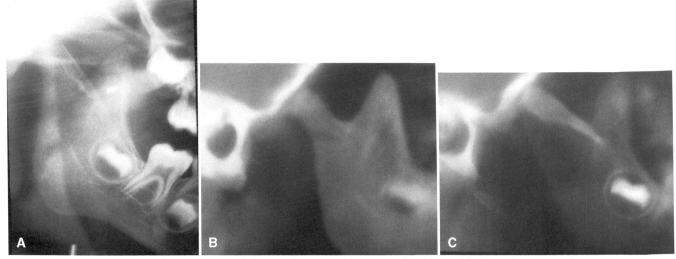

Fig. 30.33 (A) Cropped panoramic image of a neonatal fracture of the right condyle. Note the unusual shape of the coronoid notch, similar to a partially opened pair of scissors. (B) Tomographic image slice of the lateral aspect of the same joint. Note the normal-appearing coronoid notch but the lack of formation of the glenoid fossa and eminence, and the abnormal anterior position of the condyle. (C) Medial tomographic slice of the same case disclosing the fractured segment.

Differential interpretation. This condition often is not diagnosed until later in life, at which time a diagnosis of fracture may be made without a history that the fracture occurred at the time of birth. The condition must be differentiated from developmental hypoplasia of the mandible, which is unrelated to birth injury.

Management. The fracture usually is not treated, but the mandibular asymmetry may be corrected with a combination of orthodontics and orthognathic surgery.

Ankylosis
Disease Mechanism
Ankylosis is a condition in which condylar movement is restricted because of fusion of the intraarticular joint components ("true ankylosis") or a physical impediment caused by structures outside the joint. Intraarticular ankylosis may be bony or fibrous. In bony ankylosis, the condyle or ramus is attached to the temporal or zygomatic bone by an osseous bridge. In fibrous ankylosis, a soft tissue (fibrous) union of joint components occurs. Most unilateral cases are caused by mandibular trauma or infection. Severe arthritis, particularly related to rheumatic conditions, and therapeutic radiation exposure to the joint (for cancer treatment) also may give rise to ankylosis. Extraarticular ankylosis may result from conditions that inhibit condylar movement, such as muscle spasm or fibrosis, myositis ossificans, or coronoid process hyperplasia.

Clinical Features
Patients have a history of progressively restricted jaw opening, or they may have a long-standing history of limited opening. Some degree of mandibular opening usually is possible through flexing of the mandible, although opening may be restricted to only a few millimeters, particularly in the case of bony ankylosis. Patients who develop ankylosis in childhood may have an associated facial asymmetry because of altered growth of the mandible. Pain is not commonly associated with ankylosis.

Imaging Features
In fibrous ankylosis, the articulating surfaces are usually irregular because of erosions. The joint space is usually very narrow, and although the bones are not fused, the two irregular surfaces may appear to fit one

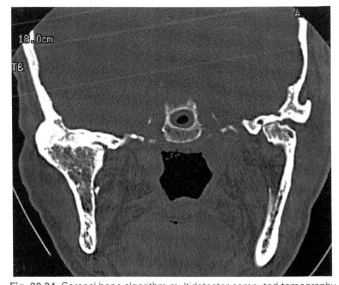

Fig. 30.34 Coronal bone algorithm multidetector computed tomography image of bony ankylosis. The right condyle and ramus are markedly enlarged. The articulating surface is irregular, and the central and lateral aspects are fused to the roof of the glenoid fossa, as evidenced by a lack of joint space. The left condylar articulating surface is eroded, and the joint space is decreased on the medial aspect; these changes are consistent with degenerative joint disease.

another like a jigsaw puzzle (see Fig. 30.25). Little or no condylar movement is seen.

Radiographic signs of remodeling occasionally are visible as the joint components adapt to repeated attempts at mandibular opening. In bony ankylosis, the joint space may be partly or completely obliterated by the osseous bridge, which can vary from a slender segment of bone to a large bony mass (Fig. 30.34). Degenerative changes of the joint components are common. Morphologic changes often occur, such a compensatory progressive elongation of the coronoid processes ar deepening of the antegonial notch in the mandibular ramus on

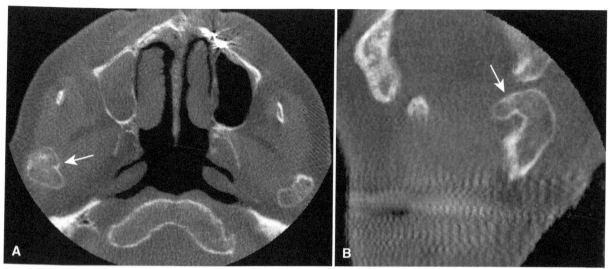

Fig. 30.35 Axial (A) and corrected sagittal (B) cone beam computed tomography reconstructions of an osteochondroma discovered incidentally. Lobulated outgrowth from anterior surface of condyle shows continuity of the cancellous and cortical bone between the normal condyle and the lesion *(arrows)*.

affected side, as a result of muscle function during attempted mandibular opening. Corrected coronal CT images are the best diagnostic imaging method to evaluate ankylosis.

Differential Interpretation

Ankylosis is a sequela to other conditions affecting the joint, and the primary cause must be determined. A history of trauma, infection, arthritis, or previous surgery may help elucidate the etiology and rule out neoplastic disease. Differentiation of fibrous ankylosis from other causes of limited condylar movement is difficult because fibrous tissue is not visible in the diagnostic image.

Management

TMJ ankylosis requires surgical intervention. Gap arthroplasty involves removal of the osseous bridge or creation of a pseudarthrosis below the original joint space. Costochondral grafts are also used. Recurrence of ankylosis after surgery may develop.

Neoplasia
Disease Mechanism

Benign and malignant neoplasms originating in or involving the TMJ are rare. Neoplasms affecting the TMJ may be intrinsic to the joint, developing in the condyle or temporal bone or soft tissue components of the joint, or they may be extrinsic, developing in the adjacent structures, such as the coronoid process or adjacent soft tissues.

Benign Neoplasia

The most common benign intrinsic tumors involving the TMJ are osteochondromas, although there have been sporadic reports of other nonodontogenic neoplasms as well, including osteomas, osteoblastomas, chondroblastomas, fibromyxomas, central giant cell lesions, aneurysmal bone cysts, Langerhan cell histiocytosis, and multiple myeloma. Benign neoplasms and cysts of the mandible (e.g., ameloblastomas, odontogenic keratocysts, simple bone cysts) may involve the entire ramus, and in ̶re cases, may extend into the condyle. In cases of extraarticular ̶osis, in which mandibular movement is restricted but the TMJs ̶ ̶ormal, hyperplasia or a tumor of the coronoid process must ̶ ̶t.

̶tures. Benign condylar neoplasms grow slowly, and may ̶le size before becoming clinically noticeable. Patients

may complain of TMJ swelling, and this may be accompanied by pain and decreased range of motion. Indeed, the symptoms often mimic TMJ dysfunction. The clinical examination may reveal facial asymmetry, malocclusion, and deviation of the mandible to the unaffected side. Tumors of the coronoid process typically are painless, but patients may complain of progressive limitation of mandibular motion.

Imaging features. A benign neoplasm involving the mandibular condyle usually manifests as an irregularly shaped enlargement of the condylar head. There may be decreased trabecular bone density owing to bony destruction or increased density owing to new, abnormal bone formed by the neoplasm. An osteoma or osteochondroma will have the appearance of being attached to, or growing from, the condyle. Osteochondromas are benign neoplasms that most often extend from the anterior surface of the condyle near the insertion of the lateral pterygoid muscle. These bony growths usually have a cartilaginous cap. To differentiate these from osteomas, it is important to note that the internal cancellous bone of the condyle is continuous with the internal structure of the osteochondroma (Fig. 30.35) while an osteoma arises from the periosteal surface and therefore does not show trabecular continuity. Because benign tumors may interfere with normal joint function, secondary bone remodeling or degenerative changes may be seen in the affected joint. Neoplasms involving the coronoid process may also affect TMJ function, which emphasizes the need to image and evaluate the coronoid process when evaluating joint abnormalities.

Differential interpretation. Condylar neoplasms may simulate unilateral condylar hyperplasia because of condylar enlargement. Osteomas and osteochondromas generally create a more irregular appearance, with a bulbous or pedunculated growth pattern, whereas the characteristic condylar shape and proportions are better preserved in condylar hyperplasia. Neoplasms involving the coronoid must be differentiated from coronoid hyperplasia, which differs from a tumor in that the coronoid process remains regular in shape.

Management. Treatment consists of surgical excision of the neoplasm, and occasionally excision of the condylar head or coronoid process.

Malignant Neoplasia

Disease mechanism. Malignant neoplasms involving the TMJs may be primary or, more commonly, metastatic. Primary intrinsic malignant neoplasms of the condyle are extremely rare and include chondrosarcoma, osteosarcoma, synovial sarcoma, and fibrosarcoma of the joint capsule.

Extrinsic malignant neoplasms may represent direct extension of adjacent parotid salivary gland malignancies, rhabdomyosarcoma (particularly in children), or other regional carcinomas from the skin, ear, and nasopharynx. Lesions of Langerhan cell histiocytosis and multiple myeloma may also involve the condyle, as well as metastatic lesions originating in the breast, kidney, lung, colon, prostate, and thyroid gland.

Clinical features. Malignant neoplasms, whether primary or metastatic, may be asymptomatic, or patients may have symptoms of TMJ dysfunction, such as pain, limited mandibular opening, mandibular deviation, and swelling. A patient occasionally is treated for TMJ dysfunction without recognition that the underlying condition is a malignancy.

Imaging features. Malignant primary and metastatic neoplasms involving the TMJ manifest with a variable degree of bone destruction with ill-defined, noncorticated and irregular borders. Most lack the ability to stimulate new bone formation, with the exception of osteosarcoma and chondrosarcoma, which may display a radiopaque component. Chondrosarcoma also may appear as an indistinct, essentially radiolucent destructive lesion of the condyle, depending on the ability of the malignant cells to produce a mineralized matrix. In some cases, the pattern of mineralization may simulate the appearances of the articular loose bodies seen in synovial chondromatosis or chondrocalcinosis (Fig. 30.36).

In the case of metastatic neoplasms, the radiographic appearance is usually nonspecific condylar destruction. Rarely, when a metastatic malignancy has the ability to stimulate bone cells locally, an osteoblastic reaction may be seen, although this does not indicate the site of origin (Fig. 30.37). Fracture of the condyle may be seen as a sequela of destruction of the bony structure of the joint (Fig. 30.38). CT imaging is the imaging modality of choice to view bone involvement, and MRI is useful for displaying the extent of involvement into the surrounding soft tissues.

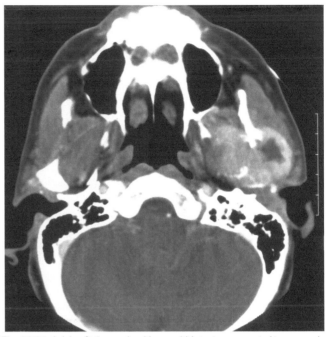

Fig. 30.37 Axial soft tissue algorithm multidetector computed tomography image of a metastatic lesion from a carcinoma of the thyroid gland that has destroyed all of the left mandibular condyle. A large soft tissue mass is also seen.

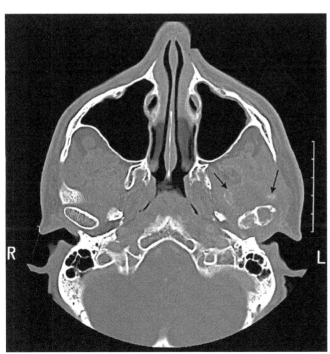

Fig. 30.36 Axial bone algorithm multidetector computed tomography image of chondrosarcoma. A radiolucent destructive lesion is present in the left condylar head, and faint radiopacities (soft tissue calcifications) are visible anterior to the condylar head *(arrows)*.

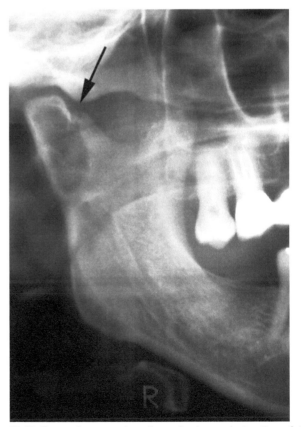

Fig. 30.38 Cropped panoramic radiograph shows destruction of the right condyle from a metastatic lung carcinoma with a secondary fracture *(arrow)*.

Differential interpretation. Joint destruction caused by a malignant neoplasm must be differentiated from the osseous destruction seen in severe DJD. Malignant neoplasm causes profound central bone destruction, whereas the bone resorption seen in DJD is more peripheral. Also, no soft tissue mass is seen in association with DJD but would be expected when a malignant neoplasm is present. Malignancies capable of stimulating local bone cells to deposit a mineralized matrix may simulate joint space calcifications, but they are also associated with severe bone destruction, in contrast to other conditions forming loose joint bodies.

Management. In the case of primary malignant neoplasms, management consists of wide surgical removal of the tumor. Tumor extension to vital anatomic structures may compromise survival. Metastatic lesions involving the TMJ rarely are treated surgically; treatment may include radiotherapy and chemotherapy.

BIBLIOGRAPHY

Disorders of the Temporomandibular Joint

Brooks SL, Brand JW, Gibbs SJ, et al. Imaging of the temporomandibular joint, position paper of the American Academy of Oral and Maxillofacial Radiology. *Oral Surg Oral Med Oral Pathol Oral Radiol Endod.* 1997;83:609–618.

Helkimo M. Studies on function and dysfunction of the masticatory system, II: index for anamnestic and clinical dysfunction and occlusal state. *Sven Tandlak Tidskr.* 1974;67:101–121.

McNeill C, Mohl ND, Rugh JD, et al. Temporomandibular disorders: diagnosis, management, education, and research. *J Am Dent Assoc.* 1990;120:253, 255, 257.

Petrikowski CG, Grace MG. Temporomandibular joint radiographic findings in adolescents. *Cranio.* 1996;14:30–36.

Rugh JD, Solberg WK. Oral health status in the United States: temporomandibular disorders. *J Dent Educ.* 1985;49:398–406.

Wänman A, Agerberg G. Mandibular dysfunction in adolescents, I: prevalence of symptoms. *Acta Odontol Scand.* 1986;44:47–54.

Anatomy of the Temporomandibular Joint

Blaschke DD, Blaschke TJ. A method for quantitatively determining temporomandibular joint bony relationships. *J Dent Res.* 1981;60:35–43.

Drace JE, Enzmann DR. Defining the normal temporomandibular joint: closed, partially open, and open mouth MR imaging of asymptomatic subjects. *Radiology.* 1990;177:67–76.

Hansson LG, Hansson T, Petersson A. A comparison between clinical and radiologic findings in 259 temporomandibular joint patients. *J Prosthet Dent.* 1983;50:89–94.

Ingervall B, Carlsson GE, Thilander B. Postnatal development of the human temporomandibular joint. II. A microradiographic study. *Acta Odont Scand.* 1976;34:133–139.

Larheim TA. Radiographic appearance of the normal temporomandibular joint in newborns and small children. *Acta Radiol Diagn (Stockh).* 1981;22:593–599.

Pullinger AG, Hohender L, Solberg WK, et al. A tomographic study of mandibular condyle position in an asymptomatic population. *J Prosthet Dent.* 1985;53:706–713.

Taylor RC, Ware WH, Fowler D, et al. A study of temporomandibular joint morphology and its relationship to the dentition. *Oral Surg.* 1972;33:1002–1013.

Ten Cate AR. Gross and micro anatomy. In: Zarb GA, Carlsson BJ, Mohl ND, eds. *Temporomandibular Joint and Masticatory Muscle Disorders.* 2nd ed. Copenhagen: Munksgaard; 1994.

Westesson P-L, Kurita K, Eriksson L, et al. Cryosectional observations of functional anatomy of the temporomandibular joint. *Oral Surg Oral Med Oral Pathol.* 1989;68:247–251.

Yale SH, Allison BD, Hauptfuehrer JD. An epidemiological assessment of mandibular condyle morphology. *Oral Surg.* 1966;21:169–177.

Diagnostic Imaging of the Temporomandibular Joint

Bag AK, Gaddikeri S, Singhal A, et al. Imaging of the temporomandibular joint: An update. *World J Radiol.* 2014;28:567–582.

Brooks SL, Brand AW, Gibbs SJ, et al. Imaging of the temporomandibular joint: position paper of the American Academy of Oral and Maxillofacial Radiology. *Oral Surg Oral Med Oral Pathol Oral Radiol Endod.* 1997;83:609–618.

Helms CA, Kaplan P. Diagnostic imaging of the temporomandibular joint: recommendations for use of the various techniques. *AJR Am J Roentgenol.* 1990;154:319–322.

Katzberg RW. Temporomandibular joint imaging. *Radiology.* 1989;170:297–307.

Diagnostic Imaging of the Temporomandibular Joint—*Hard Tissue Imaging*

Christiansen EL, Chan TT, Thompson JR, et al. Computed tomography of the normal temporomandibular joint. *Scand J Dent Res.* 1987;95:499–509.

Tsiklakis K, Syriopoulos K, Stamatakis HC. Radiographic examination of the temporomandibular joint using cone beam computed tomography. *Dentomaxillofac Radiol.* 2004;33:196–201.

Diagnostic Imaging of the Temporomandibular Joint—*Soft Tissue Imaging*

Conway WF, Hayes CW, Campbell RL. Dynamic magnetic resonance imaging of the temporomandibular joint using FLASH sequences. *J Oral Maxillofac Surg.* 1988;46:930–938.

Hansson LG, Westesson PL, Eriksson L. Comparison of tomography and midfield magnetic resonance imaging for osseous changes of the temporomandibular joint. *Oral Surg Oral Med Oral Pathol Oral Radiol Endod.* 1996;82:698–703.

Moses JJ, Salinas E, Goergen T, et al. Magnetic resonance imaging or arthrographic diagnosis of internal derangement of the temporomandibular joint. *Oral Surg Oral Med Oral Pathol.* 1993;75:268–272.

Tomas X, Pomes J, Berenquer J, et al. MR imaging of temporomandibular joint dysfunction: a pictorial review. *Radiographics.* 2006;26:765–781.

Radiographic Abnormalities of the Temporomandibular Joint—*Condylar Hyperplasia*

Gray RJM, Sloan P, Quayle AA, et al. Histopathological and scintigraphic features of condylar hyperplasia. *Int J Oral Maxillofac Surg.* 1990;19:65–71.

Rubenstein LK, Campbell RL. Acquired unilateral condylar hyperplasia and facial asymmetry: report of a case. *ASDC J Dent Child.* 1985;52:114–120.

Shira RB. Facial asymmetry and condylar hyperplasia. *Oral Surg.* 1975;40:567.

Wolford LM, Mehra P, Reiche-Fischel O, et al. Efficacy of high condylectomy for management of condylar hyperplasia. *Am J Orthod Dentofac Orthop.* 2002;121:136–151.

Radiographic Abnormalities of the Temporomandibular Joint—*Condylar Hypoplasia*

Jerell RG, Fuselier B, Mahan P. Acquired condylar hypoplasia: report of a case. *ASDC J Dent Child.* 1991;58:147–153.

Worth HM. Radiology of the temporomandibular joint. In: Zarb GA, Carlsson BJ, Mohl ND, eds. *Temporomandibular Joint Function and Dysfunction.* Copenhagen: Munksgaard; 1979.

Radiographic Abnormalities of the Temporomandibular Joint—*Coronoid Hyperplasia*

Daniels JSM, Ali I. Post-traumatic bifid condyle associated with temporomandibular joint ankylosis: report of a case and review of the literature. *Oral Surg Oral Med Oral Pathol Oral Radiol Endod.* 2005;99:682–688.

Loh FC, Yeo JF. Bifid mandibular condyle. *Oral Surg Oral Med Oral Pathol.* 1990;69:24–27.

McLoughlin PM, Hopper C, Bowley NB. Hyperplasia of the mandibular coronoid process: an analysis of 31 cases and a review of the literature. *J Oral Maxillofac Surg.* 1995;53:250–255.

Satoh K, Ohno S, Aizawa T, et al. Bilateral coronoid hyperplasia in an adolescent: report of a case and review of the literature. *J Oral Maxillofac Surg.* 2006;64:334–338.

Soft Tissue Abnormalities

Dolwick MF, Sanders B. TMJ internal derangement and arthrosis. In: *Surgical Atlas.* St. Louis: Mosby; 1985.

Helms CA, Kaban LB, McNeill C, et al. Temporomandibular joint: morphology and signal intensity characteristics of the disc at MR imaging. *Radiology.* 1989;172:817–820.

Katzberg RW. Temporomandibular joint imaging. *Radiology.* 1989;170:297.

Katzberg RW, Tallents RH, Hayakawa K, et al. Internal derangements of the temporomandibular joint: findings in the pediatric age group. *Radiology.* 1985;154:125–127.

Larheim TA. Current trends in temporomandibular joint imaging. *Oral Surg Oral Med Oral Pathol Oral Radiol Endod.* 1995;80:555–576.

Larheim TA. Role of magnetic resonance imaging in the clinical diagnosis of the temporomandibular joint. *Cells Tissues Organs.* 2005;180:6–21.

Nuelle DG, Alpern MC, Ufema JW. Arthroscopic surgery of the temporomandibular joint. *Angle Orthod.* 1986;56:118–142.

Rammelsberg P, Pospiech PR, Jäger L, et al. Variability of disc position in asymptomatic volunteers and patients with internal derangements of the TMJ. *Oral Surg Oral Med Oral Pathol Oral Radiol Endod.* 1997;83:393–399.

Sano T, Westesson PL. Magnetic resonance imaging of the temporomandibular joint: increased T2 signal in the retro-discal tissue of painful joints. *Oral Surg Oral Med Oral Pathol Oral Radiol Endod.* 1995;79:511–516.

Wilkes CH. Internal derangements of the temporomandibular joint: pathological variations. *Arch Otolaryngol Head Neck Surg.* 1989;115:469–477.

Remodeling and Arthritic Conditions—*Remodeling*

Brooks SL, Westesson PL, Eriksson L, et al. Prevalence of osseous changes in the temporomandibular joint of asymptomatic persons without internal derangement. *Oral Surg Oral Med Oral Pathol.* 1992;73:118–122.

Moffett BC, Johnson LC, McCabe JB, et al. Articular remodeling in the adult human temporomandibular joint. *Am J Anat.* 1964;115:119–141.

Remodeling and Arthritic Conditions—*Degenerative Joint Disease*

Palconet G, Ludlow JB, Tyndall DA, et al. Correlating cone beam CT results with temporomandibular joint pain of osteoarthritic origin. *Dentomaxillofac Radiol.* 2012;41:126–130.

de Leeuw R, Boering G, Stegenga B, et al. Temporomandibular joint osteoarthrosis: clinical and radiographic characteristics 30 years after nonsurgical treatment—a preliminary report. *Cranio.* 1993;11:15–24.

Helenius LMJ, Tervahartiala P, Helenius I, et al. Clinical, radiographic and MRI findings of the temporomandibular joint in patients with different rheumatic diseases. *Int J Oral Maxillofac Surg.* 2006;35:983–989.

Kurita H, Uehara S, Yokochi M, et al. A long-term follow-up study of radiographically evident degenerative changes in the temporomandibular joint with different conditions of disc displacement. *Int J Oral Maxillofac Surg.* 2006;35:49–54.

Radin EL, Paul IL, Rose RM. Role of mechanical factors in pathogenesis of primary osteoarthritis. *Lancet.* 1972;1:519–522.

Sato H, Fujii T, Yamada N, et al. Temporomandibular joint osteoarthritis: a comparative clinical and tomographic study pre- and post-treatment. *J Oral Rehabil.* 1994;21:383–395.

Remodeling and Arthritic Conditions—*Rheumatoid Arthritis*

Gynther GW, Tronje G, Holmlund AB. Radiographic changes in the temporomandibular joint in patients with generalized osteoarthritis and rheumatoid arthritis. *Oral Surg Oral Med Oral Pathol Oral Radiol Endod.* 1996;81:613–618.

Larheim TA, Smith HJ, Aspestrand F. Rheumatic disease of the temporomandibular joint: MR imaging and tomographic manifestations. *Radiology.* 1990;175:527–531.

Syrjänen SM. The temporomandibular joint in rheumatoid arthritis. *Acta Radiol Diagn (Stockh).* 1985;26:235–243.

Remodeling and Arthritic Conditions—*Juvenile Idiopathic Arthritis*

Ganik R, Williams FA. Diagnosis and management of juvenile rheumatoid arthritis with TMJ involvement. *Cranio.* 1986;4:254–262.

Hu Y-S, Schneiderman ED. The temporomandibular joint in juvenile rheumatoid arthritis. I: computed tomographic findings. *Pediatr Dent.* 1995;17:46–53.

Hu Y-S, Schneiderman ED, Harper RP. The temporomandibular joint in juvenile rheumatoid arthritis. II: relationship between computed tomographic and clinical findings. *Pediatr Dent.* 1996;18:312–319.

Karhulahti T, Ylijoki H, Rönning O. Mandibular condyle lesions related to age at onset and subtypes of juvenile rheumatoid arthritis in 15-year-old children. *Scand J Dent Res.* 1993;101:332–338.

Stoll ML, Sharpe T, Beukelman T, et al. Risk factors for temporomandibular joint arthritis in children with juvenile idiopathic arthritis. *J Rheumatol.* 2012;39:1880–1887.

Remodeling and Arthritic Conditions—*Psoriatic Arthritis*

Koorbusch GF, Zeitler DL, Fotos PG, et al. Psoriatic arthritis of the temporomandibular joints with ankylosis. *Oral Surg Oral Med Oral Pathol.* 1991;71:267–274.

Wilson AW, Brown JS, Ord RA. Psoriatic arthropathy of the temporomandibular joint. *Oral Surg Oral Med Oral Pathol.* 1990;70:555–558.

Remodeling and Arthritic Conditions—*Ankylosing Spondylitis*

Locher MC, Felder M, Sailer HF. Involvement of the temporomandibular joints in ankylosing spondylitis (Bechterew's disease). *J Craniomaxillofac Surg.* 1996;24:205–213.

Ramos-Remus C, Major P, Gomez-Vargas A, et al. Temporomandibular joint osseous morphology in a consecutive sample of ankylosing spondylitis patients. *Ann Rheum Dis.* 1997;56:103–107.

Remodeling and Arthritic Conditions—*Septic Arthritis*

Leighty SM, Spach DH, Myall RW, et al. Septic arthritis of the temporomandibular joint: review of the literature and report of two cases in children. *Int J Oral Maxillofac Surg.* 1993;22:292–297.

Sembronio S, Albiero AM, Robiony M, et al. Septic arthritis of the temporomandibular joint successfully treated with arthroscopic lysis and lavage: case report and review of the literature. *Oral Surg Oral Med Oral Pathol Oral Radiol Endod.* 2007;103:e1–e6.

Articular Loose Bodies

Ardekian L, Faquin W, Troulis MJ, et al. Synovial chondromatosis of the temporomandibular joint: report and analysis of eleven cases. *J Oral Maxillofac Surg.* 2005;63:941–947.

Carls FR, von Hochstetter A, Engelke W, et al. Loose bodies in the temporomandibular joint. *J Craniomaxillofac Surg.* 1995;23:215–221.

Chuong R, Piper MA. Bilateral pseudogout of the temporomandibular joint: report of a case and review of the literature. *J Oral Maxillofac Surg.* 1995;53:691–694.

Dijkgraaf LC, Liem RS, de Bont LG, et al. Calcium pyrophosphate dihydrate crystal deposition disease: a review of the literature and a light and electron microscopic study of a case of the temporomandibular joint with numerous intracellular crystals in the chondrocytes. *Osteoarthritis Cartilage.* 1995;3:35–45.

Lustmann J, Zeltser R. Synovial chondromatosis of the temporomandibular joint: review of the literature and case report. *Int J Oral Maxillofac Surg.* 1989;18:90–94.

Orden A, Laskin DM, Lew D. Chronic preauricular swelling. *J Oral Maxillofac Surg.* 1989;47:390–397.

Pynn BR, Weinberg S, Irish J. Calcium pyrophosphate dihydrate deposition disease of the temporomandibular joint: a case report and review of the literature. *Oral Surg Oral Med Oral Pathol Oral Radiol Endod.* 1995;79:278–284.

Yu Q, Yang J, Wang P, et al. CT features of synovial chondromatosis in the temporomandibular joint. *Oral Surg Oral Med Oral Pathol Oral Radiol Endod.* 2007;97:524–528.

Progressive Condylar Resorption

Kobayashi T, Izumi N, Kojima T, et al. Progressive condylar resorption after mandibular advancement. *Br J Oral Maxillofac Surg.* 2012;50:176–180.

Sansare K, Raghav M, Mallya SM, et al. Management-related outcomes and radiographic findings of idiopathic condylar resorption: a systematic review. *Int J Oral Maxillofac Surg.* 2015;44:209–216.

Wolford LM, Gonçalves JR. Condylar resorption of the temporomandibular joint: how do we treat it? *Oral Maxillofac Surg Clin North Am.* 2015;27:47–67.

Trauma—*Effusion*

Emshoff R, Brandimaier I, Bertram S, et al. Magnetic resonance imaging findings of osteoarthrosis and effusion in patients with unilateral temporomandibular joint pain. *Int J Oral Maxillofac Surg.* 2002;31:598–602.

Schellhas KP, Wilkes CH. Temporomandibular joint inflammation: comparison of MR fast scanning with T1- and T2-weighted imaging techniques. *AJR Am J Roentgenol.* 1989;153:93–98.

Schellhas KP, Wilkes CH, Baker CC. Facial pain, headache, and temporomandibular joint inflammation. *Headache.* 1989;29:229–232.

Westesson P-L, Brooks SL. Temporomandibular joint: relationship between MR evidence of effusion and the presence of pain and disc displacement. *AJR Am J Roentgenol.* 1992;159:559.

Trauma—*Dislocation*

Kai S, Kai H, Nakayama E, et al. Clinical symptoms of open lock position of the condyle: relation to anterior dislocation of the temporomandibular joint. *Oral Surg Oral Med Oral Pathol.* 1992;74:143–148.

Ohura N, Ichioka S, Sudo T, et al. Dislocation of the bilateral mandibular condyle into the middle cranial fossa: review of the literature and clinical experience. *J Oral Maxillofac Surg.* 2006;64:1165–1172.

Wijmenga JP, Boering G, Blankestijn J. Protracted dislocation of the temporomandibular joint. *Int J Oral Maxillofac Surg.* 1986;15:380–388.

Trauma—*Fracture*

Choi J, Oh I-K. A follow-up study of condyle fracture in children. *Int J Oral Maxillofac Surg.* 2005;34:851–858.

Dahlström L, Kahnberg KE, Lindahl L. Fifteen years follow-up on condylar fractures. *Int J Oral Maxillofac Surg.* 1989;18:18–23.

Gerhard S, Ennemoser T, Rudisch A, et al. Condylar injury: magnetic resonance imaging findings of the temporomandibular joint soft tissue changes. *Int J Oral Maxillofac Surg.* 2007;36:214–218.

Horowitz I, Abrahami E, Mintz SS. Demonstration of condylar fractures of the mandible by computed tomography. *Oral Surg.* 1982;54:263–268.

Lindahl L, Hollender L. Condylar fractures of the mandible, II: a radiographic study of remodeling processes in the temporomandibular joint. *Int J Oral Surg.* 1977;6:153–165.

Pharoah MJ. Radiology of the temporomandibular joint. In: Zarb GA, Carlsson BJ, Mohl ND, eds. *Temporomandibular Joint and Masticatory Muscle Disorders.* 2nd ed. Copenhagen: Munksgaard; 1994.

Raustia AM, Pyhtinen J, Oikarinen KS, et al. Conventional radiographic and computed tomographic findings in cases of fracture of the mandibular condylar process. *J Oral Maxillofac Surg.* 1990;48:1258–1264.

Schellhas KP. Temporomandibular joint injuries. *Radiology.* 1989;173:211–216.

Zachariades N, Mezitis M, Mourouzis C, et al. Fractures of the mandibular condyle: a review of 466 cases. Literature review, reflections on treatment and proposals. *J Craniomaxillofac Surg.* 2006;34:421–432.

Trauma—*Neonatal Fractures*

Pharoah MJ. Radiology of the temporomandibular joint. In: Zarb GA, Carlsson BJ, Mohl ND, eds. *Temporomandibular Joint and Masticatory Muscle Disorders.* 2nd ed. Copenhagen: Munksgaard; 1994.

Worth HM. Radiology of the temporomandibular joint. In: Zarb GA, Carlsson GE, eds. *Temporomandibular Joint Function and Dysfunction.* Copenhagen: Munksgaard; 1979.

Ankylosis

Ferretti C, Bryant R, Becker P, et al. Temporomandibular joint morphology following post-traumatic ankylosis in 26 patients. *Int J Oral Maxillofac Surg.* 2005;34:376–381.

Rowe NL. Ankylosis of the temporomandibular joint. *J R Coll Surg Edinb.* 1982;27:67–79.

Wood RE, Harris AM, Nortjé CJ, et al. The radiologic features of true ankylosis of the temporomandibular joint: an analysis of 25 cases. *Dentomaxillofac Radiol.* 1988;17:121–127.

Tumors—*Benign Tumors*

James RB, Alexander RW, Traver JG Jr. Osteochondroma of the mandibular coronoid process: report of a case. *Oral Surg.* 1974;37:189–195.

Nwoku AL, Koch H. The temporomandibular joint: a rare localisation for bone tumors. *J Maxillofac Surg.* 1974;2:113–119.

Pharoah MJ. Radiology of the temporomandibular joint. In: Zarb GA, Carlsson BJ, Mohl ND, eds. *Temporomandibular Joint and Masticatory Muscle Disorders.* 2nd ed. Copenhagen: Munksgaard; 1994.

Svensson B, Isacsson G. Benign osteoblastoma associated with an aneurysmal bone cyst of the mandibular ramus and condyle. *Oral Surg Oral Med Oral Pathol.* 1993;76:433–436.

Thoma KH. Tumors of the mandibular joint. *J Oral Surg Anesth Hosp Dent Serv.* 1964;22:157–167.

Worth HM. Radiology of the temporomandibular joint. In: Zarb GA, Carlsson GE, eds. *Temporomandibular Joint Function and Dysfunction.* Copenhagen: Munksgaard; 1979.

Tumors—*Malignant Tumors*

Morris MR, Clark SK, Porter BA, et al. Chondrosarcoma of the temporomandibular joint: case report. *Head Neck Surg.* 1987;10:113–117.

Rubin MM, Jui V, Cozzi GM. Metastatic carcinoma of the mandibular condyle presenting as temporomandibular joint syndrome. *J Oral Maxillofac Surg.* 1989;47:507–510.

Takehana dos Santos D, Cavalcanti MGP. Osteosarcoma of the temporomandibular joint: report of 2 cases. *Oral Surg Oral Med Oral Pathol Oral Radiol Endod.* 2002;94:641–647.

31

Soft Tissue Calcifications and Ossifications

Laurie C. Carter

Disease Mechanisms

The deposition of calcium salts, primarily calcium phosphate, usually occurs in the skeleton. When it occurs in an unorganized fashion in soft tissue, it is referred to as heterotopic calcification. Heterotopic calcifications may develop in a wide variety of unrelated disorders and degenerative processes, and they may be divided into the following three categories: dystrophic calcification, dystrophic mineralization, and metastatic calcification.

Clinical Features

Sites of heterotopic calcification or ossification may not produce signs or symptoms; they are most often detected as incidental findings during imaging examinations made for other purposes.

Imaging Features

Radiopaque entities occurring in the soft tissues are common, and can be present in about 4% of panoramic images (Fig. 31.1). In most cases, the goal is to identify the calcification correctly to determine whether treatment or further investigation is required. Some soft tissue calcifications require no intervention or long-term surveillance, whereas others may be life threatening and the underlying cause requires treatment. When the soft tissue calcification is located adjacent to bone, it can sometimes be difficult to determine whether the calcification is associated with the bone, or in the adjacent soft tissue. Therefore a second radiologic image made at right angles to the first can be useful. Important criteria to consider in arriving at the correct interpretation are the anatomic locations, number, distribution, and shapes of the calcifications. In particular, the determination of the location requires knowledge of soft tissue anatomy such as the positions of lymph nodes, ligaments, blood vessels, cartilage, and the ducts of the major salivary glands.

HETEROTOPIC CALCIFICATIONS

Dystrophic Calcification

Disease Mechanism

Dystrophic calcification results from the precipitation of calcium salts into primary sites of chronic inflammation, or in dead and dying tissue despite normal serum calcium and phosphate levels. This process is usually associated with high local phosphatase activity, an increase in local pH, and anoxic conditions within the dead or dying tissue.

Clinical Features

Common soft tissue sites include the gingiva, tongue, lymph nodes, and cheek. Dystrophic calcifications may produce no signs or symptoms, although the precipitated calcium salts may be palpated as a solid mass, and occasionally, there may be enlargement and ulceration of the overlying soft tissues.

Imaging Features

The radiographic appearance of dystrophic calcifications vary from being barely perceptible, fine, radiopaque grains, to larger, irregular, radiopaque particles that rarely exceed 5 mm in diameter. One or more of these radiopaque entities may be seen, and the calcification may be homogeneous or punctate. The outline of the calcified area is usually irregular or indistinct. Common sites are long-standing, chronically inflamed cysts (Fig. 31.2) and polyps (Fig. 31.3).

Calcified Lymph Nodes

Disease mechanism. Dystrophic calcification occurs in lymph nodes that have been chronically inflamed, and the lymphoid tissue is replaced by hydroxyapatite-like calcium salts, effacing nearly all nodal architecture. The presence of calcifications in lymph nodes implies either active disease or disease that has been previously treated. Nodal calcification is commonly ascribed to granulomatous diseases such as tuberculosis (scrofula or cervical tuberculous adenitis), sarcoidosis, cat scratch disease, bacille Calmette-Guérin vaccination as well as rheumatoid arthritis and systemic sclerosis, lymphoma previously treated with radiation therapy, fungal infections, and malignancy, including metastases from distant calcifying neoplasms (most notably metastatic papillary thyroid carcinoma).

Clinical features. Calcified lymph nodes are generally asymptomatic, and the nodes are first discovered as an incidental finding on a panoramic image. When these nodes can be palpated, they are hard, lumpy, round to oblong masses.

Imaging features

Location. The most commonly involved nodes are located within the submandibular, and superficial and deep cervical node chains. Less commonly, the preauricular and submental nodes are involved. In the submandibular region, the nodes may be located either at or inferior to the inferior border of the mandible near the angle where the image of the calcified node is sometimes superimposed over the inferior portion of the ramus. Lymph node calcifications may affect a single node or a linear series of nodes in a phenomenon known as lymph node "chaining," which is typically seen in cervical nodes (Fig. 31.4).

Periphery. The periphery is well defined and usually irregular. Occasionally, the calcified node may have a lobulated appearance similar to a cauliflower. This irregularity of shape is of great significance in distinguishing node calcifications from other potential soft tissue calcifications in the area.

Internal structure. The internal structure may vary in the degree of radiopacity, giving the impression of a collection of smaller, spherical,

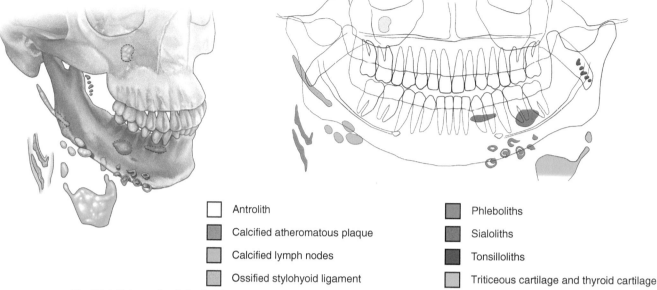

	Antrolith		Phleboliths
	Calcified atheromatous plaque		Sialoliths
	Calcified lymph nodes		Tonsilloliths
	Ossified stylohyoid ligament		Triticeous cartilage and thyroid cartilage

Fig. 31.1 Schematic of the head and neck, and panoramic image demonstrating the typical geometry and locations of selected soft tissue calcifications and ossifications.

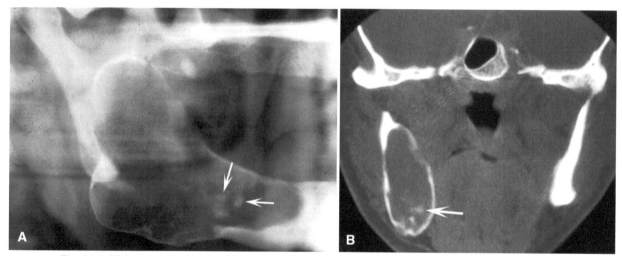

Fig. 31.2 (A) Large residual cyst with poorly defined calcifications seen in a panoramic image *(arrows)*. (B) Coronal multidetector computed tomography image with bone algorithm of the same case, which demonstrates the dystrophic calcification within the cyst *(arrow)*.

or irregular masses. Occasionally, the calcified node may have a lamellar appearance, or the radiopacity may appear only on the surface of the node. This latter appearance has been called an eggshell calcification. The pattern of nodal calcification does not reliably distinguish between benign and malignant disease.

Differential interpretation. Differentiation between a single calcified lymph node and a sialolith in the hilar region of the submandibular gland may be difficult because both may appear near or adjacent to the inferior cortex of the mandible just anterior to the angle. Usually a sialolith has a smooth outline, whereas a calcified lymph node is usually irregular and sometimes lobulated. The differentiation can be made if the patient has symptoms related to the submandibular salivary gland (see Chapter 32). Occasionally, sialography may be necessary to facilitate the differentiation. Another calcification that may have a similar appearance in this region is a phlebolith. However, phleboliths are usually smaller and multiple, with concentric radiopaque and radiolucent rings, and their shape may mimic the cross-section of a blood vessel.

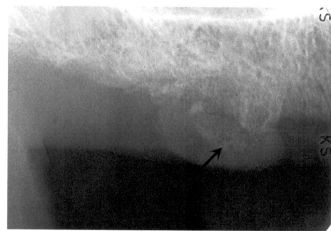

Fig. 31.3 Periapical image shows the soft tissue mass, inflammatory fibrous hyperplasia, emanating from the edentulous ridge. This soft tissue mass contains a dystrophic calcification *(arrow)*.

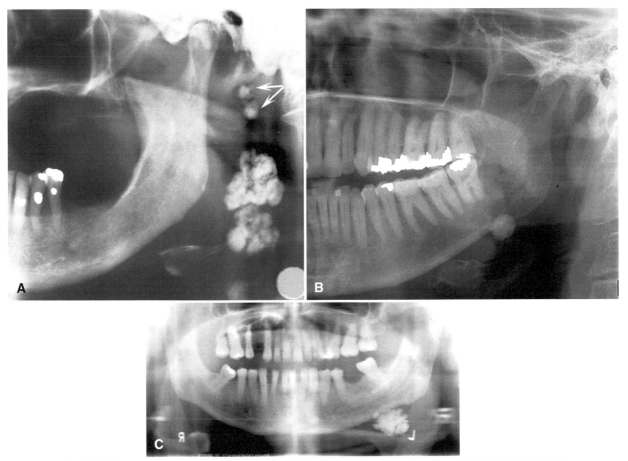

Fig. 31.4 Examples of dystrophic calcification in the lymph nodes. (A) Two large examples positioned behind the ramus with a cauliflower-like shape and two smaller examples in a more superior position *(arrows)*. (B) Submandibular lymph node superimposed on antegonial notch. (C) Larger example.

Management. Calcified lymph nodes usually do not require treatment; however, should the cause be related to an underlying disease process, that disease should be diagnosed and managed.

Dystrophic Calcification in the Tonsils

Disease mechanism. Tonsilloliths or tonsillar calculi are formed when repeated episodes of inflammation enlarge the tonsillar crypts. Incomplete resolution of organic debris (e.g., bacterial biofilms and pus, epithelial cells and food) can serve as the nidus for dystrophic calcification.

Clinical features. Tonsilloliths usually manifest as hard, round, white or yellow objects projecting from the tonsillar crypts, usually of the palatine tonsil. Small calcifications usually produce no clinical signs or symptoms. However, sore throat, swelling, halitosis due to the bacterial production of volatile sulfur compounds, dysphagia, or a foreign body sensation on swallowing have been reported with larger calcifications. Giant tonsilloliths distending lymphoid tissue, resulting in ulceration and extrusion, are much less common. Tonsilloliths have been reported to occur in individuals between 20 and 68 years old, although they are more commonly found in older age groups.

Imaging features

Location. On a panoramic image, tonsilloliths appear as single or multiple radiopaque entities that are superimposed over the mid-portion of the mandibular ramus in the region where the image of the dorsal surface of the tongue is superimposed over the ramus in the region of the oropharyngeal airspaces. Tonsilloliths may also frequently appear immediately inferior to the mandibular canal on a panoramic image (Fig. 31.5). On axial multidetector computed tomography (MDCT) or cone beam computed tomography (CBCT) images, tonsilloliths appear in the soft tissues medial to the mandibular ramus and adjacent to the lateral wall of the oropharyngeal airspace.

Periphery. The most common appearance of tonsilloliths is a cluster of multiple small, ill-defined radiopaque entities of varying sizes. Rarely, this calcification may attain a large size.

Internal structure. Tonsilloliths appear slightly more radiopaque than cancellous bone, and are approximately the same density as cortical bone.

Differential interpretation. The differential interpretation is a radiopaque entity located within the mandibular ramus, such as a dense bone island. When in doubt, a posteroanterior skull or mandible image, or an open-mouth reverse Towne image, may show that the calcification lies adjacent to the medial surface of the ramus. In some cases, MDCT or CBCT may be necessary to precisely localize the entity.

Management. No management is usually required for most tonsillar calcifications. In symptomatic patients, tonsilloliths may be expressed manually, possibly with the patient under sedation to suppress the gag reflex. Large calcifications with associated symptoms require tonsillectomy. Treatment of asymptomatic tonsilloliths may be considered in elderly

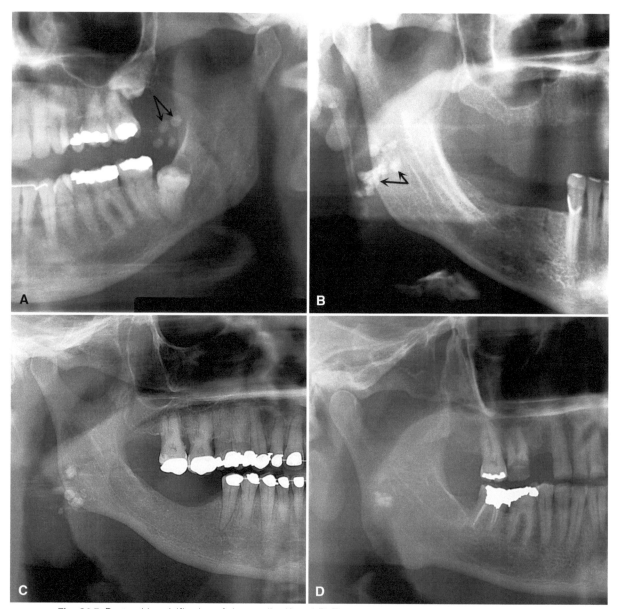

Fig. 31.5 Dystrophic calcification of the tonsils. (A and B) These two examples show positions anterior to the ramus (A) and overlapping the posterior aspect of the ramus (B; *arrows*). Note the calcified stylohyoid ligament. (C and D) Clusters of tonsilloliths superimposed on mandibular ramus.

patients with mechanical deglutition disorders and immunocompromised patients because of the risk for aspiration pneumonia.

Cysticercosis

Disease mechanism. When humans unknowingly ingest eggs or gravid proglottids from the parasite *Taenia solium* (pork tapeworm), the covering of the eggs is digested in the stomach, and the larval form (*Cysticercus cellulosae*) of the parasite is hatched. The larvae penetrate the mucosa, enter the blood vessels and lymphatics, and are distributed as cysticerci in tissues throughout the body—preferentially the brain, muscle, skin, liver, lungs, subcutaneous tissues, and heart. They are also found in oral and perioral tissues, especially the muscles of mastication. Although the glycoprotein-rich cyst wall is greater than 100-μm thick, it rarely elicits any host response when intact. However, in tissues other than the intestinal mucosa the larvae eventually die years after infection,

and are treated as foreign bodies, eliciting a strong inflammatory reaction causing granuloma formation, scarring, and calcification. There is currently an increased incidence of cysticercosis in the southwestern and urban northeastern United States, and the problem is endemic in developing countries in Central and South America, Asia, and Africa, where there is fecal contamination of agricultural soil, and where pork is a valued food.

Clinical features. Mild cases of cysticercosis are completely asymptomatic. The intensity of the signs and symptoms depends on the number of invasive oncospheres present, their location, and the immune response mounted by the host on the parasites. More severe cases have symptoms that range from mild to severe gastrointestinal upset with epigastric pain and severe nausea and vomiting. Invasion of the brain may result in seizures, headache, visual disturbances, acute obstructive hydrocephalus, irritability, loss of consciousness, and death.

Examination of the oral mucosa may disclose palpable, well-circumscribed, soft, fluctuant swellings, which may resemble a mucocele or benign mesenchymal neoplasm.

Imaging features. While alive, the larvae are not visible radiographically. Death of the parasites and development of calcifications in subcutaneous and muscular sites occurs years after the initial infection.

Location. The oral locations of calcified cysticerci include the muscles of mastication and facial expression, the suprahyoid muscles, and the postcervical musculature as well as the tongue, buccal mucosa, and lip.

Periphery and shape. Multiple well-defined elliptical entities that resemble grains of rice are seen.

Internal structure. The internal structure is homogeneous and radiopaque.

Differential interpretation. Cysticercus may appear similar to a sialolith. However, the small size of the calcified nodules of cysticerci and their widespread dissemination, particularly in brain and muscles, are highly suggestive of the diagnosis.

Management. Basic sanitation (e.g., a clean water supply for drinking and washing food that is free of fecal contamination) and proper preparation of pork are needed to eliminate this source of infection. The symptoms that accompany the initial infestation are best treated by a physician using anthelmintic drugs. Adjunctive corticosteroids help stem the inflammatory reaction, and anticonvulsants may prevent epileptic seizures. After the larvae have settled and calcified in the oral tissues, they are harmless. However, it is important to carry out a detailed investigation in each patient to rule out the presence of the parasite in other locations and to perform serologic testing on close contacts to identify a possible source of infection.

Arterial Calcifications

Two distinct patterns of arterial calcification can be identified in imaging examinations and histopathologically: medial calcific sclerosis and calcified atherosclerotic plaque.

Medial Calcific Sclerosis

Disease mechanism. Medial calcific sclerosis or Mönckeberg's medial calcinosis or arteriosclerosis is an age-related degenerative process. The hallmark of this condition is the fragmentation, degeneration, and eventual loss of elastic fibers followed by the deposition of calcium in the internal elastic lamina of the tunica intima, which extends into the medial wall (tunica media) of the vessel.

Clinical features. The vascular calcifications in medial calcific sclerosis are an independent marker of cardiovascular risk, and the highest prevalence occurs in patients with type 2 diabetes. Most patients are asymptomatic initially, although late in the course of the disease, cutaneous gangrene, peripheral vascular disease, and myositis may occur as a result of vascular insufficiency. Patients with encephalotrigeminal angiomatosis (Sturge-Weber syndrome) also develop intracranial arterial calcifications.

Imaging features

Location. Medial calcinosis may involve the facial artery or, less commonly, the carotid artery on panoramic images.

Periphery. The calcific deposits in the artery wall outline the image of the artery. A lateral projection of the artery may show a pair of thin, parallel running, radiopaque lines (Fig. 31.6). The course of these lines may be straight or their path may be more tortuous, and this has been described as a "pipe stem" or "tram-track" appearance. In cross section, the calcified artery wall may demonstrate a circular or ring-like pattern.

Internal structure. There is no internal structure because the diffuse, finely divided calcium deposits occur solely in the medial wall of the vessels.

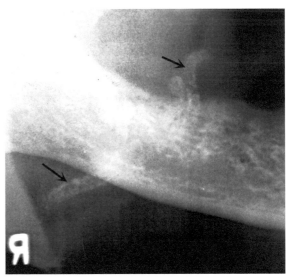

Fig. 31.6 Cropped panoramic image shows calcification of a blood vessel, probably the facial vein *(arrows)*.

Differential interpretation. The radiographic appearance of medial calcific sclerosis is so distinctive as to be pathognomonic of the condition. Clinically, hyperparathyroidism may be considered because medial calcific sclerosis frequently develops as a metastatic calcification in patients with this condition.

Management. Evaluation of the patient for occlusive arterial disease and peripheral vascular disease may be appropriate because it may be difficult to differentiate medial calcific sclerosis from a calcified atherosclerotic plaque on imaging.

Calcified Atherosclerotic Plaque

Disease mechanism. Stenotic atheromatous plaque in the extracranial carotid vasculature is the major contributing source of cerebrovascular embolic and occlusive disease. Dystrophic calcification can develop in the evolution of plaque within the intimal layer of the involved vessel.

Imaging findings

Location. Atherosclerosis first develops at arterial bifurcations as a result of increased endothelial damage from shear forces within the vessel at these sites. When calcification has occurred, these lesions may be visible in panoramic images in the soft tissues of the neck either superior or inferior to the greater cornu of the hyoid bone (where the common carotid artery bifurcates into the external and internal carotid arteries) and adjacent to the third and fourth cervical vertebrae, or the intervertebral space between them (Fig. 31.7).

Periphery. These soft tissue calcifications are usually multiple, irregular in shape, and well defined from the surrounding soft tissues, and they have a vertical linear distribution.

Internal structure. The internal structure is heterogeneously radiopaque with radiolucent voids.

Differential interpretation. Calcified triticeous cartilage and the superior cornu of the thyroid cartilage may be mistaken for an atheromatous plaque, although the uniform size, shape, and location of the calcified laryngeal cartilage skeleton identify these as normal anatomy.

Management. Patients with calcified carotid atheromas are at a heightened risk for a cerebrovascular incident. Significant carotid stenosis (≥50%) has been associated with the identification of calcified atheromata on panoramic images in 84% of cases. Furthermore, calcified atheromata on panoramic images of postmenopausal women is significantly

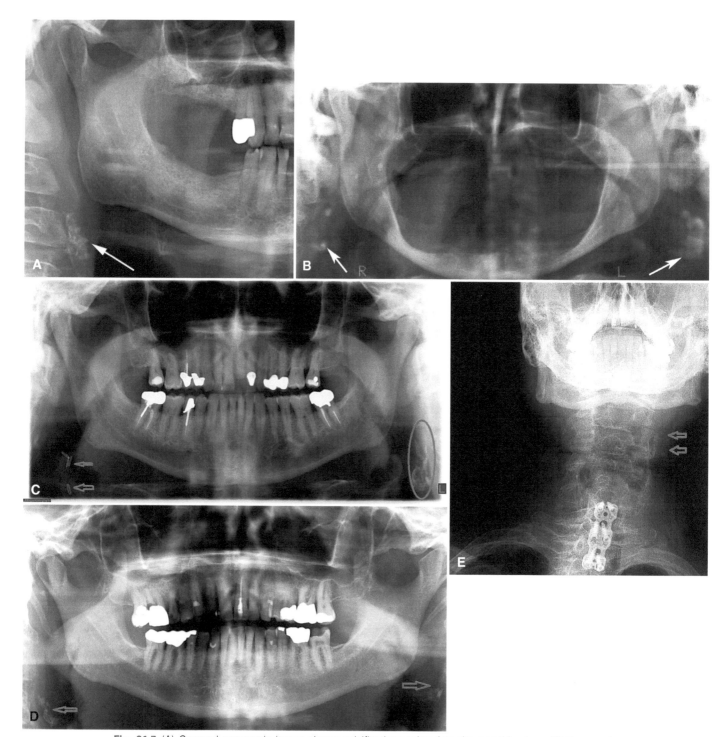

Fig. 31.7 (A) Cropped panoramic image shows calcifications related to the carotid artery. (B) Panoramic image with bilateral examples of calcifications associated with the carotid arteries *(arrows)*. (C) Calcified atheromatous plaque in the left extracranial carotid vasculature at the level of the bulb *(oval)*. Vascular staples in the right side of the neck from prior carotid endarterectomy *(arrows)*. (D) Bilateral calcified carotid atheromata *(arrows)* in a 63-year-old male with type 2 diabetes mellitus. (E) Anteroposterior cervical spine projection in the same case shown in B, displaying calcification in vascular tree *(arrows)*. The patient had fusion of the cervical vertebrae.

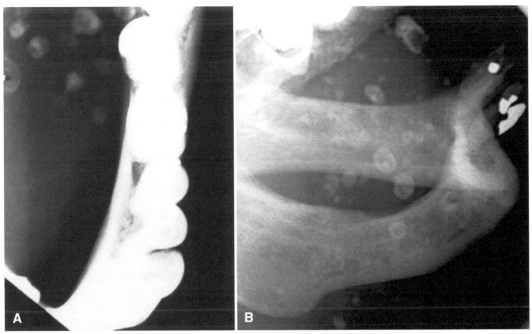

Fig. 31.8 (A and B) Phleboliths are soft tissue dystrophic calcifications found in veins. They are usually associated with hemangiomas.

associated with the presence of aortic arch calcifications, which is a validated risk indicator of adverse events.

Asymptomatic retinal arteriole emboli (ARAE) are thought to be derived from unstable plaques in the carotid bifurcation and their presence has been correlated with fatal and nonfatal strokes. Digital retinal imaging demonstrated ARAE are present in 20% of patients with calcified atheromata on panoramic images compared to 4% without. This refutes speculation that calcified atheromata on panoramic images are stable and unlikely to embolize. The ophthalmologic literature has also documented an association between ARAE, carotid plaques, stenosis, and risk of stroke; patients with retinal emboli have a hazard ratio of 2.40 for stroke-related death compared to those without. Patients with calcified carotid atheromata, especially those with established risk factors for cerebrovascular and cardiovascular disease, should be referred to their physician for further workup.

Idiopathic Calcification

Idiopathic calcification (or calcinosis) results from deposition of calcium in normal tissue despite normal serum calcium and phosphate levels. They are fairly common in the head and neck.

Sialolith

Sialoliths are calcifications found within the ducts of salivary glands, and they will be discussed in Chapter 32.

Phleboliths

Disease mechanism. Phleboliths are calcified thrombi, which can develop from venous blood stagnation in veins, venulae, or the sinusoidal vessels of hemangiomas (especially the cavernous type). Mineralization of thrombi begins in the core of the thrombus and consists of crystals of calcium carbonate-fluorohydroxyapatite.

Clinical features. In the head and neck, phleboliths nearly always signal the presence of a soft tissue hemangioma or vascular malformation. In an adult, phleboliths may be the sole residua of a childhood hemangioma that has long since regressed. The involved soft tissue may be

swollen, throbbing, or discolored by the presence of veins. Hemangiomas often fluctuate in size, associated with changes in body position or during a Valsalva maneuver. Applying pressure to the involved tissue should cause a blanching or change in color if the lesion is vascular in nature. Auscultation may reveal a bruit in cases of cavernous hemangioma, but not in the capillary type.

Imaging features

Location. Phleboliths most commonly are found in hemangiomas (see Chapter 24).

Periphery. In cross section, the shape of a phlebolith is round or oval, and they may measure up to 6 mm in diameter with a smooth periphery. If the involved blood vessel is viewed from the side, the phlebolith may resemble a straight or slightly curved sausage.

Internal structure. The internal structure has a mixed radiolucent and radiopaque appearance and is characterized by concentric laminations, giving phleboliths a bull's-eye or target-like appearance. Radiolucent flow voids may be seen, which may represent the remaining patent portions of the vessel (Fig. 31.8).

Differential interpretation. A phlebolith may have a shape similar to that of a sialolith. However, submandibular sialoliths usually occur singly. But if more than one is present, they are usually oriented in a single line. In contrast, phleboliths are usually multiple and have a more random, clustered distribution. The importance of correctly identifying phleboliths lies in the identification of a possible vascular lesion, such as a hemangioma. This is critical if surgical procedures are contemplated.

Laryngeal Cartilage Calcifications

Disease mechanism. The epiglottis and vocal processes of the arytenoid cartilages are fibroelastic cartilages, whereas all the remaining laryngeal cartilages are made of hyaline cartilage. Endochondral calcification and ossification of the hyaline laryngeal cartilages begins at the age of skeletal maturity and progresses thereafter as a physiologic process.

Clinical features. Calcified laryngeal cartilages are incidental findings on panoramic images, and the calcified triticeous and thyroid cartilages are the laryngeal cartilages that are most frequently seen.

Imaging features

Location. The small, paired triticeous cartilages are found within the lateral thyrohyoid ligaments. The calcified triticeous cartilage can be found on lateral skull or panoramic images within the soft tissues of the pharynx inferior to the greater cornu of the hyoid bone and adjacent to the superior border of the fourth cervical vertebra (C4). The superior cornu of the calcified thyroid cartilage appears medial to C4 and is superimposed on the prevertebral soft tissue (Fig. 31.9).

Periphery. The word **triticeous** means "grain of wheat," and the cartilage measures approximately 7 to 9 mm in length and 2 to 4 mm in width. The periphery of the calcified triticeous cartilage is well defined and smooth, and the geometry is exceedingly regular. Usually only the top 2 to 3 mm of a calcified thyroid cartilage is visible at the lower edge of a panoramic image. Depending on the amount of calcification of the surface, a continuous cortex may or may not be visible.

Internal structure. Calcified triticeous cartilages are generally homogeneously radiopaque, but occasionally, a peripheral cortex can be identified.

Differential interpretation. Calcified triticeous cartilage may be confused with calcified atheromatous plaque in the carotid bifurcation, but the solitary nature and extremely uniform size and shape of the former should be discriminatory.

Management. No management is needed for the calcified laryngeal cartilages, but careful attention to the differences in morphology and location enable the clinician to distinguish between calcified triticeous cartilage and calcified carotid atheromas.

Rhinoliths and Antroliths

Disease mechanism. Calcareous concretions that occur in the nose (rhinoliths) or the antrum of the maxillary sinus (antroliths) arise from the slow accretion of nasal, lacrimal, and inflammatory mineral salts such as calcium phosphate, calcium carbonate, and magnesium, around a nidus. Rarely, concretions form in the frontal or ethmoid sinus.

In the case of a rhinolith, the nidus is usually an exogenous foreign body (e.g., coins, beads, seeds, and fruit pits), especially in pediatric patients. Adult drug smugglers who carry the contraband in packets in the nose sometimes forget to remove one, and a rhinolith develops around it over time. The route of entry of the foreign body is usually anterior, but some may enter the choana posteriorly during sneezing, coughing, or emesis.

The nidus for an antrolith is usually endogenous (e.g., root tip, bone fragment, blood clot, inspissated mucus, ectopic tooth), especially in adults. Dystrophic calcification may occur within chronically inflamed mucosa of the maxillary sinus in long-standing sinusitis. The appearance is usually of small scattered and faint calcifications in the thickened mucosal lining. Occasionally, a noninvasive aspergillosis mycetoma may develop in the antrum, especially in patients with chronic sinus disease. This mycetoma may manifest as a muddy, necrotic fungus ball, or calcareous deposits may transform it into a hard mycolith.

Clinical features. Rhinoliths take approximately 15 years to form and may initially be asymptomatic. As the expanding mass begins to impinge on the mucosa, there may be pain, congestion, and ulceration. The patient may experience nasal obstruction, septal erosion, fetid unilateral purulent or blood-stained rhinorrhea, sinusitis, headache, epistaxis, anosmia, fetor, and fever.

Imaging features

Location. Rhinoliths develop in the nose near the midway point in the inferior meatus where the passage is narrowest (Fig. 31.10A). In contrast, antroliths develop in the antrum of the maxillary sinus (Fig. 31.10C).

Periphery. These stones have various shapes and sizes, depending on the nature of the nidus, but all have well-defined peripheries.

Internal structure. Rhinoliths and antroliths may manifest as mixed radiolucent and radiopaque entities, depending on the nature of the nidus, and sometimes may have laminations. Occasionally, these rhinoliths and antroliths may be homogeneously radiopaque, sometimes exceeding the density of the surrounding bone.

Differential interpretation. The differential interpretation includes osteoma, calcified polyp, odontoma, and surgical ciliated cyst.

Management. Patients should be referred to an otorhinolaryngologist for endonasal or sinus endoscopic surgical removal of the calcification. In some cases, lithotripsy has been used to debulk large rhinoliths.

Metastatic Calcification

Metastatic calcification of the soft tissues in the oral region is caused by conditions that produce elevated serum calcium and phosphate levels, such as hyperparathyroidism (see Chapter 25) or hypercalcemia of malignancy. In addition, metastatic calcification can arise from high serum phosphate concentrations that may be seen in chronic renal failure. Metastatic calcifications usually occur bilaterally and symmetrically, and they are extremely rare.

HETEROTOPIC OSSIFICATIONS

Ossification of the Stylohyoid Ligament
Disease Mechanism

Embryologically, the styloid process arises from the second branchial arch (Reichert cartilage), which consists of four sections that give rise to the styloid process and ossified ligament (the stylohyoid complex). Ossification of the stylohyoid ligament usually extends downward from the base of the skull and commonly occurs bilaterally. However, in rare cases, the ossification begins at the lesser horn of the hyoid, and in fewer still, in a central area of the ligament.

Clinical Features

The elongated styloid process and ossified ligament may be detected by palpation over the tonsil as a hard, pointed structure. Only a few patients have symptoms, and there is very little correlation between the extent of ossification and the intensity of the accompanying symptoms. Symptoms related to the elongated styloid process, which includes the ossified ligament, are termed Eagle syndrome, and they can be related to cranial nerve impingement (classic Eagle syndrome) or impingement of the carotid vessels (carotid artery syndrome). Affected individuals are usually older than 40 years.

When the symptoms are related to a recent history of neck trauma (typically tonsillectomy), the condition is classic Eagle syndrome. The ossified stylohyoid complex and local scar tissue are thought to cause symptoms by impinging on cranial nerves V, VII, IX, X, or XII, all of which pass in close proximity to the styloid process. Symptoms may include vague, nagging to intense pain in the pharynx on speaking, chewing, swallowing, turning the head, or opening the mouth widely, especially on singing or yawning; a foreign body sensation in the throat on swallowing; and tinnitus or otalgia.

Clinical findings without a history of neck trauma constitute carotid artery syndrome. The patient may describe referred pain along the distribution of the internal or external carotid artery, and the pain is the result of mechanical impingement of the involved artery and stimulation of its sympathetic nerve plexus. Symptoms when the internal carotid artery is affected may include eye pain, temporal or parietal headache, migraines, aphasia, visual symptoms, weakness, and transient hemispheric ischemia with vertigo or syncope, notably on turning the

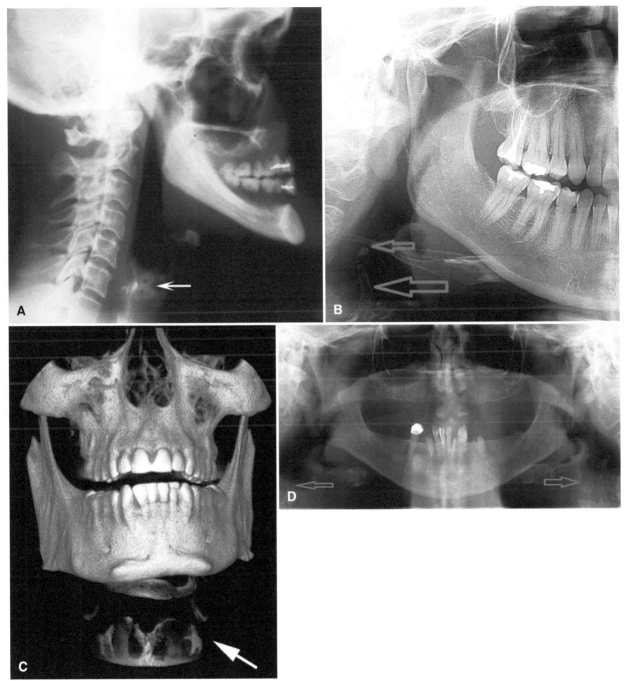

Fig. 31.9 (A) Lateral cephalometric skull image reveals calcification of the thyroid cartilage *(arrow)*. (B) Cropped panoramic image reveals calcification of the triticeous cartilage *(small arrow)* and superior cornu of the thyroid cartilage *(large arrow)*. (C) Three-dimensional reconstruction of a CBCT study shows extensive calcification of the thyroid cartilage *(arrow)*. (D) Bilateral calcification of the superior cornus of the thyroid cartilage *(arrows)*. ([C], Courtesy Dr. S. Perschbacher, Toronto, Ontario, Canada.)

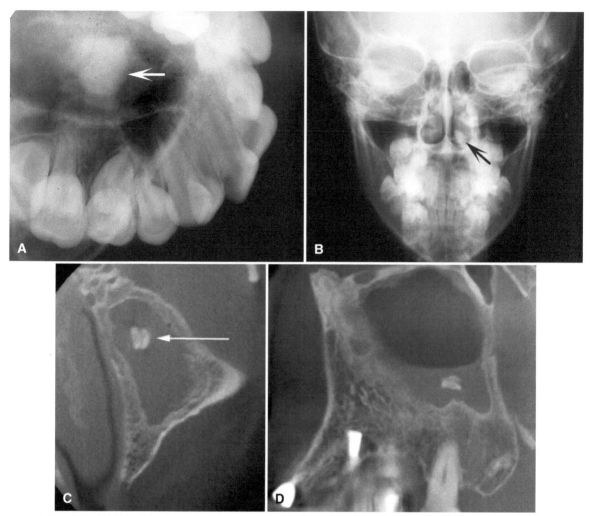

Fig. 31.10 (A) Lateral occlusal film shows a rhinolith *(arrow)* positioned above the floor of the nose. (B) Posteroanterior skull image of the same case shown in A demonstrates that the rhinolith is positioned within the nasal fossa *(arrow)*. (C) Axial cone beam computed tomography (CBCT) image reveals the presence of an antrolith *(arrow)*. (D) Coronal CBCT of the same case shown in C demonstrates the antrolith above the floor of the maxillary sinus.

head to the ipsilateral side. When the external carotid artery is impinged and stimulated, the patient may feel suborbital facial pain. Pain arises by mechanical irritation of the periarterial sympathetic nerve plexus overlying the artery, which produces regional carotidynia; this may occur even in the absence of ossification of the stylohyoid complex. Only deviation of the styloid process, usually medially, is required for the tip of the process to impinge an artery. Carotid artery syndrome is more prevalent than classic Eagle syndrome.

Imaging Features

Ossification of the stylohyoid ligament is detected commonly as an incidental feature on panoramic images. In one study, approximately 18% of a population examined showed ossification of more than 30 mm of the stylohyoid ligament. The ligament may have at least some calcification in individuals of any age.

Location. On a panoramic image, the linear ossification extends forward from the region of the mastoid process and crosses the posteroinferior aspect of the ramus toward the hyoid bone. The hyoid bone is positioned roughly parallel to, or superimposed over, the posterior aspect of the inferior cortex of the mandible.

Shape. The styloid process appears as a long, tapering, thin, radiopaque process that is thicker at its base and projects downward and

forward to almost a needle-like point (see Fig. 31.11). It normally ranges from about 0.5 to 2.5 cm in length. The ossified ligament has roughly a straight outline, but in some cases some surface irregularity may be seen. The farther the radiopaque ossified ligament extends toward the hyoid bone, the more likely it will be interrupted by radiolucent, joint-like junctions (pseudoarticulations).

Internal structure. Small ossifications of the stylohyoid ligament appear homogeneously radiopaque. As the ossification increases in length and girth, the outer cortex of this bone becomes evident as a radiopaque band at the periphery.

Differential Interpretation

When the symptoms accompanying stylohyoid complex ossification do occur, there is distinctive evidence of ligament ossification in the diagnostic images. There is little chance that the complaint will be confused with another entity.

Management

Most patients with ossification of the stylohyoid ligament are asymptomatic, and no treatment is required. Occasionally, the symptoms produced by stylohyoid complex ossification may be similar to symptoms seen with temporomandibular joint disorders. With topical anesthesia

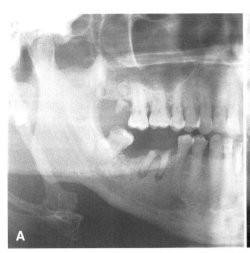
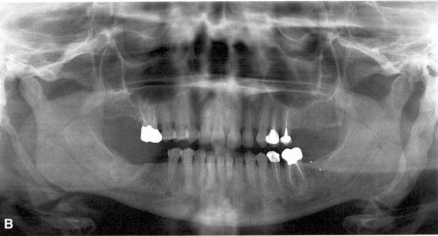

Fig. 31.11 (A and B) Examples of prominent ossification of the stylohyoid ligament. These individuals did not have any symptoms.

to suppress the gag reflex, palpation of the tonsillar fossa to reproduce the symptoms and detect the hard submucosal mass may serve as a diagnostic confirmation. For patients with vague symptoms, a conservative approach of reassurance and steroid or lidocaine injections into the tonsillar fossa would be recommended initially. However, for patients with persistent or intense symptoms, the recommended treatment is amputation of the stylohyoid process (stylohyoidectomy).

Osteoma Cutis
Disease Mechanism
Osteoma cutis is a rare soft tissue ossification in the skin or subcutaneous tissues that manifests as focal development of bone within the dermis physically removed from any original osseous tissue. Osteoma cutis may be primary, occurring in normal tissue without any preexisting condition; or secondary, developing in damaged or disrupted skin. Approximately 85% of cases are secondary and occur as a result of acne of long duration, developing in a scar or chronic inflammatory traumatic or neoplastic dermatosis. They occasionally are found in diffuse scleroderma, replacing the altered collagen in the dermis and subcutaneous septa.

Clinical Features
Osteoma cutis can occur anywhere, but the face is the most common site. The tongue is the most common intraoral site (osteoma mucosae or osseous choristoma). Osteoma cutis does not cause any visible change in the overlying skin other than an occasional color change, which may appear yellowish–white. If the lesion is large, the individual osteoma may be palpated. A needle inserted into one of the papules is met with stone-like resistance. Some patients have numerous (dozens to hundreds) of lesions, usually on the face in female patients and on the scalp or chest in male patients. This form is known as multiple miliary osteoma cutis.

Imaging Features
Location. Radiographically, osteoma cutis most commonly appears in the cheek and lip regions (Fig. 31.12). In this location, the ossified area can be superimposed over a tooth root or alveolar process, giving the appearance of an area of dense bone. Accurate localization can be achieved by placing an intraoral receptor between the cheek and alveolar process to image the cheek alone. Alternatively, a soft tissue, low (60)

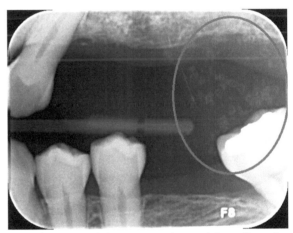

Fig. 31.12 Osteoma cutis is seen as a cluster of donut-like radiopaque calcifications in the cheek *(oval)*.

kVp posteroanterior skull image with the cheek blown outward can localize osteomas in the skin.

Periphery. Osteoma cutis are radiopaque, washer-shaped images with smooth peripheries. These single or multiple radiopaque masses are usually very small, although the size can range from 0.1 to 5 cm.

Internal structure. The internal structure may be homogeneously radiopaque but usually a radiolucent center representing normal fatty marrow may be visualized, giving the lesion a donut appearance radiographically. Trabeculae occasionally develop in the marrow cavity of larger osteomas. Individual lesions of calcified cystic acne resemble a snowflake-like radiopacity, which corresponds to the clinical location of the scar.

Differential interpretation. The differential interpretation should include myositis ossificans, calcinosis cutis, and osteoma mucosae. If the blown-out cheek technique is used, the lesions of osteoma cutis appear much more superficial than mucosal lesions. Myositis ossificans is of greater proportions, in some cases causing noticeable deformity of the facial contour.

Management. No management is required, but primary osteoma cutis is occasionally removed for cosmetic reasons. Laser resurfacing of the skin with a retinoic acid cream or curettage have been successful in treating osteoma cutis. More recently, good cosmetic results have been reported with a needle microincision-extirpation technique in patients with multiple miliary osteoma cutis.

Myositis Ossificans

In myositis ossificans, fibrous tissue and heterotopic bone form within the interstitial tissue of muscle, and associated tendons and ligaments. Secondary destruction and atrophy of the muscle occur as this fibrous tissue and bone interdigitate and separate the muscle fibers. Two principal forms have been described: localized and progressive.

Localized (Traumatic) Myositis Ossificans

Disease mechanism. Localized myositis ossificans develops from trauma or heavy muscle strain caused by certain occupations and sports. Skeletal muscle has limited capacity for regeneration after significant physical trauma, and the injury leads to considerable hemorrhage into the muscle or associated tendons and fascia. The fibrous tissue and bone form within the interstitial tissue of the muscle; no actual ossification of the muscle fibers occurs. It has been proposed that exuberant proliferation of vascular granulation tissue subsequently undergoes metaplasia to cartilage and bone during the healing process. Muscle injury from multiple injections (occasionally from the delivery of dental anesthesia) may also be a cause.

Clinical features. Localized myositis ossificans can develop at any age in either sex, but it occurs most often in young men who engage in vigorous activity. The site of the precipitating trauma remains swollen, tender, and painful for a period of time much longer than expected. The overlying skin may be red and inflamed, and when the lesion involves a muscle of mastication, opening the jaws may be difficult. After about 2 or 3 weeks, the area of ossification becomes apparent in the tissues, and a firm intramuscular mass can be palpated. The localized lesion may enlarge slowly, but eventually it stops growing. The lesion may appear fixed, or it may be freely movable on palpation.

Imaging features

Location. The most commonly involved muscles of the head and neck are the masseter and sternocleidomastoid. However, the other muscles of mastication may also be involved. The anterior attachments of the temporalis and the medial pterygoid muscles are at risk of injury on administration of mandibular block anesthesia. The ossified masses generally measure less than 6 cm in greatest dimension.

Periphery. The periphery commonly is more radiopaque than the internal structure. There is a variation in shape from irregular oval to linear streaks (pseudotrabeculae) running in the same direction as the normal muscle fibers. A radiolucent band can usually be seen between the area of ossification and adjacent bone, and heterotopic bone may lie along the long axis of the muscle (Fig. 31.13). These pseudotrabeculae are characteristic of myositis ossificans and strongly imply a diagnosis.

Internal structure. The internal structure varies with time. By 3 to 4 weeks after injury, the radiographic appearance is faint and homogeneously radiopaque. This radiopacity organizes further, and by 2 months a delicate lacy or feathery radiopaque internal pattern develops. These changes indicate the formation of bone; however, this bone does not have a normal-appearing trabecular pattern. Gradually, the image of this entity becomes more dense, more homogeneous, and better defined, maturing fully in about 5 to 6 months. Some lesions may progress more slowly and do not reach maturation until 12 months. After this period, the lesion may shrink.

Differential interpretation. The differential interpretation of localized myositis ossificans includes ossification of the stylohyoid ligament and other soft tissue calcifications. However, the form and location of myositis

ossificans often are enough to make the diagnosis. Other lesions to consider are bone-forming tumors. Although tumors, such as osteosarcoma, can form a linear bone pattern (see Chapter 26), the tumor is contiguous with the bone, and signs of bone destruction often are present.

Management. Microinjury and subsequent muscle necrosis attract macrophages, which elaborate the osteogenic growth factors. One strategy during the evolution of the lesion is bone morphogenetic protein type I receptor inhibition to reduce the heterotopic ossification. Rest and limitation of use are recommended to diminish the extent of the calcific deposit. For lesions that cause a functional restriction or neurologic impairment, surgical excision of the entire calcified mass with intensive physiotherapy to minimize postsurgical scarring is the recommended treatment. Complete maturation of myositis ossificans occurs between 6 and 12 months. Incomplete excision or excision at an immature stage can result in recurrence.

Progressive Myositis Ossificans

Disease mechanism. Progressive myositis ossificans or fibrodysplasia ossificans progressiva is a rare genetic anomaly with an autosomal dominant transmission pattern. Less commonly, it arises as a result of spontaneous mutation. The cause is a gain-of-function mutation in the bone morphogenetic protein activin A receptor type 1/activin-like kinase 2. It is more common in males and causes symptoms from early infancy. Progressive formation of heterotopic endochondral bone occurs within the interstitial tissue of muscles, tendons, ligaments, and fascia, and the involved muscles atrophy.

Clinical features. Patients display a congenital big toe deformity (hallux valgus). In most cases, catastrophically disabling heterotopic ossification starts in the muscles of the neck and upper back and moves to the extremities. The disease commences with soft tissue swelling that is tender and painful and may show redness and heat, indicating the presence of inflammation. The acute symptoms subside, and a firm mass remains in the tissues. This condition may affect tendons, ligaments, and any of the striated muscles, including the heart and diaphragm. In some cases, the spread of ossification is limited, while in others, ossification becomes extensive, affecting almost all of the large muscles of the body. Stiffness and limitation of motion of the neck, chest, back, and extremities (especially the shoulders) gradually increase. Functional deficits are progressive and handicapping. Advanced stages of the disease result in the "petrified man" condition. During the third decade, the process may spontaneously arrest; however, most patients die during the third or fourth decades. Premature death usually results from respiratory difficulties or from exhaustion of the muscles of mastication.

Imaging features. The radiographic appearance of progressive myositis ossificans is similar to the appearance of the local form. The heterotopic bone more commonly is oriented along the long axis of the involved muscle (Fig. 31.14). Osseous malformation of the regions of muscle attachment, such as the mandibular condyles, also may be seen.

Differential interpretation. In the initial stages of the disease, distinguishing between progressive myositis ossificans and rheumatoid arthritis may be difficult. However, the presence of specific anomalies suggests the diagnosis. In the case of calcinosis, the deposits of amorphous calcium salts frequently resorb, but in progressive myositis ossificans, the bone never disappears.

Management. No effective treatment exists for progressive myositis ossificans. Nodules that are traumatized and that ulcerate frequently should be excised. Interference with respiration or respiratory infection occurs in the later stages of the disease, so supportive therapy may be required. Currently, drug development is aimed at the activin A receptor mutation, which is a highly conserved target.

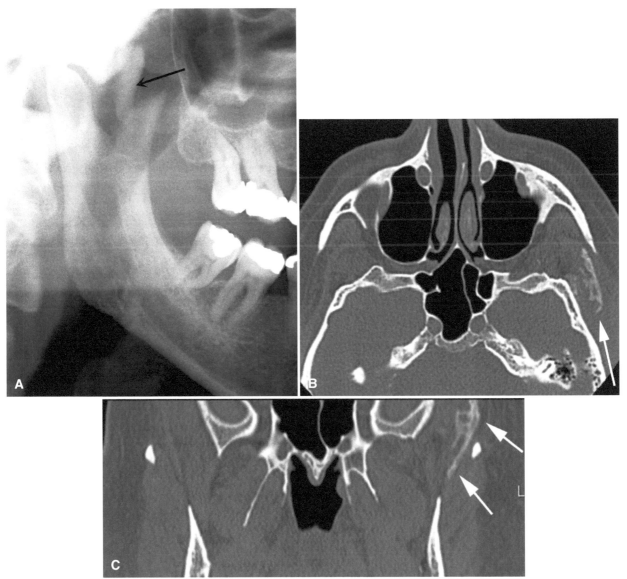

Fig. 31.13 (A) Soft tissue ossification extending from the coronoid process in a superior direction following the anatomy of the temporalis muscle *(arrow)*. This condition arose after several attempts were made to provide a submandibular nerve block, leaving the patient unable to open the mandible. (B) Axial multidetector computed tomography (MDCT) image of ossification along the temporalis muscle *(arrow)* after a surgical procedure. (C) Coronal MDCT image of the same case shown in B reveals the calcifications *(arrows)*.

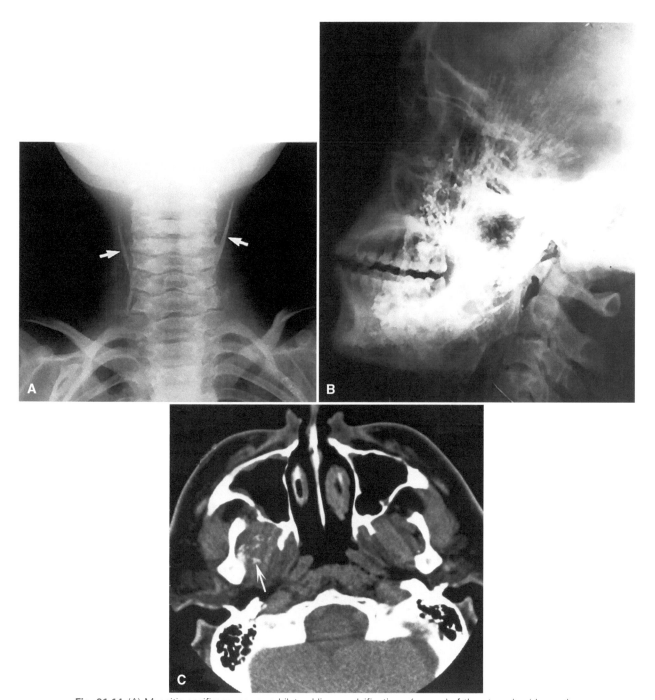

Fig. 31.14 (A) Myositis ossificans, seen as bilateral linear calcifications *(arrows)* of the sternohyoid muscle. (B) Extensive ossification of the masseter and temporalis muscles. (C) Axial computed tomography scan with soft tissue algorithm demonstrates calcifications in the lateral pterygoid muscle *(arrow)*. ([A], Courtesy Dr. H. Worth, Vancouver, British Columbia, Canada.)

BIBLIOGRAPHY

Banks K, Bui-Mansfield L, Chew F, et al. A compartmental approach to the radiographic evaluation of soft-tissue calcifications. *Semin Roentgenol.* 2005;40:391–407.

Carter L. Lumps and bumps—what is that stone? *Alpha Omegan.* 2010;103:151–156.

Ergun T, Lakadamyali H. The prevalence and clinical importance of incidental soft-tissue findings in cervical CT scans of trauma population. *Dentomaxillofac Radiol.* 2013;42:20130216.

Keberle M, Robinson S. Physiologic and pathologic calcifications and ossifications in the face and neck. *Eur Radiol.* 2007;17:2103–2111.

Worth HM. *Principles and Practice of Oral Radiologic Interpretation.* St. Louis: Mosby; 1963.

Calcified Lymph Nodes

Carter L. Decoding cervical soft tissue calcifications on panoramic dental radiographs. *Va Dent J.* 2006;83:18–19.

Eisenkraft B, Som P. The spectrum of benign and malignant etiologies of cervical node calcification. *AJR Am J Roentgenol.* 1999;172:1433–1437.

Garg A, Chaudhary A, Tewari R, et al. Coincidental diagnosis of tuberculous lymphadenitis: a case report. *Aust Dent J.* 2014;59:258–263.

Gormley K, Glastonbury C. Calcified nodal metastasis from squamous cell carcinoma of the head and neck. *Australas Radiol.* 2004;48:240–242.

Dystrophic Calcification in the Tonsils

Bamgbose B, Ruprecht A, Hellstein J, et al. The prevalence of tonsilloliths and other soft tissue calcifications in patients attending oral and maxillofacial radiology clinic of the University of Iowa, ISRN Dentistry; 2014. Article ID 839635. http://dx.doi.org/10.1155/2014/839635.

Oda M, Tanaka T, Nishida I, et al. Prevalence and imaging characteristics of detectable tonsilloliths on 482 pairs of consecutive CT and panoramic radiographs. *BMC Oral Health.* 2013;13:54. http://www.biomedcentral.com1472-6831/13/54.

Takahashi A, Sugawara C, Kudoh T, et al. Prevalence and imaging characteristics of palatine tonsilloliths evaluated on 2244 pairs and panoramic radiographs and CT images. *Clin Oral Investig.* 2017;21:85–91.

Cysticercosis

Carnero P, Mateo P, Martin-Garre S, et al. Unexpected hosts: imaging parasitic diseases. *Insights Imaging.* 2017;8:101–125.

Coral-Almeida M, Gabriel S, Abatih E, et al. Taenia solium human cysticercosis: a systematic review of sero-epidemiolgical data from endemic zones around the world. *PLoS Negl Trop Dis.* 2015;9:e0003919. doi:10.1371/journal.pntd.0003919.

Goenka P, Sarawgi A, Asopa K, et al. Oral cysticercosis in a pediatric patient: a rare case report with review. *Int J Clin Pediatr Dent.* 2016;9:156–161.

Kungu J, Dione M, Ejobi F, et al. Risk factors, perceptions and practices associated with Taenia solium cysticercosis and its control in the smallholder pig production systems in Uganda: a cross-sectional survey. *BMC Infect Dis.* 2017;17:1. doi:10.1186/s12879-016-2122-x.

Calcified Blood Vessel

Fishbein M, Fishbein G. Arteriosclerosis: facts and fancy. *Cardiovasc Pathol.* 2015;24:335–342.

Friedlander A, Giaconi J, Tsui I, et al. Meaningful correlation between asymptomatic retinal arteriole emboli and calcified carotid plaque found on panoramic dental imaging of males with diabetes. *Oral Surg Oral Med Oral Pathol Oral Radiol.* 2016;121:434–440.

Friedlander A, El Saden S, Haxboun R, et al. Detection of carotid artery calcification on the panoramic images of post-menopausal famales is significantly associated with severe abdominal aortic calcification: a risk indicator of future adverse vascular events. *Dentomaxillofac Radiol.* 2015;44:20150094.

Garoff M, Johansson E, Ahlqvist J, et al. Detection of calcification in panoramic radiographs in patients with carotid stenosis ≥50%. *Oral Surg Oral Med Oral Pathol Oral Radiol.* 2014;117:385–391.

Rhinoliths and Antroliths

Girgis S, Cheng L, Gillett D. Rhinolith mimicking a toothache. *Int J Surg Case Rep.* 2015;14:66–68.

Heffler E, Machetta G, Magnano M, et al. When perennial rhinitis worsens: rhinolith mimicking severe allergic rhinitis. *BMJ Case Rep.* 2014;doi:10.1136/bcr-2013-202539.

Shenoy V, Maller V, Maller V. Maxillary antrolith: A rare cause of the recurrent sinusitis, Case Reports in Otolaryngology; 2013. Article 527152. http://dx.doi.org/10.1155/2013/527152.

Rhinoliths and Antroliths

Atienza G, Lopez-Cedrun J. Management of obstructive salivary disorders by sialendoscopy: a systematic review. *Br J Oral Maxillofac Surg.* 2015;53:507–519.

Kraaij S, Karagozoglu K, Forouzanfar T, et al. Salivary stones: symptoms, aetiology, biochemical composition and treatment. *Br Dent J.* 2014;217:E23. doi:10.1038/sj.bdj.2014.1054.

Schapher M, Mantsopoulos K, Messbacher M-E, et al. Transoral submandibulotomy for deep hilar submandibular gland sialolithiasis. *Laryngoscope.* 2017;doi:10.1002/lary.26549.

Phleboliths

Bhat V, Bhat V. Shining pearls sign: a new identity for venous malformations on computed tomographic imaging. *Int J Angiol.* 2016;25:e21–e24.

Eivasi B, Fasunla A, Gulner C, et al. Phleboliths from venous malformations of the head and neck. *Phlebology.* 2013;28:86–92.

Gooi Z, Mydlarz W, Tunkel D, et al. Submandibular venous malformation phleboliths mimicking sialolithiasis in children. *Laryngoscope.* 2014;124:2816–2828.

Calcified Laryngeal Cartilages

Lotz M, Loeser R. Effects of aging on articular cartilage homeostasis. *Bone.* 2012;51:241–248.

Mupparrapu M, Vuppalapati A. Ossification of laryngeal cartilages on lateral cephalometric radiographs. *Angle Orthod.* 2005;75:196–201.

Naimo P, O'Donnell C, Bassed R, et al. The use of computed tomography in determining developmental changes, anomalies, and trauma of the thyroid cartilage. *Forensic Sci Med Pathol.* 2013;9:377–385.

Ossified Stylohyoid Ligament

Al Weteid A, Miloro M. Transoral endoscopic-assisted styloidectomy: how should Eagle syndrome be managed surgically? *Int J Oral Maxillofac Surg.* 2015;44:1181–1187.

Eagle WW. Elongated styloid process, symptoms and treatment. *AMA Arch Otolaryngol.* 1958;67:172–176.

Hooker J, Joyner D, Farley E, et al. Carotid stent fracture from stylocarotid syndrome. *J Radiol Case Rep.* 2016;10:1–8.

Kamal A, Nazir R, Usman M, et al. Eagle syndrome; radiological evaluation and management. *J Pak Med Assoc.* 2014;64:1315–1317.

Osteoma Cutis

Johann A, Garcia B, Nacif T, et al. Submandibular osseous choristoma. *J Craniomaxillofac Surg.* 2006;34:57–59.

Talsania N, Jolliffe V, O'Toole E, et al. Platelike osteoma cutis. *J Am Acad Dermatol.* 2011;64:613–615.

Wang J-F, O'Malley D: Extramedullary acute leukemia developing in a pre-existing osteoma cutis. *J Cutan Pathol.* 2014;41:606–611.

Myositis Ossificans

Ferra M, Costantino P, Shatzkes D. A woman with trismus. *JAMA Otolaryngol Head Neck Surg.* 2015;141:665–666.

Kaplan F. The skeleton in the closet. *Gene.* 2013;528:7–11.

Oliveira F, Fernandes C, Araujo K, et al. Clinical aspects and conservative dental management of a patient with fibrodysplasia ossificans progressiva. *J Contemp Dent Pract.* 2014;15:122–126.

Pignolo R, Bedford-Gay C, Liljesthrom M, et al. The natural history of flare-ups in fibrodysplasia ossificans progressiva (FOP): a comprehensive global assessment. *J Bone Miner Res.* 2016;31:650–656.

32

Salivary Gland Diseases

Fatima M. Jadu

Salivary glands and their secretions play a significant role in preserving the overall health of oral structures. Accordingly, conditions that affect the salivary glands and their function directly affect the teeth and mucosa. These conditions often drive patients to seek care from their dentists. Therefore it is of paramount importance that dentists understand the pathophysiology of salivary glands and be aware of the various diagnostic and management methods in order to provide optimal care for their patients.

SALIVARY GLAND DISEASE

Disease Mechanism

The salivary glands are the exocrine glands that produce and secrete saliva. There are three pairs of major salivary glands located outside the oral cavity and numerous minor salivary glands scattered throughout the oral submucosa (Fig. 32.1). Both the major and minor salivary glands can be affected by a variety of conditions that span several pathophysiologies. However, conditions affecting the salivary glands are usually divided into three major disease processes: inflammatory, noninflammatory, and space-occupying masses. Imaging plays a major role in the diagnosis, management, and follow-ups of these conditions.

Clinical Signs and Symptoms

The signs and symptoms of diseases of the salivary glands depend on the disease process and the gland affected, although swelling and pain are the two most common symptoms. Xerostomia, the subjective feeling of dry mouth, is another symptom that is often associated with pathosis of the salivary glands. Patients with xerostomia may complain of a burning sensation or soreness of the mouth and may also complain of altered taste or difficulty swallowing. Signs of xerostomia include an erythematous fissured tongue, cervical caries, and recurrent *Candida albicans* infections. The objective decrease in the quantity of saliva can be confirmed through specific tests and is termed hyposalivation.

DIAGNOSTIC IMAGING

Imaging is often used to diagnose and to plan management and follow-up of patients with salivary gland disorders. It provides crucial information regarding the nature of the disease affecting the salivary glands, the extent and severity of glandular involvement, and the effect on the surrounding structures. Many of the available imaging modalities have been used to image the salivary glands including projection radiography, high-resolution ultrasonography (HRUS), multidetector computed tomography (MDCT), magnetic resonance imaging (MRI), nuclear medicine, sialography, and most recently sialendoscopy.

PROJECTION IMAGING

Projection images, whether intraoral occlusal images or extraoral panoramic images, are helpful in identifying calcified sialoliths. Cross-sectional mandibular occlusal images are best used to identify submandibular duct sialoliths (Fig. 32.2), whereas panoramic images may be used to demonstrate both parotid and submandibular sialoliths. Parotid sialoliths appear superimposed over the mandibular rami superior to the occlusal plane, whereas submandibular sialoliths appear superior to the hyoid bone near the antegonial notch of the mandible (Fig. 32.3). Therefore these images should be considered first when the patient presents with signs and symptoms suggestive of a sialolith such as swelling and pain just prior to or during mealtime. Some of the advantages of projection images are that they are readily available, are inexpensive, and subject the patient to a relatively low dose of radiation. In addition, they allow examination of osseous structures adjacent to the salivary glands. However, projection images do fail at identifying noncalcified sialoliths, which are estimated to account for 40% of all parotid sialoliths and 20% of all submandibular sialoliths.

HIGH RESOLUTION

Ultrasonography

This technique may be used for the initial assessment of the parotid and submandibular glands, especially when an abnormality is located superficially. It may also be used to guide biopsies and further imaging choices. HRUS is helpful at differentiating cysts from neoplasms, and benign from malignant lesions (Fig. 32.4). HRUS has become more specific at detecting Sjögren syndrome, but it is still lacking in its ability to detect sialoliths. The major disadvantage of HRUS lies in its inability to detect deep salivary gland lesions, whereas its major advantage is its relative safety because it does not use ionizing radiation.

Multidetector Computed Tomography

MDCT, displayed in both hard- and soft-tissue windows, is useful in evaluating not only the salivary glands but also the structures surrounding them (Fig. 32.5). This is especially true when the images are acquired after intravenous administration of a contrast agent that renders glandular tissues hyperdense relative to the surrounding fat and muscle.

MDCT imaging is used in cases when inflammation of the salivary glands is suspected because it demonstrates characteristic features such as peripheral enhancement, thickening of the subcutaneous tissue, and lymph node involvement, some or all of which can be seen in inflammation or neoplasia. Sialoliths are well depicted on MDCT images but

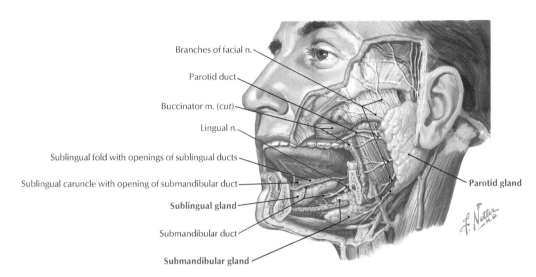

Fig. 32.1 Diagram depicting the size and location of the major salivary glands relative to the oral cavity. (Netter Images.)

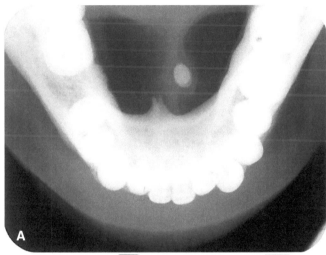

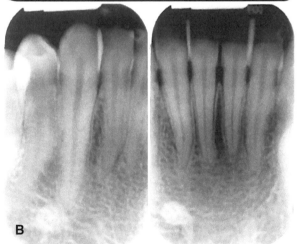

Fig. 32.2 (A) Standard mandibular occlusal and (B) periapical images demonstrating an oval-shaped radiopaque sialolith in a Wharton duct.

only if they are relatively large and significantly calcified. Smaller, less-calcified sialoliths and ductal strictures are not well depicted on MDCT images. With regards to cysts and neoplasms, MDCT imaging is excellent at detecting these lesions but may not be reliable at distinguishing benign from malignant lesions.

Magnetic Resonance Imaging

Although indications for MRI occasionally overlap with those of MDCT, MRI is the imaging method of choice for assessment of space-occupying lesions (cyst and neoplasms) of the salivary glands because of its superior soft-tissue contrast (Fig. 32.6). In addition, the use of intravenous gadolinium as a contrast agent makes MRI the imaging modality of choice for evaluation of intracranial and perineural spread of disease. Detection of sialoliths, particularly when calcified, is problematic in MRI because these calcific entities result in signal voids. Other disadvantages of MRI include long acquisition times, relatively poor spatial resolution, cost, and accessibility.

Nuclear Medicine

Nuclear medicine examinations are functional examinations of the salivary glands. This modality takes advantage of the selective uptake of specific radiopharmaceuticals such as technetium 99m (^{99m}Tc)-pertechnetate (TPT) by the salivary glands when injected intravenously. This is followed by administration of a sialagogue to evaluate the secretory capacity of the salivary glands. Pathosis may be determined on the basis of variations in the rate of TPT uptake or clearance. For example, Warthin tumor distinctively demonstrates reduced TPT clearance (Fig. 32.7).

Nuclear medicine is a highly sensitive technique that allows examination of all the major salivary glands at once; however, it lacks specificity and resolution which makes assessment of the salivary gland morphology difficult.

Sialography

First performed in 1902, sialography is an imaging technique exclusively used for the parotid and submandibular salivary glands. The technique involves infusion of the gland ductal system with an iodinated contrast agent, and then imaging the gland with projection imaging, fluoroscopy, MDCT, or cone beam computed tomography (CBCT). Sialography is the only imaging technique that can assess both the morphology of the parotid and submandibular glands in addition their function. The rate of clearance of the contrast agent from the gland, especially when prolonged, is used as an indirect indicator of reduced secretory function. MRI may be combined with sialography, but in these cases the patients' own saliva is used as a contrast agent and the imaging is done using heavily weighted T2 protocols.

The primary indication for sialography is chronic inflammatory conditions, especially when obstruction is suspected. There are two contraindications for sialography. The first of these is acute infection because injection of the contrast agent may disperse the infection into

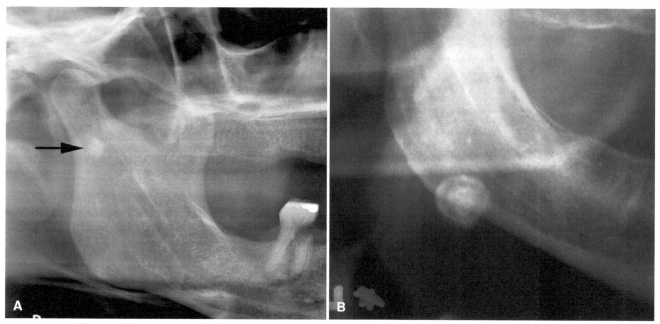

Fig. 32.3 Cropped Panoramic Images. (A) Parotid sialolith superimposed over condylar neck *(arrow)* superior to the plane of occlusion. (B) Submandibular sialolith near the antegonial notch of the mandible. Note the concentric lamellar pattern characteristic of sialoliths.

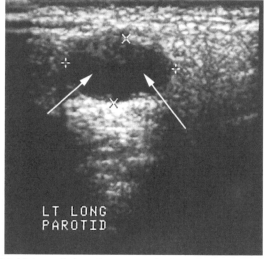

Fig. 32.4 High-resolution ultrasonography image of the parotid gland demonstrating an echo-free mass with well-defined margins, which is typical of a cystic mass *(arrows)*. (Courtesy Department of Radiology, Baylor University Medical Center, Dallas, TX.)

otherwise unaffected regions within the gland and cause further pain for the patient. The second contraindication is an immediately anticipated thyroid function test because the iodine in the contrast agent may concentrate in the thyroid gland and interfere with the results of the test.

Recently, sialography has been coupled with CBCT, and this coupling has resulted in three-dimensional images with submillimeter resolution and multiplanar capabilities that have revolutionized the visualization of the parotid and submandibular glands (Fig. 32.8).

Sialendoscopy

Since its first use in the 1990s, this examination that involves direct visualization of the parotid and submandibular major ducts (Fig. 32.9)

has transformed the diagnosis and management of obstructive conditions of these glands. The minimally invasive technique can be equipped with sialolith retrieval and stricture dilation tools that have enabled management of these common conditions with reported success rates greater than 95%. Acute inflammation is the only known contraindication for this relatively new technique because of the possible pain that may be elicited.

CONDITIONS AFFECTING THE SALIVARY GLANDS

Inflammatory Conditions

Inflammation is by far the most common disorder to affect the salivary glands in both adults and children. However, the cause of the inflammation differs between the two populations of patients. In adults, the inflammatory condition is most often due to local obstruction, whereas in children, it is often due to a viral infection. In general, inflammatory conditions of the salivary glands are either acute or chronic. Causes of acute inflammation are further subdivided into bacterial and viral infections. Chronic inflammation is most often due to chronic local obstruction.

Acute Bacterial Infections

Disease mechanism. Inflammation of the parenchymal portion of the salivary gland is termed sialadenitis, whereas inflammation of the ductal structures is termed sialodochitis or ductal sialadenitis.

Inflammation that results from an acute bacterial infection is commonly the result of reduced salivary secretion and subsequent retrograde infection of the glands by the oral flora (in particular, *Staphylococcus aureus* and *Streptococcus viridans*). Reduced salivary flow may also be the result of dehydration, certain diseases such as diabetes mellitus and bulimia, and some medications such as diuretics and antidepressants. Therefore this condition is often seen in elderly patients, postoperative patients, and debilitated patients who suffer from poor oral hygiene and low salivary secretions.

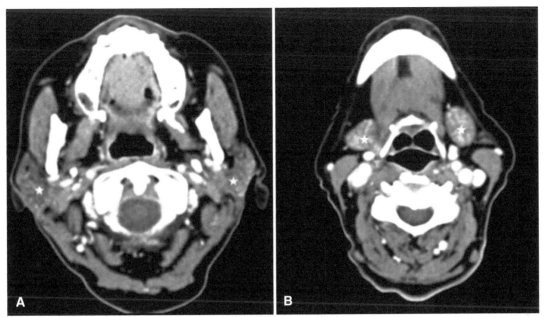

Fig. 32.5 Axial soft-tissue algorithm multidetector computed tomography images (A) at the level of the parotid glands *(stars)* and (B) at the level of the submandibular glands *(stars)*. Because the salivary glands have more fatty stroma than muscles, they appear less dense than adjacent muscles. (Courtesy Dr. K. Khashoggi, Jeddah, KSA.)

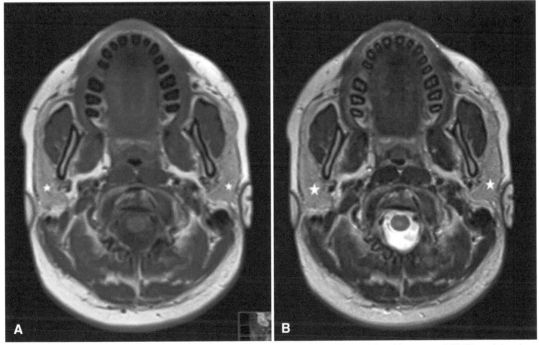

Fig. 32.6 Magnetic resonance imaging of normal parotid glands. (A) T1-weighted image and (B) T2-weighted image displaying the hyperintense signal of the parotid glands *(stars)* relative to the adjacent muscle. (Courtesy Dr. K. Khashoggi, Jeddah, KSA.)

Clinical features. The parotid glands are most commonly affected because the Stensen duct orifice is larger than that of other salivary gland orifices, and therefore it is more permissible of retrograde infections. In addition, parotid secretions are not as rich as other salivary gland secretions with respect to antibacterial substances such as immunoglobulin A (IgA). Unilateral involvement is more common than bilateral involvement, and the usual presenting sign is that of tender swelling of not only the infected gland but also the draining lymph nodes. A purulent discharge may also be noted at the orifice of the gland duct.

Imaging features. Contrast-enhanced MDCT is the imaging of choice when acute inflammation of the major salivary glands is suspected. This type of imaging demonstrates the pathognomonic features of this condition, such as enlargement of the affected gland with peripheral

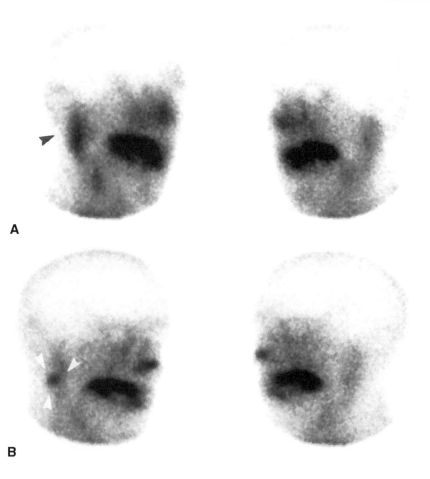

Fig. 32.7 Nuclear Medicine. (A) Technetium 99m (^{99m}Tc)-pertechnetate (TPT) scan of the salivary glands (right and left anterior oblique views) demonstrates increased uptake in the right parotid gland *(black arrowhead)*. (B) Nuclear medicine image obtained after administration of a sialagogue (lemon juice) demonstrates retention of TPT in the right parotid gland *(white arrowheads)*. This is a typical presentation of a Warthin neoplasm.

A

B

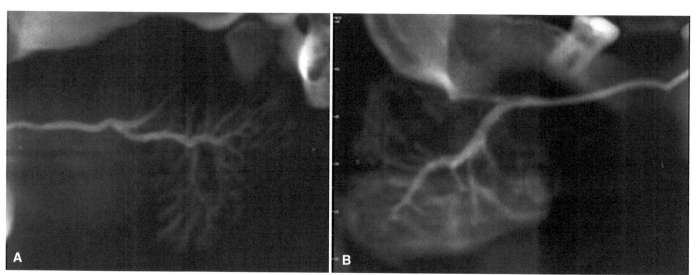

Fig. 32.8 Sialography coupled with cone beam computed tomography. (A) Corrected sagittal image of a normal left parotid gland illustrating the branching pattern of the ductal structures. (B) Corrected sagittal image of a normal right submandibular gland also illustrating the branching ducts. The outline of the gland body is displayed here due to filling of the acini with contrast material.

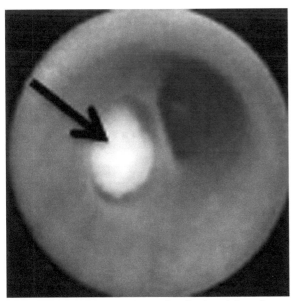

Fig. 32.9 Sialendoscopy allows direct visualization of the salivary gland ducts. This particular image demonstrates a sialolith *(arrow)* in one of the branching ducts. (Courtesy Dr. F. Marchal, Geneva, Switzerland.)

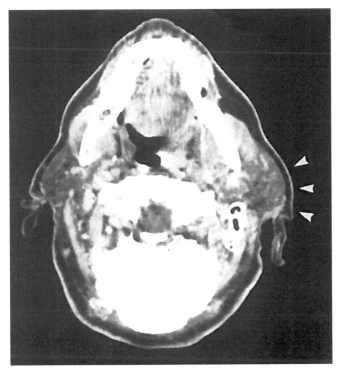

Fig. 32.10 Contrast-enhanced multidetector computed tomography image depicting a left parotid gland *(arrows)* that is larger than the right, with no suggestion of abscess formation. This appearance is consistent with acute sialadenitis. (Courtesy Department of Radiology, Baylor University Medical Center, Dallas, TX.)

enhancement, streaking of the adjacent fat tissue, and thickening of the subcutaneous tissues (Fig. 32.10). Involved lymph nodes appear enlarged with a higher attenuation than normal. If present, abscesses appear as well-defined areas of low attenuation. MRI is the second imaging modality of choice because it is unparalleled in its ability to differentiate edema from inflammatory infiltrate. Inflamed glands are usually enlarged and demonstrate a lower signal on T1-weighted MRI and a higher signal on T2-weighted images compared with the surrounding muscle.

HRUS may be helpful in distinguishing between diffuse inflammation and suppuration. It may also demonstrate abscess cavities if present in the superficial lobes of the major salivary glands. Both sialography and scintigraphy are contraindicated in cases of acute inflammation because they are minimally invasive techniques that may exacerbate the symptom of pain and may also increase the risk of introducing the infective organism further into the involved gland.

Management. Treatment of bacterial sialadenitis is typically an appropriate antibiotic regimen. This should be combined with conservative measures such as good oral hygiene and increased fluid intake. Care must be taken not to delay treatment or treat inadequately because that may result in intraglandular abscess formation and the subsequent need for more aggressive treatment and surgical intervention.

Acute Viral Infections
Disease Mechanism
Several viruses may infect the salivary glands, including Epstein-Barr virus (EBV), cytomegalovirus (CMV), coxsackievirus, parainfluenza viruses, and herpes virus, but the mumps virus is by far the most common. Mumps is an illness that usually affects children between the ages of 5 and 9 years and is caused by a paramyxovirus infection. Epidemics of this infection were common before the advent of the measles, mumps, and rubella (MMR) vaccine, thus the term "epidemic parotitis." Infected individuals usually go through an incubation period that ranges between 2 and 4 weeks, and they are considered contagious from 1 day before appearance of the clinical symptoms until approximately 14 days after resolution of the symptoms.

Clinical Features
Approximately 70% of mumps cases are symptomatic and are preceded by a prodromal period of malaise, myalgia, anorexia, and low-grade fever. This is then followed by enlargement of the parotid glands primarily and intense pain, especially during chewing. The enlargement starts unilaterally but soon after involves the contralateral side. Approximately 25% of cases demonstrate unilateral involvement, and 25% of cases develop complications such as epididymo-orchitis, meningoencephalitis, pancreatitis, thyroiditis, oophoritis, mastitis, unilateral hearing loss, and spontaneous abortion.

Imaging Features
Imaging findings are nonspecific, and the diagnosis is usually made on the basis of the clinical findings and the presence of serum antibodies to the mumps virus in the blood. MDCT images of the infected salivary glands demonstrate enlargement of the glands and a slightly higher attenuation than normal. The enlarged glands also appear to have a slightly higher T2-weighted MRI signal than normal.

Management
Treatment of mumps is palliative in nature and involves the administration of analgesics and antipyretics with bed rest. However, the best therapy is prevention, and vaccination is strongly recommended.

Chronic Inflammation
Disease Mechanism
As with acute inflammation, terms such as *sialadenitis* and *sialodochitis* are used depending on the involved salivary gland structure. Chronic inflammation is most often caused by chronic obstruction of the salivary glands. The causes of obstruction may be further subdivided into primary

and secondary causes. The primary causes include salivary stones (sialoliths), ductal narrowing (strictures), and mucous plugs, whereas secondary causes include trauma to the ductal structures or space-occupying lesions impinging on the ductal structures.

Sialoliths are not only the most common cause of chronic inflammation, but they are also the most common condition to affect the salivary glands in adults. Sialoliths begin as an inorganic nidus upon which organic and inorganic substances from the saliva are deposited. Strictures are the second most common cause of chronic inflammation, and these may occur in both the submandibular and the parotid gland ducts. Their etiology is still unknown, but the ductal narrowing is thought to be the result of fibrosis that occurs secondary to sialoliths, recurrent infections, or minor trauma.

Clinical Features

It is estimated that approximately 1% of the population have sialoliths, but the peak incidence occurs between the fourth and sixth decades of life. Approximately 83% of sialoliths form in the ducts of the submandibular glands because of their tortuous upward path that ends in a relatively narrow orifice. This, in addition to the viscous nature of submandibular saliva, its high pH and high mineral content, contribute to the higher incidence of sialoliths in the submandibular gland ducts.

Obstruction generally results in the accumulation of the saliva produced by the affected gland, proximal (i.e., closest to the gland) to the obstruction site, leading to dilatation of that segment of the salivary duct. This dilatation reaches a maximum size during mealtimes, when ample amounts of saliva are rapidly produced and excreted. Shortly after the meal, the saliva slowly finds its way around the obstruction point and into the oral cavity. However, this repeated process of saliva obstruction and buildup results in permanent dilation of

the salivary ducts (sialectasia). Stagnation of saliva in these distended portions of ducts may result in and predisposes the gland to repeated retrograde bacterial infections. Therefore patients with chronic obstruction usually present with a history of unilateral intermittent tender swelling in the area of the affected salivary gland especially during mealtime.

Imaging Features

Projection images such as panoramic images are used to identify sialoliths, which appear as well-defined, mixed radiolucent and radiopaque or completely radiopaque entities in the vicinity of the involved salivary gland. Unfortunately, up to 40% of sialoliths may not be calcified enough to appear on projection images.

Sialography is the imaging modality of choice for chronic inflammation because of its ability to depict sialoliths (even small noncalcified ones), strictures, and subtle changes in the delicate ductal structures of salivary glands. One of the typical appearances of chronic inflammation is the "sausage-like" appearance that represents alternating areas of obstruction and sialectasia (Fig. 32.11). Another typical appearance is of variably sized globular collections of contrast that represent abscess formation (Fig. 32.12). MDCT and MRI may also be used in cases of chronic inflammation, but their sensitivity for detecting small sialoliths and strictures is inferior to sialography. Sialendoscopy is quickly becoming the preferred imaging method for obstructive conditions of the salivary glands because of the added advantage it offers in terms of managing these conditions.

Management

Management of chronic inflammation depends on the type of obstruction causing it, its location, and its effect on the surrounding salivary gland

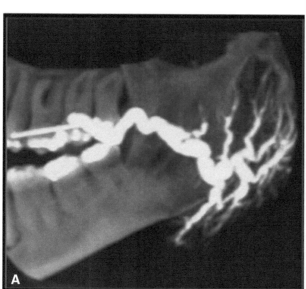
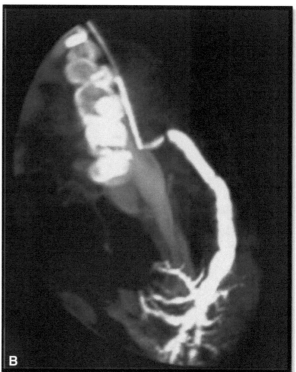

Fig. 32.11 Sialography of the left parotid gland imaged with cone beam computed tomography. (A) Sagittal and (B) axial renditions. A filling defect *(arrow)* in the proximal portion of the Stensen duct suggests a minimally calcified sialolith. Intermittent strictures and dilation of the main and secondary ducts are typical of sialodochitis.

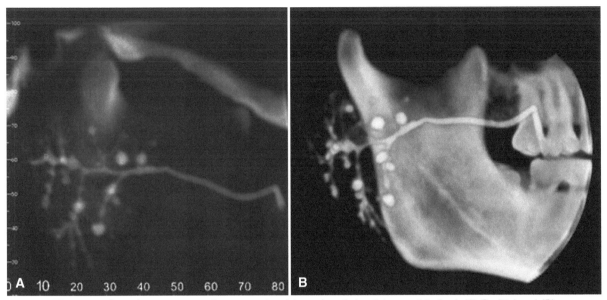

Fig. 32.12 Cone beam computed tomography sialography of the right parotid gland. (A) Sagittal and (B) three-dimensional volume images showing several variably sized globular collections of contrast material. These represent abscesses in a case of chronic sialadenitis.

structures. In general, patients are instructed to remain hydrated and to stimulate salivary production and secretion to encourage spontaneous discharge. If conservative methods fail, more invasive methods are used, such as basket retrieval of sialoliths and balloon ductoplasty for sialoliths. The last resort is complete removal of the affected salivary gland.

Noninflammatory and Inflammatory-Like Conditions

Three particular conditions (sialadenosis, autoimmune sialadenitis, postirradiation sialadenitis) are of interest because they often present with signs and symptoms that are similar to obstructive conditions of the salivary glands and thus must be differentiated from them.

Sialadenosis

Disease mechanism. Sialadenosis or sialosis is a nonneoplastic, noninflammatory enlargement of primarily the parotid glands. Causes of this condition include a variety of endocrine disorders such as diabetes mellitus, a number of nutritional abnormalities such as chronic alcoholism, and certain medications such as nonsteroidal antiinflammatory drugs (NSAIDs). The enlargement itself is due to hypertrophy of the salivary acini.

Clinical features. Because this condition is systemic in nature, bilateral involvement of the salivary glands is common. The enlargement is usually chronic or recurring and is largely painless. Patients with this condition often complain of xerostomia.

Imaging features. MDCT and MRI demonstrate nonspecific enlargements of the affected salivary glands. They may also demonstrate fibrous or fatty changes in the salivary glands, depending on the stage of the disease. Sialography provides more specific findings such as splaying of an otherwise normal ductal system (Fig. 32.13). This appearance is due to the ductal structures being pushed by the hypertrophied parenchyma.

Management. The management of sialadenosis relies on the identification and management of the primary cause of the condition. Local measures that can be taken include increased fluid intake, massage, and the use of sialagogues.

Autoimmune Sialadenitis

Disease mechanism. Sjögren syndrome, otherwise known as sicca syndrome or autoimmune sialosis, is an autoimmune disease characterized by a periductal lymphocytic infiltrate that destroys the acini of exocrine glands, resulting in a significant reduction in their ability to secrete saliva.

Clinical features. Sjögren syndrome is the second most common autoimmune condition after rheumatoid arthritis. Approximately 90% of cases are diagnosed in females between the fourth and sixth decades of life. There are two forms of the syndrome, a primary form that involves only the salivary and lacrimal glands (also known as sicca syndrome), and a secondary form that is associated with other connective tissue autoimmune conditions such as rheumatoid arthritis or systemic lupus erythematosus. The involved salivary glands are usually enlarged, but the patient's usual complaint is related to xerostomia. Patients with Sjögren syndrome are at a greater risk of developing mucosa-associated lymphoid tissue (MALT) lymphoma, a subtype of non-Hodgkin lymphoma.

Imaging features. Sialography, in the early stages of the disease, demonstrates a normal ductal system and numerous punctate (<1 mm in diameter) collections of contrast material distributed evenly throughout the gland (Fig. 32.14). These early changes are not evident on MDCT or MRI. As the disease progresses, the ducts become narrow and the collections of contrast material become globular (1 to 2 mm in diameter). This appearance is pathognomonic and is termed "pruning of the tree" or "leafless fruit-laden tree" (Fig. 32.15). Typically, these collections of contrast material remain after administration of a sialagogue, which is an indication that the material is pooled extraductally. MDCT imaging in later stages of the disease demonstrates enlarged and dense glands. On MRI, well-defined globular areas with low T1 signal intensity and high T2 signal intensity are seen throughout the gland.

Management. The management of autoimmune disorders of the salivary glands is directed toward relief of the patient's symptoms. Salivary stimulants, increased fluid intake, and artificial saliva and tears are some of the measures used to control the symptoms.

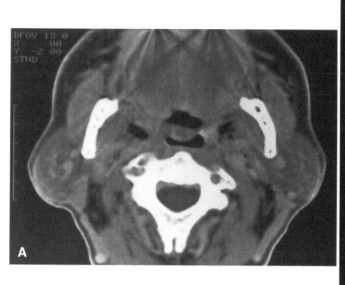
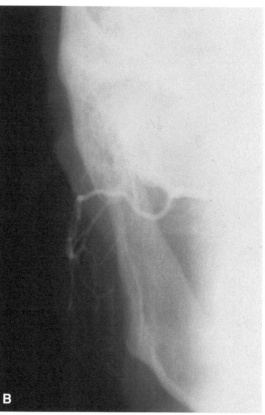

Fig. 32.13 Sialadenosis. (A) Multidetector computed tomography image demonstrating bilateral enlargement of the parotid glands. The attenuation of the parotid glands appears normal. (B) Anteroposterior skull image of a sialogram of the right parotid gland in the same patient. The size and shape of the ducts appear normal, but they are splayed laterally, a finding that is consistent with sialadenosis.

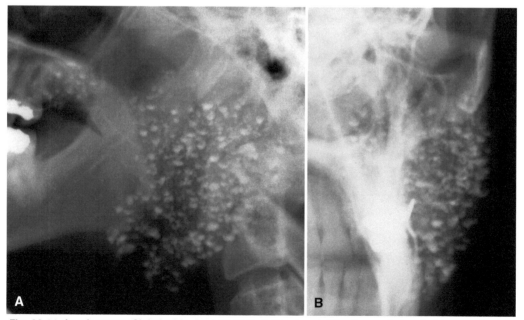

Fig. 32.14 Autoimmune Sialadenitis. (A) Lateral skull image and (B) anteroposterior skull image of a left parotid gland sialogram revealing numerous punctate collections of contrast material distributed throughout the gland parenchyma. This appearance is consistent with the early stages of autoimmune sialadenitis.

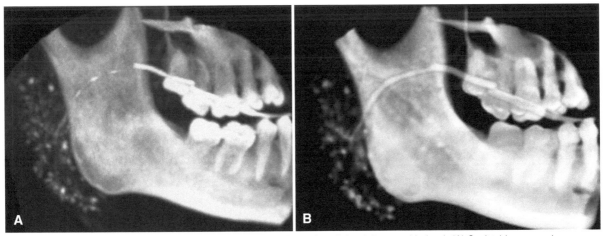

Fig. 32.15 Cone beam computed tomography sialography of the right parotid gland. (A) Sagittal image and (B) three-dimensional volume image of the same gland illustrating the typical appearance of autoimmune sialadenitis with multiple equally sized globular collections scattered homogenously throughout the parenchyma of the gland.

Postirradiation Sialadenitis

Disease mechanism. This condition is seen following both external beam radiation therapy of the head and neck and following treatment with radioactive iodine 131 (^{131}I) for management of specific thyroid conditions. Following both types of treatment, an intense inflammatory reaction arises in the salivary glands, and this causes impingement and obstruction of the ductal structures.

Clinical features. The typical presentation is tender bilateral swelling of the parotid glands because they are the most radiosensitive of all the salivary glands. This is usually accompanied by progressive xerostomia because the condition is progressive in nature, and ultimately leads to atrophy and fibrosis of the salivary glands.

Imaging features. The MDCT and MRI findings depend on the stage of the disease at the time of imaging and will likely exhibit varying degrees of gland fibrosis (Fig. 32.16). Early sialogram studies demonstrate flow voids in the parenchyma where atrophy of the acini has started to occur. Sialographic studies in late stages of the disease may not even be possible. Nuclear medicine examinations in the early stages reveal normal uptake but delayed excretion of TPT.

Management. The best management for this condition is prevention. In cases of external beam radiation therapy, measures should be taken to shield parts of the parotid glands and spare them the tumoricidal dose. These protected areas of the glands later undergo hypertrophy and compensate for the decrease in salivary flow. Unfortunately, shielding is not possible with ^{131}I treatment, but local measures (increased fluid intake, saliva substitutes) are helpful at relieving patients' symptoms.

SPACE-OCCUPYING CONDITIONS

Cystic Lesions
Disease Mechanism

Cysts of the salivary glands are rare (<5% of all salivary gland masses). They may be congenital (branchial, lymphoepithelial, dermoid) or acquired (sialocysts and acquired immunodeficiency syndrome [AIDS]-related parotid cysts [ARPCs]).

Sialocysts are true cysts that form in the salivary ducts when obstruction of these ducts results in their dilatation due to retention of saliva within them. They are known by other terms such as retention cyst,

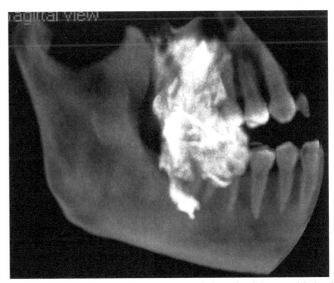

Fig. 32.16 Three-dimensional volume rendering of a right parotid gland sialogram using cone beam computed tomography. The contrast material is seen infusing only the accessory lobe of the parotid but not the ducts nor the acini of the superficial and deep lobes of the gland. These findings are consistent with fibrosis because this patient had a history of radioactive iodine therapy. Note the increased size of the accessory lobe due to hypertrophy to compensate for the lack of salivary secretions.

mucous retention cyst, ductal cyst, and salivary ductal cyst. In contrast, a sialocele or mucocoele is a pseudocyst that forms due to injury to a salivary duct and extravasation of saliva into the adjacent connective tissue. The terminology of these two conditions (sialocyst and sialocele) is often used interchangeably (and incorrectly) in the literature, but their differing pathophysiologies are well understood and documented. Finally, the term *ranula* is reserved for cysts of the sublingual glands regardless of whether the cyst is true (usually located in the oral cavity) or a pseudocyst (plunging below the mylohyoid muscle).

ARPCs are an important entity for dentists to know because they may be the first manifestation of an HIV infection. Their pathophysiology is still controversial, but their incidence has decreased with highly active antiretroviral therapy (HAART).

Clinical Features

Acquired cysts are usually identified later in life, despite being present at birth. Most cysts are unilateral except for ARPCs, which are bilateral in distribution. Similarly, most cysts affect the parotid salivary glands except for sialoceles, which are more common in minor salivary glands.

Imaging Features

Cysts may be indirectly visualized on sialography by displacement of the salivary ducts arching around them and producing an appearance termed "ball-in-hand." Cystic lesions typically appear as well-circumscribed, nonenhancing (when imaged with contrast administration), low-attenuation areas on MDCT images, whereas by MRI, they appear as well-circumscribed, high-signal areas on T2-weighted images which do not enhance after contrast administration (Fig. 32.17).

Treatment

Management of cysts of the salivary glands is typically surgical removal of the cyst or the entirety of the involved salivary gland.

Benign Neoplasms
Disease Mechanism
Salivary gland neoplasms are uncommon, accounting for less than 3% of all head and neck neoplasms. Approximately 80% of these arise in the parotid gland, 5% arise in the submandibular gland, 1% arise in the sublingual gland, and 10% to 15% arise in the minor salivary glands. The likelihood of neoplasms of the salivary glands being benign varies directly with the size of the gland. Therefore most neoplasms of the salivary glands are benign or low-grade malignancies.

Pleomorphic adenoma is by far the most common neoplasm of the salivary glands, accounting for 75% of all salivary gland neoplasms.

It is a benign neoplasm of the salivary ductal epithelium with both epithelial and mesenchymal components and hence is also referred to as a benign mixed tumor. The second most common benign neoplasm is Warthin tumor, more accurately known as papillary cystadenoma lymphomatosum. In children, the most common neoplasm of the salivary glands is the hemangioma.

Clinical Features

Benign neoplasms typically present as unilateral, slow growing, relatively painless masses. Warthin tumor uniquely affects the salivary glands bilaterally.

Imaging Features

MRI is the preferred imaging modality for salivary gland neoplasms because of its superior soft-tissue contrast resolution. MDCT is a reasonable imaging alternative, especially with contrast administration. Benign neoplasms generally appear to have well-defined margins and variable internal signal or attenuation, depending on the predominant tissue of the neoplasm (Fig. 32.18). Intravenous contrast administration causes enhancement of the neoplasm because the vascularity of the neoplasm is greater than that of the adjacent salivary gland tissue. Like cysts, sialography indirectly suggests a space-occupying mass with the ball-in-hand appearance (Fig. 32.19).

Management

The management of benign neoplasms of the major salivary glands is surgical. Benign neoplasms of the parotid gland are usually excised with the intention of preserving the gland to avoid facial nerve deficits. The submandibular and sublingual glands are invariably totally excised with the benign neoplasm.

Malignant Neoplasms

Disease mechanism. Approximately 20% of neoplasms in the parotid glands are malignant compared with 50% to 60% of submandibular

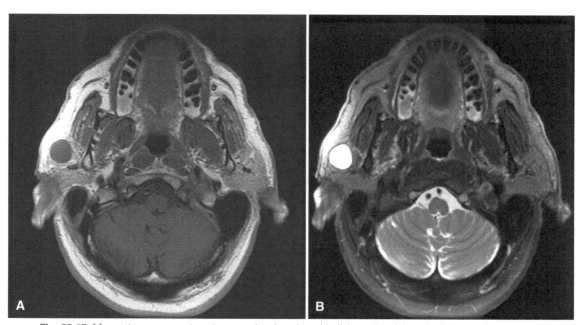

Fig. 32.17 Magnetic resonance imaging reveals a lymphoepithelial cyst involving the right parotid gland. (A) Axial T1-weighted image depicting a well-defined lesion involving the right parotid gland with an internal signal isointense to muscle. (B) Matching T2-weighted image depicting the lesion with a high signal intensity because of its fluid content.

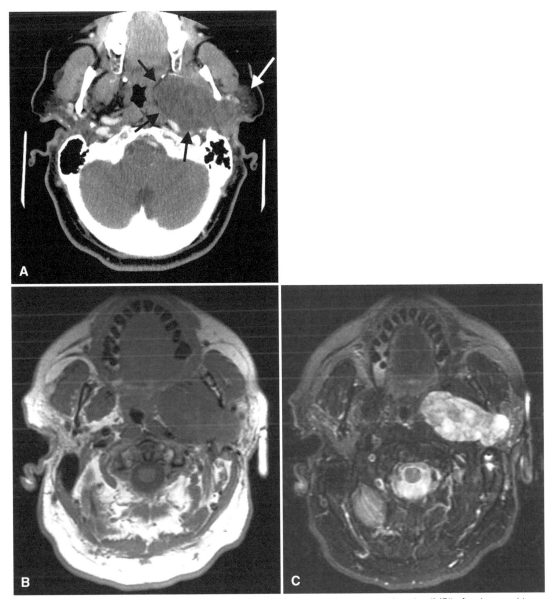

Fig. 32.18 Multidetector computed tomography (MDCT) and magnetic resonance imaging (MRI) of a pleomorphic adenoma in the left parotid gland. (A) Axial soft-tissue algorithm MDCT image. Note the well-defined periphery *(black arrows)* and the internal density that is less than surrounding muscles. The remaining parotid gland *(white arrow)* is displaced laterally. (B) T1-weighted MRI. The tissue signal of the neoplasm is isointense with muscle. (C) T2-weighted MRI. The tissue signal of the neoplasm is hyperintense to muscle.

neoplasms, 90% of sublingual neoplasms, and 60% to 75% of minor salivary gland neoplasms. The most common malignant neoplasm of the salivary glands is mucoepidermoid carcinoma, followed by adenoid cystic carcinoma. Mucoepidermoid carcinoma is composed of a variable admixture of mucous and epidermoid cells arising from the ductal epithelium of the salivary glands. Adenoid cystic carcinoma is composed of myoepithelial and ductal and has a great propensity to extend along nerves.

Clinical features. The aggressiveness of malignant neoplasms varies with their histopathologic grade. The low-grade variety presents clinically as a slowly growing, painless movable mass. These low-grade neoplasms rarely metastasize and have good prognosis, with a 5-year survival rate

greater than 95%. In contrast, high-grade neoplasms are relatively immobile and often cause facial pain and paralysis. They also spread locally via nerves, metastasize via blood and lymph, and have high recurrence rates and poor prognosis (5-year survival rate is approximately 25%).

Imaging features. The imaging presentation of malignant neoplasms is variable and is related to the grade, aggressiveness, location, and type of neoplasm. In many cases the low-grade variety has a sialography, MDCT, MRI, and HRUS presentation that is similar to benign salivary neoplasms. However, features such as ill-defined margins and invasion and destruction of adjacent structures, when seen, are considered to be typical indicators of a high-grade malignancy (Fig. 32.20).

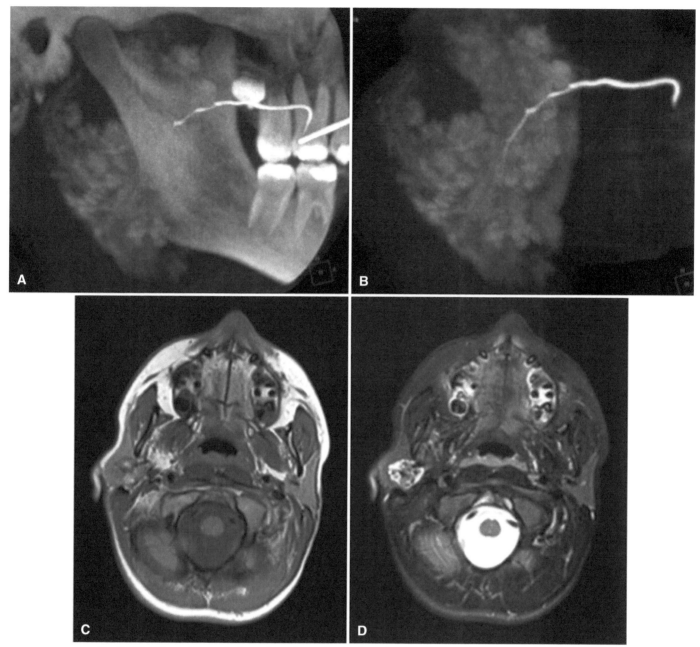

Fig. 32.19 Filling void seen in these three-dimensional volume images of a cone beam computed tomography sialogram of the right parotid gland in a 16-year-old patient. (A) With the adjacent osseous structures and (B) without the adjacent osseous structures. (C and D) Matching T1-weighted and T2-weighted magnetic resonance imaging of the same gland, respectively, demonstrating a vascular neoplasm with flow voids consistent with a hemangioma.

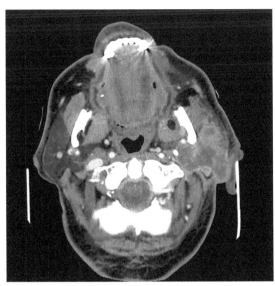

Fig. 32.20 Axial soft-tissue algorithm multidetector computed tomography image reveals an adenocarcinoma of the left parotid gland. Almost all of the gland has been replaced by this ill-defined neoplasm that has some peripheral enhancement and areas of low density internally, likely representing necrotic regions.

Management. Management of malignant neoplasms of the major salivary glands is typically surgical. Often requiring complete excision of the involved gland and a radical neck dissection. Combinations of surgery, therapeutic radiation, and chemotherapy may also be used.

BIBLIOGRAPHY

Abdel-Wahed N, Amer ME, Abo-Taleb NS. Assessment of the role of cone beam computed sialography in diagnosing salivary gland lesions. *Imaging Sci Dent.* 2013;43(1):17–23.

Abdullah A, Rivas FF, Srinivasan A. Imaging of the salivary glands. *Semin Roentgenol.* 2013;48(1):65–74.

Brown JE, Drage NA, Escudier MP, et al. Minimally invasive radiologically guided intervention for the treatment of salivary calculi. *Cardiovasc Intervent Radiol.* 2002;25(5):352–355.

Browne RF, Golding SJ, Watt-Smith SR. The role of MRI in facial swelling due to presumed salivary gland disease. *Br J Radiol.* 2001;74(878):127–133.

Burke CJ, Thomas RH, Howlett D. Imaging the major salivary glands. *Br J Oral Maxillofac Surg.* 2011;49(4):261–269.

Drage NA, Brown JE, Escudier MP, et al. Interventional radiology in the removal of salivary calculi. *Radiology.* 2000;214(1):139–142.

Drage NA, Brown JE, Escudier MP, et al. Balloon dilatation of salivary duct strictures: report on 36 treated glands. *Cardiovasc Intervent Radiol.* 2002;25(5):356–359.

Dreiseidler T, Ritter L, Rothamel D, et al. Salivary calculus diagnosis with 3-dimensional cone-beam computed tomography. *Oral Surg Oral Med Oral Pathol Oral Radiol Endod.* 2010;110(1):94–100.

El-Khateeb SM, Abou-Khalaf AE, Farid MM, et al. A prospective study of three diagnostic sonographic methods in differentiation between benign and malignant salivary gland tumours. *Dentomaxillofac Radiol.* 2011;40(8):476–485.

Jadu F, Yaffe MJ, Lam EW. A comparative study of the effective radiation doses from cone beam computed tomography and plain radiography for sialography. *Dentomaxillofac Radiol.* 2010;39(5):257–263.

Jadu FL, Lam EWN. The mystery of meal time swellings revealed. *Oral Health.* 2014;104(2):33–35.

Jadu FM, Hill ML, Yaffe MJ, et al. Optimization of exposure parameters for cone beam computed tomography sialography. *Dentomaxillofac Radiol.* 2011;40(6):362–368.

Jadu FM, Jan AM. A meta-analysis of the efficacy and safety of managing parotid and submandibular sialoliths using sialendoscopy assisted surgery. *Saudi Med J.* 2014;35(10):1188–1194.

Jadu FM, Lam EW. A comparative study of the diagnostic capabilities of 2D plain radiograph and 3D cone beam CT sialography. *Dentomaxillofac Radiol.* 2013;42(1):20110319.

Li B, Long X, Cheng Y, et al. Cone beam CT sialography of Stafne bone cavity. *Dentomaxillofac Radiol.* 2011;40(8):519–523.

Liccardi G, Lobefalo G, Di Florio E, et al. Strategies for the prevention of asthmatic, anaphylactic and anaphylactoid reactions during the administration of anesthetics and/or contrast media. *J Investig Allergol Clin Immunol.* 2008;18(1):1–11.

Ludlow JB, Davies-Ludlow LE, Brooks SL, et al. Dosimetry of 3 CBCT devices for oral and maxillofacial radiology: CB Mercuray, NewTom 3G and i-CAT. *Dentomaxillofac Radiol.* 2006;35(4):219–226.

MacDonald A, Burrell S. Infrequently performed studies in nuclear medicine: part 2. *J Nucl Med Technol.* 2009;37(1):1–13.

Mandel L. Salivary gland disorders. *Med Clin North Am.* 2014;98(6):1407–1449.

Nahlieli O, Nazarian Y. Sialadenitis following radioiodine therapy - a new diagnostic and treatment modality. *Oral Dis.* 2006;12(5):476–479.

Nahlieli O, Shacham R, Yoffe B, et al. Diagnosis and treatment of strictures and kinks in salivary gland ducts. *J Oral Maxillofac Surg.* 2001;59(5):484–490, discussion 490–492.

Ngu RK, Brown JE, Whaites EJ, et al. Salivary duct strictures: nature and incidence in benign salivary obstruction. *Dentomaxillofac Radiol.* 2007;36(2):63–67.

Shahidi S, Hamedani S. The feasibility of cone beam computed tomographic sialography in the diagnosis of space-occupying lesions: report of 3 cases. *Oral Surg Oral Med Oral Pathol Oral Radiol.* 2014;117(6):e452–e457.

Yousem DM, Kraut MA, Chalian AA. Major salivary gland imaging. *Radiology.* 2000;216(1):19–29.

33

Forensics

Robert E. Wood

SCOPE OF FORENSICS IN DENTISTRY

The scope of forensic dentistry (also called forensic odontology) includes both the identification of human remains and the associated legal responsibilities. Dental forensic investigation may involve the identification of a single individual or, in some cases, multiple individuals, as in cases of mass disaster. In the latter example, the task would be conducted by a team including forensic odontologists, forensic anthropologists, and forensic pathologists for biologic profiling and population stratification.

Multiple-fatality stratification is the sorting of individuals based on age and, to a lesser extent, ethnic background and sex. When this process is applied to a group of unidentified human remains, it increases the probability of making a positive identification between an individual and the dental records of a missing person. If an identification is not possible, at the very least an assessment of the developmental age of an individual's dentition using diagnostic imaging may allow the forensic dentist to determine chronological age. This determination involves a process where the developmental age of the dentition is compared with the corresponding dental developmental ages of a standard population to arrive at an estimate of chronological age. This process can also be performed on living individuals; for example, in identifying individuals to confirm age of majority. There are other methods (not included in this chapter) besides the developmental age of teeth to determine chronologic age, such as determining the developmental age of the bones of the wrist and hand.

All age determinations by scientific processes have an associated error rate. According to Saks in his publication, "The Coming Paradigm Shift in Forensic Identification Science," quantification of error rates in the comparative forensic sciences has been problematic. For this reason, it is imperative for the forensic dentist to understand the inherent sources of scientific errors and to be cautious in selecting the language used in the statement of official opinions.

Forensic dentists also contribute to cases involving bite-mark injuries, including the recognition, documentation, and analysis of injuries. Analysis involves the comparison of a known dentition with a bite mark in a substance, which may include human skin. Such cases may assist a dental regulatory authority or involve civil litigation. Radiology often provides objective data that are useful in supporting the opinions of the forensic dentist. This chapter focuses primarily on the role of the forensic dentist in identifying human remains.

NEED FOR IDENTIFICATION OF HUMAN REMAINS

Human remains are identified for personal, legal, and societal reasons. People place great importance on the verification of the identity of a deceased person from a personal perspective because doing so gives a measure of closure to loved ones, permits appropriate funerary rites, and allows appropriate religious ceremonies to be undertaken. In the absence of knowing for certain that a loved one has died, the grieving process may be delayed or interrupted.

From a legal perspective, certification of death is required before payment of life insurance, settling of wills and estates, dissolution of business partnerships, contracts, marriage, and settling of debts. Just as important from a legal perspective is the commencement of a suspicious death investigation. Knowing the identity of a person who has died under suspicious circumstances may instigate an investigation. Also, fulfillment of the legal requirements for the identification of an individual has importance for society as a whole. A competent forensic death investigation of human remains has four goals: determination of the means, manner, and cause of death and identification of the remains.

METHODS OF BODY IDENTIFICATION

The primary methods used in body identification are performed visually, by fingerprint, the use of DNA, the presence of unique skeletal or medical devices, and the dentition. Visual identification, although the most common method, is unpleasant and may be unreliable, given that identification is conducted at a time of high stress and in difficult circumstances. Errors in visual identification are well documented. Fingerprint identification is common but requires that the deceased individual have had fingerprints recorded before death (e.g., criminal record, military or police service), and for the cadaveric fingerprints to remain intact after death. The fingerprints may not be intact in cases where the body has undergone decomposition, maceration, or incineration. Fingerprint identification is impossible with skeletonized remains. DNA identification, accomplished by comparing an antemortem (before death) sample with an unknown set of human remains, provides confident identification except between identical twins, who have the same DNA. In addition to comparative identification, DNA analysis can be used to identify a DNA trait, which may indicate the ethnocultural group of a deceased individual. Identification by skeletal or medical

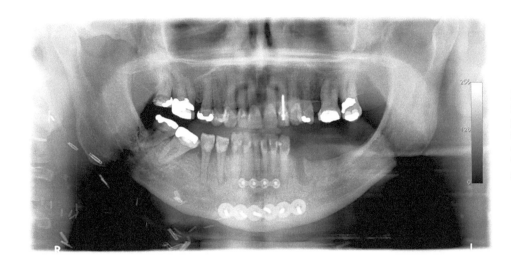

Fig. 33.1 Panoramic image revealing two fixation plates with 10 intraosseous screws placed in the anterior mandible after a mandibulotomy procedure. The shape and position of the plates and orientation of individual fixation screws provide unique information that may be used for identification.

devices can be made if these devices have serial numbers or are unusual in form (Fig. 33.1). Additionally, frontal sinus morphology is quite variable, and this may be used to compare antemortem and postmortem (after death) diagnostic images for the purpose of identification. Dental identification has many advantages over the other techniques. Empirical testing has proven that it is reliable and straightforward when antemortem images are available; it is also readily demonstrable in courts of law as well as quick and inexpensive.

UTILITY OF ORAL AND MAXILLOFACIAL RADIOLOGY FOR BODY IDENTIFICATION

Diagnostic images are used in dental identification because they provide objective evidence of the antemortem and postmortem condition. Conventional radiographs and digital images are a permanent record of the antemortem condition at the time they were made and are difficult to misinterpret. In contrast, dental charting by one dentist may not be directly comparable to dental charting of the same patient made by a second dentist. Despite the forensic utility of antemortem intraoral, oral, and maxillofacial images, most dentists (appropriately) do not expose a full mouth series of images at each appointment. Consequently antemortem images should be analyzed in conjunction with the antemortem dental chart. Antemortem dental images should never be exposed for the purpose of providing a record for later comparison, even in high-risk groups such as convicted criminals or sex-trade workers. Use of the chart and antemortem images of known date allows the forensic dentist to produce an antemortem odontogram, a record of the patient's dentition, which can be compared with the postmortem conditions for the purposes of identification.

IDENTIFICATION OF A SINGLE BODY

The process of body identification using dental criteria is relatively straightforward and is outlined by the American Society of Forensic Odontology. Using diagnostic images, the forensic dentist identifies points of agreement (concordance) between the antemortem and postmortem images and lists them numerically in a report. There is no set number of points needed for an identification to be made. A deceased person (decedent) who was edentulous before death may not have any concordant points with any other edentulous candidate. However, if teeth are present with restorations, this may provide enough unique information to eliminate all other possible candidates and provide a match for only one putative decedent (Fig. 33.2). Useful concordant

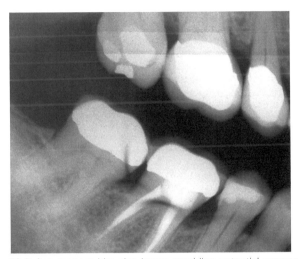

Fig. 33.2 Antemortem bitewing image providing potential concordant points because of the presence and unique shape of the restorations and root canal filling material.

points may include the specific teeth present, unique features such as the shapes of the crown and roots, and the presence of restorations, including the materials used, endodontic material, and the unique shapes of the materials.

Discordant points are also listed in the report. Such points include explainable discrepancies (e.g., points that do not match based on explainable circumstances, such as a restoration being placed after the antemortem images were exposed) and unexplainable discrepancies, where the findings cannot be explained without further investigation. An example of an unexplainable discrepancy would be a tooth missing on an antemortem examination but present on a postmortem examination. Unexplainable discrepancies, if they remain unaccounted for, preclude a positive identification using dental means. Fig. 33.3 shows antemortem and postmortem bitewing images used in the identification of an individual. After comparing images for concordant points, one may be able to determine whether this is a positive identification.

RADIOLOGIC TECHNIQUES IN BODY IDENTIFICATION

Either conventional radiographs or digital images may be used in single-person or multiple-fatality dental forensics. Using conventional

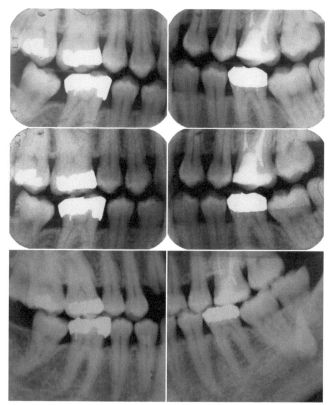

Fig. 33.3 Four antemortem conventional bitewing images *(top)* and two postmortem bitewing images *(bottom)*. A positive match can be made using the teeth present and the morphology of the teeth, such as root structure and pulp chambers, number and shape of metallic restorations, and endodontic filling material.

film-based radiographs in postmortem examinations requires the film to be processed on site. The result is a slight delay compared with using solid-state digital sensors. However, film-based images provide the flexibility of using various sizes of image receptors. For example, occlusal size (American National Standards Institute [ANSI] size 4) film can be used for bitewing images (Fig. 33.4). Furthermore, using larger image receptors such as this may permit imaging of the entire dentition with six exposures (Fig. 33.5). In cases where the remains are decomposed, receptors or specimens can readily be wrapped in polyethylene stock bags to prevent contamination (Fig. 33.6). A further advantage of using film is that the receptor latitude results in images of diagnostic quality in cases ranging from extremely bloated remains with soft tissue thickness up to five times normal to skeletonized remains, and burned and partly carbonized remains resulting from fire.

Most forensic dentists use digital imaging systems. The advantages of digital systems include the ability to make multiple images in a short period of time by modifying the angle of the incident x-ray beam to replicate the antemortem images or to augment the examination instantly, thus improving the speed of identification. However, there are some limitations to the use of digital systems. Occasionally, where there has been considerable loss of tooth structure or soft tissue coverage, the wider latitude of conventional film is superior for imaging small amounts of remaining material (Fig. 33.7).

For samples lacking soft tissue coverage, Lucite sheets can be used to mimic soft tissue, x-ray generator exposure settings can be reduced, or the x-ray tube head can be moved away from the receptor. However, in some cases there is so little tissue left that these measures may not result in more acceptable images (see Fig. 33.7). Also, digital systems can be expensive, and the image receptor and the length of the attached cord of solid-state receptors must be thoroughly protected lest they become contaminated by the human remains.

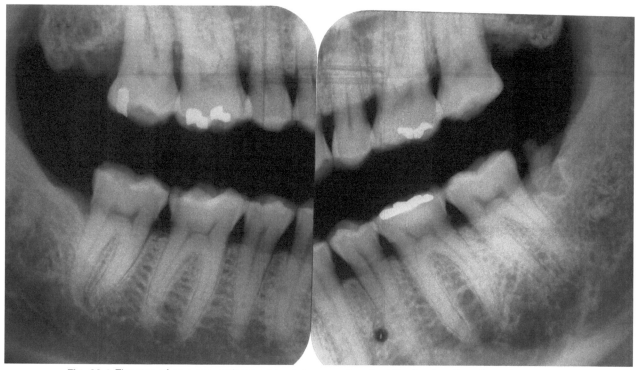

Fig. 33.4 The use of two conventional occlusal-size receptors for bitewing imaging allows for a greater amount of tissue to be imaged than if the smaller American National Standards Institute no. 2 receptors had been used.

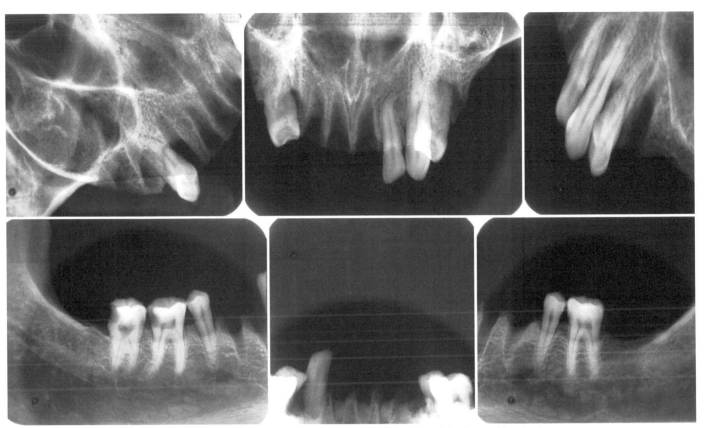

Fig. 33.5 Example of the use of occlusal images to obtain full imaging of the jaws with only six exposures.

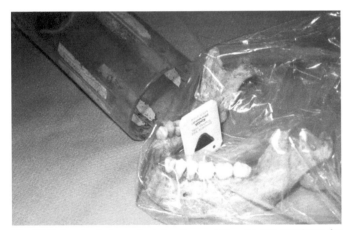

Fig. 33.6 A polyethylene stock bag is used to wrap the specimen for conventional radiographic imaging to protect the forensic dentist and others handling the material.

Regardless of which image receptor type is selected, it is imperative for the forensic dentist to operate safely by practicing body-substance precautions and radiation safety. With respect to precautions from the body being examined, it is prudent to wrap equipment in impermeable membranes to avoid contamination, and to drape bodies with disposable covers so that all government-mandated laws on the handling of body substances are obeyed.

Where available, handheld dental x-ray generators (Fig. 33.8) should be considered mandatory for dental forensics. These devices are highly portable and allow battery packs to be exchanged in cases of heavy use. Moreover, they are compatible with either film or digital receptor systems.

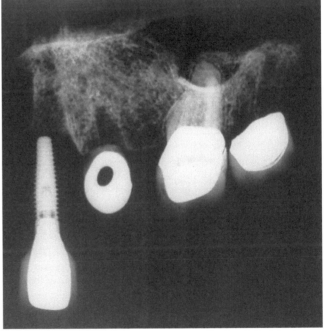

Fig. 33.7 This dark image demonstrates the difficulty of obtaining images with acceptable density when one is dealing with very small amounts of tissue.

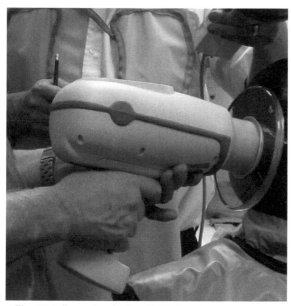

Fig. 33.8 Example of a handheld dental x-ray generator.

Finally, with regard to forensics, it is better to make too many images than too few. There is no concern with radiation dose in the deceased, so the entire tooth-bearing parts of the jaws should be imaged. Equally important, the forensic dentist or forensic radiographer should keep in mind the goal of postmortem imaging, which is to provide images of high quality for forensic comparison with antemortem images. Diagnosis of disease is not the goal of forensic imaging. Postmortem images may be made in advance of receipt of any antemortem records; therefore, with respect to radiologic imaging, the maxim "when in doubt—max out" is operative. Finally, in situations where the case is being entered into a "found-human-remains/missing persons" database such as the National Missing and Unidentified Persons System (NamUs), National Crime Information Center (NCIC), International Police Organization (INTERPOL), or others, the body may be buried or otherwise irretrievable by the time any antemortem-postmortem comparison is performed.

FORENSIC DENTAL IDENTIFICATION REPORT

After the examination is conducted, the forensic dentist writes a report for the coroner or medical examiner. Box 33.1 shows the items that should appear in the report regardless of the style of report employed.

Style of Reporting Concordant Points

It is recommended that the name of each tooth be spelled out rather than using a tooth numbering system. This procedure reduces the chance of error in the event that the report is read by persons not accustomed to using either the World Dental Federation (FDI) tooth-numbering system or the Universal (US) numbering system. For example, the report may include the following statement: "*The maxillary right third molar is present and malformed with especially stunted roots on both antemortem and postmortem radiographic examinations.*"

Materials Used in a Report

The forensic dentist must keep materials used in the examination in a secure place while they are in use. After the examination has been completed and the report submitted, it is recommended that a copy of the report be retained and all materials be returned to the coroner or medical examiner. This practice places the onus for safe, secure, and permanent storage of all materials on the coroner or medical examiner so that the chain of custody is maintained.

APPLICATIONS OF RADIOLOGIC IMAGING IN MASS DISASTERS

Forensic dental identification is very useful in multiple-fatality incidents resulting in a large number of human remains that may be commingled, macerated, burnt, or otherwise damaged. If the multiple-fatality event is small and can be managed by local providers, it may be simply a matter of undertaking multiple single identifications. However, if the incident is too large for local authorities to manage with confidence, it may be necessary to call on trained and experienced teams of forensic dentists from outside the local jurisdiction. Such situations are not the place for a well-meaning dentist lacking training or extensive case experience. Most people underestimate the stress involved with these situations, even on seasoned practitioners.

The process of identification of remains in multiple-fatality situations is the same as the individual identification except for the organization. Normally, three teams are formed: (1) an antemortem team that collects, organizes, and collates incoming data obtained by investigators; (2) a postmortem team that examines, images, and charts the remains; and (3) a comparison team that makes identifications. In all cases it is imperative to work with at least two members in each team so that errors can be identified.

In situations where the number of remains is large or fragmentation of the remains occurs, the comparisons become especially complex. Numerous computer software programs are available that can aid in the comparison (for websites, see bibliography section at the end of this chapter). These programs rank possible matches and mismatches using simple algorithms. However, all final identifications are made by experts.

APPLICATION OF RADIOLOGIC IMAGING TO LONG-TERM UNIDENTIFIED REMAINS

Methods of identification of long-term unidentified remains are limited to situations where there are antemortem records of acceptable quality for comparison with postmortem records. In the United States, there are approximately 100,000 active missing persons cases and 40,000 sets of human remains contained in depositories at any given time. This situation has been termed a silent, slow, mass disaster. In many instances, radiologic examinations of human remains can identify potential objective points of concordance and, with some degree of age stratification, can suggest a possible match of this set of human remains to a missing person. Many agencies attempt to provide this service, including NamUS, NCIC, and INTERPOL. These agencies use methods of coding the features of the dentition that facilitate the comparison process. In most cases, this comparison process is ongoing and updated at regular intervals. Once the information for a set of remains has been entered into one or more databases, it remains there until an identification is made. Similarly, antemortem records remain on the database until the person returns (in the case of a missing person) or until a match to postmortem remains is made. The information in some of these programs is available for public viewing on websites, whereas other programs keep the information exclusively for law enforcement. Generally the wider the dissemination of this information, the greater the benefit. Also, and perhaps counterintuitively, for best results, the less dental minutiae entered into the coding system, the better. The presence of excessive detail increases the chance of false rejection of a match.

BIBLIOGRAPHY

Adams BJ. The diversity of adult dental patterns in the United States and the implications for personal identification. *J Forensic Sci.* 2003;48:497–503.

American Board of Forensic Odontology. http://www.abfo.org/.

Kirk NJ, Wood RE, Goldstein M. Skeletal identification using the frontal sinus region: a retrospective study of 39 cases. *J Forensic Sci.* 2002;47:318–323.

National Research Council. Strengthening forensic science in the United States: a path forward; 2009. http://www.nap.edu/catalog.php?record_id=12589.

Saks MJ, Koehler JJ. The coming paradigm shift in forensic identification science. *Science.* 2005;309:892–895.

Wood RE, Kirk NJ, Sweet DJ. Digital dental radiographic identification in the pediatric, mixed and permanent dentitions. *J Forensic Sci.* 1999;44:910–916.

Dental Identification Websites

DVI guide. www.interpol.int/Media/Files/INTERPOL-Expertise/DVI/DVI-Guide.

WinID3. www.winid.com/.

Missing Persons Websites

British Columbia. Ministry of Public Safety and Solicitor General, Unidentified Human Remains in B.C. http://www.missing-u.ca/britishcolumbia.htm.

FBI. NCIC Missing Person and Unidentified Person Statistics for 2010. http://www.fbi.gov/about-us/cjis/ncic/ncic-missing-person-and-unidentified-person-statistics-for-2010.

National Institute of Justice (U.S.). Missing persons and unidentified remains: the nation's silent mass disaster. http://www.nij.gov/journals/256/missing-persons.html.

National Missing and Unidentified Persons System (NamUs). http://www.namus.gov/.

OPP. Missing Persons and Unidentified Bodies Unit. http://www.missing-u.ca/.

INDEX

Note: Page numbers followed by "f" refer to illustrations; page numbers followed by "t" refer to tables; page numbers followed by "b" refer to boxes.